JC, All the cats ever
thank you especially
Panda, Softie & Lady Pl
pets Carol & John Wypick

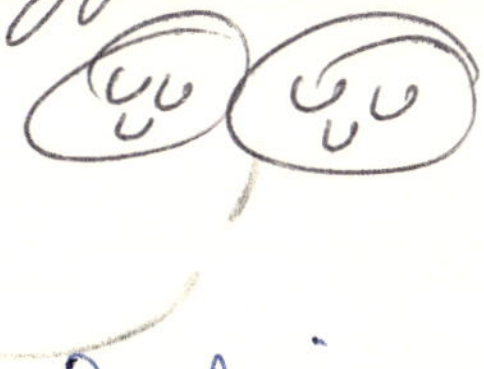

JC —
Thanks so much for helping us out when we needed that blood work. Lucy & Delilah especially thank you for not having to "shave their legs"

Janell

Sept. 1983

feline medicine

FIRST EDITION

Edited by
PAUL W. PRATT, VMD
American Veterinary Publications

AMERICAN VETERINARY PUBLICATIONS, INC.
DRAWER KK, SANTA BARBARA, CALIFORNIA 93102
1983

Library of Congress Catalog Card No. 82-082939

ISBN 0-939674-00-9

PRINTED IN THE UNITED STATES OF AMERICA

preface

For the past 5000 years, people have been privileged to have *Felis catus* as a companion and mouser. Recently the popularity of cats has greatly increased, perhaps owing to their fastidious nature, relative economy to feed and ability to live happily in apartments without need of venturing outdoors. There are over 25 million cats in the US alone, and their numbers and importance in veterinary practice are certain to increase.

Formerly *Feline Medicine and Surgery*, this first edition of *Feline Medicine* acknowledges the increasing sophistication of feline practice today. Advances in the medical aspects of feline practice have not only expanded to fill the pages formerly devoted to surgery in this book but also have increased the number of pages in the book. By concentrating on the medical aspects of feline practice, this new work reflects the more specialized nature of practice today.

As this book was designed for veterinary students and practicing veterinarians, its approach is practical. Chapters are arranged by body system and include discussions of the prevalence, cause, clinical signs, diagnosis, treatment and control of each disease. A chapter on feline behavior has been included because of the growing body of knowledge in ethology.

I am indebted to our authors for their conscientious attitude in the writing of each chapter and for their punctuality in meeting publication deadlines.

Paul W. Pratt, VMD
Editor

authors

A.L. ARONSON, DVM, MS, PhD
Professor, School of Veterinary Medicine, North Carolina State University, Raleigh, NC

M.H. ATTLEBERGER, DVM, PhD
Associate Professor, School of Veterinary Medicine, Auburn University, Auburn, AL

J.A. BARSANTI, DVM
Associate Professor, College of Veterinary Medicine, University of Georgia, Athens, GA

J. BLUE, DVM, PhD
Assistant Professor, New York State College of Veterinary Medicine, Cornell University, Ithaca, NY

P.L. BORCHELT, PhD
Director, Animal Behavior Clinic, Animal Medical Center, New York, NY

A.H. BRIGHTMAN II, DVM, MS
Assistant Professor, College of Veterinary Medicine, University of Illinois, Urbana, IL

C.C. CAPEN, DVM, PhD
Professor, College of Veterinary Medicine, Ohio State University, Columbus, OH

C.H. CLARK, DVM, PhD
Professor, School of Veterinary Medicine, Auburn University, Auburn AL

E.D. COLBY, DVM
Director, Animal Research Facility, School of Medicine, Dartmouth College, Hanover, NH

D.R. COLLINS, DVM
Practitioner, Spring, TX

W.A. CROWELL, PhD
Associate Professor, College of Veterinary Medicine, University of Georgia, Athens, GA

P. DERRICK, PhD
Clinical Pathologist, Veterinary Reference Laboratory, Salt Lake City, UT

C.E. EGER, BVSc, MSc
Assistant Professor, Murdoch University, Murdoch, Western Australia

R.J. EVANS, MA, PhD, Vet. M.B., MRCVS
Research Scholar, School of Veterinary Science, University of Bristol, Bristol, England

D.R. FINCO, DVM
Professor, College of Veterinary Medicine, University of Georgia, Athens, GA

R.B. FORD, DVM, MS
Associate Professor, School of Veterinary Medicine, North Carolina State University, Raleigh, North Carolina

P.R. FOX, DVM, MS
Cardiologist, Animal Medical Center, New York, NY

J.K. FRENKEL, MD, PhD
Professor, Medical Center, University of Kansas, Kansas City, KS

C.J. GASKELL, BVSc, PhD, DVR, MRCVS
Lecturer, School of Veterinary Science, University of Bristol, Bristol, England

T.J. GRUFFYDD-JONES, B. Vet. Med., MRCVS
Lecturer, School of Veterinary Science, University of Bristol, Bristol, England

M.R. HERRON, DVM, MS
Professor, School of Veterinary Medicine, Texas A & M University, College Station, TX

P.J. IHRKE, VMD
Assistant Professor, School of Veterinary Medicine, University of California, Davis, CA

S. KRAKOWKA, DVM, PhD
Associate Professor, College of Veterinary Medicine, Ohio State University, Columbus, OH

S.-K. LIU, DVM, PhD
Pathologist, Animal Medical Center, New York, NY

S.L. MARTIN, DVM, MS
Professor, College of Veterinary Medicine, Ohio State University, Columbus, OH

P.J. McKEEVER, DVM, MS
Associate Professor, College of Veterinary Medicine, University of Minnesota, St. Paul, MN

D.P. O'BRIEN, DVM, MS
Resident, College of Veterinary Medicine, University of Illinois, Urbana, IL

R.G. OLSEN, PhD
Professor, College of Veterinary Medicine, Ohio State University, Columbus, OH

R.L. OTT, DVM
Professor, College of Veterinary Medicine, Washington State University, Pullman, WA

A.J. PARKER, PhD, MRCVS
Associate Professor, College of Veterinary Medicine, University of Illinois, Urbana, IL

A.J. PAUL, DVM
Extension Veterinarian, College of Veterinary Medicine, University of Illinois, Urbana, IL

S.I. REINKE, DVM
Practitioner, Larkspur, CA

J.E. RIVIERE, DVM, MS, PhD
Assistant Professor, School of Veterinary Medicine, North Carolina State University, Raleigh, NC

W.R. ROSE, DVM
North Carolina Department of Agriculture, Raleigh, NC

E.J. ROSSER, JR., DVM
Resident, School of Veterinary Medicine, University of California, Davis, CA

S.A. SAWCHUCK, DVM
Resident, College of Veterinary Medicine, University of Illinois, Urbana, IL

C.A. SOUSA, DVM
Practitioner, Sacramento, CA

A.A. STANNARD, DVM, PhD
Professor, School of Veterinary Medicine, University of California, Davis, CA

B.S. STEIN, DVM
Practitioner, Chicago, IL

G. SUMNER-SMITH, BVSc, MSc, FRCVS
Professor, Ontario Veterinary College, University of Guelph, Guelph, Ontario, Canada

L.P. TILLEY, DVM
Cardiologist, Animal Medical Center, New York, NY

K.S. TODD, JR., PhD
Professor, College of Veterinary Medicine, University of Illinois, Urbana, IL

V.L. VOITH, DVM
Director, Animal Behavior Clinic, School of Veterinary Medicine, University of Pennsylvania, Philadelphia, PA

S.D. WHITE, DVM
Resident, School of Veterinary Medicine, University of California, Davis, CA

contents

5. SYSTEMIC MYCOSES

6. THE BLOOD AND BLOOD-FORMING ORGANS

7. THE IMMUNE SYSTEM

8. THE ALIMENTARY SYSTEM

14. THE NERVOUS SYSTEM

15. THE REPRODUCTIVE SYSTEM

16. THE SKIN

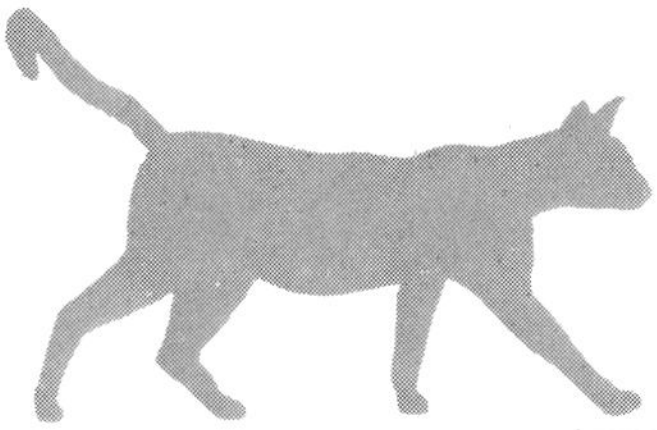

1 nutrition

D.R. COLLINS

For veterinarians, feline nutrition entails nourishing healthy cats and nourishing diseased cats. To succeed at the first, the veterinarian must understand the nutritional requirements of the cat and then must find a food adequate to provide those requirements. Nourishing diseased cats involves changing nutritionally incorrect diets, feeding anorectic sick cats, and suggesting appropriate diets to support treatment of cats with non-nutritional diseases.

A dietary history should be obtained for every patient seen, regardless of the nature of the illness. If the cat's diet is suspected of contributing to the illness, a detailed dietary history should be obtained, including formulas or recipes of diets fed or labels from food containers (Fig 1). The clinician should bear in mind that a cat's diet consists of everything it eats, not just what the owner feeds it.

FEEDING HEALTHY CATS

The daily diet of a healthy cat should be composed of energy, water, protein, fat, carbohydrates, vitamins and minerals.

Nutrient Requirements

Energy

Energy is the top metabolic priority after ingestion of food. Without energy, the vital functions of the body grind to a halt. Every day of its life, the cat must obtain enough energy to maintain its body heat and support its metabolic functions. Once the energy requirements of basal metabolism have been met, any remaining energy is used according to other priorities, such as wound repair, combatting infection, growth, exercise and storage as fat.

The ability of a food to produce energy is measured in calories (cal). Each gram of fat consumed produces about 9 cal; for each gram of protein or carbohydrate, about 4 cal.

Cats eat to fulfill their caloric requirements. This is one of the most important and fundamental principles of feeding cats. The caloric requirements for cats of various ages and conditions are listed in Table 1.

If a cat requires 350 cal daily and is fed food containing 700 cal/lb, the cat should consume ½ lb of the food daily. Similarly, if the cat is fed food containing 350 cal/lb, it should consume 1 lb of food daily. Therefore, the caloric density of the food being fed is among the most important information to be determined.

The cat is unique among mammals because it requires a portion of its energy to be supplied as protein. Most mammals do quite well using fat or carbohydrates as a source of energy, but cats seem to have both a nutritional need and a metabolic ability to handle uncommonly high quantities of dietary protein.[1]

Water

Water is used to aid in digestion and absorption of nutrients, metabolism of nutrients for energy, maintenance of body temperature, and regulation of fluid and electrolyte balance. It is the medium in which many body chemicals are dissolved and in which biochemical reactions occur. Water is necessary for the transportation of nutrients to cells and the transfer of toxic waste products from the cells to the organs of elimination. It is also required for regulation of acid-base balance. Indeed, almost any function that occurs within a cat's body has some dependency on water.

Cats require water at a rate of about 66 ml/kg (30 ml/lb) body weight daily. They require about 3 ml water for each gram of dry matter eaten and 0.8 ml water for each calorie burned.[2]

What type of food is fed? (Use brand names when possible.)

canned ____________ dry ____________ semi-moist? ____________

table scraps? (list) ____________ homemade diet? ____________

____________ recipe? ____________

____________ ____________

____________ ____________

(Labels of all commercial foods and formulas for homemade diets should be attached to cat's record.)

Comments on feeding procedure (times, amounts, containers, other cats, etc):

Does the cat eat all that is offered? ____________

What treats or supplements are fed?

- ☐ canned tuna
- ☐ canned salmon
- ☐ canned sardines
- ☐ bacon
- ☐ luncheon meats
- ☐ liver strips
- ☐ fresh fish
- ☐ cheese
- ☐ chicken breast
- ☐ giblets
- ☐ other (specify)

Is water offered? ____________ Quantity drunk daily? ____________

Is milk offered? ____________ Quantity drunk daily? ____________

Does the cat go outdoors? ____________ What have you observed cat eating outdoors? (Be specific!) ____________

____

____

Is the cat allergic to any foods? ____________ To what? ____________

General comments:

Fig 1. A dietary history.

Therefore, a 7-lb cat needs about 200 ml water daily. If that 7-lb cat is fed a canned, gourmet-type cat food containing about 75% water and 1 cal/g, it will eat 250 g food and obtain from it about 187 ml water daily. In addition, from every gram of fat in the food, the cat will metabolize another gram of water. With at least 12-15 g fat in the food, the cat is provided with all of the water it needs from canned food.

Dry foods contain only about 10% water but about 3 cal/g. If a 7-lb cat eats the 84 g dry food required to furnish the 250 cal it needs, it will get only 9 ml water from the food, plus an additional 7 ml water from fat metabolism, or a total of 16 ml water. Obviously this cat requires at least an additional 184 ml of drinking water every day to prevent water deprivation.

Protein

All mammals require dietary protein for growth, repair and replacement of tissue, and development and maintenance of immune responses. Cats, however, have a uniquely high requirement for protein. So high, in fact, that adult cats need almost 5 times more protein than do adult dogs. Kittens require about 2½ times more protein than do puppies.[3]

In addition to quantity, quality of protein is also important. Among the sources of high-quality protein are lean muscle meats (mammal, bird or fish), whole eggs, whole milk protein, organ meats, and whole grain proteins.

Fat

Although the minimum requirement for fat in the cat's diet is unknown, dietary fat must

Table 1. Caloric Requirements of Cats

Age	kcal/kg/day	kcal/lb/day
Neonate	418	190
5 weeks	275	125
10 weeks	220	100
20 weeks	143	65
30 weeks	110	50
Adult female (intact, nonpregnant)	88	40
Adult female (pregnant)	110	50
Adult female (lactating)	275	125
Adult male (neutered)	88	40
Adult female (neutered)	88	40

contain an adequate amount of linoleic, linolenic and arachidonic acids. Pragmatically, however, the cat's energy requirement is so high that most successful diets contain large quantities of fat. Since fat contains about twice the calories of either protein or carbohydrates, it is the most concentrated source of dietary energy available. Under most circumstances, successful cat diets contain 15-40% fat, calculated on a dry-weight basis. Apparently cats cannot desaturate linoleic acid and need a dietary source of linoleic as well as linolenic and arachidonic acids. This suggests that cats require a source of polyunsaturated fats of animal origin in their diets.[4]

Carbohydrates

Cats have no requirements for carbohydrates. However, as long as a proper protein:calorie ratio is maintained, carbohydrates, from such sources as boiled rice. Cream of Wheat®, bread crumbs, or boiled and peeled potatoes, can be used to supply some of the calories in the diet.

Vitamins

Vitamins neither supply energy nor form structural components; yet metabolic derangements quickly occur if they are deficient in a diet. Vitamins may be described as catalysts because they trigger many biochemical reactions without entering into the actual reaction.

Like all other mammals, cats require both fat-soluble and water-soluble vitamins in their diet. The requirement for some of these vitamins is quite high, relative to the requirements of dogs or people. The recommended vitamin allowances for cats are listed in Table 2.

Minerals

Minerals are used by the body in a wider variety of functions than any other group of nutrients. Some serve as structural elements, others as catalysts, and still others as regulators. They control the movement of other nutrients through cellular walls and help maintain acid-base balance. This diverse role leads to numerous situations in which one mineral's function depends on another's. Therefore, minerals should always be considered as an interrelated group, not as separate entities. The currently recommended daily amounts of minerals for cats are listed in Table 3.

Commercial Foods

Recommendation of a balanced diet for a cat is not nearly as difficult as it once was. Today, any commercial cat food that bears the claim "complete and balanced," "nutritional" or "adequate" must have either successfully supported the life cycle of cats in actual feeding trials or must contain the required nutrients suggested by the National Research Council.

Commercial cat foods can be divided into 3 major types according to their method of preservation and water content: dry foods, which contain 10-12% moisture; semi-moist foods, which contain 20-25% moisture; and canned foods, which contain 70-78% moisture.

Dry Foods

Dry cat foods are made by mixing raw grains, meat meal and dairy products with steam inside a blending pressure cooker. The ingredients are cooked while being whipped into a homogeneous mass. This mass is then forced through a die and expanded, by the escaping steam, into small, porous pieces. These pieces are then hot-air hardened and sprayed with a coating of liquid fat and some type of flavoring agent.

Expanded products have a couple of major disadvantages from the manufacturer's point of view. First, products designed to be expanded must contain at least 30-35% carbohydrates or the expansion process does not work. For the cat,

Table 2. Recommended Daily Vitamin Allowances for Cats[5, 26]

Vitamin	Amount/kg Dry Diet	Comments
A	10,000 IU	Cannot use carotene as source
D	1000 IU	May be synthesized in skin
E	80 IU	Fluctuates with level of polyunsaturated fats fed
K	negligible	Synthesized in intestines
B_1 (thiamin)	5 mg	Increase amount fed in lactation or fever
B_2 (riboflavin)	5 mg	Increase amount fed in lactation, fever, high-fat diet
Niacin (nicotinic acid)	45 mg	Increase amount fed in lactation or fever
B_6 (pyridoxine)	4 mg	Increase amount fed in lactation or fever
Pantothenic acid	10 mg	
Biotin	0.05 mg	Avidin in raw egg white binds biotin and makes it unavailable
Folic acid	1 mg	Increase amount fed in antibiotic therapy
B_{12} (cyanocobalamin)	0.02 mg	
Choline	2000 mg	
C (ascorbic acid)	None known	Increase amount fed in infection

such a carbohydrate level may compromise the energy or protein level. Second, fat levels must be greatly restricted or expansion cannot occur. This leaves the expanded food too low in energy content. To correct this, the liquid fat coating is added to each piece. Because of this fat coating, however, most expanded foods must be packaged in multi-walled bags having at least one ply serving as a grease barrier. This increases the cost of packaging.

Semi-Moist Foods

By adding humectants and preservatives to fresh meat and cereal ingredients cooked in a pressure blender, the amount of water in the finished product without encouraging spoiling can be higher than that in dry products. Foods so processed are called semi-moist.

Cat food containing moisture levels above 10% usually spoil if unrefrigerated, but addition of the humectants and preservatives allows moisture levels of up to 25% without spoilage. Humectants are ingredients that absorb water and prevent spoilage by microorganisms. Propylene glycol and sorbitol, 2 commonly used humectants, can also be used by the cat to supply energy. Preservatives are chemicals added to create an environment that inhibits the growth of microorganisms. Preservatives also often tend to reduce the usefulness of the water present for microorganisms. Sugars and simple syrups are used in semi-moist foods as preservatives and also serve as sources of energy.

Canned Foods

Another way of preserving fresh, wet ingredients is to seal them into containers that prevent contamination and then destroy any microorganisms of spoilage already in the food. This is the method used when cat foods are sealed in tin-plated steel cans and subjected to a heat-sterilization process.

Two varieties of canned cat foods are available: the ration type, usually found in 16-oz cans, and the gourmet type, usually found in 6-oz cans.

Table 3. Recommended Daily Mineral Allowances for Cats[5, 26]

Mineral	% or Amount/kg Dry Diet	Comments
Calcium	1%	Increase amount fed up to 1.5% during growth and lactation
Phosphorus	0.8%	Ca:P ratio should be 1:1
Potassium	0.3%	Adequate amounts in meat or fish
Sodium Chloride	0.5%	
Magnesium	0.05%	Usually present in adequate amounts
Iron	100 mg	Iron in hemoglobin available
Iodine	1 mg	May be deficient in meat
Manganese	10 mg	Usually present in adequate amounts
Zinc	30 mg	May require supplementation for diets high in soy meal
Cobalt	3 mg	Required only when vitamin B_{12} is deficient
Copper	5 mg	Adequate amounts in raw meat

In the ration-type food, the fresh meat and meat by-products are ground and then blended with ingredients that need no grinding. Animal fats, vegetable fats and water are added to the mixture. The liquid mixture is heated to about 160 F, poured into cans and sealed, then processed so the internal temperature of the mixture reaches 250 F for several minutes. With the gourmet-type food, raw animal tissues are chopped into roughly uniform pieces, in some instances are cooked by special methods before canning, then sealed in cans and processed as with ration-type foods.

From the cat owner's viewpoint, there are advantages and disadvantages to all 3 types of commercial foods (Table 4).

Noncommercial Foods

Noncommercial foods are those foods that are not sold exclusively as food for cats. Some cat owners, especially cattery owners, formulate elaborate noncommercial diets for their cats. Some of these carefully guarded formulations have been handed down from generation to generation. However, only a few have survived the test of multiple generations of cats and time. For the most part, complex formulas and elaborate mixtures of ingredients have disappeared in favor of the more convenient, less expensive and far better balanced commercial foods.

For owners who insist that their cats must be fed something other than commercial foods, either of the following 2 balanced diets can be fed:

D'Arcy Cattery Diet

4 lb raw hamburger
½ lb raw liver, ground
2 lb Purina High-Protein Dog Meal
¼ lb Theralin (Lambert-Kay) (8 tbsp)
¼ lb brewers' yeast (8 tbsp)

The dog food is soaked in enough hot water to cover it. The hamburger, liver and dry ingredients are mixed. If the mixture is too dry, a little water is added. If the mixture is too soupy, Gerber's Baby Rice Cereal can be added. The diet should be fed at ½ oz/lb body weight.

National Research Council's Diet A (Modified)

1 lb cottage cheese
½ lb whole dried milk
¾ lb raw liver
3 cups oatmeal (uncooked)
1½ oz corn oil or lard
6 oz brewers' yeast (12 tbsp)
¾ oz cod liver oil

The corn oil and cod liver oil are mixed with the cottage cheese and liver (ground or blended). The milk and brewers' yeast are mixed in, and the

Table 4. Advantages and Disadvantages of Commercial Foods

Advantages	Disadvantages
Dry Food	
1. Requires no refrigeration (moderate shelf life)	1. May contain insufficient fat (too little energy)
2. Does not spoil after package is opened	2. Processing heat may destroy vitamins
3. More nutrients and energy per pound of food	3. Insects and other vermin may contaminate
	4. Must supply adequate drinking water while feeding
	5. Spoils if wet
Semi-Moist Food	
1. Requires no refrigeration (moderate shelf life)	1. Deteriorates after package is opened.
2. Packed in convenient, portion-controlled container	2. Spoils if wet
3. More nutrients and energy per pound of food than canned	3. Expensive method of preservation
	4. Must supply adequate drinking water while feeding
	5. Some ingredients can cause digestive upsets
Canned Food	
1. Requires no refrigeration until opened (long shelf life)	1. Expensive form of preservation
2. Durable container (no tearing, no infestation)	2. Contains only 25% nutrients
3. Usually highly palatable	3. Heat processing may destroy some nutrients and vitamins
4. Ingredients usually digestible	4. Heavy, inflexible container
	5. Requires a special device to open cans

oatmeal is folded in, adding a little water if needed for a smooth blend.

FEEDING DISEASED CATS

Frank Deficiency Diseases

Frank deficiency diseases rarely involve only one nutrient. Instead, they involve multiple nutrients, each contributing its share to the overall disease pattern. As a consequence, deficiency diseases are rarely clear-cut, "textbook" pictures of disease. Instead, they cause vague and often changing clinical signs. The most insidious of these is the borderline deficiency in which one or more nutrients is present in the diet in minimal or just subminimal levels. As the resultant partial anorexia further reduces food intake, deficiencies of other nutrients may cause a new set of clinical signs.

Despite the fact that deficiencies of individual nutrients rarely are seen clinically, for convenience, each nutrient is discussed individually.

Insufficient Energy Intake

A reduction in caloric intake results in a reduction of body weight. This fact is the one upon which all weight-reduction programs are based. In moderation, reduction of caloric intake in obese animals can be a healthy and worthwhile endeavor. However, a drastic reduction of caloric intake results in energy deprivation, emaciation and malnutrition. Since the highest metabolic priority is energy production, nutrients are used for nothing else during the energy-deficient period. Therefore, during continued starvation or fasting, deficiency disease involving all nutrients usually always occurs. The nutrients the body cannot store begin to disappear first. Ultimately, levels of all nutrients become deficient, including those necessary for the maintenance of life, and the animal dies.

Water Deprivation

A cat can lose almost all of its body fat and half of its body protein and still survive. However, it will probably die if it loses only one-tenth of its body water. Although not as sensitive to water deprivation as most other mammals, cats become dehydrated if deprived of water for a long period. Uncorrected dehydration quickly causes death.

Protein Deficiency

Cats on a protein-deficient diet usually do not display the characteristic signs of protein deficiency seen in many mammals, *ie*, anemia, emaciation, reduced immune response, and hypoproteinemia, with associated edema and ascites. Protein levels must be sustained if the cat is to maintain an appetite. The anorexia produced by an even slight deficiency of protein quickly produces multiple deficiency diseases, involving most or all required nutrients.

Protein:Energy Imbalance

Protein needed for other body functions is converted to energy unless there is sufficient energy in a cat's diet. Consequently, the ratio of protein to calories is probably as important as the actual quantity and quality of the protein and energy sources. A diet containing too little fat or too much indigestible carbohydrate can be energy-deficient. A diet containing too little animal protein, too much fat or too much carbohydrate can be protein-deficient.

The signs produced by an improper protein: calorie ratio include weight loss, dull haircoat, anorexia, reproductive problems, unexplained "breaks" in vaccination programs, precipitous weight loss after injury or onset of disease, and failure to respond properly to treatment for injury, infection, endoparasitism or other disease.

Vitamin A Deficiency

The signs of chronic vitamin A deficiency include anorexia, weight loss, muscle atrophy, poor haircoat, follicular hyperkeratosis with denuded scaly patches, conjunctivitis, corneal vascularization, corneal ulceration and retinal degeneration.[6] When vitamin A deficiency progresses far enough, behavioral changes become obvious to the owner. Photophobia and a resistance to handling, especially if light is shined in the cat's eyes, may be noted initially. The pupillary reflex is greatly reduced and the pupils remain dilated in normal light. While the cat may not appear blind in its home surroundings, it demonstrates signs of vision loss when placed in a strange environment.[5]

Reproductive function is also severely affected by vitamin A deficiency. Testicular atrophy occurs in tomcats. Fetal death may occur at implantation, about halfway through pregnancy or about the 50th day of gestation. Kittens are born weak and there is a high incidence of neonatal deaths. Kittens that live past the fifth week may have ataxia, tremors, spasticity, paralysis and delay in development of activity.

Vitamin D Deficiency

Vitamin D deficiency occurs only if induced experimentally. On the contrary, oversupplementation creates the greatest problem. Excesses of vitamin D produce uneven deposition of Ca in the bones and metastatic calcification in lungs, kidneys, heart and blood vessels.

Vitamin E Deficiency

Vitamin E is an antioxidant that prevents rancidification of body fat. Deficiency of vitamin E in cats results in a yellow, brown or orange discoloration of fat deposits. The condition, known as "yellow-fat" disease or pansteatitis, is caused by accumulation of peroxides, the products of rancidification.

Pansteatitis is characterized by generalized soreness, lethargy, anorexia and fever due to inflammation of body fat. Subcutaneous pain may become so severe that affected cats crouch down to avoid touching the hanging edge of a tablecloth or bedspread. The pain may cause personality changes and gait alterations.

Affected cats usually have a history of being fed entirely or mostly canned red-meat tuna. Some affected cats have not been fed red-meat tuna but consumed diets containing large amounts of other types of fish. Occasionally a cat fed a diet containing no tuna and only small amounts of fish is affected.

Treatment includes eliminating fish and fish-based foods from the diet, and feeding an appropriate and balanced diet (see Imbalanced Diets). At least 30 mg vitamin E, in the form of alpha tocopherol, should be given PO daily until clinical signs disappear. Prednisolone, given PO at 2.0-2.5 mg every 8 hours until clinical improvement is evident, is a valuable adjunct in treatment of pansteatitis. Affected cats should be handled as little as possible.

Vitamin B_1 Deficiency

Thiamin (vitamin B_1) deficiency is caused by diets of raw or canned fish containing thiaminase. It is rare. Signs of experimentally induced thiamin deficiency in adult cats appear after a thiamin-deficient diet is consumed for about 6 weeks. The disease is divided into 3 stages.[7] The first stage is characterized by anorexia, the second by neurologic disorders, weight loss, cardiac dysfunction and convulsions of increasing severity (due to cerebral hemorrhage), and the third by ataxia, paralysis, prostration and death.[5]

In the rare event that a case of thiamin deficiency is seen, it can be treated successfully during the first 2 stages with IM injections of 1-5 mg thiamin. In fact, if a response is observed, it can be considered diagnostic. Treatment given during the third stage results in incomplete recovery due to irreversible brain damage.

Vitamin C Deficiency

Cats can synthesize vitamin C (ascorbic acid) from glucose and usually do not require a dietary source of this vitamin. However, a deficiency may develop during infectious disease because of severely impaired synthesis of the vitamin.[8] To prevent such a deficiency, in addition to other therapy, 100-200 mg ascorbic acid should be given daily during infectious disease.

Other Vitamin Deficiencies

The following vitamins rarely, if ever, produce clinical signs of deficiency as a separate entity. A brief description of signs observed in experimentally induced deficiencies is given as a matter of interest.

Vitamin B_2: Signs of experimentally induced vitamin B_2 (riboflavin) deficiency include anorexia, weight loss, cataracts, testicular hypoplasia and alopecia.[9] Death may occur.

Niacin: Experimentally induced niacin (nicotinic acid) deficiency in kittens produces diarrhea, weight loss and death. In adult cats, deficiency produces diarrhea, oral ulcers, thick saliva, malodorous breath and fever.[10]

Vitamin B_6: Signs of experimentally induced vitamin B_6 (pyridoxine) deficiency include weight loss, failure of kittens to grow, microcytic anemia and convulsions.[11] Acute renal disease may result in formation of calcium oxalate uroliths.[12] Pyridoxine deficiency should be suspected when oxalate calculi are identified since they are rare as compared to struvite crystals.

Pantothenic Acid: Experimentally induced deficiency of pantothenic acid produces fatty livers and weight loss.[13]

Folic Acid: Experimentally induced folic acid deficiency in kittens produces cessation of growth, weight loss and macrocytic anemia.[14]

Biotin: Experimentally induced biotin deficiency produces ocular, nasal and oral discharges, scaly dermatitis of the face, hemorrhagic diarrhea, marked anorexia and emaciation.[15]

Deficiencies of vitamin B_{12}, inositol and choline have not been definitively studied. Cats do not require a dietary source of vitamin K.

Calcium and Phosphorus Deficiency

The most common mineral deficiency in cats is nutritional secondary hyperparathyroidism.[16] It is most common in kittens and young cats, and usually produced by consumption of homemade meat-rich diets. Diets of cardiac and skeletal muscle are notably deficient in Ca.[17] Hyperparathyroidism is induced by an improper Ca:P ratio, sometimes as dramatic as 1:20. Such an imbalance results in osteoporosis in adult cats and osteogenesis imperfecta in growing kittens. The disease is characterized by a generalized decrease in bone density and thinning of the cortices.[18] Limping, reluctance to move, and finally spontaneous fractures may be observed. Untreated cats eventually die.

Lesions and signs of hyperparathyroidism are best reversed by feeding a diet with a Ca:P ratio of 2:1. Prevention is best accomplished by maintaining a dietary Ca:P ratio of 1:1 (Table 5).

Table 5. Calcium Carbonate Supplementation Required to Balance Ca:P Ratios

Meat	$CaCO_3$/lb
Stewed chicken	1.5 g
Raw hamburger	2.5 g
Raw liver	4.0 g
Raw shrimp (without shell)	4.0 g
Raw mackerel	6.5 g

Table 6. Quantitative Analysis of a Diet of 1/3 Canned Food and 2/3 Organ Meat[17]

		Water (%)	Protein (%)	Fat (%)	Carbo-hydrate (%)	Ash (%)	Ca (mg)	P (mg)
Step 1	Beef kidney	75.9	15.4	6.7	0.9	1.1	11	219
	Beef heart	77.5	17.1	3.6	0.7	1.1	5	145
	Beef liver	69.7	19.9	3.8	5.3	1.3	8	352
Steps 2 & 3	50% kidney	37.95	7.7	3.35	0.45	0.55	5.5	109.5
	25% heart	19.37	4.3	0.90	0.17	0.27	1.2	48.7
	25% liver	17.42	5.0	0.95	1.32	0.32	2.2	88.0
Step 4	Calculated analysis of meat mixture	74.4%	16.1%	5.20%	1.94%	1.14%	8.7 mg	246.2 mg
Step 1	Avg. of 5 canned cat foods	72.4%	14.1%	4.6%	4.5%	4.9%	1.3 mg	86 mg
	Calculated analysis of meat mixture	74.4%	16.1%	5.2%	1.9%	1.1%	8.7 mg	246.2 mg
Steps 2 & 3	33% canned food	23.9%	4.6%	1.5%	1.5%	1.5%	43.2 mg	28.4 mg
	66% meat mixture	49.3%	11.1%	3.4 %	1.3%	0.7%	5.7 mg	162.5 mg
Step 4	Calculated analysis of diet	73.2%	15.7%	4.9%	2.8%	2.2%	48.9 mg	190.9 mg
Step 5	Protein: 15.7% × 4.25 cal =				66.7 = 54%			
	Fat: 4.9% × 9.0 cal =				44.1 = 36%			
	Carbohydrate: 2.8% × 4.25 cal =				11.9 = 10%			
					122.7 cal/100 g diet			

Phosphorus, while equally as important as Ca in bone growth, is found in large amounts in meat and animal products.[17] Because of the large amount of animal protein eaten by cats, it is difficult to produce a clinical P deficiency.

Potassium Deficiency

Like P, K is found in large quantities in meats and animal products.[17] The cat's large requirement for animal protein, therefore, almost precludes any deficiency since both energy and protein deficiency develop first.

Magnesium Imbalances

Although deficiencies are the general rule with most nutrients in diets for cats, problems associated with dietary Mg are usually related to excessive intake. Most foods eaten by cats supply far more Mg than is needed. In cats prone to feline urologic syndrome, urinary excretion of excess Mg can produce insoluble urinary debris (see Chapter 12).

Other Mineral Deficiencies

Much less research has been done on experimentally induced mineral deficiencies than on vitamin deficiencies. Aside from Ca, most of the other minerals required by cats are found in more than adequate amounts in meats and other animal products, and deficiencies are rare.[25]

Imbalanced Diets

Some of the many indications, other than clinical signs of frank deficiency disease, that might lead one to suspect that the owner is feeding an imbalanced diet include obesity, weight loss, failure of kittens to gain weight, dull haircoat, loss of condition and appetite, lethargy, reproductive problems, unusually high incidence of parasitism, unexplained breaks in vaccination response, spontaneous skeletal disease, lactation failures, and a history of the owner feeding table scraps, an "all natural" diet, or a combination of natural and commercial foods.

Questions regarding the adequacy of a cat's diet often cannot be answered extemporaneously even though this is what the client usually expects. Feline dietetics is a complex subject. For this reason, when such questions arise, always obtain a detailed dietary history, including formulas and labels from containers of the diet; then delay answering until you have had time to properly evaluate the diet.

A diet can be quantitatively evaluated using the following steps (Table 6). List the quantitative analysis of all ingredients in the diet (Step 1). Then determine in what percentage each ingredient is present in the diet (Step 2). That percentage is used to determine the amount of that ingredient in the diet (Step 3). The total percentage for each ingredient represents the amount of each ingredient in the diet (Step 4). Next, the caloric density is calculated by multiplying the quantity of protein and carbohydrate by 4.15 and fat by 9.0 (Step 5). This yields the number of calories in 100 g of food. To calculate the number of calories in 1 lb of the diet, multiply the calories in 100 g by 4.54. Finally, compare the caloric density and calculated analysis to the requirements for the cat to determine the adequacy of the diet. A diet of ½ lb beef kidney, ¼ lb beef heart, ¼ lb beef liver mixed, half and half, with ration-type canned cat food is analyzed in Table 6.

In the example in Table 6, it was necessary to go through steps 1-4 twice, first to analyze the mixture of kidney, heart and liver, and then to analyze this mixture of organ meats when mixed with the canned cat food. When the evaluation of this diet was reported back to the client, it was presented something like this: "Your cat's diet contains 54% protein-derived calories, a satisfactory level. If a cat eats enough to supply it with the required calories each day (about 30 g or 1 oz/lb body weight), it will obtain adequate protein of sufficiently high biologic value. Because of this diet's low caloric density and high water content, however, some cats may be reluctant to or have difficulty in consuming a sufficient quantity. Regardless of this or any other assets of the diet, however, it is unsatisfactory because of its extremely imbalanced Ca:P ratio. While that ratio should be 1.2:1, the diet's ratio is 0.26:1, which is dangerously low, even for adult cats. Such a ratio is intolerable for reproducing queens and growing kittens."

Imbalanced or inadequate diets should be discarded and replaced with an adequate diet. Unless one is a trained dietitian and has accurate scales to measure all ingredients, trying to rearrange the ingredients of an inadequate diet to make it adequate is usually an unsatisfactory procedure. With so many adequate diets available today, the practitioner should not lack for one to suggest to his clients.

FEEDING ANORECTIC CATS

Sick cats do not eat. In fact, anorexia is the most common sign of illness in cats.[19] Even a healthy cat may suffer transient anorexia during a trip to the hospital or kennel.

When any cat does not eat, it relies upon catabolic processes to obtain the nutrients to maintain vital functions and minimal activity. When a sick cat does not eat, it catabolizes stored energy and body proteins needed for tissue repair, healing and replacement. In addition to the energy and protein, sick cats also require about 30 other nutrients, each in proper proportion to the others. Consequently, malnourishment exacerbates the effects of an infection or other disease, and disease can convert a borderline nutritional state into a full-blown deficiency disease.

A completely anorectic 8-lb cat loses weight at the rate of about 1 lb/week, at least for the first 2-3 lb.[1] This drastic wasting must be combatted by forced feeding and/or artificial alimentation. Trying a dozen different foods, to coax the cat to eat, only wastes precious time.

The first treatment, for any cat that has not eaten for 48 hours or longer, should be inserting a gastric tube and providing the animal with some nourishment. Numerous satisfactory diets for artificial alimentation can be made from ingredients found around the home or hospital, if a blender is available (Table 7). If the cat also refuses to drink water or if diarrhea, vomiting or excessive fluid loss makes dehydration a problem, the replacement of fluids and the restoration of electrolyte balance become the top priority. Most concentrated diets do not contain enough water to supply all of a cat's daily water needs. The best way to ensure adequate water intake, therefore is to mix 1 oz water with every 2-4 oz diet. Several technics for administering liquids PO have been described.[20,21]

Fluid therapy is discussed in Chapter 2.

Table 7. Diets Suitable for Artificial Alimentation

Formula	Cal/oz	Protein (%)	Fat (%)	Carbohydrate (%)	Indication
*1 jar egg yolk 1 jar water	34	5.3	8.9	0.3	Anorexia
½ jar egg yolk 1 jar water 1½ oz Karo	45	2.6	4.4	14.0	Nephritis, hepatitis, enteritis
1 jar egg yolk 1 jar water 1 tsp oil 1 tbsp Karo	46	5.0	13.0	6.0	Anorexia, febrile states, cachexia
2 oz corn oil **8 oz i/d 20 oz water	30	2.8	7.4	5.3	Nephritis, enteritis
***8 oz Dyne 8 oz cottage cheese 8 oz water	58	6.6	16.7	7.6	Anorexia, febrile states, trauma

*Swift and Co., Chicago, IL
**Hill's Div., Riviana Foods, Topeka, KS
***BioLab Corp., Kansas City, MO

DIET AND DISEASE

The final and perhaps most challenging nutritional concern of the clinician is that of prescribing an appropriate diet to support the total treatment regimen for a sick cat. While normal, balanced diets are ideal for healthy cats, they may be totally inappropriate for diseased cats. Such cats should be fed a special diet to realize maximum results from a therapeutic regimen.

Obesity

Cats become overweight for the same reason that any other mammal does—prolonged consumption of calories in excess of those needed. The first step in any weight-reduction program is determining an optimal weight for the patient. Using this figure, the caloric intake needed to maintain that weight, *ie*, maintenance intake, can be calculated. Any balanced diet can serve as a reducing diet. The calculated maintenance intake of the diet chosen should then be reduced by 30% to provide the weight-reduction intake.

The second step is to weigh the cat and begin feeding it the calculated weight-reduction intake. All tidbits and treats should be withheld. This diet should be fed until the desired weight is attained, which may take weeks or months, depending upon the activity of the cat and the degree of obesity. At that point, feeding of the maintenance intake can be resumed.

Absolute client cooperation is essential to the success of any weight-reduction program. Discussing with the client the necessity of weight control, length of time probably required for weight reduction and the importance of regular examinations is critical.

Gastrointestinal Disease

Depending upon the type, GI disease is generally characterized by vomiting, diarrhea, tenesmus or constipation. The objectives of feeding a special diet in those GI diseases characterized by the first 3 signs are to minimize irritation of the gut and maximize digestion of the food consumed. To accomplish these objectives, in addition to specific medical or surgical therapy, a commercial diet designed for use in cats with GI disease can be fed or the client can be instructed to alter the regular diet appropriately. For example, the D'Arcy diet can be altered as follows:

D'Arcy Gastrointestinal Diet

2 lb raw hamburger
2 lb cottage cheese
½ lb raw liver, ground
2 lb dry rice
¼ lb Theralin (Lambert-Kay) (8 tbsp)
¼ lb brewers' yeast (8 tbsp)

The rice is boiled and drained and the rice water is saved. The dry ingredients are sprinkled over hamburger and mixed in well; then the hamburger, cottage cheese and raw liver are mixed

Table 8. Magnesium Content of Treat Foods[17]

Food	mg/100 g Dry Matter	Food	mg/100 g Dry Matter
Shrimp	568	Corn (canned)	76
Nuts	231-269	Beef (raw)	71
Canned catfood	200	Cheese (cheddar)	71
Dry catfood	160	Rabbit	70
Semi-moist catfood	160	Dietary catfood	60
Canned meat catfood	130	Freshwater fish	56
Codfish	130	Pork liver (raw)	55
Potatoes (raw)	105	Beef liver (raw)	48
Milk (whole)	100	Whole eggs	41
Saltwater fish	93	Lamb	37
Chicken (breast)	92	Pork	36
Sardines (canned)	82	Rice	28
Beef heart	78	Carrots	0.7

together. The rice is stirred in and enough rice water is added to make the desired consistency. This diet is fed at the rate of 2 oz/3 lb body weight.

Regardless of the diet chosen, all food should be withheld for 24 hours from cats with vomiting or diarrhea. Water can be provided in the form of 1-2 ice cubes per hour. If the vomiting or diarrhea cannot be controlled, the cat is fasted another 24 hours, then fed 2-3 tbsp meat or chicken broth every 1-2 hours. If this food is not vomited, a little strained baby food can be added to the broth. Twenty-four hours later, the diet is expanded by adding cottage cheese, soft-boiled eggs, or milk puddings that contain no sugar. If vomiting and diarrhea remain under control for 48 hours, small quantities of the regular diet can be fed at every other feeding. If this causes no untoward reaction, feeding of the regular diet on a normal feeding schedule can be resumed.

Withholding food is not as important as removal of the offending fecal mass in cases of constipation. Once the fecal mass is removed, the prevention of recurrence is greatly assisted by feeding a diet containing moderate amounts of plant fiber, little or no bones, and plenty of energy, such as the basic D'Arcy cattery diet as previously discussed.

An exception to the use of moderate fiber in patients with constipation is cats with megacolon. In these cases, the diet should be highly digestible and as low in digestive residues as possible. The D'Arcy GI diet or the D'Arcy hepatic diet (see below) can be fed to cats with megacolon.

Urinary Tract Disease

The objectives of feeding a cat suffering from cystitis or the feline urologic syndrome are to minimize the urinary concentrations of Mg and possibly P while maintaining adequate blood serum levels of these minerals, and to maintain an acid urinary pH to keep urinary magnesium salts in solution.[22]

Most commercial cat foods contain relatively high levels of Mg. Items owners often add contain high levels of Mg (Table 8).[17,23]

Renal Disease

The objective of dietary therapy in renal disease is to reduce renal excretion of nitrogenous waste, thereby compensating for reduced renal function. The most practical way of reducing the level of nitrogenous waste presented to the kidney is by increasing the quality of dietary protein; this also reduces the required daily intake of protein. In diets containing a protein blend with a biologic value of 80% or greater, protein levels can be reduced to about 20% on a dry-weight basis. This is equivalent to about 6% in canned meat diets or 18% in dry diets.[24]

A satisfactory diet for cats with nephritis can be purchased or made at home by the client. An example of such a diet is another alteration of the basic D'Arcy cattery diet.

D'Arcy Nephritis Diet

3 lb raw hamburger
½ lb raw liver, ground
3 lb dry rice
¼ lb Theralin (8 tbsp)
¼ lb brewers' yeast (8 tbsp)

The rice is boiled and drained and the rice water is saved. The dry ingredients are sprinkled over the hamburger and mixed well. The hamburger, rice and liver are mixed together evenly, using as much rice water as needed to make the desired consistency. The diet is fed at the rate of 1 oz/2 lb body weight.

Because cats require some of their calories to be derived from protein, the margin between compensated and decompensated renal disease is quite narrow and the prognosis in all cases of nephritis is guarded.

Hepatic Disease

The objective of feeding a special diet to patients with liver dysfunction is to reduce the metabolic workload of the ailing liver. Two of the liver's major functions that can be influenced by diet are transamination of amino acids and conversion of purines and pyrimidines to uric acid. By restricting protein sources to those of high biologic value, the levels fed can be reduced. If the protein nucleic acid content is kept low, the need for transamination and conversion can be minimized. Sources such as whole eggs, dried skimmed milk and cottage cheese provide proteins that meet this criteria. Avoidance of commercial foods containing fishmeal, shellfish, liver or meat by-products made up largely of glandular tissues eliminates some of the largest sources of uric acid precursors.

A modification of the D'Arcy diet, incorporating the protein sources suggested, can be used as a diet for cats with hepatic dysfunction. Commercial foods designed for cats with GI disorders also are sometimes satisfactory in cases of liver dysfunction.

D'Arcy Hepatic Diet

1 lb hamburger
3 lb cottage cheese
¼ lb raw liver, ground
2 lb dry rice
¼ lb Theralin (8 tbsp)
¼ lb brewers' yeast (8 tbsp)

The rice is boiled and drained, and the rice water is saved. The dry ingredients are sprinkled over the cottage cheese and mixed well. Then the hamburger, rice and liver are mixed together evenly with the cottage cheese. If the mixture is too thick, some rice water can be added to improve the consistency. The diet is fed at the rate of 2 oz/3 lb body weight.

Pancreatic Disease

The pancreas produces digestive enzymes and insulin. While enzymes produced by the salivary, gastric and intestinal glands can replace most of the enzymes lost in pancreatic disease, nothing is available to replace insulin. Without insulin, the cat is unable to regulate glucose concentrations in the blood, resulting in diabetes mellitus. The objectives of special diets in diabetes mellitus, therefore, are to provide a uniform rate of nutrient uptake to provide a constant supply of energy, thus enabling the clinician to adjust insulin dosage. Consistent exercise patterns should also be established to maximize the effectiveness of this regimen.

Commercial diets seldom contain the consistently uniform content required to treat diabetes mellitus. Consequently, a diet must be prepared by the owner. When homemade diets are used, the owner must be convinced of the need for uniform diet. A modification of the D'Arcy diet can be used if identical ingredients and exact weights are used each time the food is prepared.

D'Arcy Diabetic Diet

2 lb hamburger
2 lb cottage cheese
½ lb raw liver, ground
1 lb dry rice
¼ lb Theralin (8 tbsp)
¼ lb brewers' yeast (8 tbsp)

The rice is boiled and drained, and the rice water is discarded. The dry ingredients are sprinkled over the hamburger and mixed well. Then the hamburger, cottage cheese and liver are mixed together evenly with the rice. If the consistency is too thick, warm tap water can be used to dilute the mixture. The diet is fed at the rate of 1 oz/2 lb body weight.

Other Diseases

In cases of fracture or soft tissue damage, feeding an adequate diet is essential. There is little to be gained by increasing the quantity of any one nutrient fed beyond that in a normally balanced diet. Because the body selectively chooses the nutrients required for tissue repair from a balanced intake, imbalancing the diet with excesses of any kind may delay healing.

Febrile animals require more energy than normal because the increased body temperature causes an increased metabolic rate. Addition of 1 tsp corn oil or lard to the diet for every 5 lb

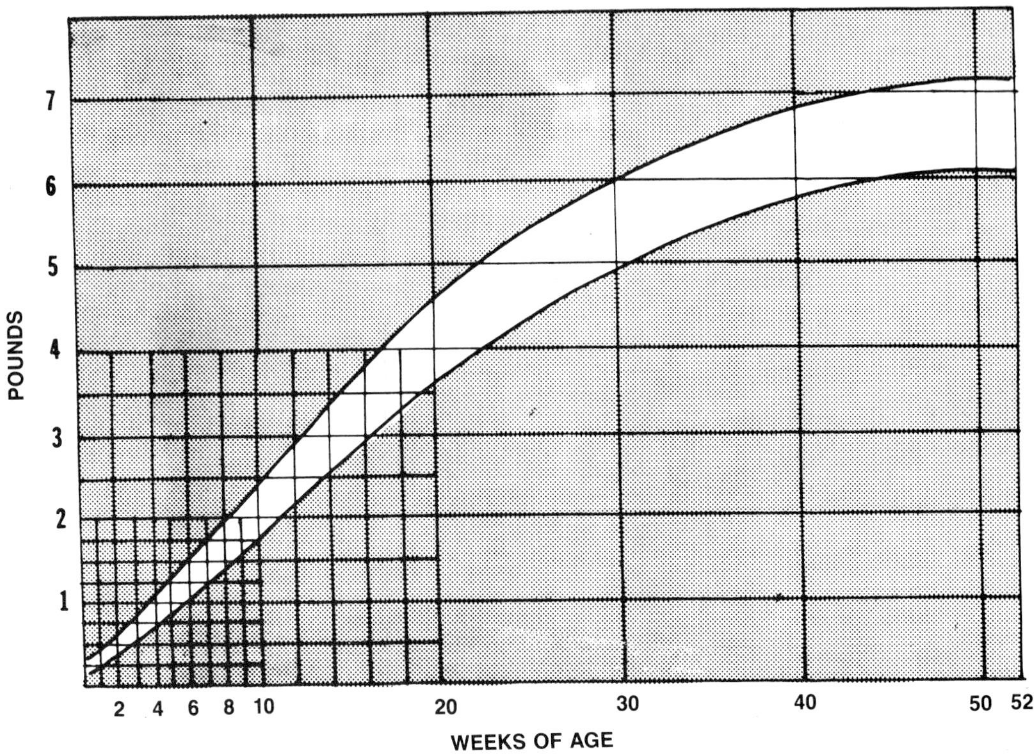

Fig 2. Normal growth rate for kittens.

body weight is sufficient to offset almost any energy losses due to fever. Forced feeding and/or artificial alimentation may be required if the animal is anorectic.

A cat should not be immunized until a dietary history has been obtained and the diet is judged adequate because the ability to develop immunity may be severely impaired if the diet is inadequate. Further, although a cat may develop a substantial level of immunity after vaccination, a cat eating an improper diet may be unable to mount an anamnestic response sufficient to prevent infection.

Table 9. Daily Quantities of Formula for Orphan Kittens

Body Weight g	Body Weight oz	Daily Quantity tbsp
93	3	1½
124	4	2½
186	6	3
248	8	4
310	10	6
372	12	7
434	14	8
496	16	9
744	24	10

FEEDING ORPHAN KITTENS

Kittens fed cow's milk or canine milk replacers suffer protein and caloric deficiencies, stop eating and eventually die. Orphan kittens should be fed a milk replacer specifically formulated for kittens (such as KMR:Borden). If this is unavailable, a substitute formula should be used, such as the following.

Orphan Kitten Formula

½ cup whole cow's milk
1 hard-boiled egg
1 tsp powdered $CaCO_3$
—liquid vitamins as per package directions

The ingredients are mixed in an electric blender until smooth. Table 9 lists the recommended quantities to be fed to kittens of various weights. The unused portion of the formula can be refrigerated for later use.

Kittens should be weighed at least weekly to determine if the dietary intake is adequate. A steady increase in weight is a sign of normal development (Fig 2).

References

1. Morris, JG and Rogers, QR. Friskies Res Dig **14 (2)** (1978) 2.

2. Collins, DR. Feline Pract **2(1)** (1972) 17.

3. Greaves, JP. Proc Symp Canine Feline Nutr Req, Br Sm Anim Vet Assoc, 1965.

4. Morris, JG. Friskies Res Dig **13(3)** (1977) 4.

5. Scott, in Catcott: Feline Medicine and Surgery. 2nd ed. American Veterinary Publications, Santa Barbara, 1975.

6. Gershoff, SN *et al.* Lab Invest **6** (1947) 227.

7. Everett, AM. Am J Physiol **141** (1944) 439.

8. Scott, PP. Gaines Sm Anim Nutr Workshop, Univ Ill, 1971.

9. Gershoff, SN *et al.* J Nutr **68** (1959) 75.

10. DaSilva, AC *et al.* J Nutr **46** (1952) 399.

11. DaSilva, AC *et al.* J Nutr **68** (1959) 213.

12. Gershoff, SN *et al.* Am J Med **27** (1959) 72.

13. Gershoff, SN and Gottlieb, LS. J Nutr **82** (1964) 135.

14. DaSilva, AC *et al.* J Nutr **56** (1955) 199.

15. Carey, CJ and Morris, JG. J Anim Sci **41** (1975) 309.

16. Bennett, D. Vet Rec **98** (1976) 313.

17. Anon. USDA ARS Handbook #8, Composition of Foods, 1969.

18. Rowland, GN *et al.* Path Vet **5** (1968) 504.

19. Siegmund, OH: The Merck Veterinary Manual. 4th ed. Merck, Rahway, NJ, 1973.

20. Teeter, SM and Collins, DR. VM/SAC **61** (1966) 1067.

21. Norsworthy, GD. Feline Pract **7(1)** (1977) 40.

22. Rich, LJ *et al.* Feline Pract **4(5)** (1974) 44.

23. Chow, FC *et al.* Feline Pract **5(5)** (1975) 15.

24. Collins, DR. Vet Clin No Am **6** (1976) 341.

25. Anon. NAS/NRC Publ #13, Nutrient Requirements of Cats, 1978.

2

fluid therapy

C.H. CLARK

Fluid therapy includes the administration of nutrients, water and electrolytes, and the correction of blood pH. Most of these alterations are corrected simultaneously by administration of of electrolytes, nutrients and $NaHCO_3$.

Cats often become anorectic during mild diseases that probably would not prevent other species from eating. The lack of nutrients and effects of starvation may become as serious as those of the primary disease. Cats seem to benefit a great deal from supplementary nutrients given during periods of anorexia. For this reason, nutrient therapy is discussed first, followed by discussions on water, electrolytes and acid-base balance.

NUTRIENT THERAPY

Nutrients are commonly used to supplement the treatment of ill animals. Use of the oral route makes it relatively easy to give cats adequate amounts of carbohydrates, fats, proteins, minerals and vitamins. Because of the large volumes required it is more difficult to meet the nutritional needs of the animal using parenteral routes. For parenteral use, the nutrients usually are confined to glucose, amino acids and vitamins. Deficiencies of some nutrients for a few days do not seem to be serious. It is, however, desirable to try to administer as complete a diet as possible.

Administration of Fluids

Fluid therapy requires administration of large volumes over longer periods than in other types of therapy. This has necessitated development of technics that enable continuous administration of large volumes of fluids. The following technics are useful in treating cats.

Oral Administration of Fluids

Pharyngotomy Tube:[1,2]: An incision is made through the cervical skin and into the pharynx. A stomach tube is placed through this into the pharynx and esophagus, and is held in place by sutures. This can be used for continuous long-term oral administration of nutrients.

The cat is first sedated with ketamine (40 mg/kg), acepromazine (0.5 mg/kg) and ketamine (20 mg/kg, or tiletamine and zolzepam (Telazol:Parke-Davis) at 5 mg/lb. Weak, debilitated cats may only require local anesthesia. The mouth is held open with a speculum and the piriform process, located caudal to the base of the tongue, is palpated. A pair of curved forceps is passed into the process and held so as to create a bulge on the lateral external surface of the cat's neck. A 5-mm incision is made in the skin and pharynx, and the point of the forceps is passed to the external surface of the animal's neck. A flexible, polyethylene plastic or rubber tube of suitable size is grasped by the forceps and pulled into the pharyngeal region. It is then directed down the esophagus into the stomach. It is important to make sure the tube is not kinked or occluded during this process and that only a sufficient amount of tubing is passed to reach the stomach. Before passing the tube, the distance from the stomach to the neck should be measured and marked with adhesive tape on the tube. After the tube is in place and the adhesive tape marker is adjacent to the skin, a nonabsorbable suture is placed through the skin and adhesive tape to secure the tube. The stomach tube is now ready for continuous oral therapy. When the animal has recovered, the sutures are snipped and the tube is removed without anesthesia.

Nasogastric Tube: A stomach tube can be passed via the nasal cavity and left in place for

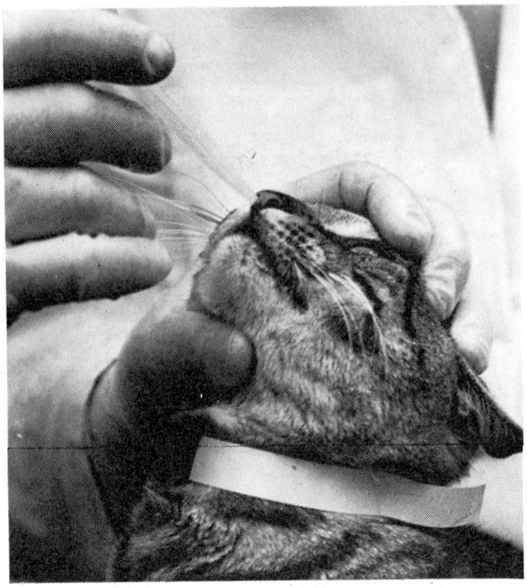

Fig 1. Before passage of stomach tube, 1-2 drops of a local anesthetic solution are instilled into one nostril.

several days. A semirigid plastic catheter is preferred for a nasogastric tube. The #8 Bard human male catheter is satisfactory. A 12-ga needle and several 20- to 30-ml syringes complete the equipment needed.

The cat must be restrained in some manner. The easiest method involves placing 1-2 drops of a topical anesthetic, such as 2% lidocaine, into a nostril (Fig 1). No more than 2 drops of local anesthetic should be applied because 4-5 drops often produce toxic signs, including mydriasis, rapid and difficult breathing, weakness and prostration. Although the cat usually recovers in 10-15 minutes, the experience further debilitates a sick animal. A second method of restraint involves giving ketamine IM at 10 mg/kg. The resultant sedation and analgesia are sufficient to enable passage of the stomach tube.

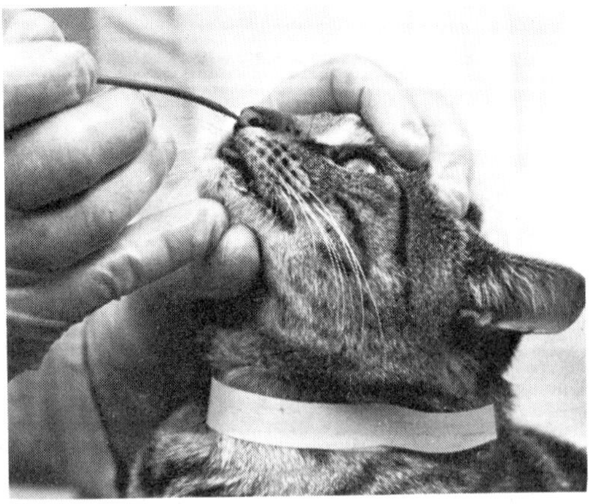

Fig 2. The end of the stomach tube (urinary catheter) is curved ventrad and inserted into the ventral part of the nostril.

To insert the catheter, the end should be bent slightly so it curves ventrad toward the esophagus when inserted into the ventral nasal passage. The cat's head usually is held with one hand as the catheter is gently inserted with the other. An assistant holds both front legs (Fig 2). A gentle touch is required until the cat swallows the catheter; thereafter it can be inserted steadily. Because of the anatomy of the pharyngeal area, there is little, if any, danger of inserting the catheter into the respiratory passage. Most cats do not bother the catheter after it is inserted; however, some cats, especially those nearly recovered from their illness, pull the tube out before it is to be removed. If the anesthetic is not effective, the cat sneezes while the catheter is being inserted. Passing a catheter intranasally can be difficult when the nasal passages are inflamed.

After the catheter is in place, a 12-ga needle is inserted into the end of it and connected to a syringe containing the mixture to be administered (Fig 3). The average 8- to 10-lb cat can accommodate 50 ml of fluid. This should be injected slowly to allow distension of the stomach; rapid distension may cause emesis.

Parenteral Administration of Fluids

Indwelling Catheter in Cephalic Vein: A technic has been described in which a catheter (Indwelling Catheter No. 416751:Sherwood Medical) is placed into the cephalic vein and the leg held rigid with a splint.[3] The vein is located and, if necessary, hair clipped to make the vein more accessible. A 22-ga, 2-inch needle is inserted a short distance into the vein with the bevel up. The plastic catheter is pushed some distance up the vein and the needle is then withdrawn. The stylette in the plastic catheter is left in place to make the polyethylene portion rigid. The catheter is held in place by tape around the leg, and the IV fluid bottle is then attached to the catheter. Because cats often withdraw the leg and obstruct the flow of fluid, a splint (Orthoplast: Johnson & Johnson) must be attached to the leg. The Orthoplast splint, after immersion in hot water, is molded around the leg.

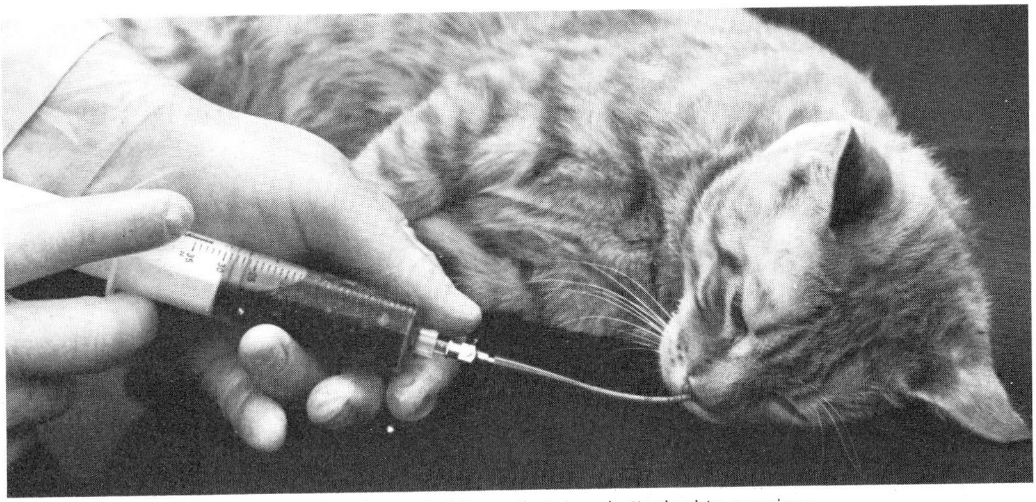

Fig 3. A 12-ga needle is inserted into the end of the catheter and attached to a syringe.

Intraperitoneal Injections

The intraperitoneal route can be used to give fairly sizable amounts of fluids. No more than 10 ml/lb body weight should be administered at any one time. Exceeding this amount often causes emesis. With the cat in lateral recumbency, a 2-inch needle is inserted into the peritoneal cavity near the umbilicus. After the needle has been inserted, the abdomen should be palpated to make sure the needle has not entered any of the internal organs. It is usually best to use nearly isotonic fluids. Some temporary dehydration occurs if hypertonic fluids are infused. All fluids injected into the peritoneal cavity should be sterile and prepared for parenteral administration, and should be warmed to body temperature before use.

Clinical Application of Nutrient Therapy

Protein and Amino Acid Therapy

Cats have a very high protein requirement of about 16-19% of the total calories for adult cats, vs only 4% for adult dogs (dry-weight basis).[4,5] Many of these amino acids are converted to carbohydrates and metabolized rather than being used in the formation of proteins. During this conversion, nitrogen is released as ammonia and must be detoxified by combining with arginine in the urea cycle; otherwise, ammonia intoxication occurs.

When 8 young-adult cats were fasted overnight and then fed a diet complete in all amino acids except arginine, they showed severe clinical signs of ammonia intoxication within 2 hours.[6] The cats exhibited lethargy, emesis, vocalization and ataxia. Severely affected cats had impaired respiration and cyanosis, and 1 cat died. Addition of either arginine or ornithine prevented these signs.

If amino acids are to be given to a cat, arginine must be added to or contained in the amino acid solutions. A dietary level of about 0.83% arginine is adequate for normal cats.[4,5,7] At least this amount should be present or added to amino acid solutions used therapeutically. Arginine powder (ICN Nutritional Biochemicals, Cleveland) is available for oral use.

Table 1 lists common sources of protein and their arginine content.[8] Fresh cow's milk and egg whites are low in arginine content. Because arginine is not as essential in people as for cats, it may not be included in amino acid solutions prepared for human use. Such solutions are not suited for use in cats. Glucose solutions can be used to meet energy requirements without the danger of ammonia intoxication.

The Urea Cycle: The urea cycle consists of 3 major constituents: ornithine, citrulline and arginine. Ornithine combines with CO_2 and ammonia released from amino acids to form citrulline. Citrulline combines with a second molecule of ammonia to form arginine. A molecule of urea is split from the arginine molecule by the enzyme arginase to reform ornithine (Fig 4.)

Ammonia Intoxication: Ammonia occurs in the blood stream as the ammonium ion (NH_4+) or ammonia gas (NH_3). Un-ionized ammonia gas penetrates nervous tissue much more readily

Table 1. Sources of Protein and Their Arginine Content

Food	Protein Content (%)	Arginine Content (%)
Cow's milk, dried		
Nonfat	35.6	1.300
Whole	25.8	0.944
Cow's milk, fresh	3.5	0.128
Casein	100.0	4.070
Cottage Cheese	17.0	0.802
Eggs, whole	12.8	0.840
Egg whites	10.8	0.634
Egg yolks	16.3	1.132
Pork or beef liver	19.7	1.201
Chicken liver	22.1	1.347

than do ammonium ions and is mostly responsible for the clinical signs of ammonia intoxication. Ammonia gas irregularly penetrates the nervous system, accumulates in certain parts of the brain and blocks the formation of energy-producing ATP and phosphocreatine.[10] Ammonia toxicity is in part due to a failure of adequate energy for function of certain parts of the brain.

There is an increased amount of ammonia gas formed when the pH rises (alkalosis).[9-12] In acidosis there are more ammonium ions formed and less toxicity. Anorectic cats often have an acidosis, which would promote ammonium ion formation and less toxicity. Before the acidosis is corrected, the ammonia should be eliminated by prior administration of arginine or amino acid hydrolysates containing arginine, such as Travasol (Travenol) or Amino-Plex (Bio-Ceutic).

In summary, anorectic cats do not develop serious ammonia intoxication. Presumably when they catabolize their body tissues for proteins during starvation, arginine is released along with other amino acids and prevents ammonia accumulation. Administration of glucose to anorectic cats does not cause ammonia intoxication and can be done safely. The problem arises only when proteins or amino acids deficient in arginine are given. Clinical signs of ammonia intoxication occur within 2-4 hours and are serious.

Ammonia intoxication can be treated in 2 ways. One is by attempting to remove the ammonia from the body with lactulose (Cephulac:Merrell Dow) and the other is to block the effects of ammonia on the CNS with sedatives, such as phenobarbital. However, correction of the cause of excess ammonia is always of prime importance, whether it is liver or kidney disease or dietary imbalance.

Use of lactulose can reduce blood ammonia levels by 25-50%. The drug is a syrup that can be given orally or by enema. Administration per rectum is probably easier than the oral route in

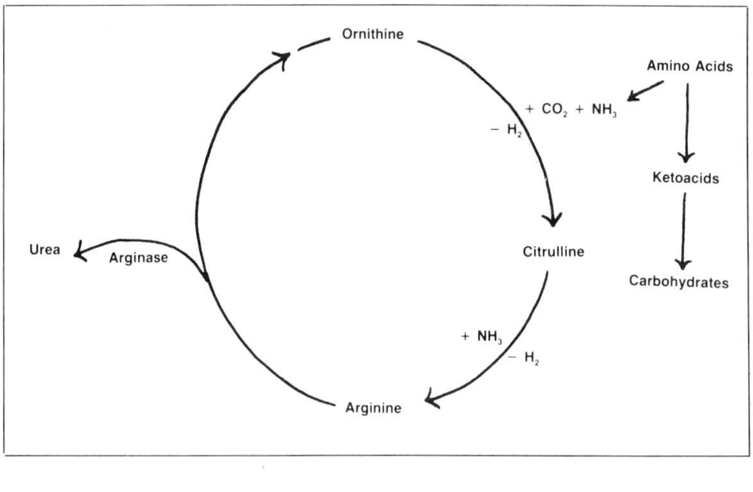

Fig 4. The urea cycle.

cats. The drug must stay in the intestine for a sufficient period to remove ammonia. When the lactulose is given as an enema, small doses given often are preferred to large doses given infrequently since large doses may stimulate evacuation of the bowels.

Lactulose acidifies the intestinal contents and is poorly absorbed from the intestinal tract. The acidification causes ammonia gas to migrate from the blood into the intestinal lumen and be converted to ammonium ions, trapping them in the intestines.

In cats with chronically elevated blood ammonia levels, lactulose can be mixed in the cat's food and be fed continuously provided the mixture is palatable. Slight sedation of chronically affected cats is another means of treating the disease. Phenobarbital, at 0.1 gr/10 lb (6 mg/10lb), provides sedation sufficient to prevent convulsions and vomiting. Although this dosage may cause excessive sleepiness and incoordination initially, the animal soon develops a tolerance for the drug. Phenobarbital should be given at meal time, when the cat consumes protein and blood ammonia levels peak. Use of phenobarbital and other sedatives is less satisfactory than use of lactulose in acute ammonia intoxication.

Oral Nutrient Therapy

Larger amounts of nutrients and electrolytes can be given with less risk of intoxicating the animal by oral administration than by other routes. Most solutions given orally have a thick consistency, with only enough water added to enable passage through the stomach tube. The cat must drink additional water to equalize its osmotic pressure; if it does not, a 5% solution of glucose may have to be given parenterally.

Oral administration of nutrients and electrolytes is indicated when an animal is completely or partially anorectic. Such therapy is provided to improve the condition of debilitated animals before surgery or administration of other medication. It is often effective when an animal is anorectic during or after an illness; cats often refuse to eat although only mildly ill or during recovery from more severe diseases. The problem, at least in part, is caused by persistent acidosis. The period of inappetence often is so prolonged that the animal's life may be threatened. Inappetence always interferes with recovery from disease.

The nutrients needed and quantities required depend on the animal's nutritional requirements and body weight. Cats require 39-95 calories/lb body weight (66-209 calories/kg). Generally, immature animals need more than adults, and sick animals require less than healthy ones. For sick animals, 30 calories/lb should be sufficient unless they are febrile. Often it is desirable to provide only minimum levels of nutrients to avoid overtreating and disturbing the animal more than necessary.

Oral medication provides nutrients to depress or delay catabolism of body tissues related to inappetence, and electrolytes and fluid to correct the pH and rehydrate tissues. Although a completely balanced diet plus electrolytes can be administered this way, the volume of fluid administered at any one time is limited; therefore, one usually attempts to correct the deficit that seems most important at the moment.

Complete Diets

These mixtures for oral administration do not require the accuracy in mixing that parenteral solutions do. Complete diet mixtures can be prepared just before use or partially mixed in advance. As some vitamin solutions are not stable, it is best to add a vitamin solution just before administering the mixture. Examples of nutrient solutions for peroral administration are shown in Table 2.

Sources of protein substitutes include amino acid hydrolysates, baby food, egg white and powdered whole milk. Sources of carbohydrate substitutes include table sugar, honey, Karo syrup and corn syrup.

Protein Preparations

Powdered whole milk, eggs, liver, fish and other good protein sources are available for oral use in anorectic animals. Because the preparation must be given through a stomach tube, its consistency is very important. In this respect, powdered milk or casein is easily added to water to make the proper consistency to pass down the stomach tube. Meat sources, such as baby food, can also be used for this purpose. On a dry-weight basis, 0.83% of the total diet should be arginine to avoid excessive ammonia formation. All of the food items in Table 2 are not on a dry-weight basis as to their arginine content; casein is, however. In addition, normal cats should have a dietary protein content of about 16% on a dry-weight basis.

Table 2. Sample Diets for Oral Use

Diet #1	Amount	Calories
Dry milk, whole protein and lactose	6 tbsp	80
Fat (Lipomul:Upjohn)	3 tbsp	270
Oral vitamins (complete)	MDR	
Note: This mixture contains ingredients that must be digested by the cat before they are absorbed.		
Diet #2		
Vivonex High Nitrogen (Tyson)		
Note: Contains amino acids 17.7%, carbohydrates 81.5%, fats 0.78%, vitamins, minerals and trace elements. All nutrients are in a readily absorbed form and do not require digestion. Comes in a powder that can be mixed with water and given by stomach tube. Each packet contains 300 calories.		
Diet #3	**Amount**	**Calories**
Egg white (protein) and egg yolk (fat)	1 egg	80
Honey (glucose, fructose)	1 tbsp	60
Complete mineral mix (*eg*. Lytrin:Mead Johnson)	as per label direction	
Oral vitamins	MDR	
Note: These high-quality nutrients are readily available. The complete mineral mix is useful for dehydrated animals.		

Amino Acid Preparations

Amino acids are prepared from acid or enzyme hydrolysis of casein or fibrin. Acid hydrolysis destroys tryptophan (an essential amino acid), but enzyme hydrolysis does not. As casein contains insufficient amounts of cystine, this essential amino acid should be added. Fibrin has adequate cystine. Amino acids may be more effective than whole proteins because GI secretions of anorectic animals may be depressed, and it is possible that whole proteins would not be adequately digested. Table 3 lists some amino acid solutions for parenteral use.

Fat Preparations

Fats usually are included in oral medications to supply calories. The same weight of this nutrient has 2¼ times the calories of protein or glucose. To supply adequate calories for thin or emaciated animals, it is important to include fats in the oral medication. Animals with adequate or excess body fat have less need for additional dietary fat. Fats should be emulsified for proper digestion and absorption. Cream and egg yolks are readily available emulsified fats. Lipomul (Upjohn) is an emulsified fat preparation providing 90 calories/tbsp. As a 10-lb cat can survive on only 300-400 calories per day, a couple of tablespoons of Lipomul substantially contribute to supplying these calories. When fats are fed, about a third of the total diet should consist of this nutrient. Methyl linoleate and linoleic acid (ICN Nutritional Biochemicals, Cleveland) are essential fatty acids that are directly absorbed and do not require digestion.

Carbohydrate Preparations

Glucose is an inexpensive source of carbohydrate that does not have to be digested for absorption; sucrose and lactose must be digested.

Electrolytes

Complete as well as special electrolyte mixtures are available for oral administration. One example of a complete electrolyte mixture is Lytrin (Mead Johnson). If indicated, a small amount of this powder can be added to solutions

Table 3. Some Commercial Amino Acid Preparations

Product	Dosage Form	Content	Manufacturer
Aminoplex	Oral powder or caps	19 amino acids, including arginine	Tyson
L-arginine or any of 20 different amino acids	Oral powder	Single amino acids	Tyson
Vivonex High Nitrogen	Oral powder	Contains 21 amino acids (arginine), vitamins and minerals	Norwich-Eaton
Travasol	Parenteral solution	Amino acids with or without electrolytes and glucose	Travenol Labs
Aminosyn	Parenteral solution	Amino acids, numerous combinations and concentrations with glucose and electrolytes	Abbott

given orally. Acidosis occurs in most diseases with concomitant starvation and is a cause of anorexia. Consequently, $NaHCO_3$ may be added to oral medication. The first time the animal is treated, $NaHCO_3$ usually is added at 1 tsp/10 lb body weight. Several hours later, the respiratory rate should decrease, indicating a reduction in acidosis. As the respiratory rate and pH approach normality, less $NaHCO_3$ should be given with each administration of fluids.

Potassium is another electrolyte that should be included in most oral medications. Usually more K can be given safely PO than parenterally. This ion is mainly responsible for maintaining the proper degree of cellular hydration. In moderate to severe dehydration, a great deal of cellular K has been lost. Potassium salt (KCl) can be given orally at ⅛ tsp/10 lb body weight in such situations.

Parenteral Nutrient Therapy

Although it is easier to give large volumes of required nutrients orally rather than parenterally, animals with vomiting, diarrhea or other contraindications to oral treatment should be treated parenterally. Even if the animal is eating, it may be desirable to supplement the nutrient intake parenterally. Wounds often heal more quickly when additional amounts of amino acids are given parenterally. Glucose injections may help prevent liver damage when vermifuges or other toxic drugs are given.

There usually is a period of anorexia associated with surgical procedures and illness. As a consequence, a cat may lose 6-25% of its body weight. Catabolism of proteins and their conversion to carbohydrates for energy, which occur during periods of inappetence, can be reduced or completely prevented by giving glucose and amino acids parenterally.[13] These solutions can be given IV, IP or SC.

Although isotonic solutions, such as 5% dextrose, are less harmful than hypertonic solutions, they provide only a small portion of the animal's caloric needs. For example, a 10-lb cat that needs 400 calories/24 hours would require 2 L 5% glucose daily to satisfy its caloric requirements. This amount of fluid is in excess of what can safely be given to a cat. A 5% glucose solution contains only 200 calories/L and some commercial preparations, such as Amigen 800 (Travenol), contain as much as 800 calories/L. This preparation contains amino acids, fructose, alcohol and electrolytes. To reach such high caloric concentrations, the fluid must be hypertonic. Alcohol is added because it contains nearly twice the calories of amino acids and fructose. The concentration of fructose is 2.5 times the isotonicity of blood.

The electrolyte composition of Amigen 800 is interesting. After the caloric portion of the solution (amino acids, fructose, alcohol) is metabolized, a hypotonic electrolyte solution remains. The excess water usually is beneficial for dehydrated animals. The only 2 electrolytes that are more concentrated than in the cat's plasma are K and Mg. They are needed to raise intracellular osmotic pressure and rehydrate the cells. The Na, Ca and Cl ions remain largely outside the cells. Therefore, this solution has a high caloric content and electrolytes needed intracellularly and extracellularly, and it supplies ample water.

When a solution, such as Amigen, is given to a cat, 500 ml are required to supply 400 calories daily. This is still an excessive amount of fluid. Recently, Beagle puppies were raised on only hypertonic nutrient solution that contained high quantities of glucose and amino acids.[14] The puppies were maintained on these IV solutions for as long as 256 days.

A mixture of 5% amino acid solution (Aminosol:Abbott), which contains 200 calories/L, and 50% dextrose, which contains 2000 calories/L, provides about 0.9 calories/ml when mixed at 1 L Aminosol to 600 ml 50% dextrose. It would require approximately 35 ml of this solution per lb daily to supply a 10-lb cat with its minimal caloric needs. Vitamins and various electrolytes would have to be added as needed. This solution is a common example of hyperalimentation fluids prepared for clinical use.

The disadvantages of hyperalimentation usually are associated with administration of solutions to uncooperative animals. The solutions must be injected slowly and continuously over 24-hour periods. In addition, they must be injected into the larger veins to obtain rapid dilution with blood; injection into smaller veins often results in thrombosis. Considerable care must be taken to prevent contamination of the solution and catheter. A 0.22 μ membrane filter should be placed in the IV setup to filter any bacteria or fungus spores. A pump is needed to force the fluids through such a filter.

The technic used to feed Beagle puppies parenterally involved implanting a Silastic radiopaque catheter in the jugular vein and passing it to the cranial vena cava or right atrium. At this point, the large blood volume dilutes the hypertonic solution thoroughly and quickly. The catheter's location was determined radiographically. The IV apparatus was arranged in the cage with a spring and swivel so the animal's movements would not dislocate it.

Another technic for parenteral feeding involves infusion into the femoral medullary cavity. A pin is inserted into the medullary cavity in the same way as for immobilization of a femoral fracture. The bone pin is then removed and a hypodermic needle is wedged into the cavity and connected to an IV infusion set. All fluids, including blood, can be given by this route. This technic is satisfactory for 2-3 days, but the danger of infection is serious.

Hypertonic nutrient solutions are also given intraperitoneally. A maximum of 10 ml/lb and preferably 5 ml/lb is given at one time. Sick animals or animals that are somewhat dehydrated should be given the lesser amount. Intraperitoneal infusions can be repeated 2-3 times daily, supplying the animal with necessary nutrients and preventing further deterioration and a negative nitrogen balance. Hypertonic solutions are absorbed from the peritoneal cavity in about 6 hours. The rate of absorption is not constant; much more of the solution is absorbed during the first portion of the 6-hour period. The rate of absorption is roughly equal to the concentration of glucose and amino acids in the peritoneal cavity and blood stream. High concentrations of glucose in the peritoneal cavity result in its rapid transfer into the blood stream. Because the solution is hypertonic, however, it tends to draw water from the blood stream into the peritoneal cavity, and thus increases the degree of dehydration. Therefore, dehydration should be corrected with isotonic and hypotonic electrolyte solutions and glucose before hyperalimentation with a hypertonic solution.

Complications of Hyperalimentation

The maximum amount of protein that could be given Beagles parenterally was 4 g/kg, even though their needs were almost twice this amount.[14] Excessive use of protein hydrolysates causes depression, emesis and sometimes convulsions. Glutamic and aspartic acids tend to promote emesis and depression. As glycine tends to prevent emesis, increasing its content in amino acid mixtures helps avoid this complication. Amino acid mixtures that do not contain glutamic and aspartic acids are less likely to cause emesis in dogs and cats.

There is danger of infection when catheters are kept in place for several days at a time. Careful aseptic procedure is necessary when implanting a catheter into a jugular vein or femoral medullary cavity. Thrombosis often occurs when catheters are left in veins for long periods. This is not a considerable problem when catheters are left for relatively short periods, as 2-3 days. Thrombosis is much less likely if the catheter empties into an area of rapid blood flow, such as the jugular vein.

Water and Electrolyte Therapy

A good beginning point in any study of fluid therapy is a brief review of water metabolism in cats. The fluid content of the cat's body is a balance between water intake and loss. Water is obtained by consuming food, by drinking water, and from metabolism or oxidation. As foods are digested, H is produced and combined with O_2 to form water. Each 100 g carbohydrate, protein or fat produce 55, 41 and 107 ml water, respectively.[15] Cats produced water by metabolism at a rate of an average of 9.3 g/kg body weight daily.[15] At the same time, these animals consumed water at 50.6 g/kg body weight daily in a combination of food and drinking water.

When the food was dry, cats drank more water than when it was moist. Dry food has a tendency to cause cats to drink more water. The lack of moisture in the mouth stimulates drinking. In a study of 13 cats, those receiving an all-dry ration consumed 198 ml water daily, while those receiving an all-meat ration consumed 158 ml water daily.[15] The mean urine volumes were 62 ml daily for cats fed the all-dry ration and 83 ml daily for cats fed the all-meat ration.

The average cat loses about 36% of the consumed water in the urine and 25% in the feces. Approximately 39% of the water is lost through insensible water losses, as in expired air and evaporation from the skin, mouth, eyes and other areas. Cats normally secrete urine of rather high specific gravity in comparison with other animals (Table 4).[15] The water intake of a cat is controlled by the composition of plasma and by extracellular fluid volume. Increased Na and protein contents increase the osmotic pressure of plasma, which affects the osmoreceptors in the hypothalamus, resulting in increased thirst and water consumption.

Kittens consume more water than do adults. Kittens 6-8 months old consumed water at an average rate of 76.9 g/kg. This decreased to the adult average of less than 60 g/kg when they reached a year of age. The total body water is less in kittens than in adults.[15]

Body Water Compartments

The body water compartments are conventionally divided into the intracellular space and extracellular space. Water readily passes among all spaces of the body, and is held in these spaces by the osmotic effects of various electrolytes and proteins. Potassium is the major cation that holds water inside the cell; proper cellular rehydration cannot occur unless adequate amounts of K are supplied, especially in kittens. The treatment of cellular dehydration in kittens should include fluids containing K.

The extracellular space compartment is divided into the blood vascular system and interstitial spaces. The interstitial spaces actually are not spaces similar to the vascular compartment but are a gel-like matrix composed of hyaluronic acid molecules, which hold the water. Subcuta-

Table 4. Water Balances and Diet in Adult Cats [15]

	Diet		
Urine Value	Dry Food	All Meat	Canned Food
Volume (ml)	49	106	69
pH	6.93	6.11	6.92
Specific gravity	1.056	1.050	1.051
Mean Values for Cats			
Mean body weight	4.4 kg		
Water consumption	50.6 g/kg/day		
Urine excretion	18.2 ml/kg/day		
Fecal water excretion	12.7 ml/kg/day		
Consumed water lost in urine	36%		

neous injections are frequently absorbed faster if the enzyme hyaluronidase is added. Sodium maintains the osmotic pressure of the extracellular space, while proteins are important in maintaining the actual portion of extracellular fluid in the blood vascular space. A reduction in the concentration of plasma proteins may reduce the plasma volume. The electrolyte content of the extracellular space is controlled primarily by the kidney.

Control of Extracellular Fluid Volumes

The volume of the extracellular fluid space, including the interstitial space and plasma volumes, are controlled by a number of physiologic systems. The importance of any one system at any particular time varies considerably and the failure of one system may not cause serious alterations of fluid volume. These systems depend upon sensory receptors located in various parts of the body.

Stretch receptors, which measure blood pressure, are located in the atria, aorta, aortic arch, carotid artery and efferent arterioles of the kidney. Osmoreceptors are located in the supraoptic nucleus of the hypothalamus. These receptors detect changes in blood pressure and osmotic pressure and make physiologic adjustments to correct defects. The osmoreceptors in the hypothalamus are sensitive to alterations of osmotic pressure and are more sensitive to alterations of osmotic pressure caused by Na changes than by sucrose, urea and other nonelectrolytes.

During dehydration there usually is a relatively greater loss of water than Na, resulting in an increased plasma osmotic pressure. The increased osmotic pressure causes the osmoreceptors to secrete antidiuretic hormone, which increases renal water retention. This helps restore normal osmotic pressure in plasma and interstitial spaces. This same mechanism is also important during fluid therapy because it helps to prevent excessive changes of osmotic pressure that may result from IV injection of fluids.

The Aldosterone System

Aldosterone secreted from the zona glomerulosa of the adrenal gland is very important in controlling plasma K and Na levels. Secretion of this hormone is controlled by the K concentration of extracellular fluid, the quantity of body Na, secretion of ACTH, and the renin-angiotensin system.

Potassium Concentration: The major control mechanism of aldosterone secretion is the K concentration in extracellular fluid. A very small increase in body K levels causes release of aldosterone, which in turn stimulates the kidney to excrete K and resorb Na. This in turn increases the plasma Na level and reduces the plasma K level. This safety mechanism helps prevent excessive plasma levels of K. This mechanism operates only when the kidneys are functioning, so that in renal disease and the feline urologic syndrome, K may accumulate in the blood in toxic levels.

Sodium Quantity: A reduction in total body Na quantity and decrease in the extracellular fluid volume results in a considerable increase in aldosterone secretion, which results in Na retention and expansion of the extracellular fluid space. This is a very important mechanism in maintaining extracellular fluid volume.

ACTH Secretion: Adrenocorticotropic hormone (ACTH), which stimulates the adrenal gland to release corticosteroids, also stimulates it to release aldosterone. This may be an important factor in stress and the accumulation of fluid in chronic congestive heart failure.

Renin-Angiotensin System: A decrease in arterial pressure or decrease in the quantity of Na in body fluids causes the juxtaglomerular apparatus of the kidney to secrete renin, which splits the vasoactive peptide, angiotensin, from plasma globulins. Angiotensin raises blood pressure by arteriole vasoconstriction and reduces the total vascular volume by mild constriction of some veins. It reduces the renal output of water and salt by constricting the renal arterioles and causes release of aldosterone, which in turn causes the kidney to resorb more Na.

All of these events reduce K levels, and increase Na levels and extracellular fluid volume.

Plasma Proteins

While water and Na are extremely important in maintaining the total extracellular volume, the plasma proteins determine the portion of extracellular fluid in the vascular space. Release of plasma proteins by the liver is mediated by the autonomic nervous system. During a serious drop in blood pressure (hemorrhage, shock), the liver releases plasma proteins into the lymph system and vascular space. This increase in plasma protein levels increases osmotic pressure, which pulls water from the interstitial and cell spaces and helps restore plasma volume.

Animals in good condition have greater quantities of plasma protein stored in the liver than do debilitated animals; therefore, healthy animals can tolerate a greater degree of blood loss. With surgery or injuries in animals in good condition, injection of saline or lactated Ringer's solution combines with the plasma protein secreted by the liver to partially restore the plasma volume. The use of saline or Ringer's solution in debilitated animals may not be as effective because of the lack of plasma proteins to hold the fluid in the vascular space. In debilitated animals, blood, plasma or plasma expanders must be used to maintain normal plasma volume.

Stretch Receptors

The stretch receptors of the atria effect the release of antidiuretic hormone. When there is a lack of stretch as a result of decreased central venous pressure, antidiuretic hormone is released and stimulates the kidney to retain water. The opposite occurs when there is excessive pressure. The stretch receptors act, through the sympathetic nervous system, on the efferent and afferent arteries of the kidney to regulate renal water excretion.

Principles of Fluid Therapy

The control of extracellular fluid volume is complex and involves the simultaneous action of a number of physiologic systems that control the K, Na and water content of the extracellular space. If fluid losses are excessive, these mechanisms fail to restore plasma and extracellular fluid volumes, and injection of fluids is required for the cat's survival. Fluid therapy is designed to supply an external source of fluid to animals to assist the physiologic control mechanisms.

Signs of Dehydration

Thirst: A cat usually is thirsty when there is cellular dehydration. Diarrhea, vomiting, polyuria, severe injuries, burns and shock may all cause thirst. The usual mechanism involves loss of water via some pathologic process, such as diarrhea, that results in increased osmotic pressure of plasma and a relatively greater loss of water than Na. The higher osmotic pressure of plasma draws water from the interstitial and cellular spaces, and loss of fluid from the cells results in K loss. This is a compensatory mechanism that helps prevent excessive osmotic pressure and distortion of the cellular enzyme systems. Cells attempt to maintain their normal architecture during water loss by excreting K to maintain near-normal osmotic pressure.

Dehydration of the cells in the supraoptic nucleus of the hypothalamus (thirst center) results in increased thirst and water consumption. Water consumption helps alleviate thirst but does not totally restore body fluid balance until K and Na levels are restored.

Another mechanism that tends to cause thirst is the renin-angiotensin mechanism. Release of renin leads to angiotensin II formation, which stimulates the thirst center and increases water consumption. During loss of whole blood, there is no alteration of osmotic pressure because all of the constituents of blood are lost in equal amounts. However, baroreceptors detect reduced blood volumes and the liver secretes plasma proteins into the circulating fluid. Large quantities of protein are found in the thoracic duct after hemorrhage. The increase in plasma protein level increases the osmotic pressure of blood, which pulls water from the interstitial cellular spaces, causing cellular dehydration. This again increases thirst and water consumption, and helps restore blood volume.

Decreased Skin Turgor: Normally when a cat's skin is pinched up over its back and released, the skin drops back into place very quickly due to sliding of tissues across one another and fluid in the interstitial space. When dehydration is greater than 2-3% of body weight, the tissues slide back into place more slowly. When water loss becomes as severe as 10% or more, tissues tend to slide back very slowly, resulting in a "tenting" effect or an elevated area where the skin was pulled. This is one of the best subjective tests of the degree of dehydration in cats.

Decreased Secretion of Body Fluids: During dehydration, secretion of natural fluids, such as saliva and ocular and nasal fluids, is markedly reduced, resulting in dryness of the eyes and mouth. Prolonged dehydration may result in dry skin and brittle hair.

Sodium and Potassium Metabolism

The Na content of extracellular fluid is about 150 mEq/L. Sodium is necessary for normal cell function. A loss of Na depresses cell function, resulting in lethargy, decreased nervous activity, and muscular weakness. Sodium is also the major ion for maintenance of osmotic pressure of the extracellular fluid. Decreases in the Na level result in decreased extracellular space volume and often decreased plasma volumes.

The extracellular K level is about 4.5 mEq/L, while intracellular levels are 150 mEq/L. Potassium is primarily excreted by the kidney. Most K is filtered in the glomerulus and then partially resorbed by the proximal tubules. Potassium is also excreted in the distal tubules in exchange for Na. After combining with an acid, Na passes through the glomerulus into the tubule. Sodium is then resorbed in the distal tubule in exchange for either K or H.

Potassium and H compete for exchange with Na. If this exchange is not made, as in some renal diseases, and Na is lost in the urine, K and H accumulate in the blood, resulting in hyperkalemia and acidosis.

Potassium cannot enter the cells unless adequate glucose and insulin are present. Both $NaHCO_3$ and lactate tend to cause K loss in the normal kidney. Excessive administration of saline solutions results in an intracellular loss of K and excretion of K into the urine. Adequate amounts of K are required for rehydration of cells. Potassium is especially important in treating dehydration associated with diarrhea in kittens, puppies and other young animals. Solutions for intracellular rehydration may contain up to 35 mEq/L of K.

Solutions containing large amounts of K (10-35 mEq/L) should be given very slowly IV, or preferably SC or IP. Solutions containing glucose should be given before or at the same time to promote passage of K into the cellular space.

Electrolyte Solutions

Potassium must be given to rehydrate the cells, while Na is primarily used for rehydration of plasma and interstitial fluids. Although normal electrolyte solutions should contain electrolytes in about the same amounts as in plasma, the proportion of electrolytes to each other is more important than the exact amounts in a solution. For example, a dilute solution containing Na at 75 mEq/L and Cl at 57 mEq/L has the proper ratio of Na and Cl. Electrolyte levels should be normal once the kidney eliminates the excess water in this solution.

In certain conditions, one or more electrolytes are lost in excess of others, creating an imbalance of electrolytes. If renal function is near normal, a complete electrolyte solution can be given and the excess amounts of various electrolytes are eliminated in urine. Sometimes it is better to give an imbalanced electrolyte solution that has the needed electrolytes in greater than normal amounts. In severe prolonged emesis, for example, Cl is lost in much greater amounts than Na. In this case, a solution that contains more Cl than Na would be superior to a normally balanced solution. Solutions containing larger amounts of K and Mg are used to correct cellular dehydration.

Table 5 lists the composition of various fluids used to treat cats.

Plasmolyte: The electrolyte composition of Plasmolyte (Baxter) is similar to that of the extracellular fluid except for the amounts of K and Mg. The moderately increased amounts of these electrolytes are designed to provide a modest degree of intracellular rehydration.

Peridial: Peridial (Cutter) is used for peritoneal dialysis in the treatment of renal disease. It has about the same composition of normal extracellular fluid except that K is excluded. This ion is not included because in oliguria or anuria, the plasma K level may be elevated to the point of toxicity.

Saline Solution 0.9%: Normal saline has been extensively used as an electrolyte fluid supplement in dehydration and other conditions. Each liter of the solution contains 154 mEq Na and 154 mEq Cl. The Na content is about the same as that for normal feline plasma; however, the Cl level is greater than in plasma. Administration of excessive amounts of Cl in relation to Na can result in excretion of plasma bicarbonate and subsequent acidosis.

Regular saline solutions are acid forming and may not be best for rehydration of acidotic animals. Use of a more balanced solution that is not acid forming, such as lactated Ringer's solution, is more desirable in acidotic animals. In renal disease and the feline urologic syndrome, it is undesirable to administer solutions containing K. Normal saline or Peridial is useful in these instances.

Ionosol-G: Ionosol-G (Abbott) was formulated to replace fluid and electrolytes in cases of severe emesis. The Na level is low and the Cl level is very high to offset severe losses of this ion in vomitus. The K level is quite high to assist intracellular rehydration. Ammonia levels may be elevated in liver and renal disease, and Ionosol-G, which contains NH_4 at 71 mEq/L, should be used carefully in such cases. The solution also contains 340 calories/L in the form of dextrose.

Dextrose 2½%, Saline 0.45%: This solution can be prepared by mixing 5% dextrose and 0.9% saline in equal amounts. Its purpose is to supply

Table 5. Composition of Various Fluids (mEq/L)

	Na	K	Ca	Mg	Cl	NH_4	HCO_3	Lactate
Plasma, cat	150	4.4	5	2.2	120	—	24	—
Plasmolyte (Baxter)	140	10	5	3	103	—	—	—
Peridial (Cutter)	140	—	5	1.5	102	—	—	—
Saline, 0.9%	154	—	—	—	154	—	—	—
Ionosol-G (Abbott)	63	17	—	—	151	71	—	—
Dextrose 2½%, saline 0.45% (Abbott)	77	—	—	—	77	—	—	—
Lactated Ringer's (Abbott)	130	4	3	—	109	—	—	28
Ringer's solution (Abbott)	147	4	5	—	156	—	—	—
Ionosol-T in D5-W (Abbott)	40	35	—	—	40	—	—	—
Multisol-M in D5-W (Abbott)	40	13	—	3	40	—	—	—

water to dehydrated patients. The fluid is isotonic and supplies some calories, water and saline. It is a beneficial, all-purpose fluid for modest degrees of dehydration.

Ringer's Solution: This solution has electrolyte levels similar to those of plasma, except for a greater amount of Cl. Because solutions high in Cl tend to cause acidosis, their use should be limited to treatment of dehydration associated with emesis.

Lactated Ringer's Solution: Lactated Ringer's solution (Abbott) is similar to Ringer's solution except that the excess Cl is replaced by lactate, which reduces the solution's tendency to cause acidosis. Lactated Ringer's solution has a balanced extracellular electrolyte composition but very little intracellular rehydrating capability.

Ionosol and Multisol: Both of these solutions contain high levels of K and are used for intracellular rehydration. The high K content can be hazardous if the solutions are given rapidly IV (Table 5). The IP and SC routes are much safer.

ACID-BASE BALANCE

Laboratory Measurement of Acid-Base Balance

The more information one has concerning the plasma concentration of bicarbonate and the blood pH, the more accurately a therapeutic regimen can be designed. Equipment for obtaining these measurements can be very expensive; however, equipment is available that is very reasonable in cost, requires only small amounts of blood or plasma, and yields a great deal of useful information.

pH Meter: The normal pH of arterial blood in cats is 7.46 and in venous blood is 7.39.[16] Values above or below these indicate alkalosis or acidosis, respectively. A pH of 7.1 indicates very severe acidosis; however, the quantity of $NaHCO_3$ necessary to treat the animal is not apparent. While the pH meter can indicate the shift in pH, it does not give very much information as to the required therapy and especially the quantity of $NaHCO_3$ needed in treating acidosis.

Oxford Titrator: The Oxford titrator (Oxford Labs, Foster City, CA) is an inexpensive instrument that requires only 50 µl (0.05 ml) of serum or plasma for its operation. The fact that it uses such small quantities of plasma makes it a desirable instrument for use in cats. The plasma bicarbonate level is measured by titrating the plasma with a standard acid until there is a color change. A calibrated wheel drops acid into the plasma until the color change is observed. The plasma bicarbonate level is indicated in mEq/L by reading the calibrations on the machine. The value obtained in the patient is subtracted from the normal value to obtain the amount of $NaHCO_3$ needed in treating acidosis. Once the bicarbonate deficiency is known, a formula can be used to compute the amount of $NaHCO_3$ needed to treat an acidotic cat: body weight (kg) x 0.3 x bicarbonate deficit (mEq/L) = total bicarbonate deficit. For example, in a 4-kg cat, a bicarbonate deficit of 12.4 mEq/L would require 14.9 mEq $NaHCO_3$ for correction of the base deficit (4 kg x 0.3 x 12.4 mEq/L = 14.9 mEq).

Harleco System: A system similar to the titrometer is marketed by Harleco (Gibbstown, NJ). The unit may be a macrosystem, which requires 1 ml of plasma, or a microsystem, which requires 100 μl (0.1 ml). The microsystem is probably more suitable for cats. The microsystem requires a shaker or agitator, which is an additional expense, but is still a reasonably priced piece of equipment.

The basic principle of this system is similar to the Van Slyke system in that CO_2 is released by adding acid to the plasma and the volume of CO_2 gas released is measured in a calibrated syringe. A standard (control) should be run simultaneously to correct for variations in barometric pressure, temperature or other factors. The instrument reads in milliosmols of CO_2 per liter, which can be considered the same as milliequivalents of bicarbonate per liter. After this value is obtained, the same procedure is used as with a titrometer in calculating the total quantity of $NaHCO_3$ in mEq/L to be administered to an acidotic cat.

Both the Oxford titrator and the Harleco system have disadvantages in that only one value is measured and the diagnosis and therapy are based on that one value. Because of the compensatory mechanisms of the body, some acid-base imbalances may resemble others. For example, chronic respiratory alkalosis may somewhat resemble, as far as the plasma bicarbonate levels are concerned, metabolic acidosis. In chronic respiratory alkalosis, the body compensates and attempts to lower the pH by reducing the plasma bicarbonate level below normal. If only one value is determined, such as the plasma bicarbonate level, there may be some confusion in such cases. However, this is very unlikely since chronic respiratory alkalosis is very rare in cats. Also, the clinical signs would be different from those of metabolic acidosis.

A similar situation would exist when comparing metabolic alkalosis with respiratory acidosis. These conditions might be confused if only one value is determined, such as plasma bicarbonate concentration. In both of these cases the bicarbonate level may be elevated; however, respiratory acidosis would primarily be due to a pathologic condition of the lungs, such as pneumonia. Metabolic alkalosis usually is caused by emesis, intestinal obstruction or some similar factor. Therefore, clinical signs would help separate the 2. The plasma bicarbonate level is reduced much greater in metabolic acidosis and the 2 methods of evaluation of the bicarbonate level would be of great value in determining the quantity of $NaHCO_3$ necessary to treat these conditions as well as some help in diagnosis.

Blood-Gas Machines: Blood-gas machines are excellent devices for determining abnormalities in acid-base balance. They determine the blood pH, from which acidosis or alkalosis can be diagnosed, and also the CO_2 level. With these 2 values and the use of a Henderson-Hasselbach nomogram, the plasma bicarbonate levels and the base deficit can be determined.

These machines also measure the O_2 content of blood. Accurate measurement of the pH and CO_2 level allows differentiation among the various types of metabolic and respiratory acidosis and alkalosis. They also are excellent for determining the quantity of $NaHCO_3$ required for therapy. Once the machine is in operation, all of these measurements can be obtained in less than a minute. The major drawback of blood-gas machines is that they are very expensive.

Acid-Base Therapy

The pH of plasma is controlled by buffer systems, of which the CO_2-bicarbonate buffer system is one of the most important. When the ratio of CO_2 to bicarbonate is 1:20, the plasma pH is 7.4. The ratio between the 2 is more important than the absolute quantities of each.

If an acid should be added to blood, it would combine with bicarbonate to form CO_2 and the Na salt of the acid. This would reduce the quantity of bicarbonate present in plasma and the pH would shift to the acid side. In this chemical reaction, more CO_2 is formed. This would increase the total CO_2 in plasma and stimulate respiration, which would increase the loss of CO_2 from plasma. This loss of CO_2 would bring the ratio back closer to 1:20. Because the ratio would not completely return to 1:20, the plasma pH would remain on the acid side for a while. The shift of pH would not be as great as would have occurred without compensation by the respiratory system.

	Normal		Acidosis		Compensated Acidosis	
	Ratio	Value	Ratio	Value	Ratio	Value
$NaHCO_3$	20	24 mEq/L	1.4	12 mEq/L	13	12 mEq/L
CO_2	1	1.2 mEq/L	1	8.2 mEq/L	1	0.9 mEq/L
pH		7.4		6.26		7.22

Fig 5. Plasma CO_2, bicarbonate and pH values in normal and acidotic animals.

As illustrated in Figure 5, the normal ratio of CO_2 to bicarbonate in plasma is 1:20 and the blood pH is 7.4. Acidosis reduces the bicarbonate content to form the Na salt of the acid and increases the amount of CO_2 present. There is a shift in the pH toward the acid side. As the respiratory rate increases, it removes this CO_2 and brings the ratio and pH back more nearly to normal. The pH is still acid since the ratio does not reach normal; however, the low pH of 6.26 is not compatible with life so the pH of 7.22 is a considerable improvement over this. After some time the kidney increases the plasma bicarbonate content of the blood stream to normal.

The pH values during acidosis and compensated acidosis in Figure 5 do not reflect the amount of $NaHCO_3$ needed to correct the condition. If only a pH meter were used at this time to measure the acid shift, it would be obvious that acidosis is present; however, there would be no way of telling the exact quantity of $NaHCO_3$ required to correct the acidosis. Use of the Oxford titrator, Harleco system or blood-gas machine would indicate the quantity of $NaHCO_3$ required.

Acid-Base Imbalances

By convention, acid-base disturbances are divided into acidosis or alkalosis when the pH is shifted below or above the normal 7.4, respectively. Usually a shift of 0.05 pH units is not considered sufficient to warrant treatment. The shift in pH of 0.2 pH units definitely requires therapy. Acidosis and alkalosis have been divided into metabolic or respiratory, depending upon whether the main causative factors are metabolic or respiratory in nature. The most common pH disturbance undoubtedly is metabolic acidosis.

Metabolic Acidosis

Metabolic acidosis develops in most diseases that cause anorexia. Carbohydrates and fats are metabolized to lactic, acetoacetic and other acids, resulting in accumulation of acids in the body. These acids are neutralized by various buffers, including the bicarbonate-CO_2 buffer system. The Na salt of the acid, such as Na lactate, is excreted by the kidney. In the renal tubules, the Na ion normally is resorbed and exchanged for K or H ions. This conserves Na and restores the plasma bicarbonate level to normal. Therefore, normal metabolism does not result in acidosis as long as the normal buffer systems continue to operate.

Metabolic acidosis is common in renal disease because of loss of Na in the urine. This results in more alkaline urine and an acid pH in blood. Metabolic acidosis is very severe in the feline urologic syndrome, in which urethral obstruction has essentially caused kidney failure. In addition, metabolic acidosis occurs in diarrhea due to loss of Na in the feces and in most diseases in which there is starvation, catabolism of body fat, and decreased or no dietary intake of Na.

Continued formation of acids reduces the plasma bicarbonate content and shifts the pH toward the acid side. Compensation by buffer systems reduces the shift of pH for awhile; however, with continued acid formation, the pH gradually decreases and acidosis becomes more severe.

Not all of the acid formed remains in the extracellular fluid. Much is absorbed by the cells and neutralized by cellular proteins. About half of the acid is in the extracellular space and the other half is inside the cells. Intracellular acid content cannot be directly calculated and can only be estimated. When pH corrections are made, one should not attempt to totally correct for all body acid at one time. Acid diffuses into cells fairly slowly and takes as long as 24 hours to leave the cells. If enough $NaHCO_3$ is given at one time to totally neutralize all body acids, it shifts the pH drastically to the alkaline side and only after 24 hours or more does sufficient intracellular acid enter the extracellular space to neutralize the excess bicarbonate. This drastic shift may harm the animal and should be avoided. The amount of bicarbonate administered at one time should be sufficient to neutralize the extracellular acid and a small amount of intracellular acid.

Treatment: To treat metabolic acidosis, information on the plasma bicarbonate level and other values is very desirable and almost necessary. Administration of $NaHCO_3$ without knowledge of the plasma bicarbonate content should be done very conservatively. A more accurate pH correction can be made when knowledge of the plasma bicarbonate content is available.

Normal reported values of the plasma bicarbonate level vary from 22 to 28 mEq/L. Different methods result in some variation, so a number of normal samples should be analyzed to establish normal values for each practice or laboratory. For this discussion, we will assume that 24 mEq/L is the normal value in cats.

We determine the plasma bicarbonate content of the patient, which in this example is 14 mEq/L. Therefore, this animal has a bicarbonate deficiency of 10 mEq/L ($24 - 14 = 10$) in its extracellular fluid. The next step is to determine the extracellular fluid volume in liters. Because about 20% of the animal's weight is extracellular fluid volume, we multiply the cat's weight (4 kg) by 20% (0.2) to determine the quantity of extracellular fluid volume ($0.2 \times 4 = 0.8$ L). The extracellular fluid volume in liters (0.8 L) is multiplied by the bicarbonate deficit (10 mEq/L) to determine the amount of $NaHCO_3$ required. Using a correction factor of 0.2 (20%) corrects only for the extracellular bicarbonate deficit. A correction factor of 0.4 instead of 0.2 would probably counteract most of the acid found in the animal's body; however, overcorrection might occur. A correction factor of 0.3 rather than 0.2 or 0.4 would be a good compromise to correct the bicarbonate deficit in the extracellular space plus some in the intracellular space. The plasma bicarbonate content should be redetermined 24 hours later and additional corrections made if necessary.

Another approach to this same problem is to calculate the bicarbonate deficit in the extracellular space using a factor of 0.02. The amount could be given slowly IV to correct only for deficits in the extracellular space. An additional equal volume could be given at intervals or slowly over the next 24 hours to allow the $NaHCO_3$ to buffer the acid in the intracellular space. The total quantity of $NaHCO_3$ given in this case would be 40% of the body weight, which would correct for extracellular and intracellular acid. This would come close to correcting for all the excess acid in the animal's body.

In the above illustration the bicarbonate deficit was calculated by measuring the plasma bicarbonate deficiency and making calculations as to the quantity needed to correct this deficit. There are other buffers in plasma, including the RBC, so the bicarbonate deficit does not accurately reflect the total amount of base needed (base deficit) to correct for the accumulation of all extracellular acids. The amount of $NaHCO_3$ given should be multiplied by 1.2 to more accurately correct for all acids (total base deficit).

Blood-Gas Machine in Metabolic Acidosis: The blood-gas machine is very accurate and useful for correction of all types of acid-base imbalances, including metabolic acidosis. Usually 3 values of the blood are measured and used to determine the base deficit on a Siggaard-Andersen nomogram (Fig 6). The pCO_2 and the pH are measured by the blood-gas machine, and hemoglobin value is determined by conventional means. With a Siggaard-Andersen nomogram, the pCO_2 and pH values are connected with a straight line and the base deficit read where this line crosses the hemoglobin value for the cat.

The same nomogram can be used to determine the base deficit by measuring the plasma bicarbonate content with the Harleco system or Oxford titrator, using a pH meter to measure the pH, and connecting these 2 points (Fig 6). The base deficit value obtained is then used in the same type formulas for the calculation of the total amount of $NaHCO_3$ needed to correct the metabolic acidosis.

Fig 6. The Siggaard-Andersen nomogram is used to calculate the amount of $NaHCO_3$ needed to correct metabolic acidosis. In this case, the patient is a 4-kg cat with a hemoglobin level of 9 g/dl, blood pH of 7.21 and pCO_2 of 35.5 mm Hg. The base deficit is determined by connecting the pCO_2 of 35.5 to the pH of 7.21 with a line and reading the base deficit (13) where the line crosses the hemoglobin value (9) line. The cat's weight (4) is multiplied by the correction factor (0.3) and by the base deficit (13) to obtain the total base deficit ($4 \times 0.3 \times 13 = 15.6$ mEq). An 8.5% solution of $NaHCO_3$ contains bicarbonate at 1 mEq/ml. Therefore, this cat would require 15.6 ml (15.6 mEq) of an 8.5% solution of $NaHCO_3$ to correct the deficit. (Courtesy of Radiometer)

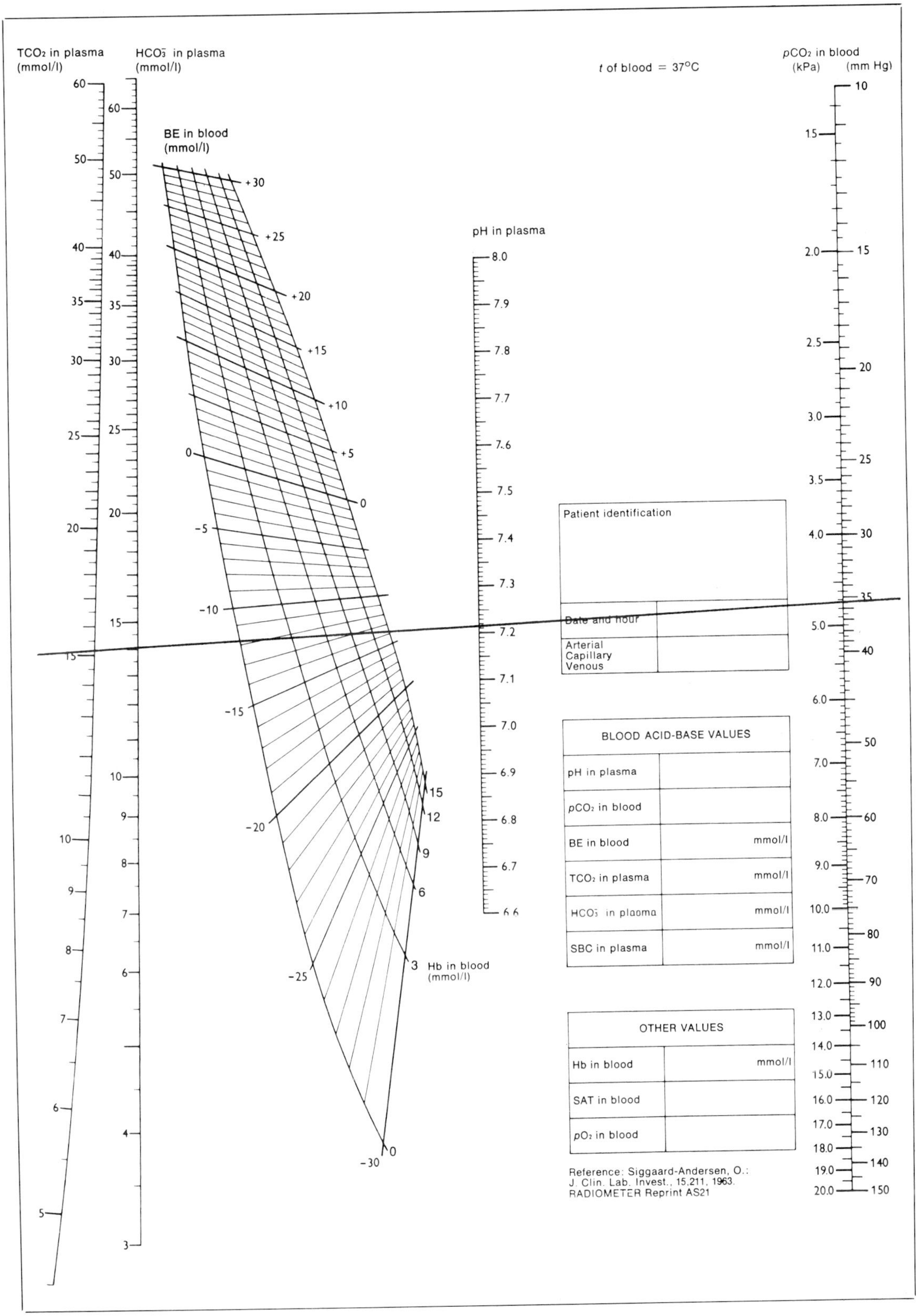
TCO₂ in plasma (mmol/l)
HCO₃⁻ in plasma (mmol/l)
BE in blood (mmol/l)
pH in plasma
t of blood = 37°C
pCO₂ in blood (kPa) (mm Hg)
Hb in blood (mmol/l)
Patient identification
Date and hour
Arterial
Capillary
Venous
BLOOD ACID-BASE VALUES
pH in plasma
pCO₂ in blood
BE in blood mmol/l
TCO₂ in plasma mmol/l
HCO₃⁻ in plasma mmol/l
SBC in plasma mmol/l
OTHER VALUES
Hb in blood mmol/l
SAT in blood
pO₂ in blood
Reference: Siggaard-Andersen, O.: J. Clin. Lab. Invest., 15,211, 1963.
RADIOMETER Reprint AS21

Respiratory Acidosis

Respiratory acidosis occurs when the respiratory system is unable to exhale sufficient quantities of CO_2. Accumulation of excessive CO_2 in plasma causes acidosis that is easily detected by a blood-gas machine. Respiratory acidosis occurs in chronic heart failure, pneumonia, pulmonary edema, allergic reactions, anaphylactic shock, pulmonary inflammation from irritants, and other conditions that interfere with CO_2 transport across the pulmonary capillaries.

The blood pH is low, the pCO_2 is elevated, and there may be a slight compensatory rise in plasma bicarbonate level. The lack of a decrease in plasma bicarbonate level and the increase in pCO_2 differentiates respiratory acidosis from metabolic acidosis.

In the bicarbonate-CO_2 buffer system, the CO_2 is the respiratory component and is a measure of respiratory function, while the bicarbonate is the metabolic component, and a measure of metabolic function. In respiratory acidosis, the pCO_2 is elevated to a considerable degree. To compensate for this, there may be some slight increase in plasma bicarbonate level. The problem is ultimately corrected by alleviating the pulmonary disease and allowing CO_2 to be exhaled more readily.

Metabolic Alkalosis

Metabolic alkalosis usually is caused by a loss of Cl during continued emesis. Pyloric obstruction and concomitant emesis cause severe depletion of Cl and metabolic alkalosis. Emesis associated with gastroenteritis usually does not cause as severe a metabolic alkalosis as does pyloric obstruction because in gastroenteritis there is a loss of intestinal Na as well as Cl in the vomitus.

Metabolic alkalosis occurs when the Cl lost is replaced by bicarbonate. The amount of bicarbonate retained is directly related to the plasma Na content. If Na also is lost, as in gastroenteritis, less bicarbonate is retained and the metabolic alkalosis is less severe. There may be some retention of CO_2 (acid) to compensate for bicarbonate retention.

Alkalotic cats tend to be very excitable. Although that clinical sign may suggest the presence of metabolic alkalosis, the condition is much more accurately diagnosed by blood-gas measurements and plasma bicarbonate determinations.

Treatment: Metabolic alkalosis is treated by alleviating the condition causing the vomiting and giving a fluid with a Cl content higher than that of normal plasma (normal = 120 mEq/L). A 0.9% saline or Ringer's solution (not lactated Ringer's) can be used. The Cl content of saline and Ringer's equals the Na content (both 150 mEq/L), but in plasma the Cl content (120 mEq/L) is less than that of Na (150 mEq/L). When equal amounts of Na and Cl are given, as with infusions of saline, there is a relative excess of Cl. This excess Cl buffers the excess plasma bicarbonate to correct the metabolic alkalosis. In severe cases of vomiting, as in pyloric obstruction, fluids containing more Cl than Na, such as Ionosol-G (Table 5) should be used.

Respiratory Alkalosis

Respiratory alkalosis occurs when rapid respiration causes an excessive loss of CO_2, which results in a shift of pH toward the alkaline side. This occurs readily in dogs when they pant excessively on hot days, and also may occur in cats. Alkalosis causes a tendency toward convulsions and hyperactivity of the nervous system. This condition apparently is rather rare in cats.

CLINICAL USE OF FLUID THERAPY

Fluid Therapy for GI Disease

Gastroenteritis usually results in 2 clinical signs that have opposite effects on acid-base balance. Diarrhea results in a loss of Na and metabolic acidosis, while emesis results in a loss of Cl and metabolic alkalosis. Whichever of these signs predominates determines the acid-base shift. Metabolic alkalosis almost always occurs in pyloric obstruction with severe emesis and may occur in moderately severe gastroenteritis, with diarrhea and vomiting.

Large quantities of fluid normally are secreted into the stomach and intestines by the digestive glands. The quantity secreted daily amounts to several times the blood volume. Practically all of this fluid must be resorbed to maintain proper hydration. In diarrhea or emesis, some of this fluid is lost and dehydration results.

Emesis

Fluids used to treat emesis should contain as much or more Cl as Na. The excess Cl is obtained by adding NH_4Cl to the electrolyte solution. The ammonium ion is very toxic and normally is converted by the liver into nontoxic urea. Because serum ammonium levels may be high in liver and kidney disease, use of ammonium-containing fluids should be avoided in such cases. High blood levels of ammonium may cause inappetence, nervousness, convulsions and coma.

Fluids used to treat severe emesis and alkalosis, as in pyloric obstruction, include Ionosol-G and 5% dextrose (Table 5).

Mild cases of emesis (not pyloric obstruction) should be treated with 0.9% saline or Ringer's (not lactated) solutions. These solutions have a high Cl content and are useful for treating animals deficient in Cl from vomiting.

Diarrhea

Acidosis usually occurs when fluids and Na are lost in diarrhea. Treatment involves providing an electrolyte solution containing more Na than Cl. Lactated Ringer's solution has some Cl replaced by lactate and is used to treat diarrhea. In severe diarrhea, the cells become dehydrated and lose K. Their hydration is more rapid when fluids containing K are administered.

Fluid Therapy for Urinary Tract Disease

Renal disease usually causes metabolic acidosis, depending to some extent on the amount of associated emesis. In renal disease, the kidneys fail to resorb Na, resulting in Na loss in urine, a decrease in the plasma bicarbonate content and consequent metabolic acidosis.

An important concept in treatment of renal disease is accurate correction of fluid deficits and acid-base balances. This almost invariably requires measurement of the plasma bicarbonate content. Accurate measurements are necessary because the kidneys normally correct for errors in fluid therapy by excreting or conserving electrolytes and water. Because diseased kidneys may not be able to compensate for errors in fluid therapy, a more accurate system of fluid therapy must be employed. If laboratory equipment is not available for measuring the plasma bicarbonate level, the fluid imbalance in renal disease should be corrected by peritoneal lavage.

Peritoneal Lavage

Peritoneal lavage involves injecting a solution containing physiologic concentrations of electrolytes into the peritoneal cavity and allowing it to equilibrate with the blood for 15-30 minutes. The lavage solution containing waste products is then withdrawn and discarded.

Diffusion of waste products and electrolytes from blood into the dialysis fluid depends on which fluid (blood or dialysis solution) contains the higher concentration. For example, if an animal has an excessive amount of plasma Cl, then Cl diffuses from the plasma into the peritoneal lavage solution. If plasma Na concentrations are low, Na diffuses from the dialysis fluid into plasma. The interchange of electrolytes tends to correct whatever imbalance may exist in the blood. In addition, waste products that diffuse into the solution are removed when it is withdrawn from the body.

Although peritoneal lavage can be performed several times daily, once a day usually is adequate. As the animal's condition improves, lavage is performed every second or third day as indicated. Usually 3-4 lavages are sufficient for animals to recover from acute nephritis.

Fluid used for peritoneal lavage should be carefully balanced and contain Na, Ca, Mg and Cl. Such solutions as 0.9% saline do not contain a sufficient variety and proper balance of electrolytes for this purpose. Peridial (Cutter) is properly balanced for peritoneal dialysis (Table 5). Inject 10-15 ml/lb IP and withdraw the remaining fluid after 15-30 minutes.

Feline Urologic Syndrome

The feline urologic syndrome essentially is renal failure caused by urinary obstruction rather than renal disease. Urethral obstruction for 24-48 hours results in severe biochemical changes, including azotemia, hyperkalemia, metabolic acidosis and dehydration. Other less life-threatening alterations are hyponatremia, hypermagnesemia, hypocalcemia, hyperphosphatemia and hyperglycemia.[17,18]

Critical abnormalities that require immediate attention are the acidosis and dehydration and the obstruction. Both clinically and experimentally, animals in which the acidosis and dehydration were treated survived, while those untreated frequently died, even though the obstruction had been removed. Relief of the obstruction alone was not as effective as relief of the obstruction and treatment for acidosis and dehydration.

Dehydration can be partially treated by administration of 50-100 ml of a saline-dextrose combination, along with sufficient $NaHCO_3$ to relieve the acidosis. Use of other fluids, such as lactated Ringer's, is not as desirable in the presence of hyperkalemia due to their K content. Additional fluids should be administered as needed over the next few days.

The degree of acidosis is very severe and, in one clinical study, an average blood pH of 7.11 ± 0.09 was found in 23 cats.[17] Acidosis of this severity requires immediate $NaHCO_3$ therapy. Laboratory measurements of the plasma bicarbonate level or base deficit are necessary to calculate the amount of $NaHCO_3$ required. The total dose of required $NaHCO_3$ is computed by the following formula: required $NaHCO_3$ (mEq) = base deficit x 0.3 x body weight (kg).[17] The base deficit can be calculated by subtracting the plasma bicarbonate concentration from 24. The total $NaHCO_3$ dose should be divided into 2 aliquots, one given immediately by IV drip and the other given IM, IP or SC over the next 24 hours along with saline therapy.

Cats with the feline urologic syndrome have high BUN and plasma ammonia concentrations.[19,20] It is inadvisable to administer amino acids or protein hydrolysates at this time because of the danger of elevating plasma urea and ammonia levels.

Most cats with the feline urologic syndrome have hyperglycemia and occasionally glucosuria. These are corrected spontaneously after the obstruction is relieved, and the acidosis and fluid deficit are corrected. This hyperglycemia may be a result of several mechanisms resulting from the stress, in that stress causes a release of the adrenal corticosteroids, which in turn convert protein to glucose and elevate blood glucose levels. In addition, an elevated plasma ammonia level stimulates release of glucagon from the liver, which also increases blood glucose levels. The hyperglycemia associated with the feline urologic syndrome does not require treatment other than that required to alleviate the urinary obstruction.

Fluid Therapy for Dehydration

Dehydration can be classified as mild, moderate or severe, based more or less on symptomatic evaluation. It cannot be stated with certainty that a specific degree of water loss causes certain signs, since the rapidity of the loss is very important. For example, a 5% water loss within a few hours might be fatal, but a similar loss over several days may not cause a problem. Mild dehydration is considered as a 5% water loss (225 ml in a 10-lb cat), moderate dehydration as a 10% loss (450 ml in a 10-lb cat), and severe dehydration as a loss of 10-15% of body water (450-775 ml in a 10-lb cat).

In mild dehydration there is loss of extracellular electrolytes (Na) from plasma and the interstitial spaces. This degree of dehydration usually can be corrected by replacing the extracellular electrolytes, water and some bicarbon-

Table 6. Fluid Therapy for Various Degrees of Dehydration

Mild Dehydration	
Lactated Ringer's solution	50 ml
Dextrose 5%	50 ml
Sodium lactate	5 mEq/10 lb
	100 ml
Moderate Dehydration	
Plasmolyte (Baxter)	40 ml
Dextrose 5%	50 ml
Multisol-M (Abbott)	10 ml
Sodium bicarbonate	5 mEq/10 1b
	100 ml
Severe Dehydration	
Plasmolyte (Baxter)	35 ml
Dextrose 5%	35 ml
Multisol-M (Abbott)	30 ml
Sodium bicarbonate	15–20 mEq/10 1b
	100 ml

Table 7. Drugs and Fluids Used To Treat Animals With Liver Disease

Drug/Fluid	Administration	Effect
Glucose	At 1 ml/kg, 15% solution given SC or IP BID; starch or sucrose may be fed PO	supplies calories
Arginine (sodium glutamate)	0.1 g/10 lb PO	decreases plasma ammonium level
Phenobarbital	6 mg/lb PO	controls neurologic signs
Whole blood	At 2-5 ml/lb, depending on need, given IV, IP or intra-medullary	supplies electrolytes, RBC, plasma proteins, nutrients, buffers
Multisol-M D5W	At 1 ml/kg, IV, IP or SC	rehydrates cells

ate. Lactated Ringer's solution is a good choice (Table 6). With moderate to severe dehydration, the signs become progressively more severe and there is a loss of extracellular and intracellular electrolytes in addition to lost fluids. Solutions with increased amounts of K, such as Plasmo-lyte, Ionosol-T or Multisol-M, should be used along with lactated Ringer's to treat moderate to severe dehydration (Table 5).

Fluid Therapy in Liver Disease

The liver converts most nutrients into a form that can be used by other tissues for energy. In the presence of liver disease, conversion of fats and proteins to metabolites used by other tissues may be inadequate. As it is not necessary for the liver to convert glucose before it can be used for energy, continuous administration of glucose is desirable during acute and chronic hepatitis. If the animal is eating, glucose can be given orally; sucrose or starch can be substituted. If parenteral administration is preferred, dextrose solution should be given SC or IP because of slower absorption. One injection in the morning and one at night provide adequate blood glucose.

The plasma ammonium level usually is above normal in liver disease because of failure of the liver to convert ammonia to urea. A temporary reduction in the plasma ammonium level usually follows administration of sodium glutamate or arginine solution at 0.1 g/10 lb.

Liver disease may also result in defective protein synthesis. Deficiency of proteins involved in coagulation results in a tendency to hemorrhage. Plasma or blood transfusion frequently alleviates these signs.

Table 7 lists drugs and fluids used in treating animals with liver disease.

Blood Transfusion

A blood transfusion supplies the animal with a completely balanced electrolyte solution, plasma proteins, antibodies, RBC and nutrients. Blood also has a considerable buffering capacity, which helps correct acid-base imbalances.

Blood can be used effectively to treat a wide variety of diseases. It is not an easy task, however, to estimate the amount of blood needed by a particular animal. The blood volume in an average cat is about 35 ml/lb body weight. A loss of 50% often is fatal unless treatment is given quickly. A 5% loss usually does not produce clinical signs. Blood transfusions at a rate of 2-5 ml/lb are sufficient in most cases. Fortunately, most cats can adapt to excessive or reduced amounts of blood and other fluids, and it is not necessary to determine precisely the volume needed for replacement.

Technics for Blood Transfusion

The following is a satisfactory method of blood transfusion. The donor cat is anesthetized with pentobarbital sodium, leaving the needle in the vein. Blood is then drawn through a cardiac puncture. Care is taken to make the puncture in the ventricle rather than the atrium. If the atrium is punctured, blood may leak into the pericardial sac, collapsing the atrium and causing death. Ventricular puncture is accomplished by palpating the thoracic wall over the the heart and introducing a 20-ga, 2-inch needle through the thoracic wall into the caudoventral portion of the heart.

Table 8. Plasma Expanders

Product	Plasma Expander	Molecular Weight	Other Ingredients	Manufacturer
Macrodex	6% Dextran	70,000	Either dextrose 5% or saline 0.9%	Pharmacia Labs
Reomacrodex	10% Dextran	40,000	Either dextrose 5% or Saline 0.9%	Pharmacia Labs
Hetastarch	6% Hetastarch	450,000	0.9% saline	American Critical Care
Dextran	6% Dextran	75,000	0.9% saline	Ceva/Abbott

The anticoagulant is 0.25 ml heparin (1000 USP units/ml) for each 10 ml blood. Unlike citrates, heparin does not appear to be significantly toxic to cats. Normally, blood can be withdrawn at 10 ml/lb without harm to the donor cat. After the blood is withdrawn, it is replaced with an equal volume of a plasma expander, such as Dextran, Hetastarch or Ringer's solution, given IV (Table 8). The latter can be injected through the same needle used to administer the pentobarbital.

Blood can be given to the recipient by various routes, each of which has advantages and disadvantages. Intravenous administration has the advantage of making the blood immediately available and, in shock, restores blood pressure and immediately improves circulation. Disadvantages of IV administration are primarily related to the rate of injection. Rapid injection can result in pronounced cardiovascular disturbances and can be fatal. Transfusion reactions from IV injections are more serious than when other injection routes are used. If blood cannot be given slowly IV, it is often better to give it IP.

Fluids can be given very rapidly by IP injection and are absorbed slowly over a period of hours. Small molecules, such as glucose, are absorbed in 4-6 hours; those the size of proteins and emulsified fat require about 24 hours; most RBC are absorbed in 2-3 days. Blood given IP must contain an anticoagulant because much of its value is lost if it clots in the abdominal cavity.

Intraperitoneal transfusion is safer than IV use because of the slower absorption. If the donor blood and recipient blood are incompatible, the reaction causes little if any harm after IP transfusion. The slowness of absorption is also the main disadvantage. When it is necessary to obtain immediate effects, as in severe shock, use of IP transfusion is not recommended.

Intramedullary transfusions apparently have limited application. Insertion of an 18-ga needle into the femur's medullary cavity was described earlier in this chapter. An IV outfit is connected with the needle and transfusion is begun. Blood enters the circulation almost as rapidly as when given IV and the needle is kept in place more easily than in a vein. Therefore, this route may be preferred when parenteral treatment is to be prolonged. A harness can be applied over the rear legs to allow the animal to walk while receiving an intramedullary infusion. The medullary cavity can also be used when it is difficult to introduce a needle into a collapsed vein. However, in intramedullary transfusion a great deal of care is required to prevent osteomyelitis.

Intramuscular and SC blood transfusions are inefficient because only about 3% of RBC are absorbed. Plasma is absorbed slowly; about 48 hours are required for absorption of most of plasma proteins after SC administration.

Blood Storage

Blood transfusions of heparinized fresh whole blood are ideal. Use of stored blood from domestic cats generally is not so satisfactory. Because domestic cats are very sensitive to citrate, there should be no more than 0.4% citrate in the transfused blood. Even this small amount may cause reactions in some recipients.

The small amount of blood withdrawn from the donor cat makes it inadvisable to use commercially available citrated blood collection bags or bottles. Addition of only a small amount of blood to the citrate in blood collection containers designed for larger quantities of blood may result in transfusion reactions in recipient cats.

Heparinized blood of domestic cats lasts only 3-4 days in the refrigerator. Experimentally, the percentage of RBC that survived, as determined by the PCV, 24 hours of refrigeration averaged 92-95%. Further, if blood stored for 24 hours is injected into a recipient cat, about 25% of the RBC are rapidly removed from the circulation. Although the RBC in stored blood appear normal, changes that occur during storage cause the phagocytic system to remove them from circulation. Refrigeration for 24 hours results in the loss of about 25% of viable RBC in the recipient cat. After storage for 3 days, the percentage of surviving RBC is less than 40%.

Platelet numbers also are adversely affected by storage. Therefore, diseases requiring platelet transfusion should be treated with fresh whole blood.

Transfusion Reactions

Although high levels of isoantibodies are not found in cats as in people, the possibility of a transfusion reaction cannot be completely disregarded. If blood from one donor is injected too often into the same recipient during a period of 7-14 days, antibodies are produced and may result in a severe reaction. As it usually requires 2-4 days for production of antibodies, multiple transfusions usually can be given safely within this period.

The incompatibility of blood varies from complete to slight. Donor RBC usually react to the plasma of the recipient; occasionally the opposite reaction occurs. Cross-matching the blood usually is of no value in detecting these incompatibilities in cats.

Interspecies Transfusions

Dog blood has been injected into cats on numerous occasions and seems to have considerable benefit at times. Canine RBC last no longer than about 3 days in cats. The same is true of RBC from sheep, goats and cattle; horse blood is incompatible. Although the plasma proteins of various species last 7-19 days in cats, there are so many different proteins it is difficult to determine exactly how long various ones last. These proteins may be of some value in expanding plasma volume.

One transfusion of dog blood into a cat seldom produces any evidence of incompatibility. A second transfusion is not advisable, however, since cats rapidly produce antibodies against dog blood in general rather than against a specific donor's blood. Another transfusion from any dog is likely to cause a severe reaction.

Plasma Expanders

These are substances that expand the plasma volume when given IV. They are a desirable adjunct in treatment of shock due to hemorrhage, burns, surgery, sepsis or trauma. Along with other fluids, they may be beneficial in treatment of diarrhea and emesis. Desirable qualities of a plasma expander are that they have the same oncotic pressure as that of plasma and diffuse slowly through capillary walls. They should not be allergenic or pyretic. Except for their physical properties, they should be pharmacologically inert. Examples of plasma expanders other than blood are electrolyte solutions, Dextran and Hetastarch (Table 8).

Electrolyte Solutions

Lactated Ringer's solution can be used to temporarily expand the plasma volume. Due to the small size of the electrolytes involved, they readily diffuse through capillary walls. Hence, the value of this type of solution is very limited. After hemorrhage, animals frequently excrete increased amounts of plasma proteins from the liver. If this occurs, the liver proteins along with lactated Ringer's may maintain the expanded plasma volume for a significant period.

Dextran Solutions

Dextrans are fairly effective plasma expanders. They are large molecules composed of glucose units that are degraded very slowly in the body. The injection of these solutions improves circulation for at least 24 hours. It takes about 2-3 weeks before the drug has been totally metabolized and eliminated. Dextran is available in 2 molecular sizes: 70,000-75,000 and 40,000. They are also combined with 5% dextrose or 0.9% saline solutions. The lower-molecular-weight Dextran solutions (40,000) reportedly improve microcirculation and prevent sludging of blood that sometimes occurs in shock better than the solutions of larger molecular size. The larger-molecular-weight solutions maintain plasma expansion longer. In general, both of these solutions are suitable for use as plasma expanders in cats. The Dextrans are antigenic and have induced antibody formation in people.

Hetastarch

This plasma expander is composed of amylopectin that has been chemically altered to decrease its rate of degradation in the body. The average molecular weight of these structures is 450,000; however, many of the molecules are much smaller than this. About 40% of the dose passes through the kidney into the urine in 24 hours in people. It requires 2-3 weeks to totally eliminate Hetastarch from the body. Hetastarch and Dextran solutions contain large molecules that do not readily pass through capillary walls and are useful in maintaining expanded plasma volumes.

Plasma expanders have the advantage that they can be purchased and stored much longer than blood and are readily available when needed.

Shock and Its Treatment

Shock may occur more often than is generally realized. It is associated not only with trauma and hemorrhage, but often develops during infectious diseases.[19] Shock was the major lethal factor in about 58% of people that died from clostridial infections, 20% of those dying from *Pseudomonas* infections, and 24% of those dying from enterobacterial infections. The failure to recognize shock during an infectious disease might result in inadequate therapy.

Shock can be divided into hypovolemic and endotoxic types. Both types are commonly treated simultaneously.

Hypovolemic Shock

Any event that reduces blood volume sufficiently can cause severe or fatal shock. The blood volume is maintained primarily by plasma proteins synthesized by the liver. Failure of the liver to synthesize these proteins, as in liver disease, starvation or vitamin deficiency, or inability of the liver to maintain sufficient quantities of protein, as a result of parasitism, bleeding ulcers or hemorrhage, may result in reduced plasma protein levels and decreased plasma volume. Animals with any predisposing factors are more likely to suffer shock during surgery or following trauma. A cat may appear normal and yet have a reduced plasma volume, and therefore be more susceptible to shock.

Treatment or prevention of hypovolemic shock involves maintaining adequate plasma volume. Intravenous administration of plasma or blood is indicated. If plasma or blood is not available, a plasma expander, such as Dextran (Abbott), or an electrolyte solution may be given.

If blood volume is insufficient, transfer of 0_2 to tissues is inadequate and lactic acid is not metabolized at the normal rate. Synthesis of glucose from lactate occurs primarily in the liver, and lack of 0_2 or chronic liver disease could interfere with this. As a result, lactic acid accumulates and causes acidosis. This is especially harmful to cats and tends to cause lethargy.

Endotoxic Shock

This condition often occurs during subacute or chronic disease, or when hypovolemic shock is accompanied by severe vasoconstriction. Toxins released by bacteria within the body produce the signs of endotoxic shock. The bacteria may be present as a result of chronic disease or may enter the blood from the intestine during hypovolemic shock. The severe vasoconstriction associated with hypovolemic shock decreases the 0_2 supply to the intestine, injuring the intestine sufficiently to allow entrance of bacteria and their toxins into the circulation. To prevent this sequence of events, the intestinal blood vessels must be moderately dilated. Before a vasodilator is given, however, it should be ensured that blood volume is adequate or blood pressure may fall so low that severe tissue hypoxia occurs.

Certain phenothiazine tranquilizers are effective vasodilators.[20] Acepromazine, at 0.5 mg/lb, provides this effect. Vasoconstrictors, such as epinephrine, should not be administered to animals in shock because they aggravate intestinal hypoxia and promote endotoxic shock.

Transfer of bacteria from the intestine to the blood can be prevented to some degree by administering a broad-spectrum antibiotic, such as tetracycline at 25 mg/lb, 24 hours before surgery. This obviously cannot be done when shock has resulted from an accident or disease. The longer administration of an antibiotic is delayed, the less effective it is since the drug is not immediately effective in controlling the growth of intestinal bacteria. As antibodies and other antibacterial substances may be beneficial, blood transfusion is of value in endotoxic shock.

Some of the effects of endotoxins can be prevented by administration of corticosteroids, such as hydrocortisone succinate at 1 mg/lb given IV. These hormones prevent penetration of endotoxins into tissues and thus avert some cellular damage. They also favor conversion of protein into glucose, which provides tissues with needed energy.

Administration of large volumes of 5% dextrose and lactated Ringer's solution may be of value in shock. These fluids increase urine volume and may help remove toxins from the body by renal clearance.

Causes of Shock

The etiology of shock is complex because there are many primary and secondary factors that combine to cause the syndrome. Primary factors generally initiate shock and secondary ones aggravate the severity of the syndrome. Primary and secondary factors cannot be clearly separated, however. Often the type of shock is referred to by a name denoting the primary cause.

Primary factors that may initiate shock include trauma (especially intestinal injury), sepsis (often a terminal event in an infection), hypovolemia due to hemorrhage or other fluid and electrolyte loss, anoxia or hypoxia, and adrenal insufficiency. Secondary factors that increase the severity of shock include liver damage, histamine and 5-hydroxytryptamine release, bacterial proteases, such kinins as bradykinin and kallidin, catecholamines, excessive vasoconstriction, electrolyte losses, hypoglycemia, serotoxins and serotonins, acidosis, anesthetics, endotoxins, lack of antibodies, and debilitation.

Although different primary causes of shock produce some variation in the signs, the course of the syndrome and basic physiologic reactions are about the same. If the physiologic reaction to a primary cause is sufficient, the animal recovers without treatment. However, if the primary cause is severe or there are multiple primary causes, progressive or reversible shock develops. Unless the animal receives proper therapy, its condition deteriorates until irreversible or terminal shock occurs. The point of irreversibility of shock is not fixed. Because vigorous treatment saves more animals than does inadequate treatment, "irreversible shock" is relative to the quality of treatment.

Although some animals recover without treatment, recovery is more rapid if therapy is given. Generally, the earlier treatment is instigated, the more successful it is.

Shock often is initiated by reduction of circulating plasma volume, as with severe hemorrhage, diarrhea, renal disease or other conditions that result in large fluid losses. Fluid losses also occur with severe tissue damage, such as crushing injuries. The injured tissues extract large amounts of fluids from the blood, reducing the circulating fluid volume and promoting shock.

Endotoxic shock is not initially accompanied by a reduction in circulating fluid volume. A shock-like syndrome results when a sufficient quantity of bacterial endotoxins enters the blood. Many of the same signs observed in hypovolemic shock are present.

Signs of Shock

When hemorrhage is the primary factor in shock, paleness of the mucous membranes, cool extremities, cyanosis, vasoconstriction, tachycardia and hemodilution are the prominent signs. When trauma is involved, edema, swelling, subcutaneous hemorrhage and intravascular clotting are additional signs. Septic shock is characterized by severe congestion of the liver and intestines, and sometimes by massive hemorrhage into the intestines, in addition to the other signs of shock. Shock resulting from dehydration (diarrhea, emesis) or thermal burns (when 25% or more of the body is burned) is characterized by hemoconcentration. When muscle is badly crushed, myoglobin released from the injured tissue precipitates in the nephrons and can cause complete renal shutdown.

Signs of shock are summarized in Table 9.

Physiologic Reaction to Reduced Circulating Fluid Volume

There usually is a reduction of circulating fluid volume in shock, resulting in a vasomotor reaction that maintains adequate circulation to vital tissues (brain and heart). This circulatory reaction consists of tachycardia and vasoconstriction of arterioles in the skin and GI tract; there is little, if any, vasoconstriction in the heart, CNS and muscles.

Several signs of shock result from cutaneous vasoconstriction. Pallor and cyanosis are a result of decreased blood flow through the skin. Whether the skin is pale or cyanotic depends on the amounts of oxyhemoglobin present. If less than 40% of the hemoglobin is in the form of oxyhemoglobin, cyanosis develops. Vasoconstriction results in cooling of the skin, especially on the extremities, and reduces loss of body heat. Early in shock, there is a tendency for the body temperature to rise, causing the animal to pant or show other signs of hyperthermia. Later in shock, especially if anesthesia is involved, hypothermia develops.

Although the vasomotor reactions in mild or moderate shock are mostly beneficial, in severe progressive shock, vasoconstriction can become so intense that it causes serious tissue hypoxia, leading to deterioration of tissues and irreversible shock.

Along with the vasomotor reactions, a series of fluid adjustments occurs. The liver releases

Table 9. Signs of Shock

Sign	Causative factors	Mechanism
Tachycardia	Hypovolemia, hemorrhage, edema, fluid losses	Reduced circulating volume is detected by stretch receptors, which effect tachycardia and vasoconstriction
Pallor, cool extremities	Hypovolemia, hemorrhage, edema, fluid losses, arteriolar constriction	Vasoconstriction primarily in skin and intestines; ischemia results in pallor, cool extremities, nausea, emesis
Thready pulse	Reduced cardiac output due to lack of venous return	Reduced stroke volume and pulse pressure
Thirst	Na retention, release of proteins from liver	Increased Na and plasma protein levels increase plasma osmotic pressure and thirst
Panting	Nervousness, fear, reduced heat loss due to cutaneous vasoconstriction	Cutaneous vasoconstriction reduces heat loss and raises body temperature during initial stages
Mydriasis	Reaction to fear	Sympathetic stimulation of iris diaphragm
Emesis	Water consumption in presence of severe GI vasoconstriction	Intestinal vasoconstriction results in accumulation of CO_2, acids and other chemicals that cause emesis
Blood clots, emboli	Endotoxic (septic) shock	Proteases released by the endotoxins cause blood clotting
Clotting deficiency	Lack of fibrinogen or clotting factors	Extensive blood clotting due to bacterial proteases consumes fibrinogen; liver disease may reduce available clotting factors
Hypotension	Release of hypotensive agents, such as bradykinin, histamine, kallidin, serotoxin; hypovolemia; damage to vasoconstrictor mechanism by hypoxia and anesthetics	Hypotensive agents cause vasodilation, capillary leakage and reduced circulating volume hypoxia
Depression, coma	Acidosis	Failure of liver to metabolize lactic acid; hypoxia interferes with liver function

a considerable quantity of plasma proteins, which raise osmotic pressure in vessels and increase the circulating fluid volume. Through the aldosterone mechanism, the kidneys retain Na, which elevates the osmotic pressure of the circulating fluid, causing the animal to consume water. The increased extracellular Na level also draws water from cells and replenishes, some of the circulating fluid volume. The increased osmotic pressure causes additional secretion of antidiuretic hormone, which increases water retention and helps restore plasma volume.

Severe vasoconstriction in the intestines results in nausea and emesis, especially after ingestion of food and water. Animals that hemorrhage tend to drink water and should be given 5% dextrose parenterally to satisfy their water needs and thus avoid emesis.

If blood loss is less than 30% of the total blood volume, most of the fluid is replaced in a few hours and the animal survives. It requires several weeks to replace all of the blood cells. Older or debilitated animals succumb to smaller blood losses than do young, vigorous ones.

Physiologic Reaction to Hypoxia

Hypoxia results in increased anaerobic metabolism, which, because of accumulation of lactic acid, can result in severe acidosis. Hypoxia also interferes with function of the reticuloendothelial system and the animal's defense against bacteria. Hypoxia may also cause cellular injury and release of proteases with detrimental effects.

With hypoxia, insufficient 0_2 is available for synthesis of glucose from pyruvic and lactic acids. This leads to a depletion of glucose stores, elevation of lactic acid levels and development of acidosis.[21,22] As dogs and cats are especially susceptible to hypoglycemia and acidosis, the pH usually drops faster in these animals than in people. A blood pH as low as 6.8 is not uncommon in dogs with severe shock. Acidosis causes depression, coma and eventually respiratory failure. The amount of 0_2 that hemoglobin can transport is also depressed in acidosis, further increasing the hypoxia. When the acidosis is corrected, the 0_2-carrying capacity of blood increases, along with blood pressure and improvement in circulation.

There is severe hypoglycemia in most fatal cases of shock.[21,22] It is important to supply glucose and treat the acidosis. Administration of more acid can be fatal. When blood stored in ACD solution 1-10 days and with an average pH of 6.4 was given to dogs in progressive shock, 85% of them died.[23] In a similar experiment in which the stored blood was treated with buffers to raise the pH to 7.6, 85% of the dogs survived. As stored blood becomes progressively more acid, addition of buffers, such as $NaHCO_3$, is important before the blood is used to treat shock.

Hypoxia also affects the reticuloendothelial system, causing a reduction in its phagocytic activities. This generally reduces the animal's ability to resist bacteria and their toxins.[24] Dogs in progressive shock have high numbers of bacteria in their mesenteric lymph nodes and are unable to destroy parenterally administered bacteria that would readily be destroyed by normal dogs. Hypoxia also results in release of proteolytic enzymes that cause blood coagulation, vasodilation and other deleterious effects.

Replacement of circulating fluid volume with whole blood corrects hypoxia. Increasing the pO_2 by giving pure O_2 is of some value, provided that bacteria and their toxins are not sufficiently involved in the shock syndrome to be lethal. Increased pO_2 is of no value in the treatment of endotoxic or septic shock.

Physiologic Reaction to Bacterial Toxins

Microorganisms and their toxins may initiate shock during an infectious disease or may be secondarily involved in shock initiated by other primary factors. Septic shock often does not begin with a reduced circulating fluid volume, but this soon develops as a result of edema, leaking capillaries and intravascular clotting.

Interest in the role of bacteria in shock was greatly increased with the discovery that the onset of progressive shock could be delayed by prior administration of antibiotics or sulfonamides. These drugs inhibited intestinal bacterial growth and thus reduced the quantity of endotoxins elaborated. As a result, less endotoxin is absorbed and progressive or irreversible shock is delayed.

If sufficient blood is removed from a dog to reduce blood pressure to 30 mm Hg and then is completely returned within 1.5-2 hours, 80% of the animals recover without additional therapy.[25] If the animals remain hypotensive (30 mm Hg) for 4 hours, only 20% recover. In the latter group (4 hours at 30 mm Hg), 40% of the animals recover if antibiotics are given during the period of shock. If the antibiotics are given 3 hours before development of shock, 80% of the animals recover after 4 hours with a 30 mm Hg blood pressure. It was concluded from these experiments that death from prolonged hypotensive shock is caused by absorbed endotoxins and that antibacterial drugs lower the death rate by reducing the quantity of intestinal bacteria and endotoxins. Gram-negative bacilli produce most of the endotoxins, and such antibiotics as neomycin and tetracyclines usually are effective in delaying shock. The failure of antibiotics to delay progressive shock has been attributed to antibiotic-resistant bacteria in the intestinal tract.

Dogs in shock cannot resist bacteria as well as normal animals. In normal dogs, the blood was cleared in 24 hours after IV injection of 5-50 billion bacteria. Conversely, dogs in shock developed bacteremia in 24 hours and died in 1-4 days when given the same doses and types of organisms. Dogs dying from shock when no bacteria have been injected have higher than normal numbers of microorganisms in the mesenteric lymph nodes and liver.

Certain barriers prevent bacteria and their endotoxins from invading tissues, including a functional intestinal wall, reticuloendothelial system, liver, antibodies and properdin, a bactericidal substance especially effective against gram-negative organisms. These barriers can destroy large numbers of bacteria and inactivate endotoxins. In shock, various factors inactivate them and allow endotoxins and bacteria to invade tissues. Both hypoxia and acidosis inactivate all of the barriers except antibodies and properdin. General anesthesia depresses the function of the liver, reticuloendothelial system and intestine wall. Anoxia and endotoxins cause cells to release proteases, kinins, serotoxin and other factors that increase the severity of shock.

Sufficient blood loss must occur to lower blood pressure enough to cause severe tissue hypoxia. This results in acidosis and impaired function of the liver, intestinal endothelium and reticuloendothelial system. Bacteria and endotoxins then enter the blood and lymph in increasing amounts. At first, these agents are destroyed by antibodies and properdin. After about 1-2 hours, stores of antibodies and properdin are exhausted and progressive shock develops. The period between the beginning of shock and development of progressive shock is much reduced in chronically ill animals in which properdin and antibody levels as well as reticuloendothelial function may already be depleted.

Proteolytic Enzymes

Both endotoxins and hypoxia cause release of a number of proteolytic enzymes that can make shock irreversible, Proteases act directly on cellular protein, causing formation of such substances as histamine and 5-hydroxytryptamine. These substances are vasodilators that increase the degree of hypotension and capillary leakage. Some proteases leave the cells and act directly on plasma proteins, causing a release of polypeptides referred to as kinins. Kinins have a hypotensive effect, thus aggravating the severity of shock. They also increase leakage of blood through capillaries, reducing the circulating fluid volume. Proteases also cause intravascular clotting, emboli formation and obstruction of capillaries.

In the early stages of shock, coagulation time is shortened because of epinephrine release. Later, proteolytic enzymes cause intravascular coagulation and formation of emboli that occlude small capillaries in the lungs, liver, nervous system and other tissues. Obviously, these emboli are a major factor in making shock irreversible. Later in shock, most of the proteins involved in blood coagulation are gone. Administration of heparin blocks the coagulating effect of proteolytic enzymes and therefore has life-saving possibilities. One of the problems with heparin therapy is knowing exactly when to administer it. It can be of considerable value, however, when given early in severe, progressive shock.

Endotoxins cause the enzyme histidine decarboxylase to convert histidine into histamine. Histamine is a vasodilator and hypotensive agent, similar to the kinins. Antihistamines have not proved to be of value in shock, however, probably because there are too many other hypotensive agents, such as the kinins, that are not inhibited by these drugs.

Another compound, 5-hydroxytryptamine, is similar to histamine. It is released in response to endotoxins and has a hypotensive effect. Other toxic substances, such as serotoxin and the "capillary permeability factor," undoubtedly are significant in some forms of shock. Serotoxin is a nonproteolytic protein that causes release of histamine. All of these substances produce vasodilation, increased capillary leakage, increased edema, hemorrhage, reduction of circulating fluid volume, and lowered blood pressure.

Fluid Therapy in Shock

The 2 most vital aspects of shock therapy are the treatment of acidosis and the expansion of plasma volume. Most cats with shock develop severe acidosis. Blood gases or the plasma bicarbonate level should be determined and the amount of bicarbonate for treatment of the acidosis calculated and administered. In severe cases this might be done every 4-6 hours. Along with the correction of the pH, large volumes of fluid are needed to adequately perfuse the capillary beds.

Fluids used in treatment of shock include electrolyte solutions, such as lactated Ringer's solution, blood and plasma expanders. Blood and plasma expanders have less tendency to produce pulmonary edema, to which cats seem to be prone to develop. Therefore, use of blood or plasma expanders is recommended in the treatment of shock. Lactated Ringer's solution can be used as an adjunct to increase the total fluid volume. The initial IV fluid dosage in treatment of cats with severe shock should be about 50 ml/kg.[26] This should consist of lactated Ringer's, plasma expanders or blood. The effect of this therapy can be monitored by testing capillary refill time in the gingivae. The speed at which the capillary bed is refilled after pressure on the gingivae is an indication of the degree of shock present. Normal capillary refill time is less than 2 seconds. The degree of pulmonary edema should be carefully monitored by thoracic auscultation. If there are increased rales, additional Ringer's solution should not be given. Additional fluid therapy should include plasma or plasma expanders, such as Dextran or Hetastarch, which contain high-molecular-weight molecules that keep fluid from entering the lungs.

In addition to fluid therapy, certain drugs are beneficial in the treatment of shock. Corticosteroids have been useful in cats in preventing the adverse effects of prostaglandins and lipozymes in shock.[27] Methylprednisolone decreases prostaglandin formation in the feline liver in shock. Both prostaglandins and lipozymes increase the seriousness of shock. In severe shock, the presence of profound metabolic acidosis warrants measurement of the plasma bicarbonate level and administration of adequate amounts of $NaHCO_3$.

References

1. Bohning, RH *et al.* JAVMA **156** (1970) 611.
2. Furneaux, RW and Kernan, F. J Sm Anim Pract **15** (1974) 129.
3. Stein, BS. Feline Pract **4(4)** (1974) 12.
4. Miller, SA and Allison, JB. J Nutr **64** (1958) 493.
5. Greaves, JP and Scott, PP. Br J Nutr **14** (1960) 361.
6. Morris, JG and Rogers, Q. Science **199** (1978) 431.
7. Anderson, PA *et al.* J Nutr **109** (1979) 368.
8. Krause, MV and Mahan, LK: Food, Nutrition and Diet Therapy. WB Saunders, Philadelphia, 1979.
9. Warren, JG and Nathan, DG. J Clin Invest **37** (1958) 1724.
10. Schenker, S *et al.* J Clin Invest **46** (1967) 838.
11. Chow, K *et al.* Proc Soc Exper Biol Med **134** (1970) 122.
12. Clifford, AJ *et al.* Proc Soc Exper Biol Med **140** (1972) 1447.
13. Miller, LL *et al.* Fed Proc **14** (1955) 707.
14. Durdick, JT. Paper presented at Am Cancer Soc Conf on Anorexia, 1969.
15. Thrall, BE and Miller, LG. Feline Pract **6(1)** (1976) 10.
16. Herbert, DA and Mitchell, RA. J Appl Physiol **30** (1971) 434.
17. Burrows, CF and Bovee, KC. JAVMA **172** (1978) 801.
18. Finco, DR and Cornelius, LM. Am J Vet Res **38** (1977) 823.
19. Ebert, RV and Abernathy, RS. Fed Proc Suppl **9** (1961) 179.
20. Millican, RC and Rhodes, CJ. J Pharm Ther **122** (1958) 255.
21. Strawitz, JC and Hift, H. Surg Forum **11** (1960) 112.
22. Cowley, RA *et al.* Surg Forum **11** (1960) 110.
23. Nahas, GG *et al.* Fed Proc **19** (1960) 54.
24. Zweifach, BW. Fed Proc Suppl **9** (1961) 22.
25. Fine, J. Fed Proc Suppl **9** (1961) 167.
26. Brasmer, TH. JAVMA **174** (1979) 475.
27. Carlson, RP *et al.* Biochem Pharm **26** (1977) 1463.

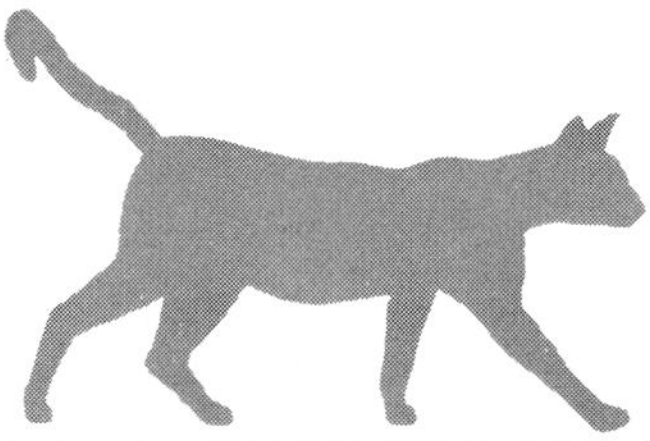

3

toxicology and pharmacology

A.L. ARONSON AND J.E. RIVIERE

Diseases in small domestic animals due to chemicals have become more frequent through increased use of potentially harmful materials in the home and in industry. Although poisonings do not constitute a major portion of the clinical problems in veterinary medicine, it is clear that cats and dogs can be poisoned by a variety of materials.[1] Moreover, cats have a reputation of responding adversely to several common therapeutic drugs.

Many chemical agents are potentially poisonous to cats. Because of the peculiarities and habits of this species, however, the incidence of poisoning in cats is not as high as in dogs and herbivores. The kind of food cats eat is somewhat limited. As a result, spoiled food, refuse, bait containing rodenticides and other sources of toxic material are given less attention by cats than by other species.

Cats are seldom gluttonous; they eat until comfortable and then desist until hungry again. Because of this, a smaller quantity of potentially toxic food might be ingested. Because most cats masticate their food well immediately after prehension, they have an excellent opportunity to taste and reject it if it is offensive. The close confinement of many cats protects them from exposure to chemical toxins.

There are several innate characteristics, however, that work adversely to the cat's interest. The average cat keeps its haircoat clean by frequent licking. This can lead to ingestion of any toxic substance on the hair. Externally applied parasiticides and dermatologic preparations may thus prove harmful. Any toxic residue in an area the cat inhabits can contaminate its paws and perhaps its body, and may be ingested. These grooming habits could lead one to believe a compound was more toxic to this species than another. When applied externally, the material could be equally toxic to a cat or dog, but appears to be more toxic in cats because the material is ingested when the cat grooms itself.

The adage "curiosity killed the cat" certainly applies to poisoning. Their natural curiosity stimulates thorough investigation of the environment, possibly leading the cat to the site of potential intoxicants. Curiosity causes cats to smell and nibble various household plants that may be toxic. Rodenticides, pesticides, open cans of antifreeze, and a host of potentially lethal agents receive their scrutiny. The hunting instinct of cats may result in capture and ingestion of rodents and insects that could be a source of a toxic agent. Secondary poisoning is thus possible, as some agents used to exterminate pests are very toxic to cats.

The tendency of cats to seek out a diet composed of fish may also predispose them to poisoning, a classic example being intoxication with methylmercury from environmental contamination (Minamata disease). In fact, cats are considered a "sentry" species for detecting outbreaks of Minamata disease in people because mercury can be detected in the blood of cats earlier than in dogs or people (see Metallic Poisonings).[2,3]

Incidence

The incidence of clinical toxicoses in cats is not readily documented. A review of 31 cases of intoxication in cats involved poisonings by ethylene glycol (6), arsenic (4), warfarin (3), insecticides (3), Vacor (3), lead (2) and miscellaneous (10).[4] In a survey limited to pesticide poisonings over a 1-year period in South Carolina, 285 poisoned cats had a 40% fatality rate, double the fatality rate reported for 804 dogs in the same survey.[5] Specific poisonings involved were organophosphate insecticides (114), chlorinated hydrocarbon insecticides (36), anticoagulant rodenticides (28), carbamate insecticides (6), metaldehyde (3), strychnine (2), unknown pesticides (96). In a survey of small animal pesticide poisonings in Los Angeles, the breakdown of 37 feline intoxications was organophosphate insecticides (14), carbamate insecticides (8), anticoagulant rodenticides (5), chlorinated hydrocarbon insecticides (3), Vacor (2) and miscellaneous (7).[6] Similar quantitative data for adverse drug reactions in cats are not available, although adverse reactions in cats to 27 drugs were reported in a review of adverse drug reactions by the FDA's Bureau of Veterinary Medicine Drug Surveillance Program for a 5-year period.[7] They included antimicrobials, antiparasitics, CNS depressants, analgesics and a hormone.

Interpretation of such retrospective studies is difficult. Since there are no data indicating the size of the cat population at risk and criteria for diagnoses are not standardized, estimates of incidence of poisonings in the general population cannot be made. However, feline poisonings must be included in the differential diagnosis of certain feline conditions.

Sensitivity of Cats to Poisoning

Veterinarians generally have the impression that cats are more sensitive than other species to the toxic effects of many drugs.[8] The same impression exists among investigators using cats as experimental subjects.[9] Inspection of toxicity data for a large number of chemical compounds reveals that cats are more susceptible than other species to many chemicals.[10]

There seem to be at least 3 reasons, in addition to the behavioral traits previously discussed (*eg*, grooming habits), for their unusual sensitivity to many chemicals and drugs: the relatively slow rate of drug biotransformation; species sensitivity to Heinz body formation, methemoglobinemia and hemolytic anemia after exposure to certain oxidant compounds; and an unusual sensitivity of certain drug receptor sites.

Drugs undergo a number of detoxication reactions in the animal that convert lipid-soluble drugs to more water-soluble derivatives, which are more easily excreted by the body. Hydroxylation and dealkylation occur at much slower rates in cats than in other species.[11,12] Moreover, the ability to conjugate foreign compounds through glucuronide formation is virtually nonexistent in cats.[13,14] Absence of this detoxication mechanism has been attributed to an insufficient quantity of the enzyme, glucuronyl transferase.[15] Compounds detoxified by this pathway in other species include alcohols, phenols, aromatic carboxylic acids, amines, amides and thiols. Common examples are acetaminophen and aspirin.[16]

Due to the relative inefficiency of the glucuronide system, compounds normally biotransformed by this route may be detoxified by other pathways. For example, phenolic compounds normally biotransformed by glucuronide conjugation are instead detoxified by conjugation with sulfate. Since the sulfate pool of the body may be easily exhausted, it is often necessary to administer an exogenous source of sulfate to allow detoxification to proceed. This is the rationale for acetylcysteine administration as an antidote for acetaminophen toxicosis in cats.[17] Cats also have unique conjugating mechanisms, an example being conjugation with phosphate as a route for phenol elimination.[18-20] Impaired elimination of acetaminophen in cats results in a greater amount of the drug being converted to hematoxic aromatic metabolites than in other species, thereby predisposing cats to methemoglobinemia and hemolytic anemia from smaller drug doses.[21-23] The biotransformation of drugs and other chemicals in cats is a complex problem that requires further research to elucidate. Any compound that undergoes extensive biotransformation should be administered with greater caution to cats than to other species.

As a species, cats appear susceptible to methemoglobinemia and Heinz body formation when oxidant drugs are given.[24,25] After administration of methylene blue, acetaminophen, phenacetin or phenazopyridine, cats will form methemoglobin more readily than will other species.[17,21,24,26] Part of this sensitivity is a result of the deficiencies in drug biotransformation described above. However, the RBC of cats are inherently more susceptible to Heinz body formation after methylene blue incubation *in vitro* than are those of people or dogs.[27] The feline RBC also have a relatively slower rate of methemoglobin reductase activity, an enzyme responsible for regenerating hemoglobin from methemoglobin, compared with those of some other species.[23] Part of the tendency for feline hemoglobin to undergo oxidation readily may be attributed to its high sulfhydryl content.[28] These factors are additive and help explain the cat's extreme sensitivity to certain drugs.

Cats may respond differently from other animals to receptor site stimulation. They become excited when given increasingly high doses of morphine, whereas most species become depressed. The pharmacologic effects of reserpine persist in most species for 1-2 days, but they persist for nearly a month in cats.[12]

Differences in feline physiology may also affect the sensitivity of the cat to drugs and other chemicals. Preliminary studies raise the possibility that cats have a "reverse" circadian rhythm of blood cortisol concentrations.[29] Peak plasma concentrations of cortisol in cats occur in the evening rather than in the morning, as in dogs and people. This cycle could potentiate adverse reactions to exogenous corticosteroid therapy administered according to canine guidelines. Cats also exhibit a unique response to decreased functional renal mass in that, unlike people and dogs, they retain the ability to concentrate urine in the face of azotemia.[30] This complicates clinical detection of drug-induced kidney damage.

Although there is a seemingly greater sensitivity of cats toward certain drugs, this does not necessarily mean these drugs cannot be given to cats. It does mean, however, that great care must be taken in the dosage regimens designed for cats; this includes the size as well as the frequency of dosage. Unfortunately, information of this kind is sparse. Excellent pharmacokinetic studies have been made of several antibiotics and analgesics, and these will be discussed. More information of this kind for other drugs is needed to establish dosage schedules that are clinically effective and safe for cats.

Diagnosis of Poisoning

The clinician may be confronted with the problem of not knowing what chemical is present in a commercial preparation that has been ingested. There are at least 3 sources of this type of information: the label on the container usually lists the names of all ingredients; the series of books entitled *Current Veterinary Therapy* contains a list of poisonous substances in common household items; and most large cities have a Poison Control Center from which information about potentially poisonous substances can be obtained. The centers usually can be reached by telephone at all times.

Unless there is a definite history of ingestion or contact with a toxic agent, one must rely on the clinical signs of poisoning. The possibility of poisoning should always be considered when the situation is puzzling and diagnosis is difficult. Ingestion, cutaneous absorption or inhalation of a toxic agent usually causes such GI disturbances as anorexia, abdominal pain, vomiting and diarrhea. Usually there is no fever. The onset of illness may be sudden and development of severe illness rapid. Signs of respiratory and circulatory disorders are also prominent at times. A diagnosis of poisoning should also be considered when one is confronted with unexplained cyanosis, shock, collapse, sudden loss of consciousness or convulsions.

Signs of poisoning can resemble those of many clinical conditions.

General Principles of Treatment

The correct diagnosis of a clinical problem is essential before one can proceed with rational treatment. In cases of poisoning, this ideal is often difficult to achieve. An evaluation of the history and signs may at best only suggest a diagnosis. An examination of the material ingested may reveal several toxic ingredients, any of which could contribute to the toxicosis. Treatment often must be started before a diagnosis is clearly established. For example, if an animal is convulsing, sedation is required, regardless of the underlying cause. Even when the toxic agent is known, often no specific antidote is available. When a specific chemical antidote is available, the patient often can be equally benefited by adequate supportive therapy.

The primary therapeutic postulate in acute poisonings in animals should be the preservation of life and stabilization of vital signs, regardless of the etiology of the toxicosis.

Rational procedures can be employed to treat a case of poisoning even though the poisonous agent is not identified. They involve preventing further absorption of the poison, enhancing the removal of absorbed poison, and providing supportive therapy to combat the effects of the absorbed poison.[31-37] When done properly, these procedures benefit the patient in any case of poisoning. The order in which these measures are taken depends on the situation. Supportive therapy must be given initially if the animal is in extreme pain, convulsing or showing signs of respiratory failure or circulatory collapse.

Although these 3 general approaches to treatment of poisoning have been discussed elsewhere, some attention will be given to the use of activated charcoal vs the "universal antidote." Activated charcoal is well established as a GI adsorbent in cases of poisoning.[38-40] The universal antidote, which includes an antacid (usually magnesium oxide), tannic acid and activated charcoal, is inferior to activated charcoal alone.[41,42] The magnesium oxide and tannic acid interfere with the adsorptive capacity of activated charcoal. Also, activated charcoal is much less expensive than the universal antidote.

Undiluted syrup of ipecac is an effective emetic in cats when given PO at 3-6 ml/kg.[43] This dosage should induce emesis in 15 (higher dose) to 60 minutes.

Finally, there recently have been many advances in use of peritoneal dialysis in small animals, making it an effective tool to increase elimination of many toxicants from the body.[44-46] Development of a functionally reliable catheter and better control of peritonitis have made this therapeutic maneuver a practical alternative.

RODENTICIDE POISONING

Warfarin

Poisoning by warfarin can be accidental or malicious. Animals may consume bait placed for rodents, or they may eat dead rodents and be poisoned. In other cases, meat or bone covered with the material is deliberately distributed to poison pets.[47] The anticoagulant rodenticides, all structurally related to coumarin, include warfarin, pindone, diphacinone and fumarin. These compounds and sulfaquinoxaline, a coccidiostat, all act similarly to warfarin and will be considered as a group.[48]

Differences would be expected in the size of the lethal dose and the duration of action. A lethal dose of warfarin varies according to the mode of ingestion. For example, rats can withstand single oral dosages of 50 mg/kg (23 mg/lb), but succumb to daily ingestion of 1 mg/kg (0.45 mg/lb) for 5 successive days. Daily ingestion of 5 mg/lb is fatal to cats and dogs in 5-15 days.[47] Others have noted that 1 mg/kg kills dogs and cats if given daily for about a week.[49] Single oral dosages of 20-50 mg/kg (9-23 mg/lb) for dogs and 5-50 mg/kg (2.3-23 mg/lb) for cats may be fatal.

The outstanding toxic effect of warfarin is reduction of the blood's ability to clot. Warfarin decreases formation of prothrombin (factor II), as well as clotting factors VII, IX and X, by interference with the action of vitamin K.[50] This vitamin is required for formation and release of these factors from the liver.[51,52] The increase in clotting time may not be apparent for several days after ingestion of warfarin. This delay is due mainly to the time required for pre-existing prothrombin and other clotting factors to be depleted. The average half-lives for factors VII, IX, X and II in dogs are about 6, 14, 16 and 41 hours, respectively.[48] Large doses of warfarin cause intense vasodilation; early death after ingestion of large quantities of warfarin may be due to vascular collapse.[53]

Clinical Signs: Hemorrhage is responsible for most of the clinical signs in warfarin poisoning. The mucous membranes usually are pale or cyanotic, and petechiae or ecchymoses may be present. The pulse is weak and rapid, breathing is labored, and weakness and prostration are common. Although hemorrhage is mainly internal, blood may be present in vomitus, urine and feces, and may ooze from external openings. Animals show no evidence of pain or discomfort and do not resist palpation.[54]

Lesions: Hemorrhage and anemia are observed at necropsy. The former is in the pleural cavity, epicardium and endocardium.[55] There may be hemorrhage into the pericardial sac and thoracic cavity. Bleeding in the abdominal cavity and skeletal muscle is less frequent. Myocarditis is common.

Treatment: Transfusion of whole blood is the most effective treatment because it provides prothrombin and other clotting factors, as well as lost RBC and fluid. A citrated whole blood mixture, consisting of 100 ml of an aqueous solution containing 2 g sodium acid citrate and 2.5 g dextrose, to which 300 ml whole blood were added, has been used.[56] This mixture was stored at refrigerator temperature for a maximum of 14 days. A minimum dosage of 20 ml/kg (9 ml/lb) was given via the radial or saphenous vein. Half the estimated volume was given rapidly and the remainder at a rate of 20 drops/minute. More blood was given if the mucous membranes were still pale. With this treatment, every poisoned animal (a total of 26 cases) partially recovered within 24 hours and fully recovered by 72 hours. Although this study involved dogs, it seems likely the treatment would prove satisfactory for cats as well.

Administration of 2.5-25 mg vitamin K_1 (*eg*, Aquamephyton:Merck) IM, SC or IV initially is indicated to promote production of prothrombin and other clotting factors by the liver.[57] Even if blood transfusions are not given, vitamin K_1 is helpful in cats.[58] One should not use synthetic vitamin K analogues, such as menadione (K_3), because they are inferior to vitamin K_1 in decreasing clotting time.

Drug Interactions: Warfarin and related coumarins are highly bound to serum proteins and can be displaced by other highly bound drugs, such as salicylates or sulfonamides. The result is an enhanced anticoagulant response. Warfarin-like drugs also undergo extensive biotransformation in the liver. Inhibitors of these detoxifying mechanisms, such as chloramphenicol, could potentiate the action of the oral anticoagulants.[59]

Strychnine

The use of strychnine as a rodenticide has decreased in recent years because of development of safer products. Deliberate poisoning of pets with strychnine is not uncommon, however.

Strychnine is readily absorbed from the small intestine but very poorly from the stomach. Thus, the presence of food in the stomach can have a definite effect on how soon clinical signs follow ingestion of the poison. In one study, clinical signs were apparent about 15 minutes after administration of a toxic dose of strychnine in a gelatin capsule to a fasted dog. However, when the same dose was administered in hamburger, clinical signs did not appear until 1-5 hours later.[60] The toxic oral dose of strychnine in dogs and cats has been reported as about 0.75 mg/kg (0.34 mg/lb).[53] However, another investigator indicates that the oral lethal dose for cats is greater, about 2.0 mg/kg.[61]

Clinical Signs: Strychnine affects the CNS, especially the spinal cord. The convulsant action is due to interference with postsynaptic inhibitory processes. Thus, the CNS becomes extremely sensitive to any sensory input. All muscles contract during a strychnine convulsion; extensor rigidity is characteristic because the extensor muscles are more powerful than the flexors.

A poisoned cat first shows a degree of anxiety and greater sensitivity to external stimuli. There is an increase in muscular tone, with twitching of the skeletal muscles. Sudden auditory, tactile or visual stimuli precipitate muscle spasms and convulsions. A clap of the hands, a jet of air, or jarring of the surface on which the animal is lying is often sufficient. At first, there are exaggerated spinal reflexes, especially of the limbs and neck. Shortly thereafter, there is tonic contraction of all voluntary muscles, causing extensor rigidity. Opisthotonus, orthotonus and risus sardonicus (grinning) are observed. Breathing ceases due to prolonged contraction of the diaphragm and thoracic and abdominal muscles. The eyeballs are fixed and the pupils are dilated.

A convulsion may last from 30 seconds to several minutes, followed by a period of relaxation. This may be due to anorexia and exhaustion from muscular contractions. Convulsions may occur repeatedly, with intermittent periods of quiescence; the frequency and severity of the seizures are increased by sensory stimulation. Death is probably due to medullary paralysis resulting from impaired breathing during convulsions. The intense muscular contractions are probably extremely painful to an animal; they are to people poisoned with strychnine.

Treatment: The treatment is purely supportive. The first objective is to control the seizures by anesthetizing the cat with IV pentobarbital. The patient should be maintained at a level of anesthesia from which it can be stimulated to show tetany only with difficulty. This may require deep anesthesia. Therefore, a cuffed endotracheal tube should be placed in the trachea to ensure a patent airway and provide positive-pressure ventilation. Inhalation anesthesia, methocarbamol (Robaxin:Robins) (150 mg/kg IM) or diazepam (Valium:Roche) (2.5-20mg IV) may be helpful.[61] Gastric lavage may be indicated to remove any strychnine not absorbed or that has accumulated in the stomach. The low pH of stomach contents favors accumulation since strychnine is an organic base.

The body temperature should be kept within the normal range during the long period of anesthesia; the body temperature can decrease or increase rapidly with the ambient temperature. If the body temperature is allowed to fall appreciably, the rate of strychnine catabolism and excretion is decreased. If the animal is warmed, the body temperature can increase markedly unless this is carefully monitored. Acidification of the urine with oral ammonium chloride enhances strychnine excretion by "trapping" of the ionized base in the urine.

The prognosis in strychnine poisoning is good if the convulsions can be controlled and care is taken that vital functions, such as respiration and body temperature, are maintained within physiologic limits during anesthesia.

ANTU

Alpha-naphthyl thiourea (ANTU) was once a popular rodenticide, but its use has decreased in recent years. The LD_{50} for cats is 75-500 mg/kg (34-227 mg/lb).[62] Daily administration of 20-50 mg/kg (9-23 mg/lb) can cause death within 2-23 days.[63] ANTU is an exception to the rule that drugs and poisons are absorbed better when the stomach is empty. If the stomach is empty, ANTU usually causes prompt emesis because it is an irritant. When taken with food, the material is retained and clinical signs appear within 10-30 minutes after ingestion.[64]

Clinical Signs: The earliest signs include dyspnea and cyanosis of the mucous membranes, especially the lips, tongue and conjunctiva. Vomiting of ingesta and frothy mucus, which may contain bile and blood, occurs early. Diarrhea also occurs soon after the onset of other clinical signs; the feces is blood-red and very watery. The legs, ears, nose, lips and gingivae become cold. The peripheral pulse becomes progressively more difficult to palpate and the heart rate is rapid. Severe pain is exhibited if pressure is applied to the thorax or abdomen. The body temperature falls as intoxication progresses.

At the terminal stage of the syndrome, the animal collapses and takes short, rapid breaths. Severe pulmonary edema and hydrothorax finally cause asphyxia. Death occurs 2-4 hours after the onset of signs.

Treatment: The treatment is symptomatic and the prognosis poor. Induction of emesis is indicated if the animal has not vomited. Prompt emesis occus after a 3- to 6-mg tablet of apomorphine hydrochloride is put into the conjunctival sac.[64] Atropine sulfate is indicated to suppress secretions in the respiratory tract. It may be helpful to give furosemide (5 mg/kg) IV. This potent diuretic has been beneficial in the treatment of pulmonary edema in people.[65] The animal should be supported in a sitting position, in which breathing is most effective. Patients that recover do so rapidly, and therapy is not required for longer than 2-3 days.

Sodium Fluoroacetate

Sodium fluoroacetate (1080) is an extremely toxic substance. The LD_{50} for cats is 0.5 mg/kg (0.23 mg/lb).[66] Cats and dogs are often poisoned secondarily by eating rats killed by 1080.[67] Although the material is quite effective as a rodenticide, its extreme toxicity and the lack of an effective treatment have resulted in laws limiting use of this compound.

Fluoroacetate is metabolized in the body to fluorocitrate, which is a potent inhibitor of aconitase, an enzyme responsible for normal citrate metabolism. As a consequence, the normal tricarboxylic acid cycle is inhibited.[68] The fact that characteristic seizures occur before an increase in citrate concentration suggests that other biochemical alterations may be even more critical.[69] Markedly elevated concentrations of ammonia in the brain have been associated with the onset of convulsions in fluoroacetate poisoning of dogs.[70] It seems likely that the increased concentration of ammonia is one of the factors contributing to the seizures. Fluoroacetate may inhibit use of ammonia in the brain.[71]

Clinical Signs: Signs referable primarily to cardiac and neural disturbances are characteristic in cats poisoned with 1080.[72] The animal initially appears restless and uneasy, and then cries out and runs wildly. Urine and feces usually are voided. After a minute or so, the victim falls and has a clonic seizure lasting 1-2 minutes. After the seizure, the animal is motionless and moans and salivates. A few minutes later another violent seizure occurs. This cycle may be repeated 3-4 times before the animal succumbs due to ventricular fibrillation.

Treatment: Administration of glyceryl monoacetate has been recommended on the basis of a competitive inhibition of fluoroacetate incorporation into the tricarboxylic acid cycle.[34,35] However, there is no specific antidote for 1080 poisoning that has been proven clinically effective in cats or dogs. Affected cats should be sedated with pentobarbital to control any convulsions.

Thallium

This was once a popular rodenticide and roach and ant bait. Because of its toxicity and propensity to cause poisoning in children and pets, the federal government restricted the use of thallium in 1965. Thallium poisoning is not frequently observed in small animals, except in metropolitan areas of the eastern US and in Chicago.[73]

Clinical Signs: Signs appear 2-3 days after ingestion of thallium.[74,75] Emesis is followed by thirst, anorexia, lethargy, progressive weakness and cachexia. There may be respiratory distress and rales. The temperature is normal early in the illness but usually falls as the intoxication progresses.

The skin around the mouth and sometimes around the eyes becomes dry, erythematous, hairless and crusted. The crusts may crack and bleed. Hair loss is not prominent except around the face. Although the hair is not shed excessively, it can be pulled out easily (see Chapter 16). An ocular discharge commonly is present, and the eyeballs are sunken and the lids partially closed. The oral mucosa usually is reddened and may become cyanotic. The breath is malodorous.

As the disease progresses, the intoxicated animal may become hyperesthetic, apprehensive and hard to handle. Incoordination, ataxia, rotation of the head, loss of landing and righting reflexes, and tremors may be seen. Palpating the skeletal muscles and opening the mouth cause pain. Plaintive, high-pitched cries are made as the patient weakens, becomes comatose and dies. The course of fatal intoxication usually is 10-14 days.

Lesions: The gross and histologic lesions have been described in detail.[75] Skin lesions are characteristic and consist of reddening, crusting, peeling and alopecia. Microscopically, there commonly is severe parakeratosis, acanthosis or dilation of hair follicles, focal purulent epidermal or perifollicular inflammation, hyperemia and edema when the lesions are advanced. Other common lesions include nephrosis, polyneuritis and necrosis of skeletal and myocardial muscle.

Diagnosis: The diagnosis is based on chemical identification of thallium in the urine or tissues, the clinical signs, typical skin lesions, and a history of exposure to the poison or poisoned rodents. Although most assays to detect thallium are performed in diagnostic laboratories, an in-hospital rapid test for detection of thallium has been described.[37]

Treatment: Induced emesis and gastric lavage are beneficial if the ingestion of thallium has been relatively recent. A number of antidotes, including diphenylthiocarbazone (dithizone), diethyldithiocarbamate, dimercaprol (BAL), potassium salts and activated charcoal, have been suggested for thallium poisoning. All of them enhance excretion of thallium from the body to some degree. Dithizone should not be used in cats because of possible toxic reactions.[75] Although occasional reports have suggested the effectiveness of these antidotes, the general experience has been disappointing.

Recently, Prussian blue (potassium ferric hexacyanoferrate II) has been studied experimentally and used clinically in people, with encouraging results.[76,77] The material is administered PO and is not absorbed from the GI tract. It binds thallium secreted into the gut and thus prevents subsequent resorption into the body. This effect appears to be due to an exchange of thallium ions for K ions on the Prussian blue molecule. As Prussian blue is not absorbed from the GI tract, the bound thallium is excreted in the feces. In this regard, Prussian blue has been far superior to activated charcoal. The total amount of thallium in the body is significantly reduced and the total excretion of thallium significantly increased after use of Prussian blue.

The efficacy of Prussian blue for thallium poisoning in cats has not been studied. However, based on the results obtained in rats and people, it is reasonable to assume that it would be effective. A suggested dosage is based on the amount of Prussian blue administered to dogs in a study dealing with cesium mobilization.[78] Dogs weighing 7-8 kg (15.4-17.6 lb) were given total daily doses of 3 g PO, divided into 3-6 fractions, for 11 days. No adverse effects ascribable to Prussian blue were reported. In human cases of thallium poisoning, Prussian blue was given PO in 10-g doses twice daily for 10-14 days, with no adverse effects attributable to Prussian blue.[77] A tentative daily dosage for cats of 0.4 g/kg, given PO in 3-6 divided doses, seems reasonable. The drug should be administered as long as there are signs of poisoning. It appears safe to administer Prussian blue for as long as 2 weeks.

For Prussian blue to be effective, the drug must pass through the GI tract and be excreted in the feces. As pylorospasm, gastric dilation and obstipation can occur in thallium poisoning, the drug would not be effective if given by capsule or stomach tube in such cases. It may be necessary to use a duodenal tube to bypass the stomach, and to administer a laxative to facilitate passage of intestinal contents.

Supportive therapy is very important and should include parenteral fluids and electrolytes, B-complex vitamins, a hematinic and an appropriate antibacterial to combat secondary infections. Ointments and lotions containing soothing, lubricating and drying agents should be used as indicated to treat skin lesions. Hand-feeding is indicated if the animal is reluctant to eat.

Vacor

Vacor (N-3-pyridylmethyl-Ń-p-nitrophenyl urea) is a recently introduced rodenticide that has been responsible for a number of feline poisonings. The LD_{50} for cats is 65-500 mg/kg, for dogs is 500-4000 mg/kg and for rats 5-20 mg/kg, which indicates that cats are a relatively susceptible nontarget species. Its mechanism of action in rats is antagonism of niacin (nicotinamide). Secondary poisoning by consumption of dead rodents has not been reported. Glycosuria occurs after Vacor consumption in animals. In people, diabetes mellitus and chronic hypotension may occur. Most animals survive an acute exposure. If the animal is presented immediately after ingestion, emesis should be induced, nicotinamide administered and measures taken to monitor for and control shock.[37,79,80] Intramuscular injection of 0.5 ml Injacom 100 + B Complex (Roche) supplies 5 mg nicotinamide.

Miscellaneous Rodenticides

Zinc phosphide is a rodenticide that reacts with water and hydrochloric acid in the stomach to liberate phosphine gas, which produces severe GI irritation 2-3 days after ingestion. The presence of food in the stomach potentiates toxicity due to the increased acidity of a full stomach. Clinical signs of acute poisoning include anorexia, colic, lethargy, emesis, increased rate and depth of respiration, coma and asphyxiation. Chronic poisoning is probably due to a combination of phosphine gas and zinc toxicity, with signs related to liver and kidney dysfunction. Treatment is supportive.[33,34,37] The incidence of zinc phosphide poisoning may be greater than reported because clinical signs vary and have a latent onset.[73]

Alpha chloralose is a rodenticide and bird repellent that acts by both depressing and stimulating the CNS. The LD_{50} for cats is 400-600 mg/kg. Fortunately, cats usually refuse bait poisoned with the compound. Clinical signs are ataxia, followed by excitement, aggressiveness, tonic convulsions and unconsciousness. Hypothermia may also occur. Supportive care is indicated but use of CNS depressants or stimulants should be avoided.[33,37]

METALLIC POISONS

Lead

Although lead poisoning is not uncommon in dogs, it seems to be rare in cats.[81,82] This probably is a reflection of the more discriminating eating habits of cats. Driveways treated with ash from a lead smelter were considered the source of lead in an outbreak involving 28 dogs and cats in Northern Rhodesia.[83] In a study of 158 cases of lead poisoning across the US, only 2 cats were reported, in contrast to 37 dogs and 102 cattle.[84] Lead poisoning of 8 cats was reported in a survey of small animal lead intoxication in New Zealand.[85] Finally, a case was recently reported in a 5-year-old male Persian cat.[86]

Clinical Signs: Signs associated with GI and neurologic disturbances are common in dogs. Only neurologic signs usually are observed in cats.[83,85] An exception is the Persian cat previously mentioned, which was presented because of lethargy, anorexia, weight loss and intermittent vomiting.[86] Clinical signs include overexcitement, hypersensitivity, intermittent hysteria, mydriasis, circling and convulsions.[83,85] Notably, blood lead concentrations in the New Zealand cats were only 20-30 μg/dl (0.2-0.3 ppm), values much lower than those in dogs in the same report.[85] The Persian cat previously discussed had a blood lead concentration of 70 μg/dl.[86]

Treatment: Procedures for treating lead poisoning in cats have not been reported. It therefore seems appropriate to describe methods that have proven effective for lead poisoning in dogs.

Both supportive and specific treatments are indicated. Supportive therapy should be directed toward removal of unabsorbed lead from the GI tract (cathartics if the animal is constipated), controlling excessive activity (sedation if hyperactive), giving mannitol and/or dexamethasone if there is evidence of cerebral edema, and parenteral feeding and fluid therapy if the animal is anorectic and dehydrated.

Specific therapy is directed toward mobilizing and increasing the excretion of lead from the body. The drug of choice is the Ca chelate of ethylenediaminetetraacetate (EDTA:Legere, Havidote:Haver-Lockhart). A regimen that produces a satisfactory clinical response in dogs consists of daily SC injections of Ca EDTA at 110 mg/kg, divided into 4 doses, for 5 days.[81] Commercial preparations of Ca EDTA should be diluted to 10 mg/ml (1% w/v) for SC injection to minimize pain at the injection site. If Havidote (6.6% Ca EDTA, Haver-Lockhart) is used, a volume of 100 ml of the 1% solution, containing Ca EDTA at 10 mg/ml, can be prepared by diluting 15 ml Havidote with 85 ml 5% dextrose solution. As this is for SC injection, strict asepsis is required when making the dilution.

Arsenic

Arsenic poisoning has been observed in cats.[37,87] Ant and snail baits containing 1-2% arsenic have been implicated as sources of the poison. As arsenical crabgrass killers are widely used in suburban environments, cats might pick up the material on their hair and ingest toxic quantities while grooming. Cats may also suffer from arsenic poisoning during therapy for *Hemobartonella felis* infection with thiacetarsamide.[37]

Clinical Signs: The signs of arsenic poisoning in cats include intense abdominal pain, staggering, extreme weakness, trembling, salivation, emesis, diarrhea, fast feeble pulse, prostration, normal to subnormal body temperature, collapse and death. Toxic arsenic nephrosis may be the primary problem in poisoned small animals.[37] In these cases, supportive fluid therapy should be directed at preservation of renal function.

Treatment: If the animal has not vomited and diarrhea is not present, administering an emetic and/or gastric and colonic lavage are indicated to remove unabsorbed arsenic from the GI tract. Dimercaprol (British Anti-Lewisite, BAL:Hynson, Westcott, Dunning) is the specific antidote. The drug should be administered IM at 3 mg/kg (1.36 mg/lb) every 4 hours for the first 2 days, every 6 hours on the third day, and every 12 hours for the next 10 days or until recovery is complete.[53] Vigorous supportive therapy is essential, including IV electrolyte solutions to combat dehydration, and vitamin B-complex. Blood transfusions may be indicated if intestinal blood loss is severe. An antibacterial agent may be indicated to control secondary infection. Morphine sulfate (0.2 mg/kg) may be indicated to control abdominal pain. Although not evaluated in cats, IM administration of 20% thioctic acid (50 ml/kg at 2-3 sites TID in calves), alone or in combination with BAL, has been somewhat effective in treating experimentally induced acute arsenite toxicosis in cattle, dogs and mice.[88,89]

Bismuth

Acute nephrosis after use of bismuth sodium triglycollamate has been observed in a cat.[90] The drug was given PO at 150 mg/day for 3 days. The cat became partially anorectic, oliguric and severely depressed. Its serum creatinine level was markedly increased and a urine specimen obtained by catheterization revealed many cellular casts. Tubular nephrosis was found at necropsy. The renal cortices contained bismuth at a concentration of 10 ppm. The renal cortices of unaffected cats did not contain detectable concentrations of bismuth.

Mercury

As discussed earlier in this chapter, cats are relatively susceptible to environmental methylmercury poisoning or Minamata disease, as compared with people or dogs, due to the large quantity of fish in their diet.[2,3] Because of this sensitivity, cats have served as sentry animals in outbreaks of the disease in people. The source of mercury in these outbreaks is water pollution from industrial wastes, which results in elevated concentrations of mercury in fish. Mercury has been used as a fungicide in seed grains.[33,37]

Clinical Signs: Experimental studies of subacute and chronic methylmercurialism in cats have been conducted.[2,91] Oral administration of methylmercury at 0.6-1.3 mg/kg produces anorexia, ataxia, hypermetria, proprioceptive impairment, blindness, vertical nystagmus and convulsions after 15-60 days of exposure. Clinical signs in natural cases included a glassy stare and profuse salivation in addition to the above signs.[3] Lesions on necropsy were similar to those seen in people, limited to the CNS and characteristic of an upper motor disease with sensory impairment. In all cases, tissues contained elevated concentrations of mercury, with highest values found in the liver and kidney (40-80 ppm).[2,91] The whole-body (excluding hair) half-life of methylmercury after a single dose was about 75 days, a value very similar to that in people.[92] Taking this and other kinetic factors into consideration, the sensitivity of cats to methylmercury poisoning must be a result of their dietary habits. In fact, blood:tissue concentration ratios suggest that people are more sensitive to poisoning than are cats.[92]

Treatment: Treatment of methylmercury intoxication in cats is futile because the neurologic lesions involved are irreversible. It is important for veterinarians in coastal communities, where industrial wastes may be present, to be alert to the signs of the disease so that outbreaks in people can be detected early.

PLANT POISONINGS

Many house plants contain highly toxic substances. Through boredom or fancy, cats may eat these plants and suffer dire consequences.

Laurel

Sheep laurel (*Kalmia augustifolia*) and mountain laurel (*Kalmia latifolia*) are indigenous in eastern North America, chiefly in the Appalachian Mountains, where they grow in wooded hillside pastures. They are frequently used in floral arrangements in homes. The toxic principle in sheep laurel is andromedotoxin.[93]

Clinical Signs: Cats intoxicated by laurel have serous ocular and nasal discharges and may salivate excessively. Emesis, intermittent convulsions and then paralysis of the limbs may occur. In severely intoxicated cats that die without showing clinical signs, the plant may be found in the stomach.[94]

Treatment: Treatment involves removing unabsorbed material from the GI tract. Sedation is indicated if the animal is excited.

Philodendron, Ivy, *Dieffenbachia*

When ingested, philodendron and large-leaf ivies can produce poisoning and death in cats.[95-97] The clinical signs include weakness, listlessness, fever, nervousness, twitching, trembling, occasional opisthotonus, and complete renal failure. The effects of repeated ingestion appear to be cumulative and the course of illness may be 1-3 months. Some authors have reported signs more confined to irritation of the oral mucous membranes, stomatitis, gastroenteritis and increased salivation.[33,98] In contrast, one group of investigators detected none of the above signs in 3 domestic cats tube-fed aqueous homogenates of *Philodendron oxycardium,* observed for 24 hours and necropsied.[99] *Dieffenbachia* spp ingestion has been associated with severe irritation of the mouth, hypersalivation, pharyngeal edema, and resultant dyspnea and dysphagia.[33,98,100] The toxic principles are Ca oxalate crystals and a proteinaceous histamine-releasing substance. This latter substance apparently is absent from *Philodendron* and is responsible for the severe systemic signs of poisoning.[98,99]

Treatment: Treatment involves removing any unabsorbed material from the GI tract and providing supportive therapy. When signs resemble those associated with a severe histamine response, specific therapy with an antihistamine may be beneficial.[99]

Pine Trees

Cats may ingest pine needles on Christmas trees or drink water from the base of the tree and become ill.[101,102] The signs are probably due to the ingested pine tar and include emesis, diarrhea, stomatitis, pharyngitis, gastroenteritis, lethargy and inanition.

Treatment: Treatment involves removing any unabsorbed material from the GI tract and providing supportive therapy.

Poinsettias

Chewing and ingestion of the leaves of certain varieties of poinsettias and other spurges of the family Euphorbiaceae may cause conjunctivitis, keratitis, stomatitis and gastroenteritis due to contact with their irritant sap.[98] However, poinsettia-feeding experiments in rats did not cause the toxic effects of ingesting the red bracts.[103]

Treatment: Treatment should be directed at removing any plant material ingested and providing supportive care.

Castor Bean, Precatory Bean

Although documented feline cases of poisoning due to consumption of seeds from the castor or precatory bean (crab's eye, rosary pea, jequirity bean) have not been reported, such poisoning in small animals is a possibility.[98] Precatory beans are bright-red seeds with a black spot, made into necklaces and brought home by US tourists in tropical areas. Both beans contain a proteinaceous phytotoxin; ricin in the castor bean, and abrin in the precatory bean.

Clinical Signs: Ingestion of castor beans may result in fever, thirst, sweating and colic, followed by profuse diarrhea, erratic heartbeat and terminal convulsions. Ingestion of precatory beans with broken seed coats may produce severe gastroenteritis, with loss of appetite, violent purgation and fever, followed by a depressed body temperature, incoordination and paralysis. Abrin is more potent than ricin in that a single precatory bean can kill an adult person.[98]

Treatment: Evacuation of the GI tract by emesis or lavage may be effective if performed early after ingestion. Otherwise, supportive fluid therapy is indicated.

Mycetism (Mushroom Poisoning)

Two varieties of mushrooms have caused intoxication in cats.[104,105] One variety, *Amanita muscaria,* produces acute poisoning. This was historically attributed to the presence of muscarine. Recent work indicates that the neurologic signs are instead caused by ibotenic acid and muscimol, while the GI signs are caused by an unidentified principle.[98] The variety *Amanita phalloides* has a delayed effect caused by the active ingredients, phallodine and amanitine.

Clinical Signs: Signs of *A muscaria* intoxication occurring about 2 hours after ingestion are typical of excessive cholinergic activity. The initial signs are excessive salivation and emesis. Hyperpnea, bradycardia, weak pulse and miosis occur later, and the cat becomes semicomatose. Signs of *A phalloides* poisoning include severe abdominal pain, emesis and diarrhea. Chronic signs are related to dysfunction of the vascular system, brain and liver.

Treatment: The treatment for *A muscaria* poisoning has historically been atropine, although IM injection of 0.25-0.5 mg physostigmine has been recommended for cats.[98] Supportive fluid therapy and B-complex vitamins also be help.

Treatment of *A phalloides* poisoning is very difficult because the signs are attributed to 2 toxic principles with independent mechanisms of action. The action of phalloidin may be antagonized by the use of thioctic acid (see Arsenic Poisoning). There is no effective antidote for amanitin; therefore, therapy must largely be supportive and the prognosis poor.[34]

MISCELLANEOUS CHEMICAL POISONINGS

Ethylene Glycol

This is a common constituent of antifreeze used in automobile radiators. Cats and other animals apparently like the taste of the material, as they are attracted to it and lick it from garage floors and accessible containers. Poisoning occurs most frequently during the winter months and is a significant problem in cats, according to recent surveys.[4,73] A fatal dosage for a cat reportedly is 1.5 ml/kg (3 ml of 50% ethylene glycol in antifreeze/kg).[106] This figure is within the range of the fatal dosages (0.9-2.7 mg/kg) reported for dogs.[107,108]

Clinical Signs: Signs of ethylene glycol poisoning include emesis, ataxia, incoordination and depression (quite similar to signs of inebriation); these signs may be followed by hypothermia, leukocytosis, loss of reflexes, convulsions, coma and death.[109,110] The signs associated with acute hepatitis, nephritis, encephalitis, uremia, head trauma and garbage intoxication can be similar to those of ethylene glycol poisoning and must be considered in the differential diagnosis.[110] Retinal detachment and edema, characteristic of toxic retinopathy, occurred from ethylene glycol intoxication in a cat.[111] This condition was believed to be an ocular manifestation of the severe uremia present and resolved after successful therapy of the underlying renal disease with intensive fluid diuresis.

Lesions: The most common gross lesions include edema and congestion of the lung, brain, liver, kidney and spleen, with occasional gastritis. Microscopic lesions include Ca oxalate crystals in the renal tubules and occasionally in the tunica adventitia and perivascular spaces of the cerebellum and hypothalamus.[112] It must be noted that it takes time for oxalate crystals to develop and successful early treatment minimizes their formation.

Ethylene glycol per se is not highly toxic (about the same as ethyl alcohol) but is metabolized by alcohol dehydrogenase to oxalic acid and a number of other intermediate metabolites (glyoxylate, glycoaldehyde, glycolate), all of which are toxic.[113] The glycolate probably is responsible for the severe anion-gap metabolic acidosis that commonly occurs 4-6 hours after ingestion of ethylene glycol.[114,115] If the animal survives this stage, precipitation of Ca oxalate crystals in the kidney may result in renal failure. Production of oxalate crystals is greater in cats than in many other species.[116] Ethylene glycol remains in the body for a relatively long period after its absorption. Appreciable quantities remain at least 24 hours in dogs and 48 hours in rats.[117,118] As long as ethylene glycol remains in the body, it can be oxidized to oxalic acid. Ethylene glycol itself is primarily responsible for the hyperosmolemia, which is a major factor in the early stages of the disease.[119] Diagnosis of ethylene glycol intoxication can be confirmed by chemical analysis of the urine using a relatively simple thin-layer chromatography procedure.[120]

Treatment: Ethyl alcohol is highly effective as treatment for acute ethylene glycol intoxication in people, dogs and cats.[114,117,121] Ethyl alcohol (ethanol) is a potent competitive inhibitor of ethylene glycol oxidation by alcohol dehydrogenase. By blocking the enzymatic conversion of ethylene glycol to oxalic acid, the metabolic acidosis and deposition of Ca oxalate crystals in tissues can be prevented. Treatment is effective if carried out properly and the disease has not progressed too far. When begun as long as 12 hours after ingestion of ethylene glycol, the treatment has been successful in people.[121] Cats given 3 times the lethal dose of ethylene glycol respond to ethanol therapy if treatment is started within 4 hours after ingestion. Delayed therapy might still be successful if a smaller dose of ethylene glycol were ingested. A decrease in incoordination and a progressive increase in alertness after each alcohol treatment indicates a favorable prognosis.[114]

Ethyl alcohol can be administered IV, IP or PO; the IV route probably allows the most satisfactory control of dosage. Although the dosage should be based on achieving a certain concentration of ethyl alcohol in the blood, such values have not been determined for dogs and cats.[121] Consequently, the most satisfactory approach seems to be administering as much ethyl alcohol as the animal can tolerate. Ethylene glycol poisoning has been treated successfully in dogs by IV injections of 50% ethyl alcohol until the animal became comatose and was insensitive to pinching the digit of a forelimb.[117] The dose was repeated whenever the dog reacted to that stimulus. When administering ethyl alcohol as treatment, one must be sure that pure ethyl alcohol and not denatured alcohol is used. It should be given for at least 3 days. In the cat study cited, IP injections of 5 ml of 20% ethanol in isotonic saline solution were given 9 times over a 56-hour period.[114]

As severe anion-gap metabolic acidosis usually is present shortly after the onset of poisoning, an attempt should be made at correction. Although rational therapy would be based on measurements of blood pH and bicarbonate concentration, a 5% solution of $NaHCO_3$ has been given IP at 6-8 ml/kg (4 ml/lb), repeated every 6 hours for 6 treatments.[107,114]

Urine formation should be carefully monitored to detect overloading with fluids should oliguria or anuria occur. Lactated Ringer's solution, given IV at 100 ml/kg/day, was successful in treating the chronic case with toxic retinopathy previously discussed.[111] If renal failure does develop, peritoneal dialysis is indicated. Such therapy has proven beneficial in human cases.[121] Dialysis may also prove effective in removing ethylene glycol and metabolites, such as glycoaldehyde, glycolate and glyoxylate, since the latter are small molecules that should be successfully removed by dialysis.[122]

Other drugs effective in treating experimental cases of ethylene glycol poisoning in laboratory animals include pyridoxine and Mg to prevent renal damage, corticosteroids, and dimethylsulfoxide. In addition, pyrazole, 1,3-butanediol and propylene glycol (alcohol dehydrogenase inhibitors), as well as disulfiram and N-butyraldoxime (aldehyde dehydrogenase inhibitors) have been employed.[120,123] Use of these additional drugs must await further laboratory trials in cats before they are adopted over traditional treatments.

Metaldehyde

This is a common constituent of snail and slug bait. Dogs and cats seem to be attracted to the bait and can consume quantities sufficient to cause poisoning. However, recent regulations by the Environmental Protection Agency have resulted in formulations relatively unattractive to dogs.[124] Spreading the material thinly over a large area, rather than applying the bait in piles, has decreased the incidence of poisoning.[125] Use of the meal formulation rather than the pellets also decreases the chances of poisoning.

Clinical Signs: The syndrome in cats is similar to that in dogs and includes incoordination, muscle tremors, hypersalivation and hyperesthesia. Muscle tremors are continuous, in contrast to the series of spasms characteristic of strychnine poisoning. Nystagmus is reportedly a prominent clinical sign in cats.[126,127] An odor of acetaldehyde often can be detected in the vomitus.[124]

Treatment: The following treatment has been described for dogs.[125] If needed, the animal is sedated to the point of general anesthesia to control the muscle spasms. General anesthesia may have to be maintained for 12-72 hours. The stomach should be lavaged to remove unabsorbed material. Acidosis can be controlled by IV administration of ⅙ M Na lactate at 22 ml/kg (10 ml/lb) during each 12 hours the animal is anesthetized.

Strong Acids and Strong Bases

Cats occasionally are exposed to strong bases or strong acids, which can cause severe skin damage unless immediate steps are taken to remove the irritant. Stomatitis, gingivitis, glossitis, pharyngitis and gastritis may result from licking the affected areas.

Treatment: Large amounts of water should be used to wash the irritant from the skin and hair, and to dilute any small amount that might remain on the surface. Regardless of whether the material is acid or base, dilution renders it less harmful.

After applying water, the remaining material should be neutralized. If the offending product is a base, vinegar or dilute acetic acid (5%) safely neutralizes it. If the material is an acid, 5% $NaHCO_3$ solution neutralizes it.

The damaged skin should be carefully cleansed and an antibiotic ointment applied. The area should be bandaged, if possible, to protect the injured skin. The animal should be examined and treated daily.

Confinement and a nutritious diet are important. Parenteral fluids and vitamin B-complex should be given if the patient becomes dehydrated or refuses to eat. Oral or gastric lesions should be flushed with 5% $NaHCO_3$ solution, followed by 1% Na perborate solution. Kaolin, bismuth, MgO_2 or mineral oil also may be given.

Benzoic Acid

Poisoning of cats due to ingestion of proprietary meat preparations containing excessive concentrations of benzoic acid has been reported.[128,129] The maximum safe level that could be fed to cats was 0.2 g/kg/day.[128]

Clinical Signs: Hyperesthesia, depression, apprehension and occasionally death were seen in cats poisoned with benzoic acid. A cumulative effect also was detected. Very large doses result in aggressiveness and convulsions.

Treatment: Supportive therapy is indicated.

Blue-Tail Lizard Poisoning

The blue-tail lizard (order Lacertilia) is common in the southeastern US. It is about 5 inches long and has a bright-blue tail that easily breaks off when handled. Cats seem to be fond of catching these lizards; when they do, the tail often breaks off and is eaten. The tail may contain a neurotoxin that is considerably more toxic to cats than to dogs.[130]

Clinical Signs: The cat becomes agitated, staggers, trembles, salivates and vomits about 2 hours after ingestion of the tail. It may display vestibular disturbances, evidenced by nystagmus, abnormal righting reflexes, tilting of the head and circling. The cat may be febrile and cry as though in pain. The signs can last for several hours. Death may ensue within 2-4 days or the animal's condition might improve after a few hours of illness. Recovery can be complete or there may be permanent vestibular damage, with a persistent head tilt.

Treatment: An emetic should be given if the animal has not vomited, and an enema can be given to remove toxic material from the colon. Thiamine hydrochloride (5 mg IM) may be given TID and lactated Ringer's solution or normal saline should be given IV if the cat appears dehydrated. Sedation may be necessary.

Toadfish (Pufferfish) Poisoning

Two natural cases of poisoning in cats by ingestion of toadfish (*Fugu*) or pufferfish (*Tetradon*) have been reported. The disease has been experimentally reproduced in cats by feeding liver and flesh from the toadfish.[131] The toxic principle is tetrodotoxin, one of the most deadly nonprotein toxins known. In Australia, the incidence of toadfish poisoning in cats apparently is increasing.[132]

Clinical Signs: Tetrodotoxin's physiologic effects include cardiovascular and respiratory depression, hypotension and flaccid paralysis. Tetrodotoxin specifically blocks Na ionic channels, which are responsible for development of action potentials in nerve synapses and neuromuscular junctions. Because of this action, it has been widely employed as a chemical probe in neurophysiology. The onset of action after tetrodotoxin ingestion in clinical cases is rapid and the prognosis in people is poor.[131,133]

Treatment: Supportive therapy should be aimed at maintaining a patent airway, sustaining adequate blood volume and urine flow by aggressive IV fluid therapy, and correcting any serious cardiac arrhythmias that develop. The cardiovascular signs are largely due to tetrodotoxin-induced depression of sympathetic innervation. Norepinephrine (diluted to a concentration of 4 μg/ml with isotonic saline and infused IV slowly to effect is reportedly successful in feline cases.[131,132] Treatment of arrhythmias or heart block with beta-adrenergic stimulators is contraindicated due to the possibility of aggravating the life-threatening hypotension, unless ventricular fibrillation occurs, at which point heroic measures must be taken.

Ciguatera Poisoning

The neurotoxin ciguatoxin (ichthyosarcotoxin) has been found in 300 species of tropical and semitropical marine fish. The red snapper, grouper, amberjack and great barracuda are prominent examples. Consumption of the viscera or roe of tropical marine fish may be hazardous to people and animals. Clinical signs in people occur after 3-5 hours and include adominal pain, nausea, emesis, muscular weakness and sometimes convulsions. Signs in severe cases occur in less than an hour, with respiratory paralysis the cause of death. Ciguatoxin is a cholinesterase inhibitor with an irreversible effect. Treatment is nonspecific and supportive.[133,134] Atropine ameliorates some of the cardiovascular and GI signs.[135] Although ciguatera poisoning in cats has not been a problem, they are susceptible and their fish-eating habits would make them particularly vulnerable.

Snakebite

Successful treatment of a cat suffering from rattlesnake bite has been described.[136] A tourniquet was applied within a half-hour after the bite was inflicted. The swelling was incised to allow escape of blood and venom, and a polyvalent antisnakebite serum was injected around the wounds and SC. The cat recovered uneventfully. Rapid improvement occurred after administration of tiger snake antivenin in a suspected case of snakebite in a cat.[137]

In a review of 41 feline cases of snakebite,[138] dilated pupils, absence of a pupillary light reflex, depression and generalized weakness were the most common signs. Other signs were vomition, dyspnea, hindlimb ataxia and flaccid paralysis. Subnormal temperature and flaccid paralysis were associated with a poor prognosis. In this Australian report, tiger snakes were identified in 7 cases and 89% of all cats recovered if given 3000 units of tiger snake antivenin, fluid therapy and nursing care.

Note that tiger snake antivenin offers protection against copperhead venom. A polyvalent antivenin effective against common North American pit vipers is available and protects against rattlesnake, cottonmouth and copperhead bites. These snakes produce venom that is hemolytic, necrotizing and anticoagulating, while the venom of the coral snake is neurotoxic. Therefore, the prognosis for recovery from the bite of a coral snake is grave.

Diagnosis of poisonous snakebite is facilitated by the occurrence of extensive swelling and tissue damage at the site of the bite.[139] The reader is urged to determine what species of poisonous snakes are indigenous to his area and keep on hand appropriate antivenin.

Supportive therapy includes a corticosteroid, IV fluids, tetanus antitoxin and broad-spectrum bactericidal antibiotic to combat the possibility of wound infection.[133,139,140] The following bacteria have been isolated from rattlesnake venom: *Pseudomonas aeruginosa, Clostridium* spp, *Corynebacterium* spp, *Staphylococcus* and *Streptococcus*.[141] When severe hemolysis, hemorrhage or defibrination is present, administration of whole blood may be necessary. When the bite is in the head or neck area, maintenance of a patent airway is essential. Shock must be aggressively treated. Supportive therapy is crucial; however, antivenin therapy is the most important part of treating snakebites.

Toad Poisoning

A digitalis-like cardiotoxin and a cholinergic toxin are present in the skin glands of *Bufo* toads (marine or cane toad, Colorado River toad) and can cause clinical disease in cats that ingest or mouth these amphibians. Numerous cases of poisoning of small animals have been reported.[73,132,133] The arrow poison frogs of Central America (*Dendrobates*) also contain these toxins.

Clinical Signs: Death can occur in 10-15 minutes in kittens exposed to *Bufo*. Signs of poisoning include profuse salivation, emesis, pulmonary edema, cardiac arrhythmia, hypertension, prostration and convulsions. Death is due to cardiac arrest.

Treatment: Treatment is directed at removing unabsorbed toxin from the mouth by flushing with large quantities of water, administration of atropine to counteract cholinergic signs, and supportive therapy as indicated. Barbiturates are effective in controlling convulsions. Alpha adrenergic antagonists, such as acepromazine given IV, SC or IM at 1.1-2.2 mg/kg, may help.

INSECTICIDE POISONINGS

Chlorinated Hydrocarbons

Cats generally are considered more susceptible than other animals to the toxic effects of chlorinated hydrocarbons. There is no doubt that externally applied DDT is more dangerous due to the licking habits of cats. In a comparative study, cats were no more sensitive than other animals when the drug was given IV or PO.[142,143] Considerable individual variation exists among cats to the toxic effects of DDT after IV administration.[144,145]

Poisoning of cats has been attributed to several chlorinated hydrocarbon compounds, including DDT, aldrin, dieldrin, endrin, benzene hexachloride and chlordane.[146-153] Clinical cases continue to be reported in the current literature;[5,6] however, curtailment of a large number of these insecticides should decrease the incidence of poisonings. Only chlordane, lindane and toxophene are readily available as of this writing.[73] These compounds have been used in dusting powders, sprays, dips and paints to eliminate insects and mites. Cats can also be exposed by walking or lying on surfaces contaminated with insecticides and become poisoned by licking their feet and fur.

Clinical Signs: Early signs of intoxication are hypersalivation, anorexia and diarrhea. Intermittent spasm of the neck muscles occurs early, causing the head to shake. Tremors of all muscles soon occur, and body movements are exaggerated. Coordination can be so poor that the animal has difficulty in eating or drinking. Severely affected cats may convulse, especially when handled.

The tendency to produce convulsions depends on the specific compound involved. The convulsion-inducing properties of various chlorinated hydrocarbon insecticides given IV to anesthetized cats were compared.[153] Dieldrin, endrin and lindane were the most rapidly acting and potent. Aldrin and heptachlor produced similar convulsions but only at 2-3 times the dose and after a delay of 20-30 minutes. The effects of DDT were variable and kelthane produced no convulsions when given at a dosage below that which caused cardiovascular collapse. Hepatoxicity, renal toxicity and myocardial toxicity may also occur.

Treatment: Phenobarbital, 15-60 mg (0.25-1 gr) given PO twice daily, has been reported to be superior to other barbiturates in controlling hyperactivity due to chlorinated hydrocarbons.[142,148] In addition to the sedative effects of phenobarbital, this drug is also a potent inducer of hepatic microsomal enzymes, which detoxify many chlorinated hydrocarbon insecticides, and, therefore, may also be beneficial in this respect. Diazepam (Valium:Roche), 2.5-5 mg given IV or PO, may be a superior anticonvulsant because it does not produce the degree of respiratory depression characteristic of barbiturates. After the animal is sedated, it may be helpful to administer 2-4 ml of a 10% solution of Ca gluconate IV.

Rotenones

These insecticides are considered relatively harmless and are contained in many preparations designed for household use. However, small amounts can induce nausea and vomiting in dogs and cats.[53] Severe liver damage occurred in cats after application of the material as a dust.[154]

Organophosphates

Insecticides with greater biologic degradability are coming into wider use. These include the organophosphate and carbamate insecticides. Although the carbamates and several organophosphate compounds are relatively safe, some of the organophosphates are highly toxic to mammals. With increased use of these compounds, the number of accidents and cases of improper use probably will increase. Thus, it is likely that more animals will be poisoned by organophosphates in the future.

The use of organophosphates in parasite control also is increasing. Whether the dermatitis associated with organophosphate flea collars is due to the drug or some "inert" ingredient is not known.[155] Malathion has been used as a 25% powder to dust cats for flea control without evidence of toxicity.[156] Chlorthion dips (0.25% solution) have been found safe for cats.[157]

Certain drugs can enhance the toxicity of organophosphate compounds by increasing the rate at which the organophosphate is activated in the body (for example, parathion, which is nontoxic per se, is metabolized by the liver to toxic paraoxon) or by decreasing the rate at which enzymes in the body break it down. Phenothiazine tranquilizers can potentiate the effect of organophosphates after the effective concentration of cholinesterase has been decreased to low levels. Organophosphates can also potentiate the effect of barbiturates.

Clinical Signs: The signs of poisoning are, to a large extent, caused by inhibition of cholinesterase (the enzyme becomes phosphorylated) at cholinergic junctions of the nervous system. These sites include postganglionic parasympathetic neuroeffector junctions (sites of muscarinic activity), autonomic ganglia and neuromuscular junctions (sites of nicotinic activity), and certain sites in the CNS. Acetylcholine is the neurohumoral mediator at these junctions. As cholinesterase is the enzyme that degrades acetylcholine after stimulation of a nerve, its inhibition allows acetylcholine to accumulate and produce excessive stimulation initially, possibly followed by depression. Virtually complete depression of blood cholinesterase activity is a useful diagnostic criterion for organophosphate intoxication.

The signs referable to excessive muscarinic activity include miosis, lacrimation, salivation, excessive respiratory secretions, bronchoconstriction, dyspnea, cyanosis, cardiac irregularities, and incontinence of urine and feces. Atropine effectively counteracts these effects. The signs referable to excessive nicotinic activity and CNS stimulation include uncontrollable muscle twitching, which can progress to paralysis, and convulsions, which can progress to coma. Although atropine can control some of the effects emanating from the CNS, especially the effects on respiration, it has little or no effect in counteracting excessive acetylcholine activity at autonomic ganglia or neuromuscular junctions.

There has also been a syndrome of ataxia and depression associated with the use of dichlorvos flea collars, believed to be a delayed neurotoxic effect of the compound.[158] This syndrome has not been confirmed.[159] Organophosphate-induced delayed neurotoxicity is not a problem in cats.

Treatment: In a severe case of organophosphate poisoning, the following steps should be taken: control excessive muscarinic activity by slow IV administration of atropine sulfate, given to effect; administer a cholinesterase reactivator (not in carbamate intoxication); institute artificial respiration if required; and decontaminate the skin, eyes or stomach as indicated. In less severe cases, procedures appropriate for the circumstances are followed.

Atropine sulfate is the preferred pharmacologic antidote.[160,161] It antagonizes the effect of acetylcholine at sites of muscarinic activity in the autonomic nervous system and also at poorly defined sites of muscarinic activity in the CNS.

Doses considerably larger than those for preanesthetic medication may be required because the action of atropine in blocking acetylcholine receptors is competitive; greater amounts of acetylcholine at the receptor sites require more atropine to block its effect. Consequently, it is not possible to state a specific dosage of atropine sulfate. If the clinical signs are mild and one is in doubt regarding the diagnosis, a dosage of 0.044 mg/kg (0.02 mg/lb) (a preanesthetic dose) given SC can help establish a diagnosis. If this dosage fails to produce signs of atropinization (mydriasis, tachycardia, dry mouth), a presumptive diagnosis of organophosphate poisoning can be made. Conversely, the occurrence of these signs casts doubt on the diagnosis or suggests that the poisoning is mild.[162]

Atropine must be given with considerable care in organophosphate poisoning because it is not difficult to overdose and thus produce atropine poisoning. Either the IV or SC routes can be used. Although the effect from IV administration is more rapid, severe hypotension can result if the injection is too rapid.

The maximal pharmacologic effect of atropine is delayed several minutes after its administration. For example, if atropine were given IV at a rate to produce evidence of atropinization in 2-4 minutes, the chances are good that signs of atropine toxicity would supervene in another 5-10 minutes. One should take at least 15-20 minutes for atropinization. Administration of atropine may have to be repeated because the drug is metabolized and excreted while cholinesterase is still inactive.

Although atropine is highly effective in counteracting the muscarinic and some of the CNS effects, it is merely a supportive treatment. It does not correct the basic biochemical lesion or antagonize the nicotinic effects associated with organophosphate poisoning. If the nicotinic effects are advanced to the point at which function of respiratory muscles is impaired, one must institute artificial respiration.

Derivatives of hydroxamic acid (oximes) can correct the biochemical abnormality. Pralidoxime chloride or 2-PAM chloride (Protopam:Ayerst) given IV, IM or SC at 20 mg/kg, is most commonly used. This compound can dephosphorylate cholinesterase, provided "aging" of the enzyme has not occurred. Fortunately, this phenomenon does not occur as rapidly with the commercial organophosphates as with some of the so-called "war gas" organophosphates. Nevertheless, oximes should be given as soon after exposure as possible because "aging" increases with time.

The drug 2-PAM is particularly valuable in that, by restoring the activity of cholinesterase, a means is provided whereby the nicotinic effects of the poisoning can be treated. However, the oximes cannot restore cholinesterase activity in the brain because their highly ionized nature precludes distribution to the brain. The dosage for 2-PAM is 44 mg/kg (20 mg/lb) given IV over a period of at least 2 minutes. It can be repeated every 12 hours if needed. The SC and IM routes also are suitable. In carbamate (Sevin) toxicity, use of 2-PAM is contraindicated.

Decontamination prevents further absorption of the organophosphate. Needless to say, the clinician must guard against becoming contaminated if there has been a severe external exposure. If indicated, the patient's skin should be cleansed thoroughly with a dilute alkaline solution (*eg*, Hilex Liquid Bleach:Sinclair); organophosphates are readily detoxified or broken down in an alkaline environment because of the presence of hydroxyl ions. Alcohol washes may have a beneficial solvent effect on some vehicles.

Treatment usually is effective if the clinical signs can be brought under control before coma develops. The usual cause of death is respiratory failure and the need for artificial respiration may develop suddenly. The patient should be observed closely for at least 24 hours, especially during the hours immediately after the beginning of treatment. Recovery usually is complete, with no undesirable aftereffects.

Paraquat

Paraquat is a relatively safe herbicide. It is noted for causing pulmonary fibrosis and renal and hepatic failure in people. A case in a cat was characterized by severe ulcerations of the tongue, anorexia, salivation and respiratory difficulties.[163] Specific therapy has not been evaluated, although corticosteroids may be beneficial. Paraquat is rapidly degraded upon contact with soil and thus ingestion of the formulation is necessary for poisoning. The LD_{50} for paraquat in cats is 30-50 mg/kg.[164]

PHARMACOLOGY AND TOXICITY OF THERAPEUTIC AGENTS

Aspirin

The fact that aspirin can produce toxicosis and death in cats has led to recommendations that the drug not be used clinically in this species. The recommendation probably is not warranted because the drug can be given safely to cats in doses that produce concentrations in blood considered to be in the therapeutic range for people.[165] No signs of toxicity were apparent when aspirin was given daily PO at 5-25 mg/kg (2.3-11.4 mg/lb) for 15 days. The safety of aspirin at those dosages is corroborated by another study in which similar daily doses of the drug were given for 4 consecutive weeks.[166]

Aspirin is commonly formulated in 5-gr (324-mg) tablets. If a 5-gr aspirin tablet is given to a 2-kg (4.4-lb) cat, the animal receives 162 mg/kg. This dosage can produce signs of toxicity in cats after 1-2 doses, and death in an average of 12 days.[167] Although it usually is not appropriate to make dosage comparisons between species, it is tempting to point out that a single 5-gr aspirin tablet given to a 2-kg cat is similar to a dose of 35 such tablets for a 70-kg man. Therefore, cat owners should be warned of the dosage restrictions of aspirin for cats. Baby aspirin tablets (1.25 gr = 81 mg) should be used, and a 2-kg cat should receive only half a tablet (40 mg) daily.

Although the efficacy of aspirin as an analgesic in cats has been questioned, others have reported that the drug has been effective.[168,169]

Clinical Signs: Daily dosages exceeding 33 mg/kg can induce signs of salicylism after as few as 1-2 doses. The signs include depression or hyperexcitability, ataxia, nystagmus, anorexia, emesis, weight loss, hyperpnea and evidence of toxic hepatitis.[167,170,171] Dosages exceeding 81 mg/kg can suppress erythropoiesis in the bone marrow, and cause anemia, gastric lesions and death. Acid-base disturbances, renal damage and electrolyte imbalances also are associated with gross overdosage.[172]

Treatment: Successful treatment has been described for acute toxicity in a 1-kg cat receiving aspirin at 162 mg/kg in a 24-hr period.[171] The cat was given 25 ml of $NaHCO_3$ solution (22.3 mEq/L) via stomach tube. Lactated Ringer's solution (150 ml) was injected IP and furosemide (10 mg) was given IM. Administration of the lactated Ringer's solution was continued the next day. Vitamin B-complex was given and supportive treatment was instituted for the diarrhea. Gastric lavage removes unabsorbed drug from the stomach and alkalinization of the urine with oral $NaHCO_3$ to effect enhances excretion of aspirin by ion trapping.

Phenylbutazone

This drug has been given to cats with cervical spondylitis at 12-16 mg/kg PO twice daily on alternate weeks for more than a year with no signs of toxicity.[173] However, at a total daily dosage of 44 mg/kg divided into 2 doses, 4 of 5 cats died after 13-20 doses.[174] The investigators advised the daily dosage not exceed 6-12 mg/kg.

Clinical Signs: In the experimental cases of phenylbutazone intoxication, death was preceded by a progressive loss of appetite, body weight and hair, dehydration, emesis and severe depression.[174] Routine hematologic examination had little value in early detection of toxicity, leading to the suggestion that the drug be withdrawn if inappetence or depression develops.

Acetaminophen

Another analgesic with marked toxicity in cats is acetaminophen (*eg,* Tylenol:McNeil), which is available in 325-mg and 500-mg tablets. Administration of 2 325-mg tablets produces clinical toxicity in cats.[21] The predilection of cats to toxicosis by this drug, addressed earlier in this chapter, is a result of deficiencies in detoxifying mechanisms and an inherent sensitivity of feline RBC to oxidative damage.

Clinical Signs: Marked cyanosis is observed within 4 hours after administration due to methemoglobin formation. A facial edema of unknown cause and anemia are also seen clinically and on necropsy. The SGPT activity is elevated within 4 hours, RBC-reduced glutathione is depleted and Heinz bodies can be seen in the RBC.[17,21,175] Hemoglobinuria and jaundice, due to intravascular hemolysis, can be detected. Histologic evidence of hepatic necrosis was documented in one study.[21]

Treatment: The most effective therapy for acetaminophen toxicosis in cats is a 10% solution of acetylcysteine (Mucomyst:Mead Johnson) given PO at 1.4 mg/kg. This treatment decreases but does not eliminate oxidative RBC damage. Its mechanism is to provide an exogenous sulfate pool for acetaminophen detoxification and thus enhance elimination. A direct protective effect within the RBC cannot be ruled out. Supportive therapy, consisting of fluid and O_2, also might be beneficial.[17,175]

Morphine

It often has been stated that morphine produces excitation in cats and should not be used in this species.[176-178] When given in large doses, morphine can excite cats. At 2-5 mg/kg, cats become shy and fearful, and at 20 mg/kg, they are restless and convulse.[179] These doses clearly are large for any species.

When morphine was given to cats at 0.1-0.2 mg/kg (0.45-0.90 mg/lb), the drug consistently caused depression.[168,179,180] A SC dosage of 0.1 mg/kg produces analgesia for at least 4 hours; therefore, dosages of 0.1-1 mg/kg should produce effective analgesia.[168,181]

Phenol

Veterinarians should be well aware of the sensitivity of cats to phenol compounds. The minimum lethal dosage of phenol to cats by IV injection is about 20 mg/kg.[182] By comparison, the lethal IV dosage in rabbits is 180 mg/kg.[10] The minimum lethal dosage by the SC route in cats is 22-80 mg/kg;[10,182] lethal SC dosages for guinea pigs and mice are 450-550 mg/kg and 420-450 mg/kg, respectively.[10]

The relatively high degree of toxicity of phenols appears to be related to the limited capacity of cats to catabolize the material, the limited binding of phenol to tissues, and the low receptor tolerance to all phenolic compounds.[183,184]

Although there is reluctance to use phenolized vaccines in cats because of their sensitivity to phenol, cats have tolerated doses of 3-5 ml of phenolized (0.5%) vaccine.[185] A 5-ml quantity of 0.5% phenol contains 25 mg of phenol. If a 4-kg cat received a 5-ml dose of phenolized (0.5%) vaccine, it would receive about 6.3 mg/kg, which is slightly less than a third of the minimum lethal dose.

Intoxication can follow application of phenolized skin preparations or use of coal-tar products as insecticidal shampoos, disinfectants and wood preservatives. The toxic agent is ingested as the cat grooms itself. The material can also be inhaled.[186] Fatal cases of poisoning in cats have been caused by exposure to pentachlorophenol in sawdust.[187] Hexachlorophene, a chlorinated phenol derivative, is also toxic to cats.

Clinical Signs: Ingestion of phenol in toxic amounts causes salivation, vomiting and sometimes diarrhea. Malaise and inappetence are common. There may be involuntary muscle twitching, head shaking, ataxia, mydriasis and a harsh voice. Body temperature often is decreased and dyspnea may be prominent. Renal tubular necrosis is a consistent finding on histologic examination.[184,188,189] Ingestion of lethal amounts can result in viciousness and violent convulsions before death.

Treatment: Every effort should be made to prevent further absorption of the poison. The cat should be bathed if the phenol is on the hair or skin. An emetic may be given if the phenol was recently ingested and the cat has not vomited. Treatment is largely symptomatic. Sedatives are indicated if the animal is convulsing. Administering GI emollients (kaolin, bismuth, mineral oil) may be helpful. Fluids (lactated Ringer's or physiologic saline) should be given IV if the cat is dehydrated.

Chloramphenicol

Chloramphenicol, given IM daily at 50 mg/kg, produced signs of toxicity characterized by inappetence and marked depression by the seventh day.[190,191] The cats were extremely ill by day 21. Examination of bone marrow revealed vacuolation in many of the early cells of both the myeloid and erythroid series by day 14. A number of lymphocytes were also vacuolated and there was a marked decrease in the percentage of erythroblasts and the total WBC count.

Chloramphenicol, given PO daily at 120 mg/kg in 3 divided doses for 14 days, produced depression, dehydration, inappetence, weight loss, diarrhea and vomiting. There was reversible bone marrow suppression, with marrow hypoplasia, maturation arrest of erythroid cells, inhibition of mitotic activity and vacuolation of lymphocytes and early myeloid and erythroid cells. Similar but less severe changes were seen at daily dosages of 60 mg/kg and 100 mg/kg.[192-194] In another study, daily dosages of 25-100 mg/kg, given only 5 days a week for 30 days, did not produce hemopoietic changes.[195]

In therapeutic doses, chloramphenicol prolongs the duration of action of many drugs by inhibiting drug-biotransformation enzymes.[196] For example, it can significantly prolong the duration of pentobarbital anesthesia in cats.[197] The duration of anesthesia was prolonged 160% when chloramphenicol was given IV at 30 mg/kg 10 minutes after administration of pentobarbital. Therefore, chloramphenicol probably should be used with caution in an animal anesthetized with pentobarbital.

Recent pharmacokinetic studies of chloramphenicol in cats have shed some light on the proper dosage for this species.[16,198-200] The half-life after IV administration was 5.1 hours. The bioavailability was judged excellent but variable after oral administration of chloramphenicol tablets (Chloromycetin:Parke Davis). Chloramphenicol palmitate suspension (Parke Davis) did not produce reliable plasma concentrations in starved cats. Peak serum concentrations after oral administration occurred at 30-120 minutes and at 30 minutes after IM chloramphenicol sodium succinate administration. A 20 mg/kg oral dosage of crystalline chloramphenicol produced peak plasma concentrations of about 10 μg/ml. The relatively prolonged half-life of this drug in cats and its susceptibility to toxicosis is a reflection of the inability of cats to eliminate chloramphenicol by conjugation with glucuronic acid, the major route of elimination in other species. In cats, 25% of chloramphenicol is eliminated unchanged in the urine in 24 hours. It may be relevant to point out that this enzyme system is deficient in neonatal kittens. The grey baby syndrome, caused by giving chloramphenicol to infants, is believed due to their inability to biotransform the drug to the glucuronide conjugate, as well as to undeveloped renal function. Thus, the drug remains in the body for a longer period.

When these data are taken into consideration and compared against the minimal effective therapeutic concentrations, some guidelines can be developed. One investigator recommends 50 mg/kg every 12 hours as a safe oral dosage.[201] In light of the relatively large volume of distribution of chloramphenicol in cats and the results of the previously mentioned toxicity studies, a more conservative dosage is 25-mg/kg every 12 hours. If a chloramphenicol-sensitive infection did not respond, the dosage could be increased. Finally, note that toxicity depends on both the dosage and duration of administration.

Aminoglycosides

Aminoglycoside antibiotics (streptomycin, kanamycin, neomycin, gentamicin, tobramycin) cause 3 toxic syndromes: proximal renal tubular damage, ototoxicosis (vestibular malfunction and deafness) and neuromuscular blockade.[202] Cats are sensitive to vestibular toxicity. This may occur before nephrotoxicity becomes apparent clinically, although subclinical nephrotoxicosis may be present.[203] Vestibular toxicity, unlike renal toxicity, is irreversible. Experimental daily dosages of gentamicin of 20-60 mg/kg produced ataxia, with toxicity occurring at a total dose of 650-800 mg.[203,204] A daily dosage of gentamicin of 10 mg/kg for 40 days did not produce ataxia or impaired righting reflexes.[204] Similarly, tobramycin at 25 mg/kg daily for 65 days did not produce vestibular toxicity.[205] These dosages are well above the recommended therapeutic dosage of gentamicin for cats of 2-5 mg/kg divided every 8 hours for 4-7 days.[206,207]

Similar considerations should hold for other aminoglycosides administered to cats with normal renal function. However, since this class of drugs is eliminated from the body solely by the kidney, dosages should be reduced, preferably by extension of the dosage interval, in renal insufficiency, as discussed in detail elsewhere, to avoid toxicity.[208,209] Significant risk of vestibular toxicity would occur in renal insufficiency, gross overdosage, volume depletion or coadministration of other ototoxic drugs, as furosemide.

Ampicillin, Amoxicillin

Both of these antibiotics are relatively safe for use in cats. Recent efficacy and disposition studies have allowed development of rational therapeutic guidelines for their use.[210,211] The half-life of ampicillin in cats was 73 minutes, twice that reported for dogs. Depending on the susceptibility of the bacterial pathogen, an adequate dosage regimen for ampicillin would be 10 mg/kg every 8-12 hours. A similar dosage of amoxicillin would be effective in most situations. The efficacy of 50 mg amoxicillin trihydrate given once daily was equal to that of 2 50-mg doses a day.[212]

Tetracyclines

Conventional doses of tetracycline and oxytetracycline given PO to cats produced diarrhea, colic, emesis, depression, fever and anorexia.[213] Doxycycline (Vibramycin:Pfizer) may be safer in cats because of its pattern of upper GI tract absorption and lack of GI effects.[214]

Griseofulvin

Griseofulvin is a fungicide used to treat dermatomycoses. It is teratogenic when given at 35 mg/kg to cats in the first trimester of pregnancy. Kittens had cleft palate and multiple congenital malformations of the brain and skeleton.[215,216]

Urinary Antiseptics/Analgesics

Methylene blue administration to cats produces methemoglobinemia and Heinz bodies and thus is contraindicated for use in cats. The urinary analgesic, phenazopyridine, also induces oxidative changes in the RBC of cats.[26] A dose of 250 mg nalidixic acid given to 7 Burmese cats every 12 hours (an inadvertent overdose) produced hysteria, dilated pupils, apprehension, salivation and ataxia in 2 of the cats.[217] This was followed by loss of consciousness and hypothermia. One cat died and the other recovered uneventfully. Therapy was supportive. Finally, ethylenediamine dihydrochloride (Chlor-Ethamine:Pitman-Moore) was ineffective as a treatment for *E coli* urinary infections in one study.[218] Depending on bacterial sensitivities, ampicillin, amoxicillin, penicillin, gentamicin, kanamycin, tobramycin or small doses of chloramphenicol would be the drugs of choice for urinary tract infections in cats. The safety of trimethoprim-sulfadiazine (Tribrissen:Wellcome) in cats has not been evaluated, although its efficacy and safety in treating canine urinary tract infections has been established.[219]

Digoxin

Digoxin disposition and toxicity were evaluated in the cat, a species alluded to as being clinically sensitive to the drug.[220,221] Plasma concentrations were greater in male cats than in female cats. Administration of 0.011 mg/kg daily for 4 days resulted in accumulation of the drug in the serum. Toxicity, as evidenced by depression, vomition, salivation and anorexia, with minimal electrocardiographic changes, occurred with a single oral dosage of 0.11 mg/kg. Complete guidelines for dosages of digoxin in cats are not available; guidelines in the literature on dogs should be consulted.[222] The above dosages can serve as a starting point. The dosage should be reduced when anorexia, vomiting or diarrhea ensues to prevent serious cardiac arrhythmias.

Megestrol Acetate

Megestrol acetate (Ovaban:Schering), a progesterone analog frequently used in cats to treat urine spraying, roaming of males, miliary dermatitis, eosinophilic granuloma, inappropriate urination, aggressive behavior, modification of estrus, endocrine alopecia, overgrooming, acne and other conditions, caused significant impairment of adrenocortical function.[223] An oral dose of 2.5-5.0 mg every day for 2 weeks resulted in functional and morphologic adrenal changes. Other adverse reactions associated with this drug in cats are obesity, endometritis, pyometra, abnormal glucose-tolerance test results, temperament changes, polyuria, mammary hypertrophy and other actions that were extensions of its physiologic effects.

References

1. Osweiler, GD. JAVMA **155** (1969) 2011.
2. Gruber, TA *et al.* Aust Vet J **54** (1978) 155.
3. Takeuchi, T *et al.* Environ Res **13** (1977) 215.
4. Stowe, CM *et al.* Proc 4th Bienn Tox Conf, Logan, UT, 1978.
5. Caldwell, ST *et al.* Vet Human Tox **19** (1977) 166.
6. Maddy, KT and Winter, J. Vet Human Tox **22** (1980) 409.
7. Aronson and Schwark, in Kirk: Current Veterinary Therapy VII. WB Saunders, Philadelphia, 1980.
8. Mardre, RB. Auburn Vet **12** (1956) 138.
9. Brodie, BB. Pharm **6(1)** (1964) 12.
10. Spector, WS: Handbook of Toxicology. Vol 1. WB Saunders, Philadelphia, 1956.
11. Glazko, AJ. Antimicrob Agents Chemother (1966) 655.
12. Brodie, in Wolstenholme and Porter: Drug Responses in Man. Little, Brown and Co, Boston, 1967.
13. McChesney, EW. Biochem Pharm **13** (1964) 1366.
14. Robinson, D and Williams, RT. Biochem J **68** (1958) 23P.
15. Dutton, in Dutton: Glucuronic Acid, Free and Combined: Chemistry, Biochemistry, Pharmacology and Medicine. Academic Press, New York, 1966.
16. Baggot, JD: Principles of Drug Disposition in Domestic Animals. WB Saunders, Philadelphia, 1977.
17. St. Omer, VV and McKnight, ED. JAVMA **176** (1980) 911.
18. Kaihara, M and Price, JM. Arch Biochem Biophys **110** (1965) 316.
19. Welch, RM *et al.* Biochem Pharm **15** (1966) 521.
20. Capel, ID *et al.* Biochem Soc Trans **2** (1974) 305.
21. Finco, DR *et al.* JAVMA **166** (1975) 469.
22. Hinson, in Hodgson *et al:* Reviews in Biochemical Toxicology. Vol 2. Elsevier-North Holland, New York, 1980.
23. Smith, in Doull *et al:* Casarett and Doull's Toxicology: The Basic Science of Poisons. 2nd ed. Macmillan, New York, 1980.
24. Fertman, MN and Fertman, MB. Medicine **34** (1955) 131.
25. Beritic, T. Blood **25** (1965) 999.

26. Harvey, JW and Kornick, HP. JAVMA **169** (1976) 327.

27. Harvey, JW and Kaneko, JJ. Proc Soc Exp Biol Med **147** (1974) 245.

28. Harvey, JW and Kaneko, JJ. Br J Haematol **32** (1973) 193.

29. Scott, DW *et al.* Cornell Vet **69** (1979) 104.

30. Ross, LA and Finco, DR. Am J Vet Res **42** (1981) 1704.

31. Aronson, in Kirk: Current Veterinary Therapy IV. WB Saunders, Philadelphia, 1971.

32. Aronson, AL. Vet Clin No Am **2** (1972) 379.

33. Atkins, CE and Johnson, RK, Vet Clin No Am **5** (1975) 623.

34. Hatch, in Jones: Veterinary Pharmacology and Therapeutics. 5th ed. Iowa State Univ Press, Ames, 1977.

35. Bailey, in Kirk: Current Veterinary Therapy VII. WB Saunders, Philadelphia, 1980.

36. Rumack and Peterson, in Doull *et al:* Casarett and Doull's Toxicology: The Basic Science of Poisons, 2nd ed. Macmillan, New York, 1980.

37. Buck, WB *et al:* Clinical and Diagnostic Veterinary Toxicology. 2nd ed. Kent/Hunt, Dubuque, IA, 1976.

38. Chin, L *et al.* Tox Appl Pharm **16** (1970) 786.

39. Decker, WJ *et al.* Tox Appl Pharm **13** (1968) 454.

40. Holt, LM and Holz, PH. J Pediat **63** (1963) 306.

41. Henschler, D and Kreutzer, P. Deutsche Med Wschr **91** (1966) 2241.

42. Picchioni, AL *et al.* Tox Appl Pharm **8** (1966) 447.

43. Yeary, RA. JAVMA **161** (1972) 1677.

44. Parker, in Kirk: Current Veterinary Therapy VII. WB Saunders, Philadelphia, 1980.

45. Thornhill, JA. Comp Cont Ed Pract Vet **3** (1981) 20.

46. Thornhill, JA *et al.* Minn Vet **20** (1980) 27.

47. Klausman, BS and Brown, HW. Vet Med **47** (1952) 235.

48. Green and Buck, in Kirk: Current Veterinary Therapy VII. WB Saunders, Philadelphia, 1980.

49. McGirr, JL. Proc 15th Int Vet Cong, 1953.

50. Biggs, R and MacFarland, RG: Human Blood Coagulation and its Disorders. 2nd ed. Blackwell Scientific Publications, Oxford, 1957.

51. Barnhart, JI and Anderson, GF. Biochem Pharm **9** (1962) 23.

52. Lowenthal, J and Birnbaum, H. Science **164** (1969) 181.

53. Clarke, EGC and Clarke, ML: Garner's Veterinary Toxicology. 3rd ed. Williams & Wilkins, Baltimore, 1967.

54. Creyke, GH. Vet Rec **68** (1956) 376.

55. Broman, U. Nord Vet Med **13** (1961) 604.

56. Lawson, J and Doncaster, RA. Vet Rec **77** (1965) 183.

57. Watt, JG and Doxey, DL. Vet Rec **73** (1961) 548.

58. Ashworth, B. Vet Rec **93** (1973) 50.

59. Hansten, PD: Drug Interactions. 4th ed. Lea & Febiger, Philadelphia, 1979.

60. Arronson, AL and Dunlop, RH, Cornell Univ: Unpublished data, 1965.

61. Osweiler, in Kirk: Current Veterinary Therapy VII. WB Saunders, Philadelphia, 1980.

62. McGirr, JL and Papworth, DS. Vet Rec **67** (1955) 124.

63. McClosky, WT and Smith, MI. Publ Health Rep **60** (1945) 1101.

64. Smith, in Kirk: Current Veterinary Therapy. WB Saunders, Philadelphia, 1964.

65. Lesch, M *et al.* N Engl J Med **279** (1968) 115.

66. Chenoweth, MB and Gilman, A. J Pharm Exp Therap **87** (1946) 90.

67. Gilcreas, FW. Bull NY State Dept Health **3** (1950) 9.

68. Peters, RA. Adv Enzym **18** (1957) 113.

69. Pscheidt, GR *et al.* Am J Physiol **176** (1954) 483.

70. Benitez, D *et al.* Am J Physiol **176** (1954) 488.

71. Lahiri, S and Quastel, JH. Biochem J **89** (1963) 157.

72. Chenoweth, MB. Pharm Rev **1** (1949) 383.

73. Osweiler, in Kirk: Current Veterinary Therapy VII. WB Saunders, Philadelphia, 1980.

74. Pile, CH. Aust Vet J **32** (1956) 18.

75. Zook, BC *et al.* JAVMA **153** (1968) 285.

76. Heydlauf, H. Europ J Pharm **6** (1969) 340.

77. Kamerbeek, HH *et al.* Acta Med Scand **189** (1971) 321.

78. Madshus, K *et al.* Int J Rad Biol **10** (1966) 519.

79. Peoples, SA and Maddy, KT. Vet Human Tox **21** (1979) 266.

80. Berg, GL: 1981 Farm Chemicals Handbook. Meister, Willoughby, OH, 1981.

81. Zook, BC *et al.* JAVMA **155** (1969) 1329.

82. Kowalczxyk, in Kirk: Current Veterinary Therapy VII. WB Saunders, Philadelphia, 1980.

83. Scott, HM. Vet Rec **75** (1963) 830.

84. Priester, WA and Hayes, HM. Am J Vet Res **35** (1974) 567.

85. McLeavey, in Kirk: Current Veterinary Therapy VII. WB Saunders, Philadelphia, 1980.

86. Jacobs, G. JAVMA **179** (1981) 1396.

87. Staples, ELJ. J Sci Tech **10** (1961) 129.

88. Grunert, RR. Arch Biochem Biophys **86** (1960) 190.

89. Hatch, RC *et al.* Am J Vet Res **39** (1978) 1411.

90. Kelley, DF *et al.* JAVMA **159** (1971) 413.

91. Davies, TS and Nielen, SW. Am J Vet Res **38** (1977) 59.

92. Hollins, TG *et al.* Tox Appl Pharm **33** (1975) 438.

93. Kingsbury, JM: Poisonous Plants of the United States and Canada. Prentice-Hall, Englewood Cliffs, NJ, 1964.

94. Wasserman, B. JAVMA **135** (1959) 569.

95. Brogger, JN. Mod Vet Pract **51(6)** (1970) 46.

96. Greer, MJ. Mod Vet Pract **42(20)** (1961) 62.

97. Pierce, JH. Mod Vet Pract **51(6)** (1970) 42.

98. Fowler, MF: Plant Poisonings in Small Companion Animals. Ralston Purina, St. Louis, 1980.

99. Sellers, SJ *et al.* Vet Human Tox **19** (1977) 92.

100. Kingsbury, in Doull *et al:* Casarett and Doull's Toxicology: The Basic Science of Poisons. 2nd ed. Macmillan, New York, 1980.

101. Sprung, C. Mod Vet Pract **51(6)** (1970) 46.

102. Kaskin, ST. Mod Vet Pract **51(6)** (1970) 46.

103. Stone, RP and Collins, WJ. Tox **9** (1971) 301.
104. Mullenax, CH and Mullenax, PB. Mod Vet Pract **43(7)** (1962) 61.
105. Rylands, JM. Vet Rec **75** (1963) 761.
106. Milles, G. Arch Path **41** (1946) 631.
107. Beckett, SD and Shields, RP. JAVMA **158** (1971) 472.
108. Kersting, EJ and Nielsen, SW. Am J Vet Res **27** (1966) 574.
109. Hadlow, WJ. JAVMA **130** (1957) 296.
110. Kersting, EJ and Nielsen, SW. JAVMA **146** (1965) 113.
111. Barclay, SM and Riis, RC. JAAHA **15** (1979) 719.
112. Kersting and Nielsen, in Kirk: Current Veterinary Therapy III. WB Saunders, Philadelphia, 1968.
113. Beasley, VR and Buck, WB. Vet Human Tox **22** (1980) 255.
114. Pneumarthy, L and Oehme, FW. Am J Vet Res **36** (1975) 209.
115. Clay, KL and Murphy, RC. Tox Appl Pharm **39** (1977) 39.
116. Gessner, PK *et al.* Biochem J **79** (1961) 482.
117. Nunamaker, DM *et al.* JAVMA **159** (1971) 310.
118. Peterson, DI *et al.*. J Am Med Assoc **186** (1963) 955.
119. Green, RA *et al.* Vet Clin Path **8** (1979) 8.
120. Maylin, GA. Cornell Vet **70** (1980) 202.
121. Wacker, WEC *et al.* J Am Med Assoc **194** (1965) 1231.
122. Parry, MF and Wallach, R. Am J Med **57** (1974) 143.
123. Cornish, in Doull *et al:* Casarett and Doull's Toxicology: The Basic Science of Poisons, 2nd ed. Macmillan, New York, 1980.
124. Mull, in Kirk: Current Veterinary Therapy VII. WB Saunders, Philadelphia, 1980.
125. Custer, in Kirk: Current Veterinary Therapy IV. WB Saunders, Philadelphia, 1971.
126. James, OD. Vet Rec **67** (1955) 248.
127. Tapernoux, A *et al.* Rev Med Vet **125** (1964) 114.
128. Bedford, PGC and Clarke, EGC. Vet Rec **90** (1972) 53.
129. Humphreys, DJ. Vet Rec **98** (1976) 219.
130. Adair, HS Jr. Auburn Vet **9** (1953) 117.
131. Atwell, RB and Stutchbury, GB. Aust Vet J **54** (1978) 308.
132. Wilkinson, GT. Proc Refresher Course, Univ of Sydney **1** (1978) 117.
133. Oehme *et al,* in Doull *et al:* Casarett and Doull's Toxicology: The Basic Science of Poisons. 2nd ed. Macmillan, New York, 1980.
134. Morse, EV. Vet Human Tox **19** (1977) 176.
135. Hughes, JM and Merson, MH. N Engl J Med **295** (1976) 1117.
136. Kroll, HM. JAVMA **129** (1956) 526.
137. Munday, BL. Aust Vet J **35** (1959) 44.
138. Hill, FWG and Campbell, T. Aust Vet J **54** (1978) 437.
139. Clark, KA. Mod Vet Pract **62** (1981) 427.
140. Hirschorn, in Kirk: Current Veterinary Therapy VII. WB Saunders, Philadelphia, 1980.
141. Goldstein, EJC *et al.* J Infect Dis **140** (1979) 818.
142. Philips, FS and Gilman, A. J Pharm Exp Therap **86** (1946) 213.
143. Smith, MI and Stohlman, EF. US Publ Health Rep **59** (1944) 984.
144. Pluvinage, RJ and Heath, JW. Proc Soc Exp Biol Med **63** (1946) 212.
145. Woodard, G *et al.* J Pharm Exp Therap **82** (1944) 152.
146. Jolly, DW. Vet Rec **64** (1952) 76.
147. Klemmer, HW *et al.* JAVMA **170** (1977) 727.
148. Easton, KL. Can Vet J **2** (1961) 310.
149. Morse, EV. JAVMA **111** (1947) 55.
150. Ressang, AA *et al.* Communis Vet **2** (1958) 71.
151. Bjotvedt, G and Wharton, MF. Feline Pract **3(4)** (1973) 44.
152. Wilkinson, GT. Vet Rec **92** (1973) 510.
153. Joy, RM. Tox Appl Pharm **35** (1976) 96.
154. Ramsay, FK *et al.* Anim Hosp **3** (1967) 221.
155. Muller, GH. JAVMA **157** (1970) 1616.
156. Cross, RF and Folger, GC. JAVMA **129** (1956) 65.
157. Bell, RR *et al.* JAVMA **126** (1955) 302.
158. Bell, TG *et al.* JAVMA **167** (1975) 579.
159. Kodama, JK *et al.* JAVMA **168** (1976) 368.
160. Douglas, WW and Matthews, PBC. J Physiol **116** (1952) 202.
161. Sudduth, JH and Kelley, ST. Vet Human Tox **20** (1978) 253.
162. Namba, T. Bull World Health Org **44** (1971) 289.
163. Johnson, RP and Hustable, CR. Vet Rec **98** (1976) 189.
164. Murphy, in Doull *et al:* Casarett and Doull's Toxicology: The Basic Science of Poisons. 2nd ed. Macmillan, New York, 1980.
165. Yeary, RA and Swanson, W. JAVMA **163** (1973) 1177.
166. Eder, H. Acta Pharm Tox **21** (1964) 197.
167. Larson, EJ. JAVMA **143** (1963) 837.
168. Davis, LE and Donnelly, EJ. JAVMA **153** (1968) 1161.
169. Cameron, DB. JAVMA **153** (1968) 356.
170. Herrgesell, JD. JAVMA **151** (1967) 452.
171. Zontine, WJ and Uno, T. VM/SAC **64** (1969) 680.
172. Davis, LE. JAVMA **176** (1980) 65.
173. English, PB and Seawright, AA. Aust Vet J **40** (1964) 376.
174. Carlisle, CH *et al.* Br Vet J **124** (1968) 560.
175. Gaunt, SD *et al.* Am J Vet Res **42** (1981) 1982.
176. Brander, GC and Pugh, DM: Veterinary Applied Pharmacology and Therapeutics. 2nd ed. Williams & Wilkins, Baltimore, 1971.
177. Jones, LM: Veterinary Pharmacology and Therapeutics. 3rd ed. Iowa State Univ Press, Ames, 1965.
178. Wilkinson, GT. J Sm Anim Pract **9(1)** (1968) 21.
179. Joel, E and Arndts, F. Morphin Arch Physiol **210** (1925) 280.
180. Whittick, W, Toronto, Canada: Personal communication, 1966.

181. Booth, in Jones: Veterinary Pharmacology and Therapeutics. 4th ed. Iowa State Univ Press, Ames, 1977.
182. Ernst, MR *et al.* JAVMA **138** (1961) 197.
183. Oehme, FW and Davis, LE. Pharm **11(2)** (1969) 63.
184. Oehme, FW. Proc Gaines Vet Symp, 1971.
185. Scheidy, SF *et al.* JAVMA **123** (1953) 330.
186. Wagener, K. JAVMA **120** (1952) 145.
187. Munro, IB *et al.* Vet Rec **101** (1977) 525.
188. Dodman, NH *et al.* Vet Rec **99** (1976) 319.
189. Liao, JTF and Oehme, FW. Vet Human Tox **22** (1980) 160.
190. Penny, RHC *et al.* Br Vet J **123** (1967) 145.
191. Penny, RHC *et al.* Br Vet J **126** (1970) 453.
192. Glauber, A and Rosenfeld, IS, Cornell Univ: Unpublished data, 1972.
193. Watson, ADJ and Middleton, DJ. Am J Vet Res **39** (1978) 1199.
194. Watson, ADJ. Am J Vet Res **41** (1980) 293.
195. Teske, RH and Mercer, HD. Can Vet J **17** (1976) 19.
196. Christenson, LK and Skovsted, L. Lancet **2** (1969) 1397.
197. Adams, HR and Dixit, BN. JAVMA **156** (1970) 902.
198. Davis, LE *et al.* Am J Vet Res **33** (1972) 2259.
199. Watson, ADJ. J Vet Pharm Therap **2** (1979) 123.
200. Watson, ADJ. J Vet Pharm Therap **2** (1979) 117.
201. Mercer, HD. JAVMA **176** (1980) 923.
202. Riviere, JE and Coppoc, GL. JAVMA **178** (1981) 508.
203. Waitz, JA *et al.* J Infect Dis **124** (Suppl) (1971) S125.
204. Black, J *et al.* Antimicrob Agents Chemother **3** (1963) 138.
205. Welles, JS *et al.* Tox Appl Pharm **25** (1973) 398.
206. Burrows, GE. JAVMA **175** (1979) 301.
207. Conzelman, GM. JAVMA **176** (1980) 1078.
208. Riviere, JE and Coppoc, GL. JAVMA **178** (1981) 70.
209. Riviere, JE and Davis, LE: Canine Nephrology. Yearbook Medical Publishers, Chicago, 1983.
210. Keefe, TJ. Feline Pract **7(1)** (1977) 30.
211. Mercer, HD *et al.* Am J Vet Res **38** (1977) 1353.
212. Keefe, TJ. VM/SAC **73** (1978) 447.
213. Wilkinson, GT. J Sm Anim Pract **9(1)** (1968) 21.
214. Aronson, AL. JAVMA **176** (1980) 1061.
215. Gillick, A and Bulner, WS. Can Vet J **13** (1972) 244.
216. Schneider, in Kirk: Current Veterinary Therapy VII. WB Saunders, Philadelphia, 1980.
217. Tiffin, RB. Vet Rec **96** (1975) 139.
218. Finco, DR. Am J Vet Res **42** (1981) 670.
219. Ling, GV and Ruby, AL. JAVMA **174** (1979) 1003.
220. Erichsen, DF *et al.* Am J Vet Res **41** (1980) 2049.
221. Bond and Tilley, in Kirk: Current Veterinary Therapy VII. WB Saunders, Philadelphia, 1980.
222. Davis, in Kirk: Current Veterinary Therapy VII. WB Saunders, Philadelphia, 1980.
223. Chastain, CB *et al.* Am J Vet Res **72** (1981) 2029.

4

systemic viral diseases

R.L. OTT

Introduction

Historical Perspective

The filterability of rabies virus was not demonstrated until 1903, although the signs of rabies had been well described in antiquity.[1] It was believed that pseudorabies was of viral etiology in 1902; however, Aujeszky was unable to filter the agent.[2] Rabies and pseudorabies were the only diseases of "proven" viral origin affecting cats until a virus was isolated from cats suffering from "infectious enteritis" in 1928.[3] It took 4 years to confirm that "infectious enteritis" or "feline distemper" was in fact a viral disease, and 10 years to confirm that the characteristic clinical laboratory picture of this disease was agranulocytosis.[4-6]

The term "feline distemper," an obvious misnomer, commonly appeared in the veterinary literature between 1928 and 1968. During the greater portion of this time, peracute, enteric and respiratory forms of feline distemper were described even though it was obvious to enlightened veterinarians that "feline distemper" was unlikely to occur in such diverse forms.

In 1942 a respiratory disease of cats caused by a member of the psittacosis lymphogranuloma group of "viruses" was described.[7,8] (This particular agent is classifed as *Chlamydia psittaci.*) The disease was called feline pneumonitis. In the same year other cases of feline viral pneumonia were described.[9] The virus isolated did not infect mice or produce elementary bodies and thus was obviously not the "pneumonitis virus." The report on feline virus pneumonia was buried in the literature for almost 20 years, during which time all contagious respiratory diseases in cats were described as pneumonitis.

Before the late 1950s and early 1960s viruses were identified by their filterability through a Berkfield porous filter, their isolation in laboratory animals or on the membranes, yolk sac or embryo of fertilized chicken eggs, and the ability of the isolated "virus" to produce disease in the original host animal. These constraints obviously restricted the number of feline diseases that could be definitively classified as being of viral etiology.

Early in 1957 a virus of feline origin was isolated in cultures of feline kidney cells.[10] Although the "kidney cell-degenerating virus" was widespread in the cat population and was also nonpathogenic, the isolation of this virus was a landmark in the new technic of virus isolation in cell culture and paved the way not only for subsequent isolation of cytopathogenic feline viruses but also for development of prophylactic vaccines using cell culture technics. A new era in feline virus isolation, identification and feline viral disease prophylaxis had begun. Later in 1957 a feline virus was isolated in cell culture.[11] This virus was subsequently shown to be different from the kidney cell-degenerating virus and also different from panleukopenia virus.

In 1958 a feline herpesvirus was isolated in cell culture and shown to produce a severe upper respiratory disease in cats.[12] The disease produced by this virus was named feline viral rhinotracheitis and has been identified as a worldwide problem of cats.

In 1960 a different feline virus was isolated from the blood and throat of a kitten with a fulminating respiratory infection and it was called the California feline isolate.[13] In the same year other workers isolated a number of antigenically different cytopathogenic viruses from the respiratory tracts of cats with various signs of respiratory disease.[14] These isolates were first classified as picornaviruses and later as caliciviruses on the basis of their electron microscopic appearance or biochemical characteristics. At least 15 serotypes of feline calicivirus have been identified.[15]

A feline reovirus, isolated from a cat in 1970, was shown to produce conjunctivitis, lacrimation and photophobia in susceptible cats.[16] Other workers have demonstrated that the canine parainfluenza virus may rarely cause respiratory disease in cats.[17] Several feline syncytia-forming viruses have been isolated from cats with respiratory infections (as well as from cats suffering from urolithiasis, intestinal diseases and neoplastic conditions.[18] *Mycoplasma* spp have been isolated from the conjunctival sac of cats suffering from conjunctivitis.[19] In 1976 feline infectious peritonitis (FIP) virus was shown to produce pneumonia in cats.[20] It would thus appear that feline respiratory diseases may well resemble, in etiologic complexity, the common cold in people.

Feline infectious peritonitis was first described as a clinical entity in 1963.[21,22] It was subsequently shown to be associated with a feline coronavirus infection, probably an immune-mediated response to a coronavirus infection.[23,24] It was recently demonstrated that there are at least 2 (and likely more) pathogenically distinct feline coronaviruses.[25,26] The FIP virus, an obvious misnomer, has been associated with pneumonia, effusive pleuritis, meningoencephalitis, hepatitis and a variety of other organ and tissue involvements, as well as the supposedly more characteristic effusive peritonitis.[20]

In 1964 a feline oncovirus (retrovirus) was shown to cause many of the syndromes associated with the feline leukemia complex.[27]

A feline viral encephalopathy has been described;[28] however, neither disease signs nor the virus has been well characterized. The herpesvirus of feline viral rhinotracheitis rarely produces signs of generalized encephalitis in immunologically suppressed, aged or very ill cats.[29]

A feline calicivirus (designated the Manx calicivirus), as well as a cell-associated herpesvirus, has been associated with the feline urologic syndrome (FUS).[30,31] A feline syncytia-forming virus also has been isolated from the urine of cats with cystitis but does not appear to be involved in the etiology of FUS.[32]

A rotavirus that causes diarrhea in young kittens was isolated in 1979.[94] Serologic surveys indicate it is widespread in the cat population.

In addition to the diseases mentioned, cats may carry Newcastle disease virus as well as the familiar, if etiologically questionable, agent of cat scratch fever.[33,34]

Virus Classification

Classification of viruses on the basis of tissue affinities is no longer valid or acceptable. Most feline viruses, as well as other animal viruses, have been classified on the basis of their immutable characteristics. In describing the clinical problems associated with various virus diseases, however, it seems somewhat less confusing to separate the diseases affecting the respiratory system from those affecting the nervous system and the body generally (panleukopenia, FIP, FeLV infection). That approach is used in this chapter.

The prevalence of many of the feline viral diseases, particularly the respiratory viral diseases, FIP and FeLV infection, has seemingly increased over the last decade. These diseases may be spread by direct or indirect contact among cats. Obviously the close contact between cats (overcrowding) in some catteries, animal shelters and veterinary hospitals increases the possibility of direct exposure of susceptible cats to infected cats. This increase in the incidence of infection in catteries has perhaps been most effectively demonstrated in the case of FeLV infection. The incidence of FeLV infection in cattery cats known to have been exposed to FeLV is 300 times greater than the incidence of FeLV infection in cats in the general population whose exposure to FeLV is unknown.[35] The possibility of indirect contact, via infected food or such fomites as contaminated bedding or grooming supplies or by persons handling an infected cat and then a susceptible cat, also increases in direct proportion to the degree of overcrowding and in inverse proportion to the sanitary standards maintained in the establishment.

Prevention of Viral Diseases

The obvious and most effective method to prevent any infectious disease is to prevent exposure to the cause of that disease. When it is impossible to absolutely prevent exposure of a cat to a given agent, such as admittance of a completely susceptible kitten into a pet shop, animal shelter or veterinary hospital, the degree of exposure can be reduced by minimizing the extent of direct and indirect contact with infected cats. This requires a scrupulous attention to sanitation and effective husbandry practices, including separation of cats, sterilization of food

Table 1. Feline Biologics

Disease	Product	Route of Administration*	Age to Start Vaccination**	Revaccination
Panleukopenia (FPL)	(1) Antiserum (feline normal serum)	SC	(Used for temporary protection only)	
	(2) Inactivated vaccine, tissue culture origin (TCO) (may be combined with FVR,FCV)	SC or IM	8 weeks	Annual
	(3) Modified live Virus (MLV) TCO (may be combined with FVR,FCV)	SC or IM	8 weeks	Annual
	(4) MLV,TCO (combined with FVR,FCV)	IN	8 weeks	Annual
Feline Viral Rhinotracheitis (FVR)	(1) Inactivated vaccine (often combined with FCV,FPL)	IM or SC	8 weeks or earlier	Annual
	(2) MLV,TCO (often combined with FCV,FPL)	IM or SC	8 weeks or earlier	Annual
	(3) MLV, TCO (usually combined with FCV and may be combined with FPL	IN	8 weeks or earlier	Annual
Feline Calicivirus Infection (FCV)	Usually combined with FVR and may be combined with FPL (see 1,2,3 and FVR)	IM, SC or IN (depending on type of vaccine)	8 weeks or earlier	Annual
Pneumonitis (chlamydial infection)	Attenuated *Chlamydia* of Chick embryo origin (CEO) (may be combined with FVR,FCV vaccines)	SC or IM	8 weeks	Annual
Rabies	See Table 2	IM only	12 weeks	Annual

* SC, subcutaneous; IM, intramuscular; IN, intranasal

** General recommendation only; specific recommendations are found in the text of this chapter

and water containers and grooming supplies between uses, and thorough washing and a change of outer protective clothing by the personnel involved after handling a potentially infected cat.

The best virucidal product against the common feline viruses for routine disinfection of cages, floors, walls, counters, food and water dishes, and other surfaces in animal facilities is a 0.175% solution of sodium hypochlorite (Clorox:Clorox Co).[36] A 1:32 dilution of Clorox (5.6% sodium hypochlorite) in water produces a 0.175% solution of sodium hypochlorite. To mask the odor of sodium hypochlorite and to increase the detergent activity of the cleaning solution, Clorox can be combined with other detergents without the loss of its antiviral activity.

In the circumstances described above, when it is difficult or impossible to prevent potential exposure of a susceptible cat to a disease agent, the adverse effects of such an exposure can often be mitigated by intelligent use of biologics (Table 1). Use of vaccines does not decrease the need for adequate sanitation and husbandry practices, and the avoidance of overcrowding. Proper attention to these factors decreases the degree of virus exposure, increases the interval between entry of the cat into the facility and exposure to infection, and may allow sufficient time for the vaccine to provide protection.

Viral Respiratory Infections

Feline viral rhinotracheitis (FVR) appears to be responsible for 40-45% of the upper respiratory infections in cats. Caliciviruses are possibly responsible for another 40-45%. The herpesvirus of FVR and various caliciviruses may exist together in a large number of cases of upper respiratory infections. The remaining 10-20% of respiratory infections may be caused by *Chlamydia psittaci*, reovirus, feline syncytia-forming viruses, parainfluenza virus, *Mycoplasma*, or bacteria acting alone or in various combinations.

Terms such as "coryza," "chronic feline respiratory disease," "influenza" and "feline distemper" have been used to describe upper respiratory infections in cats. Use of these terms, particularly feline distemper, must be discouraged because of the confusion such terminology causes to cat owners and veterinarians alike.

In the following discussion, 2 etiologically, clinically and pathologically distinct entities, feline viral rhinotracheitis and feline calicivirus infections, are described in detail. The other entities mentioned above, such as pneumonitis and reovirus infection, are not discussed in detail. Readers interested in these infections are referred to the literature cited in the introduction to this chapter.

Feline Viral Rhinotracheitis

Feline viral rhinotracheitis is a highly contagious disease characterized by sudden onset of conjunctivitis, lacrimation and nasal discharge accompanied by sneezing. The disease was first described in 1958.[12] In a comparatively short period, the identity of the virus was confirmed in widely scattered areas of the US and elsewhere in the world.

Properties of the Virus: The FVR virus has the characteristics of a herpesvirus.[37] It is an enveloped DNA virus of cubic symmetry. The organism is most stable at a pH between 6 and 7, at which it remains infective for 5 months. It tolerates a pH of 5-8 for as long as a month, however. It is heat labile and sensitive to both ether and chloroform. It is readily destroyed by many commonly used commercial disinfectants when these are diluted as recommended by the manufacturer.[36]

This organism grows readily in feline kidney cells and other feline cell cultures, and has a pronounced cytopathic effect. It produces nuclear inclusion bodies in infected cells and forms plaques in cultures.

Epizootiology: Feline viral rhinotracheitis can be a serious problem in exotic as well as domestic cats.[38] Although it appears that all Felidae are susceptible to FVR, the virus is not pathogenic for laboratory animals or fertile eggs, and grows poorly in cells from other animals. The organism has been isolated from ocular and nasal discharges, the tonsils and throat of ill cats and apparently healthy ones. It has also been isolated from the lungs of cats that died of the disease. The virus apparently multiplies predominantly in the upper respiratory tract of cats with signs of the disease and persists for some time after clinical recovery.

The infection can be transmitted by nasal instillation and nebulization of tissue culture fluids containing the virus. Parenteral injection of virus-containing media has not produced signs of disease.

Natural transmission occurs when infected cats sneeze and spray virus-containing secretions. Because of the repeated sneezing that occurs early in the disease, rapid transmission occurs when cats are closely confined.

As the virus remains active for a time at room temperature, fomites as well as persons handling an infected cat can easily be involved in the spread of FVR. In areas where cats are concentrated, such as catteries, animal shelters and veterinary hospitals, even though the cats may be individually caged, indirect contact by animal handlers is considered the most common means of transmission of FVR.

The morbidity of FVR is high, especially in young kittens and debilitated adults; in young kittens, it approaches 100%. Because the virus persists for a time in seemingly recovered cats, secondary attacks, with varying clinical signs, may occur suddenly with no history of contact, especially in stressed animals. During such a secondary attack, the virus reappears in the saliva, nasal secretions and excretions, allowing transmission to other cats.

Clinical Course: The incubation period after intranasal instillation of the virus ranges from 2 to 4 days, depending on the amount of virus inoculated. Under natural conditions, the incubation period is 2-10 days and seemingly dependent upon the degree of virus exposure.

The course and severity of FVR are extremely variable, which has led to attempts to separate one syndrome into a number of clinical entities. The duration of mild illness in older cats may vary from 5 to 10 days, and might be called coryza or pneumonitis. In severe cases, the cat may be visibly ill for 3-6 weeks. Death is often due to various complications;, and may occur 16-30 days or more after the first signs of illness. Such cases are frequently diagnosed as influenza or chronic respiratory disease.

Figure 1 lists the predominant signs and the course of FVR in 3 kittens infected by nasal instillation of the virus. These kittens were the same age (4 months) and weight, and in the same general condition at the time of exposure. All were housed and fed in exactly the same

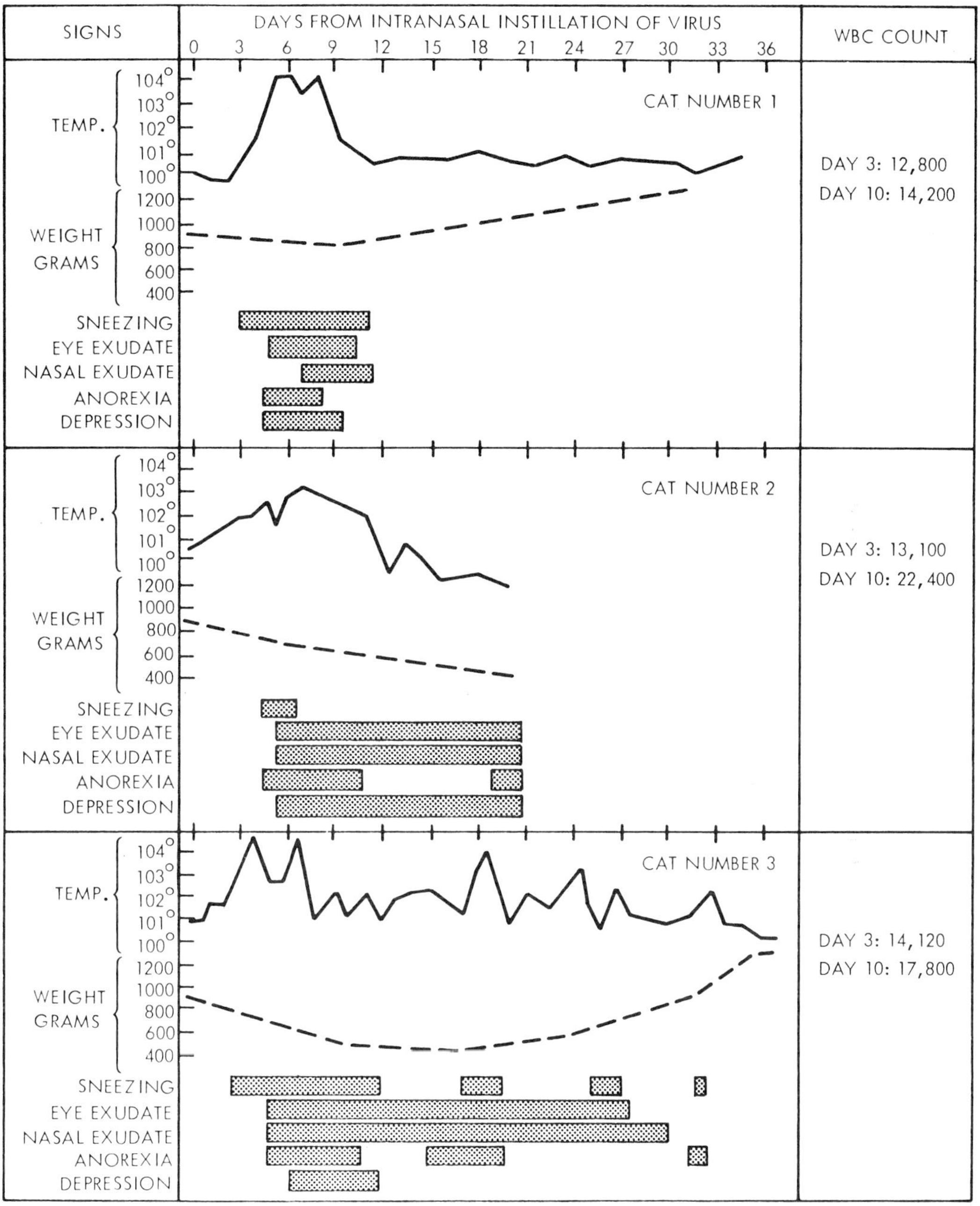

Fig 1. Characteristics of experimentally induced feline viral rhinotracheitis.

manner before and during the course of the experiment. The variety of clinical expressions of this disease is dramatically illustrated.

Clinical Signs: The onset of FVR is marked by fever, sneezing and depression (Fig 2). The fever may reach 40.6 C (105 F) and tends to fluctuate from normal to 39.4-40.0 C (103-104 F) for several days or even weeks. Profuse serous ocular and nasal discharges are accompanied by paroxysms of sneezing. The disease may be first recognized in a cattery by the constant violent sneezing that occurs when 6-10 infected cats are together. Movement or excitement seems to increase the sneezing during early stages of the

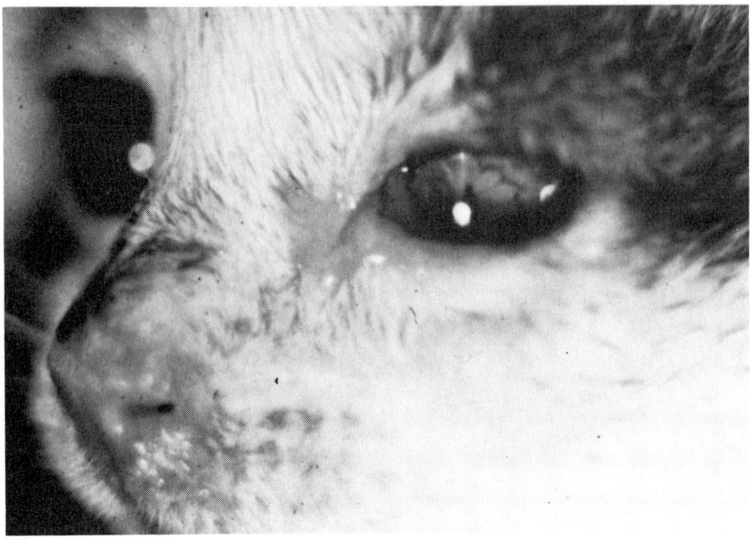

Fig 2. Early signs of feline viral rhinotracheitis include copious serous nasal and ocular discharges.

disease, resulting in rapid dispersal of the virus to nearby cats.

The serous discharges become mucopurulent within 2-3 days and tend to plug the nares and paste the eyelids together (Fig 3). Affected cats wipe their faces with their forepaws, soiling the skin and hair (Fig 4). This is especially noticeable in light-colored cats. The profuse nasal discharges cause dyspnea characterized by mouth breathing.

Anorexia and depression are pronounced by the third to fifth day of the illness. Weight loss is obvious if clinical signs persist 3 weeks or longer.

Although ulcerative lesions on the dorsal and lateral surface of the tongue may result from FVR infection, most of these lesions are a result of calicivirus infection. When ulcerative glossitis occurs in cats with the ocular and nasal signs of FVR, dual infection with herpesvirus and calicivirus should be considered.

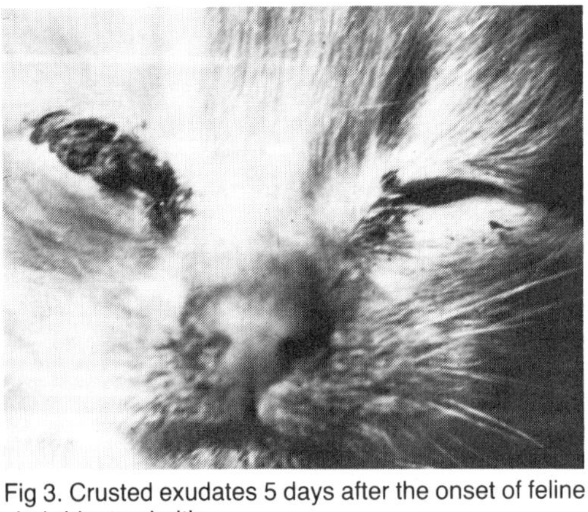

Fig 3. Crusted exudates 5 days after the onset of feline viral rhinotracheitis.

The severe purulent conjunctivitis often seen in kittens 10-14 days old, when the eyes are opening, may be a clinical manifestation of FVR acquired from the queen. This condition is often referred to as conjunctivitis neonatorum, and may also result from bacterial infections or infection with other respiratory viruses. Because the cornea at this age is soft, such complications as keratoconus, keratoglobus, other corneal deformities or even panophthalmitis may develop if the infection is untreated.

Feline herpesvirus produces superficial ulceration of the corneal epithelium in some infected cats.[39] The herpesvirus of FVR is the only one of the feline upper respiratory viruses that produces corneal ulceration.

Feline herpesvirus can infect the female genital tract. Kittens born to queens infected in the last trimester of pregnancy may suffer congenital infections. Abortion has occurred after IV or intranasal inoculation of feline herpesvirus in pregnant queens during the sixth week of gestation.[40] Abortion has also occurred in cats naturally infected with FVR.

Severe infections occur most frequently in young cats 3-18 months of age. A seemingly mild infection in an older cat may produce no fever or only a moderate temperature rise, discharges that tend to crust at the ocular canthi and edge of the nostrils, and slight sneezing.

Persistent frontal sinusitis is an occasional sequela to FVR. Affected cats have a unilateral or bilateral, rather tenacious nasal discharge. Sneezing tends to dislodge chunks and strands of thick mucus that may be accompanied by blood (Fig 5). Chronic conjunctivitis is evident and respiratory difficulty may be reflected by mouth breathing. The sinusitis seemingly lasts forever if untreated.

Empyema (necrotic or purulent pleuritis) has been considered a possible sequela to FVR. Although empyema may be associated with FIP or bacterial infections, there is no evidence to implicate FVR in the etiology of empyema.

Generalized encephalitis has been observed in cats with FVR.[29] Idiopathic vestibular neuropathy has rarely been associated with a previous or concurrent FVR infection; in most cases such an association is lacking.[41]

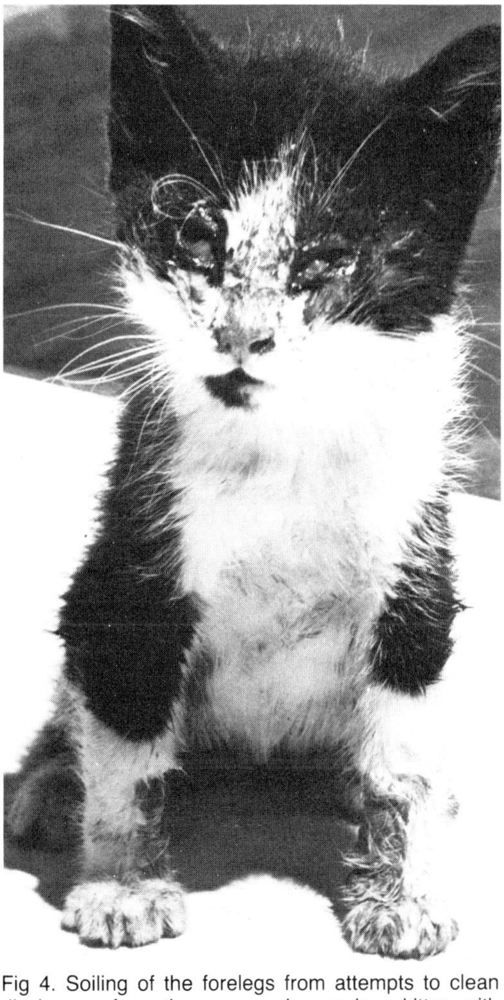

Fig 4. Soiling of the forelegs from attempts to clean discharges from the eyes and nose in a kitten with feline viral rhinotracheitis.

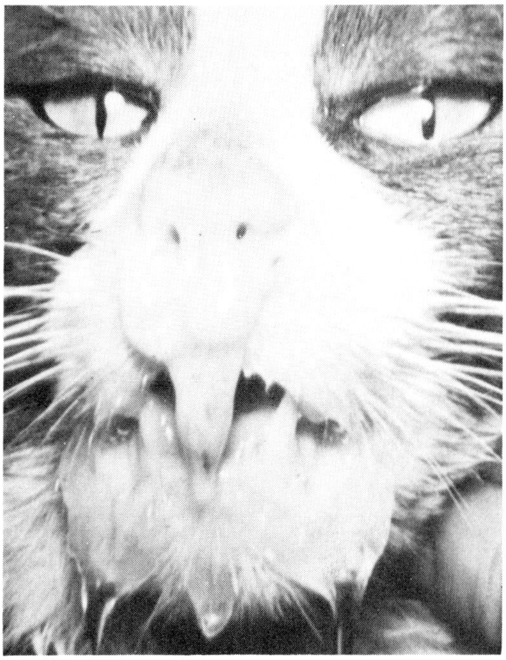

Fig 5. Persistent nasal discharge indicates possible frontal sinusitis following apparent recovery from feline viral rhinotracheitis.

Lesions: The carcass of a cat that has died from FVR is emaciated and dehydrated. Purulent nasal and ocular crusts are common. The most significant gross lesions are found in the nasal passages and turbinates, where there is focal necrosis and a mucoid or mucopurulent exudate. The larynx and pharynx may be mildly inflamed, and the tonsils somewhat enlarged and petechiated. The cervical lymph nodes may be slightly enlarged and congested, and in advanced cases the mediastinal and bronchial nodes appear congested. The lungs may be congested, with small areas of consolidation; usually the pulmonary lesions are unremarkable. In fact, one is more impressed by the lack of severe changes in the lungs.

The characteristic histopathologic feature of rhinotracheitis is the intranuclear inclusion body in epithelial cells of the nasal septum, tonsils, epiglottis, trachea and nictitating membranes. The well-formed inclusions are acidophilic and occupy a third to half of the nuclear space. There is a clear halo around the inclusion and the nuclear membrane tends to remain intact. The inclusion bodies form early in the course of the disease and tend to be most numerous about the second to fourth day of illness; some persist for 2-3 weeks. They may be difficult to find in cats that die after being ill for 3-4 weeks. The epithelial surfaces of infected tissues often are ulcerated and necrotic, with infiltration of neutrophils and lymphocytes. Actual resorption of portions of the turbinate bone may be observed microscopically.

The liver may have no glycogen; areas of cloudy swelling and other evidence suggesting chronic illness may be observed.

Diagnosis: The hemogram may be useful in differential diagnosis of FVR because leukopenia, an expected finding in viral diseases, does not occur during the course of FVR. In fact, the total WBC count often ranges from 30,000 to 40,000 cells/mm^3 and counts of 50,000 cells/mm^3 may occur. The greatest increase occurs in the polymorphonuclear series. The RBC count is not altered in the early stages of FVR. Because of inappetence and weight loss, anemia with a reduced Hb value, PCV and RBC count may be observed after prolonged illness.

A clinical diagnosis of FVR is based on the typical signs, especially the pronounced paroxysmal sneezing and nasal and ocular discharges without signs of pneumonia. Other diseases of the lungs, such as bacterial or verminous pneumonia, so-called feline asthma and space-occupying lesions of the thorax, are differentiated from FVR by their lack of profuse nasal and ocular discharges or other signs of upper respiratory involvement. The patient with lower respiratory disease tends to cough rather than sneeze. In some cases, thoracic radiographs are important in differentiation.

A definitive diagnosis of FVR is based on the typical clinical signs combined with isolation of herpesvirus from pharyngeal swabs taken from the affected cat. Since many cats carry herpesvirus, a positive virus isolation from an asymptomatic cat or a cat with signs not usually associated with FVR is of no significance. Conversely, the inability to isolate herpesvirus from a single swab of the pharynx of a cat with signs of FVR does not mean the cat does not have FVR. These factors, plus the cost and time involved before results can be reported, generally contraindicate use of virus isolation technics except for investigative epizootiology.

Clinical judgment is essential not only in the diagnosis of FVR but also in assessment of the role of herpesvirus infection in the case in question. The significant questions involve determining if FVR is the primary problem or is secondary to immunosuppressive diseases, such as FeLV infection, FIP, toxoplasmosis, prolonged stress or similar problems.

Treatment: Affected cats may be presented for treatment relatively early in the course of the disease. The owners notice sneezing, depression, anorexia, and perhaps conjunctivitis and nasal discharge. Because at this stage it is impossible to foresee the course of the disease, it is prudent to avoid giving a definite prognosis.

When possible, a kitten or cat suffering from an upper respiratory infection should be treated as an outpatient because the patient may be psychologically as well as physically stressed in the unfamiliar surroundings of a hospital. Dedicated nursing care is essential for rapid recovery. Spread of respiratory infections in the hospital is obviously reduced by treating infected cats at home.

Some exceptions to the outpatient treatment of cats with FVR are unavoidable. The owner may be unable to provide the needed care (rehydration, orogastric intubation, etc) for cats with severe, prolonged respiratory disease. Whether a patient should be hospitalized must be decided on an individual case basis by the owner and veterinarian.

Panleukopenia and FVR can occur concurrently, and the signs of rhinotracheitis may mask those of panleukopenia (Fig 6). If there is any doubt about the diagnosis, total and differential WBC counts should be made immediately. If the total count is low, with severe depletion of granulocytes, treatment for panleukopenia is essential if satisfactory results are to be obtained. If the cat does not have panleukopenia but is considered susceptible, administration of a vaccine is essential.

Regardless of where the patient is treated, it should be kept in clean, warm, well-ventilated and lighted quarters. The cat should be encouraged to eat by offering a variety of foods.

Strongly flavored or odoriferous foods may be preferred by cats whose sense of smell (and taste) may be blocked by profuse nasal discharges. Sardines, ham, smoked turkey, chicken or similar odoriferous products should be offered. Strained baby food meats may be highly palatable to anorectic cats.

Although there is no specific medication for FVR, broad-spectrum antibiotics are indicated. They can be given by injection or orally to hos-

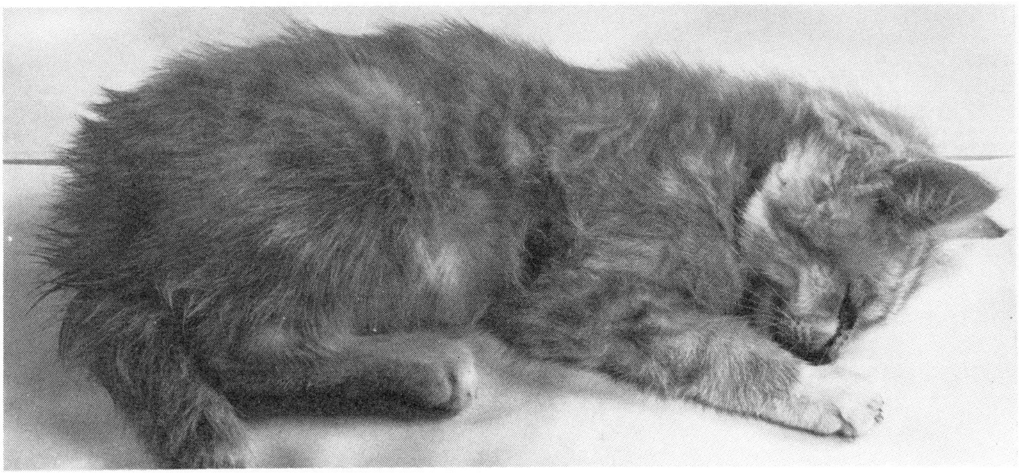

Fig 6. Cat with concurrent panleukopenia and feline viral rhinotracheitis. Note the crusted ocular discharge.

pitalized cats or as oral suspensions or tablets if the patient is treated at home. Chloramphenicol, cephaloridine, amoxicillin, ampicillin, gentamicin or similar antibiotics may be useful for this purpose. Use of tetracyclines is not recommended for pregnant or young cats since these drugs may cause a yellow to brownish discoloration of the enamel of developing teeth. If given over a protracted period, tetracyclines may cause anorexia in some cats. Neither cephaloridine nor gentamicin should be used for more than 5-7 successive days without a thorough reassessment of the patient. Use of chloramphenicol is contraindicated in anemic cats. Like the tetracyclines, chloramphenicol may cause anorexia in some cats if used for a prolonged period. It must be emphasized that secondary bacterial invaders do not play a significant role in the pathogenesis of FVR.[40] Mycoplasmal and chlamydial infections may produce signs similar to or indistinguishable from those of mild FVR; these agents are susceptible to broad-spectrum antibiotic therapy.

Antihistamines, such as chlorpheniramine maleate, may have some benefit in drying nasal secretions early in the course of FVR. Improvement is apparent within 24 to 48 hours if antihistamines are beneficial; their use should not be continued for more than 4-5 days. Corticosteroids may also aid in relieving nasal or conjunctival congestion and may stimulate the appetite. They also lower resistance to infection, however, and must be used cautiously and concurrently with broad-spectrum antibiotics if used at all.

The need for supportive medication is apparent when patients exhibit severe signs. Nasal discharges that occlude the nares must be removed frequently to ease breathing, and the surrounding skin covered with a protective salve, such as petroleum jelly. Instilling 1-2 drops of a mild decongestant twice daily reduces the amount of nasal discharge. Excessive use of decongestants can dry and irritate the mucous membranes. Phenylephrine 0.25% (Neo-Synephrine:Winthrop) or a 10-20% dimethyl sulfoxide solution in water (Domoso:Diamond) are acceptable decongestant nose drops for cats. Keeping the nasal passages clear tends to speed return of the patient's interest in food, particularly for odoriferous foods.

Vaporization with steam or nebulization with mucolytic agents, such as acetylcysteine (Mucomyst:Mead Johnson) may be beneficial when nasal discharges are profuse and tend to dry and occlude the nasal passages. A 5-10% solution of glycerine in 95% ethanol can be used for nebulization in lieu of using commercial mucolytic agents. Antibiotics may be added to the solutions to be nebulized; however, the usefulness of this has not been documented. A small closed chamber, a DeVilbis 40 nebulizer and a small motorized vacuum pump are ideal equipment for nebulization (Fig 7). Cats with extremely stubborn cases of FVR benefit from nebulization of feline normal serum. Nebulization for 20-30 minutes

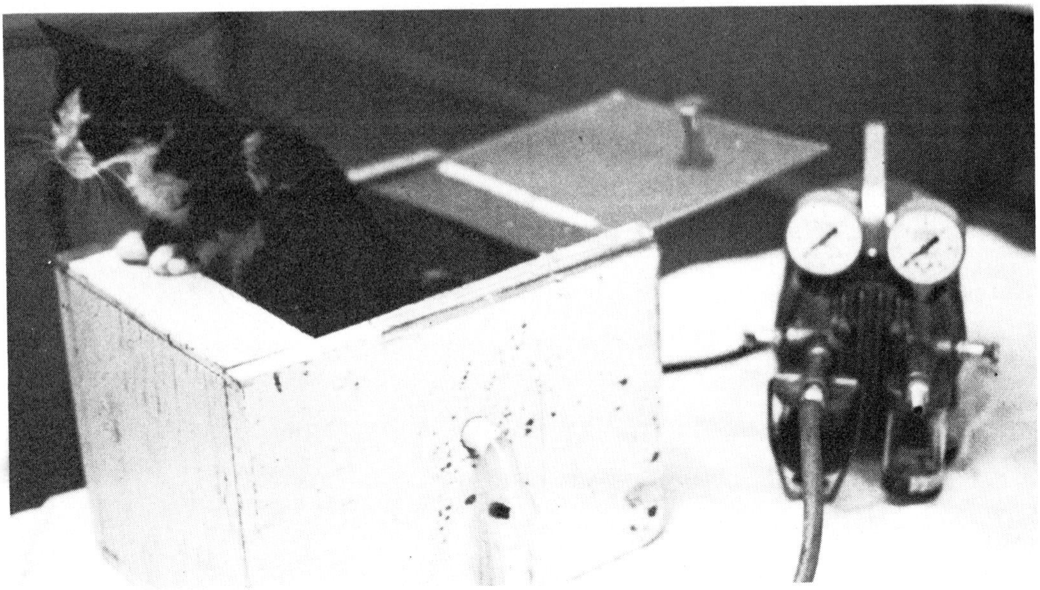

Fig 7. Simple nebulization apparatus for use in cats with respiratory disease.

twice daily is recommended. Dyspneic cats may benefit from O_2 therapy given for several days.

Ocular discharges should also be removed frequently and bland ophthalmic ointments, containing antibiotics if desired, applied as often as 5-6 times daily. Cauterization with 2% tincture of iodine may be helpful in the treatment of the infrequent herpesvirus keratitis (see Chapter 17). The effect is obtained by chemically removing the infected epithelium. Debridement may be followed by the topical administration of idoxuridine drops or ointment (Stoxil:SKF, Herplex:Allergan) or adenine arabinoside (Vira A:Parke-Davis). Antibiotic ophthalmic ointments, such as tetracycline or chloramphenicol, may be used concurrently with antiherpetic ophthalmic preparations. In stubborn cases, antiherpetics may be combined with a corticosteroid; however, use of corticosteroid ophthalmic preparations should be a avoided in FVR-induced conjunctivitis and keratitis if possible. The antiherpetics are indicated only in proven herpesvirus infections since they have no benefit in bacterial or fungal infections of the cornea.[39]

Intravenous fluids are used to correct dehydration and electrolyte imbalances that often occur after prolonged illness. A balanced electrolyte solution, such as lactated Ringer's solution or 2½% dextrose in half-strength lactated Ringer's, may be used. Supportive fluids should be administered IV but may be given SC, at no more than 50 ml per site, if care is taken to prevent laking and subsequent irritation. Supplemental vitamin B-complex should be given with parenteral fluids.

Fluids alone do not provide sufficient support nor prevent the weight loss that occurs in protracted cases. Feeding through a stomach tube is indicated in these cases. Passing the tube is relatively easy, and the results are well worth the additional effort. If it is apparent that repeated and prolonged feeding through a tube is necessary, performing a pharyngotomy to pass the stomach tube should be considered. The technic is not difficult and there is no discomfort to the patient while the tube is in place.[42]

Oral or IV administration of 250-1000 mg ascorbic acid daily has been recommended by some clinicians.[43] Although it may seemingly shorten the course of FVR, vitamin C is not a specific treatment.

There is no need for special treatment for the ulcerative glossitis that may accompany FVR or combined herpesvirus-calicivirus upper respiratory infections. This condition tends to be self-limiting and healing usually is rapid once the patient's general condition improves. Chronic ulcerative glossitis, a seemingly permanent lingual ulcer, rarely follows prolonged upper respiratory infection. Cats so affected usually prefer soft (canned) rather than dry food and frequently do not groom themselves. Recurrent bouts of excess salivation associated with a foul odor to the mouth may require a thorough cleaning of the teeth followed by antiseptic mouth washes for a few days.

If it follows FVR, frontal sinusitis may be treated conservatively using antibiotics, decongestive nasal drops and nebulization as previously described. Failing response to such treatment, the frontal sinuses may be trephined and flushed for several days postoperatively with antibiotics and proteolytic enzymes. Autogenous fat implantation in the frontal sinuses has also been described as a successful method of treating sinusitis secondary to viral respiratory disease.[44]

The veterinarian should warn owners of recovered cats that the immunity may persist for only a few months and that the cat may shed the virus for at least 2 years after recovery.[45] Other cats in the household should be vaccinated, as well as the recovered cat. Repeated (every 1-3 months) intranasal vaccination of all cats in FVR-infected catteries may eliminate that infection.

Prevention: As indicated earlier, the most effective prophylaxis against feline respiratory disease is to avoid exposure of susceptible cats to the various infectious agents. Although this may be accomplished by physical separation of cats and scrupulous sanitation, it is nearly impossible to avoid exposure in most catteries, pet shops, animal shelters and veterinary hospitals. Cats that have recovered from FVR may shed herpesvirus intermittently for at least 2 years and probably longer.[45] Stress may reactivate signs of the disease and increase the amount of virus shed; therefore, a carrier cat in apparently good health entering a veterinary hospital for elective surgery is a potential source of infection to all cats in the hospital. By maintaining scrupulous sanitation and physically separating cats in the hospital, it may be possible to delay exposure of a newly admitted, susceptible kitten or cat until it has had a chance to develop resistance following vaccination.

Parenteral and intranasal forms of FVR vaccination are available. An attenuated (modified-live virus) or inactivated (killed) form of the parenteral vaccine usually is combined with a calicivirus vaccine of broad antigenicity and may be combined with an attentuated or inactivated panleukopenia vaccine. It is generally recommended that these vaccines by given IM. Cats of any age may be vaccinated with 2 doses given 3-4 weeks apart. If the vaccinated kitten is less than 12 weeks of age, it should be revaccinated at 3- to 4-week intervals until it is 12-16 weeks of age. Annual revaccination with a single dose is recommended. The vaccine is safe when administered parenterally; however, the attenuated herpesvirus in vaccines prepared for parenteral administration produces signs of FVR if given intranasally to susceptible kittens. Inactivated herpesvirus vaccine is ineffective if given intranasally.

When administered parenterally, these vaccines produce a humoral antibody response. In susceptible kittens, an increased resistance to intranasal challenge with virulent virus (exposure) appears 2-3 weeks after the second dose of vaccine. The protection afforded by the parenterally administered vaccines is less than perfect. A successfully vaccinated cat, upon intranasal challenge or exposure to virulent virus, becomes infected, sheds the challenge virus and may have mild to moderate signs of rhinotracheitis.[45,46] Parenterally administered vaccines have the advantage of being quite safe and usually not producing reactions. Disadvantages include delay in onset of resistance after vaccination and the fact that a successfully vaccinated cat may be infected upon exposure and may have mild to moderate signs of disease. It should be noted that 50-80% of cats presented for vaccination may have been previously exposed to FVR and may have an increased humoral antibody titer and a degree of resistance as a result of that exposure. A single dose of FVR vaccine administered parenterally may produce an anamnestic response and act as a "booster" vaccination.

The intranasal vaccines are attenuated virus vaccines. As in the case of parenteral vaccines, intranasal vaccines usually are combined with a calicivirus of broad antigenicity and may be combined with an attenuated panleukopenia vaccine. One drop of the reconstituted vaccine should be placed in each eye and the remaining vaccine be placed upon the nostrils (Fig 8). One dose of vaccine is protective to cats over 12 weeks of age. In catteries with infected cats, intranasal vaccine has been used on kittens as young as 2-5 weeks and repeated at 3-week intervals until the kittens are 12-14 weeks of age. Annual revaccination is recommended.

Sneezing may be observed 5-9 days after intranasal vaccination. Mucoid ocular and nasal discharges have been observed rarely.[47,48] The calicivirus component of the vaccine may rarely produce small, transient erosions on the nose,

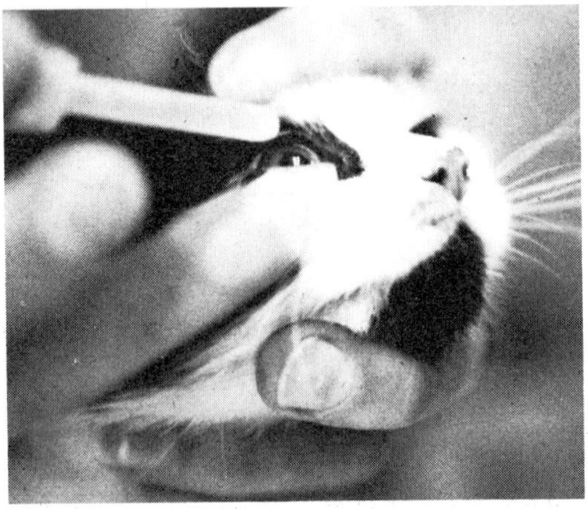

Fig 8. Use of an intranasal rhinotracheitis-calicivirus vaccine. One drop is placed in each conjunctival sac and several drops in each nostril as the cat inhales.

or lingual ulcers 8 days after vaccination.[47,48] The reactions to the intranasal vaccine usually are transient, rarely severe and usually self-limiting; however, they can be annoying to the owner.

The modified FVR virus in the intranasal vaccine may be shed by the vaccinated cat for up to 16 days after vaccination and may spread to susceptible cats closely associated with the vaccinate and produce the same transient sneezing response.[47] The calicivirus in a combined intranasal vaccine may be shed for 3-83 days postvaccination.[47] Challenge of intranasally vaccinated cats with virulent FVR virus 11 weeks after vaccination demonstrated complete protection, with no disease signs observed. In only 2 of 8 vaccinates was infection with the challenge virus demonstrated. Vaccinated cats shed the challenge virus for only 1-4 days; in contrast, unvaccinated controls shed the challenge virus for 5-8 days and again 154 days later when "stressed" by corticosteroid administration.[47]

Intranasal vaccination seems to provide immediate protection of the vaccinates against exposure to virulent FVR; 48 hours after vaccination, cats are protected against exposure to virulent calicivirus.[49] Since 7 days are required for an intranasally vaccinated cat to develop serum antibodies against FVR (14 days after parenteral vaccination), it would appear that intranasal vaccination stimulates a localized as well as a systemic humoral immune response.[50] Intranasally administered respiratory disease vaccines have the advantage of rapid onset of resistance in the vaccinates, relatively solid resistance to infection, and solid resistance to disease after vaccination. In addition, in cats over 12 weeks of age, only one initial vaccination is required, followed by yearly revaccination.

The choice of vaccines is ultimately a decision that must be made by cat owners and their veterinarians; however, it seems reasonable to suggest the use of intranasal vaccines in cats with no history of previous FVR vaccination or exposure and entering an area of potentially high risk of exposure, such as animal shelters, pet shops or veterinary hospitals. In individually owned pets and in kittens from catteries without infected cats, where immediate exposure to FVR or calicivirus infection is unlikely, either form of vaccination could be used.

Other Systemic Manifestations of Herpesvirus Infection

Increased neonatal mortality, abortions, stillbirths, fetal resorption and lowered breeding efficacy have been noted in catteries chronically infected with FVR. The herpesviruses of people, cattle, horses and dogs seem to have a predilection for both respiratory and genital tracts, and cause generalized infections of the young. Pregnant female cats inoculated intranasally with FVR virus aborted 7-14 days postinfection and the virus was isolated from the vaginas of the queens but not from the placentas.[40] Although the feline herpesvirus of FVR may be involved in genital infections and abortions, further intensive investigations are necessary to clearly demonstrate the role of the virus.

The FVR herpesvirus was isolated from moist skin ulcerations widely distributed over the body from head to tail and on the tongue and hard palate of 3 cats.[51] Two of these cats had other systemic signs suggestive of FVR, while the third had no signs other than the skin ulceration. The ulcers in one cat responded to local antiviral therapy. It seems probable that the herpesvirus infection of the skin was secondary, originating from oral secretions and transmitted by licking.

Herpesvirus encephalitis seems to be a rare sequela to FVR.[29,41] Herpesvirus encephalitis occurs in other species and further investigation into this aspect of systemic herpesvirus infections in cats is warranted.

A second feline herpesvirus, a cell-associated herpesvirus antigenically distinct from FVR, has been isolated and characterized.[31] This virus seems to be involved in FUS. The so-called "Manx calicivirus" and perhaps a feline syncytia-forming virus have also been associated with this problem.[30,32] This syndrome is discussed in detail in Chapter 12.

Feline Calicivirus Infection

Feline calicivirus infections occur among cats in about the same frequency as FVR. Numerous strains of feline calicivirus have been isolated from cats in the US and worldwide.[52]

The signs of illness produced by calicivirus infections in the cat vary markedly, depending on the strain involved, the severity of the exposure and the resistance of the host. Some strains apparently cause little or no signs of illness. Strains of low virulence produce no or only moderate pyrexia but do produce ulcers of the tongue, hard palate and nose. Strains of high virulence produce pyrexia, anorexia, depression, dyspnea or polypnea and frequently death. Ulcers of the tongue, hard palate and nose may, but do not always, occur in addition to pneumonic signs produced by the strains of high virulence.[53] A strain of the virus has also been implicated to some extent in causation of the urethritis-cystitis complex.[30]

Properties of the Virus: The feline caliciviruses contain RNA and do not produce inclusions. They are resistant to ether and chloroform, and are stable at a pH of 4. The number of virus particles drops markedly at a pH of 2-3. They are inactivated at 50 C in 30 minutes but can survive at −65 C for at least 4 years. They withstand lyophilization well.

Although FVR virus becomes inactivated by desiccation in less than 24 hours at room temperature, feline caliciviruses are much less sensitive to environmental factors and may still be infective after 10 days at room temperature.

Feline caliciviruses are rapidly inactivated by hypochlorite disinfectants. A 1:32 dilution of Clorox in water is an excellent disinfectant for cages, dishes, and other surfaces.[36]

Feline caliciviruses grow well on many feline cell cultures and have a rapid cytolytic effect that tends to distinguish them from feline herpesvirus, which has a slower cytopathic effect and also produces inclusion bodies in cell cultures. Cell cultures of heterologous species usually do not support replication of feline calicivirus, and the virus does not propagate in embryonating eggs nor in common laboratory animals. Although the virus is relatively easy to isolate from the respiratory passages of infected cats, identification of the specific serotype is time-consuming and expensive.

Since routine virus isolation from a pharyngeal swab does not include serotyping, isolation of a calicivirus from the mouth of a cat gives no indication of the potential pathogenicity of that isolate.

Although numerous serologically distinguishable feline calicivirus strains are recognized, they do have some common antigens. Cats with a demonstrable active immunity to one feline calicivirus strain often are resistant to disease if they are infected by other strains of calicivirus.[54,55] Therefore, a nonvirulent strain of feline calicivirus may be broadly antigenic against many, but perhaps not all, strains of virulent as well as nonvirulent calicivirus. That particular strain would be an excellent strain for use in vaccine production.

Feline calicivirus infection may be a problem in exotic cats as well as domestic cats. However, it does not appear to be as severe a problem as FVR.[38] A calicivirus similar to that causing feline calicivirus infection has been isolated from the tongues of dogs with severe ulcerative glossitis.[56] The significance of that finding is undetermined. Feline calicivirus infection is considered a primary problem of domestic cats.

Epizootiology: Although isolations of feline calicivirus have been made from the spleen, blood, intestine, muscles, kidney, urinary bladder and urine of infected cats, such isolations appear rare. The pathogenicity of this group of viruses generally is limited to the oral mucosa and respiratory tract. Virus isolations are commonly made from the mouth and lungs of infected cats, and less frequently from the tonsils and upper airways. This virus is shed almost continuously into the oropharynx of carrier cats, in contrast to the intermittent shedding of FVR virus by carriers. The calicivirus has been shed from the throat and in the feces of carrier cats for at least a year.[57] Because recovered cats often become carriers, shedding accounts for the persistence of the virus in nature.

Calicivirus is transmitted naturally when infected cats sneeze. Fomites can play an important role in natural transmission. The morbidity tends to be high, and mortality in young kittens with severe signs of pneumonic disease may approach 100%. The mild form of the disease, characterized by lingual ulcers, is seldom fatal.

Clinical Course: The incubation period of feline calicivirus infection is short. Signs may ap-

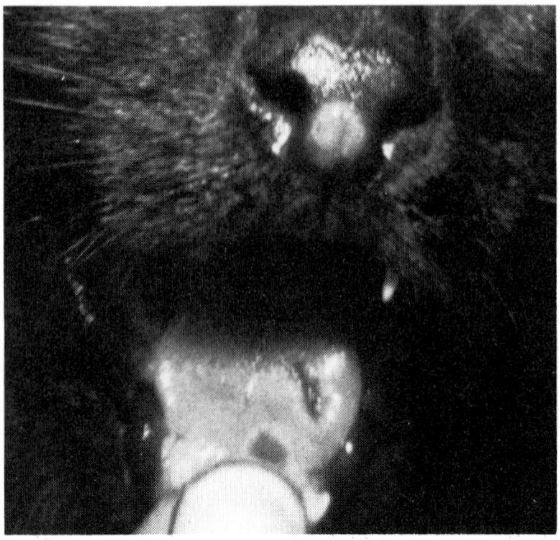

Fig 9. Nasal and glossal ulcers in calicivirus infection.

pear 1-2 days after exposure to the virus. The signs usually persist for only 3-5 days and rarely for 10 days. Death, in the pneumonic form of the disease, usually occurs within 5 days of the onset of signs.

Clinical Signs: Clinical signs may be quite variable, depending upon the strain of calicivirus involved, route of exposure, severity of the exposure and resistance of the exposed cat. Feline caliciviruses generally can be grouped into 3 types, based on their virulence. Unfortunately, there is considerable overlap and the lines of distinction among the 3 groups are not clear. The avirulent caliciviruses produce no clinical signs of infection but lead to seroconversion upon exposure.[58] Caliciviruses of low virulence produce ulcers of the tongue, hard palate and nostrils in exposed cats. Caliciviruses of high virulence produce pneumonic signs, with or without oral and nasal ulcers.

The major clinical features of the highly virulent or pneumonic caliciviruses are fever, anorexia, depression and dyspnea or polypnea. The disease is first manifested as fever (104-105 F) and anorexia. The fever tends to fluctuate after the initial elevation but the temperature tends to remain elevated through the course of the disease. Polypnea or dyspnea appears shortly after the initial fever rise, and moist rales may be ausculated. Depression tends to be marked and, except for the obvious respiratory distress, the patient may appear to be suffering from acute feline panleukopenia. Death occurs within days of the onset of signs. The pure pneumonic form of feline calicivirus infection appears to be most prevalent among neonatal (14-21 days old) and weaned kittens up to 4 months of age. Older susceptible cats exposed to the highly virulent caliciviruses may show initial signs suggestive of exudative pneumonia, which then becomes proliferative and interstitial as the cat recovers. In this age group, oral and nasal ulcers may occur concurrently with the pneumonia.

Signs of infection with caliciviruses of low virulence are confined to the oral cavity and nose. Fever is absent or of low degree and, if it occurs, lasts one day or less. Anorexia occurs only for a day or 2 as the oral ulcers develop. Cats infected with the caliciviruses of low virulence seldom show the marked depression associated with infection by highly virulent caliciviruses. The lingual lesions may begin as vesicles that rupture to produce ulcers on the edge and dorsal surfaces of the rostral part of the tongue (Fig 9). Similar ulcers may be observed on the hard palate and in the area of the nasal portion of the philtrum (Fig 9).

Paroxysmal sneezing, so common in FVR, occurs in only a few cats with feline calicivirus infection. Likewise, the copious serous-to-purulent nasal and ocular discharges so common to FVR occur rarely with calicivirus infection.

Ulcerative keratitis has not been associated with feline calicivirus infection.

Although the clinical signs of infection by a calicivirus of low or high virulence usually are quite characteristic, in some cases sneezing and nasal and ocular discharges may make it impossible to clinically differentiate calicivirus infection from FVR. Cats with respiratory signs may be concurrently infected with the herpesvirus of FVR and a pathogenic calicivirus. Such dual infection is common and has led to much confusion regarding the signs produced by calicivirus infection.

Diagnosis: The diagnosis of feline calicivirus infection is based on the typical clinical signs of oral and occasionally nasal ulcerations, with or without pneumonic signs. In neonatal kittens a rapidly fatal pneumonia with lesions of pulmonary edema is very suggestive of infection by a calicivirus of high virulence.

Transient lymphopenia may occur early in the course of calicivirus infection. The WBC count returns to a normal or high-normal level in a day or so in cats that will recover.

Virus isolation and identification of a calicivirus from lung tissue of a kitten that has died of a severe pneumonic disease is important in establishing the diagnosis of calicivirus infection in a cattery. Isolation of a calicivirus from the mouth of a cat without clinical signs of infection is of less diagnostic significance, since it is impossible to be sure that the virus isolated is a pathogenic calicivirus.

Lesions: Caliciviruses of high virulence produce severe pneumonia. Reddish-purple consolidation of the dependent aspects of the lung occurs early and later becomes diffuse. The lungs appear heavy and wet, and the cut surfaces exude fluid from the bronchioles (Fig 10). Microscopically the changes are those of exudative pneumonia, hemorrhage and pulmonary edema. In cats that ultimately recover, the exudative changes subside and the reactions become proliferative and interstitial.[53]

Ulcers on the tongue, hard palate and nose may be accompanied by mild focal lesions of interstitial pneumonia not severe enough to produce clinical signs.

Inclusion bodies are not seen with calicivirus infection; however, as the intranuclear inclusions associated with FVR are very difficult to demonstrate after the early stages of infection, finding no inclusions does not establish a diagnosis of calicivirus infection, nor eliminate a diagnosis of FVR.

Treatment: Treatment of a cat with oral ulcers associated with calicivirus infection is seldom necessary since these lesions usually resolve in a few days. Supportive therapy, vitamin supplementation and feeding of soft food may be indicated when oral ulcers are accompanied by anorexia of longer duration.

Broad-spectrum antibiotics, supportive care, bronchodilators, and O_2 therapy are indicated in cases of virulent calicivirus infection.

The treatment of combined calicivirus infection and FVR is similar to that for FVR.

Prevention: Most FVR vaccines contain a broadly antigenic feline calicivirus component. Attenuated FVR vaccines contain a nonpathogenic feline calicivirus or one of very low virulence. Feline caliciviruses, like the feline herpesvirus, if given parenterally do not produce any clinical signs of infection. However, like the feline herpesvirus, resistance to challenge after parenteral injection of calicivirus vaccine is slow to develop. A successfully vaccinated cat may become infected and subsequently shed the challenge virus.

Resistance to challenge exposure is apparent within 72 hours after intranasal vaccination with an avirulent feline calicivirus. Occasionally to rarely, small ulcers may develop on the tongue after intranasal vaccination. The intranasally applied vaccine may be shed by the vaccinate for 3-83 days after vaccination.[49]

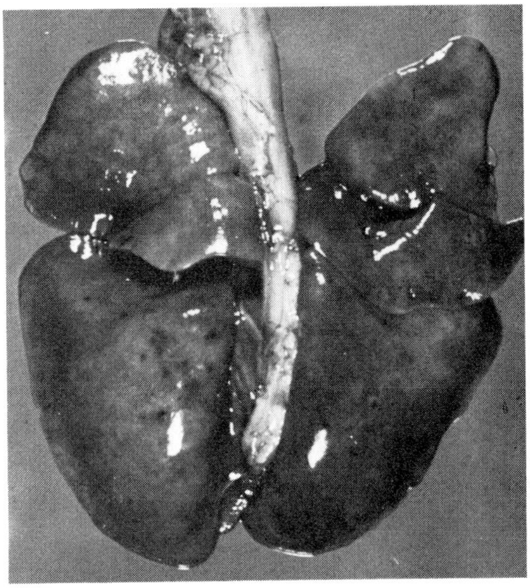

Fig 10. Gross evidence of pulmonary edema associated with fatal calicivirus pneumonia.

The types of calicivirus vaccines available and the recommendations for their use have been described in the section on FVR. Feline caliciviruses are excellent antigens and a vaccinated or previously infected cat develops high levels of systemic humoral antibodies. Kittens from such a queen receive maternal antibodies in the colostrum. Unfortunately, even kittens with high levels of passively transmitted antibodies may develop fatal pneumonic calicivirus infection when their respiratory tract is exposed to a highly virulent feline calicivirus. Apparently such a calicivirus can become well established in the lung before the circulating antibodies have a chance to diffuse to the affected area. In this type of situation, intranasal vaccination may be commenced in kittens as early as 1-2 weeks of age and repeated every 3 weeks in an attempt to provide local as well as systemic resistance. Unfortunately, this approach is not uniformly successful. Prophylaxis is then dependent on avoiding exposure to the virus by sanitation and isolation procedures discussed earlier.

Pneumonitis

Cause: In 1944 a "virus" was isolated from cats with signs of respiratory infection.[7] The

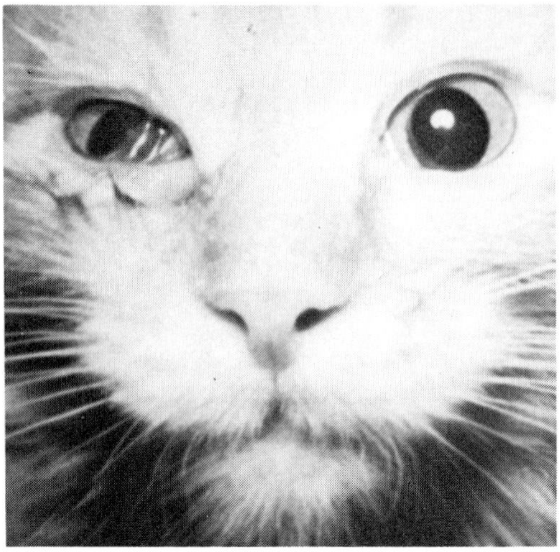

Fig 11. Serous conjunctivitis in feline pneumonitis.

agent was identified as a member of the *Miyagawanella* or psittacosis-lymphogranuloma venereum group of organisms, and the disease was named feline pneumonitis.

Properties of the Agent: The causal agent of feline pneumonitis is *Chlamydia psittaci.* Its characteristics place it in a classification among the bacteria, rickettsiae and viruses.

In suspensions of yolk sac, the agent remains infective for at least a week at room temperature and for at least a month at 4 C (39 F). Its activity is reduced after 10 minutes at 50 C (122 F) and it is destroyed after 30 minutes at this temperature or 10 minutes at 60 C (140 F). The agent remains active for at least 6 months when dried.

Chlamydia psittaci differs from other members of its group in its apparent resistance to sulfonamides. It is considered susceptible to chlortetracycline and oxytetracycline, somewhat resistant to chloramphenicol and penicillin, and completely resistant to streptomycin.[8,60]

Epizootiology: Mice, hamsters guinea pigs and rabbits were infected by nasal instillation of the agent.[7] Adult guinea pigs and rabbits become febrile and develop pneumonia after being infected with the organism. They do not die, however, in contrast to young guinea pigs, hamsters and mice. The disease is not transmitted from mouse to mouse under natural conditions.

Chlamydia psittaci, apparently of feline origin, has been isolated from a man with acute follicular keratoconjunctivitis.[61]

Transmission of pneumonitis among cats is by direct contact with secretions and droplets containing the organism. The disease is considered highly contagious. The agent is present in ocular and nasal discharges and the lungs of naturally or artificially infected cats. Suspensions of liver, spleen and kidneys usually do not contain the organism.

Tests indicate that cats that have recovered from the disease carry the organism for 1-2 months, although they are presumably immune. These cats could act as carriers.

Clinical Signs: The incubation period is 3-10 days, and the signs and course vary considerably. Generally, pneumonitis produces mild clinical signs. Affected cats seem to recover rapidly but may again show signs of illness shortly after apparent recovery. Recurrent episodes of illness may last 2-4 weeks. Such clinical observations indicate that pneumonitis tends to recur, and that infection does not produce strong or lasting immunity.

Conjunctivitis and rhinitis are the most characteristic signs of feline pneumonitis. The discharges vary from serous to mucopurulent but are never copious (Fig 11). A febrile response is uncommon, although early reports described a very short febrile period.

About 50% of infected cats suffer a mild relapse 10-14 days after the first illness; a few cats have further relapses a month or more later. This pattern may continue for up to a year.

Chlamydia produces cytoplasmic inclusions in epithelial cells of the conjunctiva, which are numerous during the first 2 weeks of infection.[62] The organisms can be stained with Giemsa stain or fluorescent antibody.

The hemogram of cats with pneumonitis tends to remain normal; there may be a slight increase in total WBC numbers.

Treatment: The treatment of pneumonitis in cats is similar to that previously described for FVR. Supportive care and broad-spectrum antibiotics, especially chlortetracycline and oxytetracycline, usually are effective.

Prevention: A modified-live *Chlamydia* vaccine of chicken embryo origin is available for vaccination of cats. Kittens should be vaccinated SC or IM shortly after weaning. Because of the possibility of the persistence of maternal antibodies, kittens less than 12 weeks of age when first vaccinated should be revaccinated at about 12 weeks of age. A single vaccination is protective in cats 12 weeks of age or older. Annual revaccination is recommended. Vaccination reduces the severity of clinical signs after challenge but may not provide solid resistance to such challenge.[63]

A combined rhinotracheitis-calicivirus-pneumonitis vaccine also is available.

Other Respiratory Viral Infections

Reovirus: Feline reovirus infection was first described in 1970.[16] Although the prevalence of the disease is unknown, a few studies suggest it is widespread in the US.[52] The importance of reovirus type 3 in the epizootiology of upper respiratory infection is not known. In one experiment, 16 of 28 kittens in contact with 2 kittens inoculated with type-3 reovirus developed (as did the inoculated kittens) lacrimation, photophobia and conjunctivitis.[16] The ocular discharges became mucopurulent in 7 of the kittens; 1 kitten developed a nasal discharge. The incubation period varied between 4 and 19 days, and the course of the illness was 1-26 days. The clinical disease was considered to be mild and of short duration, with signs usually restricted to the conjunctiva. A litter of 4 newborn kittens inoculated with type-1 reovirus died 2 days later.[59]

Feline reoviruses are double-stranded RNA viruses. The virus is resistant to heat and withstands a temperature of 56 C (133 F) for 30 minutes. It replicates in feline, bovine, hamster, canine, HeLa and human cell cultures. The virus has been isolated from the conjunctiva, pharynx, nasal passages and rectum of infected cats, and produces cytoplasmic inclusion bodies.

Although reovirus infection may complicate upper respiratory infections by other agents, it is currently thought that feline reovirus infection usually is mild, of short duration and confined to the eyes. Febrile responses, changes in the WBC count, anorexia or marked depression do not occur.

Syncytia-Forming Virus: More than 30 isolations of feline syncytia-forming viruses have been made in the US.[18] These viruses have been isolated from cats with urolithiasis, respiratory infections, intestinal infections, peritonitis and neoplasms, and from normal cats. Although inoculating these isolates into normal cats failed to produce signs of disease, the virus was recovered from inoculated cats for long periods. It is possible that a syncytia-forming virus could act in conjunction with other agents to produce disease. As these viruses apparently are widespread among cats, their potential role in disease production needs further study.

Parainfluenza Virus: Although the canine parainfluenza virus infects cats under experimental conditions, the significance of this virus in feline upper respiratory infection is unknown.[17]

FIP Virus: Feline infectious peritonitis virus may produce a severe, fatal pneumonia in cats.[20] Small, pyogranulomatous lesions are found throughout the lungs of affected cats and there may be an accompanying pleural effusion. Often there are generalized signs and lesions of FIP in these cases. This condition is described in more detail later in this chapter.

NEUROLOGIC VIRAL INFECTIONS

Rabies

Rabies is an acute contagious disease that is almost always fatal. It is characterized by neurologic signs, including increased excitability and subsequent paralysis. The virus usually is transmitted by the bite of an infected animal.

The contagiousness of rabies and the hazard associated with the bite of a rabid animal have been known at least since the time of Aristotle. Pasteur's experiments (1881-1889) proved that the virus enters the CNS; this partially solved the problem of practical immunization. The filterability of rabies virus was demonstrated in 1903, the same year in which Negri found the specific inclusion bodies that bear his name.[64]

Rabid cats usually exhibit the furious form of the disease and display a pronounced tendency to bite and claw. The transmission of rabies from cat to cat is surprisingly infrequent.

Properties of the Virus: Rabies virus contains RNA and is classified as a Rhabdovirus. The virion is a cylinder, flat on one end and round on the other, and resembles the spherical elementary bodies seen within the rabies inclusion (Negri) body (Fig 12).

The virus remains infective in tissue for several weeks at 4 C (39 F). It remains infective in glycerine for several weeks at room temperature, for months at 4 C, and for years at −12 C (10 F). In saliva it is easily destroyed by heat, most common disinfectants (formalin, phenol, alcohol, bichloride of mercury, potassium permanganate), acids and alkalies. The virus loses it virulence within a few hours in dried saliva.

Although the isolates of rabies virus may differ in virulence and immunogenicity, they are identical serologically, indicating there is only one immunologic strain. The virus isolated from a naturally infected animal is called "street vi-

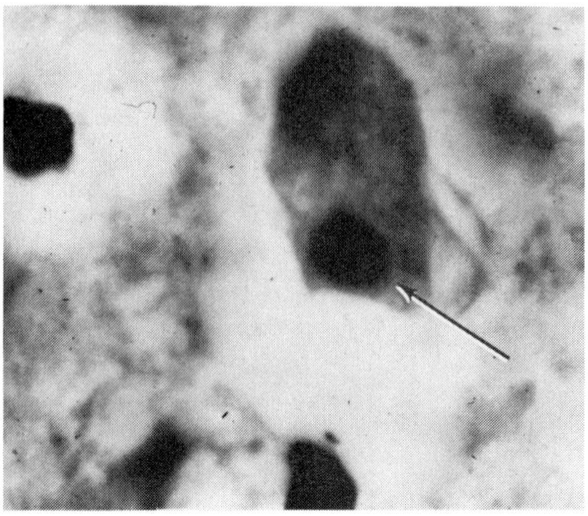

Fig 12. Negri body (cytoplasmic inclusion body) in the brain of a mouse with rabies.

rus." When street virus is passed repeatedly among animals of a particular species, it eventually becomes "fixed" for that species. The incubation period progressively shortens until it becomes constant, and the signs and course of rabies in that species tend to be constant. Fixation of the virus in the chicken embryo has been used in production of rabies vaccine; it is interesting that this fixed virus does not produce inclusion bodies. Rabies virus can also be cultivated in many cell cultures, including canine kidney cells, chicken embryo fibroblasts and hamster kidney cells. Such tissue-adapted virus often is used in production of vaccine.

Epizootiology: Rabies virus has produced disease in all mammals in which it has been inoculated and in some birds. Birds may be more resistant because of their higher body temperature. Cold-blooded animals apparently are not very susceptible. There also seems to be some difference in susceptibility to rabies virus among mammals. The opossum is highly resistant and people are thought to have a fairly high resistance.[65] Dogs, cats and skunks have medium susceptibility, whereas foxes, coyotes and cattle are highly susceptible. Young animals are thought to be more susceptible than mature or aged animals of the same species. Sylvatic rabies is difficult to control because of the wide range of species that can be infected and act as vectors.

As far as is known, only certain species of bats, such as the vampire and free-tailed species, may survive rabies virus infection and transmit the organism when infected.[66] Transmission may occur through aerosols or by casual biting. Lethal rabies also occurs in these bats; lethal infections are the rule in most species of bats.[67] The disease produced resembles that seen in dogs or cats. The bat develops encephalitis, becomes aggressive and often attacks without provocation, and dies. Rabies virus can survive for prolonged periods (as long as several months) in these bats, even though the infected bat ultimately dies of rabies. Although the spotted skunk was at one time believed to be a possible asymptomatic carrier of rabies virus, there is no evidence of this.

As rabies virus is excreted in the saliva of an infected animal, the infection can be transmitted by salivary contamination of a fresh wound. If the wound is older than 24 hours, however, usually it is covered by a scab and is not penetrated by the virus.

Rabies virus may enter the body by routes other than bite wounds and may be in other secretions or excretions in addition to saliva.[68] The excreted virus can be transmitted to susceptible animals in aerosols. It has been transmitted from bats to coyotes and foxes exposed to the air in caves densely populated by bats.[68] Transmission of rabies to cats other than by the bite of a rabid animal is unusual.

With the possible exception of certain species of bats, rabies virus generally is thought to be excreted in the saliva for several days before appearance of clinical signs, and thereafter during the course of the disease. Cats excrete virus in the saliva for only one day before the onset of signs, and for 3 days after signs are first observed.[69] There are conflicting reports, however, regarding the length of time before the onset of illness that the cat's saliva may be infective.[70]

Because cat-to-cat transmission seems unusual, the source of rabies in cats can only be postulated. The apparently increased infection rate in bats and the fact that sick bats would be easy prey for cats may be factors in the transmission of rabies among cats. Several known infections in cats have apparently resulted from skunk bites.

Clinical Course: The incubation period after IM inoculation of street virus into a large number of cats varied between 9 and 51 days, with a median of 18 days.[66] This corresponds closely to incubation periods of 14-60 days after natural exposure to the virus. In animals other than cats, incubation periods of more than 100 days have been observed occasionally and it is possible that longer incubation periods may occur in cats. The free-living habits of many cats make it difficult to obtain accurate data about exposure in naturally occurring rabies. A lacerating type of bite or multiple bites in areas with a rich nerve supply, as around the face, may result in somewhat shorter incubation periods. The incubation period in adult cats especially if they have been vaccinated, may be longer than in kittens.

After clinical signs appear, the course of rabies in cats ranges from 1 to 8 days. Most cats die 4-5 days after the onset of illness. The prodromal stage may last 1-2 days, the stage of irritability 1-4 days and the paralytic stage 1-2 days.

Apparent recovery after signs of rabies appeared has been observed, although very rarely, in dogs. This has not been observed in cats; the disease should be considered invariably fatal in this species.

Pathogenesis: Rabies virus remains at the site of its deposition for several hours before moving up the peripheral nerves to the spinal cord and then to the brain.[71] The virus does not replicate in tissues at the site of inoculation. Initial replication of virus occurs in neutral ganglia or the spinal cord. After further multiplication, the virus seems to spread centrifugally, perhaps through nerves, and can be found in many areas of the body, including the axillary, inguinal and mesenteric lymph nodes, lacrimal glands, lens, cornea and salivary glands. In immune animals, the virus apparently is destroyed at the site of deposition. Although isolation of virus from the blood of rabid animals has been mentioned, most authorities do not believe that viremia occurs often in rabies.[67]

The pathogenesis of rabies after oral or intranasal inoculation of the virus is not well understood, and the distribution of virus seems to differ from that after IM inoculation.[67]

Clinical Signs: Both furious and dumb (paralytic) forms of rabies have been observed in cats. The furious type is more common. The signs reflect encephalitis but are unpredictable because individual animals with encephalitis react differently.

The prodromal period may be easily missed. There is a change in behavior, usually marked by a tendency to hide. A fair percentage of infected cats may never be diagnosed as having rabies because the animal finds a hiding place and dies there. Although pica may be an early sign, it is less common than in dogs. Infected cats become more and more irritable during the prodromal period.

After 1-2 days, the rabid cat may suddenly attack from its hiding place, biting and scratching viciously, and may grab and hold with its teeth. If confined in a cage, the cat can easily be provoked to attack the bars of the cage or to bite at any object pushed into the cage. The irritable stage usually lasts 1-4 days. During this period the cat's voice becomes hoarse or has a peculiar tone due to developing laryngeal paralysis.

The periods of rage gradually subside and the animal's movements become uncertain, progressing gradually to complete posterior paralysis, ascending paralysis and death. The cat may live 1-2 days after the onset of the paralytic stage. Although laryngeal paralysis occurs in rabid cats, the paralysis of the masseter muscles and resultant drooping of the jaw so commonly observed in dogs occurs infrequently in cats. Drooling is also less frequent.

Dumb rabies has the same course as the furious form except that there are no vicious, aimless attacks on persons or objects. The prodromal signs may include apprehension and a tendency to hide. Posterior ataxia is followed by posterior paralysis. Paralysis becomes generalized shortly thereafter and death follows rapidly.

Because of the relatively rapid course of rabies in cats, paralysis may be the first sign observed. Often, however, paralyzed cats can be stimulated to attack moving objects. Therefore, the differentiation of dumb and furious rabies may be more hypothetic than real. This was illustrated by an 8-month-old cat that became rabid after IM infection of a live-virus vaccine modified by low egg passage.[72] Although the chicken embryo-fixed virus usually causes paralytic rabies, as it did in this cat, this animal also attacked moving objects.

All variations of encephalitis, including terminal convulsions, may be exhibited by rabid cats. The signs depend on the degree of encephalitis produced by the virus.

Lesions: There are no gross lesions characteristic of rabies. The carcass may be emaciated despite the relatively short course of the disease, and the stomach and intestines may contain foreign bodies. Neither finding occurs consistently, however.

The microscopic lesions are limited to the CNS and are quite variable. In an excellent article on the diagnosis of rabies, disseminated lymphocytic encephalitis was identified as one of the most reliable lesions of feline rabies.[73] Negri bodies usually are found in the cells of the hippocampus but also may be found in the cerebellum and midbrain. The Negri body has a rather distinct limiting membrane and may be surrounded by a slight, clear halo (Fig 12). One or several may be found in the cytoplasm of an infected nerve cell. Although Negri bodies are acidophilic, a granular and slightly basophilic internal structure (elementary body) may be present.

Unfortunately, other cytoplasmic inclusion bodies are found in normal cats and have staining characteristics essentially the same as for the Negri body.[74] Although there may be some fine points of difference, the differentiation of these cytoplasm inclusion bodies from Negri bodies is difficult and should be made by someone experienced in the field. This limits the value of a stained brain smear for diagnosis of rabies in cats. This difficulty does not occur if fluorescent antibody staining technics are used. For this reason and because of the accuracy and rapidity of the fluorescent technic, it is the preferred and standard test for laboratory diagnosis of rabies.

Diagnosis: Ante mortem clinical laboratory examination has been of no value in diagnosis. A WBC count may help to eliminate panleukopenia as a possible diagnosis, and specific laboratory tests for toxoplasmosis, intestinal parasitism and other infections might be of some value in differential diagnosis.

Diagnosing rabies is one of the most important functions performed by veterinarians. If a person has been exposed, failure to recognize the disease may jeopardize his or her life. Evidence of neurologic dysfunction alone does not justify a diagnosis of rabies. If CNS signs are recognized, however, the possibility of rabies should be considered. In these suspected cases the cat should be handled carefully but treated for other disease if such treatment seems indicated.

Toxoplasmosis, thiamin deficiency and lead poisoning are diseases with signs similar to those of rabies. Although the course of these diseases may be longer than expected with rabies, the early signs are often unnoticed by the owner. The convulsions that accompany strychnine or sodium fluoroacetate (1080) poisoning may be mistaken for the terminal convulsions seen occasionally in rabid cats. Endoparasitism, peritonitis, pleuritis or trauma may produce severe pain, causing the cat to meow pitifully and bite if handled. Trauma or arterial thrombi may produce posterior paralysis and pain. The severe weakness seen in cats with panleukopenia, FIP, FeLV infection and a variety of other infectious diseases may simulate the paralysis of rabies and its rapid course.

A combination of signs, including unprovoked, vicious attacks on people or moving objects, followed or accompanied by paralysis and especially a voice change, should suggest the strong possibility of rabies. Unfortunately, differential diagnosis is very difficult in the late stages of the disease and in moribund cats with little or no history of previous signs of illness.

The diagnosis of rabies can be made by fluorescent antibody examination or inoculation of laboratory animals. Because of the reliability of the fluorescent antibody technic for demonstrating rabies virus antigen in brain tissue of infected animals, most diagnostic laboratories use only this test, and no longer inoculate laboratory animals for diagnosis of rabies.

If a cat has bitten people or other animals before dying and after exhibiting signs suggestive of rabies, laboratory confirmation of the diagnosis should be sought. Other diseases that produce signs suggestive of rabies occur frequently and account for the large percentage of negative examinations obtained in laboratories performing rabies tests.[73] This cannot be avoided, however, when definite exposure of people or other animals has occurred.

Treatment: There is no treatment of value after clinical signs of rabies have appeared. The effect of postexposure prophylactic treatment of cats bitten by known rabid animals has not been determined. If a cat is exposed to an animal subsequently proven rabid and has been vaccinated within a year before the exposure, the cat should be immediately revaccinated and confined by the owner for 30 days. In these circumstances the booster dose of vaccine should provide adequate protection. A bat bite or exposure to erratically acting bats, as a cat catching and eating a bat in the daytime, should be considered as an exposure to rabies unless proven otherwise by examination of the bat.

If an unvaccinated cat or a cat that has not been vaccinated within the last year is exposed to a rabid animal as described above, the cat should either be destroyed or isolated (strict cage confinement) for 6 months in such a manner that it cannot be in contact with people or other animals. At the end of 5 months of such confinement, the cat may be vaccinated with an approved rabies vaccine.

Table 2. Rabies Vaccines For Cats [75]

Vaccine	Manufacturer	Trade Name	Dose	Age at Primary Vaccination	Booster Recommended
Modified-Live					
Canine cell origin, high egg passage, Flury strain	Norden	Endurall-R	1 ml	3 months	Annually
Inactivated					
Murine origin	Rolynn	Trimune (Fort Dodge)	1 ml	3 months	Annually
Murine origin	Rolynn	Annamune (Fort Dodge)	1 ml	3 months	Annually
Murine origin	Douglas	SMBV	1 ml	3 months	Annually
* Murine origin	Douglas	Pan-Rab	1 ml	3 months	Annually
Hamster cell origin, high cell passage, Kissling strain	Beecham	Rabcine	1 ml	3 months	Annually
Hamster cell origin, high cell passage, Kissling strain	Beecham	Rabcine-Feline	1 ml	3 months	Annually
Porcine cell origin	Norden	Endurall-K	1 ml	3 months	Annually

* combination vaccine

Again it must be emphasized that the efficacy of postexposure treatment of cats positively exposed to rabies is unknown.

Prevention: Vaccination of cats against rabies should be encouraged by veterinarians for protection of not only the cat but of people and other animals in the vicinity. Inactivated and attenuated rabies vaccines are available for use in cats (Table 2).[75] Since no vaccination program is perfect, cats suspected of being rabid should be observed carefully whether or not they have been vaccinated previously.

No vaccine is licensed for use in exotic cats. It is strongly recommended that exotic cats not be kept as household pets. If vaccination of wild or exotic animals is necessary (zoologic collections, etc), only inactivated (killed) rabies vaccines should be used.

All rabies vaccines must be administered IM at one site in the thigh muscles.

Because they may cause rabies in cats even when properly administered, neither the low egg-passage, Flury strain nor the SAD (ERA) strain of attenuated vaccine are licensed for use in cats.

Cats should be revaccinated against rabies each year. Tests in progress may later lead to different recommendations.

Public Health Responsibilities of the Veterinarian: Even though the rabid cat may not be an important vector of rabies, it does pose a risk to the owners and other human contacts. As a consequence, the practicing veterinarian and public health authorities in the area should cooperate closely. The public should be educated in a factual rather than an emotional manner. Such education should be continuous rather than delayed until a rabies epizootic occurs and public concern becomes disproportionate to the seriousness of the threat.

Animal bite wounds suffered by people should be, as required by law in most of the US, reported to the appropriate public health official. This official should then order the impounding of the biting animal for veterinary observation. The veterinarian that impounds such an animal should obtain the names and addresses of the cat's owners, the persons bitten, and the physician that treated the victim's wounds. Also to be noted are the date and circumstances of the biting, the vaccination status of the animal, and any unusual behavior exhibited by the suspect during the past few days.

The period for which the biting animal must be observed is established by law in most areas. Although it is doubtful that an infected cat sheds rabies virus in its saliva for more than a few days before the onset of clinical signs, the prodromal manifestations of rabies may be difficult to recognize in a cat. A suspect should be confined and closely observed for at least 10 days. If there are any signs suggestive of rabies, the veterinarian should promptly notify the physician and public health officials. Any decision concerning the treatment of persons bitten is the physician's responsibility. If no signs suggestive of rabies are observed during the required observation period, the physician and public health official should be notified and the cat released to its owner.

The purpose of confining the cat is to determine whether it was capable of transmitting virus in the saliva at the time of the biting incident, and not to determine whether it is in the incubation period of the disease. The veterinarian should explain this to the owner.

The World Health Organization has suggested that cats or other animals that bite without provocation may be destroyed for immediate examination by the FA technic to avoid antirabies treatment if the suspect's brain is found negative. This is now recommended in cases involving all wild animals. In cases involving domestic cats, the owner must agree to this course. This procedure can be recommended for unowned or unvaccinated cats in areas where rabies is enzootic. The suspect's head must be sent to a laboratory that performs the FA test for rabies diagnosis. If the fluorescent antibody test is negative, it can be assumed that rabies virus is not present in the brain and was not present in the saliva at the time of the bite. Conversely, if rabies virus is found in the brain by the FA test, it can be assumed that the cat could have been shedding rabies virus in its saliva at the time of the bite. If a cat that has not bitten a person is presented to a veterinarian while showing clinical signs suggestive of rabies, the owner should be calmly informed of the possibility of rabies. It is prudent for the veterinarian in this instance to contact the owner's physician and appropriate public health authorities. The owner can be told that the diagnosis is not positive and that the cat will be treated until a more definite diagnosis can be made.

Most public health laboratories specify that no live animals and only the suspect's head should be sent for diagnosis of rabies. Under these circumstances, after the animal is carefully euthanized, the veterinarian should sever the animal's head close to the shoulders with a sharp knife. Rubber gloves should be worn and care taken to avoid lacerations by bone splinters. Sufficient tissue should be left with the head to ensure inclusion of the salivary glands. The head should be put in a metal watertight container with a tight-fitting lid and the lid further secured with waterproof tape. This container is placed in a larger watertight one and packed with cracked ice. Dry ice should not be used because it freezes the tissues and makes microscopic examination impossible.

Before sending the head of a rabies suspect to a laboratory, a call should be made to inform the laboratory of its imminent arrival.

If the laboratory is located nearby, the head can be delivered by messenger; if not, it must be sent by air express, rail express or bus. Postal regulations do not permit mailing of heads of rabies suspects. As transportation services are sufficiently rapid today, there is no reason for the veterinarian to risk exposure to rabies virus by attempting to remove the brain for shipment.

A label reading "CAUTION: This package contains the head of a cat suspected of having rabies." should be affixed to the outer container before shipment. The head should be kept refrigerated until it is sent to the laboratory and should be sent so that it reaches its destination on a weekday.

The following information should accompany the head: the owner's name and address; the species, breed, age and sex of the animal; whether the animal had been confined and observed before death and for how long; clinical signs, if any; vaccination history; names and addresses of persons bitten; and the names of the physician or public health officials involved.

The importance of following the recommendations noted above (obtaining complete histories, close observation of clinical signs, rapid delivery of rabies-suspect heads, when warranted, to the laboratory) cannot be overemphasized since the rapid diagnosis of rabies means that treatment of exposed persons can commence soon after exposure, increasing the chance of success.

Pseudorabies

Pseudorabies is an acute infectious disease that affects cats infrequently. It is characterized by signs of encephalomyelitis and frequently by a severe localized pruritus. Usually it is lethal. It is also known as Aujeszky's disease, mad itch and infectious bulbar paralysis.

Aujeszky, a Hungarian physician and veterinarian, is credited with first reporting pseudorabies in 1902. However, farm journals in the US had carried descriptions of "mad itch," which undoubtedly was pseudorabies, almost 100 years earlier. Aujeszky demonstrated that the disease occurs naturally in cattle, dogs and cats, and is transmissible to rabbits.

Properties of the Virus: Pseudorabies virus contains DNA and is in the herpes group. The virus survives under field conditions for 30 days in the summer and 46 days in winter, and is stable at a pH of 4-9. Pseudorabies virus is rapidly destroyed by heat above 60 C (140 F) and by 0.5% sodium hydroxide, 5% phenol or 0.5% formaldehyde.

Pseudorabies virus can be propagated in fertile eggs and a variety of tissue cultures, including chick, rabbit, guinea pig and dog tissues. The virus produces cytopathic effects and plaques in tissue culture. Intranuclear inclusion bodies can be found in virus-infected tissue cultures and fertile eggs.[76]

Epizootiology: Pseudorabies occurs worldwide. In some areas like the midwestern US, the disease appears to be enzootic in pigs. Although pseudorabies apparently is a naturally occurring infection in cats and is prevalent in pigs in the US, there have been no descriptions of naturally occurring cases in cats in the US that have been authenticated by virus isolation. However, there is reason to believe that natural infections do occur in native cats. In areas of Europe, the disease is more common in cats than in dogs.[77]

Pseudorabies occurs naturally in cattle, sheep, rats, cats, dogs and swine. Rare cases, characterized by mild pruritus and early recovery, have occurred in people. In all species except pigs and people, natural infections are highly lethal. Nearly all warm-blooded animals, including birds, can be infected by inoculation.

As in most species other than swine, pseudorabies apparently is not directly contagious from cat to cat. It can be produced by SC, IM or IV injection and by intraconjunctival instillation or spraying the virus on abraded areas of skin. Ingestion is believed to be the natural route of infection in cats. As there is a relatively high infection rate in rats and pigs in the US, it is likely that unrecognized cases of pseudorabies occur in cats in the US.

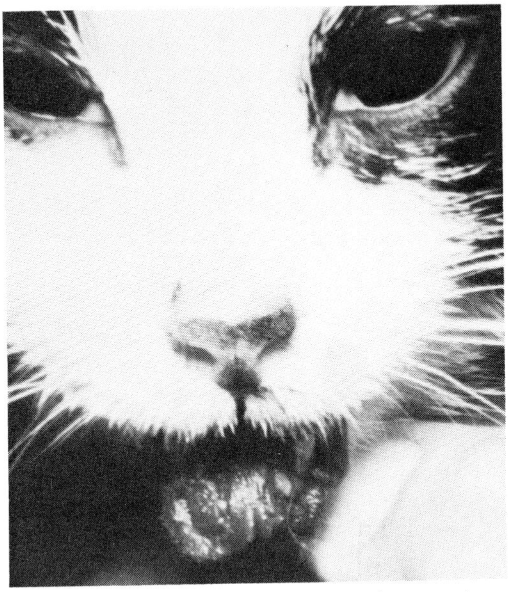

Fig 13. Protrusion of the tongue from pharyngeal paralysis associated with pseudorabies.

Course of the Disease: The incubation period varies, depending on the route of infection, from 24 hours when the virus is injected intracerebrally, to 3-4 days when it is ingested. Under natural conditions, the incubation period is believed to be 2-9 days. Cats invariably die within 24-36 hours after the onset of signs.

Pathogenesis: After ingestion, the virus apparently is absorbed and may be found in blood and various organs. The organism is thought to reach the CNS via peripheral nerves. In some animals it may be found in the brain, spinal cord, lung, skin, subcutaneous tissue, several internal organs, nasal secretions, blood and urine. In other cases, the virus may be found only in the brain or spinal cord, and sometimes cannot be isolated from the brain.

Clinical Signs: The onset of the disease may be associated with a change in behavior, lassitude and a tendency to bite. As in rabies, the cat may meow plaintively as if in pain. Anorexia is early and complete, and vomiting has been noticed. These early signs may be easily overlooked. Pharyngeal paralysis appears early in the course of illness and results in drooling and inability to swallow (Fig 13).

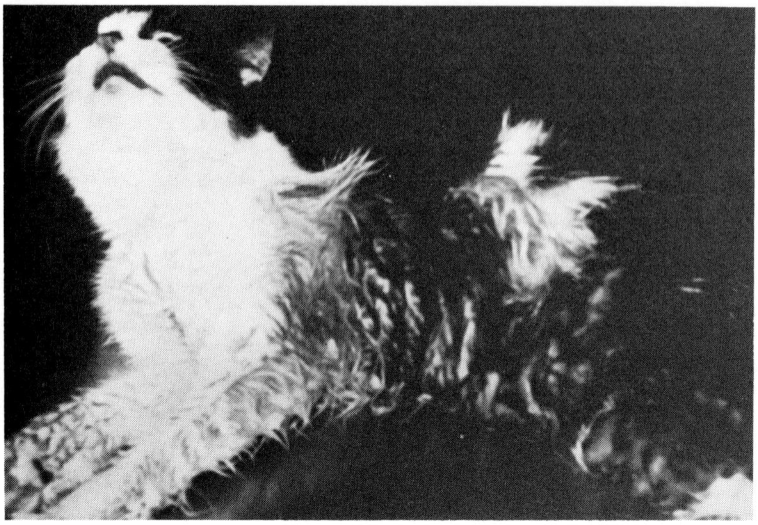

Fig 14. Experimental infection with pseudorabies virus. The abrasions over the thorax were caused by licking of pruritic areas.

Evidence of pruritus is characteristic, and affected cats lick incessantly at some area of skin (Fig 14). As the irritation increases, the animal gnaws, scratches and rubs the area, producing a rather extensive lesion. In peracute cases, death may occur before pruritis is noticed.

Twitching of the lips or other facial muscles may be observed and terminal convulsions occur in some cases. Respiration tends to be labored; the body temperature is not raised and soon becomes subnormal.

Lesions: If pruritus has occurred, there are large areas of inflammation and focal necrosis in skin and subcutaneous tissue. Otherwise, gross lesions are not prominent. The cerebral meninges and the brain may be congested or petechiated.

The important microscopic changes in the nervous system vary somewhat with the course of the disease. The extremely short duration of pseudorabies in cats limits pathologic changes to slight evidence of meningitis and neuronal damage in the cord and brain. There may be focal necrosis, perivascular cuffing and an increased number of glial cells.

Diagnosis: Specific laboratory examinations for diagnosis of pseudorabies in a living cat or characteristic changes in blood and urine of sick animals have not been described.

In many respects, pseudorabies in cats resembles rabies. The shorter course, absence of vicious attacks on animals and people, absence of progressive posterior paralysis, and the intolerable pruritus of pseudorabies tend to distinguish the 2 diseases.

Conclusive diagnosis of pseudorabies depends on virus isolation. Rabbits are susceptible to pseudorabies virus injected intracerebrally or SC. The SC route has 2 advantages: contaminated samples or samples from animals with intercurrent infections are less likely to kill the rabbit, and the localized pruritus at the area of SC injection helps identify the nature of the virus. Its definite identification can be made by a serum virus-neutralization test, using known antiserum against both the new isolate and known pseudorabies virus. Fluorescent antibody tests are also used for virus identification.

Although inclusion bodies are found in infected rabbits, it is questionable that they can be found in naturally infected cats. Because of the varied distribution of virus in affected animals, the brain, subcutaneous tissue in and about the scratched areas, and portions of the spinal cord nearest the affected skin area should be submitted for virus isolation.

Treatment: Treatment of cats with pseudorabies is uniformly unsuccessful. If the cat shows evidence of severe pruritus, pain or convulsions, general anesthesia is indicated to relieve the signs and supportive treatment should be given.

Prophylaxis: An attenuated virus vaccine is available for use in swine in known infected areas. This vaccine produces lethal pseudorabies in dogs and probably would in cats as well. Its use in swine is strictly regulated. Since naturally occurring pseudorabies has not been diagnosed in cats in the US, there is currently no demand for a cat vaccine.

Other Neurologic Viral Infections

Herpesvirus encephalitis has been described as a rare sequela to FVR.[29] The association of the feline herpesvirus of respiratory disease (FVR) to the idiopathic vestibular syndrome of cats is dubious.[41]

Viral encephalopathy has been described; however, the virus associated with this disease has not been characterized nor has the disease been reproduced or the clinical signs well elucidated.[28]

Lesions of meningoencephalitis often are associated with fatal cases of FIP. Signs of posterior or generalized ataxia, paralysis, anisocoria, tremors, personality changes, and radial, facial or trigeminal nerve paralysis have been associated with FIP.[78] The neurologic signs exhibited by a cat with FIP depend upon the distribution of lesions. Differential diagnosis may be difficult with only vague neurologic signs; however, most frequently the neural lesions occur in conjunction with lesions elsewhere in the body. It is unusual to find only neurologic lesions in cats with clinical FIP.

Posterior paralysis and tetraplegia have occurred in cats infected with FeLV.[79] Some cats with these signs have focal areas of lymphosarcoma compressing the spinal cord; however, other cats similarly affected have no evidence of such compressive lesions of lymphosarcoma. In these latter cases, it is postulated that the FeLV may have damaged nerve tissue.

Cerebellar ataxia (granuloprival cerebellar hypoplasia) is a common result of panleukopenia virus infection of the feline fetus *in utero* or at birth. Signs of mild to severe cerebellar cortical deficiency become evident as affected kittens begin to walk at about 4 weeks of age.[41]

Canine parainfluenza virus infection of the CNS has been associated with paralysis in dogs.[80] It is quite conceivable that in the next few years, viruses other than those previously described will be found to produce neurologic lesions and signs in cats.

MULTISYSTEMIC VIRAL INFECTIONS

Feline Panleukopenia

Feline panleukopenia is a highly contagious disease characterized by an explosive, short course and high mortality. The disease is worldwide in distribution.

Panleukopenia has variously been described as feline distemper, infectious enteritis or gastroenteritis, feline agranulocytosis, cat plague or fever, show fever, pseudomembranous enteritis, maladie du jeune chat, Katzenstaube and other more colorful terms. Feline panleukopenia is, however, the most acceptable name.

Properties of the Virus: Feline panleukopenia virus is a single-stranded DNA-containing virus currently classified in the parvovirus group. It is very stable and may remain infectious at room temperature for as long as a year.[52] It is resistant to ether, chloroform, phenol, trypsin, many acids and other chemicals, but can be activated by 0.175% sodium hypochlorite.[36] The virus resists heating at 56 C (133 F) for 30 minutes but can be destroyed after one minute at 100 C (212 F).

Feline panleukopenia virus is a single immunogenic type. It has been adapted to grow on cultured feline kidney cells.[81] The virus has an affinity for rapidly dividing cells and its growth is optimal in cell cultures inoculated with the virus within a few hours after cell seeding. The virus produces intranuclear inclusions in cells of the culture.

Epizootiology: Although the domestic cat is the principal host for the disease, any felid may be affected.[82] In addition, the binturong in the Viverridae family, the raccoon, coati and possibly the kinkajoe and lesser panda in the Procyonidae family are susceptible to panleukopenia. Mustelidae, such as the mink, ferret, marten, skunk, badger and otter, are susceptible to disease produced by mink enteritis virus, very closely related to panleukopenia virus. All Mustelidae in zoologic collections should be vaccinated against panleukopenia. All attempts to transmit panleukopenia virus to species other than those mentioned above have failed.

Cats may be infected by practically all routes. Although transmission of the virus usually is by direct contact among susceptible and infected cats, transmission can also occur via fomites on food dishes, bedding, infected cages, and the hands and clothing of handlers. Arthropods, such as fleas, may serve as mechanical vectors of the virus.

Recovered cats may shed the virus in their feces and urine for long periods after recovery. Neonatally infected cats may harbor the virus in their kidneys for a year or more and shed the virus periodically in the urine.[83]

The prolonged period of virus shedding, which may occur after subclinical infection or recovery from frank clinical disease, combined with the

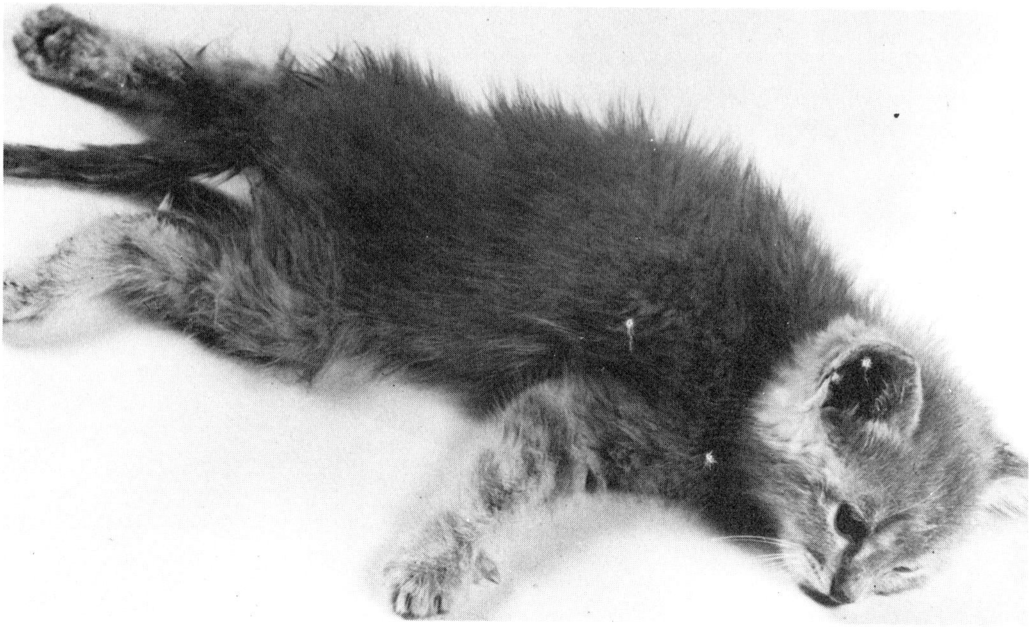

Fig 15. Severe depression, rough haircoat and soiling of the perianal hair in a kitten with panleukopenia.

stability of the virus, is undoubtedly responsible for maintenance of the disease in nature.

Feline panleukopenia is principally a disease of young cats but it can affect cats of any age. Morbidity and mortality vary markedly from one outbreak to another. In a completely susceptible cattery, the incidence of infection may approach 100%, with most infected cats exhibiting clinical signs of disease; however, in another susceptible cattery, only 25% of infected cats may show frank clinical signs. The other 75% are subclinically infected and develop strong resistance to the disease.[52]

Clinical Course: The incubation period after natural exposure to the virus is 2-10 days and usually 5-7 days. It may be shorter after experimental exposure. The course is rapid. In peracute cases, death occurs within 12-24 hours after signs of illness are noticed. The course in acute cases seldom exceeds 5-7 days.

The mortality is highest (approaches 90%) among untreated kittens less than 6 months old. Affected older cats are more resistant, but 50-60% may succumb. The outcome seems to be resolved during a crisis that usually occurs 3-4 days after the first elevation of body temperature, or sooner in younger cats. Persistent diarrhea may follow the crisis in animals that recover. These cats are often eating and much less depressed than before the crisis. In germfree cats, there are no signs of enteritis after experimental challenge with panleukopenia virus, although other signs, such as depression, fever and leukopenia, are present.[84] The course of experimental panleukopenia in such gnotobiotic cats is short and recovery rather than death is the rule. It thus seems reasonable to assume that the severe signs and the enteric signs and lesions seen in most cats are caused by microbial flora of the intestines.

Clinical Signs: The signs of feline panleukopenia vary from none in a subclinical infection of an adult cat to those of a peracute, fulminating disease in an 8- to 10-week-old kitten.

The initial sign is fever (104-105 F) that may persist for 24 hours. The temperature usually is almost normal for the next 24 hours and then rises again. Although the fever is often diphasic, the patient may die during the first febrile period. Afebrile affected cats have been reported.[85,86] The temperature usually drops abruptly to subnormal levels before death.

Depression is apparent during the first febrile period and often is profound during the second temperature rise. The cat's head may be dropped between the outstretched forepaws as it lies prostrate. Weight loss and dehydration commence with the first temperature rise and become pronounced by the second febrile period. Dehydration becomes quite severe, especially when emesis or diarrhea occurs.

Anorexia is complete within 48 hours after the onset of fever, although polydipsia or at least the desire for water remains throughout the course of the disease. Vomiting is frequently an early sign. Initially the vomitus consists of the last meal eaten but rapidly changes to a white or yellow frothy fluid. Emesis may occur only in about a third of clinical cases and may be less common in hospitalized cats not forced to move.

If the patient survives the initial febrile period, diarrhea may occur 2-4 days later. It is due to inflammation and degeneration of the epithelial lining of the small intestine. The affected animal may eliminate large quantities of liquid feces that are dark with partially digested blood; there may be evidence of frank hemorrhage and/or shreds of intestinal mucosa in the feces. It is noteworthy that diarrhea does not occur early in the course of the illness and frequently does not occur at all in fatal cases.

Affected cats may meow plaintively, especially when handled, due to the pain that accompanies intestinal inflammation. Because of the pain and fever, the cat often prefers to lie with its abdomen on a cool surface.

Peracute or fulminating panleukopenia usually affects recently weaned kittens. A kitten may be found dead after having been seen healthy and active 8-12 hours previously; the owner is often sure that the kitten has been poisoned. Physical examination of affected kittens is apt to be unrewarding because characteristic signs of the disease have not yet developed. If the kitten is alive, a blood count should be made. Other kittens that may have been in close association with the sick one should be carefully examined.

When presented to the veterinarian, older affected cats have a body temperature varying from high to subnormal. The animal's chin may be moist from vomitus or attempts to lap water, the haircoat is rough and unkempt, and feces may soil the hair (Fig 15). These patients are severely dehydrated and depressed. Their mucous membranes may appear somewhat pale. The eyes are sunken and the nictitating membranes may be prominent; there may be excessive mucus about the eyes. Contrary to earlier opinion, a nasal discharge is not present in the absence of concurrent respiratory disease (Fig 5). When placed in a cage, the patient stretches out in ventral recumbency and lies with its head hanging over the water dish.

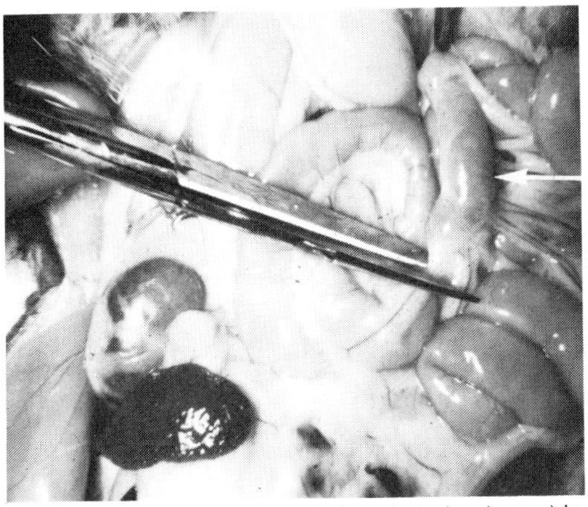

Fig 16. Edematous mesenteric lymph nodes (arrow) in a cat with panleukopenia.

Germ-free cats infected with feline panleukopenia virus are febrile, anorectic and leukopenic, and lose weight. They have no signs of enteric disease and recover completely.

The virus can penetrate the placental barrier in pregnant queens. Infection of the fetus in the early stages of pregnancy may result in abortion, stillbirth or early fetal death and resorption. Infection of the fetus in the last trimester of pregnancy results in cerebellar hypoplasia.[87] The virus replicates in placental cells; transplacental infection may not occur in all of the fetuses of an infected pregnant queen.[83] Clinical signs of cerebellar hypoplasia usually are not apparent in affected kittens until they are about 4 weeks of age, when they become ambulatory.

Lesions: The cadaver usually is dehydrated and emaciated, except in peracute cases in which gross changes are not apparent. In such cases, careful examination may reveal lesions in the small intestines, particularly in the jejunum and ileum. The intestines usually are dilated and somewhat edematous, thickened and inflamed. The serosal surface is hyperemic and contains petechial hemorrhages. The mucosal surface is often covered with hemorrhagic exudate and shreds of sloughed mucosa. The mesenteric lymph nodes are somewhat enlarged and edematous, and may be hemorrhagic (Fig 16). On breaking a long bone, the lack of hematopoietic marrow often is obvious. The marrow appears greasy, is yellowish white and has a semifluid consistency.

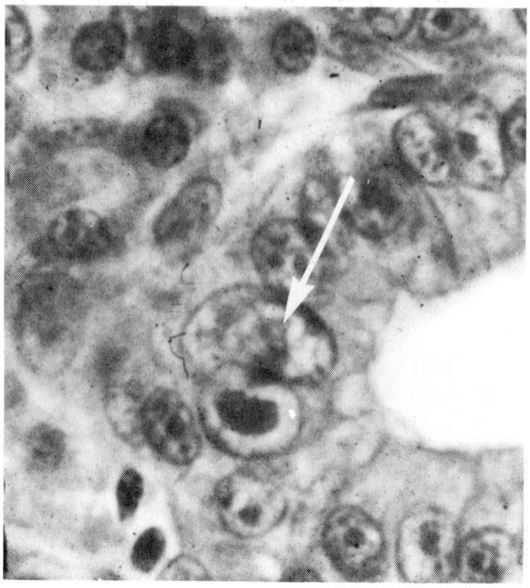

Fig 17. Intranuclear inclusion body (arrow) in an intestinal epithelial cell of a cat with panleukopenia.

In experimentally infected germ-free kittens, the only gross lesion of significance is a reduction in size and weight of the thymus.[84]

The degree of cerebellar hypoplasia in ataxic kittens may vary from a reduction by a fifth to a half of normal size, a lack of convolutions, to no gross change in cerebellar size but a loss of granular cells and a deficit in Purkinje cells.

The principal microscopic changes are found in bone marrow, the lymphoreticular system and, in naturally occurring cases, the intestinal mucosa. The changes involve cells undergoing active replication (mitosis). There is myelodestruction of bone marrow and resultant depression of myeloid activity, and a decrease in all stages of neutrophilic leukocytes from promyelocytes onward. Often there is total diminution of cellular elements, vacuolation, and replacement of normal hematopoietic marrow by fat. The degree of change varies from a slight loss to almost complete obliteration of cellular elements.

Intestinal lesions are marked by necrosis of the mucosa, particularly of the jejunum and ileum; the duodenum and colon occasionally may be necrotic. In some cats the necrotic mucosa is sloughed and replaced with a fibrinonecrotic membrane.[88]

The crypts of Lieberkühn are distended and may be filled with debris. This is the most consistent and prominent lesion in naturally occurring cases of panleukopenia. Intranuclear inclusion bodies are present in epithelial cells where the intestine is eroded. Although these inclusions are found most consistently in experimental animals, they may be found in 75% of naturally occurring cases (Fig 17).[88]

Edematous, hyperemic mesenteric lymph nodes are depleted of lymphocytes in the follicles, and there is reticuloendothelial cell proliferation. Intranuclear inclusions have been found in a small proportion of monocytic cells. Depletion of lymphocytes and proliferation of reticuloendothelial cells also occur in other lymph nodes, Peyer's patches, spleen and thymus. Petechial hemorrhages are present in the thymus of cats that die, and thymic atrophy has been found in germfree cats.[84]

Diagnosis: Feline panleukopenia has been likened to canine distemper in that both diseases can be manifested by a wide range of signs, depending on the virulence of the virus, resistance of the host, and type and severity of other viral and bacterial complications.[89] Fortunately for the clinical diagnostician, signs of feline panleukopenia tend to be somewhat more characteristic than those of canine distemper, and the changes in the WBC count in feline panleukopenia tend to be significant. The clinical diagnosis depends on recognition of the clinical signs and demonstration of the characteristic changes in the hemogram.

The total WBC count may be reduced to 500 cells/μl blood or even lower. If there are fewer than 5000 cells/μl, predominantly of the lymphoid series, and clinical signs of panleukopenia are present, a presumptive diagnosis of feline panleukopenia is warranted.

Both gradual and precipitous declines in the WBC count can occur.[86] There usually is a progressive decline in WBC numbers, with a precipitous drop at the time of the crisis (Table 3). The neutrophils are affected chiefly and may disappear at the rate of about 4000 cells/μl daily. Because of this, the numbers of other WBC are disproportionate. Lymphocyte numbers decrease but not as rapidly as neutrophils, resulting in an absolute lymphopenia and a relative lymphocytosis. Monocytes seem to follow the same pattern. Bone marrow changes reduce the production of eosinophils, but because their normal life span is 2-6 days, they may be absent or relatively increased in number.

If the cat recovers, after the crisis WBC return to the circulation at the rate of 4000-6000/μl

Table 3. Hemogram of a Cat Experimentally Infected With Panleukopenia Virus [90]

	RBC	Hb		WBC		Differential Leukocyte Count (%)				
Day	($x10^6$)	(g/dl)	PCV	($x10^3$)	Band	Neut	Lymph	Mono	Eos	Temp
0	7.5	12	37	16.4	1	60	32	2	5	101.5
(Inoculation)										
1	7.5	12	37	15.6	1	60	32	2	5	101.2
2	7.5	12	37	11.5	0	50	40	4	6	105.2
3	7.4	11	36	7.6	0	30	60	5	5	101.8
4	7.3	11	36	3.7	0	15	75	5	5	105.6
5	7.3	11	35	.75	0	10	77	8	5	105.0
6	7.1	10.5	35	.35	0	4	80	9	7	104.5
(Crisis and Recovery)										
7	7.1	11	37	4.5	35	40	20	3	2	102.3
8	7.1	11.4	37	10.5	39	39	16	3	3	101.8
9	7.2	11	36	16.7	34	41	20	2	3	101.5
10	7.4	11.5	36	22.8	20	55	20	3	2	101.0
Normal Values										
Mean	7.5	12	37	17.0	0.5	59	32	3	5.5	
Range	5.5-10	8-14	24-45	8-25	0-3	35-75	20-55	1-4	2-12	
(Basophils are rare)										

daily. The total count may reach 35,000 cells/μl in 3-4 days due to neutrophilia; this usually is accompanied by a shift to the left.

Depletion of the bone marrow during the illness curtails the production of RBC, but their relatively long life (100-120 days) compensates, and anemia is mild as reflected by the hemoglobin level, PCV and RBC count. In fact, the severe dehydration may result in an apparent increase of RBC numbers.[90]

Enteritis produced by *E coli* in cats has been described as being characterized by diarrhea and leukopenia, and closely resembling feline panleukopenia clinically.[91] The total WBC count in this disease may be as low as 2000 cells/μl. The severe enteritis and leukopenia seen in many clinical cases of panleukopenia may, in fact, be related to secondary *E coli* endotoxemia. A necrotic colitis from *E coli* septicemia has been described as affecting older vaccinated cats. Counts of 1500 WBC/μl and typical signs of feline panleukopenia are reported.[92] Although a severe *E coli* infection often accompanies feline panleukopenia, not all cases of bacteremia and septicemia in the cat are secondary to feline panleukopenia. Many severe and/or prolonged diseases produce bone marrow depression and subsequent leukopenia.

Acute toxoplasmosis may be difficult to differentiate from feline panleukopenia. Affected cats may have a WBC count of less than 3000 cells/μl. Usually there is a relative neutrophilia and left shift in toxoplasmosis, however.

Normal cats or kittens carrying FeLV may develop a panleukopenia-like syndrome after the animal has been stressed by hospitalization, abscesses as a result of cat fights, or upper respiratory disease.[79] The panleukopenia-like syndrome is characterized by diarrhea, dehydration and leukopenia. Clinically it is indistinguishable from feline panleukopenia; however, it may occur in cats known to be resistant to feline panleukopenia. In contrast to feline panleukopenia, anemia may be present in the FeLV-induced panleukopenia-like syndrome.

A rotavirus may produce diarrhea in young kittens; however, the syndrome tends not to be the peracute, severe type that would be expected with typical panleukopenia in young kittens.[94] A reovirus has been isolated from the intestinal tract of cats; however, it is not considered to be primarily an intestinal pathogen. The feline enteric coronavirus (see Feline Infectious Peritonitis) may produce mild to severe enteric signs in young kittens. The characteristic changes in the hemogram in panleukopenia are not seen in kittens infected with the enteric coronavirus.

Sudden changes in food, intestinal parasitism (ascarids, coccidia, *Giardia*), or other stresses may produce severe diarrhea in young kittens and these conditions must be differentiated from panleukopenia.

Because feline panleukopenia may be superimposed on other acute or chronic infections, this must be considered when a sick cat is examined. The differential diagnosis of feline panleukopenia is based on the history, involvement of an unvaccinated cat, presence of characteristic signs, and a hemogram that reveals leukopenia without another obvious cause.

Treatment: Strict isolation of the patient is essential to minimize transmission of feline panleukopenia. Scrupulous sanitation and warm, draft-free quarters are important in preventing secondary infections in debilitated patients. As affected cats often seem to lose the "will to live," they should be given compassionate care. Provision of heating pads, frequent petting, hand-feeding and other nursing care are essential for recovery. The patient should be returned to its owner as soon as possible.

Treatment is aimed at combating extreme dehydration, providing nutrients and electrolytes, and preventing secondary infection. Because most affected cats vomit, the therapeutic agents must often be administered parenterally for the first few days of treatment.

Whole-blood transfusions are an important treatment. As determined by the animal's response to therapy, whole blood should be given at the rate of 20 ml/kg body weight daily or on alternate days. The blood should be given slowly IV, best accomplished with a butterfly catheter. Affected cats should not be forcibly restrained, and struggling is minimized by using the infusion set. Although blood can be administered through an 18- 20-ga needle inserted into the medullary cavity of a femur, there is little to recommend this route of administration. Blood should not be administered intraperitoneally (see Chapter 2).

In addition to whole blood, buffered lactated Ringer's solution (10 ml 7.5% $NaHCO_3$/L lactated Ringer's) should be given for rehydration. The amount of fluid administered depends on the cat's maintenance needs (age, weight, etc) and degree of dehydration (see Chapter 2).

The usual dosage of lactated Ringer's solution is 20-40 m/kg and should be administered IV as often as necessary. If the patient is in shock when presented, short-term, high-dosage corticosteroid therapy, such as hydrocortisone succinate (Solu-Delta Cortef:Upjohn) at 25 mg/kg, may be given IV daily for 2-3 days with other fluids. Urine output or central venous pressure should be monitored when large amounts of fluids and corticosteroids are given IV.

In less life-threatening situations, the supportive fluids can be given SC or IP. However, only isotonic fluids should be given by these routes. If given SC, the fluids should be given at multiple sites over the body to prevent laking and delayed absorption. Care should be taken to ensure that all of the fluid is absorbed before additional amounts are injected.

Adding dextrose to the electrolyte mixture has been advocated to provide nourishment. The few calories provided in this manner, however, are unimportant. Unless given IV, 5% is the maximum concentration of dextrose that should be given; 2.5% in half-strength lactated Ringer's is the solution of choice. Greater concentrations tend to increase dehydration.

Vitamin B-complex supplementation is indicated and especially important when fluids are administered. In addition, IV administration of 1000-2000 mg ascorbic acid has been recommended. There is no good evidence, however, of any increased efficacy of IV doses of vitamin C as compared to older recommendations for peroral adminstration of 500 mg ascorbic acid 3 times daily. Supplementation of vitamin A may be indicated during the recovery period to assist healing and regeneration of severely damaged intestinal mucosa.

Broad-spectrum antibiotics should be injected during the acute phase of the disease. As noted earlier, *E coli* is the most serious secondary invader, but other organisms may be implicated. Therefore, a broad-spectrum antibiotic is indicated. An extended-spectrum penicillin, such as ampicillin, may be administered SC or IM at 10 mg/kg every 6 hours. Gentamicin may be used at 4 mg/kg every 12 hours for the first 24 hours, then at 2 mg/kg every 12 hours. Other broad-spectrum antibiotics may be equally effective.

The efficacy of antiserum is questionable. Its value is greater when given in the very early stages of the disease; use of at least 8 ml/kg daily, given SC is recommended.

The judicious use of injectable antiemetics and anticholinergics to prevent further dehydration caused by vomiting and diarrhea may be indicated early in the course of feline panleukopenia. Intestinal protectants, such as kaolin and pectin preparations, or astringents may be administered to control diarrhea after vomiting has ceased. Sloughing of a portion of the intestinal mucosa can be expected during the recovery stage, but the associated diarrhea should last only 2-3 days.

If the cat survives for 48 hours, the chances for its complete recovery are much better. After this period of therapy, emesis usually ceases to be a problem, and oral feeding and medication can commence. An orogastric tube has proved convenient for feeding convalescent cats (see Chapter 2). Strained baby foods, such as egg yolk, chicken or beef, diluted with water so they can be administered easily through the tube, with vitamin-caloric supplements are satisfactory. The baby food—vitamin mixture should be given at 1-2 oz/kg body weight twice daily for 2-3 days or until the cat is eating a normal ration. The quantity given by stomach tube should be small initially and gradually increased as the cat learns to tolerate this method of feeding.

Although it is difficult to make an accurate prognosis for each cat with feline panleukopenia, recent refinements in methods of treatment have markedly decreased the fatality rate. Practitioners have reported an overall recovery rate of 72% for all patients treated and of over 75% for affected cats that were 16 weeks and older. The prognosis for kittens less than 8 weeks of age generally is poor but usually is favorable for cats more than 16 weeks old if adequate treatment is provided early in the course of disease.

During the treatment period and after the patient's recovery or death, all litter should be burned and the cage thoroughly cleaned with an effective disinfectant, such as a 1:32 solution of Clorox. Susceptible cats should not be placed in cages used by infected cats for at least 3-4 days after the cages have been disinfected. After a cat has died of feline panleukopenia, the owners should be advised that any replacement kitten or cat should be immunized before being placed in the home.

Prevention: One attack of panleukopenia apparently confers lasting immunity. Because many cats have been found resistant to experimental infection, mild unnoticed infections apparently occur and also produce immunity. Sufficient antibody may be transferred from immune dams to kittens to limit natural infections in such young kittens to inapparent but immunizing episodes. Kittens younger than 2 months from immune dams have been exposed to feline panleukopenia virus and did not become ill.[93] All were immune when subsequently exposed to the virus; however, this is not recommended as a method of prophylaxis.

Temporary protection may be conferred by use of immune serum.[4,5,93] Commercial antiserum, given SC at 2.0 ml/kg, protects for 5-10 days. It is most effective if given 1-2 days before exposure but may protect susceptible kittens even when the virus is injected simultaneously. Antiserum is indicated when the danger of immediate exposure is high; it may be useful for cats recently exposed but showing no signs of disease. In the latter situation, doses larger than those recommended for prophylaxis should be given.

Normal feline serum may be used if antiserum is not available since it usually contains feline panleukopenia antibodies. A larger dose than that used for antiserum should be given, however, because the panleukopenia antibody content of normal serum is not determined before it is marketed and thus cannot be guaranteed.

Another possible use of antiserum is in colostrum-deprived kittens, which should be given the serum as soon as possible after birth. Vaccine is given later at appropriate intervals.[95]

Antiserum is not indicated in the usual vaccination program for feline panleukopenia. There is evidence that prophylactic use of antiserum to passively immunize kittens is less effective than multiple doses of vaccine.[96] Antiserum interferes with subsequent response to vaccine for at least 3 weeks after the serum's administration.[95] Such interference is apparently the same as that imposed by passively transferred maternal antibodies.

Use of antiserum is thus recommended for susceptible cats or kittens exposed to feline panleukopenia virus, for susceptible cats or kittens that may soon be exposed to the virus, and for colostrum-deprived kittens.

Although tissue-origin vaccines for the protection of cats against panleukopenia have been effective for many years, use of only cell culture-origin vaccines, either attenuated or inactivated, is recommended. Attenuated feline panleukopenia vaccines have been combined with attenuated herpesvirus (rhinotracheitis) and calicivirus vaccines for parenteral or intranasal administration. Inactivated feline panleukopenia vaccines have also been combined with inactivated or attenuated herpesvirus/calicivirus vaccines for parenteral use. Attenuated feline panleukopenia vaccine should not be given to pregnant queens, those of breeding age that could possibly be pregnant, or kittens less than 4 weeks of age because the virus can cross the placenta and has an affinity for actively dividing cells, especially in the cerebellum of fetuses and neonates.

Queens immune to feline panleukopenia transfer antibodies to their kittens via colostrum; within 24 hours after birth a kitten's antibody titer approaches that of the queen.[97] Maternal antibodies that persist in the kitten are directly proportional to the amount of these antibodies received from the queen. Kittens from susceptible queens are susceptible to feline panleukopenia at birth. If the queen has a low titer, the kittens are susceptible at 4-8 weeks of age. Kittens from a queen with a very high antibody titer are not susceptible until they are 12-16 weeks old.

Either attenuated or inactivated vaccine should be administered SC or IM in 2 doses, starting when the kittens are 9-10 weeks of age. The second dose of inactivated vaccine should be given 2 weeks later. For maximum protection, a third vaccination should be given when the kitten is 16 weeks old. For modified-live vaccines, the second vaccination should be given at 14-16 weeks of age. If the kittens are older than 12 weeks at the time of the first vaccination with modified-live vaccines, a second vaccination is not necessary. Annual revaccination is recommended for maximum protection. Unvaccinated kittens should not be admitted to an area of possible exposure to feline panleukopenia virus without immediate vaccination or preferably the administration of antiserum.

Where feline panleukopenia has been a serious problem in catteries or similar areas, vaccination can be started as early as 5 weeks of age and repeated at frequent intervals until the maternally derived immunity is lost. Regardless of the method of vaccination, every effort should be made to prevent exposure of kittens to virulent feline vaccination virus until the vaccination program is completed.

Susceptible cats vaccinated with cell culture-origin feline panleukopenia vaccine, either attenuated or inactivated, are consistently protected against challenge administered 3 days after vaccination. There have been indications that susceptible kittens vaccinated with the attenuated vaccine resist clinical exposure to virulent feline panleukopenia virus, through exposure to diseased cats, immediately after vaccination. Results of such experiments are not uniform and a great deal of further work must be done regarding the onset of resistance after vaccination.

Feline Infectious Peritonitis

Feline infectious peritonitis (FIP) was first described in 1963 as chronic fibrinous peritonitis.[22,23] In 1966 a series of cases was described and the syndrome was named FIP.[98]

Cause: Although, as described later, the disease has been associated with a coronavirus infection, it is now hypothesized that the clinical signs of naturally occurring FIP are a consequence of the host's immune reaction rather than being caused by viral cytopathogenicity.[24]

Clinically apparent FIP is characterized by a prolonged, progressively debilitating course marked by fever, anorexia, depression, loss of weight, and anemia. Approximately half of all cats affected by clinically apparent FIP exhibit peritoneal and/or pleural effusions. Signs associated with noneffusive FIP, such as jaundice, ataxia, paralysis, anterior uveitis or pneumonia, depend upon the location of the lesions. Although the disease usually is fatal in cats that exhibit marked clinical signs, most infections with feline coronavirus are subclinical.

Wild as well as domestic Felidae are affected.[99] The disease is worldwide in distribution.[100]

Properties of the Virus: The infectious nature of FIP was demonstrated in 1966 when the disease was transmitted by inoculation of abdominal exudates from naturally infected cats into susceptible cats.[99] Later, both filtered and unfiltered, bacteriologically sterile abdominal exudates or organ homogenates from affected cats were found to produce the disease. In 1970 the agent was tentatively identified as a coronavirus and its identity was confirmed in 1977-78.[101-103] The FIP coronavirus has been cultivated in monolayer feline cell cultures.[104-106]

The FIP coronavirus is an RNA virus. Antigenically it is related to canine coronavirus, transmissible gastroenteritis virus of swine, and human coronvirus 229E. It is unrelated to mouse hepatitis virus type 3, hemagglutinating encephalomyelitis virus 67N of swine, calf diarrhea coronavirus and human coronavirus OC43.[103]

The FIP coronavirus replicates by budding from the endoplasmic reticulum. The agent is stable for many months in organ homogenates frozen at −70 C and resists repeated freezing and thawing. It is inactivated by ether, chloroform, formalin, chlorhexidine and benzalkonium chloride, although it is relatively resistant to acidic conditions, phenol and trypsin. The virus is heat labile, being inactivated at 59 C (138 F) in one hour and within 24 hours at room temperature.

The FIP virus has been propagated in suckling mice and suckling rats, and hamsters supported replication of FIP virus after intracerebral inoculation.[107] The rabbit and chicken embryo appear refractory to infection. Different isolates of feline coronaviruses vary widely in their pathogenicity for cats. A recent isolate, a feline enteric coronavirus, antigenically indistinguishable from FIP coronavirus, may cause inapparent or mild to severe enteritis in young kittens but does not cause the peritonitis, pleuritis or granulomatous disease usually associated with clinical FIP.[25,26] Some isolates of FIP virus consistently produce severe disease only if injected IP, IV or IM, whereas other isolates consistently produce severe clinical FIP when administered PO or by nebulization or nasal drops as well as by injection.[106] These various isolates of feline coronavirus cannot be differentiated serologically.

Epizootiology: Cats may be infected through the intraperitoneal, intravenous, intranasal, intratracheal, intrathoracic, intracerebral, subcutaneous and oral routes. Some isolates of FIP virus produce disease consistently only when injected, whereas other isolates consistently produce severe disease when administered PO. The rapidity of onset of disease signs and severity of disease signs after administration of the challenge virus is directly proportional to the dose of the challenge virus administered and to the antibody titer of the challenged cat. Seropositive kittens (those with a positive antibody titer) developed viremia 2 days after aerosol challenge and developed severe clinical disease 7 days postchallenge, whereas seronegative kittens did not develop viremia until 6 days after challenge and severe signs were not seen until 16 days or more after challenge.[108] Other investigators consistently report similar findings.[109] The signs of disease tend to be much more severe and the clinical course of the disease until death tends to be much shorter in cats that are seropositive at the time of challenge with FIP virus. These factors, plus the fact that FIP viral antigen, IgG bound to antigen, and complement have been demonstrated in focal FIP lesions in the liver, strongly suggest that FIP is immunologically mediated.[109,110]

Cats may be exposed to moderate amounts of FIP virus by the oral or respiratory route. A WBC-associated viremia develops and an antibody response follows. Perhaps in most naturally infected cats, the infection subsides and the viremia disappears. A more severe exposure to the virus (or to a more virulent strain) or re-exposure to the virus may lead to persistent or recurrent viremia, excessive antibody production, and formation of immune complexes and their precipitation in vascular beds, with resultant disease. Such a hypothesis presupposes that an antibody excess occurs in the clinical disease; antibody tests in diseased cats indicate that this occurs. Viremia does not occur in cats infected with the feline enteric coronavirus; however, such cats develop antibodies to the enteric virus that are indistinguishable from FIP antibodies.[25] Whether these antibodies sensitize the cat to subsequent FIP infection or whether local resistance in the intestine blocks the absorption of FIP virus following oral infection remains in doubt and requires further investigation.

Although the natural route of infection with FIP virus is unknown, it is logical to assume that it is by the oral or respiratory route. The role of ectoparasites, blood transfusions from viremic cats, improperly sterilized needles or the bites of infected cats in the natural transmission of FIP virus is not known but would seem to be of minor significance. Infected cats shed the virus in the feces, urine and saliva.[111]

There is no apparent seasonal incidence of FIP nor does there appear to be a breed or sex predilection. The disease seems to be most prevalent in cats less than 3 years of age; however, there is another slight rise in incidence in cats over 10 years of age.[78] There is some indication that the classic effusive form of FIP occurs less frequently than other forms and that various parenchymal forms are being recognized more frequently.

Under natural conditions, as in catteries or households with more than one cat, FIP is transmissible. The morbidity rate is widely variable, however. In one household, all 3 closely related Siamese cats were clinically affected with FIP simultaneously. Conversely, in other households with 3-5 cats, only one was clinically affected and no signs appeared in the other cats that were in close contact with the sick one. In catteries, 1-4 of every 10 cats may develop FIP over

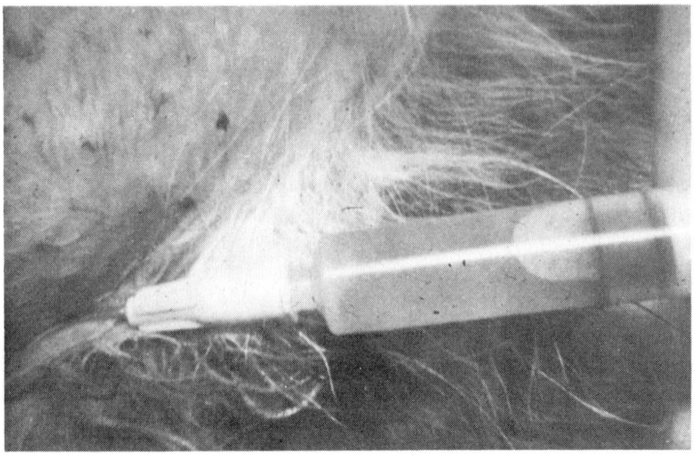

Fig 18. Peritoneal effusion evident on abdominocentesis in a kitten with effusive FIP.

a period of a year. In a few catteries, newly introduced young cats develop the disease but resident adult cats are unaffected. The relatively low morbidity of FIP compared to upper respiratory infections or panleukopenia may represent acquired resistance, inefficient transmission of the virus, or an over-responsive immune system in affected cats.

Of the cats in a multiple-cat household, cattery or research colony where there is relatively close association among cats, 80-90% have an antibody titer against feline coronavirus.[112,113] Whether these antibodies represent a response to enteric coronavirus or to virulent FIP antigen is currently unknown. Also, it is not known if cats with a high antibody titer shed virus or if they are resistant or highly susceptible to clinical FIP.

A disproportionate number (up to 50%) of cats with FIP are positive for FeLV group-specific antigen by the IFA test or the enzyme-linked immunosorbent assay (ELISA) test. This may be related to immunosuppression of suppressor T-cells by the FeLV, resultant depression of immune-mediated surveillance, and excessive FIP antibody formation. It does not represent a direct causal relationship between the 2 viruses.

Course of the Disease: Little is known regarding the incubation period of FIP under natural circumstances. Cases have been reported in households 3-4 months after removal of an infected cat.[114] This may reflect a prolonged incubation period, a latent period or a prolonged course of disease with no recognizable early signs. Seropositive experimental cats develop severe clinical disease within 3-5 days after challenge with virulent FIP virus, whereas seronegative kittens similarly challenged may not show signs of disease for 14-33 days.[108,114] The natural incubation period of FIP probably is prolonged, with an insidious onset of clinical signs.

The course of naturally occurring FIP is prolonged. The early clinical signs of FIP often are so innocuous that they do not attract the owner's attention; therefore, the veterinarian sees the terminally ill patient and may not be aware of the prolonged course of the disease. Some affected cats seem to respond temporarily to therapy and these remissions may last for 1-2 months. Some cats have lived for 4-6 months after FIP was diagnosed. A very few cats have apparently recovered fully after definitive diagnosis of FIP. The usual interval from the onset of clinical signs until death is 2-5 weeks.[99]

The course of experimentally induced FIP from the initial febrile episode to death is 5-7 days. This short course may be related to the overwhelming challenge and/or the previously acquired high antibody levels.

Clinical Signs: Feline infectious peritonitis may be manifested in one or more of several clinical forms. The classic or effusive form is characterized by accumulation of fluid in the abdominal and/or thoracic cavity. This form often is referred to as exudative or "wet" FIP. There are several clinical types of noneffusive or "dry" FIP. The clinical signs reflect involvement of specific organs, such as the spinal cord and brain (pyogranulomatous meningoencephalitis), eyes (pyogranulomatous uveitis), lungs (pyogranulomatous pneumonia), or liver, spleen, kidneys, pancreas or other abdominal organs. Thus, several subtypes of noneffusive FIP may be described: the ocular FIP when the eyes are involved and the neural form when signs reflecting neurologic involvement are seen. Pneumonic parenchymal FIP or abdominal parenchymal FIP reflects involvement of the lungs or various abdominal organs, respectively. The forms described are clinical; the basic histopathologic lesions are identical regardless of their location and they occur in both effusive and noneffusive forms of the disease.

Several clinical forms of FIP can exist simultaneously. For example, the ocular form and the abdominal effusive form may coexist. Therefore, the term "feline infectious peritonitis" is a misnomer. It has become so well established, however, that this name undoubtedly will continue to be used for many years. Feline infectious vascularitis would be a more logical name.

Regardless of the clinical type of FIP, certain features of the disease are consistent. Although an affected cat may be of any breed or either sex, it is likely to be a young adult between 6 months and 3 years of age. The history indicates an insidious onset, with rather vague signs of fever (103-106 F), depression and intermittent or constant anorexia. As the disease progresses, the body temperature may fluctuate; weight loss and dehydration tend to be progressive. Nonregenerative anemia may develop, resulting in pallor of the mucous membranes. Jaundice is observed occasionally. A few patients vomit or have diarrhea. The hemogram is altered rather consistently (see Diagnosis).

Cats with effusive FIP usually are presented because the owners have noticed a gradual enlargement of the abdomen (peritoneal effusion) or respiratory distress suggesting pleural effusion. The classic signs of effusion, along with a history of a prolonged wasting illness, should suggest a diagnosis of FIP. The diagnosis is confirmed by abdominocentesis or thoracentesis and examination of the characteristic exudate (see Diagnosis) (Fig 18).

The parenchymal forms of the disease are more difficult to diagnose. Histologically, parenchymal FIP is characterized by multifocal pyogranulomatous lesions. The disease usually involves many organs, but the presenting signs often are referable to only 1 or 2 of them.

In the abdominal form of parenchymal FIP, debility and fever are characteristic but the usual effusion is lacking. The omentum may be involved, resulting in adhesions and vague signs of digestive disturbances, discomfort and pain on abdominal palpation. The kidneys may be enlarged and irregular due to pyogranulomatous lesions. The BUN level may be elevated, accompanied by proteinuria. Because these cases can resemble renal lymphosarcoma, renal biopsy may be necessary to differentiate the 2 diseases. The liver may be affected, with signs of liver failure. Involvement of the pancreas can lead to signs of pancreatic enzyme deficit, diabetes mellitus or acute pancreatitis.

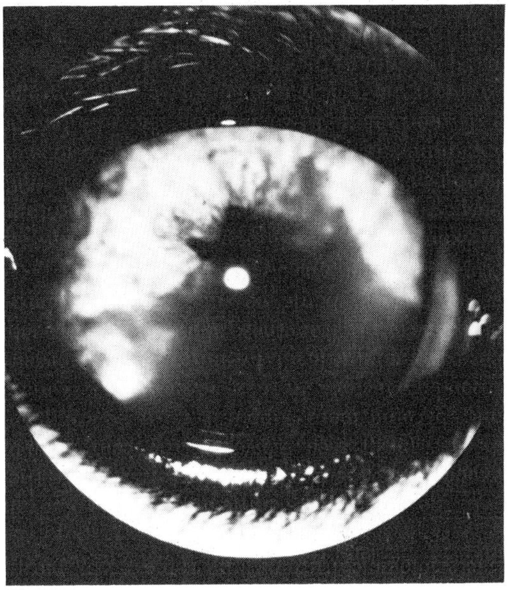

Fig 19. Hyphema in a cat with FIP.

In the thoracic parenchymal form of FIP, the pleura, diaphragm, lungs or heart may be affected. Usually there are no signs directly referable to lesions in the thoracic cavity in the absence of effusions. Effusive pericarditis occurs occasionally. If this is the only lesion, diagnosis of the disease is difficult.

Cats with ocular FIP have a bilateral, severe anterior uveitis, with extensive flare, keratic precipitates and, in some cases, hemorrhage in the anterior chamber (Figs 19, 20).[115] Characteristic flame-shaped retinal hemorrhages may be seen early in the course of the disease.[78] The iris may be edematous and lose its characteristic striations. The intraocular exudate appears as a hypopyon or an organized fibrinous mass in the anterior chamber. The pupil is miotic and secondary synechiae often develop rapidly. Mild conjunctival inflammation may accompany some degree of corneal edema. The lens tends not to be primarily affected. If the fundus can be visualized through the clouded media, signs of cho-

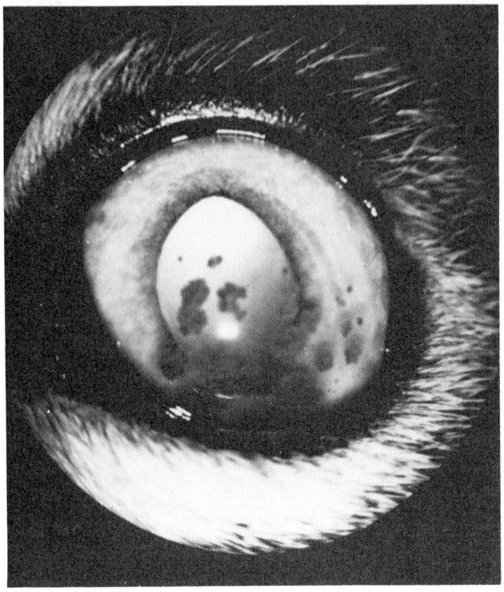

Fig 20. Keratic precipitates are all that remain about 2 weeks after most of the blood in the anterior chamber has been absorbed in a cat with FIP.

roiditis and retinitis may be observed. Fluid exudate associated with choroiditis can cause retinal detachment. Conditions to be differentiated from ocular FIP include panophthalmitis of bacterial origin, ocular lymphosarcoma, toxoplasmosis and systemic mycoses.

Involvement of the CNS may occur as a noneffusive form of FIP. The most frequent evidence of this form of the disease is incoordination of the rear limbs, often progressing to generalized ataxia. Tremors, convulsions, anisocoria, personality changes and radial, facial and trigeminal nerve paralysis have all been described in cases of pyogranulomatous meningoencephalitis.[78] Diagnosis may be aided if the patient exhibits signs referable to involvement of other organs, especially when a typical effusion is present in the abdominal or thoracic cavity. Without other signs of disseminated FIP, diagnosis of the CNS form depends on recognition of the prolonged debilitating course, signs of encephalitis, hemogram and analysis of CSF.

Feline infectious peritonitis has been incriminated in a disease referred to as "kitten mortality complex." This so-called complex includes reproductive failures, endometritis, pyometritis, repeat breeders, fetal resorptions, abortions, stillbirths, congenital malformations and neonatal deaths (weak, small kittens that do not nurse well and ultimately "fade away" and die). Acute congestive cardiomyopathy has also been observed in a few affected kittens.[116] There is no conclusive evidence that FIP is the cause of such a gamut of problems; however, further investigation is warranted.

Lesions: The cadaver of a cat that has died from FIP is emaciated and dehydrated. In the effusive form, the most obvious finding is copious amounts of straw-colored, serum-like fluid within the abdominal and/or thoracic cavity. Similar effusion occasionally is found within the pericardial sac. A granular, greyish-white, fibrinous exudate or whitish strands of fibren often are suspended in the fluid (Figs 21, 22).

The fibrinous exudate gives the peritoneal or pleural surface a dull, granular appearance that may be especially prominent on the surfaces of the liver and spleen. The omentum may be granular and irregularly thickened. In severe cases, it may be contracted and seemingly consist of several walnut-sized masses. Occasionally the testes appear enlarged as a result of inflammation of the surrounding tunics.[117]

Areas of necrosis, apparent as discrete, white foci 1-3 mm in diameter, may be seen on the surface of the liver, spleen, pancreas, kidneys, lung, brain, iris and testes. These are characteristic lesions of the parenchymal form of FIP and are necrotic pyogranulomatous lesions. They extend into the parenchyma of involved organs and appear to be located predominantly around blood vessels, especially venules.[118] These ne-

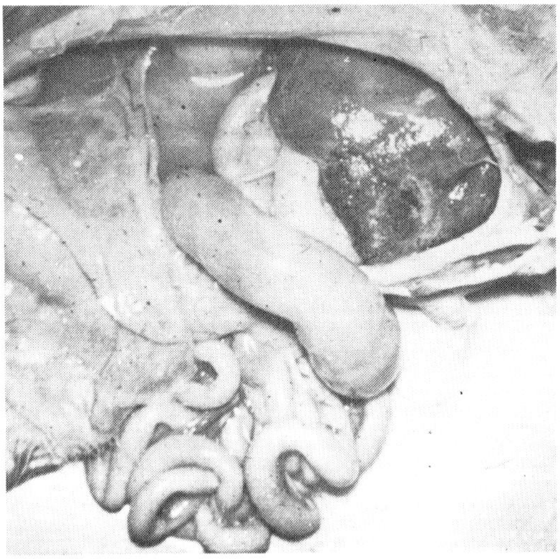

Fig 21. Typical exudate and fibrin strands on the liver of a cat that died of FIP.

crotic foci seem to be less noticeable in the effusive form of FIP.

The gross appearance of ocular lesions of FIP have been described in the section on clinical signs.

In the effusive form of FIP, there is microscopic evidence of fibrinous peritonitis or pleuritis involving practically all of the abdominal or thoracic organs. The cellular infiltrate consists of neutrophils, plasma cells, lymphocytes, and histiocytes; it may appear focally or diffusely within the exudate on the serosal surfaces.

The necrotic pyogranuloma of the parenchymal form of FIP is relatively typical, regardless of the organ in which it is located. There is an exudate composed of protein-rich fluid and fibrin, along with necrotic debris. Among the inflammatory cells, neutrophils usually predominate but macrophages, lymphocytes and plasma cells also are present. The amount of necrosis and exudation and the predominant cell type may vary somewhat among the lesions. Often there is a cellular reaction, with little or no necrosis. A typical pyogranuloma involving the ciliary body is shown in Figure 23.

In the thoracic parenchymal form of the disease FIP, the pleura, diaphragm, lungs or heart may be affected.

Cats with ocular FIP have a bilateral, severe anterior uveitis, with extensive flare.

Diagnosis: In all types of FIP, a CBC may demonstrate alterations from severe leukopenia to moderate to marked leukocytosis. Toxic leukopenia often is present in terminally ill cats. Typically there is a relative or absolute neutrophilia and an absolute (as well as relative) lymphopenia. Total lymphocyte counts may range from 0 to 250 cells/µl.[119]

Moderate to severe anemia is common in cats with FIP. The anemia tends to be progressive, becoming more severe toward the termination of the disease. In about 50% of the cases, the RBC count is below 5 x 10^6 cells/µl, the hemoglobin level is below 8.0 g/dl and the PCV is below 24%. These figures represent the minimum normal values for cats. The RBC in anemic cats are normocytic and normochromic; the anemia is a result of depressed erythrogenesis. The anemia of FIP is difficult to distinguish on the basis of RBC morphology from that of the feline leukemia complex. The RBC in these nonregenerative anemias differ from those of the regenerative forms of anemia seen in hemobartonellosis and similar hemolytic infections.

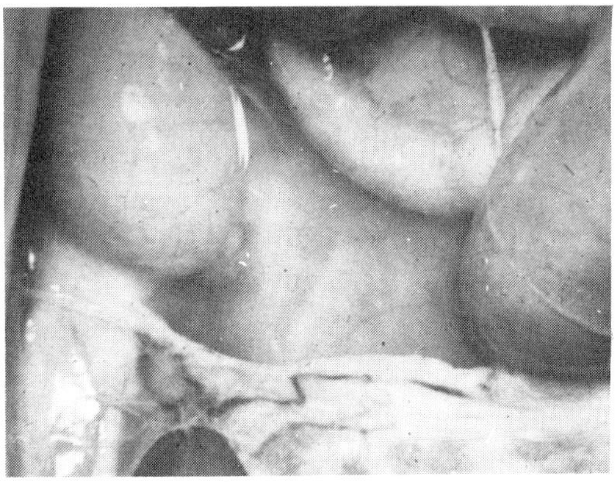

Fig 22.Peritoneal effusion in a cat that died of FIP.

Focal hepatic necrosis in FIP may result in an increase in the icterus index to a range of 10-50 units. (Normal icterus index is 2.5-5 units or up to 7.5 units in severely dehydrated cats.)

Hyperproteinemia (total plasma protein level exceeding 7.8 g/dl) occurs in a significant number of cats with FIP. Characteristically the hyperproteinemia is due to a hyperglobulinemia; electrophoresis indicates the elevation in globulin levels involves the beta or gamma fraction. Although the significance of the hyperglobulinemia is unknown, serum electrophoresis may provide useful information when considered with other diagnostic data. About 20% of cats with FIP have a plasma fibrinogen level above 400 mg/dl.[78] (The normal plasma fibrinogen level in cats is 50-300 mg/dl.)

Significant clotting abnormalities may be observed in terminally ill cats or when the liver is severely affected. These clotting abnormalities include prolongation of prothrombin and partial

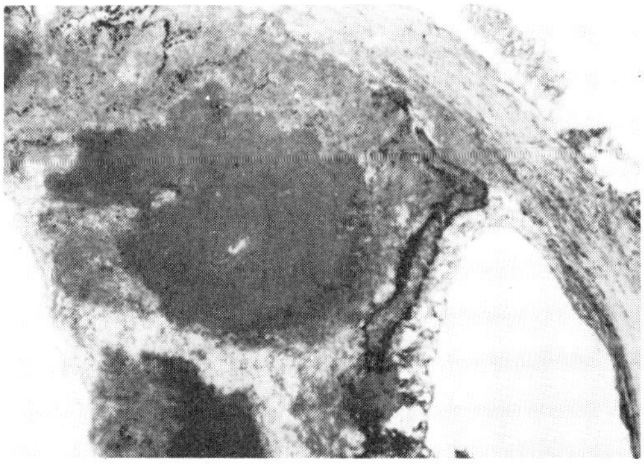

Fig 23. Pyogranuloma in the ciliary body of a cat with the ocular form of FIP.

thromboplastin times, depression of coagulation factors VII, VIII, XI and XII, elevation of fibrinogen and fibrin-fibrinogen degradation product levels, and thrombocytopenia.[119] These clotting abnormalities suggest that disseminated intravascular coagulopathy may be involved in the pathogenesis of FIP and may contribute significantly to mortality.

Radiographs of cats with thoracic or abdominal effusion may reveal the presence of the exudate. After it has been determined that an effusion is present, some of the exudate should be collected for examination.

The exudate is straw colored and serum-like in consistency. It often contains flakes of fibrin and may clot on exposure to air. The specific gravity of the exudate varies between 1.017 and 1.027. The protein content may range from 3.4 mg/dl to as high as 11.8 mg/dl, with an average protein content of about 5 mg/dl. Electrophoretically, the exudate's protein spectrum roughly parallels that of the serum; globulin is the main protein.[107,119,120]

White blood cells are always present in the fluid, but the total count may be as low as 100/μl or less; this is in contrast to the high numbers found in suppurative peritonitis or pyothorax. The predominant cells in FIP effusions are neutrophils, with a smaller proportion of mononuclear cells and detached mesothelial cells. Bacteriologic culture of fluid removed by paracentesis is negative.

In the early stages of the disease, the pleural exudate has the typical characteristics. As the disease progresses, however, the composition may become more suppurative, depending on secondary factors. In these later stages, it may be extremely difficult to differentiate thoracic effusions of FIP from those of pyothorax. In such cases, tissues should be submitted for microscopic examination.

Examination of CSF is indicated in cats with suspected FIP and neurologic signs. The protein content of the CSF may be elevated to 90-2000 mg/dl in cats with neurologic manifestations of FIP (normal is 10-20 mg/dl). The number of WBC in the CSF is also elevated, with a range of 90 to 2500/μl (normal is 0-8/μl) and predominantly neutrophils.[78]

In cats with ocular lesions, analysis of the aqueous humor reveals an increase in neutrophil and macrophage numbers. Although these changes are not specific for FIP, the absence of *Toxoplasma* organisms, systemic fungal elements or blast forms of lymphocytes should be helpful in differentiation.

The spectrum of alterations in serum enzyme activity varies according to the severity of the lesions and organs affected. With severe liver necrosis, hyperbilirubinemia and increased levels of SGPT and SGOT may be observed. Renal lesions may lead to increased BUN and serum creatinine levels. If the pancreas is involved, variable elevations in the serum lipase and/or amylase level may occur. Cases of diabetes mellitus secondary to FIP-induced pancreatitis have been reported.[20] Although there is little specific value in screen testing of serum enzyme levels, specific tests as indicated may be helpful in more firmly establishing a diagnosis.

Histopathologic examination of formalin-fixed biopsy samples or FA or IFA tests run on frozen biopsy samples is probably the most reliable method of establishing a diagnosis of parenchymal noneffusive FIP before death. Laparotomy and careful punch biopsy of organs are preferred to percutaneous needle biopsy since the discrete lesions can be identified and biopsied using the former procedures.[121]

Serologic evaluation for antibodies against feline coronaviruses may be helpful in evaluation of patients with suspected FIP. Both IFA and ELISA tests are available. The IFA test, using canine kidney cells infected with canine coronavirus or porcine cells infected with TGE virus as antigen, is more commonly used. The IFA test is strongly positive, at titers of 1:1600 to 1:25,000 or greater, in cases of clinical FIP. Unfortunately, high titers may also occur in normal cats and signify only that the cat has been exposed to a feline coronavirus. Therefore, results of serologic examination must be interpreted with caution.

Feline infectious peritonitis should be considered in the differential diagnosis of any chronic wasting disease of cats. The effusive form of FIP is not difficult to diagnose. Characteristic ocular lesions in a cat with a history of prolonged illness and typical hematologic changes affords a greater diagnostic challenge. Most difficulty in diagnosis is presented by cats that are weak, lethargic, and febrile, with only slight evidence of specific organ involvement and no effusions or alterations of the hemogram. Organ biopsies, serum enzyme evaluation and serologic examination may be indicated in such cases.

Treatment: Although temporary remissions occasionally occur in affected cats after treatment, relapses are almost inevitable and the patient ultimately dies. Very few affected cats recover completely. These latter cases usually are of the ocular noneffusive form or abdominal parenchymal form, with minimum organ involvement. An occasional cat with the abdominal effusive type has recovered completely. At best, the prognosis is poor, and one wonders if the affected cats that recovered did so because of or in spite of treatment. The prognosis for a cat with clinical signs of FIP and concurrent FeLV infection is very poor and treatment of such cats usually is not warranted.

Treatment of cats clinically affected with FIP is largely supportive. In the thoracic effusive cases, removal of the exudate is essential and a chest drain should be placed. It is far less essential to remove abdominal effusions, unless they compromise respiration by pressure against the diaphragm. Older therapeutic regimens that involve peritoneal lavage are of very questionable value.

Since FIP is an immune-mediated disease, the most logical therapy should be aimed at immunosuppression. The most successful therapy combines prednisone or prednisolone tablets, at 2 mg/kg BID, with melphalan tablets (Alkeran: Wellcome), at 0.2 mg/kg every third day.[122] The dosage must be adjusted based on evidence of myelosuppression as determined by serial CBC. Use of broad-spectrum antibiotics is indicated during the early stages of treatment.

Although intensive therapy with immunosuppressants, antibiotics and supportive care may prolong the clinical course of FIP, cures are rare. Plasmaphoresis, aimed at removal of the immune complexes, may ultimately provide a successful means of therapy and certainly warrants further investigation.

Prevention: The exact pathogenesis of FIP is unknown. Further investigation into the role of enteric coronaviruses as a possible sensitizing agent is indicated. Potential vaccines are under investigation.[123]

Reasonable husbandry procedures, including isolation of obviously affected cats in the household or cattery, are indicated. Removal of cats that are not clinically diseased merely because they have an antibody titer against FIP is unwarranted and contraindicated.[124]

More research must be done before suggestions on prevention of FIP can be made.[124]

Feline Leukemia Virus Infection

The term feline leukemia virus infection is used in the broadest sense to denote any disease process caused by or closely associated with infection with feline leukemia virus (FeLV), whether or not the changes associated with the disease are evident in the circulating blood. The common viral etiology of the malignant proliferative and degenerative diseases of the hematopoietic system, reproductive disorders, and the immunosuppression associated with this infection justify the broad use of the term feline leukemia virus infection or feline leukemia complex.

Table 4 illustrates the many possible manifestations of FeLV infection. With the possible exception of mast-cell sarcoma, FeLV has been found in cats with all of the syndromes listed in Table 4 and is the presumed cause of those syndromes. Sometimes it is impossible to demonstrate that an individual with the characteristic signs is infected with FeLV; however, this difficulty in isolating the virus does not mean that the signs are not caused by FeLV infection. On the other hand, demonstration of FeLV by use of the indirect fluorescent antibody (IFA) or enzyme-linked immunosorbent assay (ELISA) does not mean that all signs of illness in that patient are a direct result of FeLV infection.

The feline leukemia complex includes both lymphoreticular and myeloproliferative malignant processes. Either type of disease may occur as a proliferative or degenerative process. The proliferative neoplastic processes arising from lymphoid tissue are commonly referred to as lymphosarcomas or malignant lymphomas. Many types of feline lymphosarcomas occur in various locations: lymphocytic leukemia (blood and bone marrow), thymic or cranial mediastinal, gastrointestinal, multicentric, renal, neurologic, ocular, osseous and cutaneous.

The degenerative disease resulting from FeLV infection of the lymphoreticular tissues is manifested by thymic atrophy. This occurs in neonatal kittens and is a cause of the so-called fading kitten syndrome (see Chapter 15). Malignant neoplasms arising from cells derived from bone marrow generally are classified as myeloproliferative diseases. A nonregenerative anemia and a panleukopenia-like syndrome caused by FeLV are degenerative processes involving erythroid cells and granulocytes, respectively; they are classified as degenerative diseases of the myeloid cells.

In addition to the lymphoreticular, myeloproliferative and degenerative processes noted above, FeLV causes infertility, fetal resorption and abortion.[125] Autoimmune hemolytic anemia has been associated with some FeLV infections, as has an immune-mediated membranous glomerulonephritis.[126,127]

Feline leukemia virus suppresses the immune responses, which is manifested as an increased susceptibility to and higher mortality from viral and bacterial diseases. The incidence of such unrelated infections as hemobartonellosis, FIP, chronic nonhealing abscessees, chronic rhinotracheitis and generalized bacterial disease appears to be much higher in FeLV-infected cats than would be expected in the general population of uninfected cats.[125,128,129]

The immunologically indistinct feline sarcoma virus produces fibrosarcomas of the skin, usually in young cats.[130]

Incidence: Although it is extremely difficult to determine the true incidence of FeLV infection, this is among the most prevalent and devastating diseases of domestic cats.[131] The annual incidence of lymphosarcoma was once estimated as 41.6 cases/100,000 cats in the population at risk.[132] This figure included only the lymphoreticular malignancies and was based on a survey in a restricted geographic area. The percentage of lymphosarcoma in all cases of FeLV infection has been estimated at between 75% and 90%. In the area around Pullman, Washington, however, lymphoreticular neoplasms constitute less than 50% of all cases of FeLV infection. If this incidence were applicable nationwide, the annual incidence of FeLV infection could well be more than double the reported 41.6 cases/100,000 cats.

Another factor that must be considered is the increase in morbidity among cats exposed to the virus, as occurs in infected catteries or multiple-cat households.[133-135] It has been suggested that of 100,000 cats in the general population whose exposure to FeLV is unknown, 100 are infected with the virus; however, 33% or 33,000 cats of 100,000 cats known to have been exposed to FeLV may be infected with the virus.[136] A more recent report indicates that half or more of the free-ranging pet cat population appears to become infected with FeLV, at least in a transient manner.[137] Most of these infected cats respond immunologically and apparently eliminate the infection; however, about 1.8% are unable to respond and become chronically viremic (persistent infection).[138] This means that about 1% of pet cats harbor (and excrete) FeLV. The incidence of disease is less. The same report estimates an annual incidence of 76 lymphosarcomas and 127 non-neoplastic FeLV-associated diseases per 100,000 cats in the population at risk, or an annual incidence of about 0.2%.

Feline leukemia virus infection is worldwide in distribution.

Properties of the Virus: Feline leukemia virus was first isolated from a cluster of cats with lymphosarcoma in 1964.[27] It is an exogenous oncogenic RNA virus currently classified as a retrovirus. It is distinct from the endogenous feline retroviruses, such as RD-114, which are not oncogenic. The FeLV can synthesize a DNA transcript (provirus), which is inserted into the DNA of infected cells. The integrated provirus may code for the replication of more virus, may cause cell transformation (to neoplastic cells) or both. The provirus may also seemingly remain latent in the cell. The integrated FeLV DNA also may combine with cellular genes to generate the highly oncogenic feline sarcoma virus. The FeLV isolates are all capable of infecting susceptible cells and thus contain the genes for virus replication. Feline sarcoma virus isolates contain a mixture of replication-defective feline sarcoma virus genes and replication-competent FeLV genes.

Ultrastructural examination of the FeLV reveals spikes protruding from the virion envelope. The envelope of the virus consists of glycoproteins assembled onto the nucleocapsid as it buds through the infected cell membrane. There are 3 FeLV subgroups or strains, designated A, B and C, that reflect slight differences in the envelope antigens. Infected cats may develop neutralizing antibodies against specific envelope antigens. Thus a cat may develop resistance against strain A but still be susceptible to infection with strain B or C.

Each FeLV subgroup may induce a different type of disease. For example, subgroup A may produce thymic lymphosarcoma and nonregenerative anemia, whereas subgroup B may produce myeloproliferative disease. Most FeLV isolates consist of a mixture of A and B subgroups, and several isolates consist of a mixture of all 3 subgroups. Much more research is needed before this can be fully established.

The internal core of the virion consists of viral RNA in a tight coil and several additional protein subunits. All FeLV and feline sarcoma virus strains share a common species-specific antigen, which is tested for using the various FeLV tests.

All FeLV isolates grow in feline cell cultures and various of the subgroups A, B and C grow in cells of guinea pig, bovine, canine, porcine and human origin. Subgroup A has the most restricted host range.[139] There is no evidence that FeLV has a role in the natural occurrence of leukemia in people, dogs, cattle or pigs.

Feline sarcoma virus produces fibrosarcomas experimentally in a variety of hosts including kittens, puppies, neonatal sheep, neonatal rabbits, subhuman primates, guinea pigs and pigs.[79] However, the tumors so induced tend to regress rather than progress. Feline sarcoma virus grows in a wide variety of cell cultures. It transforms human cells in cell culture.[79]

Three types of antigens are associated with FeLV and infected cells: virion antigens, cell-surface antigens and soluble antigens. Virion antigens include the envelope antigens (type specific) and the internal antigens (group specific). The virion antigens have been described previously. Although the infected cat may produce protective levels of neutralizing antibodies against the envelope antigens, antibodies against the internal or core antigens are produced in very small amounts and do not appear to be protective.

The virus-specific cellsurface antigen produced by an FeLV-infected and transforming cell is seemingly analogous to the tumor-specific transplantation antigens that occur in other, possibly virus-induced cancers. Cells infected with FeLV produce a feline oncornavirus-associated cell membrane antigen (FOCMA) that is not a structural component of the virion. Cats infected with FeLV can produce specific anti-FOCMA antibody that, in high levels, enables the cat to resist or even reject an FeLV-induced tumor. The FeLV is not neutralized by anti-FOCMA antibody; cats with high anti-FOCMA antibody levels may be healthy carriers of FeLV.

Soluble antigens may be found in the body fluids of cats infected with FeLV; however, their biologic significance is unknown.

Epizootiology: The FeLV often is present in the blood and bone marrow of infected cats. The virus is shed in the saliva, urine, feces, milk and nasal secretions of some infected cats.[136] It can be transmitted through saliva by biting, through urine or feces by use of common litter pans, via aerosol transmission by sneezing, through milk from the infected dam to her offspring, and possibly by bloodsucking insects. The virus also may be spread by blood transfusions.

Clustering or multiple cases of FeLV infection in unrelated cats suggest the infectious nature of the disease.[135] Saliva from chronically viremic cats appears to be the major source of infection for susceptible cats. Spread appears to occur during close contact, such as an infected cat biting or licking (grooming) a susceptible cat. Aerosol transmission appears to be rare.[138]

Although genetic transmission of the endogenous feline retrovirus, RD-114, occurs, genetic transmission of FeLV does not occur. The FeLV is spread by horizontal (cat-to-cat) transmission and epigenetic vertical transmission (transplacentally, via the colostrum, or in the saliva as the queen grooms her kittens).

Two to four weeks after infection with FeLV, acute disease develops, manifested by fever, lymphadenopathy and malaise. However, these signs are seldom significant and are demonstrable only in laboratory settings with the cats under close observation.[140,141]

At the time of the acute disease, the host immune response to infection becomes critical and determines which animals recover and eliminate the virus and which animals ultimately die of FeLV infection or diseases related to the immunosuppression of chronic FeLV infection. Humoral immune responses, assisted by cell-mediated immune responses to the virus envelope antigens and to the cell-surface antigens (FOCMA), correlate with resistance to chronic viremia and tumor progression respectively. The quantitative production of these antibodies (neutralizing antibody directed against virion envelope antigens and anti-FOCMA antibody) seems to depend on the age of the cat at the time of infection, the dose of virus received, and perhaps the strain of the virus. Kittens tend to respond poorly and have a significantly increased incidence of chronic viremia and virus-induced lymphoreticular and myeloproliferative diseases compared to cats infected at older ages.[142]

Cats that fail to respond immunologically become chronically viremic, are immunosuppressed by the FeLV infection and have an increased risk of dying of FeLV infection or other diseases. As noted earlier, about 1.8% of cats infected with FeLV fail to respond immunologically and become persistently viremic.[138]

The time from the onset of viremia and the appearance of the later signs of FeLV infection is termed the induction period. This period is extremely variable and obviously difficult to determine in most clinical situations since most cats are first tested for viremia at the time clinical signs develop. Induction periods ranging from 2 to 52 months have been reported, with an average induction period of 22.9 months.[138] Many cats have been persistently viremic for more than 5 years without overt signs of disease.[143] The factors that bring about signs of FeLV infection in persistently infected cats after a prolonged disease-free period are unknown.

The fact that a cat can mount a seemingly effective immune response at the time of initial infection with FeLV and does not become persistently viremic does not entirely preclude later development of FeLV infection. About 33% of all cats with naturally occurring FeLV infection are virus negative at the time the diagnosis is made.[144] This could possibly be a result of a "hit and run" type of oncogenesis in response to the infection or could represent the integrated DNA of the FeLV (provirus) coding for transformation of cells without coding for virus replication. Bone marrow cells taken from nonviremic but previously infected cats and grown in cell culture free of the inhibitory action of that cat's serum may allow replication of FeLV.

Course of the Disease: The clinical course of FeLV infection varies widely and depends on a number of factors, including the type of disease (*eg,* lymphosarcoma, myeloproliferative disease) present, the success of therapy if therapy is initiated, and the immune response of the cat.

Reticuloendotheliosis, a myeloproliferative disease involving the stem cells, tends to be refractory to treatment. A profound, nonresponsive anemia often accompanies the disease. The clinical course, unless the patient is repeatedly transfused, tends to be short. Panleukopenia-like manifestation of FeLV infection, thymic atrophy in neonatal kittens, and many of the cases of nonregenerative anemia often respond poorly to therapy. The affected cat usually dies shortly after a diagnosis has been made.

Lymphosarcoma tends to be more amenable to treatment. Figures 27-29 are radiographs of a cat with a cranial mediastinal lymphosarcoma before and after treatment with cyclophosphamide, vincristine and prednisone. This animal responded well to treatment, the mass disappeared and treatment was ultimately discontinued. However, the cat remained persistently viremic and died from thoracic effusive FIP about a year after the mediastinal lymphosarcoma was first diagnosed and treated. Successful treatment of various lymphosarcomas (gastrointestinal, renal, multicentric) has produced periods of remission averaging 105-130 days, with many patients surviving much longer. Myeloproliferative disorders and lymphocytic leukemias tend to respond poorly to treatment, although survival for 316 days in response to chemotherapy of myeloproliferative disease has been reported.[145]

Many cats with reproductive diseases, such as infertility and fetal resorption caused by FeLV infection are persistently viremic for years without showing other signs of disease. As noted previously, several infectious diseases appear to be more common and more severe in persistently viremic cats. Since they tend to be more severe, the course of these diseases also tends to be shorter in FeLV-infected cats.

Questions regarding the course of FeLV infection can only be answered in generalities. About 80% of persistently FeLV-viremic cats die within 2½-3½ years; 10% of uninfected cats of similar ages die within that period.

Clinical Signs: The clinical signs of disease associated with FeLV infection are extremely varied. Unfortunately, there are no classic clinical signs common to all forms of the disease complex. The patient often has a rather vague history of prolonged anorexia with clinical signs of weight loss, depression, some degree of anemia and perhaps recurrent fever. Young adults are typically affected (the mean age of cats with lymphosarcoma is 2 years) and the major immediate complaint may be dyspnea, vomiting, diarrhea, noticeable swellings of lymph nodes or extreme lethargy.

For descriptive purposes it is useful to divide the diseases in the feline leukemia complex into 2 categories: neoplastic and non-neoplastic diseases (Table 4). Classification of neoplastic diseases is based on the cell type that has undergone malignant transformation. They are further subclassified on the basis of location of the lesion. The clinical signs depend on the location of the lesion.

Non-neoplastic diseases in the feline leukemia complex are not easily classified and frequently are confused with other diseases. Nonregenerative anemias and reproductive disorders may be caused by a variety of agents. Infections may persist because of immunosuppression caused by FeLV infection, but this association may not be immediately apparent.

Two or more clinical forms of FeLV infection may coexist. Thus a cat may be presented with

Table 4. Diseases Associated with Feline Leukemia Virus and Feline Sarcoma Virus

Feline Leukemia Virus

Neoplastic Diseases

- Lymphoreticular Cell
  - Lymphosarcoma
    - Cranial Mediastinal (thymic)
    - Alimentary
    - Multicentric
    - Renal
    - Ocular
    - Osseous
    - Dermal
    - Neurologic
  - Lymphocytic Leukemia
  - Reticulum-Cell Sarcoma
- Myeloid Cell (myeloproliferative disease)
  - Stem Cell
    - Reticuloendotheliosis
  - Erythroid Cell
    - Erythremic myelosis
    - Erythroleukemia
  - Granulocytic Cell
    - Myelogenous leukemia
    - Granulocytic leukemia
    - Eosinophilic leukemia
    - Basophilic leukemia
  - Mast Cell
    - Mast-cell leukemia
  - Monocyte
    - Monocytic leukemia
    - Myelomonocytic leukemia
  - Megakaryocyte
    - Megakaryocytic leukemia
  - Myelosclerosis
  - Myelofibrosis
- Fibroblast
  - Multicentric Fibrosarcoma (FeSV)

Non-Neoplastic Diseases

- Thymic Atrophy (fading kittens)
- Panleukopenia-like syndrome
- Anemia (usually nonregenerative)
- Pancytopenia
- Reproductive Disorders (infertility, abortion, fetal resorption)
- Immunosuppression
- Immune-Mediated Disease
  - Hemolytic anemia
  - Glomerulonephritis

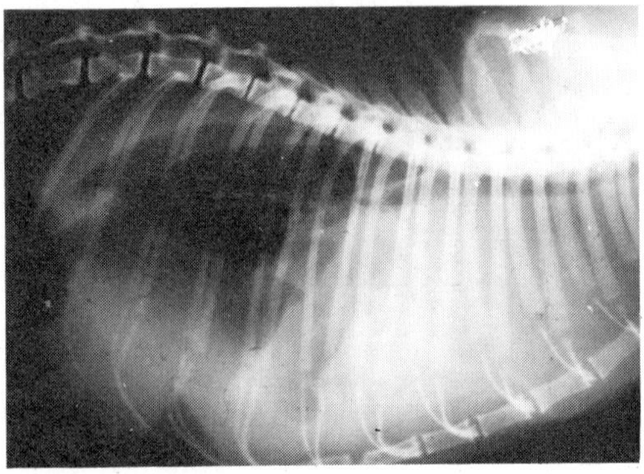

Fig 24. Lateral pretreatment radiograph of a cat with cranial mediastinal lymphosarcoma.

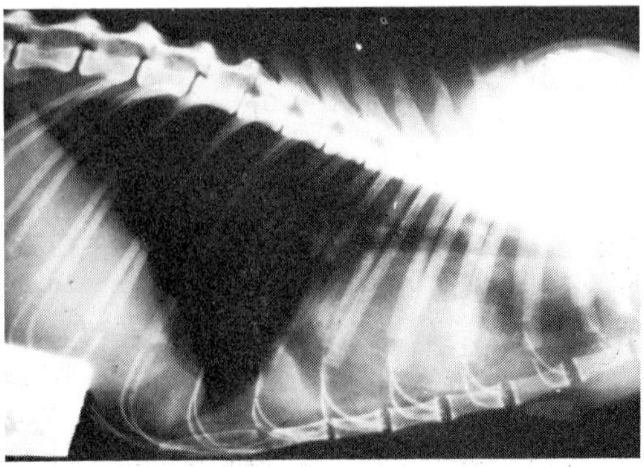

Fig 25. The cat in Figure 24 8 days after treatment was initiated. Note the decreased amount of effusion.

ocular lymphosarcoma, myelomonocytic leukemia and nonregenerative anemia. The following is only a very brief description of the more common clinical entities in FeLV infection. A more complete description of these disorders is given in chapters on various organ systems and in several excellent texts.[146-148]

Neoplastic Diseases: Lymphocytic leukemia occurs most frequently in young adult cats. Anorexia, lethargy and depression are the common presenting signs. Anemia, fever, splenomegaly and hepatomegaly are common physical findings. A blood count reveals leukocytosis (often 30,000-300,000 cells/mm^3), usually with predominantly lymphocytes, blast forms and prolymphocytes. The anemia often is myelophthisic; marrow examination reveals infiltration with abnormal lymphocytes.

The lymphosarcomas represent a common manifestation of FeLV infection. Classification of the lymphosarcomas is based on their location. Although the nonspecific signs common to many of the diseases in FeLV infection, such as anorexia, depression, lethargy, weight loss and fever, occur with lymphosarcomas, anemia tends to be less pronounced than with myeloproliferative disorders, nonregenerative anemias or lymphocytic leukemias.

Thymic (cranial mediastinal) lymphosarcomas produce signs of respiratory embarrassment or, rarely, regurgitation due to pressure on the esophagus (Figs 24-27). The onset of respiratory signs tends to be acute and may be precipitated by a pleural effusion that develops as the tumor reaches a critical size. Microscopic examination of the pleural effusion reveals a predominance of lymphoblasts. Thoracic radiographs help to establish the diagnosis (Fig 24).

Gastrointestinal lymphosarcomas cause vomiting, diarrhea, melena, anorexia and weight loss. Bowel thickening may be palpated; mesenteric lymphadenopathy is common and often palpable (Fig 28). Diagnosis is established by biopsy since about 50% of these cases are FeLV negative by blood test.

Peripheral lymphadenopathy, often with hepatomegaly, splenomegaly and mesenteric lymphadenopathy, is classified as multicentric lymphosarcoma. It may not cause the classic prolonged anorexia and weight loss of other forms of lymphosarcoma. Diagnosis is by excisional biopsy of an affected peripheral node.

Cats with renal lymphosarcoma are presented because of signs of renal failure (Fig 29). Both kidneys usually are involved. The enlarged kidneys are smooth and symmetrically enlarged or nodular on palpation. Radiographs usually demonstrate the renomegaly. Azotemia usually is

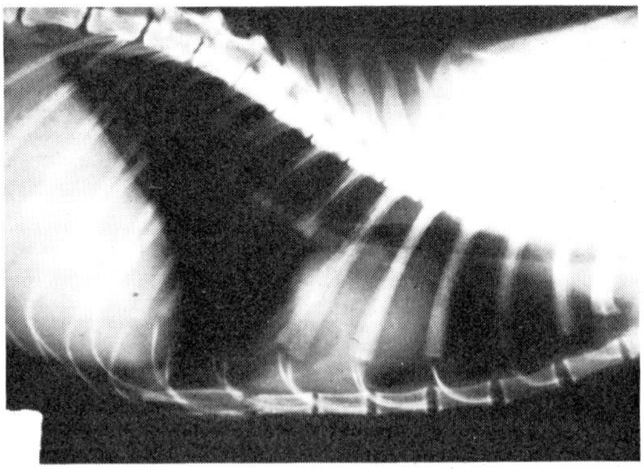

Fig 26. Lateral radiograph of the cat in Figure 24 15 days after treatment was initiated. There are no radiographic signs of the tumor or an effusion.

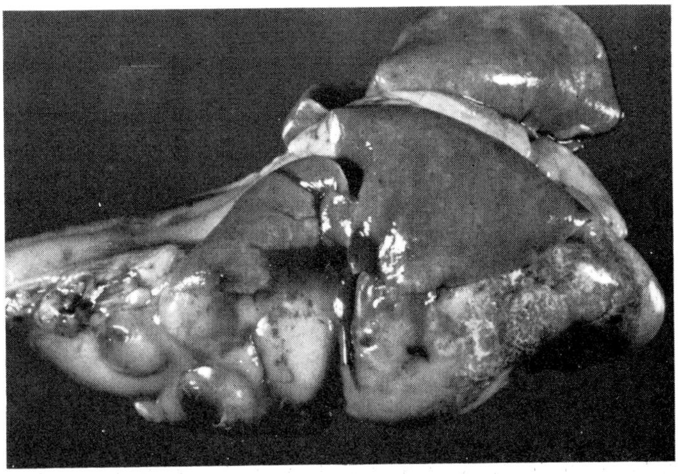

Fig 27. Cranial mediastinal (thymic) lymphosarcoma.

present when these cats are presented. Percutaneous biopsy confirms the diagnosis.

Neurologic lymphosarcoma is rare. Signs vary from paraplegia to convulsions, depending upon the location of the lesion. A non-neoplastic feline neurologic syndrome, manifested by a slowly progressive ascending paralysis and occasionally by convulsions, occurs in some persistently viremic FeLV-infected cats.[149] Lymphosarcomas are not found in such cases. At necropsy, there are demyelinating lesions in the cord and brain, but FeLV has not been isolated. This disorder may be an immune-mediated response to FeLV infection.

Ocular lymphosarcoma usually causes anterior uveitis, with hypopyon (Fig 30). The lesion often is bilateral and not easily differentiated from the ocular lesions of FIP or toxoplasmosis by external examination. Keratocentesis reveals lymphoblasts and prolymphocytes in ocular lymphosarcoma. Ocular lymphosarcoma often coexists with lymphocytic leukemia or other lymphosarcomas.

Osseous lymphosarcoma causes lameness and limb pain. Any bone may be involved. Radiographs reveal lytic lesions, with some evidence of new bone formation. Diagnosis is confirmed by biopsy.

Cutaneous lymphosarcoma, manifested by multicentric cutaneous masses, has been observed in young cats.[146] Diagnosis is by cutaneous punch biopsy. Cutaneous lymphosarcoma often coexists with other lymphosarcomas or lymphocytic leukemia.

The clinical findings in cats with myeloproliferative disease tend to be similar, regardless of the cell type affected. These diseases affect the bone marrow, causing progressive replacement of normal bone marrow elements with proliferating neoplastic cells. A progressive, severe, nonregenerative myelophthisic anemia develops. The mucous membranes are pale and the cat is lethargic, weak and depressed. Heart murmurs associated with anemia may be detected. Petechiae, ecchymoses and excessive bleeding from venipuncture sites occur if thrombocytopenia results from the disease. Splenomegaly, hepatomegaly, lymphadenopathy and jaundice may be detected on clinical examination. Examination of the blood and bone marrow reveals abnormal cells, with the type of abnormal cell found characterized by the type of myeloproliferative disease present. Reticuloendotheliosis, granulocytic leukemia, eosinophilic leukemia, myelomonocytic leukemia, erythremic myelosis and erythroleukemia are all classifed as mye-

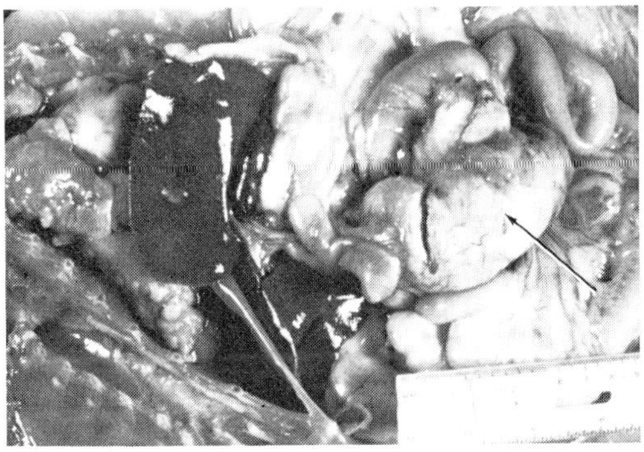

Fig 28. Alimentary lymphosarcoma. Note the enlarged mesenteric lymph node (arrow).

loproliferative disorders (Fig 31). Pancytopenia occurs with myelofibrosis and myelosclerosis. In these cases, trephine biopsy of the bone marrow reveals intramedullary fibrosis.

Feline sarcoma virus-induced fibrosarcomas are not common. Cats 3 years of age or less usually are affected. Although they may occur as a single dermal or subcutaneous mass, usually they are multicentric. The lesion often grows rapidly, ulcerates on the surface and tends to recur soon after surgical removal. The head is a common site of tumor growth. Diagnosis is established by excisional biopsy, with a histologic diagnosis of fibrosarcoma, combined with a positive blood test for FeLV.

Non-Neoplastic Diseases: Thymic atrophy is a degenerative disease of the lymphoid tissues in neonatal kittens caused by transplacental infection or infection early in life with FeLV from an infected queen. The FeLV apparently destroys the developing T-lymphocytes in the thymus. The affected kitten has a defective cell-mediated immune response, rendering it highly susceptible to other infectious diseases. These affected kittens literally fade away. They do not gain weight and tend not to nurse vigorously. Hence the term "fading kitten syndrome." Death usually occurs within a few weeks of birth. Necropsy reveals little or no thymic tissue and microscopically there is atrophy of the thymus. Because thymic atrophy may also be induced by panleukopenia virus, FIP and possibly other infections, it is not, in itself, diagnostic of FeLV infection.

The so-called "panleukopenia-like" form of FeLV infection is a myeloblastopenia. The disease resembles panleukopenia, hence the name. Clinical signs include diarrhea, which may be hemorrhagic, vomiting, severe depression and anorexia. Examination of the peripheral blood reveals severe leukopenia (100-3000 WBC/mm^3) and, in contrast to findings in panleukopenia, often an anemia. This syndrome often is difficult to distinguish from feline panleukopenia unless it occurs in a cat adequately immunized against feline panleukopenia.

Degenerative diseases of the erythroid elements are perhaps the most common and confusing diseases of FeLV infection. Although FeLV-induced erythroblastosis (regenerative anemia) is rare in cats, the most common form of anemia induced by FeLV infection is nonregenerative anemia (erythroblastopenia). Either of these forms may terminate in pancytopenia (aplastic anemia), in which all hematopoietic cells, erythroid precursors, granulocytes and megakaryocytes are reduced in numbers. Affected cats are listless and the mucous membranes are pale. Fever is variable. The total WBC count may be normal or increased in cases of erythroblastopenia or erythroblastosis; however, it is markedly decreased in the pancytopenic form of the disease. An FeLV-induced erythroblastosis is marked by a regenerative response, ie, polychromasia, anisocytosis, poikilocytosis and increased numbers of reticulocytes and nucleated RBC in peripheral smears. An FeLV-induced erythroblastopenia produces a nonregenerative anemia, characterized by few or no reticulocytes or nucleated RBC and no polychromasia in peripheral blood smears. Hemobartonellosis and autoimmune hemolytic anemia cause regenerative anemia, whereas FIP causes nonregenerative anemia. However,

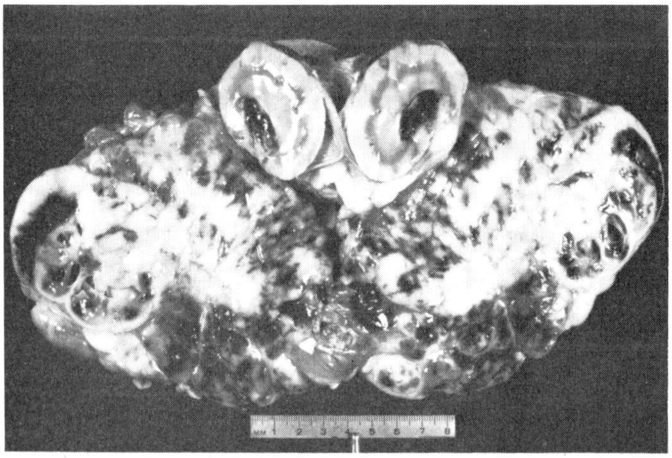

Fig 29. Cut surface of a kidney affected by lymphosarcoma.

in all patients with anemia, the possibility of FeLV infection must be strongly considered.

Infertility, fetal resorption or abortion late in gestation is very common in catteries containing cats infected with FeLV. A dramatic reduction in the number of kittens born in a cattery is a strong indication that the FeLV status of the cats should be assessed. The FeLV is thought to damage the maternal-fetal attachment *in utero*, leading to death and resorption or occasionally abortion of the fetuses.[149]

At least 2 immune-complex diseases associated with FeLV infections have been described: glomerulonephritis and autoimmune hemolytic anemia.[146] More FeLV-infected cats probably die as a result of chronic diseases caused by FeLV-induced immunosuppression than from lymphosarcoma, myeloproliferative disease or FeLV-induced degenerative diseases.[125,129] There is no doubt that FeLV infection induces immunosuppression of cell-mediated immunity.[150] As a result of this immunosuppression, cats infected with FeLV are more susceptible to and suffer more severe responses to hemobartonellosis, chronic nonresponsive gingivitis, recurrent abscesses, fever, septicemia, FIP, toxoplasmosis, chronic upper respiratory infections and the like. Although FeLV does not cause these infections, it does render the infected cat more susceptible to secondary infection because of its immunosuppressive effects.

Diagnosis: Diagnosis of FeLV infection should be based on the clinical findings, plus cytologic or histologic examination of body fluids and tissues. Diagnosis of lymphosarcoma requires a combination of blood studies, bone marrow aspiration or biopsy and cytologic examination of other fluids or tissues. Myeloproliferative diseases usually are diagnosed by a combination of blood and bone marrow examinations. Cytologic or histopathologic study of sections from splenic red pulp or the liver may be helpful because these organs often are involved in myeloproliferative diseases. In cases of nonregenerative anemia, panleukopenia-like syndrome, thymic atrophy or other degenerative processes associated with FeLV infection, a definitive diagnosis cannot be made. Only presumptive diagnoses can be made on the basis of the history, possibility of exposure, clinical signs and laboratory findings.

The indirect fluorescent antibody (IFA) test, performed by experienced personnel with properly prepared specific antisera, enables accurate identification of FeLV antigen in blood smears of infected viremic cats. When properly performed, the IFA test is sensitive, reliable and specific for FeLV. The test detects specific FeLV antigens rather than antibody to FeLV. A positive result means that the cat is infected (viremic) with FeLV. Although this is not a specific diagnostic test for any disease, the IFA test can aid in diagnosis of FeLV infection when other laboratory examinations are inconclusive.

An enzyme-linked immunosorbent assay (ELISA) has been developed to provide practitioners with a rapid, sensitive method to test for the FeLV antigen in blood, saliva, secretions or excretions of cats suspected of harboring FeLV.[151] Although there is some controversy regarding the use of ELISA, if properly performed by experienced personnel, the ELISA is more sensi-

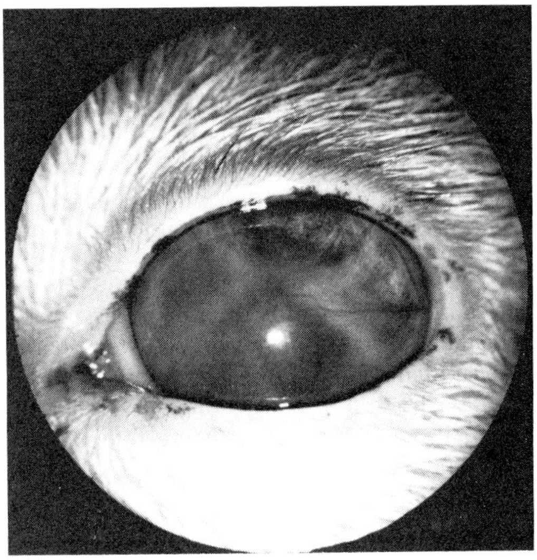

Fig 30. Ocular lymphosarcoma.

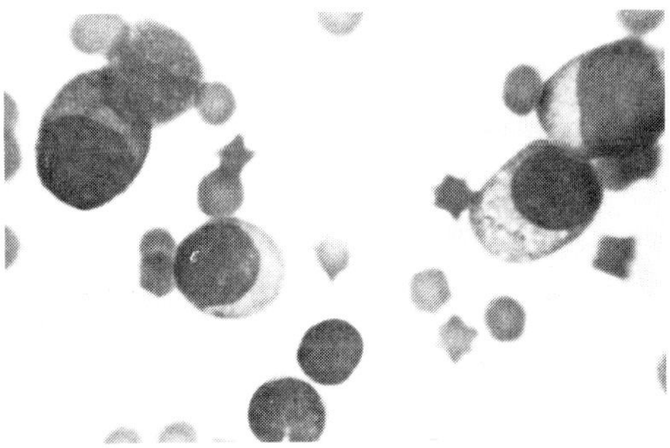

Fig 31. Blood smear from a cat with reticuloendotheliosis. Note the large, bizarre cells with eccentric nuclei.

tive than the indirect fluorescent antibody test for the detection of FeLV antigen.

A cat may be infected with FeLV and not have a positive IFA test or ELISA. This is not a false-negative reaction but an indication that the cat was not viremic when the test was run. A cat may be infected with FeLV, have a positive IFA test or ELISA, and be asymptomatic. This is not a false positive reaction because the cat is infected and possibly shedding the virus. The IFA test and ELISA thus enable detection of healthy FeLV carrier cats and aid in prevention of FeLV transmission.

Treatment: A positive diagnosis of FeLV infection, whether based on cytologic evaluation, virus isolation, or IFA test or ELISA, should not automatically dictate a recommendation for euthanasia. Both the short-term and long-term prognoses for the patient should be discussed in detail with the client.

It is not within the scope of this chapter to detail the treatment protocols for all of the various types of disease that occur within the feline leukemia complex. Detailed discussions of treatment protocols can be found in chapters dealing with the various organ systems and in the references cited in this chapter.[146,147]

Although progress is being made in efforts to convert asymptomatic FeLV-positive cats or FeLV-positive cats in clinical remission to an FeLV-negative status by appropriate immunotherapy, it is too early to predict the long-term results of such therapy.[143]

Prevention: Although progress is being made in development of an FeLV vaccine, such a vaccine probably will not be available for at least several more years. Any comments on the efficacy of the vaccine or a vaccination program would be inappropriate at this time.

Until an effective vaccine is available, the following suggestions for the control of FeLV infection can be made:

1. All FeLV-infected cats, whether healthy or sick, should be isolated from other cats. Euthanasia is an alternative. If the owner elects to have the cat treated, it should be isolated from other cats as described below.

2. All cats with diseases known to be caused by FeLV (lymphosarcoma, myeloproliferative diseases, nonregenerative anemia, panleukopenia-like syndrome, thymic atrophy) should be isolated from healthy cats. Euthanasia is an alternative if the owner wishes. The recommendations for cats with leukemia but not proven to harbor the FeLV are the same as for FeLV-infected cats. This is based on the consideration that most cats with leukemia are viremic with FeLV or may become viremic and potential shedders of the virus.

3. Cats infected with FeLV should not be allowed to contact other cats and should be confined indoors.

When a case of FeLV infection is diagnosed in a multiple-cat household or cattery, the other cats on the premises should be tested and the positive cats should be handled as suggested for the original cat. The FeLV-negative cats should be tested in 3 months and at appropriate intervals as long as additional cats are IFA or ELISA positive.

Since cats can be transiently infected with FeLV, final recommendations concerning disposition of infected cats should not be made until a persistent viremia is proven. If a cat is positive on 2 tests at intervals of 3 months, it can be assumed with a sufficient degree of reliability that the cat is persistently viremic.

In multiple-cat households (not catteries), the decision to test the remaining cats is up to the owner. The owner may decide to consider them as infected and to isolate them, or he may have them tested. An FeLV test (IFA or ELISA) and an anti-FOCMA antibody test should be done. If the remaining cats are FeLV negative and anti-FOCMA antibody positive (greater than 1:8), or FeLV positive regardless of the anti-FOCMA antibody titer, the originally infected cat may be safely returned to the household. If FeLV-negative cats with non anti-FOCMA antibody are found in the household, infected cats should not be returned. The owners should be advised not to bring new cats into the household until all FeLV-positive cats have been removed. A 30-day interim period should be observed.

When an FeLV infection is diagnosed in a cattery, the other cats on the premises should be tested and the positive cats should be handled as suggested for the original cat. The remaining negative cats should be retested in 3 months and at appropriate intervals as long as additional cats become positive. The owners should be advised to test all incoming cats and to quarantine them for 3 months and retest them. No cats should be allowed into the cattery until the post-quarantine test is negative. Although this procedure is not perfect, it has been very effective in clearing a cattery of FeLV infection.

Perhaps as many as 30-50% of all cats are infected with the FeLV "provirus," are negative to FeLV tests and show no signs of disease. It is possible that under conditions of stress, the "provirus" in such cats could initiate virus replication or cell transformation and a cat would then become FeLV positive or diseased and a potential shedder of FeLV. Cattery owners should be warned of such possibilities so that a false sense of security is not developed after a single FeLV-negative test of the cats in the cattery. The proven value of a "test and removal program" in FeLV-infected catteries should be strongly stressed to cattery owners.

FeLV Infection and Human Disease: No relationship has been shown between FeLV and human disease. New and more sensitive methods may be developed for detection of such a relationship. Although there is no cause for alarm, it seems prudent to advise that women of child-bearing age and children should avoid close contact with cats infected with FeLV or showing signs of an FeLV-associated disease.

OTHER MULTISYSTEMIC INFECTIONS

Toxoplasmosis
by P. Derrick

Although toxoplasmosis is not a viral disease, it is included in this chapter because of its multisystemic effects.

Many serologic surveys, epidemiologic studies and current reviews confirm a high rate of *Toxoplasma* infection in people and animals.[153] More than a third of the world's population have antibodies, indicating past infection with *Toxoplasma gondii*. Still, clinical infections are relatively uncommon.

Life Cycle: Toxoplasma is a coccidian parasite and, like most other coccidia, has an enteroepithelial cycle in a specific host, resulting in the formation of oocysts. Before 1970, gaps existed in our knowledge of the life cycle. With identification of the fecal stage of *T gondii* in the cat as coccidian oocysts, a major gap in the life cycle has been filled.[154] Other studies have since added much to our understanding.[155-159]

The various stages and types of *Toxoplasma* organisms have been placed into 5 major categories.[155] Three of these stages occur only in the feline enteroepithelial cycle: enteroepithelial multiplicative stages (types A through E organisms), the gametocyte stage, and the oocyst stage (Fig 32).[160] The fourth and fifth stages occur in the extraintestinal (tissue) cycle in intermediate as well as feline hosts: the tissue group stage formed during acute infection (tachyzoites) and the tissue cyst stage formed during chronic infection (bradyzoites).

Details of asexual reproduction (schizogony) and sexual reproduction (gametogony and sporogony) have been described in detail.[155,157,158]

The life cycle consists of the enteroepithelial phase and the systemic phase. The cat is the only known definitive host (having both sexual and asexual stages in the same animal). All other animals harboring *Toxoplasma* are intermediate hosts with only asexual stages. In the cat, the asexual ȧnd sexual stages occur in the intestinal mucosa (enteroepithelial phase) and result in the formation of oocysts, which are shed in the feces. The oocysts are not infective when first shed, but must mature and sporulate. This process takes 2-5 days and results in an oocyst that is 12 x 10 μ in diameter, with 2 sporocysts containing 4 sporozoites in each sporocyst.[155]

Oocyst production lasts about 14 days and can result in the shedding of millions of oocysts in a single stool. Cessation of oocyst production is generally concurrent with development of immunity to *T gondii*.[159] Oocyst production commences with the cat ingesting sporulated oocysts from fecal contamination or infected tissue (such as an infected mouse) containing zoites.[155,157,158]

The prepatent period (time elapsed until oocysts appear in the feline feces) after ingestion of cysts (bradyzoites) is only 3-5 days, but it is 5-10 days or longer after ingestion of tachyzoites and 20-24 days or longer after ingestion of oocysts. Cats can occasionally shed oocysts a second time (recrudescent infection). This is tied closely to the cat's immunity.

Oocysts may remain infective if kept moist and cool. Freezing, drying and high temperatures decrease infectivity. Environmental influence can be observed in the geographic distribution frequency of infections with *Toxoplasma*. Warm, moist temperate climates, as opposed to freezing or hot, dry climates, are more conducive to viability. These influences can be seen in the local epizootiology of the organism also. Dry cat litter, which absorbs moisture, helps reduce the viability of oocysts. Uncovered, moist children's sand boxes are a potential hazard when infected cats are around.

Concurrent with the sexual phase of oocyst production in the cat is the asexual stage, which is responsible for the generalized or systemic infection. After infection of the intestinal epithelium, the deeper tissue layer, the lamina propria, becomes involved and the tachyzoites (asexual) are spread by the portal circulation to the liver, through the venous circulation to the lungs and into the arterial circulation, to be distributed throughout the body. Lymph from the lamina propria also carries the tachyzoites to the lymph nodes and, by way of the thoracic duct, to the heart and lungs as another means of systemic spread. After systemic spread, the organism may encyst (bradyzoites) in the tissues and the animal enters a chronic or carrier stage. The tachyzoite stages that have found their way throughout the system originally infect the animal through ingestion of the sporulated oocysts, ingestion of tachyzoites from another animal with an acute infection, or ingestion of bradyzoites encysted in tissues of a chronic carrier. This is the familiar form of the disease that occurs in people and many other host species in addition to felids.

A partial list of naturally infected animal species in which the organism has been found illustrates the broad spectrum of intermediate hosts: wombats, moles, shrews, hedgehogs, gondi (the North African rodent in which the organism was first discovered), a variety of mice, rats, guinea pigs, rabbits, squirrels, chinchillas, marmots, dogs, foxes, cats, swine, sheep, cattle, elk, moose, pigeons, chickens and various primates, including people.

Toxoplasma tachyzoites have been found in milk from infected women, as well as from cows, goats, sheep, pigs, dogs, cats, rabbits, guinea pigs and mice.[156] This is another avenue of infection. Possible venereal transmission in goats was evidenced by prolonged excretion of *Toxoplasma* in semen.[161]

Clinical Signs: Important manifestations of acute feline toxoplasmosis are fever, interstitial and alveolar pneumonia accompanied by dyspnea, hepatitis and associated bilirubinemia, adenitis (mainly in mesenteric lymph nodes), and sometimes myositis and myocarditis.[159] When it occurs, diarrhea may be mucoid and bloody. Strong immunity develops in cats that recover but the disease can be fatal. Acute disease with clinical signs is rare in cats; most infections are asymptomatic and result in shedding of oocysts.

In subacute and chronic infections, leukopenia, anemia, retinochoroiditis, iritis and encephalitis may occur. Oocyst shedding usually has ceased by the time these signs appear, and the tissues have also developed viable and persistent cysts (bradyzoites). Occasionally bradyzoite cysts rupture, causing hypersensitivity responses that lead to necrosis. These lesions occur mainly in the brain, retina and heart. Intestinal smooth muscle granulomata are seen occasionally in older cats with recurrent toxoplasmosis. These can lead to intestinal obstructions and have been attributed to decline in immunity associated with aging.

In people, toxoplasmosis is easily mistaken for other ailments. Frequently it causes a slight fever, "washed-out" feeling and swollen lymph glands, much like a case of "flu" or infectious mononucleosis. A few unfortunate people may suffer heart attacks, blindness or damage to the brain or other parts of the CNS.[162]

The most serious danger to people is congenital toxoplasmosis, which is passed on by the mother during the last 5-6 months of pregnancy. Severe birth defects, including blindness and brain damage, stillbirths and possibly miscarriages may occur in toxoplasmosis. Many congenitally infected people do not have physical abnormalities but carry the encysted form of the organism throughout life in a harmless cyst in their tissues. Occasionally, sometimes years after birth, the cysts rupture, and the parasites invade and destroy body cells, especially in the nervous system.[162]

*Treatment:**[163,164] Indications for treatment are clinical signs and lesions of toxoplasmosis, whereas the mere presence of antibody without illness does not necessitate treatment. Acute infection in most cats is asymptomatic and followed by immunity. However, very young kittens, aged cats and those with debilitating diseases or immunosuppression may develop toxoplasmosis with illness. Prophylactic treatment might be considered to prevent oocyst shedding by an indoor cat returning after an escapade during which infected birds or rodents may have been eaten. Once oocyst shedding has started, therapy is less effective.

Optimal treatment combines the synergistic action of sulfamerazine (or sulfamethazine, sulfamethoxazol or sulfadiazine) and pyrimethamine (Daraprim:Wellcome). The sulfonamide

---

*by J.K. Frenkel

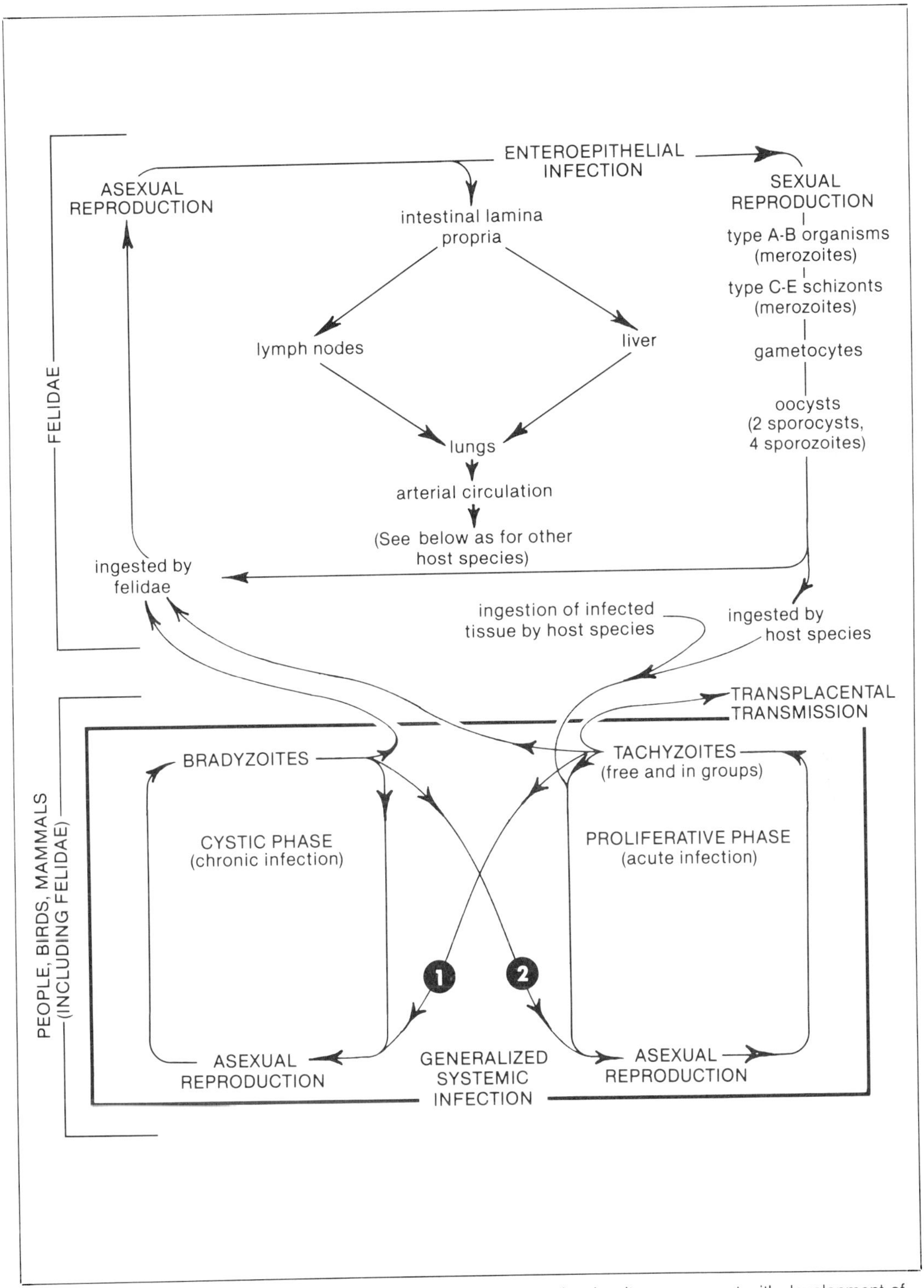

Fig 32. Life cycle of *Toxoplasma gondii*. 1. Tachyzoites encyst as bradyzoites concurrent with development of immunity. 2. Upon ingestion of tissues containing cysts, tachyzoites proliferate. Waning immunity or immunosuppression may convert a chronic latent infection to an active one.

dosage is 60-120 mg/kg daily in 4 divided doses. The sulfonamide can be given alone at the higher dose. The pyrimethamine dosage is 0.5-1.0 mg/kg once daily. The larger dose of pyrimethamine is used as a loading dose during the first 3 days of therapy. Both drugs are effective by mouth, but IV preparations can be used, such as sodium sulfamerazine. Use of sulfonamides not tested by sensitivity tests for efficacy against *Toxoplasma* should be avoided in that only those that reach a high intracellular concentration are effective. Pyrimethamine has a bitter taste and should be given by gavage with canned meat.

Treatment is continued until signs of illness subside. With prolonged treatment, WBC and platelet counts should be determined. If these are markedly reduced, folinic acid (Leucovorin:Lederle), at 1 mg/kg daily PO, or fresh bakers' yeast, at 100 mg/kg daily PO, can be added to the treatment regimen without harm.

Public Health Guidelines: Many reports have created widespread concern about toxoplasmosis in people, especially pregnant women. Many cats have met an untimely death because of the threat, real or imagined, that cats could be a source of infection in people. However, the direct role of cats in the transmission of toxoplasmosis is very difficult to substantiate. An indirect role for fecal contamination of soil with oocysts and eventual transmission to people by soil contact or through the food chain (people consume meat of herbivores) is plausible and has supportive evidence.[165] Recommendations for prevention of toxoplasmosis in people, especially pregnant women, include:[155]

1. Heat meat throughout to 66 C (151 F) before eating.
2. Wash hands after handling raw meat.
3. Feed indoor cats only dry, canned or boiled food and prevent them from hunting.
4. Flush cat feces down the toilet and scald litter pans daily, or incinerate disposable litter trays daily.
5. Cover children's sand boxes when not in use and dispose of contaminated sand as required.
6. Wear gloves when handling litter pans and contaminated soil. Pregnant women should not change cat litter pans at all.
7. Avoid cats whose food source is unknown (emphasized for pregnant women).
8. Control numbers of cockroaches, flies, stray cats and rodents.

Periodic fecal examination and serologic surveillance of cats are not effective in detecting the infectious shedding period of infective oocysts.[166] Control of diet is the only effective and practical method of preventing infection in cats.[166] Oocysts are resistant to acids, alkalies and common disinfectants but are killed by heat and by 10% ammonia.[167]

The hypothetical degree of vulnerability of pregnant women with pet cats has been reported.[168] The following situations are generalizations to which exceptions may occur. The highest degree of vulnerability to infection with *Toxoplasma* occurs when the woman has no *Toxoplasma* titer nor does her cat but exposure to *Toxoplasma* may have occurred. Both the woman and the cat have no antibody protection and are completely susceptible. In most of these situations, the woman and cat are healthy, and no infection should occur if proper preventive management is maintained. However, if the cat is ill but has no titer, it could have acute toxoplasmosis and could be shedding oocysts. The titer would only begin to slowly rise after the dangerous period of oocyst shedding has ceased.

In a situation of lesser vulnerability, the woman has no titer but the cat does. The cat has previously been infected and has gained some immunity. By this time the oocyst shedding state has passed. The cat has immunity to further infection unless immunosuppressed for some reason and a recrudescent infection occurs. The woman is in danger because she is susceptible to oocyst contamination from the environment. If a recrudescent infection occurs, oocysts can again be shed. Also, a cat not shedding oocysts but with an acute systemic infection may, upon close contact, (sneezing or coughing), infect the woman by active tachyzoite spread.

In a situation of least vulnerability, both the woman and her cat have a stable titer. In this case both woman and cat have immunity against further reinfection. If the woman was immune before pregnancy, the fetus should be protected. If the titer was obtained during pregnancy, there could be possible danger to the fetus.

Serologic Testing[155]

Serologic tests for detecting toxoplasmosis include the Sabin-Feldman dye test and the indirect fluorescent antibody (IFA) test.[169,170] These 2 tests detect early antibodies of the IgM class and are positive 8-10 days after *Toxoplasma* infection.[171,172] They also detect antibodies of the IgG class (past infection).

The indirect hemaglutination (IHA) test and the complement-fixation (CF) test detect antibodies that appear 14 days or more after *Toxoplasma* infection.[172-174] The CF test titers indicate recent or active infection and usually disappear within 1-2 years, whereas the IFA, IHA and dye test titers usually persist indefinitely after infection.[172]

There has been misunderstanding concerning the significance of various antibody titers and the differences in titers between people and animals. Cats develop titers to *T gondii* more slowly than do other animals.[175] Emphasis should be placed upon paired titers and a 4-fold titer increase in cats. In people, low titers (1:4 on CF test, 1:64 on IFA, IHA and dye tests) generally indicate past infection, intermediate titers (1:8 on CF test, 1:256 on other tests) indicate recent infection, and high titers (1:32 on CF test, 1:1024 or 1:4096 on other tests) suggest active or recent infection.

Negative titers in sick animals should be interpreted cautiously. The initial serum sample, although negative, may have been obtained during early infection, when the cat was actively shedding oocysts. For this reason, another serum sample should be evaluated 2-3 weeks later.

In general, as the antibody titer rises, the cat gains immunity to further infection. By the time the titer reaches protective level, the cat is no longer shedding oocysts. However, the humoral (serum) antibody titer does not reflect the entire immune system since cell-mediated responses are also active. The latter have not been evaluated in toxoplasmosis.

Animals with protective titers and that ingest infective oocysts and/or tissue forms normally do not become reinfected. However, recrudescence may occur in stressed or immunosuppressed animals through conversion of encysted bradyzoites to proliferative tachyzoite (Fig 32). Such animals become ill and again shed oocysts.

Serologic methods of differentiating IgM from IgG make testing more valuable. Various methods for IgG and IgM determinations have been used for *Toxoplasma* testing.[170,171] Antibody profiles in people with toxoplasmosis have been published.[172-175]

References

1. Remlinger, P. Ann L'Inst Past **17** (1903) 834.
2. Aujeszky, A. Zbl Bakt **132** (1902) 353.
3. Verge, J and Cristoforoni, N. C Soc Biol Paris **99** (1928) 312.
4. Hindle, E and Findlay GH. J Comp Path Therap **45** (1932) 11.
5. Leasure, J *et al.* No Am Vet **15** (1934) 30.
6. Lawrence, J and Syverton, J. Proc Soc Exp Biol **38** (1938) 914.
7. Baker, JA. J Exp Med **79** (1944) 206.
8. Hamre, D and Rake G. J Inf Dis **75** (1944) 206.
9. Blake, FG *et al.* Yale J Biol Med **15** (1942) 139.
10. Fastier, LB. Am J Vet Res **18** (1957) 382.
11. Bolin, VS. Virol **4** (1957) 389.
12. Crandell, RA and Maurer, FO. Proc Soc Exp Biol **97** (1958) 487.
13. Crandell, RA and Madin, SH. Am J Vet Res **21** (1960) 551.
14. Bittle, JL *et al.* Am J Vet Res **21** (1960) 547.
15. Kahn, DE. Vet Clin No Am **1** (1971) 313.
16. Scott, FW *et al.* Am J Vet Res **31** (1970) 11.
17. Scott, FW. Cat Fancy **12(10)** (1969) 9.
18. Scott, FW. JAVMA **158** (1971) 944.
19. Cello, RM. Am J Ophth **43** (1957) 296.
20. Pedersen, NC. Feline Pract **6(3)** (1976) 42.
21. Feldman, BM. JAVMA **144** (1963) 1409.
22. Holzworth, J. Cornell Vet **53** (1963) 157.
23. Ward, JM. Virol **41** (1970) 191.
24. Horzinek, MC and Osterhaus, ME. J Sm Anim Pract **19** (1978) 623.
25. Pedersen, NC *et al.* Am J Vet Res **42** (1981) 368.
26. McKiernan, AJ *et al.* Feline Pract **11(3)** (1981) 16.
27. Jarrett, WFH *et al.* Nature **202** (1964) 567.
28. Magrassi, F *et al.* Boll Soc Ital Biol Sper **27** (1951) 1233.
29. Povey, in Kirk: Current Veterinary Therapy VI. WB Saunders, Philadelphia, 1977.
30. Rich, LJ *et al.* Cornell Vet **61** (1971) 542.
31. Fabricant, CG and Gillespie JH. Inf Immun **9** (1974) 460.
32. Fabricant, CG *et al.* Cornell Vet **59** (1969) 667.
33. Moses, HF. JAVMA **119** (1951) 213.
34. Fashay, in Hull: Diseases Transmitted from Animals to Man. 4th ed. Charles C Thomas, Springfield, IL, 1955.
35. Hardy, WD Jr *et al.* Nature **224** (1973) 266.
36. Scott, FW. Am J Vet Res **41** (1980) 410.
37. Crandell, RA. Adv Vet Sci Comp Med **17** (1973) 201.
38. Laughlin, in Kirk: Current Veterinary Therapy VII. WB Saunders, Philadelphia, 1980.
39. Bistner, SI *et al.* JAVMA **159** (1971) 1223.
40. Hover, EA and Griesemer, RA. JAVMA **158** (1971) 929.
41. de Lahunta, A. Veterinary Neuronanatomy and Clinical Neurology. WB Saunders, Philadelphia, 1977.
42. Bohning, RH *et al.* JAVMA **156** (1970) 611.
43. Edwards WC. VM/SAC **63** (1968) 696.
44. Tomlinson, MJ and Schench, NL. JAVMA **167** (1975) 927.
45. Ford, RB. Comp Cont Ed **1** (1979) 337.
46. Orr, CM *et al.* Vet Rec **103** (1978) 200.
47. Orr, CM *et al.* Vet Rec **105** (1980) 164.
48. Clark, WB *et al.* VM/SAC **75** (1980) 415.
49. Davis, EV and Beckenhauer WH. Norden News **52** (1977) 30.
50. Scott, FW. Feline Pract **5(1)** (1975) 17.

51. Flicknell, PA *et al.* Vet Rec **104** (1979) 313.
52. Gillespie, DH and Scott, FW. Adv Vet Sci Comp Med **17** (1973) 163.
53. Hoover, EA and Kahn, DE. JAVMA **166** (1975) 463.
54. Kahn, DE and Hoover, EA. Vet Clin No Am **6** (1976) 599.
55. Kalunda, M *et al.* Am J Vet Res **36** (1975) 353.
56. Evermann, JF *et al.* Canine Pract **8(2)** (1981) 36.
57. Stein, in Kirk: Current Veterinary Therapy VII. WB Saunders, Philadelphia, 1980.
58. Ott, in Catcott: Feline Medicine and Surgery. 1st ed. American Veterinary Publications, Santa Barbara, 1964.
59. Hong, C. Master's thesis, Cornell Univ, 1970.
60. McKercher, DG. Am J Vet Res **14** (1953) 105.
61. Schacter, J *et al.* Lancet **1** (1969)1063.
62. Cello, RM. JAVMA **158** (1971) 968.
63. Kolar, JR and Rude, TA. VM/SAC **76** (1981) 1171.
64. Negri, A. Z Hyg Infek Kr **43** (1903) 507.
65. Beamer, PD. Am J Vet Res **21** (1960) 507.
66. Constantine, in Nagano and Davenport: Rabies. University Park Press, Baltimore, 1971.
67. Johnson, in Nagano and Davenport: Rabies. University Park Press. Baltimore, 1971.
68. Constantine, DG Publ Health Rep. **77** (1962) 287.
69. Vaughn, JB. J Am Med Assoc **184** (1963) 705.
70. Anon. Ohio Dept Health Newsletter **67(9)** (1960) 3.
71. Kogher, IJ and Bernkopf, H. Br J Exp Path **24** (1943) 15.
72. Communicable Disease Summary. Vol XII No. 43, Oregon State Board of Health, Portland, 1963.
73. Mitchell, FE and Monlux, WS. Am J Vet Res **23** (1962) 435.
74. Szlachta, HL and Habel, RE. Cornell Vet **42** (1953) 207.
75. Anon. JAVMA **178** (1971) 16.
76. Bruner, DW and Gillespie, JH: Hagen's Infectious Diseases of Domestic Animals. 6th ed. Cornell Univ Press, Ithaca, 1973.
77. Galloway, LA. Vet Rec **50** (1938) 745.
78. Pedersen, NC *et al.* Proc 41st Ann Conv AAHA, 1974.
79. Hardy, in Hardy *et al.* Feline Leukemia Virus. Elsevier/North-Holland, New York, 1980.
80. Evermann, JF *et al.* JAVMA **177** (1980) 1132.
81. Johnson, RH. Vet Rec **76** (1964) 1008.
82. Goss, L. Am J Vet Res **9** (1948) 65.
83. Csiza, CK *et al.* Am J Vet Res **32** (1972) 419.
84. Rokovsky, MW and Fowler, EH: JAVMA **158** (1971) 872.
85. Gochenour, WS. No Am Vet **24** (1943) 104.
86. Lawrence, J *et al.* Am J Path **16** (1940) 333.
87. Kilham, L *et al.* JAVMA **158** (1971) 888.
88. Langkeinrich, KA and Nielson, SW. JAVMA **158** (1971) 863.
89. Carpenter, JL. JAVMA **158** (1971) 857.
90. Schalm, OW: Veterinary Hematology. Lea & Febiger. Philadelphia, 1961.
91. Irwin, WF. Vet Med **45** (1950) 353.
92. Cello, RM. JAVMA **158** (1971) 861.
93. Enders, JF and Hammon, WD. Proc Soc Exp Biol **43** (1940) 194.
94. Snodgrass, DR *et al.* Vet Rec **104** (1979) 222.
95. Scott, FW and Gillespie, JH. Vet Clin No Am **1** (1971) 231.
96. Gillespie, JH *et al.* JAVMA **158** (1971) 835.
97. Scott, FW *et al.* JAVMA **156** (1970) 439.
98. Wolfe, LG and Griesemer, RA. Path Vet **3** (1966) 255.
99. Robison, RL *et al.* JAVMA **158** (1971) 981.
100. Horzinek, MC and Osterhaus, ADME. Am J Vet Res **40** (1979) 1487.
101. Ward, JM. Virol **44** (1970) 191.
102. Horzinek, MC *et al.* Zbl Vet Med B **24** (1977) 398.
103. Pedersen, NC *et al.* Arch Virol **58** (1978) 45.
104. O'Reilly, KJ *et al.* Vet Rec **104** (1979) 348.
105. Black, JW. VM/SAC **75** (1980) 811.
106. Evermann, JF *et al.* Vet Path **18** (1978) 256.
107. Osterhaus, ADME. Zbl Vet Med B **25** (1978) 301.
108. Weiss, RC and Scott, FW. Am J Vet Res **42** (1981) 382.
109. Pedersen, NC and Boyle, JF. Am J Vet Res **41** (1981) 868.
110. Horzinek, MC and Osterhaus, ADME. Arch Virol **59** (1979) 1.
111. Ott, RL. Paper presented at 4th Ann Symp World Assoc Vet Microbiol Immun Spec Infect Dis, Alfort, France, 1977.
112. Pedersen, NC. Am J Vet Res **37** (1976) 1449.
113. Loeffler, DG *et al.* Fel Pract **8(1)** (1978) 43.
114. Hardy, WD Jr and Hurvitz, AI. JAVMA **158** (1971) 994.
115. Doherty, MJ. JAVMA **159** (1971) 418.
116. Scott, FW *et al.* Fel Pract **9(1)** (1979) 44.
117. Wolf, LG and Griesemer, RA. JAVMA **158** (1971) 987.
118. Slauson, DO and Finn, JP. JAVMA **160** (1972) 729.
119. Weiss, RC and Scott, FW. Fel Pract **10(2)** (1980) 16.
120. Hardy, WD Jr and O'Reilly, WJ. JAVMA **155** (1969) 1728.
121. Abel, DL and Johnson, JJ. Fel Pract **5(2)** (1975) 44.
122. Madewell, BR *et al.* JAVMA **172** (1978) 169.
123. Ott, RL, Washington State Univ: Unpublished data, 1982.
124. Scott, FW. JAVMA **175** (1979) 1164.
125. Cotter, SM *et al.* JAVMA **166** (1975) 449.
126. Scott, DW *et al.* JAAHA **9** (1973) 530.
127. Mackey, L. Vet Rec **96** (1975) 5.
128. Essex, M *et al.* Infect Immun **11** (1975) 470.
129. Bech-Nielsen, S *et al.* JAAHA **17** (1981) 759.
130. Snyder, SP and Thielen, GH. Nature **221** (1969) 1074.
131. Gilmore, CE and Holzworth, J. JAVMA **158** (1971) 1013.
132. Dorn, CR *et al.* Am J Vet Res **28** (1967) 993.
133. Brody, RS *et al.* Bibl Haemat **36** (1970) 333.
134. Schneider, R *et al.* Cancer Res **27** (1967) 1316.
135. Cotter, SM *et al.* Cancer Res **34** (1974) 1061.
136. Hardy, WD Jr *et al.* Nature **224** (1973) 266.
137. Essex, in Klein: Viral Oncology. Raven Press, New York, 1980.

138. Francis and Essex, in Hardy *et al:* Feline Leukemia Virus. Elsevier, New York, 1980.
139. Jarret, in Hardy *et al:* Feline Leukemia Virus. Elsevier, New York, 1980.
140. Pedersen, NC *et al.* Am J Vet Res **38** (1977) 1523.
141. Grant, CK *et al.* Cancer Res **40** (1980) 823.
142. Hoover, EA *et al.* J Nat Cancer Inst **57** (1976) 365.
143. Ott, RL, Washington State Univ: Unpublished data, 1982.
144. Francis, DP *et al.* Cancer Res **39** (1979) 3866.
145. Theilen, GH *et al.* Proc 43rd Ann Mtg AAHA, 1976.
146. Olson, RG. Feline Leukemia. CRC Press, Boca Raton, FL, 1981.
147. Theilen, GH and Madewell, BR: Veterinary Cancer Medicine. Lea & Febiger, Philadelphia, 1979.
148. Hardy, WH Jr *et al:* Feline Leukemia Virus. Elsevier, New York, 1980.
149. Hardy, WD Jr. JAAHA **17** (1981) 941.
150. Perryman, LE *et al.* J Nat Cancer Inst **49** (1972) 1357.
151. Kahn, DE *et al.* Feline Pract **10(2)** (1980) 41.
152. Derrick, P. Vet Ref Lab Newsletter **5(2,3)** (1981) 1.
153. Frenkel, JK. Bio Science **23** (1973) 343.
154. Frenkel, JK *et al.* Science **167** (1970) 893.
155. Jones, SR. JAVMA **136** (1960) 1038.
156. Frenkel, in Hammond and Long: Coccidia: Eimeria, Isospora, Toxoplasma and Related Genera. Univ Park Press, Baltimore, 1973.
157. Dubey, JP and Frenkel, JK. J Protozool **9** (1972) 155.
158. Hutchinson, WM *et al.* Tr Roy Soc Trop Med Hyg **65** (1971) 380.
159. Jacobson, in Kirk: Current Veterinary Therapy VII. WB Saunders, Philadelphia, 1980.
160. Dubey, JP. Am J Vet Res **40** (1979) 1634.
161. Dubey, JP and Sharnma, SP. Am J Vet Res **41** (1980) 794.
162. Anon: Questions and Answers About Toxoplasmosis. AVMA, Schaumburg, IL, 1971.
163. Frenkel, in Kirk: Current Veterinary Therapy VI. WB Saunders, Philadelphia, 1977.
164. Frenkel, JK. Curr Topics Path **54** (1971) 28.
165. Reif, JS. Comp Cont Ed Pract Vet **6** (1980) 810.
166. Frenkel, JK. J Infect Dis **126** (1972) 664.
167. Dubey, JP *et al.* J Parasit **56** (1970) 447.
168. Krick, J and Remington, J. N Engl J Med **298** (1978) 550.
169. Anon: Serodiagnosis of Toxoplasmosis, Rubella, Cytomegalic Inclusion Disease, Herpes Complex. HEW Immunology Series #5, US Govt Printing Office, Washington, DC, 1974.
170. Johnson, RB and Libby, R. J Clin Microbiol **10** (1980) 451.
171. Pyndiah, N *et al.* J Clin Microbiol **9** (1979) 170.
172. Carmago, ME *et al.* Rev Inst Med Trop S Paulo **18** (1976) 215.
173. Carmago, ME and Leser, PG. Rev Inst Med Trop S Paulo **18** (1976) 227.
174. Carmago, ME *et al.* Rev Inst Med Trop S Paulo **20** (1978) 41.
175. Carmago, ME *et al.* Infect Immun **21** (1978) 55.

5

systemic mycoses

M.H. ATTLEBERGER

Causes

With the exception of cryptococcosis, systemic mycoses are rare in cats. The etiologic agents involved are dimorphic. The tissue or parasitic form is a yeast (*Histoplasma capsulatum*, *Blastomyces dermatitidis* and *Sporothrix schenckii*) or a spherule (*Coccidioides immitis*). Their saprophytic form in nature is mycelial. Because some contaminants closely resemble some of these fungi morphologically and microscopically, both forms should be isolated when culturing; if only the mycelial form is isolated, then they should be converted to the parasitic form.

Some opportunistic fungi, present as contaminants, may invade the tissues of immunodeficient or debilitated animals. The aspergilli and phycomycetes are often opportunistic pathogens.

Clinical Signs

A fungal infection should be considered or suspected if one or more of the following signs are present: chronic disease that fails to respond to treatment; chronic nasal discharge; granulomas; pale mucous membranes; enlarged lymph nodes; draining or nondraining fistulous tracts; abscesses that heal and recur; and shallow ulcers. Most of the infections occur when spores are inhaled or enter through wounds.

Diagnosis

The success of treatment frequently depends upon a rapid diagnosis. With the exception of sporotrichosis, nearly all of these infections may be tentatively diagnosed in the practitioner's laboratory by direct smears, especially if skin lesions and enlarged lymph nodes are present. Examination of skin lesions, nasal discharge, pus, transtracheal washings and especially lymph node biopsies may be made in 20% KOH or 20% KOH with Parker's ink (Parker Pen Co.) under the low or high-dry objective of the microscope. The ink-KOH combination outlines the fungus, thus aiding in identification. An India ink and water preparation should be used in suspected cases of cryptococcosis and a gram stain for nocardiosis and actinomycosis. Smears for histoplasmosis from lymph node biopsies or peripheral blood in severe cases should be stained with an appropriate hematologic stain.

Except for sporotrichosis, the diseases discussed here are not considered transmissible.

Systemic Mycoses

Cryptococcosis

Cause: Cryptococcosis is caused by the encapsulated yeast *Cryptococcus neoformans*, which occurs worldwide, and is generally considered the most common systemic mycosis of cats.

The organism is frequently associated with pigeon nests and roosts. It passes through the gut of the pigeon but does not affect the pigeon, probably because of its body temperature of 42 C (107.6 F). The yeast survives but does not grow at 44 C (111.2 F) and remains viable for 2 or more years in moist or desiccated pigeon excreta. Increased humidity enhances its survival in sheltered sites not in contact with soil, such as barn lofts and attics. *Cryptococcus neoformans* is usually nonencapsulated in its saprophytic environment and becomes virulent after it acquires a capsule.[1]

In people the disease frequently is associated with leukemias, debilitating diseases and diseases in compromised hosts after drug therapy, especially with immunosuppressants.[1]

It is not known if benign infections occur in cats or if cats recover from systemic infections. Cats are affected by respiratory, cutaneous, neurologic and ocular forms. One or more syndromes may occur in the same cat.

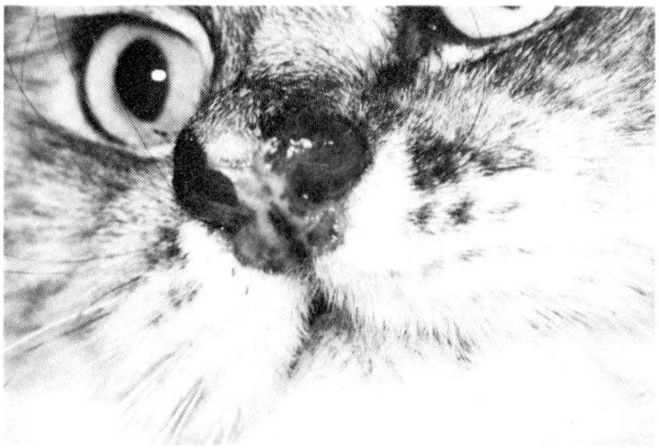

Fig 1. Swollen nose and granulomas in a cat with cryptococcosis.

Clinical Signs: Infection is usually chronic and associated with a great variety of signs.[2-10] Affected cats may show a weight loss, pale mucous membranes, listlessness and fever. Cryptococcosis should be suspected if chronic rhinitis is present. Respiratory signs include sneezing, snuffling, nasal discharge, swelling over the bridge of the nose, and granulomatous tissue in the nasal cavity (Fig 1). Inappetence and firm, enlarged lymph nodes also may be present.

Muscular incoordination, paralysis and blindness are evidence of neurologic involvement.

Ocular involvement, if present, may be an extension of neurologic involvement. One cat with progressive pupillary dilation, on examination of the eye, had mydriasis, pupillary areflexia, bilateral papilledema and retinal hemorrhages.[6] Another cat had a light-yellow mass in the anterior chamber of the left eye, with peripheral corneal vascularization and aqueous flare. Several small and 2 large masses with focal hemorrhages were seen in the right retina. The aqueous and vitreous humor of both eyes contained inflammatory exudate.[7]

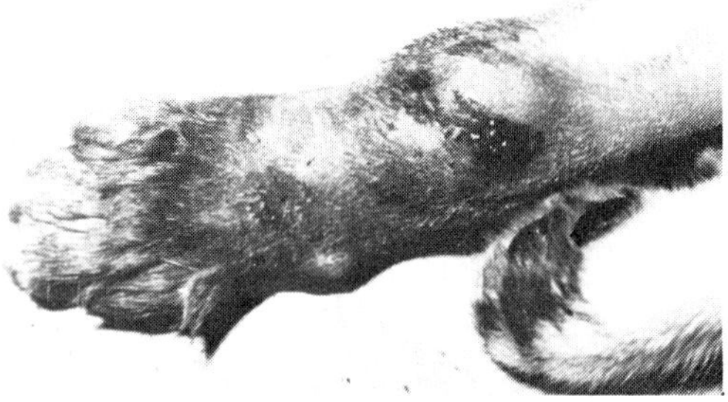

Fig 2. Single subcutaneous abscess in localized cryptococcosis.

There may be single or multiple cutaneous lesions, such as abscesses or ulcerated tumor lesions (Fig 2). The exudate is frequently mucoid.

Diagnosis: Exudates, scrapings from granulomas, CSF and other tissues should be examined in India ink and water preparations for encapsulated yeasts (Fig 3). Occasionally yeasts may be nonencapsulated. The above may be performed in the practitioner's laboratory but specimens for culture and identification should be sent to a diagnostic laboratory for confirmation.

Serologic tests, such as the tube agglutination test for antibody, the slide latex agglutination test for antigen, and the direct fluorescent antibody test, are available.

Treatment: Treatment for systemic cryptococcosis often fails although there have been some reports of success.[9,12-14] It involves many weeks of IV injections and is costly. Localized cutaneous cryptococcosis, however, responds to treatment.

Amphotericin B (Fungizone:Squibb) is the drug of choice. A polyene antibiotic, it binds sterols to the cell membrane, resulting in leakage of the cell content. Unfortunately, it also causes nephrotoxicosis, hypokalemia and anemia.[11]

A fluorinated pyrimidine, 5-fluorocytosine (Ancobon:Hoffman-La Roche), which acts by inhibiting nucleic acid synthesis, has been used in conjunction with amphotericin B. It is well absorbed from the intestines but may cause bone marrow depression, especially in people with underlying lymphoreticular disorders. It also may cause mild hepatotoxicosis, especially with preexisting liver disease. Because the drug is excreted through the kidneys, the dosage should be reduced if the patient's renal function is impaired. Unfortunately, cryptococci often develop resistance to 5-fluorocytosine.[11]

A cat with a nasal tumor, which caused chronic discharge and sneezing, was treated IV with amphotericin B at 0.3 mg/kg body weight 3 times a week intermittently because of BUN elevations.[9] Biopsies during treatment showed progressively fewer and then finally no cryptococci. There was no recurrence over 3 years. Another cat treated showed signs of improvement initially but finally was euthanized.

Amphotericin B has been used successfully in combination with 5-fluorocytosine to treat a cat with nasal involvement.[12] Over a 30-minute period, 1.7 mg amphotericin B (0.5 mg/kg) dissolved in 17 ml 5% dextrose in water (0.1 mg amphotericin B/ml) were given IV, followed by 150 ml lactated Ringer's solution. This was administered 3 times weekly on an outpatient basis. This cat also was given 375 mg 5-fluorocytosine PO daily (100 mg/kg/day) in 3 divided doses every 8 hours. Treatment continued 32 days. Serum creatinine and BUN concentrations were determined before each treatment. Serum K content and glutamic-pyruvic transaminase activity were determined every 2 weeks and a hemogram was obtained weekly. Treatment was stopped when the BUN reached 70 mg/dl and the serum creatinine reached 4.8 mg/dl. The cat had an initial latex agglutination titer for antigen of 1:16, which decreased to 1:1 after treatment. This test has diagnostic and prognostic values, especially when several samples are assayed.

Cryptococcosis has been treated successfully with amphotericin B at 1 mg/day in 10 ml 5% dextrose and water injected rapidly IV 3 times a week.[13] Healing was evident at 2 weeks and the dosage was reduced to 0.25-0.50 mg/day depending on BUN level. Because of depression, anorexia and a BUN level above 70 mg/dl, treatment was discontinued for 10 days. The feet, which were also infected, were treated with amphotericin B cream. Treatment was stopped when impression smears showed no organisms and all lesions were well epithelialized. When a new ulcer appeared on the foot, treatment was begun again and continued until the cat was normal. The entire treatment period was 4 months and the cat received a total of 16.25 mg amphotericin B. Although the cat was polydipsic and polyuric during treatment, it usually ate and generally seemed well, and was normal 20 months after treatment.

A cat with a nasal granuloma was treated initially with 5-fluorocytosine at 125 mg/kg divided BID.[14] The lesion decreased in size after 40 days treatment, then began to enlarge. Clinical signs reappeared even though the dosage of 5-fluorocytosine was increased to 250 mg TID. A new treatment was begun in which 0.25 mg atropine and 1.0 mg piperacetazine were given SC initially, followed 30 minutes later by 2 mg amphotericin B in 5% dextrose given IV, then 100-200 ml 5% dextrose in water given SC. This was repeated 3 times a week for 12 weeks, at which time the cat was asymptomatic and cultures negative. The BUN level ranged from 25 mg/dl to 40 mg/dl, except twice when it was 70 mg/dl and above. Treatment was discontinued at these times and then resumed when BUN levels dropped.

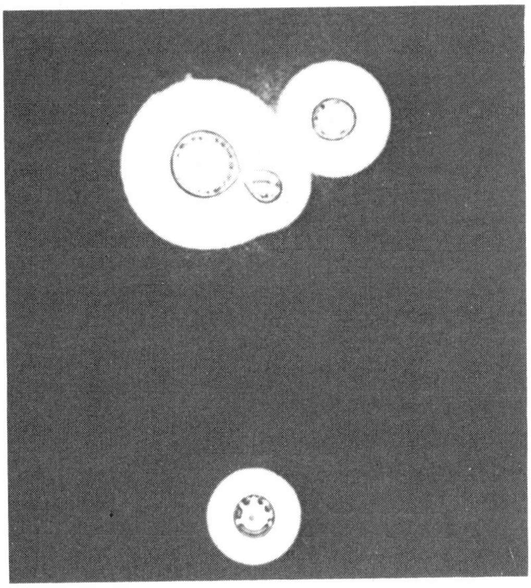

Fig 3. *Cryptococcus neoformans* in nigrosin stain. Note capsules, budding cell and internal granules in yeast. Nigrosin gives a better background than India ink.

The regimen for using amphotericin B in cats at the Auburn University Small Animal Clinic is to dilute the amphotericin B powder with 20 ml diluent, then administer 0.8 mg amphotericin B added to make a volume of 10 ml with 5% dextrose in water, injected slowly IV over 5 minutes every 3-4 days. Treatment is continued until signs regress and cultures are negative. Lactated Ringer's solution is used to aid in reducing high BUN levels. One cat with a localized abscess was treated successfully. Another cat with nasal granulomas in both nares and swelling over the bridge of the nose responded favorably at first. The granulomas disappeared from the nares and the bridge of the nose returned to normal. Cultures always grew cryptococci and the latex agglutination test for antigen was over 1:1064. Lesions in the nares returned and the cat failed to respond to further treatment.

Blastomycosis

Cause: Blastomyces dermatitidis, a dimorphic fungus, is the etiologic agent of blastomycosis. In the US, the enzootic areas follow the drainage pattern for the Mississippi and Ohio River basins, and to some extent the Missouri River. The enzootic area also extends into sections of Manitoba and Ontario, Canada. Another enzootic area in western New York and eastern Ontario follows the St. Lawrence River through Quebec.[1] Isolation from soil is rare and the natural habitat is not definitely known. Spores are inhaled but wound infection must be considered as a mode of infection. Benign cases may occur but proof of this is lacking.

Clinical Signs: With the respiratory form of blastomycosis there is dyspnea, nasal discharge and occasionally coughing and sneezing. Slight to dry, pronounced rales, fever, listlessness and emaciation may occur.[15,16]

Paronychial infection, which began as a red papule with a serosanguineous discharge, was the only lesion in one cat.[17] Body temperature, pulse rate and respiratory rate were normal and there was no lymphadenopathy.

Cutaneous blastomycosis was detected in a cat presented for vaccination, at which time a small puncture wound was noted in the right foreleg.[18] Several weeks later the leg had enlarged to 3 times its normal diameter and had multiple fistulous tracts with a serosanguineous discharge. The cat became lethargic, anorectic and the body temperature was 39 C (102.2 F). The leg was amputated and the cat made an excellent recovery, ate well and gained weight. Radiographs showed no lung involvement and no other treatment was given.

Diagnosis: Exudates, transtracheal washings and skin scrapings should be examined in 20% KOH or 20% KOH and Parker's ink for large, thick-walled budding yeasts with internal structure and a broad base where the bud attaches to the mother cell. Plates should be held several weeks when culturing and both the yeast and mycelial phase should be recovered to confirm the presence of *B dermatitidis.*

An agar-gel and a complement-fixation test are available but results may be misleading. Therefore, samples for culture should always be obtained. Diagnosis should not be made on the basis of serologic results alone.

Treatment: If infection is systemic, use of amphotericin B may be beneficial. Systemic treatment may not be needed but the cat should be closely monitored if there is a localized or primary cutaneous infection. The following treatment was given to the cat with paronychial infection. The cat was considered "cured" but the possibility of spontaneous healing was considered.[17] For 4 days, 325 mg potassium iodide solution (Fisher) were given IV once daily as a bolus injection. The dose was decreased to 195 mg for the next 7 days, and for the final 7 days of treatment, 325 mg potassium iodide were given PO as tablets.

The prognosis is guarded to poor in systemic blastomycosis but fair to good in localized or primary cutaneous infection.

Histoplasmosis

Cause: Histoplasmosis is caused by the dimorphic fungus, *Histoplasma capsulatum.* In the US, the highly enzootic area is the eastern part of the country, especially the Ohio-Mississippi River Valley. The organism is found in association with avian and bat roosts. Spores (2-5 μ) sprout when inhaled into alveolar spaces, then transform into yeasts, which are found in cells of the reticuloendothelial system. Wind, birds and bats aid in dissemination of spores. The disease is rare in cats but there has been an increase in reported cases in the past 5 years. Benign cases may occur. In a study on 50 cats in Virginia, *H capsulatum* was isolated from 22 cats, primarily from the peribronchial and cervical lymph nodes but also from abdominal organs.[19] The organism was isolated from 4 of 6 pregnant cats and from 5 of 11 cats that recently had delivered kittens. The cats showed no agglutinins or complement-fixing antibodies.

Clinical Signs: Respiratory distress is one of the most common signs reported. Cats may show dyspnea, abdominal respiration or rapid, shallow respiration. Respiratory signs in some cats are not severe. Some have a nasal discharge and may have a nonproductive cough. Pale mucous membranes, indicating anemia, are present in most cases. Depression, lethargy, emaciation and dehydration may be seen. Some cats have a rapid pulse and the body temperature is elevated in most cases. Lymphadenopathy, hepatomegaly and splenomegaly occur in some disseminated cases. Cutaneous and subcutaneous granulomatous lesions with draining tracts may be present. Lameness may occur.[19-23] Choroiditis in the posterior segment of the eye and bilateral granulomatous chorioretinitis have been reported.[23] Radiographs show diffuse miliary opacities throughout the lung.

Diagnosis: The tissue or parasitic phase of *H capsulatum* is a small, intracellular yeast found in the macrophages. Peripheral blood from severely affected cats or a biopsy of an enlarged lymph node stained with a hematologic stain may contain the intracellular yeasts. Transtracheal washings and urine, centrifuged and the sediment stained, may be examined also. Any of the above specimens are suitable for culture, which may involve up to 6 weeks' incubation.

Specimens for culture should be kept refrigerated because yeasts die rapidly at room temperature. The agar-gel and/or complement-fixation tests may be tried.

Treatment: Treatment is generally not successful but amphotericin B may be tried. The prognosis is poor and affected cats usually die or are euthanized.

Coccidioidomycosis

Cause: Coccidioides immitis, a dimorphic fungus, appears as a spherule with endospores in the tissues and in the mycelial form in nature. The highly enzootic areas are the southwestern US and northern Mexico, and some areas in Central and South America. It is a soil organism, often associated with rodent burrows, where it can survive. Windstorms, construction work, farming and digging in contaminated soil result in dust aerosols, thus spreading the spores that may be inhaled or enter through skin lesions.[1]

Clinical Signs: Primary cutaneous coccidioidomycosis occurred in a cat with an abscess lanced on the left rear foot.[24] Three weeks later, several draining tracts, with a serosanguineous exudate, opened up on the medial side of the foot, followed by induration and multiple draining tracts in the left popliteal and ischial areas. The cat's appetite, activity, CBC and serum blood chemical profile were normal. Radiographs showed no pulmonary or bone involvement. The precipitin test was positive and the complement-fixation test negative, which would indicate no dissemination. The cat was observed for 1 month with no treatment and 1 month later, the draining tracts had disappeared and the enlargement in the popliteal area had decreased. Results of serologic examination remained the same.

Disseminated coccidioidomycosis was observed in a 4-year-old spayed female that developed an abscess between the tuber coxae and tuber ischii.[25] The cat was anorectic and lost weight but had no fever or abnormal respiratory sounds. After death, organisms were found in the soft tissue, lung and thoracic lymph nodes.

A 3-year-old intact male cat, lame for 3 months, had a persistent cough, progressive weight loss and a firm swelling on the thigh, with 3 openings discharging small amounts of serous exudate.[25] At necropsy, numerous *C immitis* organisms were found in the lungs, thoracic lymph nodes, liver, kidney and subcutaneous tissue.

Diagnosis: Exudate, tissues, transtracheal washings or lymph node biopsies should be examined in 20% KOH or 20% KOH and Parker's ink for spherules with and without endospores. Biopsies for histopathologic examination should be stained with a fungal stain. When handling the mycelial phase after culture, the fungus should be wetted with sterile saline or water prior to microscopic examination to prevent the spread of arthrospores. Reliable serologic tests, the agar-gel test and the complement-fixation test are available.

Treatment: The primary cutaneous form may heal without treatment and prognosis is probably favorable. Use of amphotericin B may be beneficial but the prognosis is poor in the disseminated form.

Sporotrichosis

Cause: Sporotrichosis is caused by the dimorphic fungus, *Sporothrix schenckii,* which is a yeast in the tissues and mycelial in nature. It is found in soil, decaying vegetation, sphagnum moss, wood, water and straw. It has also been isolated from people and the mouth of a normal rat. The organism usually enters through wound contamination. Infected cats are often positive for feline leukemia virus and the Siamese breed appears to be most often infected.

Clinical Signs: Various clinical signs have been reported.[26-29] Cutaneous lesions may be single or multiple and appear as papules, nonhealing ulcers, granulomas or irregular, crust lesions. The hair and skin may slough in some lesions, leaving necrotic areas. Affected cats may appear listless and unkempt but the appetite usually remains good, especially if only cutaneous lesions are present. The body temperature may remain normal or increase to 39 C (102.2 F). Lymph nodes may enlarge but thickening of the lymphatics in cats has not been reported. When the disease progresses and becomes systemic, the cat becomes more depressed, the appetite diminishes and the animal usually dies or is euthanized. Organisms were found in the macrophages in the lamina propria of the palpebral conjunctiva in one cat.[26]

A Siamese cat treated by the author had numerous skin lesions in the form of ulcers, granulomas and a large necrotic area on the foreleg (Fig 4). It was depressed, had a poor appetite and did not respond to treatment with IV sodium iodide. At necropsy, *S schenckii* was isolated

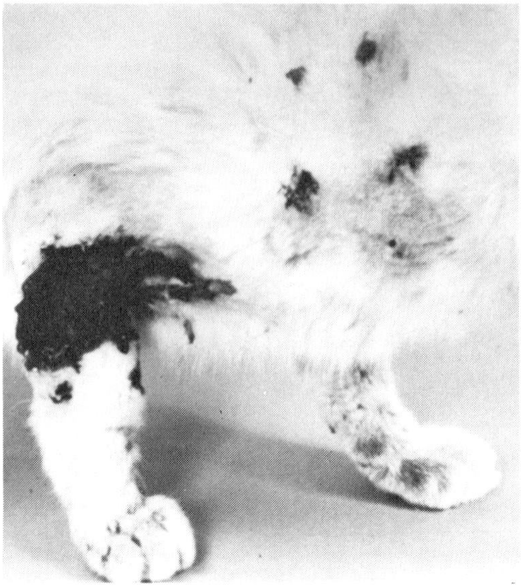

Fig 4. Cat with sporotrichosis, showing scattered cutaneous lesions and large necrotic area on foreleg.

from the lungs and liver. The cat had a positive feline leukemia virus test.

Diagnosis: Stained smears or wet mounts in KOH are unsatisfactory because so few yeasts are present in the exudates. Use of impression smears of cutaneous lesions for fluorescent antibody study is recommended. Diagnosis is frequently made by culture. Both the yeast and mycelial phases should be recovered to confirm the presence of *S schenckii*. Biopsy for histopathologic examination is not recommended as it may result in spread of the infection.

Treatment: Treatment is usually ineffective in disseminated sporotrichosis but amphotericin B should be tried. Potassium iodide is usually not successful and cats may vomit after its use. Topical application of amphotericin B ointment (Fungizone Cream:Squibb) is effective for cutaneous lesions in cats with a good appetite and that appear normal otherwise. Moist hot dressings may help also. Surgery is contraindicated as it may result in spread of the disease.

Transmission: People may develop sporotrichosis just from handling infected cats; a scratch or bite wound is not necessary for infection. A student with a history of allergies handled an infected cat and developed a shallow ulcer on one finger, from which *S schenckii* was isolated. At no time was he bitten or scratched. Care should be taken in handling infected cats; gloves should be worn and hands washed thoroughly.

Aspergillosis and Phycomycosis

Cause: Panleukopenia virus infection may be a predisposing factor to infection with the aspergilli or phycomycetes. Both groups are ubiquitous, frequently found as contaminants on laboratory culture media. Spores are inhaled and swallowed daily. Mycotic pneumonia and mycotic enteritis or colitis are probably secondary infections to the panleukopenia.

In a review of 9 cases of aspergillosis and phycomycosis in cats, the diseases were associated with panleukopenia in 7 cases, hookworms in 1 case and an upper respiratory tract infection in the other case.[30]

Clinical Signs: Clinical signs include anorexia, lethargy, depression, nasal discharge, coughing and sneezing. Mucous membranes are pale, the body temperature may rise to 41 C (105.8 F), and conjunctivitis occurs. Vomiting and diarrhea may lead to dehydration.[30-34]

Diagnosis: Diagnosis of aspergillosis and phycomycosis is usually made during histopathologic examination of tissues obtained at necropsy; the fungi frequently are not identified. Direct scrapings of necrotic areas or granulomas found in lung or intestine should be examined in KOH for hyphae. Pieces of tissue should be submitted for culture before the rest is placed in formalin for histologic examination. Because these fungi are frequent contaminants on culture media, proof of tissue invasion must be made by direct smears or histopathologic examination.

Nocardiosis and Actinomycosis

Cause: The aerobic actinomycetes most frequently involved in animal infections are *Nocardia asteroides, N brasiliensis* and *N caviae*. They are found in soil, occur worldwide and enter the body through inhalation or skin lesions.

Some pathogenic anaerobic actinomycetes naturally inhabit the oral cavity. The habitat of others is unclear.

Clinical Signs: A 5-year-old castrated male cat had several abscesses and lacerations typical of cat-bite wounds on the left hindfoot.[35] A month later, fistulous openings had developed on the hip of the lame leg. During this time the cat had not responded to antibiotics. It was hospitalized 1 month later and failed to respond to antibiotics and proteolytic enzymes. Microscopic examination of pus revealed branching filaments and a tentative diagnosis of actinomycosis was made. However, the organism was later identified as *N brasiliensis*. The cat did not respond to further treatment and died. Icterus and bilirubinuria were observed just before death.

A 4-year-old cat infected with *N asteroides* was anorectic, constipated and had a body temperature of 41 C (105.8 F) for 2 weeks.[36] Three weeks later there was thoracic pain, listlessness and the body temperature decreased to 38.5 C (101.3 F). Radiographs revealed lung lesions and an increased amount of thoracic fluid. The cat was euthanized.

Three cases of nocardiosis in cats have been seen at Auburn University. *Nocardia asteroides* was isolated from wounds caused by trauma from a fan belt in one cat and from a subcutaneous mass and draining tracts in another cat. In the third case, a 4-year-old cat first developed abscesses on the skin of the thorax, with subcutaneous tracts. One week later, tracts had developed on the abdominal area. *Nocardia brasiliensis* was isolated from the lesions.

A case of actinomycosis in the spinal canal of a cat has been reported.[37] A 15-month-old male was presented with hindleg weakness, depression and poor appetite of 3 days' duration. One month previously an abscess had developed at the base of the tail but the abscess was now considered healed. The cat was hyperesthetic when touched anywhere along the dorsum, abdomen or rear legs. Within 48 hours the cat had improved with no treatment and was returned to its owners. Four days later the cat was returned with hindleg paraplegia. A myelogram showed a diffuse extradural mass causing spinal cord compression. At surgery an extradural fatlike mass, lightly adhered to the spinal cord dorsad and extending around to the right side, was removed. The cord was not involved. Bacteriologic examination of swabs taken from the affected tissue yielded an *Actinomyces* sp. On histopathologic examination, a single bacterial colony containing gram-positive rods was seen. The authors felt the findings were compatible with actinomycosis. The cat regained neurologic function after surgery and chloramphenicol was dispensed. The animal recovered uneventfully.

Diagnosis: Exudates should be gram stained and examined under oil for gram-positive, branching, beaded filaments, which are suggestive of nocardiosis and actinomycosis. If the above are seen, a Hank's or Kinyoun acid-fast stain should be made. Some *Nocardia* organisms are acid-fast, some are partially acid-fast and some are not acid-fast, as are the *Actinomyces*. An organism should not be judged as *Nocardia* on the basis of this stain alone.

Culturing is necessary to positively identify the organism. Exudate should be examined carefully for small flakes or granules, which are colonies of *Nocardia* or *Actinomyces*. These should be cultured on blood agar and/or brain-heart infusion agar at 35 C (95 F) under aerobic, microaerophilic and anaerobic conditions. Another set of plates should be incubated at room temperature. Cultures should be held at least 2-3 weeks. Inclusion of flakes is essential when culturing. In several instances in our laboratory, the exudate alone did not yield organisms. As soon as growth is visible, it should be gram stained and examined for filaments and coccobacillary forms. It is essential to differentiate *Nocardia* sp from other actinomycetes since the recommended treatments are different.

Serologic tests are available for diagnosis of nocardiosis.

Treatment: Nocardia organisms are sensitive to sulfa drugs; large doses of penicillin are preferred for actinomycosis. Chloramphenicol also may be used to treat actinomycosis. Single, localized lesions that do not contain numerous tracts may be removed surgically. Wounds may be flushed with triple-sulfa solutions.

Nocardial empyema in one cat was treated successfully using pleural lavage and antibiotics.[38] After aspiration of the thoracic exudate, a mixture of 50,000 IU penicillin G and proteolytic enzyme (Kymar:Armour) was infused into the thoracic cavity. Procaine penicillin G (20,000 IU/lb IM) and sulfadimethoxine (12 mg/lb PO) were given once daily. Supportive therapy included vitamin supplementation and lactated Ringer's solution as warranted by the state of hydration. When thoracentesis samples were clear and pleural exudation ceased, the cat was sent home with sulfadimethoxine to be given PO for 2 months. The cat was normal a year later.

References

1. Rippon, J: Medical Mycology—The Pathogenic Fungi and the Pathogenic Actinomycetes. 1st ed. WB Saunders, Philadelphia, 1974.
2. Trautwein, G and Nielsen, SW. JAVMA **140** (1962) 437.
3. Clark, L and Roubin, GS. Aust Vet J **46** (1970) 544.
4. Johnson, LAY *et al.* Aust Vet J **39** (1963) 306.
5. Lau, RE *et al.* VM/SAC **66** (1971) 777.
6. Wanner, RA and Baird, JD. N Zeal Vet J **22** (1974) 78.

7. Gwin, RM *et al.* JAAHA **13** (1977) 680.
8. Rutman, MA *et al.* Feline Pract **5(3)** (1975) 36.
9. Palumbo, NE and Perri, S. VM/SAC **70** (1975) 553.
10. Wilkinson, GT. J Sm Anim Pract **20** (1979) 749.
11. Abernathy, RS. Medicine **52** (1973) 385.
12. Weir, EC *et al.* JAVMA **174** (1979) 507.
13. Thall, MA *et al.* Feline Pract **3(5)** (1976) 15.
14. Barrett, RE and Scott, DW. JAAHA **11** (1975) 511.
15. Jasmine, AM *et al.* VM/SAC **64** (1969) 33.
16. Sheldon, WG. Lab Anim Care **16** (1966) 280.
17. Easton, GL. Can Vet J **2** (1961) 350.
18. Campbell, KL *et al.* Feline Pract **10(3)** (1980) 28.
19. Rowley, DA *et al.* J Inf Dis **95** (1954) 98.
20. Weissman, S and Acampado, EE. Feline Pract **5(5)** (1975) 28.
21. Breitschwerdt, EB *et al.* JAAHA **13** (1977) 216.
22. Mahaffey, E *et al.* JAAHA **13** (1977) 46.
23. Gwin, RM *et al.* JAVMA **176** (1980) 638.
24. Wolff, AM. JAVMA **174** (1979) 504.
25. Reed, RS *et al.* JAVMA **143** (1963) 953.
26. Werner, RE *et al.* JAVMA **159** (1971) 407.
27. Anderson, NV *et al.* JAAHA **9** (1973) 526.
28. Anon. Animal Disease Trends. Ohio Dept Disease Trends. Ohio Dept Ohio Dept 31. McCausland, IP. N Zeal Vet J **20** (1972) 10.
32. Saulter JH *et al.* JAVMA **127** (1955) 518.
33. Pakes, SP *et al.* JAVMA **151** (1967) 950.
34. Stokes, R. Aust Vet J **49** (1973) 499.
35. Ajello, L *et al.* JAVMA **138** (1961) 370.
36. Langham, RF *et al.* MSU Vet **19** (1959) 102.
37. Stowarter, JL *et al.* Feline Pract **8(1)** (1978) 26.
38. Campbell, B and Scott, DW. JAAHA **11** (1975) 769.

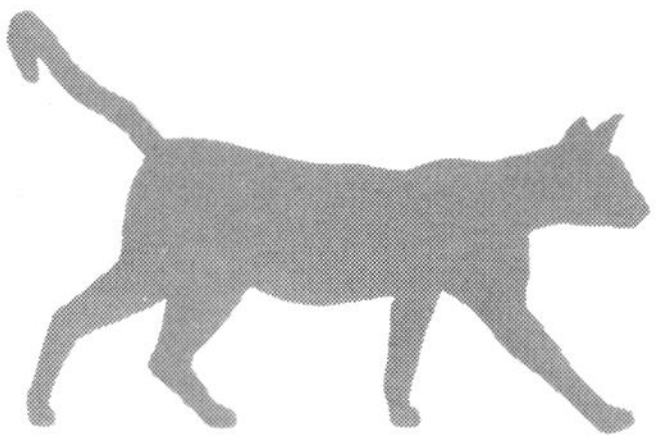

6

the blood and blood-forming organs

J. BLUE

Diseases of the hematopoietic system are frequently encountered in feline patients, largely due to the ubiquitous feline leukemia virus (FeLV) that plagues this species. Diseases of other systems, moreover, frequently are reflected by hematologic abnormalities. To the clinician armed with an understanding of normal hematopoiesis and the expected response to stimuli and injuries, the hematologic evaluation can provide clues into the nature of disease in many patients and guide the steps toward a correct assessment of the condition. Without an examination of the formed elements in blood, clinicians are seriously handicapped in their efforts to diagnose problems and manage them appropriately. In this chapter, emphasis is placed on the pathogenetic mechanisms of hematologic abnormalities and on the key features that aid in recognition of their significance. A great deal of information concerning regulation of hematopoiesis has been produced in recent years. Because this information is fundamental to understanding hematopoietic responses, a review of the anatomy and physiology of hematopoietic tissue is included.

ANATOMY AND PHYSIOLOGY OF HEMATOPOIETIC TISSUE

Anatomy of Bone Marrow[1-3]

Hematopoiesis in postnatal life is localized in the bone marrow, a tissue uniquely specialized to harbor hematopoietic stem cells and permit the growth, differentiation and orderly release of their progeny. Although the spleen of the adult cat contains a few megakaryocytes and scattered foci of erythropoiesis, extramedullary hematopoiesis does not normally contribute many cells to circulating blood. Hematopoietically active marrow in adults of most species, including cats, is restricted to the bones of the axial skeleton and the proximal ends of long bones. In conditions of great and persistent need for blood cells, hematopoiesis is extended into the shafts of the long bones and, to some extent, into the liver and spleen.

Bone marrow consists of a system of venous sinuses and hematopoietic cords lying between them (Fig 1). The blood supply of the marrow is derived from arterial vessels that pass through bone before entering the marrow and connect with sinuses, which subsequently empty into the large veins that leave the marrow. Blood circulating through marrow is separated from hematopoietic tissue by the walls of blood vessels. Newly produced blood cells enter the circulation by passing through the walls of the sinuses. Normally only blood cells at the appropriate stage of maturation are released; however, such conditions as myelofibrosis, metastatic tumor and hematopoietic neoplasms can disrupt sinus walls and allow release of immature blood cells.

Hematopoietic cords consist of a delicate stromal meshwork, macrophages and hematopoietic cells. The meshwork is formed by branched cells called reticular cells, which are a special type of fibroblast. The broad, outstretched cytoplasmic processes of one reticular cell are joined to the branches of other reticular cells and support macrophages and developing hematopoietic cells. Reticular cells next to sinuses extend some of their processes around the sinus endothelium to form an adventitial cover. These adventitial reticular cells can accumulate lipid to become the marrow fat cells. Since the medullary cavity is a fixed space that must be filled, decreased volume of hematopoietic cells is balanced by increased volume of fat cells. Under steady-state conditions of normal hematopoiesis, the ratio of

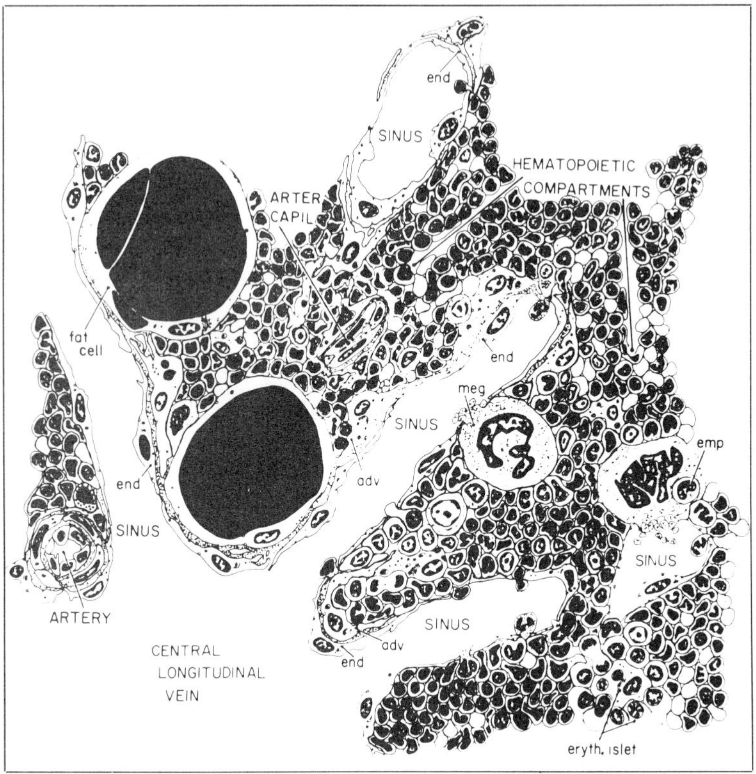

Fig 1. Schematic view of a cross section of bone marrow of a long bone, showing sinuses and cords of hematopoietic tissue.

fat to hematopoietic cells in active marrow is approximately 1:1. This fat is readily mobilized during accelerated hematopoiesis and the ratio decreases. Reticular cells synthesize the small amount of extracellular material in marrow, which constitutes reticular fibers and the basement membrane of sinuses. The extracellular material can be demonstrated in sections of bone marrow by the periodic acid-Schiff (PAS) reaction or by precipitation of silver salts. This PAS- or silver-stained material is called reticulin; an increased amount is called reticulin fibrosis. Mature collagen is not present in normal marrow but is produced in the pathologic condition called myelofibrosis.

Macrophages are integral elements of bone marrow and participate in marrow functions. They store iron and phagocytize defective hematopoietic cells. Macrophages are closely associated with developing erythroid cells in clusters called erythroblastic islets.[4] Erythroblasts are nestled in the surface folds of these voluminous cells. The erythroblast matures in the islet and when it reaches the reticulocyte stage extrudes its nucleus. The extruded nucleus and rim of cytoplasm are then phagocytized by the central macrophage. Defective erythroblasts are phagocytized by their macrophage before they mature. If a large proportion of developing erythroblasts are phagocytized, the condition is called ineffective erythropoiesis. Marrow macrophages also assist in clearing circulating blood of aged or damaged blood cells and other particulate material. Macrophages next to sinuses thrust pseudopodia between endothelial cells into the lumen, where they can be exposed to circulating material. Entire macrophages may lie within the lumen. Because macrophages have access to circulating blood, the bone marrow is one of the organs of the reticuloendothelial system, a functional grouping of the organs, including spleen, liver and lymph nodes, that bear most of the responsibility of removing particulate material (microorganisms, damaged blood cells, injected particles) from circulating blood and lymph. It should be noted that macrophages, endothelial cells and fibroblastic cells are structurally associated in these organs but developmentally unrelated. The term "reticuloendothelial cell" is inappropriate now and dates from the time of light microscopic studies, which were unable to distinguish the cells that ingested particles (macrophages) from the reticular cells and endothelial cells upon which they lay.

The nonhematopoietic cells in marrow help create an environment in which normal hematopoiesis can proceed. The bone marrow provides an ecologic niche necessary for hematopoietic stem cells to express their full capacity for self-renewal.[5] Furthermore, local environmental factors seem to influence the direction of commitment of hematopoietic stem cells.[6,7] A microenvironment capable of supporting hematopoiesis can be created *in vitro* by cultured marrow stromal cells and in extramedullary sites by transplantation of marrow fibroblastic cells.[8,9] In certain strains of mice and in some people with congenital anemia, the marrow microenvironment is defective and unable to support normal hematopoiesis.[10] The hematopoietic cell lines are segregated to some extent within the marrow, probably reflecting the effect of local factors. Megakaryocytes áre located against the walls of sinuses and erythroblasts are concentrated near sinuses.[2] Granulocytopoiesis takes place away from sinuses and is concentrated near bone.[11]

From its position against the sinus wall, a megakaryocyte releases its platelets directly into the sinus lumen.[12] Elongated processes of megakaryocyte cytoplasm penetrate the endothelial cell and break free in the lumen. These long strips, called proplatelets, later fragment to release up to 1200 platelets. Reticulocytes released from erythroblastic islets are temporarily motile and able to reach and penetrate the sinus endothelial cells.[4] Granulocytes become motile as they near full maturation and likewise migrate to the sinus wall and enter the lumen by transendothelial passage.[4] Blood cells cross the sinus wall at areas not covered by adventitial reticular cells. Normally about 60% of the outer surface of the endothelium is covered, but this area can be reduced to 20% during heightened release of cells.[13] Endotoxin and increased erythropoietin concentration can effect a decrease in adventitial cover and enhance release of marrow reticulocytes and granulocytes.[2,14]

Hematopoiesis[15,16]

Hematopoiesis is the process in which mature red cells, neutrophils, eosinophils, basophils, monocytes and platelets are made. The maintenance of appropriate numbers of each type of blood cell results from complex cellular and humoral interactions that regulate proliferation, differentiation and maturation. Lymphopoiesis in the postnatal animal takes place mainly in the lymphoid tissues rather than in bone marrow. However, because lymphocytes circulate in blood and share a progenitor with other blood cells, their production will be briefly discussed in this section. Hematopoiesis is a continuum but can be considered as progressing through 4 major stages represented by the following groups of cells: pluripotential stem cells, hematopoietic and lymphopoietic stem cells, committed precursor cells, and cells in terminal differentiation (Fig 2). A stem cell is a cell with both the capacity to renew itself and the capacity to provide cells for further differentiation to serve the functions of the tissue. Only cells in the first 2 stages fulfill these criteria.

Pluripotential Stem Cells

The pluripotential stem cell can provide precursor cells for both lymphocyte and hematopoietic cell differentiation. The existence of a pool of pluripotential stem cells in mice has been demonstrated, but it is doubtful that a functioning pluripotential stem cell pool exists after birth in people or other animals. The infrequent occurence of coexisting primary disorders of hematopoiesis and lymphopoiesis is circumstantial evidence against a functional pluripotential stem cell in adult animals other than mice.

Hematopoietic Stem Cells

Red cells, granulocytes, monocytes and platelets arise from a common stem cell pool. Cells in this compartment replicate themselves and give rise to daughter cells, which differentiate into cells committed to a single cell line. Most of our knowledge of the biology of hematopoietic stem cells comes from experimental studies in mice. Mouse bone marrow contains cells that reestablish normal hematopoiesis after lethal irradiation. If moderate numbers of bone marrow cells are injected into an irradiated mouse, 10 days later the spleen of the recipient contains discrete colonies of hematopoietic cells. Some of the colonies are mixtures of granulocytes, erythroblasts and megakaryocytes; others contain cells of a single type. If a colony is excised and made into a cell suspension that is injected into another recipient, more colonies are formed, indicating that the original colony contained cells

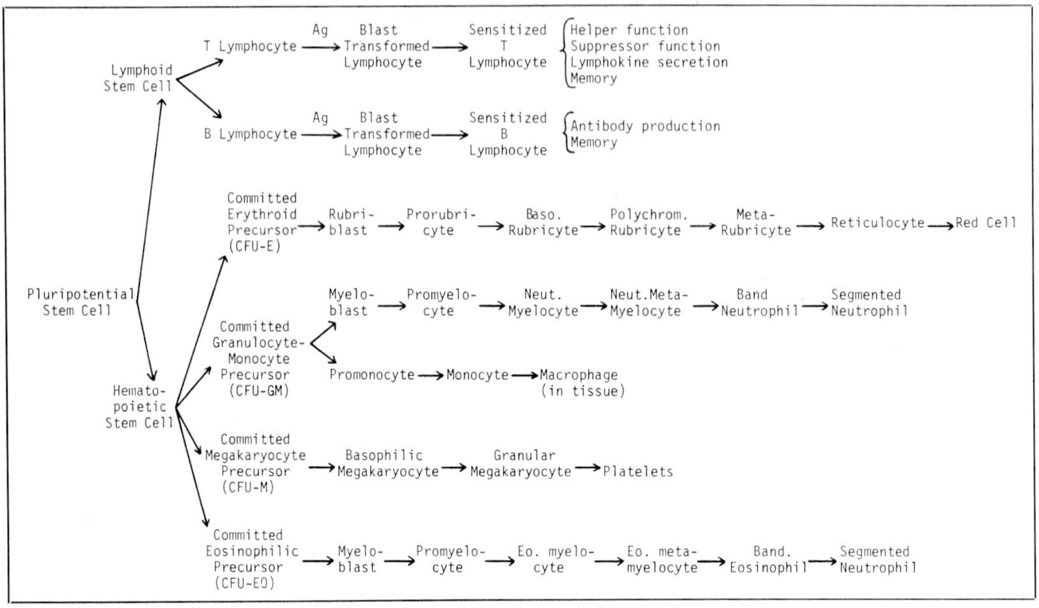

Fig 2. Stages in the production of blood cells.

that could replicate themselves and provide cells for differentiation into all hematopoietic cell lines. The hematopoietic stem cell, as demonstrated in the mouse spleen assay system, is called the colony-forming unit-spleen. Evidence in other species of a hematopoietic stem cell is found in the clonal disorders of hematopoiesis. For example, in people with various neoplastic hematopoietic conditions, the disease may be expressed predominantly in one cell line; however, cytogenetic or enzyme studies demonstrate that cells in other lines originate from the same malignant clone.

Hematopoietic stem cells in normal animals have an unlimited capacity for self-renewal, which can be diminished by irradiation and some cytotoxic drugs.[5] In steady-state conditions, few hematopoietic stem cells are synthesizing DNA; this pool of cells is therefore less susceptible than actively proliferating cells to agents that interfere with DNA synthesis. Hematopoietic stem cells can be induced into rapid proliferation by maneuvers that depopulate the marrow or create sudden demands for differentiated cells. Under such circumstances, hematopoietic stem cells respond by proliferation and increased flow into committed cell compartments to restore normal cell numbers.[5] Day-to-day regulation of blood cell production takes place at more differentiated levels.

Lymphopoietic Stem Cells

Precursor cells that provide cells for differentiation into T- and B-lymphocytes arise in primitive hematopoietic tissue. During fetal development they migrate from the yolk sac to liver and finally to marrow.[17] That this stem cell pool is separate from the hematopoietic stem cell pool is indicted by observations that immune deficiency states in which there is failure to produce both T- and B-lymphocytes are not accompanied by hematopoietic failure.

Committed Precursor Cells

Stem cell progeny that enter the compartment of committed precursor cells are set into a program of differentiation that takes them along one or another of the cell lines. The step from multipotential to committed cell seems to be mediated by humoral factors and local environmental influences that are not yet fully understood. With commitment, cells become responsive to the specific hormones that regulate their proliferation and drive their differentiation. The number of committed precursor cells in marrow is small; amplification in each cell line is achieved by mitotic divisions within this compartment and during later maturation stages. Committed precursor cells have considerable proliferative capacity but cannot maintain their numbers indefinitely as can true stem cells. Committed precursor cells are unrecognizable by morphologic means but their number and behavior can be assessed by their functional ability to produce colonies of differentiated cells when cultured in appropriate media. The cells that produce colonies in culture are called colony-forming units.

There are at least 2, and probably more, intermediate stages of precursor cells committed to the erythroid line. The burst-forming unit-erythroid gives rise to very large colonies of erythroblasts and represents an earlier cell than the colony-forming unit-erythroid, which produces smaller colonies but in a shorter interval. Growth of erythroid colonies requires erythropoietin, a glycoprotein hormone that regulates erythropoiesis *in vivo*. Erythropoietin is produced chiefly in the kidney and released in an inactive form that is activated as it circulates in plasma. Tissue hypoxia sensed by the kidney is the stimulus for increased erythropoietin production. Impaired O_2 delivery to the kidney may result from decreased red cell mass (anemia), decreased O_2-carrying capacity of the hemoglobin molecule, or decreased renal blood flow. Erythropoietin stimulates erythroid-committed cells to proliferate and induces them to enter terminal differentiation, resulting in increased production of red cells.[18] With restoration of normal tissue oxygenation (in the case of anemia, restoration of the normal red cell mass), erythropoietin release and red cell production return to normal.

Other bone marrow cells produce colonies of neutrophilic granulocytes, macrophages or mixtures of both. This cell, the progenitor of blood neutrophils and monocytes, is called the colony-forming unit-granulocyte monocyte. A group of glycoprotein hormones, called colony-stimulating factors, supports proliferation and differentiation of colony-forming unit-granulocyte monocytes.[18,19] The most important physiologic source of colony-stimulating factors seems to be macrophages. The negative arm of the feedback loop controlling neutrophil and monocyte production is in the form of inhibitors, which are derived from macrophages and neutrophils.[10,19] These inhibitors include lactoferrin and other, unidentified substances in neutrophils and prostaglandins from macrophages.

The eosinophil-committed precursor cell is distinct from the colony-forming unit-granulocyte monocyte and probably regulated by factors specific for it.[19] Both T-lymphocytes and macrophages are needed for elaboration of eosinophil colony-stimulating factors. In rats, baseline numbers of eosinophils can be maintained without T-lymphocytes, but appropriately sensitized T-lymphocytes must be present for increased eosinophil production in response to infection by a parasite, such as *Trichinella*.[20]

Megakaryocytes can also be grown in culture from their precursors, the colony-forming unit-megakaryocyte. Regulatory factors have not been defined clearly yet, but a humoral substance, called thrombopoietin, stimulates megakaryocytopoiesis. In general, megakaryocytopoiesis and platelet production are related inversely to total platelet mass.

Culture systems for lymphocyte precursors, analogous to those for hematopoietic cells, are being developed only now. Other methods of investigation have indicated that precursors of T- and B-lymphocytes are present in bone marrow during fetal and neonatal life. It is not clear whether lymphocyte precursors become committed to T- or B-lymphocyte differentiation while still in marrow or whether the commitment is determined elsewhere. For a cell to become a T-lymphocyte, it must travel from bone marrow to the thymus. There, under the influence of thymic epithelial cells, it proliferates and matures to a cell with the functional characteristics of a T-lymphocyte.[17,21] In birds, differentiation of precursor cells into B-lymphocytes takes place in another epithelial organ, the bursa of Fabricius. Bone marrow is probably the functional equivalent of the bursa in mammals.[17,21]

Cells in Terminal Differentiation and Mature Blood Cells

Red Cell Series: The nomenclature system used in this chapter for the various stages of erythroid maturation conforms to that in general use in the veterinary literature. The term "erythroblast" is used as a generic term for all nucleated cells recognizable as belonging to the red cell line of differentiation.

Maturation of erythroblasts from the earliest to the latest stage is associated with a decrease in nuclear size due to progressive condensation of chromatin, a decrease in cell size due to successive cell divisions, and an increase in cytoplasmic acidophilia due to hemoglobin accumulation. At all stages, erythroblasts are decidedly round and have centrally located nuclei, features that help distinguish them from other cells with which they might be confused.

The youngest cell in marrow smears recognizable as an erythroid cell is the rubriblast, a large cell with a rim of deep-blue cytoplasm. The chromatin is coarse but uniformly distributed, and 1-2 nucleoli may be visible. Rubriblasts are scarce in normal marrow and greatly outnumbered by cells in later stages of maturation. This represents amplification resulting from an average of 4 mitotic divisions during the maturation process. An estimated 16 red cells may arise from a single rubriblast. A rubriblast becomes a reticulocyte in approximately 4 days.

The next cell in the sequence is the prorubricyte, which has a slightly denser nucleus and lacks visible nucleoli.

The rubricyte stage includes a spectrum of cells. Early rubricytes, called basophilic rubricytes, are larger and have bluer cytoplasm than later rubricytes, called polychromatophilic rubricytes, which contain enough hemoglobin to impart a grey tint to the cytoplasm. During the rubricyte stage, the chromatin becomes more clumped until at the end of this stage the nucleus has a cartwheel pattern of dark chromatin clumps separated by unstained areas. Early rubricytes divide several times; however, by the end of the rubricyte stage, a critical concentration of hemoglobin is reached and mitosis ceases. Metarubricytes have pyknotic nuclei and cytoplasm that is close to the color of red cells. The nucleus may be extended either at the end of the polychromatophilic rubricyte stage or during the metarubricyte stage. The resulting anucleate cell is the reticulocyte.

Reticulocytes usually remain in the marrow for 2-3 days before entering the circulation. Reticulocytes contain mitochondria and ribosomes, and continue to synthesize hemoglobin for a brief time after the nucleus is lost. Nevertheless, they contain enough hemoglobin to function effectively in O_2 transport should sudden demand for red cells induce their early release. Reticulocytes are larger than mature red cells and possess more surface membrane. After leaving the marrow, reticulocytes pause in the spleen, where they lose their excess membrane and are remolded into the size and shape of mature red cells. The RNA in reticulocytes can be stained by supravital dyes, such as new methylene blue. The loss of this stainable material as the cell matures is independent of the function of the spleen.

Normal marrow responds to increased red cell loss or destruction by increasing the rate of red cell production up to 6-8 times the normal rate. The condition of increased numbers of erythroblasts in marrow is called erythroid hyperplasia. If it represents effective erythropoiesis, it is accompanied by rising reticulocyte counts in the blood. Increased erythropoietin levels in anemia stimulate erythroid precursor cells to proliferate and mature.[18] High erythropoietin levels probably stimulate the rate of hemoglobin synthesis per cell.[22] As a result, the critical hemoglobin concentration that shuts off mitosis is reached sooner and a final cell division may be skipped. Such reticulocytes, produced under intense erythropoietic stress, are larger than normal and contain large amounts of reticulum. This phenomenon is most apparent in the early phase of response to severe, acute anemia.

A rising reticulocyte count produced by erythroid proliferation can be detected approximately 3 days after the onset of acute anemia. The interval between erythroid commitment and release of reticulocytes is shorter than usual because of erythropoietin-induced shortening of intervals between mitoses, reduced maturation time, and early release of reticulocytes. Reticulocytes in marrow at the onset of sudden severe anemia are released immediately through the effects of increased erythropoietin levels, accounting for a small rise in blood reticulocyte numbers several hours after a drop in circulating red cell mass.[14]

The mature red cell of the cat circulates for approximately 70 days.[23] It is shaped like a disc with shallow central depressions, a shape that provides a surface area:volume ratio that allows the cell to deform as it flows through the microvasculature. Structural proteins arranged in lattice formation beneath the plasma membrane maintain the disc shape and provide the elasticity that allows recovery of the original shape after deformation. Glycolysis provides most of the energy, in the form of ATP, needed to keep the structural membrane proteins in their proper configuration and to maintain normal concentrations of intracellular ions. Loss of surface membrane, alterations in structural proteins, and osmotic swelling each may cause the cell to become spherical, unable to deform, and more susceptible to lysis and fragmentation.

At the end of its life span, the red cell is removed from circulation by macrophages in the spleen, liver and bone marrow. As the red cell ages in the circulation, IgG attaches to its surface until enough IgG is present to mediate recognition and binding of the red cell by a macrophage.[24,25] After ingestion, the red cell is degraded rapidly within the macrophage and most of its components made available for reuse. Degeneration is so rapid that few macrophages in normal individuals contain red cells recognizable by light microscopy. However, in hemolytic anemia, macrophages engorged with red cells are found easily in smears or sections of bone marrow, liver and spleen as evidence of an increased rate of erythrophagocytosis. After red cells are digested, iron is stored within macrophages as hemosiderin and ferritin or released from the macrophage to be bound by the plasma protein transferrin and transported to marrow. Globin is catabolized to amino acids, which are returned to the body pool. The protoporphyrin ring of heme is split, releasing carbon monoxide, and converted to bilirubin, which is carried to the liver bound to albumin. Liver cells take up bilirubin, conjugate it to glucuronide and excrete it in bile.

Granulocyte Series: The 3 types of granulocytes (neutrophils, eosinophils, basophils) do not arise from the same committed precursor cell nor is their production regulated by the same factors. However, the maturation sequence is parallel in all 3 lines and can be described simultaneously. As in erythroid maturation, terminal differentiation is a continuous process arbitrarily divided into stages on a morphologic basis. There are at least 4 sequential divisions during maturation, producing 16 or more mature granulocytes from one myeloblast if all of the cells survive to maturity. In people, dogs and probably other species, 15-20% of granulocytes die in the marrow at the myelocyte or later stages.[26]

The youngest granulocyte is the myeloblast, a cell with a large, round or oval nucleus and cytoplasm that is less intensely blue than that of the rubriblast. The next stage, the promyelocyte, is recognized by the small red granules in its cytoplasm. In cat marrow, some promyelocytes are larger than others. Nucleoli are visible in myeloblasts and promyelocytes. The granules of the promyelocyte contain peroxidase and other enzymes, and are called primary or azurophilic granules. Peroxidase-positive granules are produced only at the promyelocyte stage. These granules lose their affinity for routine blood stains as the cell matures and consequently are not visible in later stages.

The myelocyte stage is indicated by the presence of secondary granules specific for the cell line. Depending on the specific granule present, myelocytes and more mature cells are designated as neutrophilic, eosinophilic or basophilic. Primary granules are still visible in some early myelocytes. Specific granules in feline neutrophils are not clearly stained by routine blood stains; neutrophilic myelocytes and later stages are therefore recognized by their apparent lack of granulation. Eosinophil granules are small, rod-shaped and orange. Basophil myelocytes contain small, light-pink granules and a few large, dark-purple granules (Fig C12). The latter either change or are lost during cell maturation since only the dull-pink granules are visible in mature basophils. The cytoplasm becomes less blue as the cell matures through the myelocyte stage, the nucleus becomes oval, and the chromatin more condensed.

Early myelocytes are proliferating cells but mitosis ceases at the late myelocyte stage. As the cell continues to mature, the nucleus is indented (the metamyelocyte) and then elongated with parallel sides (the band). The nucleus of the mature feline neutrophil is not segmented into discrete lobes connected by filaments but is twisted and pinched at several places. The eosinophil nucleus is bilobed. Chromatin in mature granulocytes is uniformly dense or arranged in dense plaques slightly separated by lighter areas. The cytoplasm of mature neutrophils is off-white or light-grey and agranular; that of eosinophils and basophils is light-blue but almost obscured by specific granules. The light-blue cytoplasm and pink granules of the basophil give it an overall lavender hue. Functional maturity of neutrophils and eosinophils is associated with increased motility, increased phagocytic capacity, and increased numbers of surface receptors for complement components and the Fc portion of IgG.

Myelocytes, metamyelocytes, bands and mature cells compose a postmitotic pool of maturing and stored granulocytes in marrow. Normally 6-7 days are required to reach the metamyelocyte stage and an equivalent time is spent in the marrow postmitotic pool.

After leaving marrow, mature neutrophils circulate 6-7 hours and are lost from blood in a random fashion, owing either to migration into tissues or removal by macrophages in reticuloendothelial organs. Egress from blood is enhanced at sites of inflammation where neutrophils, responding to local factors, stick to the walls of capillaries and postcapillary venules, then migrate between endothelial cells into the tissue.

Increased demand for neutrophils, as in inflammation, is met in 2 ways. First, release of late-stage neutrophils from marrow increases the number in the blood within a few hours. Second, continued demand for neutrophils increases the production rate, a state recognized as myeloid hyperplasia. Colony-stimulating factors produced by macrophages at the site of inflammation mediate the proliferative response. With colony-stimulating factors, more granulocyte-committed precursor cells enter the differentiation pathway, maturing cells divide more and fewer die, the interval between divisions is shortened, and less time is spent in the postmitotic pool.[26] Concomitantly, RNA and protein synthesis is stepped up to provide the neutrophil with its complement of granule enzymes in a shorter time.[26] As peripheral demand is met, the system is damped by various inhibitors derived from macrophages and granulocytes, and neutrophil production subsides to normal.[18,19]

Mature eosinophils circulate for several hours, then migrate into tissues, where they reside for several days. Eosinophils in tissue outnumber circulating eosinophils several hundred to one. They tend to localize beneath epithelium exposed to the external environment and are therefore found in skin, the mucosa of the respiratory and GI tracts, the vagina and wall of the uterus, and in lactating mammary glands.[27] Heightened eosinophil production is mediated by soluble factors produced by T-lymphocytes sensitized by exposure to certain antigens. With stimulation, all phases of the cell cycle are shortened and eosinophil production can be increased 16- to 64-fold.[28]

Very little is known about the regulation of basophil production.

Monocyte-Macrophage Series: Monocytes in blood, like granuloctyes, are in transit from their site of origin, the bone marrow, to their sites of function, the peripheral tissues. Unlike granulocytes, monocytes are not end-stage cells destined to die soon, but are partly differentiated cells capable of mitosis and extensive protein synthesis.

Promonocytes, the youngest cells of the monocyte series, can be detected in marrow by electron microscopy, cytochemical methods or functional assays but are rarely recognizable in routinely stained smears. They are few compared with granuloctye numbers; there is no marrow reserve of promonocytes or monocytes. Granule production begins in the promonocyte with the formation of peroxidase-positive granules and continues in circulating monocytes and macrophages with the formation of peroxidase-negative granules.[29] Receptors for complement components and the Fc portion of IgG are also synthesized as the cell differentiates.[30] After release from marrow, monocytes circulate for several days before entering tissues, where they may survive several months unless destroyed in an inflammatory process. Blood monocytes are larger than granulocytes and lymphocytes. The nucleus in some is elongated and folded, but in others it is kidney-shaped or ameboid. The chromatin is fine and evenly dispersed. The cytoplasm is blue to grey and may contain vacuoles and/or fine pink granules.

After migrating into tissues, the cell assumes the features of a macrophage, becoming larger, with more abundant cytoplasm and a rounded nucleus. In some diseases, monocytes circulating in blood have morphologic features of macrophages, a change that represents stimulation and activation. Activation of macrophages, as in inflammation, refers to a state of enhanced metabolism, mobility and phagocytic capacity. Macrophages are activated by many agents, including endotoxin and lymphokines from sensitized T-lymphocytes, and by ingestion of particulate matter.[31] Activated macrophages produce colony-stimulating factors, which in turn stimulate monocyte and neutrophil production. Lymphokines and other chemotactic factors recruit monocytes to sites where they are needed. Mitotic division of macrophages at the site of inflammation also increases their number.

If the agent that initiated the inflammatory response can be removed and degraded, monocytopoiesis returns to normal and the lesion resolves. Persistence of some agents, either extracellularly or within macrophages, can lead to prolonged and widespread macrophage activation that results in inappropriate phagocytosis of circulating blood cells in the liver, spleen and marrow.[31] This phenomenon is evident in some patients with granulomatous diseases, such as histoplasmosis.

Resident macrophage populations, such as Kupffer cells of the liver and the peritoneal and alveolar macrophages, are derived from bone marrow cells but probably do not depend on continued influx of monocytes to maintain their numbers under normal conditions.[30] Resident macrophages are long-lived and capable of maintaining their population by cell division.[32] Monocytes from blood rapidly supplement resident macrophages in areas of inflammation.

Neutrophils, eosinophils and macrophages are capable of phagocytosis, the process of ingestion and degradation of particles and macromolecular complexes. Whereas phagocytosis is the chief function of neutrophils, it is only one of many macrophage functions and has a secondary role in eosinophil functions. All 3 cells are motile and capable of directed migration toward the source of chemotactic factors.

Phagocytosis is initiated by the attachment of a particle, for example a bacterium, to the plasma membrane of the phagocyte, a process facilitated by opsonization of the organism by complement and antibody. Microorganisms coated with C3 or IgG are bound to the surface of the phagocyte by C3 and Fc receptors. Subsequent to binding, the particle is surrounded by pseudopodia and enclosed in a phagocytic vacuole. Granules then fuse with the vacuole and discharge their enzymes into it. The major microbicidal mechanism involves the reaction of peroxidase in combination with hydrogen peroxide and a halide ion. Ingestion also triggers a burst of oxidative metabolism that produces hydrogen peroxide and unstable, high-energy products that are lethal to many microorganisms.[33] Other granule proteins participate in the killing and digestion of microorganisms. Granule enzymes are released into the tissue upon the death of neutrophils or through granulation stimulated by binding immune complexes or binding to antigens on a nonphagocytizable surface. Extracellular degranulation causes tissue damage and contributes to the pathogenesis of disease, such as rheumatoid arthritis and glomerulonephritis.

Macrophages perform an imposing assortment of extracellular functions.[34] They contribute to tissue inflammatory response by releasing hydrolytic enzymes, collagenase, elastase, plasminogen-activating factor and other enzymes. They contribute to host defense by secreting interferon and complement components. Macrophages participate in immune responses by presenting antigens in a form that facilitates lymphocyte response and by cooperating with lymphocytes in cell-mediated immune responses against virus-infected cells, transplanted cells and tumor cells.

Eosinophils are less effective phagocytes than neutrophils and macrophages. They function mainly to modulate immediate hypersensitivity reactions and to defend against metazoan parasites.[27] Eosinophils are attracted to areas of mast cell degranulation and there release granule contents that counteract the effects of mast cells by degrading substances released by mast cells and suppressing further mast cell degranulation. Eosinophils also are major components of the reaction against tissue-migrating stages of parasites, a function that depends on sensitization of T-lymphocytes. Eosinophils attach to the parasites by complement and Fc receptors, and release enzymes into and around the parasite that damage or kill it. Noninvasive stages of parasites do not evoke an eosinophil response.

Neutrophils, eosinophils and monocytes all are involved to some extent in many inflammatory lesions. The predominant cell involved and the tempo and duration of the response are affected by the chemotactic factors released. In general, neutrophils predominate in the first day or 2 and monocytes predominate thereafter. Some chemotactic factors, such as products of activated complement, are strongly attractive to all 3 cell types. Other factors, such as collagen degradation products, attract monocytes more than neutrophils. Some bacteria, such as staphylococci and streptococci, are more chemotactic for neutrophils, while others, such as mycobacteria, are more chemotactic for monocytes. Separate lymphokines have been demonstrated to be preferentially chemotactic for each cell.[34]

Megakaryocyte-Platelet Series:[35] Megakaryocyte differentiation and platelet production are strikingly different from differentiation and amplification in other cell lines in that megakaryocytes increase their DNA content without cell division. In the megakaryocyte line, only the morphologically unrecognizable, diploid (2N) committed precursor cell proliferates and increases its numbers by mitosis. Between the level of the 2N megakaryocyte precursor cell and the earliest recognizable megakaryocyte, the cell becomes polyploid by simultaneous replication of all DNA until the chromosome content is 4N to 128N. Most megakaryocytes stop replicating DNA at 8N, 16N or 32N. The higher the ploidy, the greater the amount of cytoplasm and number of platelets produced per cell. Cytoplasm begins to increase and mature before DNA synthesis ceases but nuclear lobes are formed only after DNA synthesis is completed.

The basophilic megakaryocyte is the earliest recognizable cell of the series.[4] Its nucleus is large and spherical and its cytoplasm is scant and deep-blue. Granular megakaryocytes, the next stage, are the most numerous cells of the series. The nucleus has multiple lobes and the cytoplasm contains many pink-red granules. At approximately 100 μ in diameter, it is the largest of the hematopoietic cells. As cytoplasmic maturation continues, granules are arranged in groups surrounded by light areas, which represent demarcation membranes destined to be platelet membranes upon fragmentation.[12] Platelets are released from the fully mature megakaryocyte and the bare nucleus is phagocytized. Platelets circulate for 7-10 days and are removed from blood by phagocytosis or consumption in coagulation.

Little is known about the regulators of platelet production. A stimulating factor, thrombopoietin, is present in the plasma of thrombocytopenic individuals. On the other hand, platelet production is suppressed when an individual is transfused with enough platelets to raise the platelet mass above normal. The factors that balance platelet production against platelet mass are not defined yet. In response to a decrease in platelet mass, megakaryocytes show compensatory increases in cell number and in the DNA content and cytoplasm of individual cells. They also mature more rapidly than normally. Rising platelet counts are detectible several days after the induction of thrombocytopenia. In the acute phase of platelet regeneration, many platelets are larger than normal.

Lymphocyte Series:[17,21,36] The peripheral lymphoid tissues, not bone marrow, are the sites of lymphocyte proliferation in postnatal animals. Proliferation is driven by antigen and results in clonal expansion of lymphocytes bearing surface receptors for the antigen. After exposure to antigen, lymphocytes transform into large cells, with deep-blue cytoplasm, that divide and produce daughter cells, some of which are effector cells and others that are long-lived memory cells. In the case of T-lymphocytes, the effector cells may have helper function and suppressor activity, may be cytotoxic, or may produce lymphokines. In the case of B-lymphocytes, effector cells produce immunoglobulin and differentiate into plasma cells. Memory cells of either lymphocyte line circulate as small lymphocytes.

EVALUATION OF HEMATOPOIESIS

The first step toward the detection and diagnosis of primary hematologic disorders is the quantitative and qualitative assessment of the cells in peripheral blood. However, this procedure should not be reserved only for patients in which clinical signs and physical findings seem to indicate a hematopoietic disease but should be included as a routine part of the evaluation of any patient. Many diseases of other systems are reflected by changes in the numbers and morphologic characteristics of circulating blood cells. Valuable insight into the nature, severity and progress of a patient's disease often is provided by examination of its blood. As with all diagnostic procedures, the usefulness of hematologic tests depends on the use of correct sampling and testing methods and the interpretative skill of the clinician.

Fortunately, blood is the easiest tissue to sample and can be prepared for examination within minutes. The basic hematologic tests—determination of packed cell volume (PCV), total white cell count, differential white cell count, and examination of a stained blood smear—can be performed in a practitioner's laboratory equipped with a microhematocrit centrifuge and a microscope. Alternatively, blood samples can be sent to a commercial laboratory for evaluation. The hemogram report from most laboratories includes PCV, total and differential white cell count, hemoglobin concentration, red cell count, and red cell indices. Reticulocyte and platelet counts are done on request.

Collecting and Handling Blood for Hematologic Evaluation

Although most laboratories request that blood sample volume be at least 2-3 ml, for in-office tests a volume of 1 ml or less is sufficient to make several blood smears and to measure the PCV and WBC numbers. The external jugular vein is the best site for collection of several milliliters of blood from a cat. It is accessible and has a diameter large enough to allow withdrawal of 2-3 ml of blood without prolonged compression. Jugular venipuncture is best accomplished using a 21- or 22-ga needle, either attached to a syringe or fitted for direct attachment to a vacuum tube containing anticoagulant. The cephalic vein and marginal ear vein are convenient sites for collection of a smaller quantity of blood for procedures done in the office. Several heparinized microhematocrit capillary tubes and a diluting pipette can be filled directly from a needle inserted into the cephalic vein or from drops of blood that well up after the marginal ear vein is punctured with a lancet or scalpel blade. Spreading a thin coat of petroleum jelly over the ear prior to lancing the marginal vein enhances the formation of large drops and facilitates blood collection.

Blood collected into a syringe should be transferred immediately to a tube containing anticoagulant and mixed thoroughly. No advantage is gained by dropping blood onto slides for smears before mixing it with anticoagulant since even the small delay may allow time for clotting that invalidates test results. Clotted samples should be discarded.

Ethylenediamine tetracetic acid (EDTA) is the preferred anticoagulant for hematologic tests because cellular artifacts develop comparatively slowly in it. Blood smears should be made as soon as possible after blood is drawn but acceptable smears can be made up to 2-3 hours later if the sample is refrigerated. The 3-ml vacuum tube containing EDTA is best for blood samples from cats. Using 5-ml tubes for 2- to 3-ml samples is unwise since the excess EDTA can cause shrinkage of red cells, thereby decreasing the PCV. A rule of thumb is that the PCV of a 0.5-ml sample in a 5-ml tube containing liquid EDTA is 75% of the actual PCV, that of a 1-ml sample is 84%, that of a 2-ml sample 93% and that of a 4-ml sample 96%. Heparin is less satisfactory than EDTA because it tends to cause clumping of white cells and platelets, which interferes with cell counting, and because it does not preserve white cell morphology well. However, heparin does not affect the size of red cells or the PCV as EDTA may.

After blood is collected and smears made, the sample must be kept refrigerated at 4 C (39.2 F) until other tests are performed, whether the sample is to be sent out to a laboratory or evaluated in the office. Even if the sample is to be sent to a laboratory, it is wise to make blood smears at the time of collection and send them with the sample. If blood is anticoagulated with EDTA and stored at 4 C, the white cell count, PCV, hemoglobin concentration, red cell count, red cell indices, reticulocyte count and platelet count remain stable for up to 24 hours.[37] However, many of the white cells in smears made of 24-hour-old blood are broken and smudged beyond recognition, making an accurate differential white cell count impossible.

Table 1. Normal Range for Hematologic Determinations in the Cat[23]

PCV	24-45%
Hb	8-15 gm/dl
RBC	5-10 × 10^6/μl
MCV	39-55 fl
MCHC	30-36%
Reticulocytes[38]	
Aggregate	0-0.4%
Punctate	1-10.5%
WBC	5.5-19.5 × 10^3/μl
Neut	2.5-12.5 × 10^3/μl
Band Neut	0-1.5 × 10^3/μl
Lymph	1.5-7.0 × 10^3/μl
Eosino	0-1.5 × 10^3/μl
Mono	0-0.8 × 10^3/μl
Platelets	300-700 × 10^5/μl

Quantitative Determinations

Reference values for quantitiative hematologic tests are shown in Table 1.

Packed Cell Volume

The PCV, or hematocrit, of a blood sample is the concentration of red cells in whole blood, expressed as a percentage. The PCV can be easily and quickly measured by centrifuging microhematocrit tubes filled with well-mixed blood for 5 minutes at 10,000 g. The length of the whole column and the length of the red cell column are then measured with a microhematocrit reader and the result is reported as the percent of the total column length that is composed of red cells.

A falsely high PCV may result from failure to allow adequate duration and speed of centrifugation. If extending the time of centrifugation reduces the PCV, then the original time was inadequate for maximal packing of red cells. A falsely low PCV may result from red cell shrinkage in excess EDTA. Other technical errors include failure to mix the blood and inaccurate reading of column lengths.

The color of the plasma should be noted when the PCV is measured. Normal feline plasma is light yellow. Red discoloration indicates hemolysis and release of hemoglobin either in the sample or in the patient. A deep-yellow color indicates hyperbilirubinemia. Pale, almost colorless plasma often is seen in cats with severe hypoplastic anemia, perhaps owing to decreased red cell turnover and bilirubin production. The concentration of total protein in the plasma column can be easily measured with a refractometer. A high total protein concentration suggests hemoconcentration and indicates that the PCV as measured is higher than it would be if the patient were in a normal state of hydration. In the absence of dehydration, a high total protein concentration indicates an absolute increase in plasma solids, often an increase in globulin concentration.

Hemoglobin Concentration

Hemoglobin (Hb) concentration is expressed in g/dl blood. This determination is done routinely in commercial laboratories but few clinic laboratories are equipped to measure Hb concentration accurately. Since the usual method of measuring Hb concentration involves spectrophotometry, falsely high values are produced if the sample contains substances that increase light absorbance. Lipemia or the presence of Heinz bodies is the common cause of falsely high Hb concentration. Bilirubin does not interfere with Hb measurement since it absorbs light at a different wavelength. Hemolysis, either in the sample or in the animal, lowers the PCV without changing the Hb concentration, resulting in a PCV to Hb ratio of less than 3:1.

Cell Counting

Red cells, white cells and platelets can be enumerated by manual methods or by electronic cell counters. Cells can be counted in a hospital laboratory by mixing blood with the proper diluting solution and counting the cells in a hemacytometer. This procedure has been facilitated by development of the Unopette system (Becton-Dickinson). Plastic vials containing the appropriate type and volume of diluent and plastic micropipettes of the appropriate volume are provided for each cell type. Explicit instructions are included with the Unopette components. The results compare favorably with cell counts from electronic counters and are accurate enough for diagnostic purposes.

Clinical laboratories handling many samples use electronic cell counters. Some of these instruments measure the volume of red cells as they are counted and determine the size of the average red cell (mean corpuscular volume). The mean corpuscular volume and the red cell count are then automatically used to calculate the PCV. This calculated PCV frequently is lower than the PCV of the same sample as measured by the microhematocrit method since in the latter method small amounts of trapped plasma contribute to the height of the red cell column. The presence of abnormally large platelets or platelet clumps can spuriously increase both the red cell count and the white cell count measured electronically. Clumping of platelets lowers the platelet count. Since feline platelets are often clumped in the sample, this possibility should be checked by examining a stained blood smear.

Differential White Cell Count

The differential count represents the percentage distribution of the different types of white cells. The usual procedure is to examine 100 white cells in a stained blood smear and classify appropriately each cell that is encountered. This percentage is then multiplied by the total white cell count to give the absolute number of each cell in a volume of blood. The differential count arrived at in this manner is at best an estimation of the actual differential count in whole blood. Sampling errors can cause disagreement between differential counts done on 2 blood smears from the same sample. The accuracy of the differential count can be improved by using well-made blood smears, in which the white cells are randomly distributed, and by increasing the size of the population examined. Counts based on 500 or 1000 white cells are more representative of the actual distribution in blood than counts based on 100 white cells, but the increased accuracy is seldom worth the time required to classify additional cells. Because of the error inherent in the method, small fluctuations in the differential count from one time to another should not be overinterpreted. Interpretation of the differential white cell count should be based on the absolute numbers rather than on percentages.

Red Cell Indices

The red cell indices are expressions of certain properties of red cells and are usually derived by computations based on measured values of PCV, red cell count and Hb concentration. The mean corpuscular volume (MCV) is the volume of the average red cell expressed in femtoliters (fl) or cubic microns (μ^3). The mean corpuscular hemoglobin concentration (MCHC) is the average concentration of Hb per red cell, expressed as a percentage. The mean corpuscular hemoglobin (MCH) is the amount of Hb in the average red cell.

Table 2. Classification of Anemias in the Cat According to Cause and Typical Red Cell Indices

Normocytic, normochromic anemia - Normal MCV, MCHC
Anemia of chronic disease
Anemia of renal failure
Anemia of FeLV-associated erythroid suppression
Hypoplastic and aplastic anemia not associated with FeLV
Acute blood loss or hemolytic anemia prior to reticulocytosis
Chronic blood loss or hemolytic anemia with mild anemia and modest reticulocytosis
Macrocytic anemia - increased MCV, usually normal MCHC
Acute hemolytic or blood loss anemia with intense reticulocytosis
FeLV-associated hematopoietic neoplasia with megaloblastoid erythropoiesis
Folate deficiency
Microcytic hypochromic anemia-decreased MCV, MCHC
Iron deficiency anemia

The MCV, MCHC and MCH provide a quantitative basis for describing red cells as normocytic, macrocytic or microcytic and as normochromic or hypochromic. Because they are derived from measured values, the red cell indices more accurately represent the average red cell than does a subjective impression gained by examining a stained blood smear. However, calculation of red cell indices should not be used in place of visual inspection of red cells. Red cells of abnormal size or pigmentation, although too few to cause abnormal indices, may have great interpretative importance. The value of recognizing red cells with abnormal size or Hb content, either by calculation or visual inspection, lies in the correlation of certain abnormalities with certain types of anemia. Table 2 shows the relationship of morphologic and etiologic classifications of feline anemia.

Reticulocyte Count

Reticulocytes are young red cells that contain RNA, which can be demonstrated by certain staining methods. The reticulocyte count is the number of RNA-containing red cells per 100 red cells, reported as a percentage. A total of 500 or 1000 red cells is counted to derive the reticulocyte count. For the purpose of counting reticulocytes, blood is stained supravitally, *ie*, without fixation, by such a stain as new methylene blue.[23] Equal parts of blood and stain are incubated for 15-20 minutes and smears are made of the mixture. New methylene blue precipitates RNA into readily seen blue-green granules. Cat blood prepared in this fashion contains 2 types of reticulocytes: punctate reticulocytes, in which the granules are sparse and discrete, and aggregate reticulocytes, which contain heavier, clumped granules (Fig C1). Reticulocyte counts of cat blood should include the percentage of each type, as well as the total. In normal cats the aggregate reticulocyte count is less than 0.5% and the punctate reticulocyte count is 1.0-10.5%.[38] An alternative method of demonstrating reticulocytes is to place a drop of new methylene blue on a dry blood smear and cover the drop with a coverslip.[23] Only aggregate reticulocytes are discernible by this method.[39] Smears prepared this way are not permanent and cannot be kept for later examination. Aggregate reticulocytes contain enough RNA to impart a diffuse blue tint (polychromasia) to the red cell stained with routine blood stains (Fig C2). The percentage of polychromatophilic red cells agrees closely with the aggregate reticulocyte count.[39]

Some confusion exists regarding the interpretation of reticulocyte counts in cats because of the 2 types of reticulocytes. Following the onset of acute, severe anemia, aggregate reticulocytes begin to increase in number after 24 hours, peak around the fourth day and decrease to normal levels 8-10 days later. Punctate reticulocytes are increased in number at the fourth day, peak by the twelfth day and thereafter decrease slowly. The rise of the punctate reticulocyte number is closely parallel to the increase in PCV.[40] Although the punctate reticulocyte count may exceed 50%, the aggregate reticulocyte count is rarely above 5%. The early appearance of aggregate reticulocytes after the onset of anemia may reflect premature release of reticulocytes from marrow during the time when PCV is lowest, hypoxic stimulus strongest and erythropoietin levels highest. Although the aggregate reticulocyte count is used by many as the indicator of erythropoietic activity in anemic cats, the punctate reticulocyte count is a truer indication of the efficacy of the erythropoietic response in restoring the PCV to its former level.[40]

The reticulocyte count should be correlated with serial determinations of PCV. Failure of the PCV to rise steadily despite increased numbers of reticulocytes implies either continued blood loss or hemolysis or a primary bone marrow disorder. Some cats with FeLV-associated hematopoietic neoplasia, especially erythremic myelosis or erythroleukemia, at times have reticulocytosis but unremitting severe anemia.

Influence of Physiologic Factors

Various physiologic factors must be considered when interpreting the results of quantitative hematologic tests. Age influences several hematologic variables. Newborn kittens have fewer red cells than adult cats but the red cells are much larger; therefore, PCV and Hb concentration are equivalent to adult values. During the first month of postnatal life, normally sized red cells replace the large cells, and the PCV and Hb concentration fall to approximately 75% of adult values, returning again to the normal range by puberty.[23] Total white cell counts are not affected by age but kittens typically have more lymphocytes than do adult cats.[23] Cats at high altitudes, because of the stimulatory effect of low O_2 concentration, have higher red cell values than do cats living at low altitudes.[23] Excitement or fear can induce increases in both red cell and white cell values. Mental stress or physical exertion results in contraction of the spleen and increased blood flow in small vessels. The cat, like other domestic animals, possesses a muscular spleen which, in a relaxed state, contains a third of the total platelet mass and a concentrated mass of slowly moving red cells amounting to 10% of the total body red cell mass. Splenic contraction ejects these platelets and red cells and immediately raises the platelet count and PCV of peripheral blood. Conversely, barbiturate anesthetics lower the PCV by increasing the size of the splenic red cell pool. The hemodynamic changes effected by excitement alter the distribution of neutrophils in the vascular system. In a calm cat, approximately one-fourth of the total neutrophils in blood are circulating in large vessel blood while the rest are moving slowly along the walls of small vessels.[41] In an excited cat, many of these marginating neutrophils are flushed into large vessels, producing a transient physiologic leukocytosis. The white cell count returns to normal within 20-30 minutes if the cat is allowed to regain its equanimity.

Morphologic Evalution of Blood Cells

The examination of a properly prepared blood smear is an essential part of the hematologic evaluation. The primary purpose of this procedure is to determine the differential white cell count and to detect morphologic abnormalities of diagnostic importance. Additionally, the white cell and platelet counts can be estimated from the smear if these cells are evenly distributed. The white cell count can be estimated by calculating the average number of white cells per field in a minimum of 10 fields, using the 43X (high-dry) objective and multiplying this number by 1000. A platelet count within the normal range is indicated by the presence of 1 platelet per 10-20 red cells or at least 5 platelets per oil-immersion field. These estimates are crude but allow one to detect marked deviations from the normal range.

The examination of a blood smear should follow an orderly and consistent sequence. First, the smear is scanned at low magnification to judge the quality of the smear, to detect nonrandom distribution of white cells and clumping of platelets, and to form an impression of white cell numbers. A thin area of the smear in which cells touch but do not overlap is selected and the high-dry objective is used to estimate the white cell count. The differential count may be done at this magnification or at the higher magnification provided by the oil-immersion objective. Using the oil-immersion objective, red cells are examined for excessive variation in size (anisocytosis) and shape (poikilocytosis), for the presence of increased numbers of polychromatophilic red cells and nucleated red cells, and for erythroparasites and red cell inclusions. Next, platelet numbers are noted and platelets are examined for abnormalities in size, shape or granulation. Finally, white cells are examined for morphologic abnormalities. The rewards yielded by this procedure are proportional to the care with which the smears are made and the ability of the examiner to recognize and interpret morphologic abnormalities. Misleading information is likely to result from sloppy preparation or superficial examination.

Preparing Blood Smears

The standard preparation for morphologic evaluation of blood cells is the blood smear stained by one of the Romanowsky-type stains, such as Wright, Wright-Giemsa or Giemsa. These stains are readily available and come with step-by-step instructions for use. The staining time is usually less than 10 minutes. A 3-solution rapid-staining method (Diff-Quik:Harleco) is available. If care is taken to precisely time the staining steps and to use fresh solutions, this stain produces smears with tinctorial properties similar to those of standard stains.

Blood smears can be made by spreading a drop of blood between 2 glass microscope slides or 2 coverslips.[23] Either method is satisfactory if performed with skill. Satisfactory blood smears are thin and quickly dried, and have large areas in which the cells form a monolayer. White cells should be evenly dispersed rather than concentrated at the edges of the smear. In smears that are thick or slowly dried, red cells are shrunken and crenated and white cells look like small, dark dots that are impossible to classify.

Morphologic Abnormalities of Blood Cells

Red Cells: Slight anisocytosis is normal in smears of feline blood. Marked anisocytosis is most common in strongly regenerative anemia, owing to large numbers of reticulocytes, and in FeLV-associated megaloblastoid erythropoiesis. Red cells should be round and smooth but artifactual changes often produce red cells with scalloped edges or surface projections (Fig C3). Central pallor is most evident in thick areas of the smear rather than at the edges, where cells are more flat. Poikilocytosis is not common in feline blood and is usually associated with red cell fragmentation or Heinz-body formation. Rouleau formation is usually present in thick areas and is accentuated in severe anemia and inflammatory disease (Fig C3).

Feline red cells may contain a variety of inclusions. Howell-Jolly bodies are small, round, dark-purple bits of nucleus that may be present in a few red cells in normal cats; the number increases during response to anemia. Nucleated red cells, usually metarubricytes, likewise are occasionally present in normal cats and increase in number during response to anemia. The appearance of many nucleated red cells in blood without appropriate reticulocytosis implies a bone marrow problem involving release of cells and/or abnormal production. Very large numbers of nucleated red cells, sometimes more than 50-100 per 100 white cells, may circulate in the blood of cats suffering the erythremic myelosis or erythroleukemia forms of FeLV-associated hematopoietic neoplasia.

Heinz bodies, aggregates of denatured Hb, are frequently present in a few or many red cells in nonanemic cats. These small Heinz bodies, also called erythrocyte refractile (ER) bodies, do not noticeably affect red cell life span. Small Heinz bodies are not visible in Romanowsky-stained blood smears but appear as round, blue-green inclusions in red cells stained with new methylene blue. Large Heinz bodies produced by exposure to oxidant drugs cause hemolytic anemia, a topic discussed in another part of the chapter. Crystalloid bodies, composed of crystalline Hb, are curious, rarely seen inclusions in feline red cells.[42] Red cells bearing crystalloid bodies are recognized in smears as rectangular or square red cells. Basophilic stippling is the presence of multiple fine blue granules in red cells stained with Romanowsky-type stains and represents aggregates of RNA. Punctate basophilia of young red cells, although common in some species during response to anemia, is rare in cats.

Neutrophils: Cytoplasmic and nuclear abnormalities, collectively called toxic changes, include vacuolation of the cytoplasm, Doehle bodies, diffuse cytoplasmic basophilia, bizarre nuclear shapes, and loose chromatin pattern. Cytoplasmic vacuolation, which may appear as diffuse foaminess or as discrete vacuoles, represent intracellular release of granule enzymes. The presence of a few vacuolated neutrophils or a few vacuoles in otherwise normal neutrophils has little diagnostic importance. Similarly, the presence of Doehle bodies, which are light-blue patches representing aggregated RNA, is not an important finding since they are present in many mildly ill cats.

Extensive vacuolation and diffuse cytoplasmic basophilia in most circulating neutrophils are highly noteworthy toxic changes and usually accompanied by nuclear abnormalities (Fig C3). Some neutrophils bearing such toxic changes are larger than normal cells. The presence of severe toxic changes in many neutrophils often indicates serious infectious disease, usually involving gram-negative bacteria and endotoxemia.

Plate 1

Fig C1. Feline reticulocytes in blood, new methylene blue stain. The 5 heavily granulated red cells are aggregate reticulocytes; the rest are punctate reticulocytes.

Fig C2. Primary hemobartonellosis. The parasitemia is unusually heavy and some intravascular hemolysis has occurred. Parasites, most of which are ring forms, are clearly visible on the ghosts of lysed red cells. Some lie between red cells. Two polychromatophilic red cells (aggregate reticulocytes) are in the center of the field.

Fig C3. Blood from a cat with FIP. The white cell at the left is a toxic neutrophil with vacuolated cytoplasm and abnormally segmented nucleus. The white cell at the right is an activated monocyte. Red cell rouleaux in this area of the smear reflect the high plasma fibrinogen concentration in this cat. The crenation of red cells is a common artifact.

Fig C4. Bone marrow in the hypoplastic stage of panleukopenia. This field was representative of the entire marrow. The large cells with grey, vacuolated cytoplasm are macrophages. A nucleolus is visible in the smudged nucleus of the macrophage at the left side of the cluster. The other cells are small lymphocytes and an eosinophil.

Fig C5. Bone marrow in the hyperplastic stage of panleukopenia. The large cells with fine chromatin and prominent nucleoli are granulocytes that have not passed the myelocyte stage. The small, dark nuclei belong to lymphocytes. This marrow pattern might be mistaken for that of granulocytic leukemia.

Fig C6. Bone marrow of erythremic myelosis. A cluster of abnormal erythroblasts fills the field. Three polychromatophilic megaloblastoid rubricytes, one in mitosis, are at the right. The large cell at the top is a prorubricyte. Asynchronous maturation is also evident in the other rubricytes with basophilic cytoplasm but condensed, mature nuclei. Note also the variation in cell and nuclear size in the basophilic rubricytes.

Fig C7. Bone marrow of erythroleukemia. Abnormal maturation in erythroid, granulocytic and megakaryocytic lines was prominent in this marrow. The 2 cells at the left of the field are erythroid. The 2 large granulated cells at the right of the field, one binucleate and one with prominent nucleoli, are probably granulocytic. The cell near the center that contains a small round nucleus and heavily granular cytoplasm is a dwarf megakaryocyte. The other cells lined up top to bottom through the center are more mature granulocytes.

Fig C8. Monocytic leukemia, blood. The granules in the leukemic monocytes were reactive for nonspecific esterase, a monocyte marker. Similar cells packed the marrow, spleen, liver and lymph nodes.

Fig C9. Myelomonocytic leukemia, blood. The neutrophil is markedly hypersegmented as were most neutrophils in this cat's blood.

Fig C10. Myelomonocytic leukemia, bone marrow, same cat as in Figure C9. Blast cells surround a dwarf megakaryocyte.

Fig C11. Leukemia of undetermined cell type (reticuloendotheliosis), bone marrow. The appearance of the neoplastic cells give no clue to their lineage, although cells similar to those pictured here contained pink granules.

Fig C12. Lymphoma, bone marrow. This marrow particle contained a nearly uniform population of neoplastic lymphocytes. Other particles contained a normal population of hematopoietic cells. The hematopoietic cells in this field include several polychromatophilic rubricytes, a band neutrophil and a partially disrupted basophilic myelocyte.

Severe toxic changes also are associated with feline infectious peritonitis (FIP), some staphylococcal infections and some systemic fungal infections. Severe toxic changes are a warning that the disease is a serious one and should be treated intensively. Cats recovering from feline panleukopenia pass through a stage in which most of their neutrophils are intensely blue and have bizarre nuclei.[23] In contrast to the toxic neutrophils of bacterial infection, these neutrophils usually are not vacuolated.

Monocytes: Monocytes activated while in the circulation develop the morphologic characteristics of macrophages. Activated monocytes have round to oval nuclei and large amounts of blue cytoplasm (Fig C3). They are usually much

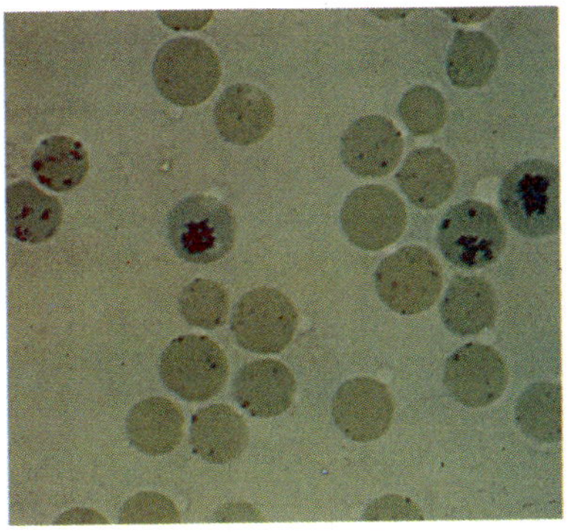
C-1

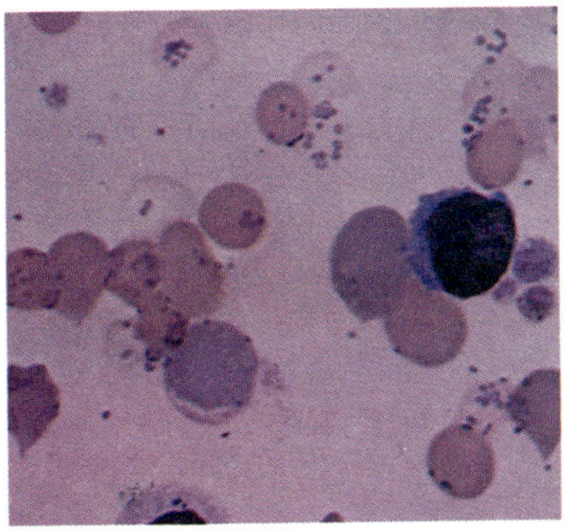
C-2

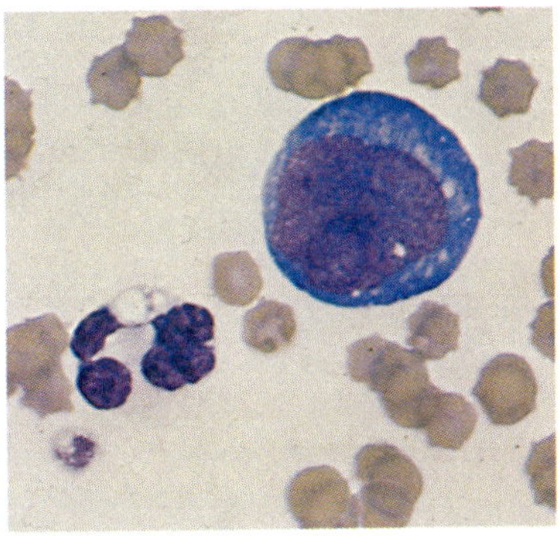
C-3

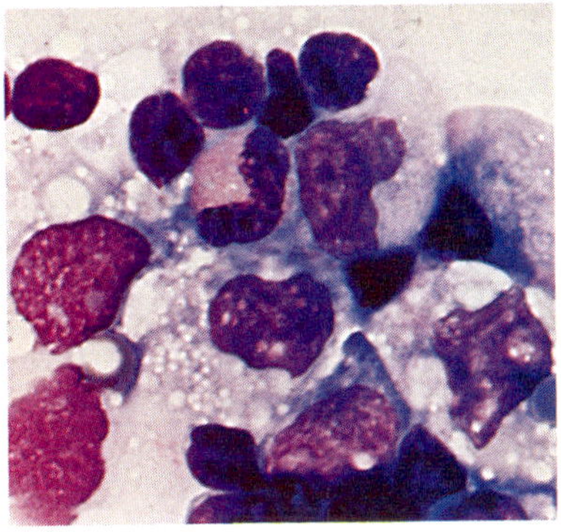
C-4

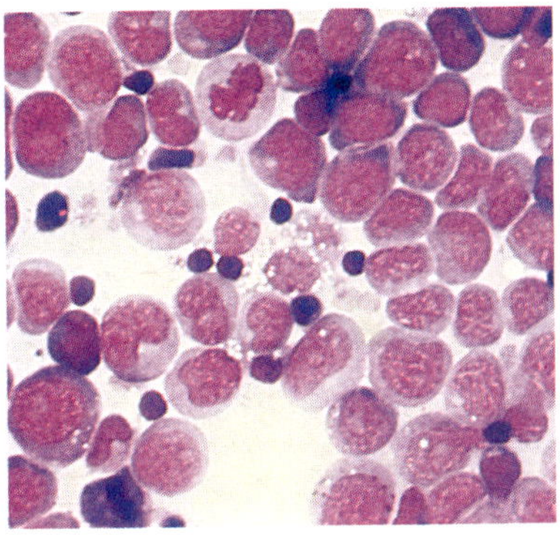
C-5

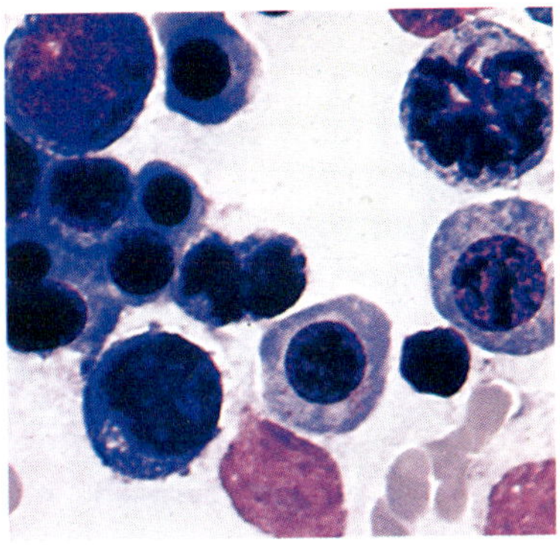
C-6

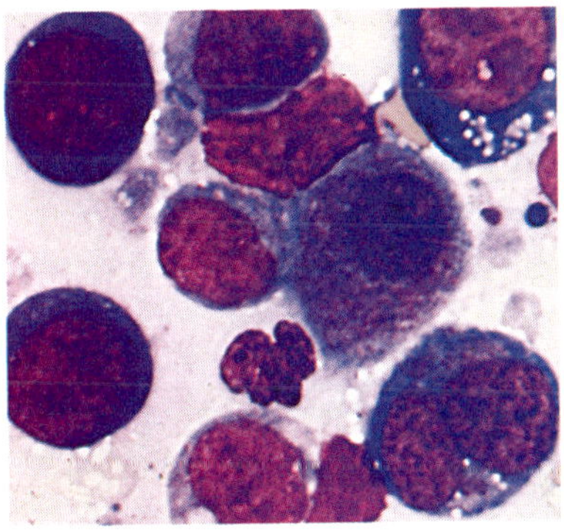
C-7

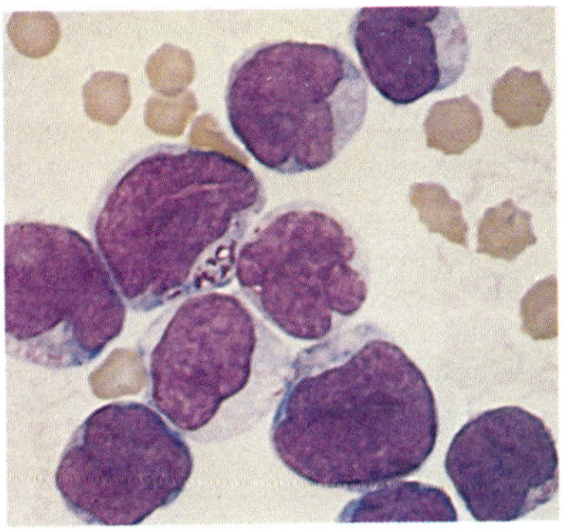
C-8

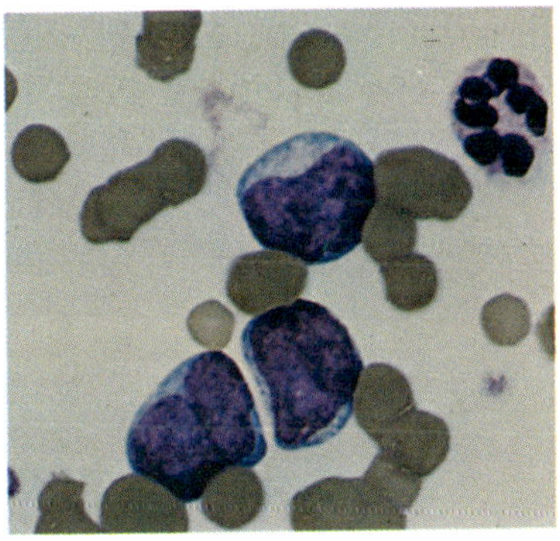
C-9

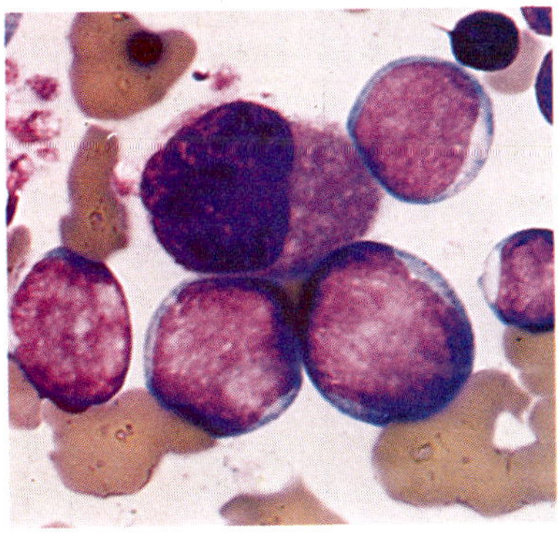
C-10

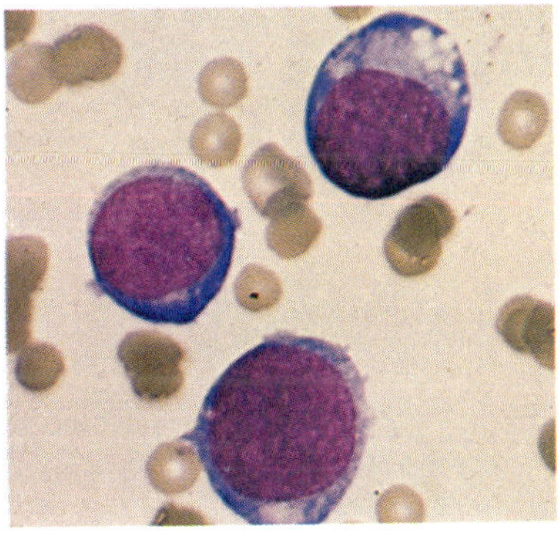
C-11

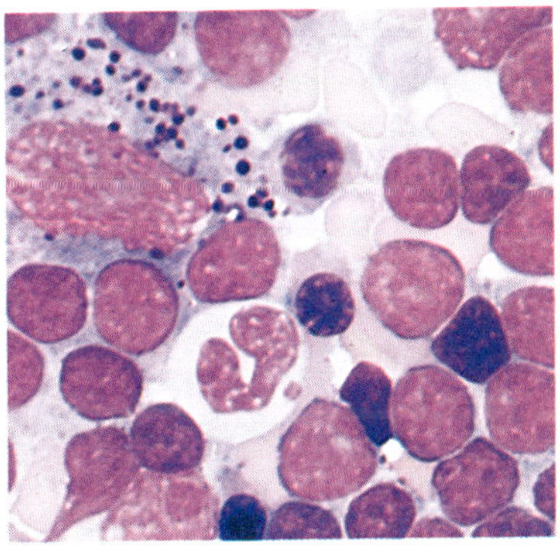
C-12

larger than normal monocytes. Activated monocytes frequently are present in blood from cats with FIP and activated monocytes containing phagocytized red cells often can be found in blood from cats with hemobartonellosis or autoimmune hemolytic anemia.

Lymphocytes: Normal feline lymphocytes have round to oval nuclei, which may be indented, and chromatin that is dense and smooth. The cytoplasm may be abundant or barely visible as a rim around the nucleus. Some lymphocytes contain paranuclear clusters of coarse pink granules. Some lymphocytes in animals with chronic infections or other conditions involving strong antigenic stimulation are larger than normal and have deep-blue cytoplasm, a high nucleus to cytoplasm ratio and fine chromatin. These reactive lymphocytes account for only a small fraction of the total lymphocyte count.

Platelets: Platelets in blood smears are round to oval or irregularly shaped, with multiple points of filamentous projections. The latter configuration is assumed as platelets spread on the surface of the glass slide. Normal platelets have grey to blue cytoplasm seen as a narrow rim around a central cluster of tiny purple granules. The demarcation between granules and cytoplasm is accentuated in activated platelets. Platelets tend to aggregate in blood samples and appear as clumps in the smear. In some smears, platelet clumps are amorphous masses in which individual platelets are not discernible. There is considerable variation in platelet size in normal blood; however, most, if not all are smaller than red cells. During regeneration after acute thrombocytopenia or in pathologic conditions that stimulate a reactive thrombocytosis, many platelets are larger than normal and some may be as large as red cells. Increased numbers of large platelets are a common finding in cats with some forms of FeLV-associated hematopoietic neoplasia.

Bone Marrow Examination

The decision to examine bone marrow as part of the hematologic evaluation should be based on peripheral blood findings. The following are the usual indications for bone marrow examination: persistent leukopenia, thrombocytopenia or nonregenerative anemia, the presence of abnormal circulating cells, or any combination of these conditions. A sample of peripheral blood must be collected at the time of bone marrow collection to facilitate interpretation of the bone marrow pattern.

Bone marrow samples are conveniently collected from cats by aspiration of the dorsal iliac crest or proximal part of the femur through the trochanteric fossa. Bone marrow cores for preparation of sections are collected at the same sites with special biopsy needles; this procedure is done infrequently in cats. Sections of bone marrow cores are useful for estimating overall marrow cellularity and for detecting disturbances of marrow architecture or the presence of focal lesions, such as granulomas or neoplasms, that might not be detected in aspirate smears. Fibrotic marrow or marrow packed with neoplastic cells sometimes cannot be aspirated; bone marrow biopsy is the only way to collect samples of such marrow. The technics of marrow aspiration and biopsy are described and illustrated elsewhere.[23,43-45]

Successful aspiration yields many translucent flecks of marrow that are gently crushed between 2 slides or 2 coverslips to make bone marrow smears. As in the preparation of blood smears, the marrow smears must be thin and quickly dried since thick smears are almost useless for evaluation. Bone marrow smears are stained as blood smears but a longer staining time usually is required.

Bone marrow smears should be examined with the same methodic routine applied to blood smears. The slides are first scanned at low magnification to estimate the cellularity of particles, to evaluate megakaryocyte numbers and to detect focal lesions. During scanning, one also forms an impression of the nature of the cell population, whether it is a normal, heterogeneous population or a monotonous pattern of nuclei having the same shape and size. After scanning many particles, areas in which the cells are well spread are selected for examination with the oil-immersion objective and cytologic details are noted.

Estimates of overall marrow cellularity, based on the cellularity of particles in smears, are rough guesses but must suffice in the absence of sections of bone marrow cores. At least 6 different particles should be observed before an opinion is made. Particles that have at least normal cellularity should contain enough cells to obscure the stromal elements and should be surrounded by a zone of well-spread, individual cells. The proportion of fat to hematopoietic cells should be approximately 50%. Particles of low cellularity have few hematopoietic cells and consist mostly of stromal cells and blood vessels. Hypocellular particles are often, but not always, fatty. Hypocellular marrow, resulting from acute marrow injury, may contain little fat. Hypercellular marrow contains markedly increased numbers of hematopoietic cells and few fat vacuoles.

If all particles are of normal or increased cellularity, the marrow itself probably is normo- or hypercellular. If all particles are deficient in hematopoietic cells, the marrow probably is hypocellular. Variation in cellularity from one particle to another may reflect patchy distribution of hematopoietic cells within the marrow. The cellularity of such marrow can be estimated only from sections of a marrow core.

Normal megakaryocytes are seen easily at low magnification as large cells with multilobed nuclei and blue to pink cytoplasm. To note that the megakaryocyte number is abnormal, there should be either markedly increased megakaryocyte numbers or almost none.

The periphery of a particle is the best area to identify and evaluate individual cells using the oil-immersion objective and to estimate the ratio of granulocytes to erythroblasts, or myeloid to erythroid (M:E) ratio. Differential counts of marrow cells are time-consuming and unnecessary for most interpretative purposes, but an estimated M:E ratio is a useful determination and quicky done. To accommodate for nonrandom distribution of cells in the smear, the overall estimate of the M:E ratio should be derived by looking at many fields in different areas. The interpretation of the M:E ratio is influenced by the cellularity of the marrow. The M:E ratio of normal feline marrow is approximately 1:1. An M:E ratio of 3:1 or greater in hypercellular marrow indicates myeloid hyperplasia, whereas the reverse indicates erythroid hyperplasia. An M:E ratio of 3:1 or greater in normo- or hypocellular marrow indicates probable erythroid suppression, whereas the reverse indicates probable myeloid suppression. An M:E ratio close to 1:1 in hypocellular marrow indicates suppression of both series.

After the M:E ratio is estimated, cells of each series should be examined for morphologic evidence of disturbed maturation and production. In unstimulated marrow, cells in late maturation stages should greatly outnumber early cells. About three-fourths of the erythroblasts should be rubricytes and metarubricytes, and an equivalent proportion of granulocytes should be metamyelocytes, bands and mature neutrophils. Hyperplasia of either series usually is accompanied, at least initially, by an increased percentage of cells in early maturation stages, a shift to the left. A predominance of cells in early stages may have any of several meanings and should be interpreted in light of peripheral blood counts at the time of bone marrow sampling and several days later. A marrow pattern of hyperplasia and shift to the left in either series may be seen at the beginning of an appropriate response to a stimulus, such as acute anemia or acute inflammation, or in the early phase of recovery from a prior state of suppression. Effective erythroid hyperplasia should be evident in rising reticulocyte counts and PCV; effective myeloid hyperplasia should be reflected by rising neutrophil counts. If there is no increase in the numbers of mature cells in blood within several days, 2 possibilities must be considered. Either the mature cells are being consumed at an excessive rate or the hyperplasia represents ineffective hematopoiesis and arrested maturation. In cats, the most frequent cause of peripheral cytopenia in the face of marrow hyperplasia is FeLV-associated hematopoietic neoplasia. Further evidence of disturbed hematopoiesis in such cats almost always can be found as morphologic abnormalities in a few or many cells. Characteristic morphologic abnormalities are described in the section on FeLV-associated hematopoietic neoplasia.

Cells other than hematopoietic cells are constituents of smears of normal marrow. Lymphocytes may be as many as 20% of the nucleated cells in feline bone marrow. These are small lymphocytes with scant cytoplasm and are dispersed among the hematopoietic cells. Plasma cells should be less than 5% of all marrow cells. Increased numbers of plasma cells indicate either an immune response or myeloma, a neoplastic proliferation of plasma cells. Bone marrow macrophages appear in smears as cells with voluminous, palely stained cytoplasm and oval nuclei (Fig C4). They are most easily recognized when filled with the debris of phagocytized cells. Many macrophages are smudged as the smear is made; their disrupted nuclei have ropy chromatin and visible nucleoli. Macrophages are particularly numerous in hyperplastic or neoplastic marrow and in acutely injured marrow. Osteoclasts and osteoblasts sometimes are included in the smear. These cells are most commonly present in marrow from young cats or cats with conditions involving active bone formation and remodeling. Osteoclasts are cells comparable in size to megakaryocytes and have multiple separate nuclei of uniform size. Their cytoplasm is blue, with pink areas and large pink granules. Osteoblasts have eccentric nuclei and trailing blue cytoplasm. They frequently form small clusters.

Smudged cells with slightly disrupted nuclei are the most commonly misinterpreted artifacts in bone marrow smears (Figs C4, C10). Some broken cells are completely disrupted, leaving only nuclei that appear as pink, amorphous or stringy masses stripped of cytoplasm. Other broken cells, less severely damaged, appear as nuclei surrounded by cytoplasm. The chromatin of partially disrupted cells is more pink and coarse than that of intact cells and forms a stippled pattern, a loose network or linear strands. The nucleoli of such cells are no longer hidden by uniformly dispersed chromatin and are highly visible. Myeloblasts, promyelocytes, rubriblasts, macrophages, osteoblasts and osteoclasts, in particular, are likely to be disrupted when the marrow particle is crushed. Smudged cells with ropy chromatin and visible nucleoli should not be interpreted as more primitive or more active than their intact counterparts.

Ferric iron, stored as hemosiderin in marrow macrophages, can be demonstrated by staining smears with Prussian blue.[43] Stored iron is evident as blue deposits of variable size and heavily concentrated in the thick areas of the marrow particle. Normal marrow should contain hemosiderin. The absence of stainable iron may indicate an iron-deficiency state, but many nonanemic cats have little bone marrow hemosiderin. Excessive marrow iron is characteristic of the anemia of chronic disorders and hemolytic anemias.

ANEMIA

A state of anemia, although it may be suspended on the basis of clinical signs and physical findings, is detected only by laboratory evaluation. A cat with a PCV less than 25%, with a correspondingly lowered Hb concentration and red cell count, is anemic. A PCV between 25% and 30% in an adult cat may reflect a pathologic decrease in red cell mass, although the anemia is so mild as to go unnoticed unless the PCV is measured. Once anemia is detected, all reasonable efforts should be made to determine the type and probable cause since prognosis and choice of treatment depend on these considerations. The diagnostic precedures should include examination of a Romanowsky-stained blood smear, reticulocyte count, white cell count, thorough physical examination to detect concurrent diseases or source of hemorrhage, and examination of bone marrow if indicated by other findings. All anemic cats, regardless of the apparent cause of anemia, should be tested for the presence of FeLV antigen.

The clinical signs and physical findings of anemic cats are related to the severity of the anemia, the rate of development, and the cause. Cats suffering acute anemia may be prostrate and gasping for breath. In contrast, cats with slowly progressing anemia show only subtle signs easily overlooked by the owner until the anemia is severe. Such cats, when finally presented for medical attention, may have a PCV below 10% yet be in little distress while calm. The clinical signs of chronic anemia are nonspecific and include lethargy, weakness and partial anorexia. An occasional cat may develop pica. Tachycardia, with heart rates of 200 beats/minute or more, shallow rapid respiration, soft systolic murmur, and pale oral mucous membranes are typical physical findings in cats with moderate to severe anemia. Retinal vessels are pale and small retinal hemorrhages may be present. The body temperature may be low, normal or high. Icterus and/or splenomegaly may be evident in cats with hemolytic anemia.

Transfusions

Cats with marked distress related to anemia may need transfusions of whole blood or packed red cells to sustain them until specific therapeutic measures can take effect or to prolong life when the disease cannot be corrected by available treatment. A blood sample for laboratory evaluation should be drawn before the patient is transfused. Blood donors should be young, healthy cats negative for FeLV antigen and FIP antibody, and splenectomized to reveal inapparent *Hemobartonella* infection. Blood for transfusion can be collected at the time of need or collected and stored at 4 C (39.2 F) for 2-3 weeks. Heparin is a satisfactory anticoagulant for blood to be transfused immediately; acid-citrate-dextrose solution should be used for stored blood.[45]

Little is known regarding blood group antigens in cats and blood typing is not done. Cats that have never been exposed to foreign red cells apparently do not have isoantibodies; therefore, no reaction is expected at the first transfusion. Crossmatching donor and recipient blood to detect incompatibility prior to subsequent transfusion is the safest procedure, but serious acute hemolytic reactions are rare, even in cats receiving multiple transfusions. Nevertheless, an immune response to the transfused red cells is implied by the short life span of donated red cells after several transfusions. Reactions to plasma proteins may occur during transfusion and are indicated by shivering, fever, vomiting or urticaria. Should this occur, administration of the transfusion should be slowed and the patient given hydrocortisone.[47]

The decision to use transfusion therapy is based on the PCV and the severity of clinical signs. A useful rule of thumb is to transfuse cats with regenerative anemias if the PCV is below 10% or cats without reticulocytosis if the PCV is below 15%.[46] These limits should be adjusted according to the obvious need for additional O_2 carrying capacity in the individual patient. A transfusion of packed red cells rather than whole blood often is advisable for normovolemic cats to avoid volume overload. The amount of red cells to be transfused is determined by either of 2 approaches. Since 40-50 ml of blood is the most that can be drawn safely from a donor cat at one time, this volume may be given arbitrarily as frequently as indicated by clinical signs. Alternatively, the amount of blood required to raise the PCV to the desired level (usually to a PCV of 18-20%) can be calculated by the following formula:[46,48]

$$\text{donor blood in anticoagulant needed (in ml)} = \frac{\text{recipient wt (lb)} \times 30 \times \text{PCV desired} - \text{PCV recipient}}{\text{PCV of donor in anticoagulant.}}$$

Classification of Anemia

The etiologic classifications of anemia can be conveniently grouped as anemias due to decreased red cell production, due to blood loss, and due to increased rate of red cell destruction. Anemias in the first category typically are normocytic normochromic and lack reticulocytosis, *ie*, they are nonregenerative, and develop over a period of weeks. Anemias in the last 2 categories are regenerative anemias that usually are acute in onset and associated with reticulocytosis. The prognosis for cats with chronic, nonregenerative anemias generally is poor. The outlook for cats with acute, regenerative anemias is considerably more optimistic.

Anemias Due to Decreased Production of Red Cells

Anemia of Chronic Disease

Cancer and chronic infections and inflammation are accompanied by mild to moderate anemia, with a PCV usually not less than 20%. Abscesses, FIP, pyometra and lymphoma are frequently associated with this type of anemia. The clinical signs are more attributable to the primary disease than to the anemia. Neutrophil and platelet counts are normal or increased, indicating that granulocytopoiesis and thrombocytopoiesis continue despite a relative failure of erythropoiesis. The bone marrow typically is normo- or hypercellular, with an increased M:E ratio, owing to decreased numbers of erythroblasts. The erythroid maturation sequence is normal and cells in the different maturation stages are present in normal proportions. The amount of marrow iron, demonstrated by Prussian blue staining, is increased.

Several factors are implicated in the development of anemia secondary to chronic diseases: slightly shortened red cell life span, impaired release of stored iron, and resistance of erythroid cells to stimulation by erythropoietin.[49] Red cell survival is modestly decreased, perhaps due to the increased phagocytic efficiency of activated macrophages. Normally functioning bone marrow would easily compensate by increasing red cell production. Instead, in the anemia of chronic disease, erythropoiesis is not stimulated and may even be less than the normal rate. The major fault in erythropoiesis appears to be the unavailability of stored iron for Hb synthesis despite the large quantities present in macrophages. The failure of iron release is reflected in low serum iron concentration (normal in cats is 68-216 g/dl).[50] The hypoferremia of chronic disease is accompanied by a low concentration of transferrin, measured as unbound iron-binding capacity (normal in cats is 105-205 g/dl) and normal to low saturation of transferrin.[50] The reduction in serum iron level prevents the appropriate increase in erythropoiesis when red cell life span is shortened. Most cats with lymphoma, even without replacement of hematopoietic tissue by extension to bone marrow, are anemic and have low reticulocyte counts.[51] Whether erythropoietic suppression in these cats is produced by the mechanism described here or by other mechanisms is not certain.

Treatment for the anemia of chronic disease is rarely necessary. The erythropoietic abnormality is corrected by resolution of the primary disease, such as removing the tumor or eliminating the infection.

Anemia of Renal Failure

A moderate anemia nearly always accompanies the decrease in functional renal tissue of advanced renal disease. The cellularity and M:E ratio of bone marrow are normal and the anemia is normocytic normochromic. The anemia develops from a slightly decreased red cell life span in an animal unable to secrete appropriate amounts of erythropoietin. The relative lack of erythropoietin precludes erythroid hyperplasia to compensate for shortened red cell survival. Treatment is supportive and directed toward relieving the metabolic abnormalities of renal disease. The anemia usually is too mild to necessitate transfusion.

Anemia Due to Deficiency of Vitamin B_{12} or Folic Acid

Vitamin B_{12} and folic acid are required for the synthesis of thymidylic acid, one of the 4 deoxyribonucleotides of DNA. Actual or functional deficiencies of these vitamins and the action of drugs that interfere with DNA synthesis, such as the anticancer agents 6-thioguanine, hydroxyurea and methotrexate, produce disturbances in hematopoietic cell maturation and peripheral cytopenias. In people, vitamin B_{12} and folic acid deficiences are common causes of anemia. The disturbed DNA synthesis results in morphologic abnormalities or erythroid cells that are described as megaloblastic changes. Affected cells are larger than normal erythroblasts. Nuclear maturation lags behind Hb synthesis. Megaloblasts with abundant Hb typically have nuclei in which the chromatin is less compact than that in a normal erythroblast. The bone marrow is quite cellular but hematopoiesis is ineffective and many developing cells die with the marrow. Red cells that are produced are oval macrocytes. Thrombocytopenia and neutropenia are common; some neutrophils are hypersegmented.

It is highly unlikely that simple deficiency of vitamin B_{12} or folic acid is ever responsible for anemia in cats. Cats fed a folate-deficient diet developed megaloblastic erythropoiesis but not anemia or macrocytosis.[52] A few anemic cats with megaloblastic changes in marrow have shown apparent response to vitamin B_{12} and folic acid treatment by a rise in PCV.[23,43,53] In most instances, where follow-up was available, the cats subsequently developed overt FeLV-associated hematopoietic neoplasia. Serum levels of vitamin B_{12} and folic acid were not measured in any of the cats. Such cases indicate that, although anemic cats with megaloblastic erythropoiesis may benefit temporarily from treatment, the primary cause is not due to vitamin deficiency but rather to the effect of FeLV on hematopoietic cells.

Aplastic Anemia, Hypoplastic Anemia and Selective Erythroid Suppression

Aplastic anemia, more correctly called aplastic pancytopenia, is a condition in which the bone marrow fails to produce red cells, granulocytes and platelets. A less complete failure of hematopoiesis is called hypoplastic anemia. Infections and bleeding tendencies due to neutropenia and thrombocytopenia usually are the first clinical manifestations of hematopoietic failure. Anemia develops later because of the longer life span of red cells. As the hematopoietic tissue diminishes, the volume of marrow fat increases. A diagnosis of aplastic or hypoplastic anemia is strongly suggested by peripheral pancytopenia and bone marrow smears that consist mainly of fat vacuoles, stroma and lymphocytes. The morphologic diagnosis should be confirmed by bone marrow biopsy.

Aplastic anemia in people is considered to represent a fault at the level of the hematopoietic stem cell. Aplastic anemia may develop via either of 2 postulated pathways: too few hematopoietic stem cells available for proliferation and differentiation because of an intrinsic defect or an extrinsic factor that reduced their number, and failure of stem cells to develop because of some suppressive substance or lack of necessary humoral factor.[54] The re-establishment of hematopoiesis after transplantation with compatible bone marrow cells indicates that most aplastic anemias in people are the result of too few stem cells.

The cause of the aplastic anemia cannot be determined in many people. Radiation, many drugs and chemicals, or immune reaction is the cause in other patients. Radiation and most of the drugs and chemicals known to cause aplastic anemia produce a dose-dependent, often reversible bone marrow suppression. The list of drugs and chemicals is long and includes chloramphenicol, phenylbutazone, benzene, DDT, lindane and many anticancer drugs. Chloramphenicol, in addition to its consistent, dose-dependent effect, can cause a rare, irreversible idiosyncratic reaction in some individuals. Circulating inhibitors of hematopoiesis and cell-mediated cytotoxic reactions directed against hematopoietic stem cells are thought to be causes of aplastic anemia in some patients. In particular, the aplastic anemia that develops in some people after viral hepatitis apparently is the result of an autoimmune response.

Selective suppression of erythropoiesis, or pure red cell aplasia, in people can be either a congenital or acquired disease.[55] Pure red cell aplasia has occurred as a secondary disorder in patients with thymoma, lymphoma and many other diseases. In other patients, pure red cell aplasia is the primary disorder. Circulating IgG, capable of inhibiting erythropoiesis, has been identified in a few patients but in most the pathogenetic mechanism has not been defined.

Any agent or mechanism capable of producing aplastic anemia in people must be considered a potential cause of aplastic anemia in cats. Chloramphenicol can suppress hematopoiesis in cats but the effect is relatively mild and reversible after cessation of use of the drug.[56] The chief cause of hematopoietic suppression and selective erythroid suppression in cats appears to be FeLV. Transient bone marrow hypoplasia may occur in most, if not all, cats at the time of infection. In one study in which FeLV was transmitted to the subject cats by contact with infected cats, the PCV, white cell count and platelet count dropped during the initial viremic period and then returned to normal.[57] The marrow during the stage of peripheral cytopenia had decreased cellularity and decreased numbers of erythroblasts and granulocytes. In other studies, certain strains of the virus inoculated into kittens produced a progressive suppression of erythropoiesis without markedly affecting neutrophil or platelet production.[58,59] A panleukopenia-like syndrome noted in some FeLV-infected cats apparently is a type of hypoplastic or aplastic anemia in combination with GI disease.[60] Affected cats display clinical signs similar to those of feline panleukopenia. These signs include anorexia, fever and dehydration often accompanied by vomiting and bloody diarrhea. The bone marrow is hypocellular, with an M:E ratio near normal;[44] the blood is anemic and neutropenic. It may be that the FeLV-mediated hematopoietic suppression renders these cats vulnerable to disease involving enteric bacteria and endotoxemia. Hematopoietic suppression likely worsens the severity of anemia in FeLV-infected cats with chronic or recurrent bacterial infections.

Erythroid suppression and nonregenerative anemia induced by FeLV is not reversible by therapeutic agents available. However, some cats may recover spontaneously and resume red cell production if given supportive therapy and blood transfusions.[61] Androgens and prednisone are of doubtful benefit, although they may be tried. Iron deficiency is not a component of the disorder and iron injections should not be given.[61] Vitamin preparations are harmless but are of no value in the treatment of hypoplastic anemia.

Anemia Due To Blood Loss

Anemias of blood loss occur from acute hemorrhage or chronic blood loss. The physical and laboratory findings in these 2 conditions are quite different.

Acute Hemorrhage

Sudden loss of blood amounting to more than 25% of the total blood volume precipitates a clinical syndrome of hypovolemic shock, with cold extremities, pale mucous membranes, prostration, tachycardia and labored breathing. Trauma and surgical procedures are the most common causes of acute blood loss in cats. Massive bleeding also may result from erosion of blood vessels in tumors and disorders of coagulation. External bleeding should be obvious; internal bleeding may be detected by paracentesis.

In the period immediately following acute hemorrhage, the PCV may be normal because of a proportional loss of plasma and red cells. Over 2-3 days, blood volume is restored by mobilization of extravascular albumin and fluid but red cells are replaced at a slower rate. The PCV drops as the red cell mass is diluted. Volume replacement therapy accelerates the drop in PCV. Erythroid hyperplasia develops and about 3 days after hemorrhage, the regenerative response is evident in a peripheral blood smear as increased numbers of polychromatophilic red cells. The PCV should return to normal about 2 weeks after a single episode of bleeding. Persistent anemia and reticulocytosis imply continued blood loss. Neutrophilic leukocytosis and thrombocytosis usually are present during the early period of acute blood loss anemia.

The urgent goals of treatment are prevention of further blood loss and restoration of blood volume to prevent shock. Lactated Ringer's solution, in a volume 2-3 times the estimated volume of blood loss, should be infused without delay. Intravenous corticosteroids are also indicated. When estimating the volume of blood loss, it should be remembered that blood volume in an adult cat is about 30 ml/lb body weight. Clinical signs of acute blood loss are apparent after 20% of the total blood volume is lost and increase in severity until 50% is lost. A loss of greater than 50% quickly causes death. Once blood volume is sufficient to avert hypovolemic shock, the red cell mass can be supplemented with blood transfusions. The PCV should not be raised higher than 20% to avoid suppression of the erythropoietic response.

Chronic Blood Loss

Continuous, slow loss of blood may not be obvious until body iron stores are depleted and iron-deficiency anemia develops. Iron for Hb synthesis is provided by food and by degradation of aged red cells. Iron is stored in macrophages and released as needed. Normally, very little iron is lost from the body and iron absorption is determined by body needs. Chronic loss of red cells upsets the normal balance. The amount of dietary iron absorbed in the intestine increases to compensate for iron loss. In cats, which are usually fed a diet rich in iron, this mechanism may avert the development of iron-deficiency anemia. However, in a few cats the iron loss may be too great or the diet too low in iron for this mechanism to be fully effective. Nursing kittens are especially susceptible to iron deficiency because of the low iron content of milk.

The hallmark of iron-deficient erythropoiesis is the microcytic hypochromic red cell. As anemia develops, the MCV and MCHC fall below the normal range. Iron deficiency should be considered if even a small portion of the red cells in a blood smear are excessively pale. Hypochromic red cells have pronounced central pallor, pale rims and are often misshapen and fragmented. Erythroid hyperplasia and a low M:E ratio are characteristic of the marrow in iron-deficiency anemia. Erythropoiesis is largely ineffective and few reticulocytes reach the peripheral blood.

Fully developed iron-deficiency anemia is rare in cats. Chronic GI or urinary tract bleeding is a possible cause in adult cats. Heavy flea infestation or hookworm burden are likely causes in kittens.

Treatment includes correcting the cause of blood loss and supplementing the diet with iron. Parenteral administration of iron should be used sparingly and only when iron deficiency is documented because of the hazards of iron overload. Iron injections should never be given on the chance that iron may improve an anemia of unknown cause. Overenthusiastic use of injectable iron can result in hemosiderosis and compromised function of many organs, including the heart and endocrine glands.

Hemolytic Anemia

Destruction of circulating red cells is accomplished by phagocytosis of red cells by macrophages in the organs of the reticuloendothelial system and by rupture of the red cell membrane, with release of Hb into the plasma. Although erythrophagocytosis takes place within vascular channels, removal by macrophages is termed extravascular hemolysis. Red cell rupture is called intravascular hemolysis. Hemolytic anemia develops when the rate of red cell destruction exceeds the rate of red cell production. In acute hemolytic anemia, the sudden destruction of many red cells causes a sharp drop in PCV. Several days later, compensatory erythroid hyperplasia is evident in peripheral blood as a rising reticulocyte count. In chronic hemolytic anemia, the PCV may be maintained at near-normal levels by increasing red cell production as much as 8 times the normal rate. Persistent reticulocytosis is expected in such circumstances.

Presumptive diagnosis of hemolytic anemia is based on finding actively erythropoietic bone marrow, appropriate peripheral reticulocytosis, and no evidence of blood loss. Icterus and hyperbilirubinema are valuable clues to the hemolytic nature of the anemia but may not be present if the rate of red cell destruction is increased only slightly. Intravascular hemolysis is indicated by hemoglobinemia and/or hemoglobinuria. Free Hb appears in urine only if the amount released from damaged red cells exceeds both the capacity of plasma haptoglobin to bind Hb and the capacity of renal tubular cells to take up filtered Hb. Serum iron concentration and marrow iron stores are normal or increased in hemolytic anemia.

Hemobartonellosis

Severe, even fatal hemolytic anemia can result from infection by *Hemobartonella felis*. Infection can be transmitted experimentally by inoculation or parasitized red cells. Natural transmission probably is via fleas or ticks. A recent study provided insight into the clinical course of the disease.[62] After infection there is a prodromal period of 2 weeks or less, followed by a second stage featuring anemia and cyclic episodes of parasitemia. During this phase, which may last a month or longer, the PCV consistently is below normal but fluctuates with sharp rises and falls. The extent of parasitemia may change abruptly; at one moment many red cells may be parasitized but within hours the parasites may be extremely scarce. The PCV does not always fall with the parasitemia as would be expected if the parasitized red cells were removed. Instead, the PCV may rise after the drop in parasitemia. Apparently, splenic macrophages can remove some organisms from the surface of the red cells, thereby decreasing the parasitemia and releasing the parasite-free red cells back to the circulation.[63] However, many parasitized red cells are phagocytized and even red cells cleared of their parasite burden probably do not circulate for long. Parasitized red cells become spherical, which makes them more susceptible to osmotic lysis and more likely to be trapped in the spleen.[64,65] The efficiency of macrophage recognition and ingestion of parasitized red cells probably is increased by production of antibodies against either the parasite or, more likely, the parasite-red cell complex. About 2 weeks after the appearance of parasites, experimentally infected cats become Coombs-positive, *ie,* their red cells are coated with antibody that can be demonstrated with feline antiglobulin.[66] Eventually the recurrent parasitemia ceases and the PCV rises to normal. The cat then becomes a carrier and later may have transient episodes of parasitemia and moderate anemia.

The clinical syndrome of naturally occurring, primary hemobartonellosis is one of acute hemolytic anemia. Anorexia, fever, splenomegaly, icterus and pallor are frequent findings. Polychromasia, metarubricytes, anisocytosis, neutrophilic leukocytosis and thrombocytosis typically are evident in blood smears. The parasites, which appear as rod-shaped, coccoid or ring-shaped bodies on red cells, may be numerous or scarce (Fig C2). If parasites are not detected in the first blood sample, more samples should be drawn later in hope of detecting a parasitemic episode. Monocytes and lymphocytes often appear reactive; some monocytes in the blood smear may contain red cells.

Blood transfusion may be necessary for severely anemic cats. Tetracyclines and arsenical compounds are helpful in reducing the parasitemia. Tetracycline is given for 3 weeks at 8 mg/lb TID or thiacetarsamide is given IV at 0.5 ml/lb once and repeated 2 days later for a total of 2 injections.[67] These drugs hasten recovery from the acute phase of the illness but the parasites rarely are completely eliminated. Recovered cats should be considered carriers.

Latent infections often become apparent when carrier cats are subjected to stress, splenectomized or infected with FeLV. In fact, *Hemobartonella* parasitemia is a fairly common finding in FeLV-infected cats. The anemia in cats with concurrent infection by *H felis* and FeLV typically is nonregenerative. Treating such cats with tetracycline or arsenical agents is not likely to result in hematologic recovery since the erythroparasite is a minor component of the disease.

Heinz-Body Hemolytic Anemia

Feline Hb is particularly susceptible to oxidative denaturation, probably because it contains a larger number of reactive sulfhydryl groups than does the Hb of other species.[68] Consequently, the normal red cell mechanisms that maintain these groups in a reduced state are relatively easily overwhelmed by oxidant drugs. In the face of oxidant stress, disulfide bonds are formed that link various parts of the Hb molecule, altering its conformation and causing it to precipitate. Oxidant drugs simultaneously may convert the ferrous iron of oxyhemoglobin to the ferric state, thereby producing methemoglobin, which cannot carry O_2. The enlarged Heinz bodies alter the shape of red cells, rendering them rigid and susceptible to intravascular lysis or phagocytosis.[69]

Chlorates, nitrates and aromatic compounds, containing amino, nitro or hydroxy functional groups, are potential causes of methemoglobinemia and Heinz-body formation. Methylene blue, phenacetin, acetaminophen and phenazopyridine can cause Heinz-body hemolytic anemia and/or toxic methemoglobinemia in cats.[70-74] Methylene blue is a component of some urinary antiseptics used to treat cystitis and urolithiasis. Phenacetin and acetaminophen are nonsalicylate analgesics available without prescription. Well-intentioned owners, aware of the toxic affects of aspirin on cats, may give preparations containing these compounds instead. Even one 325-mg tablet of acetaminophen can produce Heinz bodies and methemoglobin.[73] Serious liver damage is an additional complication of acetaminophen and phenacetin poisoning. Phenazopyridine, a urinary tract analgesic, likewise causes methemoglobinemia, Heinz-body anemia and liver damage in cats.[74] Benzocaine, a local anesthetic in some ointments, has been implicated as the cause of methemoglobinemia and Heinz-body formation in 3 dogs.[75] Although benzocaine is not readily absorbed through intact skin or oral mucosa, sufficient amounts apparently were absorbed through inflamed skin of the affected dogs to produce clinical illness. It is easy to see that an owner wishing to relieve his cat's itching might liberally apply such ointments with similar disastrous results.

Heinz-body hemolytic anemia is typically acute and usually severe. The severity of the anemia is directly related to the amount of the drug absorbed. Icterus and splenomegaly are frequent but not constant physical findings. Red cells are destroyed both by intravascular hemolysis and by erythrophagocytosis. Hemoglobinemia and hemoglobinuria are prominent in some cats. The significance of red urine as a sign of intravascular lysis may be overlooked in cats that were previously hematuric. Cyanosis and dark-brown blood due to methemoglobinemia are common signs in cats poisoned by acetaminophen, phenacetin or phenazopyridine.

The blood smear is typical of acute regenerative anemia and shows polychromasia, neutrophilic leukocytosis and thrombocytosis. Heinz bodies usually are visible in Romanowsky-stained blood smears as irregular, bulbous projections on red cells or as pale, unstained areas within the red cell. Heinz bodies are clearly demonstrated by staining blood with a supravital stain, such as new methylene blue, either by mixing blood and stain or placing a drop of stain on a dried blood smear. In wet preparations, Heinz bodies are dark-blue or green and slightly refractile. In smears of the blood-stain mixture, the Heinz bodies are light blue-green.

Patients with Heinz-body hemolytic anemia and toxic methemoglobinemia are best treated by removing the drug and giving supportive treatment until the signs abate. Methylene blue and ascorbic acid have been recommended for the treatment of toxic methemoglobinemia in people. Methylene blue should never be used in cats since it potentiates Heinz-body formation. Ascorbic acid has not been shown to be effective.[73] A recent report indicates that acetylcysteine may be a safe and effective treatment for methemoglobinemia in cats when used early in the course of acetaminophen poisoning.[76]

Autoimmune Hemolytic Anemia

Autoimmune hemolytic anemia develops when an individual produces antibodies that bind to antigens on its own red cells, thus accelerating the rate of red cell destruction. Anti-red cell antibodies are either of IgG or of IgM class of immunoglobulin. The IgG autoantibodies bind to red cell membrane antigens but usually do not cause spontaneous agglutination of red cells; IgM autoantibodies frequently agglutinate red cells. To produce agglutination, an antibody must bind to 2 or more red cells simultaneously. The IgG molecules are too small to span the distance between red cells maintained by the repulsive electronegative charges on the red cell surface. In contrast, IgM antibodies are large enough to bind to adjacent red cells. *In vitro* autoagglutination of washed red cells almost invariably indicates the presence of an IgM antibody. The presence of IgG or nonagglutinating amounts of IgM on red cells is demonstrated in the Coombs test. Antibody-coated red cells are agglutinated when incubated in serum containing antibody to the immunoglobulin of the species being tested. The anti-immunoglobulin in the Coombs serum binds to the immunoglobulin on the red cells, causing agglutination. Similarly, complement-coated red cells are agglutinated by anticomplement antibody. Complement is fixed to the red cell membrane by IgM autoantibodies and only rarely by IgG. Only one molecule of IgM need be bound to the red cell surface to fix complement. In contrast, 2 IgG molecules must be bound close together and in the proper spatial configuration to fix complement. With most IgG-red cell interactions, the immunoglobulin molecules are not close enough to fix and activate complement.[77]

In vivo, IgG-coated red cells are recognized and bound by macrophages through their receptors for the Fc portion of the IgG molecule. The bound red cells are phagocytized either wholly or in part. Prolonged contact between red cells and macrophages in the splenic red pulp makes the spleen the major site of removal of red cells coated with relatively few IgG molecules. At high antibody titers and many IgG molecules per red cell, Kupffer cells in the liver assume a more important role in the hemolytic process.[78]

Because autoantibodies of the IgG class bind most avidly to red cells at physiologic temperature (37 C), they are called warm-reacting antibodies.

The IgM autoantibodies typically have greatest affinity for red cells at temperatures below 37 C and are called cold-reacting antibodies, or cold agglutinins. Cold agglutinins attach to red cells in vessels in the cool extremities, fix complement, then elute from the red cells as they are carried into the warm interior. Intravascular hemolysis results if complement is completely activated. More often, complement activation is incomplete and C3 is left on the red cell membrane. The C3-coated red cells are cleared primarily by macrophages in the liver; splenic clearance is inefficient.[78] The presence of cold agglutinins is indicated by autoagglutination in a chilled blood sample that disperses as the sample is warmed to 37 C.

These pathogenetic mechanisms have important implications regarding treatment. Splenectomy benefits patients with a low titer of IgG autoantibodies but has little effect in patients with IgM autoantibodies or a high titer of IgG. Glucocorticoids act first to interfere with macrophage binding and ingestion of red cells; eventually, they reduce antibody production. Glucocorticoids are most effective in preventing phagocytosis of IgG-coated red cells but are unable to reduce clearance of IgM- and complement-coated red cells.[78]

Autoimmune hemolytic anemia in the cat almost always is associated with FeLV infection, either as the primary manifestation or as a secondary complication of lymphoma, hematopoietic suppression or hematopoietic neoplasia.[67,79,80] Presumably, FeLV either induces antigenic changes in red cells that stimulate antibody production or causes disturbances in the immune system that allow production of antibodies against normal red cell antigens. Antibody-mediated thrombocytopenia is an additional problem in some cats with autoimmune hemolytic anemia.

Most cats with autoimmune hemolytic anemia uncomplicated by concurrent erythroid suppression are presented for examination with a history of 5-10 days of anorexia, lethargy and other nonspecific signs of illness.[79] Pallor, icterus, splenomegaly and hepatomegaly are usual physical findings. The anemia is moderate to severe (PCV less than 20%) and accompanied by a modest reticulocytosis. Monocytosis, with reactive monocytes, is common.

The clinical and hematologic findings of autoimmune hemolytic anemia are very similar to those of hemobartonellosis. A diagnosis of autoimmune hemolytic anemia should be based on a positive Coombs test or autoagglutination of washed red cells, evidence of effective erythropoiesis (reticulocytosis with or without circulating nucleated red cells), and failure to find *H felis* after examining sequential blood smears. The autoantibody usually is IgG but a few patients have an IgM autoantibody. Failure to find reticulocytosis in a Coombs-positive cat implies a concurrent disturbance of hematopoiesis; a bone marrow examination is indicated.

Affected cats should be treated with glucocorticoids and supportive care as indicated. Some cats respond well to glucocorticoids and make a full recovery, at least temporarily. Some live long and healthy lives even though infected with FeLV. Most affected cats experience recurrences or develop other FeLV-associated disorders that prove fatal. Cats with autoimmune hemolytic anemia should be examined thoroughly to detect concurrent lymphoma that might be amenable to treatment.

Congenital Erythropoietic Porphyria

Congenital porphyria is the only known inherited defect of Hb synthesis in cats. The disorder is characterized by an accumulation of the type-I isomers of uroporphyrin and coproporphyrin in red cells and other tissues. The disease is extremely rare; 2 families of affected cats have been studied.[81,82] The disease was mild in one family and quite severe in the other. Porphyrins are red pigments that discharge energy when exposed to ultraviolet light, causing fluorescence and photochemical reactions. Bones and teeth of porphyric animals are red-brown and fluoresce pink under ultraviolet light.

The anemia is hemolytic, with compensatory erythroid hyperplasia and reticulocytosis. The excessive porphyrin content of red cells apparently makes them rigid and subject to fragmentation. Schistocytes and polychromatophilic macrocytes are characteristic findings in blood smears. Many red cells contain Pappenheimer bodies, coarse blue granules that represent iron-loaded mitochondria, as evidence of the abnormal incorporation of iron into heme.

LEUKOCYTOSIS AND LEUKOPENIA

Leukocytosis refers to a total white cell count higher than the upper limit of the range established for healthy cats. A white cell count exceeding 19,500/μl is a useful numeric definition of leukocytosis; leukopenia is a white cell count less than 5500/μl, the lower limit of the normal range. In almost every instance, alterations in the neutrophil count are responsible for the abnormal white cell count. Increases and decreases in the absolute number of other white cells rarely shift the white cell count out of the normal range. Nevertheless, quantitative changes in lymphocytes, monocytes and eosinophils are of importance to the interpretation of leukocyte patterns. The white cell count, the differential count expressed as absolute numbers, and an assessment of morphologic characteristics are used to identify an abnormal leukocyte pattern as resulting from physiologic response, stress response, inflammatory response or hematopoietic suppression or neoplasia.

Neutrophilia and Neutropenia

Neutrophilic leukocytosis can be due to shifts in neutrophil distribution within the vascular system, prolonged circulation time, release of marrow reserves, or increased marrow production of neutrophils.

Physiologic leukocytosis is recognized as an increased white cell count, usually less than 25,000/μl, with increased neutrophils and normal to increased numbers of lymphocytes, eosinophils and monocytes. The mechanism of redistribution of neutrophils from marginated pool to circulating pool has been described in an earlier section.

Stress leukocytosis, produced by the effect of endogenous or exogenous glucocorticoids, is a neutrophilic leukocytosis, with lymphopenia and eosinopenia. The monocyte count is normal or increased. The acute response to glucocorticoids is evident within 8 hours of a dose of prednisone and is due mainly to the release of mature neutrophils from the marrow.[23] The chronic response to continued glucocorticoid stimulation may represent a combination of increased effective granulocytopoiesis and decreased rates of egress of neutrophils from the vasculature. Leukocytosis subsides within 24 hours of a single dose of glucocorticoids but persists for several days after cessation of long-term glucocorticoid administration.[83] Stress leukocytosis is expected in any cat treated with glucocorticoids or subjected to such physical stress as surgery, trauma, pain, exposure to heat or cold, or electric shock. Hyperadrenocorticism produces a similar pattern. Stress leukocytosis is a component of most debilitating conditions and serious metabolic disturbances.

Mild, nonpurulent inflammatory conditions may elicit a modest neutrophilic leukocytosis difficult to distinguish from stress leukocytosis on hematologic findings alone. However, the lymphocyte count often is normal rather than decreased. Animals in the convalescence stage of infections or inflammatory disease may have a slightly elevated white cell count and neutrophil count, with a normal lymphocyte count.

More severe inflammation that involves numerous bacteria or tissue injury, resulting in necrosis, denaturation of serum and tissue protein, and complement activation, evokes a greater neutrophil response. The white cell count may go as high as 75,000/μl. Neutrophils and monocytes are attracted to the site of inflammation and are lost from the circulation. The need for neutrophils is initially met by release of marrow reserves. If the inflammation and accelerated loss of neutrophils persists, myeloid hyperplasia develops and neutrophils are produced at an increased rate. Immature neutrophils often are released during the inflammatory response. Neutrophilic leukocytosis with a significant left shift (more than 1000 immature neutrophils/μl) is characteristic of the leukocyte pattern of inflammation.[83] Monocytosis usually is evident after several days. Lymphopenia and eosinopenia reflect concurrent stress.

Some infections are so severe and acute that bone marrow and blood are depleted of neutrophils. In such an instance, the white cell count and neutrophil count may be normal or decreased but the number of immature neutrophils may exceed 300/μl, considered a significant left shift when present with neutropenia or normal neutrophil count.[83] This pattern is most likely to occur during the early stages of infection due to gram-negative bacteria, with endotoxemia. Endotoxin effects release of marrow neutrophils but also damages neutrophils, causing them to be sequestered in the spleen and microvasculature. Sequential hematologic evaluation should show a rising neutrophil count, with marked toxic changes in neutrophils.

A leukocyte pattern of inflammation is produced by a variety of infectious and noninfectious diseases. Abscesses, FIP, pyoderma, pyometra, pneumonia, peritonitis and pleuritis are among the common infectious diseases of cats. Pancreatitis, aspiration pneumonia, necrotic tumors, foreign bodies and acute hemolytic anemias are among the noninfectious causes of neutrophilic leukocytosis with a significant left shift.

Persistent neutropenia usually is caused by FeLV-associated hematopoietic suppression or neoplasia. Transient neutropenia of feline panleukopenia is discussed below.

Lymphocytosis and Lymphopenia

The lymphocyte count in healthy, calm cats should fall between 1500 and 7000/µl. Counts below and above this range constitute lymphopenia and lymphocytosis, respectively. Most of the lymphocytes in blood are long-lived T- and B-lymphocytes that are part of a recirculating pool of lymphocytes. Recirculating lymphocytes leave blood vessels as they pass through lymphatic tissue, migrate to T- and B-lymphocyte areas of the tissue, and return to blood via lymphatic vessels and the thoracic duct. Since these lymphocytes amount to only a small fraction of the total body lymphocyte mass, changes in the blood lymphocyte count do not necessarily reflect changes in lymphocyte mass. Conversely, changes in production of lymphocytes are not always associated with alterations in the blood lymphocyte count. The size of the recirculating pool is fairly constant; alterations in blood lymphocyte count usually are due to shifts in the distribution of the recirculating pool.

Lymphocytosis is often a part of the leukocyte pattern of excitement in cats. This physiologic lymphocytosis may be due to an influx of thoracic duct lymphocytes or a transient failure of lymphocyte migration into tissue.[41] The lymphocyte count is high but the cells are morphologically normal, small lymphocytes. Increased, antigen-driven production and release of lymphocytes from lymphatic tissue account for lymphocytosis following immunization, infection and autoimmune or hypersensitivity reactions. In such circumstances, the lymphocytosis is due to increased numbers of short-lived lymphocytes traveling through blood from their sites of production to other tissues. Some of these lymphocytes appear reactive and sometimes are called immunocytes. Lymphocytosis also may be a feature of lymphoid neoplasia. Neoplastic lymphopoiesis should be suspected if many blood lymphocytes are large and have a low nucleus to cytoplasm ratio. Confirmation should be sought by examination of bone marrow and biopsy of masses or enlarged lymph nodes.

Lymphopenia most frequently is due to stress. Glucocorticoids induce sequestration of lymphocytes in tissue compartments.[84] Lymphopenia also follows irradiation or the administration of cytotoxic drugs capable of killing intermitotic cells. Such drugs as azothiaprine and methotrexate, which are selective for actively proliferating cells, do not have an immediate effect on blood lymphocyte count. The recirculating lymphocytes are spared because of their low turnover rate. Some viruses induce lymphopenia by lysing cells, causing sequestration, or other mechanisms not yet determined. Lymphopenia is a frequent finding in FIP, panleukopenia and many FeLV-associated diseases. Lymphocyte loss is another cause of lymphopenia. Repeated drainage of fluid from the pleural cavity of a cat with a ruptured thoracic duct could profoundly deplete the recirculating lymphocyte pool. Loss of lymphocytes from intestinal lymphatic vessels would have the same effect. Lymphopenia due to congenital immunodeficiency has not been noted in cats.

Monocytosis

The monocyte count is usually lower than 850/µl; higher counts constitute monocytosis. Monocytosis may be part of the stress response or of the response to inflammation. Monocytosis with activated monocytes is particularly evident in diseases involving antibody-mediated hemolysis or cell-mediated immune response. Specific disorders in which monocytosis and/or activated monocytes is expected include hemobartonellosis, autoimmune hemolytic anemia, histoplasmosis, toxoplasmosis and FIP.

Eosinophilia and Eosinopenia

Eosinophilia, blood eosinophil counts greater than 1500/µl, usually implies an immediate hypersensitivity reaction involving release of mast cell granules or a T-lymphocyte-mediated immune response. The skin, respiratory tract and GI tract are the tissues most often affected by conditions that evoke an eosinophil response. Eosinophilia may be present without signs of the underlying disease and the cause may go undetermined.

Internal parasites are a major cause of eosinophilia but the eosinophil response occurs only at certain stages in the host-parasite interaction. In general, eosinophilia in parasitic diseases coincides with the period when parasite antigens are exposed to sensitized T-lymphocytes, which then release factors that increase eosinophil production and attract eosinophils to the parasite. Intestinal helminths produce eosinophilia as larvae migrate through tissue but not while adult parasites reside in the intestinal lumen. Eosinophilia in lungworm (*Aelurostrongylus abstrussus*) infection is most pronounced during the time larvae are shed.[85] The eosinophilia wanes as the worms are walled off by a granulomatous inflammatory response. Eosinophilia is evident at certain stages of heartworm (*Dirofilaria immitis*) infection in cats.[86]

A recent report describes 6 cats with marked eosinophilia and eosinophilic gastroenteritis and compared the findings with the hypereosinophilic syndrome in people.[87] The hypereosinophilic syndrome in people is characterized by persistent eosinophilia and diffuse organ infiltration by mature eosinophils.[88] The syndrome covers a spectrum of disorders varying in severity and extent of tissue involvement. The cause is unknown but thought to be a hypersensitivity reaction to an unknown antigen or group of antigens. The extreme eosinophilia in some patients has been called eosinophilic leukemia by some. Of the 6 cats in the report mentioned above, 2 had eosinophilic infiltration restricted to the GI tract and 4 had disseminated eosinophilic infiltration of other abdominal organs. One was considered to have eosinophilic leukemia on the basis of immaturity of blood eosinophils and the extent of infiltration in various organs. The disorder was fatal in all cats.

Eosinopenia almost always is a reflection of increased serum concentration of glucocorticoids, either due to administration or due to endogenous release during stress or as a result of hyperadrenocorticism.

Feline Panleukopenia

Feline panleukopenia is caused by a parvovirus that requires actively proliferating cells for its own replication and cytolytic activity.[89,90] In postnatal cats, cells in bone marrow, lymph nodes and intestinal crypts fulfill the needs of the virus and are most affected in the pathogenesis of the disease. Soon after infection, the virus produces an almost complete depletion of differentiating hematopoietic cells. Stem cells and slowly proliferating committed precursor cells are spared. The sudden decrease in the volume of hematopoietic tissue allows congestion of venous sinuses; many of these fragile vessels rupture, producing hemorrhage and edema. Marrow at this stage examined grossly is red but hypocellular, an exception to the rule that red marrow is active marrow. Hemorrhage and cell destruction evidently stimulate marrow macrophages. Smears of marrow collected in this early stage are devoid of hematopoietic cells but contain many lymphocytes and large, vacuolated macrophages (Fig C4). Mature eosinophils are also present. Peripheral blood is markedly leukopenic; the white cell count often falls below 1000/μl. Lymphocytes and eosinophils are the only cells left in peripheral blood. The white cell count remains low until the marrow repopulates and a wave of granulocytes is released.

Marrow in the hypoplastic stage of feline panleukopenia appears different from aplastic or hypoplastic marrow associated with FeLV infection. In the latter condition, fat is more evident, there is no macrophage response, and the few hematopoietic cells present are in various stages of maturation. The leukopenia is usually less severe and anemia frequently present.

Marrow regeneration after panleukopenia virus infection begins quickly and is recognized by the presence of a uniform population of myeloblasts and promyelocytes. Early regeneration is evident in histologic sections of marrow as scattered foci of myeloblasts. The marrow becomes uniformly hypercellular as the wave of granulocyte regeneration continues (Fig C5). If marrow is sampled before the first cohort has reached later maturation stages, the pattern may be misinterpreted as arrested maturation or neoplasia since band and mature neutrophils are not present. However, within another day or 2 the regenerative nature of the abnormal pattern is evident in rapidly climbing white cell and neutrophil counts.

The first neutrophils to reach the blood during recovery from panleukopenia are strikingly abnormal in appearance. The cytoplasm is blue but not vacuolated and nuclei take many strange forms. Many neutrophils are larger than normal cells. The white cell count may reach 50,000/μl before dropping back to the normal range. If the recovery is uncomplicated by secondary infections, the white cell count and neutrophil appearance become normal in several days.

The course of bone marrow depletion and regeneration covers about 5-7 days from infection by the virus to return of neutrophils to peripheral blood. A cat may be presented for examination any time during that period. It is important to remember that a patient may be seriously ill from the metabolic disturbances of dehydration and diarrhea at the time when bone marrow recovery is advanced and the white cell count is high. The morphologic features of the neutrophils are a more important aid to the correct diagnosis in such a cat than the white cell count.

Thrombocytosis and Thrombocytopenia

The platelet count in healthy cats is between 300,000 and 700,000/μl. High-normal or slightly increased platelet counts most often accompany the leukocytosis of inflammation or are seen during a regenerative response to anemia. Thrombocytopenia, although defined as a platelet count less than 300,000/μl, does not assume clinical significance until the platelet count is much lower. Abnormal bleeding due to thrombocytopenia is not apparent unless the platelet count is below 50,000/μl if platelet function is normal. Thrombocytopenia may be due to peripheral destruction or decreased production of platelets.

Autoimmune thrombocytopenia has been observed in cats and may be more common than previously recognized.[91] Enough platelets may be consumed in severe disseminated intravascular coagulation to result in thrombocytopenia. Perhaps the most frequent cause of thrombocytopenia in cats is decreased production. Megakaryocyte numbers and platelet production are markedly decreased in some forms of FeLV-associated hematopoietic neoplasia. Replacement of hematopoietic tissue by intramedullary lymphoid neoplasms likewise curtails megakaryocytopoiesis.

Cats with thrombocytopenia and bleeding tendencies should be transfused with fresh, whole blood since stored blood contains too few platelets to be beneficial. Prednisone should be given if destruction by macrophages is the probable cause. This would be indicated by thrombocytopenia, many megakaryocytes in marrow, and no evidence of diffuse intravascular coagulation.

NEOPLASTIC DISEASES OF BONE MARROW

Current Classification of Hematopoietic Neoplasia in People

In people, neoplastic disorders of hematopoietic stem cells can be grouped into 3 major categories on the basis of clinical syndrome and hematologic patterns: myeloproliferative disorders, hematopoietic dysplasia ("preleukemia"), and acute myelogenous leukemia. During the past decade, evidence has accrued to support the hypothesis that hematopoietic neoplasms in all categories are clonal in nature, *ie,* they arise from single hematopoietic stem cells. Each category comprises several subclassifications.

Myeloproliferative Disorders[16,92-95]

The myeloproliferative disorders include polycythemia vera, chronic myelocytic (granulocytic) leukemia, primary thrombocytosis, and myelofibrosis/myeloid metaplasia. These disorders represent a clonal proliferation of hematopoietic stem cells that results in overproduction of mature cells. The marrow is hypercellular, at least initially, in each disorder. Splenomegaly is a consistent feature. Overproduction of red cells is the predominant feature of polycythemia vera but thrombocytosis and neutrophilic leukocytosis are also typical. Neutrophilic leukocytosis is extreme in chronic myelocytic leukemia but megakaryocytic hyperplasia and thrombocytosis accompany the granulocyte hyperplasia. Thrombocytosis, with platelet counts in excess of 1,000,000/μl, is the chief feature of primary thrombocytosis; neutrophilia is common. Myelofibrosis-myeloid metaplasia begins as a panhyperplasia in marrow but hematopoietic tissue is rapidly replaced by fibrosis and the spleen becomes enlarged with extramedullary hematopoiesis. The proliferative disorders typically have an indolent course and patients survive for several years. Myelofibrosis often develops and any of the disorders may terminate as hematopoietic failure due to replacement of marrow hematopoietic tissue with collagen. Acute leukemia, in which the marrow is packed with blast cells that fail to mature, is the terminal event in some patients. Patients in terminal "blast crisis," like those with myelofibrosis and hematopoietic failure, succumb to infection, bleeding and anemia.

Hematopoietic Dysplasia[96-100]

Hematopoietic dysplasia, or preleukemia, is a stem cell disorder resulting in underproduction of mature blood cells. The marrow typically is cellular, with all 3 cell lines represented, but production apparently is ineffective and disproportionately few mature red cells, granulocytes and platelets reach the circulating blood. The hallmark of hematopoietic dysplasia is the presence of qualitative abnormalities in 2 or more cell lines. In most patients, the diagnosis is based mainly on morphologic abnormalities visible in Romanowsky-stained bone marrow smears. Typical abnormalities in the erythroid line include megaloblastoid features (asynchrony of nuclear and cytoplasmic maturation), multinucleated erythroblasts, nuclear fragmentation, disproportionately high numbers of very young erythroblasts, and ringed sideroblasts (erythroblasts in which iron-laden mitochondria encircle the nucleus). Dysplastic megakaryocytes may be small megakaryocytes containing one round nucleus or several discrete nuclei (dwarf or micromegakaryocytes) or large megakaryocytes containing many separate nuclei. Dysplastic granulocytopoiesis is evident as a left shift in which early myelocytes or younger cells predominate. Dysplastic hematopoiesis is reflected in peripheral blood as macrocytes, neutrophils with hypersegmented nuclei or Pelger-Huët nuclei (oval or bilobed), and giant platelets with abnormal granulation. Other abnormalities in the cells of the abnormal clone can be detected by electron microscopy, cytochemistry, functional assays and bone marrow culture.

There is some variation in the bone marrow patterns among patients with hematopoietic dysplasia. The cellularity usually is normal or increased but may be decreased. In some patients the erythroid line predominates and granulocytes are few; the reverse is present in other patients, and in still others there is a near-normal mixture of erythroblasts and granulocytes. Megakaryocytic hyperplasia is a striking feature in some patients. Different morphologic diagnoses have been used for the different patterns, including primary acquired sideroblastic anemia, refractory megaloblastic anemia, refractory anemia with excess myeloblasts, red cell aplasia with excess myeloblasts, erythremic myelosis and erythroleukemia, and chronic myelomonocytic leukemia, in which peripheral blood cells appear to have morphologic features of both monocytes and neutrophils. The trend among hematologists is to recognize that these patterns, rather than representing discrete disease entities, are various manifestations of a stem cell disorder and should be grouped together.

In many patients with hematopoietic dysplasia, the disease progresses to acute myelogenous leukemia. For this reason, some hematologists prefer the term "preleukemia." However, years may pass before acute leukemia emerges. Many patients die of the complications related to anemia, neutropenia and thrombocytopenia before acute leukemia develops. Since most patients are elderly, death due to age-related disorders may supervene. Nevertheless, bone marrow culture studies indicate that hematopoietic dysplasia, or preleukemia, is a neoplastic disorder in which the malignant clone is established; precursor cell maturation becomes progressively impaired until there is termination in the severe maturational block recognized as acute myelogenous leukemia.[100]

Acute Myelogenous Leukemia[101,102]

Acute myelogeneous leukemia is an hematopoietic neoplasm characterized by accumulation of blast cells in blood and bone marrow and a failure to produce mature blood cells. The predominant manifestation is in the granulocyte-monocyte series but erythroid and megakaryocyte series are also involved. A block in maturation at the myeloblast-promonocyte stage, rather than proliferation, is responsible for the accumulation of neoplastic cells. The growth of normal hematopoietic clones is suppressed by the neoplastic clone.

The bone marrow in patients with acute myelogenous leukemia is packed with immature cells of the granulocyte-monocyte series. Many neoplastic cells circulate and infiltrate other tissues. Acute myelogenous leukemia is subclassified according to the direction of differentiation and the extent of maturation apparent in bone marrow smears. Cytochemical technics are of great value in appropriately classifying the variants of the disease.[103] The most useful reactions are those that demonstrate myeloperoxidase, chloroacetate esterase and nonspecific esterase. Myeloperoxidase activity is present in granulocytes and monocytes. Chloroacetate esterase activity is specific for neutrophils. Nonspecific esterase, with alpha-naphthol butyrate as the substrate, is specific for monocytes and macrophages. Using these special stains, acute myelogenous leukemia can be differentiated from acute lymphoblastic leukemia (myeloblasts are practically indistinguishable from lymphoblasts in Romanowsky-stained smears) and subclassified as myeloblastic with or without slight maturation, myelomonocytic (in which the neoplastic population comprises both granulocytes and monocytes or cells that contain both granulocyte and monocyte enzymes), or monocytic (in which cells with monocyte enzymes predominate).

FeLV-Associated Hematopoietic Neoplasia (Feline Myeloproliferative Disorders)

The various patterns of disturbed hematopoiesis in FeLV-infected cats that are discussed in this section have been called feline myeloproliferative disorders.[23] However, in view of current knowledge concerning the variants of hematopoietic neoplasia in people and cats, it is clear that the disease in cats is more closely analogous to hematopoietic dysplasia and acute myelogenous leukemia than to myeloproliferative disorders in people. The syndrome in cats is not one of overproduction of mature blood cells but rather of underproduction from disturbed maturation of hematopoietic cells. Affected cats are consistently anemic and often neutropenic and thrombocytopenic. Abnormal cells of all 3 series often are present in blood and/or marrow. The appropriate studies have not yet been performed to show whether FeLV-associated hematopoietic neoplasia is indeed a clonal hemopathy. However, the morphologic parallels between the species are strong. It is reasonable to assume, until research indicates otherwise, that hematopoietic neoplasia in cats also reflects a fundamental defect in a hematopoietic stem cell, in this case probably induced by FeLV.

FeLV-associated hematopoietic neoplasia includes 4 major hematologic patterns (Table 3), although a degree of overlap suggesting transition may be evident in some cats. The clinical signs and physical findings in affected cats are remarkably uniform. At the time of initial examination, most cats with FeLV-associated hematopoietic neoplasia have a history of illness of fairly short duration and manifested as listlessness, anorexia, weight loss and, frequently, vomiting. Dehydration, splenomegaly and signs of severe anemia are consistent physical findings. Hepatomegaly and enlarged lymph nodes are present in some cats. Nearly all are positive for FeLV group-specific antigen on immunofluorescence. The PCV typically is less than 15%. The diagnosis and classification of hematopoietic neoplasia are based on the cellular patterns in blood and bone marrow.

Erythremic Myelosis

In this form of hematopoietic neoplasia, erythroid hyperplasia dominates the marrow pattern but ineffective erythropoiesis is implicit in the persistent anemia and lack of reticulocytosis. Morphologic abnormalities, such as megaloblastoid erythroblasts, may be evident but need not be prominent (Fig C6). In some cats, the erythroid maturation sequence appears complete and the smear contains approximately normal proportions of early and late erythroblasts. In others, rubriblasts and prorubricytes are present in excess. Granulocytes and megakaryocytes often are not noticeably abnormal.

The chief abnormalities in blood smears are the absence of polychromatophilic red cells and the presence of numerous erythroblasts, which may be megaloblastoid rubricytes or apparently

Table 3. Classification of Bone Marrow Neoplasms

FeLV-associated hematopoietic neoplasia (myeloproliferative disorders)
Erythremic myelosis
Erythroleukemia
Myelogenous leukemia
Granulocytic
Myelomonocytic
Monocytic
Leukemia of undetermined cell type (reticuloendotheliosis)
FeLV-associated lymphoid neoplasia
Lymphocytic (lymphoblastic) leukemia
Lymphoma with extension to bone marrow
Metastatic tumors, especially mastocytomas
Miscellaneous conditions, possibly neoplastic
Polycythemia vera
Eosinophilic leukemia

normal polychromatophilic rubricytes and metarubricytes. Circulating erythroblasts may outnumber the white cells. In cats with megaloblastoid erythropoiesis, macrocytes may be numerous enough to raise the MCV above normal.

Erythroleukemia

Obvious disturbances in granulocytopoiesis accompany the abnormal erythropoiesis in this variant of hematopoietic neoplasia (Fig C7). The division between erythremic myelosis and erythroleukemia is not distinct; the choice of the appropriate classification for an individual patient often is a matter of personal judgment. In general, the morphologic abnormalities in erythroblasts, granulocytes and megakaryocytes are more pronounced in erythroleukemia. Many erythroblasts show evidence of asynchronous maturation of nucleus and cytoplasm. In some cells the nucleus is immature but the cytoplasm is pink with Hb. In other cells the nucleus may be dense and clumped but the cytoplasm is still blue. Nuclei may appear deficient in chromatin and have large nucleoli. Giant erythroblasts and multinucleated erythroblasts may be present. Many of the immature cells may have the deep-blue cytoplasm and coarse chromatin of rubriblasts and prorubricytes but contain pink granules suggestive of granulocytic differentiation. Cells obviously belonging to the granulocyte series often have bizarrely shaped nuclei and retain cytoplasmic basophilia in later stages. Megakaryocytes may be scarce or plentiful but at least some are morphologically abnormal. Some of these are small and contain one or 2 nuclei (Figs C7, C10); others are more normal in size but contain multiple nuclei or bizarrely lobulated nuclei.

The peripheral blood of cats with erythroleukemia contains a variety of abnormal cells. In some cats, megaloblastoid erythroblasts are numerous and the MCV is high. In others, abnormal red cell precursors are found only after careful searching. Granulocytes with hypersegmented nuclei or odd nuclear shapes may be interspersed with granulocytes of normal appearance. Platelet counts generally are high and many platelets are large and pleomorphic. Most cats with erythroleukemia have few to many of the very immature cells that resemble rubriblasts with granules. Additional examples of blood and bone marrow cells in erythremic myelosis and erythroleukemia are shown elsewhere.[23,43,104,105]

Myelogenous Leukemia

Myeloid hyperplasia and diminished numbers of erythroblasts and megakaryocytes characterize the bone marrow pattern in the variants of this form of hematopoietic neoplasia. The condition is said to be subleukemic if the white cell count is low and few abnormal cells circulate, and leukemic if abnormal cells are numerous in the blood. The neoplastic growth may involve predominantly granulocytes (granulocytic leukemia), predominantly monocytes (monocytic leukemia), or both (myelomonocytic leukemia).

In granulocytic leukemia, the marrow is hypercellular with cells of the neutrophilic granulocyte series. Myeloblasts and promyelocytes predominate, but more mature cells are also present. The peripheral blood in leukemic forms has a high white cell count and many myeloblasts and promyelocytes.

In monocytic leukemia, the predominant cell in the blood and marrow is monocytic in appearance (Fig C8). The cytoplasm is blue and may contain granules and/or vacuoles. The nucleus is elongated, folded or indented and composed of fine chromatin.

In myelomonocytic leukemia, the neoplastic cells are a mixture of neutrophilic granulocytes and monocytes (Fig C9). Blast cells may be numerous in marrow but most circulating neutrophils are later-stage cells, with hypersegmented or long, ribbon-like nuclei (Fig C10).

There is considerable variation among cats in the number of erythroblasts and megakaryocytes remaining in the marrow in the variants of myelogenous leukemia. Megakaryocytes may be strikingly increased in number but more often are scarce.[106] Many may have abnormal morphologic features. Erythroblasts almost always are few, but diligent searching of a bone marrow smear often shows some megaloblastoid erythroblasts. Erythroblasts and giant, bizarre platelets may be present in blood smears; their number and appearance there reflect the number and quality of erythroblasts and megakaryocytes in marrow.

Case histories and additional examples of blood and marrow cells in myelogenous leukemias are reported elsewhere.[105-113]

Reticuloendotheliosis

This term has been applied to the form of hematopoietic neoplasia in which the bone marrow and blood contain few differentiated cells but many cells that share the morphologic characteristics of round nuclei, with evenly dispersed chromatin and blue cytoplasm that may contain pink granules (Fig C11). The cytoplasm usually extends to one side of the nucleus and may be drawn into a tail. Many may contain ingested red cells or other cell debris. A population of cells of abnormal erythroid or granulocytic differentiation may be present as well.

The lineage of these cells has not been determined. Some have suggested that they are pluripotent cells; others have suggested that they belong to the erythroid series.[114] The term "reticuloendotheliosis" should be discarded. It was introduced many years ago to designate the condition in cats in which cells of this type were present in large numbers in spleen, bone marrow, liver and lymph nodes, the organs of the reticuloendothelial system, and to distinguish this condition from lymphoid neoplasia.[115] Because the cells lacked features that would allow classification into differentiated hematopoietic cell lines, they were called reticulum cells or reticuloendothelial cells. Until the nature of these cells is more clearly understood, it is perhaps preferable to call the condition leukemia of undetermined cell type. Several reports of cats with this form of hematopoietic neoplasia are available.[116-118]

The blood and bone marrow patterns in most cats with hematopoietic neoplasia conform fairly closely to one or another of the general descriptions given above. However, in one cat the megakaryocyte line was the most remarkably abnormal series.[119] In addition to the severe anemia typical of all forms, this patient had extreme megakaryocytic hyperplasia and thrombocytosis. Large blast cells, thought to be megakaryocytic, circulated in increasing numbers as the disease progressed.

By the time hematopoietic neoplasia is diagnosed, the spleen is infiltrated with hematopoietic cells and often the liver and lymph nodes also are involved. Imprint smears of these organs made at necropsy contain cells similar to those in the blood and marrow. The presence of hematopoietic cells in these and other tissues represents extension of the neoplastic process rather than compensatory extramedullary hematopoiesis by normal cells.

An autoimmune response is evident in some cats. A positive Coombs test and agglutination of red cells and erythroblasts in smears has been reported.[23,120] Phagocytosis of red cells and/or platelets by circulating neutrophils or monocytes occurs in some cats and implies production of anti-red cell and antiplatelet immunoglobulin. Lupus erythematosus cells, which indicate production of antinuclear antibody, have also been noted.[104]

Precise classification of the form of hematopoietic neoplasia is of little importance with regard to patient management. No program of treatment has produced permanent or even good temporary remission.[120-122] Various cytotoxic drugs may decrease the number of abnormal cells for a time but normal hematopoiesis is not restored and serious side effects may even hasten death. Successful therapy, if it is ever developed, probably will be directed toward eliminating the virus, perhaps through enhancement of the immune response, rather than toward suppressing the growth of abnormal cells.[123] Transfusions and intensive supportive care, including prompt treatment of infections, remain the most useful means of prolonging survival and improving the quality of life. Despite the best of care, affected cats usually die of infections, hemorrhage or organ dysfunction within a short time after the disease is discovered.

Most owners of affected cats, when informed of the improbability of long-term survival, may decide on euthanasia. However, a bit of cautious optimism can be offered with some justification. Some cats may remain fairly stable for a period of months if transfused periodically. The disease appears to progress from a pattern of moderately abnormal maturation to a pattern of greater immaturity and atypia.[105,120,124] Therefore a cat with erythremic myelosis or granulocytic leukemia, in which there is a residual population of fairly normal-appearing cells and a PCV of 15% or higher, may be expected to survive longer than a cat with more markedly abnormal maturation and more severe anemia and leukopenia. A few cats may experience temporary or prolonged spontaneous remission if maintained with transfusions after the diagnosis is made.[125]

Myelofibrosis

Myelofibrosis, the replacement of hematopoietic tissue with collagen, has been noted in cats with hematopoietic neoplasia.[23] At one time, popular thought held that marrow fibroblastic cells were derived from pluripotential hematopoietic stem cells. Cytogenetic, enzymatic and antigen-typing methods have shown clearly that fibroblastic cells are unrelated to hematopoietic cells.[126-128] Proliferation of fibroblasts and abnormal production of extracellular material during the course of hematopoietic neoplasia in people now is considered to be a reactive phenomenon, perhaps induced by the intramedullary release of growth factors mitogenic for mesenchymal cells by malfunctioning platelets produced in the neoplastic disease.[129] Collagen or increased amounts of reticulin are best seen in specimens stained to show these elements. Myelofibrosis may be suspected if attempts to aspirate marrow produce nothing more than bloody fluid. However, marrow packed with immature cells also may be difficult to aspirate. Bone marrow biopsy or necropsy is needed to confirm a diagnosis of myelofibrosis.

Intramedullary and subperiosteal proliferation of bone has been observed in one cat with naturally occurring FeLV-associated hematopoietic neoplasia and has been induced in kittens by inoculation of FeLV.[130-131] In the latter, C-type virus particles were found in osteoblasts and osteocytes, providing presumptive evidence of a direct effect of the virus on bone-producing cells. Marrow was neither obliterated by the bone reaction nor shown to be fibrotic. It cannot be ruled out, however, that myelofibrosis in FeLV-infected cats is a result of a virus effect on marrow fibroblasts.

Lymphoid Neoplasia

Like the various forms of hematopoietic neoplasia, lymphoid neoplasms have a consistent association with FeLV. Nearly all cats with lymphoid neoplasia of any form are FeLV-positive. Bone marrow may be either the primary site of the neoplastic lymphocytic or lymphoblastic leukemia, or secondarily infiltrated by neoplastic lymphocytes from tumors in other sites, in which case the condition is called lymphomatous involvement of marrow. For practical purposes, lymphocytic leukemia is the diagnosis used in the absence of masses elsewhere.

Lymphocytic Leukemia

Lymphocytic leukemia is reportedly a common form of lymphoid neoplasia in cats.[51,132] The clinical syndrome is similar to that of hematopoietic neoplasia and involves listlessness, anorexia, weight loss and anemia. Neutropenia is common and increases susceptibility to concurrent infections. The white cell count of affected cats may be normal or above or below the normal range. A few or many of the white cells in a blood smear may be abnormal lymphocytes with a high nucleus to cytoplasm ratio, fine chromatin pattern and visible nucleoli. Red cells and other white cells should have a normal appearance. Thrombocytopenia may be present.

The anemia, leukopenia and thrombocytopenia are due primarily to the replacement of normal hematopoietic tissue by the neoplastic lymphocytes. At the time of diagnosis, bone marrow smears typically are hypercellular and composed of a uniform population of neoplastic lymphocytes.[133] Normal elements are scarce or absent. The spleen, liver and lymph nodes likewise may be diffusely infiltrated.

It may be difficult or impossible to determine, on the basis of Romanowsky-stained blood and marrow smears, whether the neoplasm in a particular cat is of lymphopoietic or hematopoietic origin when the cells present are undifferentiated, blast-type cells. A presumptive diagnosis of hematopoietic neoplasia, rather than lymphocytic leukemia, should be considered if remaining hematopoietic cells show abnormal morphologic features. This dilemma may be resolved if cytochemical technics are used more often.

Lymphoma

Lymphomatous involvement of marrow may be either diffuse or focal. If the pattern is diffuse, the marrow smears are hypercellular and contain increased numbers of lymphocytes mixed with normal hematopoietic cells. The infiltrating lymphocytes may be small and fairly normal in appearance or large with large nuclei and abundant cytoplasm. Focal collections of neoplastic lymphocytes may escape detection unless many particles are examined or sections of bone marrow cores are scanned (Fig C-12).

Affected cats may have normal hematologic values or may be anemic, neutropenic and thrombocytopenic, depending on the extent of replacement of hematopoietic tissue. Lymphocytosis and circulating abnormal lymphocytes may be detected in the blood of some cats whether or not there is extension to the marrow. The primary lymphoma may be in the mediastinum, alimentary tract or other tissues. More specific clinical signs and physical findings are referable to these tumors.

Chemotherapy has had more success in the treatment of lymphoid neoplasia than of hematopoietic neoplasia. Use of various regimens involving combinations of cytotoxic drugs has been recommended.[51,122,132] Partial or complete remissions are achieved in many patients but relapses unfortunately are frequent. Severely anemic patients may need transfusions. Patients treated with cytotoxic drugs should be monitored closely for excessive suppression of hematopoiesis and treated appropriately for complications, such as infections and hemorrhage.

Myeloma

Myeloma is another neoplasm of lymphoid origin but so rare in cats that an association with FeLV has not been determined. Myeloma is the neoplastic growth of a clone of B-lymphocytes having the morphologic features of plasma cells. The myeloma cells produce immunoglobulin in quantities related to the size of the tumor cell mass. Because all of the myeloma cells in a particular patient are the offspring of a single cell, the immunoglobulin produced is monoclonal, *ie,* it contains one type of heavy chain, mu, alpha or gamma, and one type of light chain, either kappa or lambda. When serum containing a monoclonal immunoglobulin is subjected to electrophoresis, the abnormal protein, also called paraprotein, is evident as a tall, narrow-based peak. Immunoelectrophoresis or radial immunodiffusion demonstrates the homogeneity of the paraprotein with regard to light and heavy chains. Light chains are produced in excess by some myelomas and spill into urine as Bence-Jones protein. The electrophoretic pattern of polyclonal immunoglobulins, produced in response to antigenic stimulation, has a broad outline and represents increased amounts of several immunoglobulin types. Myeloma cells are confined to the marrow at first but may extend to other tissues as the tumor grows.

A diagnosis of myeloma is suggested by the presence in marrow smears of increased numbers of plasma cells, which may be normal in appearance or markedly atypical. Since marked plasmacytosis may also be evident in marrow of patients experiencing antigenic challenge, the diagnosis of myeloma must be confirmed by demonstrating a monoclonal immunoglobulin.

Myeloma has been observed in a few cats.[134,135] The paraprotein in all contained gamma heavy chains. Osteolytic lesions, typical of myeloma in people and dogs, were not detected in the feline patients.

Miscellaneous Neoplasms

Polycythemia Vera

Erythrocytosis, analogous in part to polycythemia vera in people, is extremely rare in cats. There is only one report of such a patient in the literature.[136] Four other cases are included in a table in another source but the specifics of the illness were not provided.[122] Polycythemia vera in people is a clonal proliferative disorder in which the predominant feature is excessive erythropoiesis and increased red cell mass. Platelets and granulocytes are also produced in excess of normal. Splenic enlargement and extramedullary hematopoiesis are other components of the disease. Hypoxia and abnormal erythropoietin production must be ruled out to diagnose a patient with erythrocytosis as having polycythemia vera.

The one cat for which details of the disease are available had an increased red cell mass, normal arterial O_2 saturation and leukocytosis. Thrombocytosis and extramedullary hematopoiesis were not present. The report predates the availability of the FeLV fluorescent antibody test and methods of assaying erythropoietin levels. The available evidence is still too scant to determine if polycythemia vera, as recognized in people, actually exists in cats or to establish an association with FeLV.

Eosinophilic Leukemia

There are 4 reported cases of a hematologic disorder in cats considered to be a neoplastic growth of eosinophils.[87,108,137,138] In each cat the diagnosis of eosinophilic leukemia was based on a marked eosinophilia in the blood and marrow and an eosinophil infiltrate of various organs, particularly of the liver, spleen, lymph nodes and GI tract. Splenomegaly was present in all cats; vomiting and diarrhea were reported in 3. Anemia was absent or mild. Circulating eosinophils were, for the most part, mature cells and eosinophil maturation in marrow was not markedly abnormal. Other hematopoietic cells had a normal appearance. None of the cats was reported as FeLV positive but 2 of the 4 were reported before the availability of the FeLV test.

There have been too few cats with extreme hypereosinophilia to assume that these and similar patients are affected by an FeLV-associated disease. Indeed, the syndrome may not represent a primary hematopoietic disorder at all but rather an extremely exaggerated eosinophil re-

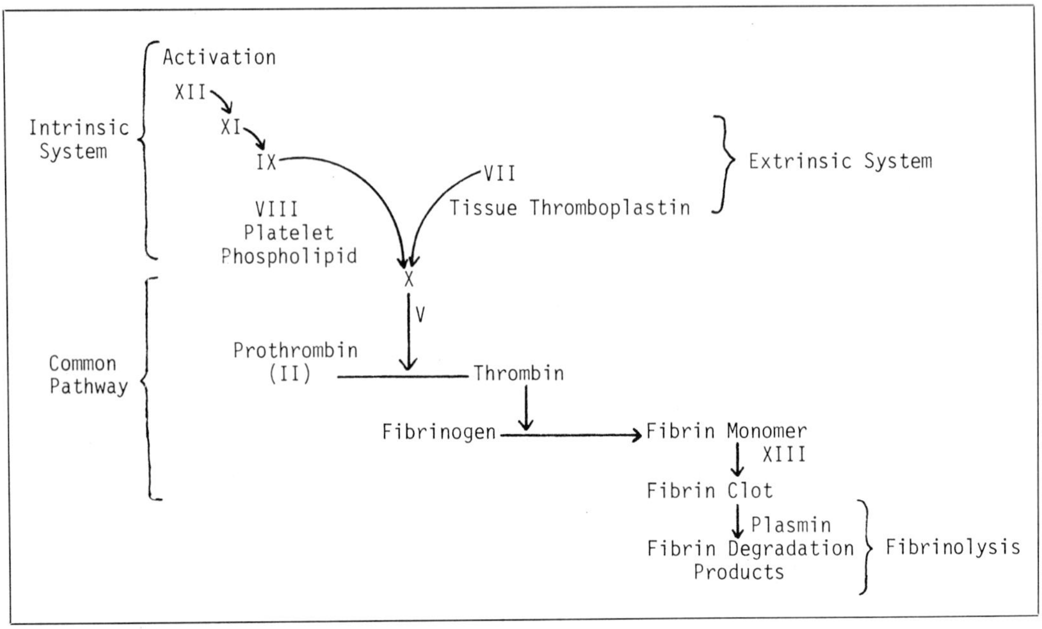

Fig 3. Simplified diagram of coagulation and clot lysis.

sponse stimulated by hypersensitivity to an undetermined antigen. The existence of eosinophilic leukemia in people as a true neoplastic growth of eosinophils is a matter of controversy.[27,88] Patients with persistent, extreme eosinophilia do not die a leukemic death, *ie,* death due to anemia, infection or hemorrhage. Death is the result of organ damage and fibrosis associated with the eosinophil infiltrate or endothelial damage and thrombosis.[27] Prednisone and hydroxyurea have controlled the hypereosinophilia in some people.

Disorders of Coagulation

Disorders of the blood-clotting mechanism resulting in clinically apparent bleeding are not common in cats. However, both congenital and acquired coagulation defects have been recognized in this species.

For convenience, the blood-clotting mechanism can be considered as 2 sequential pathways with a common terminal sequence (Fig 3). The extrinsic system is activated when circulating factor VII forms a complex with tissue thromboplastin from damaged endothelial cells. The intrinsic system is initiated by contact with any of a variety of substances, including collagen and endotoxin. Kaolin, glass and ellagic acid are substances that initiate the intrinsic system cascade *in vitro.* The laboratory tests most often used to detect abnormal clotting are the one-stage prothrombin time and the activated partial thromboplastin time. The prothrombin time is prolonged by defects in the extrinsic system or common pathway; the partial thromboplastin time is prolonged by defects in the intrinsic system or common pathway. Since special equipment is needed for these and other coagulation tests, most veterinarians must rely on outside laboratories. The appropriate sample for coagulation tests is either fresh citrated blood or the frozen plasma of fresh citrated blood. Citrated blood is 9 parts whole blood in 1 part 3.8% sodium citrate. Tubes containing citrate may be purchased (Vacutainer:Becton-Dickinson). A similar sample from a normal animal should accompany the patient's sample to serve as a normal control. More information regarding coagulation tests and their application to veterinary patients is available elsewhere.[139,140]

Congenital deficiencies of factors VIII and XII have been reported.[141,142] Factor XII deficiency is not clinically apparent but prolongs the partial thromboplastin time. Deficiency of factor VIII procoagulant activity (hemophilia A), in contrast, produces a clinical syndrome of abnormal bleeding after minor injury or surgical procedures.[143] Affected cats have normal bleeding times because of formation of a platelet plug; however, a normal clot fails to form and bleeding begins again some hours later and may be life-threatening. Deficiency of factor VIII or another intrinsic system factor should be suspected if the prothrombin time is normal but the partial thromboplastin time is prolonged. Special assays are necessary to identify the factors involved.

Bleeding due to factor VIII deficiency is treated most practically and effectively by transfusions of fresh whole blood or fresh frozen plasma. The recommended regimen for fresh frozen plasma is 6-10 ml/kg body weight given 2-3 times daily until bleeding is controlled.[143] If equipment to process plasma is not available, transfusions of whole blood repeated for 2-5 days should be adequate. Blood stored for several days is useless.

Acquired coagulation defects and bleeding tendencies may be the result of ingestion of rodenticides containing vitamin K antagonists, such as warfarin. Vitamin K in an active form is necessary for a critical step in the hepatic synthesis of factors VII, IX, X and II (prothrombin). Depletion of active vitamin K by the action of warfarin and related compounds produces a deficiency of these factors that may result in severe hemorrhaging. Both the prothrombin time and partial thromboplastin time typically are prolonged because of multiple factor deficiencies. Treatment should consist of vitamin K_1 administered IV in 10-mg doses twice daily for 1-2 days, followed by daily oral doses of 5-10 mg for 5 days.[139,140] After discontinuation of vitamin K_1 therapy, the patient should be watched closely for signs of recurrent bleeding. Severely affected patients may require infusion with fresh blood or plasma to control bleeding until synthesis of clotting factors resumes.

Since the liver is the source of many coagulation factors, bleeding tendencies may be observed in patients with severe liver disease. The prothrombin time and partial thromboplastin time are prolonged as in vitamin K deficiency but the defect is not reversible by vitamin K therapy.

Severe bleeding may accompany many serious diseases owing to a vicious cycle of intravascular clotting and clot lysis known as disseminated intravascular coagulation (DIC). Although DIC is always a secondary disorder, it can contribute to the pathogenesis of such primary conditions as septicemia, tumors, shock, trauma and FIP. In DIC, the coagulation mechanism is inappropriately activated by one or more agents, such as endotoxin, tissue thromboplastin, tumor products, immune complexes or viruses. Regardless of the initial stimulus, thrombi form, circulate, and lodge in small arterioles, occluding them and producing ischemic damage to various organs. Platelets, fibrinogen and clotting factors are consumed in widespread coagulation. The presence of thrombi stimulates endothelial cells to release plasminogen activator, which results in fibrinolysis and dissolution of thrombi. Fibrinolysis, while re-establishing blood flow in the microcirculation, results in the release of fibrin degradation products with anticoagulant activity. The combined effect of fibrin degradation products, thrombocytopenia and hypofibrinogenemia is to produce a hemorrhagic state.

The presence of DIC is reflected in abnormal results in many tests. The prothrombin time and partial thromboplastin time are prolonged, the platelet count is low, the plasma fibrinogen concentration is low but the level of fibrin degradation products is high. The last can be measured by a latex-agglutination test available as a kit (Thrombo-Wellco Test:Burroughs Wellcome). A positive test at a serum dilution of 1:25 is considered evidence of heightened fibrinolysis.[144]

For a patient with clinical and laboratory evidence of DIC, the first priorities of treatment are to correct the primary disease, if possible, and to interrupt thrombus formation. Continuous IV fluid therapy helps maintain tissue perfusion and averts sludging and stasis in small vessels. Platelet function inhibitors, such as aspirin, help prevent further clotting.[140] Heparin is an anticoagulant often used to treat DIC but it should be used with caution and only if facilities are available to monitor therapy with coagulation tests. Heparin therapy should be continuous and is accomplished by administering it in an IV drip or by SC injection. The patient's prothrombin time and partial thromboplastin time should be maintained at about 2 times the normal time.[141] The dosage of heparin should be adjusted accordingly. Severe hemorrhages during treatment necessitate discontinuation of heparin therapy and administration of blood or plasma.

References

1. Weiss and Brookoff, in Dietschy: The Science and Practice of Clinical Medicine. Vol 6. Grune and Stratton, New York, 1980.
2. Weiss, L. Blood Cells **1** (1975) 617.
3. Weiss, L. Anat Rec **186** (1976) 161.
4. Bessis, M: Blood Smears Reinterpreted. Springer International, Berlin, 1977.
5. Schofield, R. Clin Haemat **8** (1979) 221.
6. Trentin, JJ. Am J Path **65** (1971) 621.

7. Wolf, N. Clin Haemat **8** (1979) 469.
8. Dexter, TM. Clin Haemat **8** (1979) 453.
9. Friedenstein, AJ *et al.* Transplant **17** (1974) 331.
10. Bernstein, SE *et al.* Ann NY Acad Sci **149** (1968) 475.
11. Westen, H. and Bainton, DF. J Exp Med **150** (1979) 919.
12. Tavassoli, M. Blood **55** (1980) 537.
13. Weiss, L. Blood **36** (1970) 189.
14. Chamberlain, J *et al.* Blood Cells **1** (1975) 655.
15. Lichtman and Brennan, in Dietschy: The Science and Practice of Clinical Medicine. Vol 6. Grune and Stratton, New York, 1980.
16. Quesenberry, P and Levitt, L. N Engl J Med **301** (1979) 755, 819, 868.
17. Winkelstein, in Dietschy: The Science and Practice of Clinical Medicine. Vol 6. Grune and Stratton New York, 1980.
18. Lord, BI. Clin Haemat **8** (1979) 435.
19. Moore, MA. Clin Haemat **8** (1979) 287.
20. Basten, A *et al.* J Exp Med **131** (1970) 1271.
21. Micklem, HS. Clin Haemat **8** (1979) 395.
22. Adamson, in Dietschy: The Science and Practice of Clinical Medicine. Vol 6. Grune and Stratton New York, 1980.
23. Schalm, OW*et al:* Veterinary Hematology. 3rd ed. Lea & Febiger, Philadelphia, 1975.
24. Kay, MMB. J Supramol Struct **9** (1978) 555.
25. Szymanski, IO *et al.* Blood **55** (1980) 48.
26. Cronkite, EP. Clin Haemat **8** (1979) 351.
27. Bass, in Spivak: Fundamentals of Clinical Hematology. Harper and Row, Hagerstown, 1980.
28. Spry, CJF. Cell Tissue Kinet **4** (1971) 351.
29. Bainton, DF and Golde, DW. J Clin Invest **61** (1978) 1555.
30. Van Furth, R. Ann NY Acad Sci **278** (1976) 161.
31. Groopman, JE and Golde, DW. Ann Int Med **94** (1981) 95.
32. Volkman, A. J Reticuloend Soc **19** (1976) 249.
33. Tsan, in Spivak: Fundamentals of Clinical Hematology. Harper and Row, Hagerstown, 1980.
34. Dannenberg, in Spivak: Fundamentals of Clinical Hematology. Harper and Row, Hagerstown, 1980.
35. Ebbe, S. Clin Haemat **8** (1979) 371.
36. Anderson and Anderson, in Spivak: Fundamentals of Clinical Hematology. Harper and Row, Hagerstown, 1980.
37. Nelson, in Henry: Clinical Diagnosis and Management by Laboratory Methods. Vol 1. WB Saunders, Philadelphia, 1979.
38. Cramer, DW and Lewis, RM JAVMA **160** (1972) 61.
39. Alsaker, RD *et al.* JAVMA **170** (1977) 39.
40. Fan, LC *et al.* JAAHA **14** (1978) 219.
41. Duncan, JR and Passe, KW: Veterinary Laboratory Medicine. Iowa State Univ Press, Ames, 1977.
42. Altman, NH *et al.* Blood **39** (1972) 801.
43. Lewis, HB and Rebar, AH: Bone Marrow Evaluation in Veterinary Practice. Ralston Purina, St. Louis, 1979.
44. Duncan, JR and Prasse, KW. Vet Clin No Am **6** (1976) 597.
45. Maggio, L. Compend Cont Ed **1** (1979) 114.
46. Greene, CE. Proc 47th Ann Mtg AAHA, 1980.
47. Young, K, Univ Penn: Personal communication, 1981.
48. Norsworthy, GD. Feline Pract **7(9)** (1977) 29.
49. Zucker, in Dietschy: The Science and Practice of Clinical Medicine. Vol 6. Grune and Stratton, New York, 1980.
50. Kaneko, in Kaneko and Cornelius: Clinical Biochemistry of Domestic Animals. Academic Press, New York, 1970.
51. Cotter, in Kirk: Current Veterinary Therapy VI. WB Saunders, Philadelphia, 1976.
52. Thenen, SW and Rasmussen, KM. Am J Vet Res **39** (1978) 1205.
53. Schalm, OW. Feline Pract **4(5)** (1974) 16.
54. Goldstein, M. Hosp Pract **15** (1980) 85.
55. Krantz, in Dietschy: The Science and Practice of Clinical Medicine. Vol 6. Grune and Stratton, New York, 1980.
56. Watson, ADJ and Middleton, DJ. Am J Vet Res **39** (1978) 1199.
57. Pedersen, NC *et al.* Am J Vet Res **38** (1977) 1523.
58. Mackey, L *et al.* J Nat Cancer Inst **54** (1975) 209.
59. Hoover, EA *et al.* J Nat Cancer Inst **53** (1974) 1271.
60. Norsworthy, GD. Feline Pract **7(9)** (1977) 38.
61. Cotter, SM. JAVMA **175** (1979) 1191.
62. Harvey, JW and Gaskin, JM. JAAHA **13** (1977) 28.
63. Maede, Y. Am J Vet Res **40** (1978) 691.
64. Jain, NC and Keeton, KS. Am J Vet Res **34** (1973) 697.
65. Maede, Y and Sonoda, M. Jap J Vet Sci **37** (1975) 209.
66. Maede, Y and Hata, R. Jap J Vet Sci **37** (1975) 49.
67. Hathaway, J. Vet Clin No Am **6** (1976) 495.
68. Harvey, JW and Kaneko, JJ. Proc Soc Exp Biol Med 147 (1974) 245.
69. Jain, NC and Keeton, KS. Am J Vet Res **36** (1975) 1691.
70. Schechter, RD *et al.* JAVMA **162** (1973) 37.
71. Boon, GD and Rich, LJ. Feline Pract **4(6)** (1974) 49.
72. Schalm, OW. Feline Pract **7(6)** (1977) 30.
73. Finco, DR *et al.* JAVMA **166** (1975) 469.
74. Harvey, JW and Kornick, HP. JAVMA **169** (1976) 327.
75. Harvey, JW *et al.* JAVMA **175** (1979) 1171.
76. St. Omer, VV and MacKnight, ED. JAVMA **176** (1980) 911.
77. Winklestein, in Criep: Allergy and Clinical Immunology. Grune and Stratton, New York, 1976.
78. Frank, MM *et al.* Ann Int Med **87** (1977) 210.
79. Scott, DW *et al.* JAAHA **9** (1973) 530.
80. Madewell, BR and Feldman, BF. JAVMA **176** (1980) 419.
81. Glenn, BL *et al.* Am J Vet Res **29** (1968) 1653.
82. Giddens, WE *et al.* Am J Path **80** (1975) 367.

83. Prasse, KW and Duncan, JR. Vet Clin No Am **6** (1976) 581.
84. Winkelstein, in Dietschy: The Science and Practice of Clinical Medicine. Vol 6. Grune and Stratton, New York, 1980.
85. Lautenslager, JP. Vet Clin No Am **6** (1976) 353.
86. Donahoe, JMR *et al.* JAVMA **168** (1976) 413.
87. Hendrick, M. Vet Path **18** (1981) 188.
88. Reison, B and Benisch, B. NY State J Med **80** (1980) 89.
89. Kahn, DE. JAVMA **173** (1978) 628.
90. Carlson, JH and Scott, FW. Vet Path **14** (1977) 173.
91. Joshi, BC *et al.* JAAHA **15** (1979) 585.
92. Gilbert, HS. Med Clin No Am **57** (1973) 355.
93. Laszlo, J. Sem Hemat **12** (1975) 409.
94. Fialkow, PJ *et al.* Am J Med **63** (1977) 125.
95. Adamson, JW and Fialkow, PJ. Br J Haemat **38** (1978) 299.
96. Brecher, in Baldwin and Ebbe: Platelets: Production, Function, Transfusion, and Storage. Grune and Stratton, New York, 1974.
97. Geary, CG. *et al.* Br J Haemat **30** (1975) 289.
98. Linman, JW and Bagby, GC. Blood Cells **2** (1976) 11.
99. Dreyfus, B. Blood Cells **2** (1976) 33.
100. Koeffler, HP and Golde, DW. Ann Int Med **93** (1980) 347.
101. Bennet, JM *et al.* Br J Haemat **33** (1976) 451.
102. Cline, MJ *et al.* Ann Int Med **91** (1979) 758.
103. Beckstead, JH *et al.* Blood **57** (1981) 1088.
104. Schalm, OW. Feline Pract **5(5)** (1975) 20.
105. Schalm, OW. Feline Pract **5(6)** (1975) 31.
106. Sutton, RH *et al.* N Zeal Vet J **26** (1978) 273.
107. Fraser, CJ *et al.* JAVMA **165** (1974) 355.
108. Schalm, OW. Feline Pract **6(5)** (1976) 36.
109. Stann, SE. JAVMA **174** (1979) 722.
110. Henness, AM *et al.* JAVMA **170** (1977) 1325.
111. Loeb, WF *et al.* Vet Path **12** (1975) 464.
112. Schalm, OW. Feline Pract **6(3)** (1976) 32.
113. Schalm, OW. Feline Pract **6(7)** (1976) 44.
114. Hurvitz, AI. Am J Vet Res **31** (1970) 747.
115. Gilmore, CE *et al.* Path Vet **1** (1964) 161.
116. Schalm, OW. Feline Pract **5(4)** (1975) 16.
117. Crow, SE *et al.* JAVMA **170** (1977) 1329.
118. Giles, RC *et al.* JAVMA **165** (1974) 456.
119. Michel, RL *et al.* JAVMA **168** (1976) 1021.
120. Madewell, BR *et al.* Vet Path **16** (1979) 510.
121. Henness, AM and Crow, SE. JAVMA **171** (1977) 263.
122. Theilen, GH and Madewell, BR: Veterinary Cancer Medicine. Lea & Febiger, Philadelphia, 1979.
123. Jones, FR *et al.* Cancer **46** (1980) 675.
124. Harvey, JW *et al.* Vet Path **15** (1978) 437.
125. Lester, SJ and Searcy, GP. JAVMA **178** (1981) 471.
126. Van Slyck, EJ *et al.* Blood **36** (1970) 729.
127. Jacobson, RJ *et al.* Blood **51** (1978) 189.
128. Golde, DW *et al.* Br J Haemat **44** (1980) 183.
129. Groopman, JE. Ann Int Med **92** (1980) 857.
130. Zenoble, D and Rowland, GN. JAVMA **175** (1979) 591.
131. Hoover, EA and Kociba, GJ. J Nat Cancer Inst **53** (1974) 1277.
132. Cotter, SM. Vet Clin No Am **6** (1976) 367.
133. Cotter, SM and Essex, M. Am J Path **87** (1977) 265.
134. Farrow, BR and Penny, R. JAVMA **158** (1971) 606.
135. Kehoe, JM *et al.* J Immun **109** (1972) 511.
136. Reed, C *et al.* JAVMA **157** (1970) 85.
137. Silverman, J. JAVMA **158** (1971) 199.
138. Simon, N and Holsworth, J. Cornell Vet **57** (1967) 579.
139. Dodds, in Ettinger: Textbook of Veterinary Internal Medicine. WB Saunders, Philadelphia, 1975.
140. Dodds, WJ. Mod Vet Pract **58** (1977) 680, 756.
141. Didisheim, P *et al.* J Lab Clin Med **53** (1959) 866.
142. Green, RA and White, F. Am J Vet Res **38** (1977) 893.
143. Cotter, SM *et al.* JAVMA **172** (1978) 166.
144. Kociba, in Kirk: Current Veterinary Therapy V. WB Saunders, Philadelphia, 1974.

7

the immune system

S. KRAKOWKA AND R.G. OLSEN

The cat, like other domestic animals, has developed, by evolutionary pressures, a complex system of adaptive immunity in response to noxious or foreign influences on life processes. This system is designed to operate in conjunction with various nonspecific body defenses, including the physical barriers of intact skin and mucous membranes, the natural antibacterial acidity of sebaceous secretions and stomach, such soluble factors as lysozyme, enzyme inhibitors, interferon, complement and blood coagulation factors, such cellular factors as the phagocytic capability of neutrophils, monocytes and the monocyte-origin cells of the reticuloendothelial system, and a complex inflammatory response, including both humoral and cellular elements, teleologically designed to provide protection and tissue repair following tissue damage.

Fortunately, the immunologic defense system is a conservative evolutionary adaptation and, as such, many of the features of the system are common to all mammals. This fact permits the extrapolation of observations made in intensively studied species, such as rodents and people, to such species as cats, in which comparable studies are fragmented or incomplete. The basic principles of immunity in cats were reviewed and delineated in 1971.[1] Significant advances in our understanding of both basic and applied immunologic phenomena in this species have been made in the last decade. It is the objective of this chapter to update and review these data and to provide insights into application of these principles to the practice of feline medicine.

Components of the Immune System

Like that of other animals, the feline immune system can be divided into humoral and cellular components. Both subdivisions are ultimately derived from a common stem cell progenitor population during embryonic development. *In utero,* immunocompetent cells first appear in the yolk sac and then in the liver. At about mid-gestation, the bone marrow assumes primacy and this function is continued in postnatal life. The feline thymus, a source of thymus-dependent or T-lymphocytes, is populated by lymphocytes from the bone marrow at about 40 days of gestation.[2] Consequently, advanced development and subsequent peripheralization of T-lymphocytes to secondary lymphoid organs (*eg,* spleen and lymph nodes) are thought to be well advanced prior to birth. Thus, postnatal removal of the feline thymus as an experimental method of T-cell depletion does not have major adverse influences on this component of immunity.[3] This is in marked contrast to rodents, in which post-thymic peripheralization occurs after birth and, therefore, thymectomy at birth profoundly influences lymphocyte patterns of movement and subsequent immunologic differentiation. Lymphocytes that differentiate in the thymus (T-cells) play the major role in allograft rejection, specific immunologic protection against obligate intracellular parasites, such as certain bacteria and viruses, and immunity to cancer.

The second subdivision of lymphocytes does not play major roles in the above phenomena but rather exerts its effects by secretion of specific antibodies into the circulation or at body surfaces. These cells do not require a thymic environment for differentiation and apparently arise in bone marrow throughout postnatal life. This cell population is referred to as the B-lymphocyte (bursal-equivalent or bone marrow-derived) population and subsequently differentiate into immunoglobulin-secreting plasma cells in secondary lymphoid organs or areas of chronic inflammation after antigenic stimulation.

The functional integrity of both lymphocyte subpopulations is intimately dependent upon a third accessory cell, the bone marrow-origin monocyte or macrophage. Regarding a developing immune response, macrophages apparently digest and present the immunogen in question in cell membrane-bound form to immunocompetent lymphocytes. This critical role, in addition to that of phagocytic defenses, has received only limited attention in cats. Unfortunately, little is known about subsets of macrophage regulator functions and changes as they relate to disease susceptibility or immunity.

Feline macrophages lack lysozyme activity.[4] The *in vitro* phagocytic properties, however, of feline macrophages are well established.[5] Macrophage function is correlated with resistance to neoplastic disease. Macrophages from young kittens, highly susceptible to FeLV infection, are also more susceptible to infection with oncogenic virus.[5] This susceptibility apparently does not correlate with phagocytic ability.[5] Factors that diminish macrophage functions *in vivo,* such as administration of hydrocortisone or silica dust, increase the susceptibility to oncogenic disease. In contrast, factors that enhance macrophage function, such as glucan, appeared to promote resistance to disease.[5] Cytotoxic effector feline peritoneal macrophages have been detected in cats vaccinated intraperitoneally with tumor cells;[6] yet no differences in cytotoxicity were seen in healthy cats exposed to feline leukemia virus (FeLV) and normal, unexposed cats.

Humoral Immunity

Immunoglobulins

Traditionally, biochemical and functional properties of various immunoglobulins have been delineated by study of serum proteins. Normal cat serum contains at least 6 major electrophoretically distinct serum fractions, including albumin, alpha$_1$, alpha$_2$, beta$_1$, beta$_2$ and gamma globulin.[7] There are many similar characteristics of feline serum components and those of other species. Specific antibody activity is largely restricted to the gamma globulin fraction of serum. At least 3 major immunoglobulin (Ig) classes have been identified in the cat: IgG, IgM and IgA.[8] These proteins have been identified by both heavy-chain antisera specific to them and by virtue of serologic cross-reactions with antisera to comparable human Ig.[1,8] Two subclasses of IgG, designated as IgG$_1$ and IgG$_2$, have been identified. In addition, 3 feline IgG-secreting myelomas (neoplastic plasma cells) have been described.[10] Presumptive evidence for feline reaginic antibody (IgE) has been obtained by demonstrating cross-reactivity with bovine antireaginic serum.[9] It is likely, but not proven, that the structure and function of feline Ig classes are similar to those of other species. Adult cat serum, colostrum, tears and nasal secretions contain all 3 major immunoglobulins.[8] Intestinal contents contain IgG and IgA, whereas only IgA and IgM have been found in bile.

Passive Immunity: Immediate postnatal immunologic protection for most domestic animals is provided by oral ingestion of colostrum during the first 24-36 hours of life. Although several investigators have reported that serum from fetuses or kittens that have not suckled is devoid of immunoglobulin, others have reported the presence of IgG, indicating either *in utero* immunoglobulin synthesis by the fetus or limited *in utero* transfer of maternal origin IgG, as has been documented for dogs, a species with similar maternal-fetal placentation.[7,8,11,12] Others have shown that serum from kittens that have not suckled contained significant quantities of antibodies to *Salmonella montevideo* after vaccination of pregnant queens with the organism.[13]

Although queen colostrum contains IgM, suckling kitten serum lacks this protein.[8] Colostrum-origin protection in cats is similar to that in other species. For example, maternal-origin feline panleukopenia virus antibody appeared in kittens 24 hours after birth, with subsequent decline in titers thereafter.[14] In another study, young cats were protected against a lethal viral challenge by feline sarcoma virus if they had nursed queens vaccinated with feline sarcoma virus.[15] Maternal-origin specific antibody interferes with vaccination against various viral pathogens in immediate postnatal life.[16,17]

Induction of Active Immunity: The humoral immune responses of cats to foreign immunogens, as either experimental inanimate substances or products from selected viral, protozoal or bacterial pathogens, have been widely studied in the last decade. Much of the work has been directed toward documenting the appearance of specific antibodies to feline viral pathogens of clinical importance. Virus-specific protective antibodies have been demonstrated in cats after infection with or vaccination for feline panleukopenia virus, feline rhinotracheitis virus, rabies virus, feline reovirus, feline leukemia virus, feline sarcoma virus, feline oncornavirus membrane antigen, feline infectious peritonitis virus and feline caliciviruses.[15,18-25] In the last instance, serologic typing and classification procedures have been used to identify an isolate that induced the best cross-protective responses for subsequent use in a vaccine.[26] In addition to these feline viral diseases, cats have been shown to respond immunologically to Aujeszky's disease herpesvirus, canine distemper virus, canine parainfluenza virus and *Brucella canis*.[18,27-29]

The kinetics of developing immune responses have also been evaluated by a series of immunization-response experiments. Tolerance (*ie*, a specific lack of a detectible immune response) has been induced in newborn kittens by IV inoculation with bovine serum albumin or bovine gamma globulin.[30] Other investigators have also indicated that bovine serum albumin was not immunogenic for cats.[31] The immune response to ovine RBC has been documented in cats with or without concurrent FeLV infection.[32] Hemagglutinating antibodies were detected in serum of both groups of cats 7 days after immunization.

The ability to demonstrate specific antibody activity to an immunogen depends upon the assay technic used. The direct complement-fixation (CF) test may not demonstrate antibodies to the immunogen in question.[28,33,34] Further investigation of this phenomenon demonstrated that a heterologous CF reaction depends upon development of antibody in one IgG subclass and is antigen-dependent.[35] To avoid false-negative reactions, a composite complement source, consisting of early feline-origin complement components plus late-acting guinea pig complement components, has been developed and is recommended for investigation of feline humoral immune responses by complement fixation.[36]

Complement System

The close biochemical and temporal interrelationships between humoral antibodies and the serum complement system has prompted a number of studies on feline complement. Total hemolytic complement levels in cats are somewhat low when compared with those in other species. Values of 70-150 complement hemolytic units/ml under optimal test conditions have been reported.[37] The functional activity of individual components C1, C6, C7, C8 and C9 is readily titrated using guinea pig-origin complement intermediates.[38] The functional activity of other components in the complement cascade (C4, C2, C3 and C5), while detected with standard intermediates, may lead to underestimates of activity. The third feline complement component (C3) has been purified from normal cat serum.[39] Deposits of C3 and IgG in renal glomeruli have been detected in cats with suspected feline infectious peritonitis-related immune complex disease.[39] Similar phenomena have been reported in FeLV-infected cats.[40] In the latter instance, FeLV-infected viremic cats had low blood levels of complement.[41] *In vitro* purified FeLV activates the complement system via the classic pathway.[42]

Interferon: Interferon is a low-molecular weight protein produced by animal cells in response to viral infection. It confers nonspecific resistance to infection in adjacent cells and, as such, constitutes an important nonimmune body defense mechanism. The potential uses of interferon in veterinary medicine have been reviewed.[43] Newcastle disease virus and polyriboinosinic:polyribocytidylic acid stimulate interferon production in cats.[44] The latter was very toxic for cats and an inconsistent inducer of interferon formation. In contrast, Newcastle disease virus was a potent inducer of interferon formation. *In vitro*, Crandell feline kidney cells produced interferon after Newcastle disease virus infection and this induced interferon-inhibited FeLV infection.[45] More recently, a synthetic chemical induced interferon production in cats *in vivo*.[46]

Cellular Immunity

Lymphocyte Subpopulations

The array of available *in vivo* manifestations of cell-mediated immunity documented in other species probably also exists in cats. Detailed *in vivo* documentation of these phenomena are lacking, however. Draining lymph nodes of cats immunized with either oxazalone or ovalbumin have been examined for morphologic evidence of developing cellular immunity.[47] Oxazalone stimulates T-cell-dependent cellular proliferation in the paracortical regions of feline lymph nodes similar to that reported for guinea pigs and mice. In contrast, immunization with ovalbumin, an antigen capable of activating both T- and B-lymphocytes, resulted in the appearance of prominent germinal centers (B-cell-dependent areas), as well as paracortical stimulation in draining nodes. During the course of the response, dramatic increases in the number of mast cells in lymph nodes were observed. In this regard, feline cutaneous mastocytomas may reflect a variant form of dermal cellular hypersensitivity (Jones-Mote reaction) and not a neoplasm.[48]

Cats are clearly capable of rejection of foreign allogeneic skin grafts, a manifestation of cellular immunity. Normal rejection times of 13.1 ± 1.4 days have been reported.[32] Postnatal thymectomy marginally prolonged this rejection time to 14-18 days, as did infection with FeLV (rejection time 18 days) and exposure to a single noncarcinogenic dose of methylnitrosourea (rejection time 41-84 days).[3,33,49]

Attempts to establish delayed hypersensitivity to a number of antigens emulsified in complete Freund's adjuvant in cats have met with some success. A positive 24-hour skin test response was demonstrated in most cats tested, although corneal responses were quantitatively superior to those obtained in skin.[31] However, unlike that in other species, the feline response to tuberculin is poor.[1,31] Cats naturally infected with tuberculosis have a negative skin test.[50] Nine cats injected with viable *Mycobacterium bovis* developed fever, leukocytosis, neutrophilia and regional lymphadenopathy.[51] A transient (present at 21 days postinoculation and absent by 49 days postinoculation) cutaneous response to tuberculin was noted. Histologic evaluation of skin test sites revealed cellular infiltrates, chiefly of neutrophils and mononuclear cells. Many mast cells were present in the lesion. Skin test responses to specific fungal or bacterial pathogens probably can be obtained in actively infected cats. All positive tests of this nature should, however, be confirmed by biopsy and histopathologic examination of the skin test site.

Lymphocyte Isolation and Culture

Feline peripheral blood lymphocytes are readily isolated from heparinized or defibrinated blood by centrifugation over ficoll-diatrizoate.[52] Cells collected at the interface are virtually free of RBC and consist of 80-90% mononuclear cells, with some contamination by neutrophils. Cellular suspensions from spleen, lymph nodes and thymus are obtained by finely mincing these organs and pressing the resultant slurry through stainless-steel mesh.[53] Short- and long-term *in vitro* culture of feline lymphocytes has been achieved with various culture media.[52,53]

In Vitro Lymphocyte Functions

Lymphocyte Blastogenesis: The overall range of feline lymphocyte blastogenesis to well-characterized T-cell mitogens is limited.[52] Significant responses were reported with concanavalin A and pokeweed mitogen but not with the well-characterized T-cell mitogen phytohemagglutinin and B-cell mitogens, purified protein derivative and lipopolysaccharide.[52-54] Subsequent studies showed that feline lymphoid cells respond to protein A of *Staphylococcus aureus*.[55,56] Responding lymphocytes were of T-cell origin.[56]

Lymphocyte blastogenic responses to these mitogens are controlled by immune regulator cells.[57] These suppressor cells in the peripheral blood are functionally short-lived *in vitro*. During leukemogenesis these cells disappear from the circulation, reflecting the overall immunodysfunction observed in feline leukemia.[57]

Suppressor lymphocytes are generated *in vitro* by incubation of peripheral blood cells with low doses of the mitogen concanavalin A.[58] Moreover, the selective elimination of this cell population permits feline lymphocytes to respond vigorously to mitogens, such as phytohemagglutinin, that normally fail to induce blastogenesis of feline lymphocytes.[58]

Mixed Lymphocyte Reaction: The mixed lymphocyte reaction is a powerful tool in delineating lymphocyte-defined histocompatibility antigens. Current knowledge relates these antigens with phenotypic products of the immune-responder genes in the major histocompatibility complex. The mixed lymphocyte reaction of feline peripheral blood WBC can be detected with as little as 1 x 10^5 responder cells and 1 x 10^5 stimulator cells. Optimal *in vitro* conditions require 5% rabbit serum, an 8-day incubation and 18-hour pulse with tritiated thymidine.[58]

Cytotoxic Effector Lymphocytes: Effector T-lymphocytes in all species are characterized by antigen-specific cytotoxic effects against allogeneic cells, tumor cells and isogeneic virus-infected target cells.[21] Cytotoxic effector cells are present in the spleen, peripheral lymph nodes and peripheral blood.[6] A prerequisite for effector cytotoxicity is histocompatibility restriction (the "self" recognition process involves major histocompatibility antigens) mediated by lymphocyte-defined antigens. The lack of knowledge about major histocompatibility antigens in cats, along with the unavailability of inbred cats, limits the scope of cytotoxic lymphocyte studies.

Natural Killer Cells: Natural killer-cell activity has been demonstrated in lymphoid cell populations in peripheral blood, lymph node cells and spleen in normal cats.[6] The highest degree of activity occurred in spleen cells.

Characterization of Feline Lymphocytes

Fully differentiated feline lymphocytes possess nearly the same surface markers and receptors as on lymphocytes of other species. Feline thymus-derived lymphocytes spontaneously form E rosettes with both guinea pig and rat RBC.[3,59,60] The guinea pig RBC react with a broader spectrum of T-lymphocytes than do rat RBC. Feline peripheral blood contains approximately 17% and 13%, respectively, of guinea pig E rosettes and rat E rosettes.

Peripheral blood contains approximately 36% erythrocyte-antibody-complement rosettes and 30% immunoglobulin-bearing lymphocytes.[60] Thymocytes lack both erythrocyte-antibody-complement rosettes and surface immunoglobulin. Thus, it is assumed that cells with these cell markers are B-lymphocytes.

Feline lymphocytes contain concanavalin A receptors similar to those on human and mouse lymphocytes.[61] Interreaction of concanavalin A with lymphocyte receptors results in coalescence of concanavalin A at one polar area of the lymphocyte (capping), indicating that the concanavalin A receptor is motile on the cell surface membrane. Treatment of cat lymphocytes with colchicine, a microtubular-dispersing agent, augments the capping reaction. Colchicine treatment dramatically increased capping compared to that in untreated controls.[61] Neoplasia of the hemopoietic system results in immune dysfunctions. Concanavalin A receptor motility of feline peripheral blood lymphocytes is greatly diminished during the preleukemic and leukemic stages of feline leukemia.[61]

The cell surface markers on feline T- and B-lymphocytes are quite dynamic. Continuous feline lymphoid cell lines have been useful models in evaluating the appearance and expressing the E rosette markers during the cell cycle.[62] Lymphoid cells grown to saturation density *in vitro* exhibit variation in the presence of cell-surface markers, implying that some null cells (lymphocytes without T- or B-lymphocyte markers) within a population may be influenced by the stage of cell cycle at the time the markers are assayed.

The influence of exogenous factors, such as viral infection, on lymphocyte cell-surface markers is thought to be a relevant factor in lymphocyte integrity. The erythrocyte-antibody-complement and E rosette markers are apparently continually shed as the mitotically active lymphoid cell proceeds through its cycle. This phenomenon permits the recovery of biochemically active receptor for further purification and characterization.[63]

Feline B- and T-lymphocytes have also been identified and separated by electrophoresis.[64] In cats, as in other mammals, B-lymphocytes possess a lower electrophoretic mobility than do T-lymphocytes.

Immunopathology

Drug-Induced Immunosuppression

The use of corticosteroids in symptomatic treatment of inflammatory diseases in both human and veterinary medicine is widespread. In corticosteroid-sensitive species (mouse, rat, rabbit), administration of corticosteroids results in direct lympholysis and resultant systemic lymphoid depletion.[65] In corticosteroid-resistant species (people, guinea pig, dog) peripheral lymphopenia occurs via redistribution of recirculating lymphocytes to the bone marrow. In both instances, however, corticosteroids are markedly immunosuppressive. The susceptibility of cats to corticosteroids has not yet been determined, although methyl prednisolone causes severe lymphoid depletion.[66] Administration of corticosteroids enhances susceptibility of cats to development of FeLV-related disease and toxoplasmosis.[66,67]

Methylnitrosourea, although not carcinogenic in cats, is a potent resorptive carcinogen in a variety of animal species.[68] A single dose of this chemical (15 mg/kg) resulted in a prolonged and profound immunodepressive effect in cats.[49] This effect was manifested as prolonged retention of skin grafts, depressed responses to phytomitogens or antigen, and T-lymphocyte lymphopenia. Like corticosteroids, methylnitrosourea potentiates the cat's susceptibility to FeLV-related neoplastic disease.[69]

Virus-Induced Immunosuppression

One well-established effect of systemic viral diseases is virus-associated immunosuppression. Immunodepressive viral diseases of veterinary medical importance have been reviewed.[70,71] In this regard, a number of mechanisms or combinations thereof have been identified. General features include requirements for a systemic phase of infection and concomitant hemolymphatic trophism. A direct virolytic effect on lymphoid tissues is one recognized mechanism of suppression. Abrogation of lymphocyte function in the absence of virolysis occurs and has been attributed to viral effects on cellular membrane receptors, competition between viral protein and cells for protein of DNA-synthetic machinery, generation of interferon, disruption of T-lymphocytes, B-lymphocytes and macrophage interactions, and virus-associated activation of suppressor T-lymphocytes. Two viral diseases of cats, FeLV-infection and feline panleukopenia, are immunosuppressive in cats.[71]

Feline panleukopenia virus is a parvovirus that attacks rapidly dividing cells.[18] A prominent feature of infection is dramatic reduction of peripheral blood WBC numbers, including lymphocytes.[72] Concomitant lesions in lymphoid tissues consist of thymic atrophy and systemic lymphoid depletion.[72,73] This effect is transient and rapidly followed by marked hyperplasia or lymphopoietic proliferation in these tissues.[73] Kittens infected *in utero* with feline panleukopenia virus had delayed skin graft rejection times.[74] Infected adult cats had a transient depressed response to concanavalin A and phytohemagglutinin but not to pokeweed mitogen. The humoral antibody responses to foreign RBC were not affected.[74] This study suggests that feline panleukopenia virus has a transient suppressive and rapidly reversible effect on T-lymphocyte function.[70]

A prominent feature of FeLV infection in cats is generalized immunosuppression. This preneoplastic deficit is responsible for several FeLV-related disorders, including a wasting disease, increased susceptibility to unrelated secondary infections, abortion and increased mortality rates.[75] Infection with FeLV causes multiple defects in various immunologic mechanisms. Atrophy of the thymus and concomitant paracortical (T-) lymphocyte depletion precede the onset of lymphosarcoma by several months.[76] Functional correlates include delayed skin graft rejection and depressed peripheral blood phytomitogen responses.[32,77] Appearance of these deficits coincides with onset of FeLV-associated persistent viremia. Two explanations have been proposed that would account for these phenomena. Direct viral infection of lymphocytes, with subsequent malignant transformation or virolysis and simultaneous loss of function, has been suggested but no convincing evidence for the presence of intact virus in these cells has been obtained. Recent studies have suggested that an FeLV virion polypeptide modulates lymphocyte function, resulting in immunosuppression.[78] Subsequent studies have confirmed this mechanism and suggest that release of this virion polypeptide from productive sites of viral infection in the bone marrow or epithelial tissues is the source of this material.

Systemic Anaphylaxis

Systemic anaphylaxis and related hypersensitivity reactions are uncommon naturally occurring diseases. The reaction is initiated by contact of the immunogen with tissue-bound specific antibodies. Subsequent release of pharmacologically active substances, including histamine, serotonin and slow-reacting substance of anaphylaxis, is responsible for the lesions observed (bronchogenic and vascular smooth-muscle contraction) and the attendant clinical signs of cardiovascular collapse, dyspnea, cyanosis, urination and defecation, all of which may culminate in death.

Cats appear particularly resistant to development of systemic anaphylaxis.[1,79] However, they can be rendered hypersensitive to certain antigens. Of 15 immunized cats, 9 developed anaphylaxis after IV challenge with antigen.[80] The lung is apparently the target organ in cats. Clinical signs referable to respiratory distress (dyspnea and restlessness), along with gross pulmonary lesions (emphysema, hemorrhage, edema) and microscopic pulmonary lesions (alveolar wall thickening, infiltration by neutrophils, hemorrhage, edema, reduced numbers of mast cells), have been observed.[80] Although feline pulmonary tissue is more sensitive to serotonin, anaphylaxis can be ameliorated by treatment with the antihistamine, halopyramine.[79]

Cutaneous Anaphylaxis and Hypersensitivity Reactions

Cutaneous hypersensitivity reactions have been elicited in immunized cats by intradermal inoculation of the antigen in question.[81] Acute reactions, presumably mediated by interaction of antigen with mast cell-bound antibody and subsequent histamine release, and Arthus reactions, characterized by precipitation of antigen-antibody complexes in blood vessels with subsequent neutrophilic infiltration, have been recorded.[81] Salient histologic features of the acute reaction included edema and mast cell degranulation. Feline serum-mediated passive cutaneous reactions to milk protein and *Otodectes cynotis* antigen have been documented.[82,83]

Allergies

Food allergies apparently occur in cats, although less frequently than in dogs. Hypersensitivities are manifested clinically as vomiting and diarrhea after exposure.[1,84] Acute dermatitis may accompany this event. Foods incriminated include cow's milk, meat products of bovine, rabbit or chicken origin, and oral penicillin.[85] Diagnosis can be established by skin testing with food allergen extracts.[1] Allergic dermatitis has also been linked to allergens in carpets, bedding, pollens and to tapeworm, bacterial or mycotic infections in affected cats.[85]

Cutaneous allergic responses to a haptenic salivary protein of fleas (*Ctenocephalides felis*) is a well-recognized clinical entity.[1,86,87] Flea-allergy dermatitis has been successfully treated by environmental control of fleas (extermination on premises, plus twice weekly dusting with flea powder), and hyposensitization therapy with commercial flea antigen extract.[86] Fair to excellent responses to therapy were noted in 19 of 20 cases treated in this manner.

Feline ear mite (*Otodectes cynotis*) infestation may lead to development of an immunopathologic response to mite antigens. Naturally occurring otoacariasis is characterized chiefly by chronic proliferative inflammation of the external auditory canal.[88] Both immediate and Arthus-like reactions to extracts of the mite have been found in afflicted cats.[88] Most, if not all, affected cats, including those without clinical involvement, have been exposed to ear mites. The inference from this finding is that only cats that develop allergy to mite antigens develop clinical manifestations of auditory involvement. A more recent study confirmed the allergic nature of this disorder experimentally.[83]

Immune Complex Disease

Soluble circulating complexes of specific antibody and antigen can initiate acute and chronic inflammatory responses in tissues. Pathologic effects are largely restricted to the renal glomerulus, chiefly because of the blood filtration function of that structure. Complexes are deposited in extravascular spaces in areas of increased capillary vascular permeability. These immobilized complexes activate the complement system and result in generation of chemotactic substances that attract both neutrophils and macrophages to the area. The blood coagulation system is also activated, which subsequently leads to fibrin deposition in glomeruli.

Immune complex-mediated glomerulonephritis in cats is relatively uncommon. Several investigators have demonstrated the deposition of IgG in feline glomeruli.[89-92] Clinical signs in affected cats are those of chronic and progressive renal dysfunction, including weight loss, weakness, depression, anorexia, polydipsia, polyuria, proteinuria and nocturia.[89,92] The nephrotic syndrome may also be caused by immune complex glomerulonephritis.[93] The predominant histologic change observed in affected glomeruli is membranous glomerulonephritis, with minimal cellular proliferation.[92]

Most cases of immune complex disease are associated with FeLV infection.[40,94,95] Both soluble FeLV antigen-antibody complexes and a low level of complement are present in the sera of FeLV-viremic cats with lymphosarcoma.[41,96]

In one instance, the leading cause of death of cats in a closed FeLV-infected household was glomerulonephritis and not lymphoma.[96] Some of the lesions observed in feline infectious peritonitis (FIP), a coronavirus infection of cats, have also been attributed to *in vivo* immune complex phenomena.[39,97,98] Seropositive cats subsequently infected with FIP rapidly developed the effusive form of the disease.[98] This was confirmed by treating seronegative kittens with immune serum or IgG before inoculation with FIP virus. In another study, 12 of 14 cats with FIP had deposits of IgG and the third component of complement in renal glomeruli.[39]

Arteritis

A syndrome characterized by polyarteritis of medium- to small-sized arterioles has been observed in cats. The disease, polyarteritis nodosa or periarteritis nodosa, is characterized by fibrinoid necrosis of muscular arteriole walls, with subsequent neutrophilic and lymphoplasmacytic infiltration.[1,99,100] The disease is a suspected immune complex-mediated immunologic disorder analogous to that in people.

Arthritis

Chronic progressive rheumatoid-like polyarthritis has been observed in cats.[101] Unlike the comparable condition in dogs, affected cats were negative for both rheumatoid factor and antinuclear antibody. Of 18 cats tested, 10 were positive for FeLV infection. An immunopathologic disease mechanism was suspected on the basis of characteristic histologic findings, responsiveness to corticosteroids and attendant glomerulonephritis at necropsy.[101]

Autoimmune Hemolytic Anemia

Anemia is a common feline medical disorder. In most cases, the anemia is normocytic normochromic and can be attributed to concurrent FeLV-mediated bone marrow suppression or myelosclerosis.[102,103] Coombs-positive hemolytic anemia, clinically characterized by autoantibody-mediated premature destruction of RBC, occurs in cats, although infrequently when compared with dogs.[1] Clinical and hematologic findings in 7 cases of autoimmune hemolytic anemia in cats have been published.[104] Salient findings included corticosteroid-responsive anemia and the erythroagglutination with a Coombs reagent in 6 of 7 cases. The FeLV status of these cats was not determined.

Plasma-Cell Myeloma

Neoplasms of plasma-cell origin are rare in cats. Monoclonal gammopathies have been observed in 3 cats.[10] All were of IgG origin.

Lymphoma and Lymphosarcoma

Cancer of the lymphatic system is the most common neoplastic disorder of cats. The cause of most of these tumors is FeLV. The biology of FeLV infection and subsequent neoplastic transformation is covered in Chapters 4 and 6.

Four clinical forms (alimentary, multicentric and thymic lymphosarcoma plus leukemia) are recognized.[105] In spite of the non-T-cell dependent distribution in the alimentary form, virtually all lymphomas of cats are felt to be of T-lymphocyte origin. The transformation event probably occurs in the bone marrow during the preleukemic phase. As described elsewhere in this chapter, preleukemic FeLV-infected cats are markedly immunosuppressed; this feature of the disease is responsible for FeLV-related diseases of intercurrent infection and wasting syndrome.

The occurrence of FeLV-negative feline lymphosarcoma and related disease has been documented.[106] Failure to demonstrate FeLV in these cats can be attributed to technical problems or to the thought that a low proportion of feline lymphomas are not induced by FeLV.

References

1. Gorham, RJ *et al.* JAVMA **158** (1977) 846.
2. Ackerman, GA. Anat Rec **158** (1967) 387.
3. Hoover, EA *et al.* Am J Vet Res **39** (1978) 99.
4. Hoover, EA, Ohio State Univ: Personal communication, 1981.
5. Hoover *et al*, in Hardy *et al:* Feline Leukemia Virus. Elsevier, North Holland, 1981.
6. McCarty and Grant, in Hardy *et al:* Feline Leukemia Virus. Elsevier, North Holland, 1981.
7. Okoshi, S *et al.* Jap J Vet Sci **29** (1968) 337.
8. Schultz, RD *et al.* Infect Immun **9** (1974) 391.
9. Nielson, KH. Can J Comp Med **41** (1977) 345.
10. Kehoe, MJ *et al.* J Immun **109** (1972) 511.
11. Tomoda, I. Jap J Vet Sci **24** (1964) 337.
12. Krakowka, S and Long, D. J Infect Dis **137** (1978) 605.
13. Harding, SK *et al.* Cornell Vet **51** (1961) 535.
14. Scott, FW *et al.* JAVMA **156** (1970) 439.
15. Schaller, JP *et al.* J Nat Cancer Inst **59** (1977) 144.
16. Jarret, O *et al.* Vet Rec **101** (1977) 304.
17. O'Reilly, KJ *et al.* Vet Rec **84** (1969) 376.
18. Povey, C. Vet Rec **98** (1976) 293.
19. Crandell, RA. JAVMA **158** (1971) 922.
20. Bettle, JL and Rubic, WJ. Am J Vet Res **36** (1975) 89.
21. Wardley, RC *et al.* Can J Comp Med **40** (1976) 257.
22. Csiza, CK. Infect Immun **9** (1974) 159.
23. Essex, M *et al.* Int J Cancer **8** (1971) 384.
24. Pederson, NC. Am J Vet Res **37** (1976) 1449.
25. Povey, RC. Infect Immun **10** (1974) 1307.
26. Kalunda, M *et al.* Am J Vet Res **36** (1975) 353.
27. Appel, M *et al.* Am J Vet Res **35** (1974) 803.
28. Black, LS and Lee, KM. Cornell Vet **60** (1970) 120.
29. Randhawa, AS *et al.* JAVMA **171** (1977) 167.
30. Miller-Ben Shaul, D. Israel J Med Sci **1** (1965) 563.
31. McCusker, HB and Aitken, ID. Res Vet Sci **8** (1967) 265.
32. Perryman, LE *et al.* J Nat Cancer Inst **49** (1972) 1357.
33. Otten, E. *et al.* Ztschr Tropenmed u Parasit **5** (1954) 187.
34. Olsen, RG *et al.* J Nat Cancer Inst **49** (1972) 395.
35. Perryman, LE *et al.* Am J Vet Res **34** (1973) 1529.
36. Olsen, RG *et al.* Am J Vet Res **35** (1974) 1389.
37. Barta, O and Oyekan, PP. Am J Vet Res **42** (1981) 378.
38. Barta, O and Habbert, NL. Am J Vet Res **39** (1978) 1303.
39. Jacobse-Geels, HEL *et al.* J Immun **125** (1980) 1606.
40. Glick, AD *et al.* Am J Path **92** (1978) 321.
41. Kobilinsky, L *et al.* J Immun **122** (1979) 2139.
42. Kobilinsky, L *et al.* Infect Immun **29** (1980) 165.
43. Krakowka, S. Mod Vet Pract **62** (1981) 191, 275, 367, 447.
44. McCullough, B. J Infect Dis **125** (1972) 174.
45. Rodgers, R *et al.* Nature New Biol **237** (1972) 270.
46. Stringfellow, DA and Weed, SD. Am J Vet Res **38** (1977) 1963.

47. Anderson, LJ and McKeating, FJ. Immun **19** (1970) 935.
48. Holzinger, EA. Cornell Vet **63** (1973) 87.
49. Tarr, MJ *et al.* Chem Biol Interactions **28** (1979) 181.
50. Snider, WR *et al.* Am Rev Resp Dis **104** (1971) 866.
51. Legendre, AM. Am J Vet Res **40** (1979) 1613.
52. Cockerell, GL *et al.* Am J Vet Res **36** (1975) 1489.
53. Rojko, JL *et al.* Work in progress, 1982.
54. Olsen, RG, Ohio State Univ: Unpublished data, 1981.
55. Rojko, JL *et al.* Work in progress, 1982.
56. Rojko, JL *et al.* Work in progress, 1982.
57. Olsen *et al*, in Hardy *et al*: Feline Leukemia Virus. Elsevier, North Holland, 1981.
58. Stiff-Torvik, M and Olsen, RG, Ohio State Univ: Unpublished data, 1981.
59. Taylor, D *et al.* J Immun **115** (1975) 862.
60. Cockerell, GL *et al.* J Nat Cancer Inst **57** (1976) 907.
61. Dunlop, JE *et al.* Cancer Res **39** (1979) 956.
62. Krakowka, S *et al.* In Vitro **13** (1977) 119.
63. Krakowka, S *et al.* J Immun Methods **14** (1977) 257.
64. Damont, F and Reichart, E. Comp Immun Microbiol Infect Dis **2** (1979) 23.
65. Glau, JN *et al.* Immun **15** (1968) 561.
66. Rojko, JL *et al.* Cancer Res **39** (1979) 3789.
67. Dubey, JP and Frenkel, JP. Vet Path **11** (1974) 350.
68. Koestner, A *et al.* Prog Exp Tumor Res **17** (1972) 9.
69. Schaller, JP *et al.* Cancer Res **38** (1979) 966.
70. Cockerell, GL. Vet Clin No Am **8** (1978) 613.
71. Rouse and Babiuk, in Osburn and Schultz: Basic and Clinical Aspects of Veterinary Immunology, Academic Press, New York, 1979.
72. Rohovsky, MW and Griesemer, RA. Vet Path **4** (1967) 391.
73. Carlson, JH *et al.* Vet Path **15** (1978) 383.
74. Schultz, RD *et al.* Cornell Vet **66** (1976) 324.
75. Mackey, L. Vet Rec **96** (1975) 5.
76. Hoover, EA *et al.* Cancer Res **33** (1973) 145.
77. Cockerell, GL *et al.* J Nat Cancer Inst **57** (1976) 1095.
78. Mathes, LE *et al.* Nature **274** (1978) 687.
79. Szilagyi, L *et al.* Z Immun Forsch **145** (1973) 201.
80. Aitken, ID and McCusker, HB. Vet Rec **84** (1969) 58.
81. McCusker, HB and Aitken, ID. Res Vet Sci **8** (1967) 265.
82. Parish, in Rook and Walton: Comparative Physiology and Pathology of the Skin. Blackwell Scientific, Oxford, 1965.
83. Powell, MB *et al.* Am J Vet Res **41** (1980) 877.
84. Piermattei and Gowing, in Catcott: Feline Medicine and Surgery. 1st ed. American Veterinary Publications, Santa Barbara, 1964.
85. Walton, GS. Vet Rec **81** (1967) 709.
86. Reedy, LM. VM/SAC **70** (1975) 703.
87. Criep, LH: Allergy and Clinical Immunology. Grune and Stratton, New York, 1976.
88. Weisbroth, SH *et al.* JAVMA **165** (1974) 1088.
89. Osborne, CA and Vernier, RL. JAAHA **9** (1973) 101.
90. Slauson, DO *et al.* J Path **108** (1971) 131.
91. Thornburg, LP *et al.* Vet Path **16** (1979) 604.
92. Slauson, DO and Lewis, RM. Vet Path **16** (1979) 135.
93. Farrow, BRH and Hurtable, CRR. J Comp Path **81** (1971) 463.
94. Saegusa, K *et al.* Arch Path Lab Med **103** (1979) 475.
95. Francis, DP *et al.* Am J Epidem **111** (1980) 337.
96. Day, NK *et al.* J Immun **126** (1980) 2363.
97. Pederson, NC and Boyle, JF. Am J Vet Res **41** (1980) 868.
98. Weiss, RC and Scott, FW. Am J Vet Res **42** (1981) 382.
99. Campbell, LH *et al.* JAVMA **161** (1972) 1122.
100. Altera, KP and Bonasch, H. JAVMA **149** (1966) 1307.
101. Pederson, NC *et al.* Am J Vet Res **41** (1980) 522.
102. Cotter, SM. JAVMA **175** (1979) 1191.
103. Hoover, EA *et al.* J Nat Cancer Inst **53** (1974) 1271.
104. Scott, DW *et al.* JAAHA **9** (1973) 530.
105. Mackey, LJ and Jarrett, WFH. J Nat Cancer Inst **49** (1972) 853.
106. Hardy, WD *et al.* Nature **288** (1980) 90.

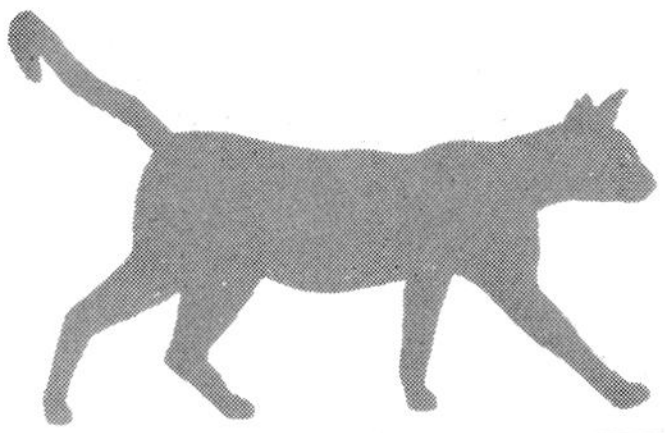

8

the alimentary system

THE ALIMENTARY SYSTEM

by T.J. Gruffydd-Jones, R.J. Evans and C.J. Gaskell

Analysis of the records of 992 cats referred to the School of Veterinary Science of the University of Bristol revealed that 19% had a primary disease of the alimentary system. Of these, 8% had oral or pharyngeal disease, a major component of this classification being primary or secondary gingivitis, and 11% had primary digestive disorders. Of the 992 cats, 5% were presented with diarrhea and 8% with vomiting. These signs frequently arose from disease of other body systems.

Further analysis revealed that 6% of the cats had oral or pharyngeal lesions other than those arising from acute upper respiratory tract viral infection. Only 1% had idiopathic regurgitation and 1% had other conditions. Gastric disease was noted in 2% of the animals. Small intestinal disease was noted in 5% of the animals. In our experience, liver disease is also rare in cats; in only 0.4% of the animals was any nonincidental liver condition conclusively diagnosed.

Another 3.3% had peritoneal disease characterized by accumulation of peritoneal fluid; 89% of these had the classic effusive form of feline infectious peritonitis (see Chapter 4). These figures are for a highly selected population seen at the major feline referral center in the United Kingdom. Nonetheless, they resemble those noted elsewhere.[1,2]

ANATOMY AND PATHOPHYSIOLOGY

The anatomy and physiology of the alimentary tract of the cat reflect its specialization as an obligate carnivore. The alimentary anatomy of cats resembles that of dogs, but its carnivorous specialization is carried to a greater extreme.

Notable differences occur in the relatively increased importance of the canine teeth in the cat and in the presence of lingual papillae directed caudad, both of which assist in prehension of prey in feral cats. The relatively wider bite of cats also contributes to their greater ability in this respect. The cat's dentition reflects its tendency to rapidly swallow prey whole. There is reduction of the premolar and molar tooth series compared with those of dogs. The dental formula of cats is as follows:

$$\text{Deciduous teeth} = 2 \times \left(\mathrm{I}\,\frac{3}{3}\;\mathrm{C}\,\frac{1}{1}\;\mathrm{M}\,\frac{3}{2}\right) = 26$$

$$\text{Permanent teeth} = 2 \times \left(\mathrm{I}\,\frac{3}{3}\;\mathrm{C}\,\frac{1}{1}\;\mathrm{PM}\,\frac{3}{2}\;\mathrm{M}\,\frac{1}{1}\right) = 30$$

The teeth of cats are considerably more brittle than those of dogs, a point of considerable importance when undertaking extraction. Because of the wide bite and the retractability of the lips, the entire buccal cavity can be examined easily.

The esophagus has longitudinal and circular muscle layers. In the middle and distal thirds, the muscle is smooth rather than striated. Bolus transition is therefore relatively slow.[3] The musculature is innervated by the vagus nerve, the axons originating from cells of the dorsal motor nucleus and the nucleus ambiguus.[4] The lower esophageal musculature forms a functional sphincter. Experimentally induced esophagitis interfered with gastroesophageal sphincter competence.[5] Interestingly, hydrochloric acid-induced esophagitis did not cause stricture formation.

The stomach of cats resembles that of dogs. It is large but less protected by the rib cage than that of dogs. Thus, palpation of gastric foreign bodies is easier.

The small intestine is relatively larger in cats than in dogs and fills the ventral portion of the abdomen caudal to the liver and stomach. The large intestine resembles that of dogs but the cecum is only a small, straight, blind pouch.

The anal glands of cats are discrete, saccular structures.[6]

SIGNS OF ALIMENTARY SYSTEM DISEASE

Accurate diagnosis of disorders of the alimentary system requires a careful and precise assessment and record of the signs encountered. The source of many misdiagnoses is failure to adequately discriminate between closely related signs. All systems must be examined, even if the disease is apparently clearly related to the gut.

Dysphagia

In taking the clinical history and in assessing hospitalized cats, it is important to distinguish adequately between anorexia, and dysmasesis and/or dysphagia. Anorexia applies only to loss of appetite, revealed by the animal showing no interest in food or turning away before beginning to eat. This is a very nonspecific sign and may be associated with disease of any system. By contrast, dysmasesis refers to difficulty in chewing and dysphagia to difficulty in swallowing. Because it is difficult to distinguish between these functions in cats, the term dysphagia is used to describe both abnormalities in this species. Dysphagia is characterized by pain or disability in attempts to chew or swallow. It also may be characterized by the prompt rejection of food, lip-slapping, quidding or salivary overflow. There also may be repeated and abortive attempts to swallow. Care must be taken to distinguish these conditions from failure of mastication secondary to fifth or seventh cranial nerve palsies, or of swallowing due to ninth or tenth cranial nerve dysfunction. In dysphagia, careful examination of the mouth and pharynx usually reveals disease of the lips, buccal cavity or pharynx. Halitosis is a common sign. If there is any uncertainty, the function of the cranial nerves should be assessed (see Chapter 14).

Vomiting and Regurgitation

Regurgitation and vomiting must be clearly differentiated. Cats have marked control over esophageal function, and regurgitation is a common clinical sign. Vomiting is usually characterized by marked effort, with involvement of the abdominal musculature. Food in the vomitus may be obviously partially digested and pH paper confirms admixture with acid. Cats rarely attempt to ingest vomited food. In contrast, regurgitation of esophageal contents requires little effort. The material is clearly not digested nor is it admixed with acid, and cats often avidly eat it. In some cases of regurgitation, the cat may move backward, producing a sausage-like esophageal cast of regurgitated material. The time at which regurgitation or vomiting occurs in relation to feeding is also of considerable significance. In pyloric stenosis, vomiting usually occurs ½-1 hour after feeding. Esophageal regurgitation is much more variable in relation to time of feeding and may occur when the animal is asleep. Vomiting due to pyloric dysfunction often is very forceful and may be projectile, the vomitus being propelled some distance in front of the cat.

The presence of dark-brown granules of acid hematin ("coffee grounds") in the vomitus indicates gastric hemorrhage and is a useful indicator of organic gastric disease. Fresh blood in vomitus is often regarded as pregastric in origin, but in our experience is more frequently an indication of gastric lesions.

Diarrhea

The term "diarrhea" is also used in an imprecise fashion to describe an increase in the volume, fluidity or frequency of passage of feces. Accurate definition of the owner's use of this term is essential. It is also important to assess the color, consistency and odor of feces. The presence of melena, free blood or mucus in the stool is also of considerable significance in determining the site of origin of the diarrhea.

Jaundice

Jaundice is uncommon in cats and may be prehepatic, hepatic or posthepatic in origin. It is most commonly of hepatic origin, in which case it is usually a consequence of an acute hepatic intoxication.

Constipation

Owners may be excessively concerned about their pet's bowel habits as a reflection of their own anxieties. The consistency of cat feces is as variable as the frequency of defecation. Constipation is significant only when it clearly represents a change in a consistent bowel habit or, alternatively, the failure to establish a consistent habit. In the absence of other abnormalities, cats void fecal balls of a very hard consistency unless they are concreted into a continuous fecal column within the colon and rectum.

EXAMINATION OF THE ALIMENTARY SYSTEM

Mouth

In examining the mouth, attention should be paid to all features of the buccal cavity, as well as to the lips and perioral skin. The dentition should be assessed to confirm the reported age. The teeth should be examined for calculus, loose or misaligned teeth, broken or cracked crowns, and periodontal pyorrhea. Jaw apposition is usually accurate but prognathism or brachygnathia may be encountered occasionally.

The gingivae should be carefully inspected for evidence of hyperemia, ulceration, hemorrhage, retraction from tooth roots, proliferation or tumor formation. Capillary refill also should be assessed by applying pressure to the gingivae. The gingivae are a poor site for assessment of mucous membrane color in cats; the tongue is a much better site.

The tongue should be carefully inspected, including its undersurface, for symmetry, mobility and color. Attention should also be paid to the glossal base and frenulum if a foreign body is suspected. Careful note should also be made of the presence of ulcers and glossal inflammation.

The palate should be carefully inspected for congenital and acquired defects. The same features should be noted as with the tongue and special care taken if a foreign body is suspected.

Careful attention should also be paid to the mucous membrane of the fauces and to the tonsils. It may be necessary to administer a general anesthetic and to examine the nasopharynx and dorsal surface of the palate with a dental mirror and palate lever if a foreign body, palatal tumor or nasopharyngeal polyp is a possible diagnosis.

The oral odor should be evaluated. The ammoniacal odor of uremia may suggest this as the cause of ulceration. A fetid odor may be caused by dental disease, gingivitis, ulceration of the lips or mucosa, or pulmonary disease. Ketosis due to diabetic ketoacidosis is rare.

Esophagus

Examination of the esophagus usually is not helpful and only the proximal third is directly accessible. Nonetheless, palpation of the neck may reveal a foreign body or accumulation of food. Examination of the esophagus is best achieved by radiography and esophagoscopy when a sufficiently small endoscope is available.

Stomach and Intestines

Examination of the abdominal viscera should be made from behind the standing animal. With the exception of palpation of the kidneys, a gentle, single-handed technic of drawing the hand ventrad, starting at the sublumbar musculature, is most appropriate in cats. Palpation should be preceded by percussion to determine the presence of excessive peritoneal fluid, characterized by a fluid thrill, or of excessive visceral gas, characterized by tympany. The degree of relaxation or tone of the abdominal muscles should be noted. Guarding denotes abdominal pain. With patience and gentle continuous pressure, it is usually possible to examine the viscera of all cats but those with a most painful abdomen. Guarding is reflected in a "tucked-up" appearance of the abdomen.

The size, position and shape of stomach, liver and spleen should be noted. The consistency of the abdominal and colonic contents should also be evaluated. The colon and rectum of cats are more mobile than those of dogs and may sit low in the abdomen. The feces of some individuals may be very hard and require considerable pressure to mold them. Such masses should not be misinterpreted as enlarged abdominal lymph nodes. Caution is required in assessing the gut wall in emaciated cats since there may be a false impression of increased gut thickness. Gut thickening can only be recognized reliably when it is localized and associated with lymphadenopathy. In young animals with abdominal pain and a history of vomiting, particular attention must be paid to the possibility of intussusception. This may be palpated as a distinct sausage-shaped mass in the right cranial quadrant, in the vicinity of the ileocecocolic junction.

Examination of the alimentary system is not complete without inspection of the anal ring and the perineum. Rectal palpation in cats should be performed only under general anesthesia and even then with great care.

Diagnostic Technics

Abdominocentesis

In animals with ascites, abdominocentesis should be performed for biochemical and cytologic examination to determine the nature and origin of the fluid. The viscous, high-protein (globulin-rich), straw-yellow fluid of feline infectious peritonitis, containing fine clots, is most commonly encountered. Bile, urine, low-protein transudates, chyle or frank pus may be obtained occasionally.

Abdominocentesis can be performed without general anesthesia. An area 4 cm square in the ventral midline, centered 1 cm caudal to the umbilicus, is shaved and surgically prepared. The operator should be gowned and gloved. If a needle of 20 ga or smaller diameter is used, local analgesia is not necessary; if required, local analgesia may be induced with 2% lidocaine administered from a dental syringe. The animal is supported at the edge of a table in a standing position by an assistant. A standard hypodermic needle and syringe may be used. The needle is introduced through a raised fold of skin and the point moved 1 cm caudad or craniad to create a flap valve on withdrawal. It is then introduced into the peritoneal cavity through the linea alba. Continual suction is maintained on the syringe plunger. Once fluid begins to flow, the needle is advanced no further. This minimizes the risk of penetrating a viscus.

Fluid for cytologic examination is dispensed into tubes containing EDTA. For biochemical assessment, heparin is used as anticoagulant. Samples for cytologic examination may be prepared as direct smears. Recently we have found that examination of smears of pelleted cells, with or without fixation, yields the most information about cell types and proportions. In particular, small numbers of neoplastic cells are more readily detected by this method than by others.

Radiography

For full details of the radiographic technic and of radiologic interpretation as applied to the feline alimentary system, textbooks of radiography and radiology should be consulted.[7-9]

Differentiation of structures depends upon the variation in radiographic density of air, fat, soft tissue, fluid and mineral. Thus, the composition of organ contents and material surrounding them is of considerable relevance to their radiographic resolution. The small intestine of cats usually contains considerably less gas than that of dogs, which renders its resolution difficult.[7,8] Contrast technics are required in many cases to clearly delineate components of the GI tract or for functional studies in the form of barium swallows or of pneumoperitonography. Soluble iodinated contrast media may be of value in rare occasions.[7-9]

Because of the relatively limited range of radiographic density in the abdomen and the small size of cats, care must be taken to avoid overexposure, particularly with emaciated animals, in which the absence of abdominal fat greatly reduces intraabdominal contrast. Some authorities recommend starvation and administration of an enema before GI radiography.[7] In our experience, the presence of ingesta in the gut may aid in interpretation of plain films in cats. Starvation is of course mandatory for contrast studies. Sedation should be avoided.

Emaciation may cause loss of detail on abdominal films and may mimic the ground-glass abdominal appearance associated with the presence of peritoneal fluid. In difficult cases, standing lateral views may determine if fluid is present; however, no fluid line is evident unless there is also pneumoperitoneum.[7] It is impossible to distinguish the nature of fluid by radiography. Abdominocentesis is essential if fluid is detected in the peritoneal cavity. Diffuse peritonitis and the mottling of fat encountered in pansteatitis may also reduce abdominal detail. Pancreatitis may result in localized loss of detail over the cranial part of the small intestine.[7]

Evidence of intra-abdominal masses should be sought. Enlarged mesenteric or sublumbar lymph nodes may be detected in lymphosarcoma. Occasionally masses may be masked by the presence of fluid; abdominocentesis to remove all of the fluid is required for their radiographic demonstration.

If ventral herniation is suspected but no clear discontinuity in abdominal wall muscles can be detected, SC injection of water-soluble iodinated contrast medium may clarify the disposition of the viscera.[7]

Esophagus: Megaesophagus may be delineated on plain films by the presence of air or accumulated food.[7,8] If this is secondary to vascular ring anomalies, the accumulation is precardiac.[7,8] In true megaesophagus, the accumulation is both pre- and postcardiac, as confirmed by contrast studies. Contrast studies are also helpful in postanesthetic stricture, suspected foreign body or in compression of the esophagus by extrinsic masses, particularly thymic lymphosarcoma. The animal should be starved for 24 hours prior to administration of 5-10 ml barium sulfate suspension. The transverse rugae of the esophageal mucosa create a fishbone pattern of the prediaphragmatic esophagus in such studies and must not be interpreted as an abnormality.[7] Should liquid barium reveal no abnormality, the investigation may be repeated 24 hours later using barium admixed with meat or canned cat food. Radiographs obtained immediately and 5, 15, 30, 60 and 120 minutes later are required.[10] Longer time intervals should be used as required.

In hospitals equipped to safely perform the procedure, study of peristalsis by fluoroscopy may be of help in diagnosing disease of the esophagus or stomach.

Esophageal foreign bodies are frequently fishhooks or needles and may therefore be apparent on plain films. In the pharyngeal region, care should be taken to avoid confusion with components of the hyoid apparatus.[7] If contrast studies are required and esophageal perforation is suspected, water-soluble iodinated contrast medium should be used since it is absorbed from the mediastinum, whereas barium is not.

Stomach: The stomach presents particular difficulties in radiographic investigation. Gastritis probably is never definitely recognized by radiography. The appearance of rugae should never be overinterpreted. Neoplasia of the stomach is rare in cats and is usually a diffuse lymphosarcomatous infiltration; neither masses nor filling defects are detectible in most cases.

Contrast studies may be of some value in evaluation of pyloric function.[11] Displacement of the stomach by extrinsic masses may occasionally be recognized.

Small Intestine: The small amount of small intestinal gas in cats means that contrast media are required for all detailed and critical investigations of the small intestine. Fluoroscopy for assessment of peristalsis may also prove helpful in hospitals equipped to safely perform the procedure. In assessing the small intestine, attention should be paid to its caliber and disposition. In paralytic ileus, the small intestine is distended with ingesta and/or gas. Cats frequently swallow linear foreign bodies, such as string. In such cases, the gut takes up a characteristic accordion-like plication as it contracts around the foreign body.[12] Alimentary tumors are usually lymphosarcomas and are frequently diffuse. Nodular lymphosarcoma occasionally produces filling defects as observed in contrast studies; however, usually it is not possible to detect alimentary lymphosarcoma radiographically.

Large Intestine: The large intestine is visualized because of the presence of gas and feces. In constipation, a continuous compacted column of feces may be evident. The presence of old pelvic injuries or of multiple bone fragments may indicate the cause. A true equivalent of Hirschsprung's disease (megacolon) occurs in cats and may be diagnosed radiographically by the presence of a terminal constricted (aganglionic segment) and a rectum empty of feces.[7]

Foreign bodies in the large intestine are usually subsequently voided and are likely to be of little clinical significance.

Liver: The edge of the liver shadow on the lateral abdominal radiograph is formed primarily by the left liver lobe.[7] The liver size may be revealed directly or by abnormal placement of the gastric image; administration of barium may help. Hepatomegaly may occur in cardiac incompetence, primary or secondary liver neoplasms, and hepatitis. Decreased liver size may be noted in portosystemic vascular shunt syndromes or cirrhosis. Unequivocal detection of portosystemic shunts requires portal venography.

Biliary System: Disease of the biliary system is rare in cats. The gallbladder is not detectable on plain films. Contrast studies of the biliary system are rarely indicated in cats.

Pancreas: The pancreas is not evident radiographically. A localized increase in cranial abdominal density suggests pancreatitis.[7]

DISEASES OF THE MOUTH AND PHARYNX

Oropharyngeal problems are commonly encountered in feline practice. Despite their common occurrence, many of these conditions are remarkably unresponsive to treatment. No rational therapy is available for a large proportion of these conditions because of the present incomplete understanding of their etiology.

A number of oropharyngeal diseases may be secondary to systemic disease, particularly chronic renal failure, leukopenia, immunosuppression subsequent to FeLV infection, and occasionally diabetes mellitus. In such cases, therapy is not successful unless the underlying cause is treated. A full medical history and clinical investigation is therefore required in all cases of oral disease.

The presenting signs of oropharyngeal disease are dysphagia, with or without inappetence, excessive salivation, halitosis and in some cases bleeding. Clawing at the mouth and head-shaking may also be noted with markedly irritating lesions or foreign bodies. Weight loss may occur as a consequence of anorexia or dysphagia.

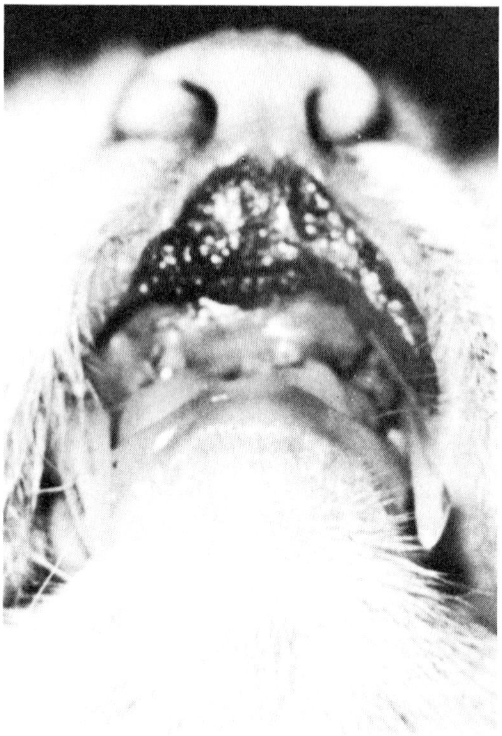

Fig 1. Eosinophilic granuloma of the lip. (Courtesy of Vet Ann)

The Lips

Eosinophilic Granuloma

Eosinophilic granuloma (rodent ulcer, labial ulcer) is a chronic ulcerative lesion of the lips, usually at the mucocutaneous junction (Fig 1). The lesion is localized, progressive, often bilateral and usually found in the region of the philtrum or of the canine tooth on the upper lip. The edges of the lesion are irregular and indurated and the base of the ulcer is a salmon-pink color. Occasionally lesions may occur on the tongue, lower lip, palate or nose. Other components of the so-called eosinophilic granuloma complex occur on the limbs or flanks. Lip and mouth lesions are disfiguring and more of cosmetic than clinical significance in most cases. Some lesions may progress to involve deep structures and cause pain, reluctance or inability to eat and inability to groom.

Cause: The cause of eosinophilic granuloma is obscure. The condition has no marked age or sex incidence, although it is more common in females than males and tends to occur in adult cats.[13] The condition may be a consequence of food allergy, infection or continual irritation by the papillae of the tongue. More than one cat in a household may be affected.

Histologically the lesions are characterized by proliferation of granulation tissue and infiltration with eosinophils, macrophages and lymphocytes. The overlying skin is ulcerated. Although eosinophils are a feature of the lesions, circulating eosinophilia is not a common finding.

Treatment: Various medical and surgical treatments have been applied in cases of eosinophilic granuloma, reflecting the unsatisfactory prognosis of these lesions. Treatments have included antibiotics, corticosteroids, chemical and electrical cautery, radical excision and radiotherapy. In our hands the most successful approach has been an initial 4- to 6-week course of prednisolone (1 mg/kg). This may be followed by radical cryosurgery, using a double freezing and thawing cycle, in cases not fully responsive to prednisolone.[14] Although this inevitably leads to some scarring, recurrence is infrequent. Some authors have recommended intralesional injection of corticosteroids. Use of oral progestogens is also reportedly successful and certainly worthy of trial as initial conservative therapy.[15]

Recurrence of the lesions is common and repeated treatment may be required.

Squamous-Cell Carcinoma

Squamous-cell carcinoma (see below) may affect the lip and is an important differential diagnosis of eosinophilic granuloma.[13] In cases of doubt, the diagnosis may be established by biopsy. Cryosurgery is the treatment of choice. Fibromata also occur, but much less commonly.

Mycobacterial Granulomas

Proliferative lesions, containing acid-fast organisms, occur occasionally. These mycobacterial granulomas may ulcerate. Excision or cryosurgery is the treatment of choice.

Harelip

Harelip is a congenital anatomic malformation that may be associated with cleft palate. Surgical intervention is impractical and euthanasia is the most appropriate course.

Wounds

Wounds of the lip are a common result of fighting, particularly in intact toms, and also as a consequence of traffic accidents. Abscess formation may follow.

The Mouth

Acute Stomatitis and Ulcerative Glossitis

Cause: Acute stomatitis may be caused by a variety of organisms but most commonly is a consequence of infection with one of the common feline upper respiratory tract viruses. Both feline calicivirus and feline viral rhinotracheitis virus produce stomatitis, with feline calicivirus much more commonly so.

Within the single serotype of feline calicivirus, a number of strains vary in antigenicity and pathogenicity.[16] Certain strains of feline calicivirus produce mouth ulceration only. The ulcers typically occur on the dorsum of the tongue but may also be encountered on the gingivae, palate and nasal cavity. Depending upon the strain of infecting virus, ulceration may occur in combination with relatively mild signs of upper respiratory tract disease.

Feline viral rhinotracheitis is a much more severe disease, with typical upper respiratory tract signs and associated pharyngitis and tonsillitis.[17] Glossitis, with small ulcers on the tongue, is rare.

Stomatitis is occasionally due to ingestion of irritants. This rare cause is overdiagnosed.

Treatment: In the absence of systemic antiviral drugs, treatment must be aimed at the control of secondary bacterial infection with broad-spectrum antibiotics, such as ampicillin or amoxicillin. Pediatric syrup preparations are of particular value because of the local action in the mouth and their ease of administration.

Supportive therapy with multiple-vitamin preparations is claimed to be of value. Diligent nursing, with attention to removal of secretions, is important. The cat should be offered liquid preparations of aromatic foods, with strongly flavored fish being particularly valuable. If inappetence or dysphagia is particularly marked, insertion of a pharyngostomy tube may be lifesaving. In dehydration, a mixture of 4% glucose and 0.18% saline should be given SC or IV.

Dental Disease

True dental caries is very rare in cats but such lesions of the tooth tables are encountered from time to time, particularly involving the molars. Affected teeth should be extracted.[13,18]

A more common problem is erosion of the crown-root junction, which may lead to the crown shearing off from the root under normal wear or when an attempt is made to extract the tooth. The root is likely to be infected and should be extracted.

Focal periapical abscesses may occur around any tooth. Diagnosis is by demonstration of periapical bone lucency on radiography. The tooth should be extracted to establish drainage. Abscessation around the roots of the upper carnassial tooth may, as in dogs, present as malar abscessation, a fluctuant swelling below the orbit, or as a discharging sinus in the same site. Radiographic demonstration of bone lysis confirms the diagnosis. Extraction is indicated.

Dental Calculus, Periodontitis and Gingivitis

Dental calculus, also called tartar, consists of bacterial plaque impregnated with a deposit of the mineral hydroxyapatite. Tartar may occur on any tooth but is most common on faces near the openings of salivary ducts. Accumulations occur especially on the lateral aspects of the molars and premolars, and on the lingual aspect of the mandibular incisors. Calculus accumulates with age and is more common in animals fed soft food. Calculus formation tends particularly to involve the gingival sulcus. As calculus is deposited, a niche is produced in which bacterial infection can be established. The adjacent gingiva becomes inflamed, retracts from the base of the teeth, and may become ulcerated and infected, leading to bacterial gingivitis. Recession of the gingival margin from the tooth roots predisposes to periodontal infection and frank pyorrhea. In addition to this infection of the alveolar membrane, the tooth root itself may become eroded and infected.

In early cases, removal of calculus is the only treatment required. Systemic antibiotic therapy, based on the results of culture and sensitivity tests, is required in advanced cases and should be maintained for at least a month. All involved teeth should be extracted after antibiotic therapy has been instituted for at least 3 days to avoid consequent septicemia.

Calculus usually reforms after the scaling of teeth and is predisposed to by surgically created microabrasions on the enamel. Dental attention is therefore likely to be required with increasing frequency once it has been initiated. Feeding dry cat food may help limit the problem.

Hyperemia of the Gingival Margin

A narrow zone of hyperemia adjacent to the gingival margin is common in kittens. It appears to present no problem and resolves without any

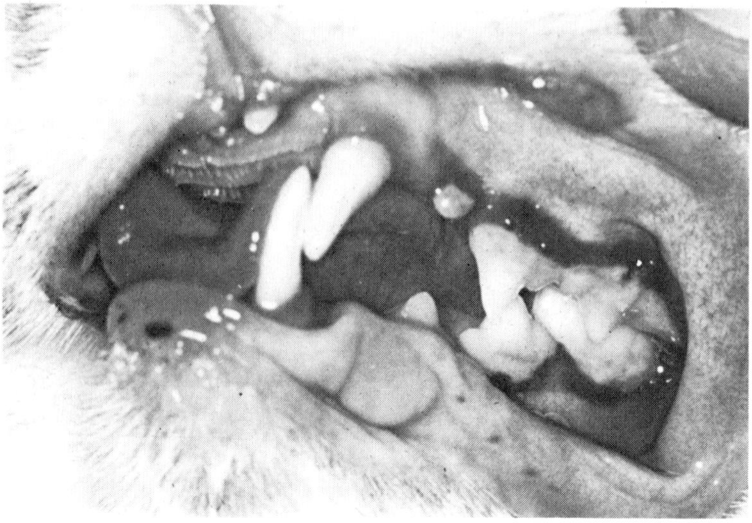

Fig 2. Primary, nonspecific gingivitis. Note the ring of hyperemia around the gingival margin. (Courtesy of Vet Ann)

treatment. Owners are, however, often excessively concerned about this.

A specific gingivitis has been reported in kittens aged 3½-7 months.[19] The cause is unknown and the condition often fails to respond to therapy. Spontaneous resolution may occur when the permanent dentition is established.

Nonspecific Gingivitis and Stomatitis

Nonspecific gingivitis and stomatitis constitute a large group of oral inflammatory lesions unrelated to dental disease and extremely refractory to treatment.[20] The condition causes chronic inflammation, vesiculation and ulceration of the oral mucosa (Figs 2, 3). This is most frequently noted at the angle of the mandible, extending to the fauces. Lesions occur less commonly on other parts of the oral mucosa.

Cause: The etiology of this condition is not clear. Spirochetes and organisms of the genera *Fusiformis*, *Bacteroides* and *Actinomyces* are commonly isolated, although their significance remains uncertain. Feline calicivirus and occasionally feline rhinotracheitis virus cause acute stomatitis lasting 2-3 weeks. However, feline calicivirus may have a significant role in the etiology of chronic stomatitis and gingivitis with ulceration of the fauces. In a recent survey conducted by the authors, the incidence of gingivitis was very much higher in pedigreed cats than in

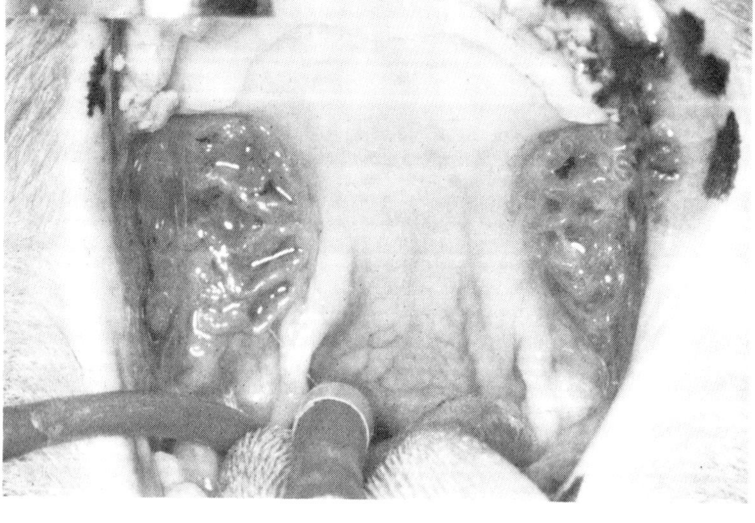

Fig 3. Ulceration of the fauces. (Courtesy of Vet Ann)

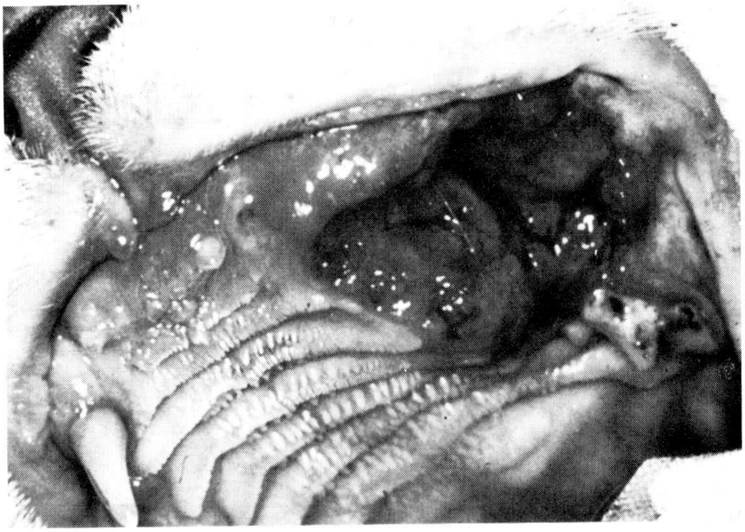

Fig 4. Gingival squamous-cell carcinoma, with invasion of the maxilla. (Courtesy of Vet Ann)

cats of mixed breeding. All of the cases in pedigreed cats were of the nonspecific form but many in cats of mixed breeding were associated with dental disease. The difference in the incidence of gingivitis in the 2 groups was reflected in the difference in the isolation rate of feline calicivirus. Furthermore, there was a strong correlation between the presence of feline calicivirus and gingivitis in both groups.

Intractable stomatitis and gingivitis also may be secondary to infection with FeLV and consequent immunosuppression.[21]

Treatment: Treatment is long-term systemic antibacterial therapy based on the results of bacterial culture and sensitivity testing. If spirochetes, *Bacteroides* spp, *Fusiformis* or anaerobes are involved, metronidazole (*eg*, Flagyl:Searle) is a valuable drug. The value of systemic or intralesional corticosteroids in reducing inflammation must be carefully balanced against their inhibitory effects on healing, and on phagocytosis and inactivation of bacteria and the danger of underlying viral infection. The use of antiseptic mouth washes or cream applied locally has been advocated but may not be practical. Some clinicians advocate use of chemical cautery and thermocautery. Supportive measures as recommended for acute stomatitis are of value. Despite the lack of apparent involvement of dental disease in this syndrome, refractory cases may respond to removal of any teeth surrounded by lesions, or even removal of all teeth. The molars and premolars usually are removed.

Gingival Hyperplasia

Cause: Gingival hyperplasia may arise from the area of the fauces and spread to involve the gingivae around the molars and premolars. The cause of this condition is obscure. It remains unclear whether it is a progression of the ulceration encountered in the same region or whether it is a distinct clinical entity.

Clinical Signs: The proliferating tissue becomes traumatized during mastication, yielding an extensive, bleeding, ulcerated mass that may lead to marked pain, ptyalism and inappetence.

Treatment: Removal of the teeth may reduce trauma to the tissue mass. Because the tissue is very vascular and hemostasis is a major problem, sharp incision of the mass should be avoided. Electrocautery or cryosurgery is more successful initially but may provoke excessive formation of granulation tissue. Intralesional or systemic corticosteroids are of little value. The lesions tend to recur regardless of treatment.

Neoplasia

The proliferative lesions of nonspecific gingivitis must be differentiated from those of oral neoplasia. In cases of doubt, biopsy may be indicated. Malignant tumors of the oral cavity are relatively common in cats and most are squamous-cell carcinomas.[13] Fibrosarcomas are another commonly encountered tumor, and benign fibromas (epulis) occasionally may be encountered on the gingivae.

Tumors are encountered mainly in older cats, commonly on the ventral surface of the base of the tongue or between the lingual frenulum and the gingivae. They may also be found on the gingivae, tonsils and palate. In the early stages, the lesions appear as firm white or pink nodules or lobulated masses (Fig 4). Often the animal is presented in an advanced stage of disease, when the mass is ulcerated, hyperemic and difficult to differentiate from gingival hypertrophy.

Because oral tumors often invade underlying bone, radiographic examination may help distinguish them from gingival hyperplasia. The diagnosis should be confirmed by biopsy.

Oral tumors rarely metastasize but local recurrence is common after surgical excision.[88] Cryosurgery is useful alone or as an adjunct to excision, but all measures are palliative. Tonsillar squamous-cell carcinomas frequently metastasize and have a poor prognosis. In cases of benign fibromas on the lips, removal is unnecessary unless the lesion is extensive. Nasopharyngeal polyps arising from the palate are readily amenable to excision.

The Salivary Glands

Primary disease of the salivary glands is rare in cats. Occasionally cats exposed to people with mumps may develop similar signs of salivary gland enlargement and discomfort.[22] Supportive treatment should be instituted using the regimen described for viral upper respiratory tract infection (see Chapter 10).[22]

Ranula and salivary mucocele may occur. They resemble the conditions in the dog and the same treatments may be applied.

The Palate

Cleft Palate

Cleft palate occurs in kittens as a developmental anomaly of genetic, teratogenic or idiopathic origin.[23] It may occur alone or associated with harelip. The condition is manifested soon after birth by difficulty in suckling and regurgitation of milk via the nostrils, with consequent sneezing, respiratory noise and distress. Affected kittens become weak and may develop aspiration pneumonia. Cleft palate is also a common cause of sudden neonatal mortalities. Treatment of congenital cleft palate is impractical and euthanasia is the most appropriate course of action.

Cleft palate also occurs as a consequence of trauma, most commonly following traffic accidents or falls from high places. The practicality of repair depends upon the severity of any other injuries sustained. Surgery texts should be consulted for details on repair.

Shortened Soft Palate

Congenital shortening of the soft palate may be encountered in kittens. The signs resemble those of cleft palate. Treatment is impractical.

The Pharynx

Pharyngeal and tonsillar disease have signs similar to those of oral disease but retching may be an additional feature. Pharyngitis commonly occurs as a component of upper respiratory tract viral infection.

Pharyngeal tumors are usually squamous-cell carcinomas.[24]

In any cat with signs of pharyngeal dysfunction, the possibility of a foreign body should be considered, as should the possibility of neuropathies involving the glossopharyngeal or vagus nerves. Foreign bodies commonly encountered include small bones, fish scales, needles, fish hooks and fibrous or filamentous material.

The Tonsils

Tonsillitis

Primary tonsillitis is extremely rare other than as a component of viral upper respiratory tract infections. Squamous-cell carcinoma of the tonsil is discussed above.

DISEASES OF THE ESOPHAGUS AND STOMACH

The importance of obtaining a thorough history in cats with signs suggestive of esophageal or gastric disease has already been stressed. Differentiation between vomiting and regurgitation, the cardinal signs of such disorders, and obtaining details of the nature of vomition are particularly important since they may provide useful clues to the underlying cause.

Vomiting and Regurgitation in Kittens

A number of congenital disorders may lead to persistent vomiting and regurgitation in young kittens. Certain clinical features are likely to be present, irrespective of the underlying cause. Most affected kittens manage to retain fluids and therefore clinical signs may not appear while they are still suckling the queen. Even after weaning, vomiting or regurgitation may be overlooked in a single kitten of a large litter.

Therefore, the problem is often first apparent in the newly acquired kitten.

Initially, affected animals have a good appetite and show few clinical signs apart from the vomiting or regurgitation. However, in time the kitten may become inappetent and depressed. Affected kittens grow poorly and appear stunted in comparison with normal littermates. Some owners report that the kitten may be able to retain certain foods, particularly of a softer, semiliquid consistency.

Although the cause of the vomiting or regurgitation may be suspected on the grounds of the history and clinical signs, radiographic examination is essential to confirm the diagnosis.

Pyloric Dysfunction

This is the most common cause of persistent vomiting in young kittens. There is a marked predisposition in the Siamese breed and evidence of hereditary transmission.[11]

Clinical Signs: The vomiting may be of a characteristic projectile nature, the vomitus being deposited some distance from the kitten. Vomiting of partially digested food may occur consistently half an hour to a few hours after feeding, but in other cases it may be unrelated to the time of feeding. Some kittens with pyloric dysfunction develop an associated megaesophagus and are presented with a history of regurgitation rather than vomiting.

Diagnosis: The major radiographic features of this disease are gastric dilation and prolonged gastric emptying time (Fig 5). In normal cats the gastric emptying time ranges from 2 to 6 hours. Barium may still be present in the stomach of cats with pyloric dysfunction after 24 hours. Any contrast material that passes into the duodenum appears in small, discrete spurts. Associated megaesophagus may also be demonstrated by contrast radiography.

Treatment: The treatment of choice is pyloromyotomy, even though true stenosis is not present. This surgical technic is difficult to perform in very young kittens and should ideally be delayed until the age of 6 months. Clinical signs may recur after cicatrization of the pylorus and a guarded prognosis should be given.

In mild cases, conservative treatment may be of some help. Frequent, small meals of semiliquid or pureed food should be provided. The owner should be advised to experiment with different types of food since affected kittens may retain certain foods more readily than others.

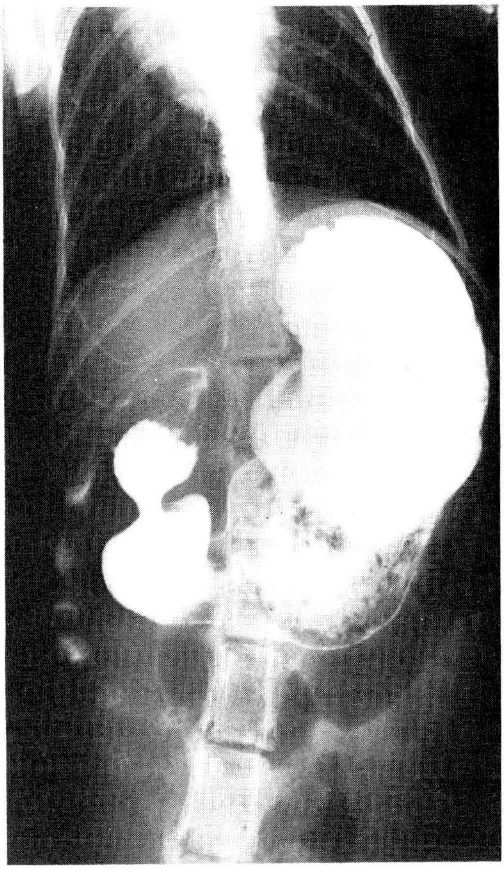

Fig 5. Ventrodorsal radiograph of a cat with pyloric dysfunction after administration of barium meal. Note the gastric dilation and small, discrete spurts of contrast material in the duodenum. (Courtesy of Dr C. Gibbs and J Sm Anim Pract)

Administration of atropine 5-10 minutes before feeding, either by injection or orally in the form of drops, tablets or commercial "chews," may aid dilation of the pylorus and gastric emptying. These conservative measures may be of value in maintaining a kitten's bodily condition until it is of a more suitable size for pyloromyotomy.

Primary Megaesophagus

Cause: Primary megaesophagus or achalasia is uncommon in cats. It has been seen in related cats and may be inherited as a simple-recessive factor.[25] It has been suggested that the disorder primarily results from a failure of innervation. The condition can be reproduced by sectioning the vagal nerves but there is no reduction in the number of cells of the myenteric ganglia, dorsal motor nuclei or nucleus ambiguus as in naturally occurring cases.[4,26]

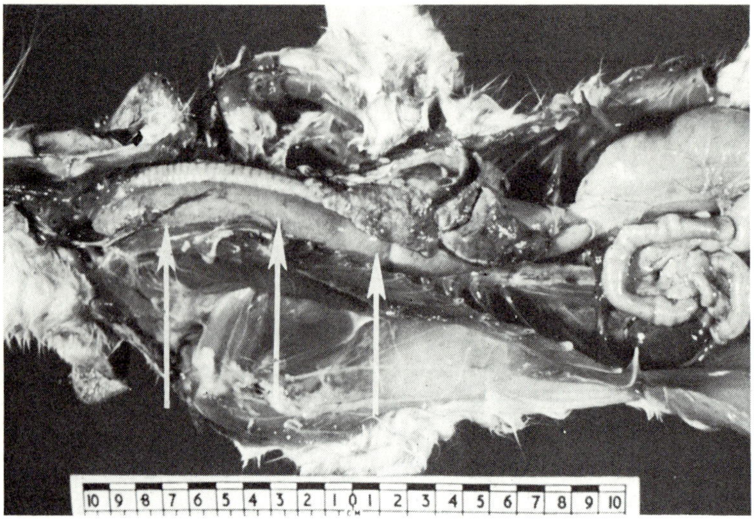

Fig 6. Primary megaesophagus in a kitten. The arrows indicate the dilated esophagus.

Clinical Signs: Primary megaesophagus is characterized by a dilated, atonic esophagus, ineffective peristalsis and failure of the terminal esophageal musculature ("cardiac sphincter") to dilate (Fig 6). This leads to retention of food within the distended esophagus and subsequent regurgitation. Most affected kittens have a history of regurgitation of a sausage-shaped bolus of undigested food, which has assumed the shape of the esophagus. This usually occurs within a few minutes of feeding but in some cases, particularly if there is marked esophageal dilation, the food may be retained within the esophagus for some time. The kitten or other cats may attempt to eat the regurgitated food. As in pyloric dysfunction certain foods, especially of a soft consistency, may be retained satisfactorily.

Diagnosis: Dilation of the thoracic esophagus can be readily appreciated on plain radiographs and after administration of a barium meal. In the normal kitten no appreciable amount of contrast material is retained in the esophagus after a few minutes. Care should be taken not to confuse the herringbone pattern that may persist for some time due to the corrugations of the mucosal surface with the abnormal retention of barium in megaesophagus (Figs 7, 8). It is also important to appreciate that the esophagus may

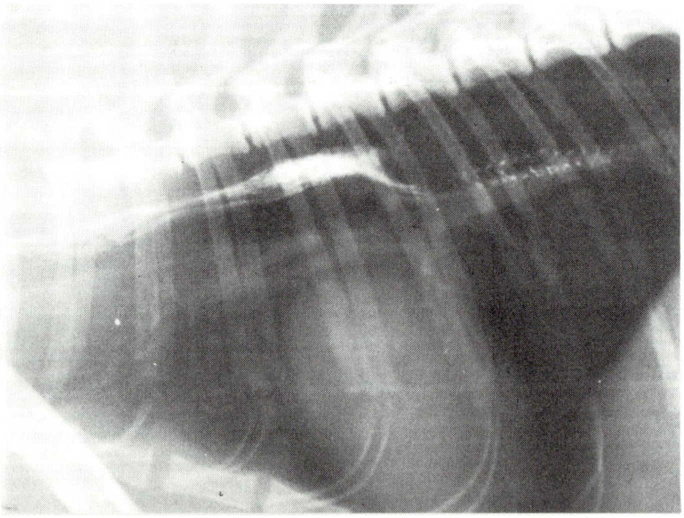

Fig 7. Lateral radiograph of a normal cat after administration of barium meal. Note the corrugated herringbone appearance of the esophagus. (Courtesy of Dr C. Gibbs)

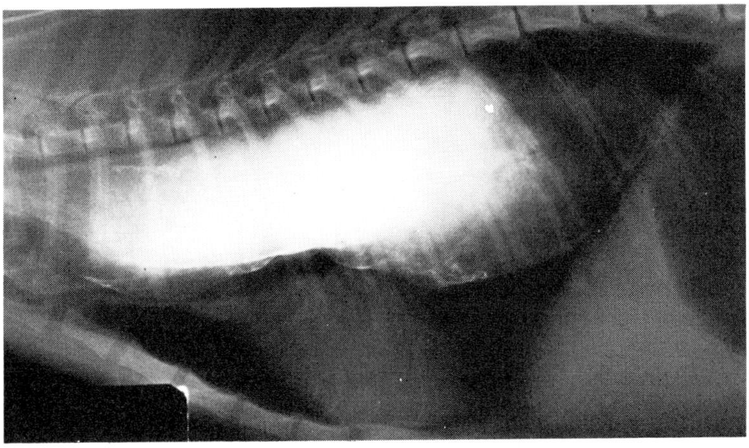

Fig 8. Lateral radiograph of a cat with primary megaesophahgus after the administration of barium meal. (Courtesy of Dr C. Gibbs)

appear dilated in anesthetized cats; therefore, radiographic examination of the esophagus should be performed only on conscious cats.

Treatment: Treatment of this condition is not usually successful. An attempt can be made to institute postural feeding, which entails feeding the animal in an upright position to aid passage of food through the esophagus into the stomach with gravity. It is most satisfactorily achieved by one person holding the kitten in an upright position, with paws resting on his shoulders, while a second person feeds the cat (Fig 9). This is not usually well tolerated by cats. Feeding frequent, small meals of semiliquid or pureed food may aid retention. Preprandial administration of atropine, used in the same way as for pyloric stenosis, may be of value in dilating the gastroesophageal sphincter. Unfortunately, these measures are likely to meet with only limited success. A serious secondary complication, rhinitis, develops in most cases due to regurgitation of food down the nasal passages. This may be so severe as to necessitate euthanasia.

Secondary Megaesophagus

The megaesophagus associated with pyloric dysfunction has already been described. Megaesophagus may also occur secondary to the vascular ring anomaly, persistent right aortic arch (see Chapter 9). This is an uncommon condition that causes the same signs as primary megaesophagus. The 2 conditions can be readily differentiated by contrast radiography of the esophagus. In primary megaesophagus, the dilation extends throughout the length of the thorax, as far caudad as the diaphragm. In persistent right aortic arch, it does not extend beyond the base of the heart (Fig 10).

The only satisfactory treatment for this condition is surgical division of the vascular ring structure. The prognosis for recovery is fair.

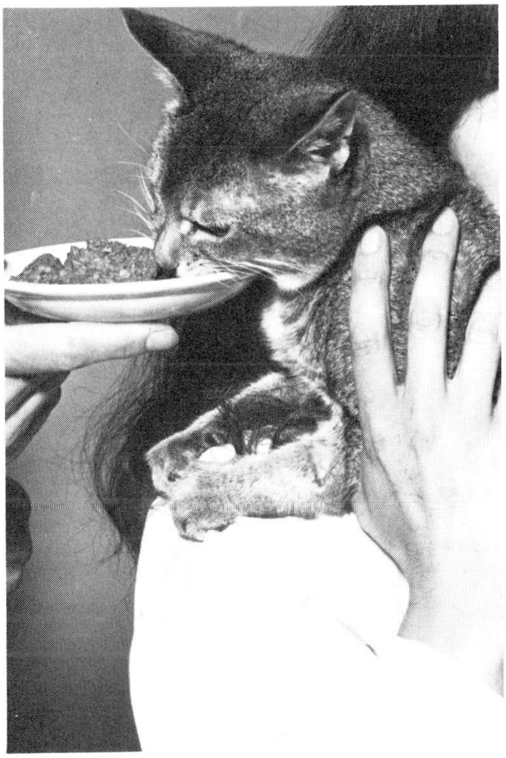

Fig 9. Postural feeding.

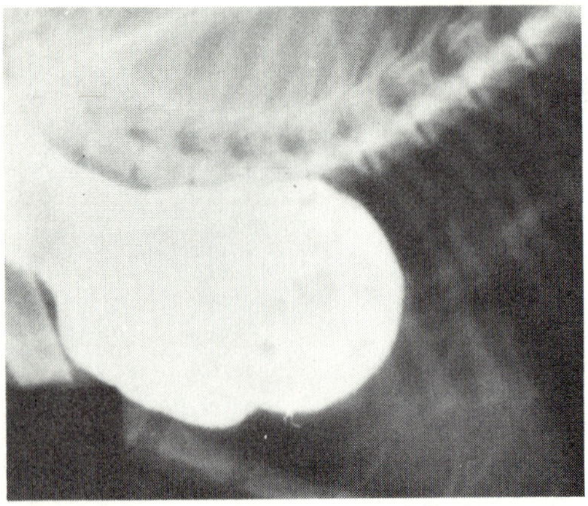

Fig 10. Lateral radiograph of a cat with megaesophagus secondary to persistent right aortic arch, after administration of barium meal. Note that the contrast material extends caudad only as far as the base of the heart. (Courtesy of Dr C. Gibbs)

Regurgitation in Adult Cats

Regurgitation is not common in adult cats. Occasionally the congenital conditions described as causes of regurgitation in kittens may not be recognized until later in life. It is not certain whether they have remained masked earlier or are acquired in such cases. A number of other conditions must be considered in the differential diagnosis of regurgitation in older animals.

Cranial Mediastinal (Thymic) Lymphosarcoma

This FeLV-related tumor is the most common form of lymphosarcoma in young cats, usually under 3 years of age. There is a marked predisposition in oriental breeds.[27]

Clinical Signs: The major presenting sign in this condition is dyspnea. However, in a significant proportion of cases, persistent regurgitation, alone or in combination with dyspnea, may be the main reason for presentation. The tumor may be palpable as it protrudes through the thoracic inlet and a lack of compressibility of the cranial thorax usually can be detected. There may be other evidence of lymphosarcoma in the form of superficial lymphadenopathy.

Diagnosis: The diagnosis can be readily confirmed by radiographic identification of a cranial thoracic mass that displaces the carina caudad and causes marked elevation of the trachea. The thoracic mass is usually smaller and associated with less thoracic fluid in cats presented with regurgitation than in those with dyspnea. The regurgitation results from external pressure by the tumor on the esophagus, which can be demonstrated by contrast radiography. In cases with equivocal radiographic signs, the presence of lymphoblasts in the thoracic fluid can be relied upon for confirmation of the diagnosis.

Treatment: No treatment is effective for this condition.

Esophageal Stricture

Cause: Esophageal stricture is a rare complication of general anesthesia.[28] The condition may result from reflux of gastric acids into the esophagus during anesthesia. This may lead to esophagitis and subsequent stricture formation. However, the precise cause is unknown. Use of atropine, which relaxes the gastroesophageal sphincter, might be a predisposing factor; however, in a series of cases in dogs and cats, there was no common factor in the type of premedication or anesthetic agents used.[28]

Clinical Signs: Affected cats develop regurgitation 3-14 days later. They retain a good appetite initially, but if untreated become depressed and inappetent, and lose condition.

Diagnosis: The stricture can be demonstrated by contrast radiography and endoscopy (Fig 11).

Treatment: The most satisfactory treatment is repeated, progressive, slow and gentle dilation of the esophagus under anesthesia, using probes of appropriate size. Initially a male canine urinary catheter may be a suitable size. Care should be taken not to perforate the esophagus. Administration of corticosteroids may help minimize fibrosis.

The prognosis depends to some extent on the length of the stricture. This may be difficult to determine and the apparent length determined radiographically may be misleading. Prompt diagnosis and use of corticosteroids in the early stages are probably critical in improving the prognosis. We have achieved a satisfactory outcome in approximately half of our cases using the measures described above. Surgical correction is to be avoided since postoperative wound breakdown is almost inevitable.

Idiopathic Intermittent Regurgitation

Cause: The authors have observed a syndrome of idiopathic intermittent regurgitation in nearly 20 middle-aged cats. Extensive radiographic investigation, involving administration of barium meals and fluoroscopic assessment of the esophageal passage of barium-coated boluses of food, failed to reveal any abnormality. Furthermore,

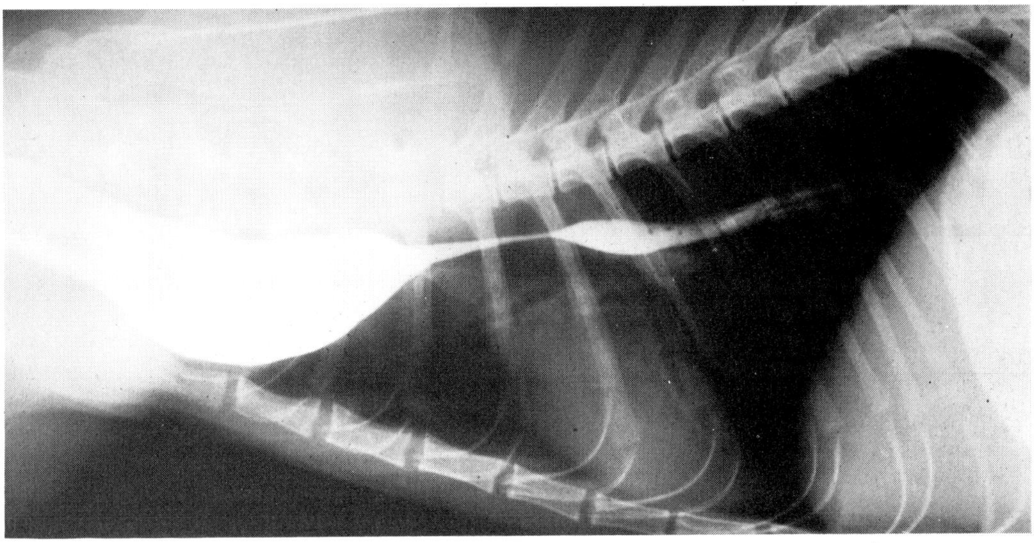

Fig 11. Lateral radiograph of a cat with esophageal stricture, after administration of barium meal. (Courtesy of Dr C. Gibbs and J Sm Anim Pract)

following hospitalization no regurgitation has been noted. Most affected cats have been of a nervous temperament and the first evidence of regurgitation has coincided with some stress factor, such as introduction of a new cat into the household or a change in the feeding routine. Stress has been shown to influence esophageal motility in people and we therefore suspect the problem is psychogenic in some cases.[29]

Clinical Signs: Affected animals regurgitate undigested food within a few minutes to half an hour after feeding, several times weekly. The regurgitation appears as typical "sausage vomiting," the cat backing away from a large, long bolus of food. Affected cats usually do not suffer from any distress or loss of condition but the regurgitation is unacceptable to the owner.

Treatment: The regurgitation can be markedly reduced in some cats by implementing the conservative measures described for managing primary megaesophagus. Small oral doses of phenobarbital may also be of value.

Miscellaneous Conditions

Regurgitation may occasionally be associated with other conditions. Foreign bodies in the esophagus are rare in cats. However, cats may swallow needles attached to thread, which may become twisted around the base of the tongue, preventing further passage of the needle. Esophageal rupture and development of an esophagobronchial or esophagotracheal fistula may be seen as secondary complications of foreign bodies. Mediastinitis may also occur.

Primary esophagitis is rare.

Squamous-cell carcinoma was a relatively common tumor in a series of cats with neoplasia from the London area.[24] However, the condition is rare in America and elsewhere in Great Britain. We have seen just one case. The tumor occurs at the thoracic inlet and causes partial obstruction leading to regurgitation. Ulceration usually develops and may lead to the regurgitated food being streaked with fresh blood. Administration of barium results in patchy esophageal retention at the thoracic inlet.

Megaesophagus has been observed in cats with myasthenia gravis, a rare condition in cats, but did not result in regurgitation.[30]

Vomiting

It is important to differentiate "normal" vomiting from pathologic vomiting. Cats readily vomit and simple overeating or a change of diet may be responsible. Occasional vomiting in the absence of any other clinical signs usually is not a cause for concern. In many cats vomiting is associated wtih eating grass. The reason for consumption of grass is not known. It is possible that cats deliberately eat grass for its emetic effect or grass may provide some important dietary component.

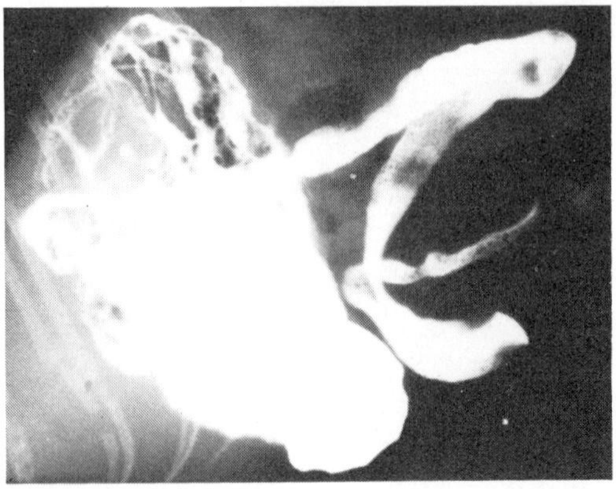

Fig 12. Lateral radiograph of a cat with gastric lymphosarcoma, after administration of barium meal. Note the filling defect. (Courtesy of Dr C. Gibbs)

Nonspecific Vomiting

In most cases of vomiting, the underlying cause is not clear but the condition resolves within a few days. Many of these cases may result from such factors as stress, change of diet or eating spoiled food. Treatment can only be empiric. A period of starvation, followed by feeding of a bland diet and administration of astringents, is indicated.

Gastritis

Primary gastritis is rare in cats. The most likely cause of gastritis is ingestion of an irritant. Bacterial gastritis akin to food poisoning in people is unusual, perhaps because of the highly discriminatory feeding behavior of cats.

Other Causes of Vomiting

Hairballs are almost certainly overdiagnosed as a cause of vomiting in cats. Retention of hair within the stomach and periodic vomiting of a hairball is a normal physiologic process. Occasionally the hairball may cause impaction of the stomach, especially in longhaired cats shedding heavily. Abnormal retention of hairballs, with impaction, may signify a more serious underlying condition. Esophageal hairballs have been observed in a cat with a suspected functional anomaly of the esophagus.[31] The single case of esophageal squamous-cell carcinoma we have encountered was presented with impaction of the stomach by a hairball.

Lubricants, such as white petroleum jelly or liquid paraffin, usually facilitate passage of the hairball. Regular grooming is obviously important as a preventive measure.

Cats, particularly young kittens, occasionally may vomit roundworms. If the worms enter the stomach, they may irritate the gastric mucosa and provoke vomiting.

Vomiting may also be associated with other conditions, such as feline panleukopenia, and alimentary lymphosarcoma or chronic renal failure in old cats. Toxemia, as in serious cat bite abscesses, intestinal obstruction or pyometra, may also result in vomiting.

Foreign bodies are uncommon in cats and are unlikely to lodge in the stomach.

Primary gastric neoplasia is virtually unknown in cats. Occasionally lymphosarcoma may affect the stomach. It is unlikely that such tumors could be palpable but they may occasionally be identified radiographically as a filling defect (Fig 12).

Torsion of the stomach has been reported but appears to be rare in cats.[32] The main presenting signs are abdominal distention and ascites.

DISEASES OF THE SMALL INTESTINE

The cardinal clinical sign in diseases of the small intestine, whether primary or secondary, is diarrhea. The normal behavior of cats tends to mask many clinical signs, particularly diarrhea. Cats are fastidiously clean animals and normally secretive about their defecatory habits. Diarrhea is therefore only noticed if the cat uses a litter tray, defecates in the house, or soils its perineal area.

The causes of diarrhea will be considered under the headings of acute and chronic. This is an artifical division and there is considerable overlap between the 2 groups, but it is the most clinically relevant approach to diarrhea in cats. There may be other signs of systemic illness in cats with acute diarrhea, but most animals with the chronic form have few other clinical signs apart possibly from some associated weight loss.

Acute Diarrhea

Panleukopenia

Panleukopenia is considered fully in Chapter 4 and will only be discussed briefly here in relation to diarrhea. In peracute infections, sudden death occurs and there may be no evidence of diarrhea. The virus has a predilection for rapidly dividing cells and one of the major sites of viral replication is in the epithelial lining of the intestinal mucosa. Therefore, diarrhea is one of the main presenting signs in panleukopenia infections, together with vomiting, dehydration, depression and fever.

It is primarily a disease of young, unvaccinated cats and is a particular problem in cat shelters and large breeding establishments. Most practitioners are familiar with the dilemma of managing diarrhea in young, newly acquired unvaccinated kittens. Most such cases are the result of stress associated with the change of environment and diet, and require no treatment other than dietary adjustments and possibly astringents. However, some such kittens are showing the first signs of panleukopenia infection and require a more vigorous approach, incorporating broad-spectrum antibiotics and fluid therapy. In this situation, hematologic examination to check for leukopenia is valuable. Cat breeders should be advised not to sell kittens before vaccination at 12 weeks of age.

Necropsy findings may be misleading and although there may be the classic red-rose serositis, the intestines may appear grossly normal. Histologic identification of epithelial loss, villus damage and particularly duodenal intranuclear inclusion bodies is the most reliable and practical method of diagnosis.

Some cats that have recovered from panleukopenia infection have a long-term or permanent predisposition to diarrhea, which may be due to irreversible damage to the villi, leading to malabsorption.[33]

Feline Leukemia Virus Infection

An association between FeLV and a syndrome of acute enteritis that closely resembles panleukopenia infection has been recognized for some time.[34] Panleukopenia is a highly infectious disease and if a susceptible colony is infected, a number of cases are likely to be seen in a short period. In contrast, FeLV-related acute enteritis occurs sporadically.

Acute enteritis has been the most common cause of death in one of our colonies of FeLV-positive cats. Antibody concentrations have not been determined in these animals but long-term persistence of viremia and failure to develop tumors suggest they are feline oncornavirus-associated cell membrane antigen-antibody (FOCMA) positive, and serum-neutralizing antibody negative. Most cases occur shortly after stress, such as surgery or change in household.

The disease runs a very rapid course, with severe depression, dehydration and hypothermia leading to collapse and death, often within 24 hours of appearance of the first clinical signs. The feces may be heavily tinged with fresh blood and mucus, or frank blood may be passed. Hematologic examination reveals a profound nonregenerative anemia and leukopenia, providing further confusion with panleukopenia.

The pathogenesis of this syndrome is not clear and a variety of pathologic lesions of the intestines has been observed. Ulcers in the GI tract and evidence of a hemorrhagic diathesis have been found. The latter may be associated with disseminated intravascular coagulation, which is also sometimes seen in feline infectious peritonitis.[35] Attempts to isolate panleukopenia virus and demonstrate inclusion bodies have been unsuccessful. A possible explanation for the pathogenesis of this syndrome is an FeLV-related hypoplastic marrow crisis, with immunoincompetence leading to overgrowth of gut organisms and endotoxic shock.

There may be a temporary response to blood transfusion, fluid therapy and broad-spectrum antibiotics; however, euthanasia is the most satisfactory approach. The presence of sporadic cases of acute panleukopenia-like enteritis in a vaccinated cattery is clearly an indication for FeLV screening.

Salmonellosis

Because cats, even of a young age, have a high natural resistance to infection by *Salmonella* spp, salmonellosis is not a common cause of diarrhea.[36] However, there are 2 situations in which salmonellosis may be of importance. First, stressed or immunocompromised adult cats may become susceptible. Salmonellosis has occurred in some adult cats immunosuppressed with concurrent FeLV infection and in show animals exhaustively used for breeding and exhibition. Second, *Salmonella* spp may cause diarrhea and neonatal mortality in young kittens in catteries, particularly if the standard of hygiene and husbandry is unsatisfactory.

Diagnosis depends on isolation of the organism from rectal swabs or preferably feces. *Salmonella typhimurium* is the organism most frequently encountered.[37] Unless the infected animal is profoundly ill and showing systemic signs, use of antibiotics is not advisable because antibiotics may prolong the period of excretion of bacteria and increase the risk of carrier status developing.[38] It has been suggested that prior antibiotic therapy predisposes cats to infection with *Salmonella* spp and that there is more

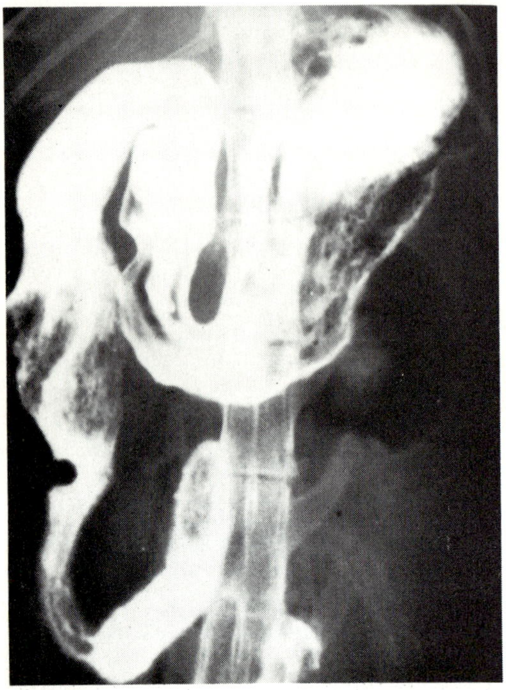

Fig 13. Ventrodorsal radiograph of a cat with a cellophane candy wrapper foreign body in the duodenum, after administration of barium meal. (Courtesy of Dr C. Gibbs)

likely to be systemic invasion with injudicious use of such drugs.[36] Most affected cats respond to supportive treatment, including provision of a bland diet and use of astringents and fluid therapy. Owners should be warned of the zoonotic potential of infection.

Infection may arise from feeding contaminated food or by contact with other infected animals, directly or indirectly. The importance of carriers in the epizootiology of this disease is not known. Our experience is that adult cats excrete the organism for only a short time. We have not encountered recurrences or later excretion.

Yersiniosis

In view of the apparent rarity of infection and frequent exposure to *Yersinia* spp through predation of wild animals, cats probably have a high natural resistance to this bacterium. Occasional cases have, however, been reported. If infection is by the oral route, the GI form of the disease, with diarrhea, may be seen.[39,40] There is usually rapid emaciation, depression and enlargment of the mesenteric lymph nodes. Hepatic abscessation, with jaundice, may also occur.

Diagnosis is only likely to be made with certainty at necropsy.

Tetracycline is the drug of choice, but the prognosis is poor in established cases.

Tyzzer's Disease

Tyzzer's disease, caused by *Bacillus piliformis*, has occasionally been observed in cats and is characterized by anorexia, depression and diarrhea.[41,42] The disease is more acute in young cats, often resembling panleukopenia and leading to death within a day or so. The course may be more protracted in adults. Infection is spread to susceptible animals by the fecal-oral route.

As with salmonellosis, infection is most likely to occur in immunosuppressed animals, as in FeLV infection, or those subjected to a poor standard of husbandry.[42]

Diagnosis is complicated by the difficulty in isolating the organism and demonstrating its presence in tissue sections.

Treatment is unlikely to be effective.

The authors have also encountered an outbreak of *Bacillus cereus* infection in a cattery. Contaminated food was soaked for 24 hours before feeding. Diarrhea and depression were the main presenting signs. The response to antibiotics and fluids was poor and the mortality rate was high once clinical signs developed.

Tuberculosis

Tuberculosis is now uncommon in cats but is of importance due to its zoonotic potential. If infection occurs by the oral route, the alimentary form may be seen. Affected cats show progressive weight loss and enlarged mesenteric lymph nodes. The disease may therefore be misdiagnosed as alimentary lymphosarcoma.[43]

Foreign Bodies

Cats are discriminatory feeders and foreign bodies are uncommon in the GI tract. However, when they do occur they are often linear in nature, presenting difficulties in diagnosis. The linear nature of the foreign body may also cause only partial obstruction of the gut; therefore, there may be a history of persistent diarrhea and weight loss.

Demonstration of the foreign body depends on contrast radiography (Fig 13). One of the most common foreign bodies in cats is a length of string. It may not be possible to visualize this radiographically but the gut may display a characteristic plicated appearance (Fig 14).

Treatment is surgical removal of the object.

Intussusception

Intussusception is an occasional sequel to diarrhea. It is more common in young cats and it is not unusual to see several kittens affected in the same litter. The intussusception may occur at any point along the gut but the most common site is the ileocecocolic junction.

Affected kittens initially show severe abdominal pain and may resent abdominal palpation. Depression with collapse rapidly ensues and prompt surgical correction is required.

Diagnosis is by palpation of a cylindric, doughy swelling in the abdomen, confirmed by radiographic examination.

The prognosis depends on the severity and duration of the lesion. It is important to treat the cause of the underlying diarrhea. Recurrence of intussusception is not uncommon.

Chronic Diarrhea

Feline Infectious Peritonitis

Some cats with histologically confirmed feline infectious peritonitis (FIP) have a history of chronic diarrhea. The intestine may be the primary site of infection. The importance of other coronaviruses as a cause of diarrhea in other species has recently been recognized.[44] In addition, a coronavirus that appears to be distinct from that causing FIP has been isolated from the feces of cats.[45] Further studies on the relationship between these coronaviruses and diarrhea are in progress.

Other Viral Infections

There is an increasing awareness of the role of recently recognized enteropathogenic viruses in the etiology of diarrhea in people and animals. Until appropriate serologic tests become more readily available and electron microscopic examination of feces is performed more regularly, the importance of such agents cannot be accurately assessed. Many cases almost certainly pass undiagnosed and resolve spontaneously. Rotavirus has been isolated from kittens with diarrhea but some workers have found a high incidence of this virus in the feces from normal cats.[46-48] Attempts to demonstrate viral particles by electron microscopy in approximately 20 cats with diarrhea of undetermined cause were unsuccessful.[49]

Bacterial Infection

Although bacteria may cause acute rather than chronic diarrhea, other clinical signs usually are not evident. Several enteropathogenic bacteria, particularly *E coli* and *Clostridium welchii*, have been incriminated as a cause of diarrhea in cats.[1] However, such organisms are normal gut inhabitants and assessment of their role in diarrhea is difficult. Their isolation in profuse growth may merely reflect multiplication secondary to some other cause of intestinal disease.

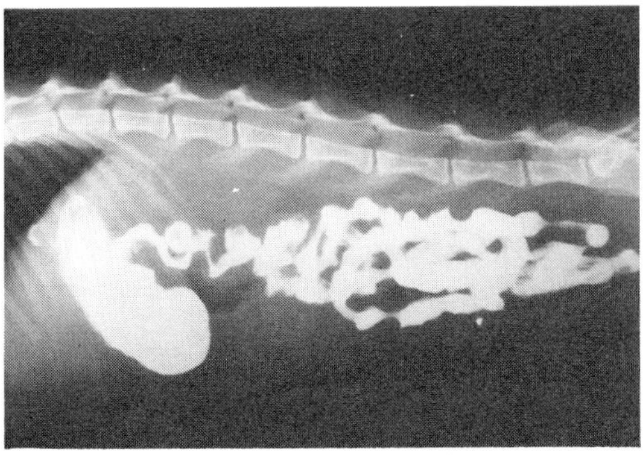

Fig 14. Lateral radiograph of a cat with a string intestinal foreign body, after administration of barium meal. Note the plicated appearance of the gut. (Courtesy of Dr C. Gibbs)

Attempts have been made by the authors to relate hemolytic strains of *E coli* to diarrhea. However, there was no significant difference in the relative frequency of different serotypes of 57 isolates from cats and kittens with diarrhea and 108 isolates from other sites. In both groups, serotypes 02, 025, 04 and 06 have predominated (10%, 9%, 17% and 28%, respectively, of cats with diarrhea, 13%, 20%, 8% and 20%, respectively, from other sites). These findings suggest that the importance of hemolytic *E coli* as a cause of diarrhea has been exaggerated in the past.

Attention has recently been focused on the importance of *Campylobacter* spp, particularly *C jejuni* and *C coli*, as enteropathogens. There have been conflicting reports on the isolation rates from normal and diarrheic cats.[50] This may partly result from differences in technics in isolating these fastidious organisms and the screening of cats from different environments.

Some authors claim *Campylobacter* is common in both normal and diarrheic cats. However, the authors' experience is that this organism is rarely responsible for diarrhea in cats.[51] This is supported by experimental studies demonstrating that even young kittens have a high natural resistance to infection.[52] Cats have been incriminated as a source of campylobacteriosis in people, but reverse transmission cannot be discounted.[53,54]

Diagnosis of *Campylobacter* infection is by isolation of the organism from selective media.

Infections usually are self-limiting, but in severe cases erythromycin therapy is indicated.

Other bacterial agents are occasionally isolated from cats with diarrhea. We have encountered *Plesiomonas shigelloides* in several cats. However, the significance of these isolates is difficult to assess.

Endoparasitism

Roundworm and tapeworm infections are common in cats. However, unless a very heavy burden is present in a young or debilitated animal, diarrhea is unlikely to result.

The importance of *Coccidia* as a cause of diarrhea in cats is uncertain. These protozoa, especially *Isospora felis,* are frequently found in the feces of normal cats. However, in catteries with a poor standard of husbandry, they may be pathogenic, particularly in young kittens. If oocysts are identified in feces, the possibility of multiplication secondary to some other problem must be considered.

The cat is the primary host for *Toxoplasma gondii,* but even heavy infestations are unlikely to cause intestinal disturbances.[55]

Other GI parasites are rare in cats, such as whipworms and *Capillaria,* but they do not appear to be a significant cause of diarrhea.[56,57]

Fluke infestation occurs occasionally but mainly in tropical countries. Infection is derived from eating lizards.

Neoplasia

The lower intestinal tract is one of the most common sites of neoplasia in cats, particularly of lymphosarcoma and carcinoma. There is considerable geographic variation in the incidence of alimentary lymphosarcoma judging from the proportion of all cases of lymphosarcoma this represents in different areas. The alimentary form of lymphosarcoma has been the most common in some reported series.[58,59] Feline leukemia virus is inconsistently isolated from these cats and can be recovered from only approximately a third of all affected cats.[34] However, recent epidemiologic surveys of large households in which the virus is enzootic suggest that FeLV-negative lymphosarcomas are associated with exposure to FeLV.[60,61]

Neoplasia is primarily a disease of old cats. Affected animals usually have a history of variable appetite and progressive weight loss, with occasional vomiting and diarrhea. The major differential diagnosis is chronic renal failure. However, in some old cats that become cachectic, no evidence of underlying disease can be identified and the loss of condition is presumed to represent "senile degeneration." Such cats may live with reasonable comfort for several years.

In alimentary lymphosarcoma and carcinoma, swellings of the gut and possibly also of the mesenteric lymph nodes are usually palpable. The prime site for both tumors is the ileocecal junction. Such cases present little difficulty in diagnosis. However in other cats there may be a more diffuse thickening throughout the gut, which may be difficult to appreciate on abdominal palpation. A false impression of gut thickening may be obtained on palpation of a thin cat and care must be taken to avoid any consequent confusion. It may only be possible to confirm a diagnosis of alimentary neoplasia in cases of diffuse infiltration by histologic examination of gut biopsies.

Chronic Renal Failure

Chronic renal failure is common in old cats and, together with alimentary lymphosarcoma, is the major differential diagnosis of the wasting syndrome so common in old cats. As with alimentary lymphosarcoma, affected animals may have a variable appetite, pale mucous membranes, and intermittent diarrhea and vomiting. Examination of the mouth may reveal stomatitis, oral ulcers, uremic halitosis and ptyalism.

Since cats are often secretive about their drinking and urination patterns, the owner may not report any polydipsia or polyuria. Some cats prefer to drink from puddles or pond water. A previously housebroken cat may begin to urinate in the house, particularly if confined indoors at night. Abdominal palpation may reveal small, shrunken, fibrotic kidneys, but this is not a consistent finding.

The most significant change in blood chemistry is an elevated BUN level. This must be differentiated from any prerenal or postrenal uremia, particularly if the cat is dehydrated. Serum phosphate and creatinine determinations may help assess the extent of renal damage and help formulate a prognosis. Most affected cats have an associated nonregenerative anemia.

However, this is also a common feature of alimentary lymphosarcoma.

Chronic renal disease is fully discussed in Chapter 12.

Glomerulonephritis

The characteristic presenting feature of glomerulonephritis is the nephrotic syndrome. However, some cats may have chronic diarrhea at an early stage, which is probably due to edema of the gut wall that may develop prior to generalized subcutaneous edema. Further details of this condition are contained in Chapter 12.

Diet-Related Diarrhea

Although cats are generally conservative feeders, dietary factors may be an important cause of diarrhea. There is considerable individual variability in the capacity of cats to adjust to dietary changes. Some animals may tolerate sudden variations without difficulty and consume apparently unsuitable foods with impunity. Others may develop diarrhea in response to the smallest change of diet.

Food allergy in cats has been reported but is much less common than in dogs.[62] Confirmation of this diagnosis is complicated by the reluctance of most cats to accept a bland, allergen-free diet. Therefore, diagnosis and management depend on trial-and-error adjustment of the diet.

Intolerance of cow's milk is probably the most common dietary cause of diarrhea. Many cat breeders, particularly those who keep oriental cats, report that their animals cannot tolerate cow's milk. This has been ascribed to a lactase deficiency, although no laboratory studies have been documented to support this.[13,63] Our experience is that this is more likely due to an allergy to the proteins in cow's milk. Most cats tolerate milk from other species and addition of lactose to the diet does not induce diarrhea.

Nonspecific Diarrhea

In most cases of diarrhea unassociated with other clinical signs, the underlying cause is not determined. Because most cases resolve spontaneously within a few days with empiric treatment, extensive laboratory investigations are not justified. However, in other cats, the diarrhea persists and, despite fecal examinations, blood analysis and other laboratory tests, the diagnosis may prove elusive.

Over-treatment, particularly with antibiotics during the initial stages of the disease, may be partly reponsible for this situation. There is no indication for empiric use of antibiotics in the treatment of nonspecific diarrhea, particularly if the cat has no other clinical signs. Such treatment may further compromise the normal gut flora, compounding the problem.

The most suitable approach to these cases is to provide astringents, such as kaolin and pectin, and a bland diet. The authors favor a diet of white meat (chicken and fish) or canned food and water. Provision of a bulking agent may also be of value. Feeding live-culture yogurt in an attempt to re-establish normal gut flora is sometimes advocated, but the value of this measure is uncertain.

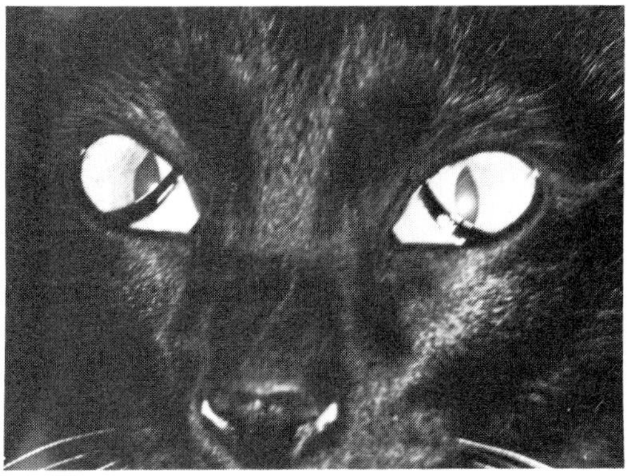

Fig 15. Burmese cat with protrusion of the nictitating membranes associated with chronic diarrhea.

Other Causes of Diarrhea

Some other diseases may cause diarrhea on rare occasions. Ingestion of irritant toxins and exposure to organophosphates may lead to diarrhea. Organophosphate intoxication may respond to treatment with atrophine and is discussed more fully in Chapter 14.

Sprue, villous atrophy and eosinophilic enteritis are rare in cats.[63] The only form of malabsorption seen with regularity is associated with lymphosarcoma.

The syndrome of chronic diarrhea with protrusion of the nictitating membranes has been observed in apparently otherwise healthy cats (Fig 15).[64,65] Affected cats show no other clinical signs and appear bright, with a good appetite. The protrusion of the third eyelid may be the only abnormality detected by the owner and the reason for presentation of free-living cats. However, if the cat is confined indoors, diarrhea is invariably discovered.

Despite extensive investigation of nearly 50 affected cats, the authors have been unable to determine any common factor. No organisms have been consistently identified by light and electron microscopic examination or culture of feces, and attempts to demonstrate serum antibodies to FIP, using cross-reactivity with TGE virus of pigs, have been unsuccessful. The ocular manifestations do not appear to be related to dehydration or loss of retrobulbar fat since the cats retain good bodily condition.

No form of treatment has been effective but all affected cats have recovered spontaneously. This, however, may take several months and in large catteries affected animals may show recurrence. This may be related to stress, particularly at the time of parturition, and the condition may subsequently appear in the litter. These epizootiologic observations and the presence of lymphocytosis in most affected cats lead us to suspect a viral etiology.

DISEASES OF THE LARGE INTESTINE

Apart from constipation, large intestinal disease is not a major problem in cats.

Congenital Malformations

Congenital deformities of the terminal rectum and anus occasionally occur in cats. The most common of these is atresia ani. Affected kittens are usually presented at a few days of age with a bloated abdomen, continual crying and restlessness. Surgical correction may be possible.

Failure of neurogenic control of the rectum may occur in young kittens, leading to fecal incontinence or retention. This is a particular problem of Manx cats, rumpies and stumpies, all of which have spina bifida and other spinal deformities to some extent. Dietary measures may help but the prognosis should be guarded.

Colitis

Colitis is rare in cats and only occasional isolated cases have been recorded. A case of necrotic colitis, involving partial sloughing of a segment of colon, has been described.[66] Other similar cases were mentioned and a history of depression, pyrexia and bloody feces, rapidly leading to collapse and death, was reported. Although most affected cats died, 2 cats were successfully treated with enemas of an antifungal agent. The cause of this syndrome was not determined, although a viral etiology was postulated. The description bears many similarities to the FeLV-related hemorrhagic enteritis. Marked leukopenia was a consistent feature.

Ulcerative colitis, with numerous punctate ulcers of the colon, has been reported.[67] The affected cat was thin and had bloody feces, although this sign had been overlooked by the owner. The cat responded favorably to salicyl azosulfapyridine treatment. The etiology was not determined.

Histiocytic ulcerative colitis, characterized by granulomatous infiltration of the mucosa, has been reported.[68] The affected cat had a long history of bloody diarrhea. An uncharacterized *Bacillus* organism was detected in the macrophages and the cat improved after prolonged antibiotic therapy.

Mycotic colitis associated with *Aspergillus* has been reported.[69] However, this was considered to be secondary to panleukopenia infection and antibiotic therapy.

The authors have seen a single case of colitis in an aged cat with a long history of tenesmus and passage of thin, misshapen masses of feces streaked with blood and mucus. There had been no diarrhea. A colonic stricture was identified on proctoscopy and contrast radiography. The cause of the colitis and stricture was not clear.

Constipation

Chronic constipation is common in cats, particularly in older, debilitated animals and long-haired cats during shedding. It may also be a long-term complication of previous pelvic injuries. The problem may be successfully managed by dietary adjustment, particularly by adding bulking agents, such as Metamucil (Searle) and feeding high-fiber foods, such as brown bread and bran. Regular administration of lubricants may also be of value.

Extreme care must be exercised in forced administration of liquid paraffin or mineral oil. This is the most common cause of aspiration pneumonia. A safer alternative is to instruct the owners to deposit some white petroleum jelly on the cat's tongue with a wooden spatula. If the cat is receiving regular dosing with such agents, it is important to ensure that deficiencies of fat-soluble vitamins do not result; if necessary, appropriate supplementation should be implemented. Daily grooming with a fine-toothed comb is important.

An enema is required in extreme cases of fecal retention. Severe loss of colonic muscle tone may occur with time, leading to frequent recurrences of fecal retention. Oral administration of bethanechol, in a dose of up to 1.25 mg twice daily, may be of some value in such cats. The owner should be warned of possible side effects due to parasympathetic over-stimulation, although these can be readily reversed by atropine.

Technics for partial colonic resection have been described, but these drastic measures should be reserved as a final resort.[70,71]

Miscellaneous Diseases

Cats have anal sacs that may perform some role in territorial marking. Although associated problems are much less common in cats than in dogs, anal sac impaction and abscessation may occasionally occur and should be considered in cats with perineal irritation.

Rectal prolapse is sometimes a complication of diarrhea, particularly in young kittens. It usually resolves after treatment of the underlying diarrhea but, in extreme cases, surgical repair may be necessary.

Perineal hernia usually occurs secondary to constipation.[72,73] Surgical correction may be performed in the same fashion as for dogs.

Ascites

Ascites is not as common in cats as in dogs. Several differential diagnoses should be considered.

Feline Infectious Peritonitis: The most common cause of ascites in cats is the classic or "wet" abdominal form of FIP. The associated fluid is typically straw-colored, clear, viscid and rich in globulin (see Chapter 4).

Peritonitis: Peritonitis is uncommon in cats but may result from rupture of abdominal organs from trauma or may be iatrogenic. We have encountered a few cases of bacterial peritonitis apparently related to gut rupture. Evidence of foreign bodies is usually found. *Salmonella typhimurium* has been isolated in such cases.

Glomerulonephritis: The hypoalbuminemia of glomerulonephritis may lead to accumulation of transudate within the abdominal cavity, but subcutaneous edema is likely to be a more prominent feature.

Heart Disease: In contrast to dogs, cats with heart failure rarely have obvious ascites.[74] Accumulation of a thoracic transudate is much more common. The reason for this unusual response to heart failure is not understood.

DISEASES OF THE PANCREAS

Pancreatic disease is not a major problem in feline medicine. Pancreatic lesions are frequently identified at necropsy as incidental findings but rarely can be associated with prior presence of clinical signs.

Pancreatitis

Pancreatitis has been divided into acute and chronic forms according to the clinical presentation, or into a number of types on the basis of the underlying pathologic changes. However, no system of classification is ideal and there is considerable overlap among the different groups.

Cause: The cause of pancreatitis in cats is unknown. Cholangitis is often associated with pancreatitis.[89] The bile and pancreatic ducts fuse in the cat before entering the duodenum and this raises the possibility of ascending infections originating in the gut. Trauma may also cause pancreatitis.[90]

Clinical Signs: The main presenting signs in pancreatitis are depression and weight loss, possibly with vomiting, diarrhea, polydipsia and cranial abdominal pain.[75-77] Because these signs are rather nonspecific, the possibility of pancreatitis may be overlooked. In acute cases there is usually leukocytosis and a rise in serum liver enzyme levels, but serum amylase levels may not be increased.[77]

Diagnosis: Radiographic examination may help in diagnosis, but the main change of haziness and poor contrast in the cranial abdomen may be difficult to appreciate.

Treatment: Treatment with antibiotics and corticosteroids has been advocated. Reports suggest a survival rate of approximately 50% in acute cases.

Exocrine Pancreatic Insufficiency

Exocrine pancreatic insufficiency is rare in cats, judging from the paucity of reported cases. It has been a sequel to pancreatitis in some cats but few clinically significant cases have been reported.[75,78,79] We have occasionally encountered low fecal trypsin levels (<20 azocasein units) in cats presented for investigation of chronic diarrhea and weight loss. However, these have been isolated low values and subsequent serial fecal samples from the same cats have shown normal values (>50 azocasein units).

Endocrine Pancreatic Disease

Endocrine pancreatic disease is discussed in Chapter 11.

Neoplasia

Neoplasia of the pancreas is not uncommon. The most frequently encountered tumor is squamous-cell carcinoma, the prime site being the head of the pancreas. This often leads to obstruction of the bile duct and posthepatic jaundice, with elevated serum liver enzyme levels. There is usually marked weight loss and the mass is readily palpable. Metastasis, particularly to the liver, is common.

DISEASE OF THE LIVER

Liver disease is not common in cats. In contrast to most other species, no specific viral or bacterial organisms are recognized as causes of hepatitis. Cats appear to be naturally resistant to leptospirosis.

The major presenting signs in liver disease are depression, inappetence, weight loss and jaundice. Vomiting, diarrhea and neurologic signs occasionally occur. In most normal cats, it is only possible to palpate the caudal portion of the liver lobes. In cats with hepatic disease, the liver usually is readily palpable and swelling of the individual lobes can be detected. Radiography may be of value in confirming the presence of hepatomegaly.

Biochemical examination of the blood is crucial in the evaluation of suspected liver dysfunction. Elevated serum bilirubin levels are usually detected only if jaundice is apparent. Determination of the relative proportions of conjugated and unconjugated forms of bilirubin may help differentiate among prehepatic, hepatic and posthepatic jaundice. However, the distinction among these 3 types is often not clear.[80]

Serum glutamic pyruvic transaminase (SGPT) levels provide a sensitive indication of acute, hepatocellular necrosis.[81] Glutamic oxaloacetic transaminase (GOT) is found in high concentrations in a variety of tissues and is therefore thought to be a less sensitive guide to hepatic damage.[82] For many years it was suggested that serum alkaline phosphatase (SAP) concentrations are seldom elevated in cats due to efficient renal excretion. It has now been shown that SAP levels may rise in biliary obstruction; however, the half-life of this enzyme is very short.[80,83]

Comparison of the relative increase in SGPT and SAP levels appears to provide a more reliable method of differentiating between hepatic and obstructive jaundice than differential serum bilirubin levels. In hepatic disease, SGPT levels rise more dramatically than SAP levels; in posthepatic disease, the reverse is true.[80] Blood ammonia levels and BSP retention tests may also help assess liver function but have not been used extensively.

Discussions of the main types of liver disease follow.

Toxic Hepatitis

A number of toxins, particularly coal tar derivatives and phenolic compounds, may cause toxic hepatitis in cats. Cats are particularly sensitive to these compounds due to their poor ability to conjugate them with glucuronic acid.

Use of sawdust or woodshavings, derived from previously treated wood, as litter is probably the most likely cause of exposure. Affected cats are depressed, anorectic and jaundiced. Some assessment of prognosis may be determined from the degree of increase in SGPT level.

Cholangiohepatitis

Cholangiohepatitis, with or without pancreatitis, is a relatively common necropsy finding. Associated clinical disease is recognized less often but this may merely reflect the vagueness of clinical signs and the difficulty in confirming this diagnosis in the live animal.

The main clinical signs are fever, anorexia, weight loss and jaundice. These are often intermittent in nature. Blood examination reveals leukocytosis, with a left shift and a moderate increase in SGPT levels. Some cats respond to treatment with fluids, corticosteroids and antibiotics. In such animals, the diagnosis must be considered presumptive.

Neoplasia

Hepatic neoplasia occasionally is encountered in cats. Lymphosarcoma of the liver occurs as a feature of disseminated lymphosarcoma and as an isolated entity. Bile duct carcinoma has been observed in cats, and the liver may be a site for metastasis of carcinomas from other primary sites, particularly the intestines.[84]

Cats with hepatic neoplasia usually have weight loss and possibly jaundice, mainly due to a rise in conjugated bilirubin levels, with vomiting and diarrhea. Hepatomegaly can be demonstrated on abdominal palpation. Serum levels of liver enzymes may be elevated, but this is not a consistent feature.

Miscellaneous Conditions

Fluke infestation of the biliary tree and liver by *Platynosomum concinnum* is rare but may occur in tropical countries. Infection is probably derived from eating lizards. In an experimental study, even inoculation with large numbers of flukes resulted in only mild clinical signs of inappetence and lethargy.[85]

Three cases of portacaval shunts in cats have recently been described.[86,87] The main presenting signs were seizures and stunting. High blood ammonia levels occurred in 2 cats, although in only one was abnormal retention of BSP observed.[87] The diagnosis was confirmed by contrast portosplenography. In both cats the shunts were congenital, with no portohepatic communication. Treatment was not attempted.

Hepatic cysts are occasionally associated with polycystic renal disease. They are rarely important clinically. There may be hereditary basis to this condition, as in people. In the authors' experience most cases occur in longhaired cats.

The liver is often involved in other diseases. In FIP, fibrinous plaques may be deposited on the visceral peritoneal surface. Fatty infiltration and congestion may be sequels to endocrine diseases, particularly diabetes mellitus and cardiac failure. Cirrhosis of the liver is also occasionally encountered. However, in all of these conditions, the hepatic lesions rarely contribute significantly to the clinical picture.

Hepatic abscessation is a relatively common cause of neonatal mortality. It is a sequel to umbilical infection, in which organisms ascend the umbilical vessels. Several kittens in the same litter may be affected.

Jaundice

Jaundice is an unusual clinical sign in cats and is not in itself a disease. Although it is a common finding in hepatic disease, there are other causes to consider. It is most readily appreciated by noting the color of the sclera in natural daylight. In cats of the semialbinistic series (*ie*, Burmese, Siamese), the color of the iris may change from blue or yellow to green.

Feline Infectious Peritonitis: Jaundice is common in the later stages of FIP, both in its classic abdominal and extraperitoneal forms. The origin of this jaundice is not always clear. Although there may be hepatic involvement in some cats with FIP, this is usually confined to the visceral peritoneal surface and there is often little elevation of the serum level of hepatic enzymes. In others, there is no evidence of hepatic lesions. Most cats with FIP have anemia of a nonregenerative nature. Therefore, there is often no obvious explanation for the jaundice.

Liver Disease: An increase in the serum level of both forms of bilirubin occurs in primary hepatic diseases, usually associated with hepatocellular toxicity. The SGPT level is significantly raised. In obstruction of the biliary tree, as in cholangiohepatitis and neoplasia, most circulating bilirubin is conjugated.

Hemolytic Anemia: Increased destruction of RBC may result in a rise in the serum level of unconjugated bilirubin and, hence, jaundice. However, cats have a considerable capacity to conjugate bilirubin and jaundice is only seen after an acute hemolytic crisis, as in severe infections with *Hemobartonella felis*. We have also seen prehepatic icterus in Heinz-body anemias presumed to be of toxic origin.

References

1. Osbaldiston, GW *et al.* Feline Pract **2(5)** (1972) 8.
2. Evans, RJ, Univ Bristol: Unpublished data, 1980.
3. Strombeck, DR. Vet Clin No Am **8** (1979) 229.
4. Clifford, DH *et al.* Br Vet J **136** (1980) 74.
5. Eastwood, GL *et al.* Gastroent **69** (1975) 146.
6. Greer, MJ and Calhoun, ML. Am J Vet Res **27** (1966) 773.
7. Kealy, JK: Diagnostic Radiology of the Dog and Cat. WB Saunders, Philadelphia, 1979.
8. Douglas, SW and Williamson, MD: Veterinary Radiological Interpretation. Heineman Veterinary Books, London, 1970.
9. Douglas, SW and Williamson, MD: Principles of Veterinary Radiography. 3rd ed. Baillière Tindall, London, 1980.
10. Morgan, JP. J Am Vet Rad Soc **18** (1977) 134.
11. Pearson, H *et al.* J Sm Anim Pract **15** (1974) 487.
12. Root, CR and Lord, PF. J Am Vet Rad Soc **12** (1971) 45.
13. Wilkinson, GT: Diseases of the Cat. Pergamon Press, Oxford, 1966.
14. Lane, JG. J Sm Anim Pract **15** (1974) 715.
15. Dillon, in Kirk: Veterinary Therapy VII. WB Saunders, Philadelphia, 1980.
16. Gaskell, CJ and Gaskell, RM. In Practice **2** (1980) 5.
17. Povey, RC. Vet Rec **98** (1976) 293.
18. Ross, in Ettinger: Textbook of Veterinary Internal Medicine. WB Saunders, Philadelphia, 1975.
19. Joshua, JO: The Clinical Aspects of Some Diseases of Cats. William Heineman Medical Books, London, 1965.
20. Gaskell, RM and Gruffydd-Jones, TJ. Vet Ann **17** (1959) 195.

21. Barrett, RE *et al.* Feline Pract **5(6)** (1975) 34.
22. Catcott, EJ: Progress in Feline Practice. American Veterinary Publications, Santa Barbara, 1971.
23. Loewy, HT. J Dent Res **53** (1974) 453.
24. Cotchin, E. Vet Rec **69** (1957) 425.
25. Clifford, DH *et al.* JAVMA **158** (1971) 1554.
26. Clifford, DH. Am J Vet Res **34** (1973) 1333.
27. Gruffydd-Jones, TJ *et al.* Vet Rec **104** (1979) 304.
28. Pearson, H *et al.* J Sm Anim Pract **19** (1979) 507.
29. Rubin, J *et al.* Psychosomatic Med **24** (1962) 170.
30. Mason, KV. J Sm Anim Pract **17** (1976) 467.
31. Van Stee, EW *et al.* VM/SAC **75** (1980) 1873.
32. Turner, T. J Sm Anim Pract **9** (1968) 231.
33. Carpenter, J. JAVMA **158** (1971) 857.
34. Cotter, SM *et al.* JAVMA **166** (1975) 449.
35. Weiss, RC *et al.* Am J Vet Res **40** (1980) 663.
36. Timoney, JF *et al.* Cornell Vet **68** (1978) 211.
37. Fox, JG and Beaucage, CM. J Infect Dis **139** (1979) 362.
38. Nelson, JD *et al.* Pediat **65** (1980) 1125.
39. Mair, NS *et al.* Vet Rec **81** (1967) 461.
40. Obwolo, MJ and Gruffydd-Jones, TJ. Vet Rec **100** (1977) 424.
41. Kovatch, RM and Zebarth, G. JAVMA **162** (1973) 136.
42. Bennett, AM *et al.* Vet Microbiol **2** (1977) 49.
43. Orr, CM *et al.* J Sm Anim Pract **21** (1980) 247.
44. Pederson, NC and Boyle, JF. Am J Vet Res **41** (1980) 868.
45. Hoshino, Y and Scott, FW. Arch Virol **63** (1980) 147.
46. Snodgrass, DR *et al.* Vet Rec **104** (1979) 222.
47. Chrystie, IL *et al.* Vet Rec **105** (1979) 404.
48. McNish, WC. Paper presented at Br Sm Anim Vet Assoc Ann Cong, 1980.
49. Gruffydd-Jones, TJ and Chrystie, IL, Univ Bristol: Unpublished data, 1980.
50. Skirrow, MB. Vet Res Comm. *In press*, 1982.
51. Gruffydd-Jones, TJ *et al.* Lancet **2** (1980) 366.
52. Prescott, JF and Karmali, MA. Can Med Assoc **119** (1978) 1001.
53. Svedhem, A and Norkrans, G. Lancet **1** (1980) 713.
54. Skirrow, MB *et al.* Lancet **1** (1980) 1188.
55. Dubey, JP. JAVMA **169** (1976) 1061.
56. Hass, DK. Feline Pract **8(2)** (1978) 31.
57. Endres, WA. VM/SAC **71** (1976) 1553.
58. Crighton, GW. Vet Rec **82** (1968) 122.
59. Meincke, JE *et al.* JAVMA **160** (1972) 1093.
60. Francis, DP *et al.* Cancer Res **39** (1979) 3866.
61. Hardy, WD *et al.* Nature **288** (1980) 90.
62. Walton, GS *et al.* Vet Rec **83** (1968) 35.
63. Reed, in Catcott: Feline Medicine and Surgery. 2nd ed. American Veterinary Publications, Santa Barbara, 1975.
64. Gruffydd-Jones, TJ *et al.* Vet Rec **101** (1977) 413.
65. Ott, RL *et al.* Feline Pract **5(3)** (1975) 16.
66. Erbeck, DH and Hagee, JH. VM/SAC **69** (1974) 603.
67. Ewing, GO. JAAHA **8** (1972) 64.
68. Van Kruiningen, HJ and Dobbins, WO. Vet Path **16** (1979) 215.
69. Bolton, GR and Brown, TT. VM/SAC **67** (1972) 978.
70. Yoder, JT *et al.* VM/SAC **63** (1968) 1049.
71. Leighton, RL. Feline Pract **8** (1978) 31.
72. Ashton, DG. J Sm Anim Pract **17** (1976) 473.
73. Leighton, RL. Feline Pract **9** (1979) 44.
74. Liu, SK *et al.* JAVMA **156** (1970) 1319.
75. Duffell, SJ. J Sm Anim Pract **16** (1975) 365.
76. Owens, JM *et al.* JAAHA **11** (1975) 83.
77. Schaer, M. JAAHA **15** (1979) 681.
78. Colles, CM. Vet Rec **96** (1975) 323.
79. Sheridon, V. Vet Rec **96** (1975) 229.
80. Everett, RM *et al.* Am J Vet Res **38** (1977) 963.
81. Cornelius, CE and Kaneko, JJ. JAVMA **137** (1960) 62.
82. Nilkumhang, P and Thornton, JR. J Sm Anim Pract **20** (1979) 169.
83. Hoffman, WE *et al.* Am J Vet Res **38** (1977) 1637.
84. Feldman, BF *et al.* Feline Pract **6(1)** (1976) 33.
85. Taylor, D and Perri, SF. Am J Vet Res **38** (1977) 51.
86. Hornbuckle and Allan, in Kirk: Current Veterinary Therapy VII. WB Saunders, Philadelphia, 1980.
87. Vulgamott, JC *et al.* JAAHA **16** (1980) 915.
88. Bostock, DE. J Sm Anim Pract **13** (1972) 119.
89. Kelly, DF *et al.* J Sm Anim Pract **16** (1975) 163.
90. Suter, PF and Olsen, SE. J Am Vet Rad Soc **10** (1969) 4.

METAZOAL AND PROTOZOAL PARASITES OF THE ALIMENTARY SYSTEM by K.S. Todd, Jr. and A.J. Paul*

The following discussion concerns only endoparasites of the alimentary system that are found in North America. Parasites of other organs are discussed in the appropriate chapters. This information is intended to be of practical use to veterinary students and clinicians. Those who desire more detailed knowledge about parasites and parasitic diseases can refer to textbooks on veterinary parasitology.[1-9]

General Comments

Endoparasites are ubiquitous in nature, but their pathogenicity for their hosts varies and depends on many complex host-parasite interactions, including the species and number of par-

*The authors thank Anne E. Casassa and Edward V. McGinnis for their assistance with the literature.

asites present, the age and general health of the host, the organ or tissue infected, and whether or not the parasite is in its normal host. Endoparasites may injure the host in many ways, such as causing irritation, removing nutrients, ingesting blood, cells and tissue, producing stenosis, producing toxic substances, and causing hypersensitivity. These effects may lead to host reactions that result in loss of organ functions and reduce resistance to other infectious agents. Cats fed an adequate diet are much less susceptible to parasitic diseases than those that are malnourished or fed a marginal diet.

Depending on the conditions just listed, clinical manifestations of parasitic infections may range from undetectible to severe. When compared with diseases caused by other infectious agents, metazoal and protozoal parasitisms often are slower in producing clinical signs.

Types of Internal Parasitisms

Two types of internal parasites infect cats: single-celled organisms (Protozoa) and multicellular organisms (Metazoa). The latter include Trematoda (flukes), Cestoda (tapeworms) and Nematoda (roundworms). The life cycles vary, depending on the species of parasite. Their reproduction may be sexual and/or asexual, and the life cycle may be direct or indirect.

With direct life cycles, only one host is involved; in indirect life cycles, one or more intermediate hosts and a definitive host are required to complete the cycle. Transport hosts may be present in both direct and indirect life cycles. In general, transmission of parasites with a direct life cycle is by the definitive host's ingestion of infective stages of the parasite or by penetration of the host's skin by infective larvae. Parasites with an indirect life cycle may infect the definitive host when the intermediate host is ingested or when infective stages of the parasite are introduced into the definitive host's body while the intermediate host is sucking blood.

Some endoparasites of cats can be transmitted by vectors. Mechanical vectors are objects that transmit the parasite by carrying the infectious agent to the host. Biologic vectors are living organisms in which the parasite multiplies.

All flatworms (Platyhelminthes) that infect cats have an indirect life cycle. Snails serve as intermediate hosts for trematodes; some trematodes have a second intermediate host that may be either a vertebrate or invertebrate animal. All tapeworms have intermediate hosts that are either vertebrates or invertebrates. The nematodes are a diverse group that includes many parasitic and free-living species with direct and indirect life cycles.

Immunity

The antigenic characteristics of parasitic protozoa and metazoa usually are more complex than those of viruses and bacteria. Although immunity to protozoan and metazoan parasites may result in a response similar to that to other infectious agents, the mechanisms often are not as well understood and the host's response may be different. The immunologic responses to protozoan and metazoan parasites usually involve both a humoral antibody response and a cell-mediated response. A comprehensive review of parasite immunology has been published.[10]

Host specificity also is important in determining resistance to parasites. Animals may be naturally resistant to certain organisms because of their genetic properties, as well as those of the parasite. Some parasites are restricted to a narrow range of hosts or to a single host and experimental infection of abnormal hosts is not possible. Other parasites have a wide range of natural hosts and an even broader range of hosts can be established artificially. Another group of parasites has a narrow host range and is rarely found under natural conditions; artificial infections may be established, however, in experimental hosts.

In general, older animals are more resistant to parasitic infections than younger ones. Although this may be the result of prior infections that have produced immunity, physiologic factors and changes that result in different feeding and behavioral patterns may also influence resistance in older animals. Some evidence indicates that young animals of certain species may derive immunity to certain protozoal and metazoal parasites from colostrum.

Although animals may be protected from further parasitic infections by active immunity produced by prior infections, the degree of immunity varies. It can be affected by such factors as genetics, age, stress and presence of other parasitic species and other infectious agents that may exacerbate disease. Nutrition plays an important role in development of immunity.

Prevention and Control

Proper sanitation and preventing contact with intermediate hosts, transport hosts and vectors can minimize or eliminate most endoparasitic diseases. Because most endoparasites are transmitted through feces containing infective eggs or cysts, prompt removal of feces and thorough cleaning of litter pans are essential in controlling parasites. Most eggs and cysts require some time after passing in the feces before they become infective. For some parasites this is about 2 days under ideal temperature and moisture conditions. Therefore, feces should be removed and litter pans cleaned daily.

The survival times of eggs, cysts and larvae that are infective to cats vary and depend on several factors. Some parasites are better adapted to survive adverse environmental conditions because the infective stages are highy resistant to extreme temperatures, drying and sunlight. Others are extremely sensitive to these same environmental factors. The eggs and cysts of some parasites are not affected by any of the commonly used disinfectants. Cats kept indoors are not exposed to most of the intermediate and transport hosts and vectors as frequently as unconfined cats. Unconfined cats also have a greater chance of contacting infective parasite eggs and cysts. Control of fleas prevents infection by one of the common tapeworms (*Dipylidium caninum*) that infects cats.

A few parasites (*eg, Toxoplasma gondii, Sarcocystis* spp) can be transmitted by feeding cats raw or undercooked meat. To avoid transmission of these parasites, all meat fed to cats should be cooked thoroughly.

Any cat to be added to a cattery or home should first be examined for parasitic and other diseases, and any infected animal properly isolated and treated. Kittens' feces should be examined as soon as a specimen can be collected and again about 3-4 weeks after treatment for parasites.

Hazards to Human Health

Cats and other pets often are maligned as the source of parasites that infect people. Although there is a long list of parasites that are shared by people and domestic animals, many examples are based on a single case report, and little information has been acquired about prevalence and pathogenicity.[11] The fallacy still persists that cats and dogs can be sources of pinworm infections for children. Cats and dogs do not have pinworms.

Several endoparasites can be transmitted from cats to people. Although *Dipylidium caninum,* a common cestode of dogs and cats, can be transmitted to people, the incidence of infection is low. Children are most commonly infected. The parasite is transmitted when a child ingests fleas containing infective larvae or kisses dogs that have infective larvae on their lips after chewing infected fleas.

Visceral larva migrans in people is caused primarily by *Toxocara canis.*[12] Other species of ascarids may be involved in this disease.[13] This condition should not be confused with cutaneous larva migrans, which is caused by migrating hookworm larvae. Visceral larva migrans usually is caused by infective larvae of *Toxocara canis* migrating through somatic tissues of abnormal hosts, including people. The migrating larvae are found in granulomatous lesions, often in the liver, lungs or eyes. This disease is most common in young children with a history of pica and close association with dogs.

Dogs and cats infected with *Strongyloides stercoralis* are reportedly sources of this infection in people. Their importance as a source of human infections is not clearly understood.

Research has implicated cats as a source of *Toxoplasma gondii* infections in people and other animals. The importance of cats in the epidemiology of this parasite will be discussed later.

Clinical Examination

Signs of internal parasitism may be vague and easily confused with those of other diseases. Emaciation, diarrhea, alternate diarrhea and constipation, rough haircoat, edema, ascites, vomiting, eosinophilia, abdominal discomfort, coughing, dyspnea, anemia and other signs indicate the possible presence of endoparasites. Laboratory procedures usually are needed, however, to confirm a tentative diagnosis.

Detection of parasites of the GI tract usually requires fecal examination. Because some helminth eggs may embryonate and hatch in a short time, fresh feces should be examined.

The feces should be inspected grossly to determine if intact specimens or fragments of helminths are present. Tapeworm proglottids usually are passed intact and can be identified without microscopic examination; proglottids may also be found in the perianal region. Pet owners occasionally present material found in the animal's bedding for identification, including dehydrated tapeworm proglottids (Fig 16). When placed in water, they are rehydrated and resemble the fresh proglottids found in feces or in the perianal region (Fig 17).

Feces should also be examined microscopically for parasite eggs or cysts. Examining a fecal smear is the simplest method. This is often not reliable, however, because of the small quantity of feces examined. When a few eggs or cysts are present, they may not be detected in a smear. The smear technic is useful when searching for motile forms of intestinal protozoa. Gastrointestinal protozoa, other than coccidia, are rarely found in cats, however, and fecal smears are not routinely prepared. Concentration technics are used to detect coccidial oocysts.

Because of the high incidence of parasites in young cats, their feces should be examined when they are given their first physical examination or earlier. The number of parasite eggs or cysts found by fecal examination often is not indicative of the number of adult parasites present or their pathogenic effects. Some species of parasites produce large numbers of eggs or cysts, and others relatively few; some have intermittent periods of egg or cyst production. The pathogenicity of some parasites is caused by immature stages when eggs or cysts are not produced.

Concentration methods should be used routinely to confirm a tentative diagnosis of parasitism. Detection of parasites and their products by flotation technics involves placing feces in a solution with a high specific gravity. Many solutions have been used for this purpose; each has certain advantages and disadvantages. The most common flotation solutions are:

1. NaCl solution: NaCl is added to water in excess of that which dissolves to produce a saturated solution.
2. Sodium nitrate solution: sodium nitrate is added to water in excess of that which dissolves to produce a saturated solution.
3. Zinc sulfate solution: composed of 331g $ZnSO_4 \cdot 7\ H_2O$ in 1 L H_2O.
4. Magnesium sulfate solution: composed of 350 g $MgSO_4 \cdot 7\ H_2O$ in 1 L water.
5. Sucrose (Sheather's) solution: composed of 500 g sucrose (granulated sugar) and 6.5 g (5 ml) melted phenol in 320 ml H_2O. This is heated until the sugar is in solution.

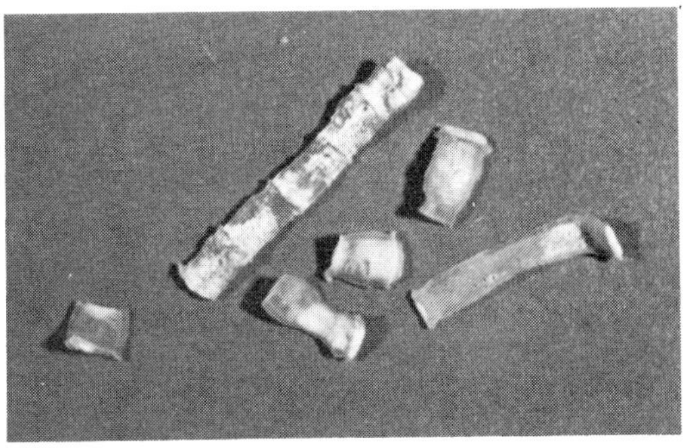

Fig 16. Dehydrated tapeworm segments of *Taenia* spp.

The concentrated salt solutions have a low viscosity and enable a more rapid examination of samples than Sheather's solution. Because salt solutions dry rapidly, the preparations must be examined within a short time or the parasite eggs or cysts may become desiccated and unidentifiable.

Although feces is best examined shortly after it is eliminated, this is often impractical. If samples must be stored for a short time, they should be placed in fully-filled, air-tight containers and preferably refrigerated. This inhibits embryonation and hatching of helminth eggs. If the sam-

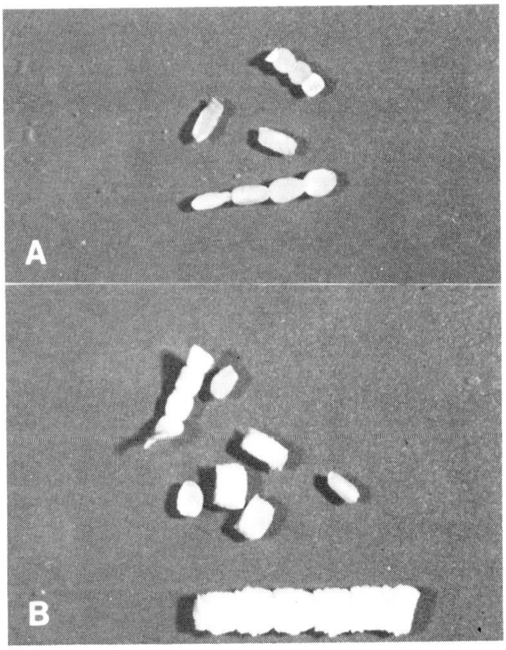

Fig 17. Proglottids of *Dipylidium caninum* (A) and *Taenia* spp (B).

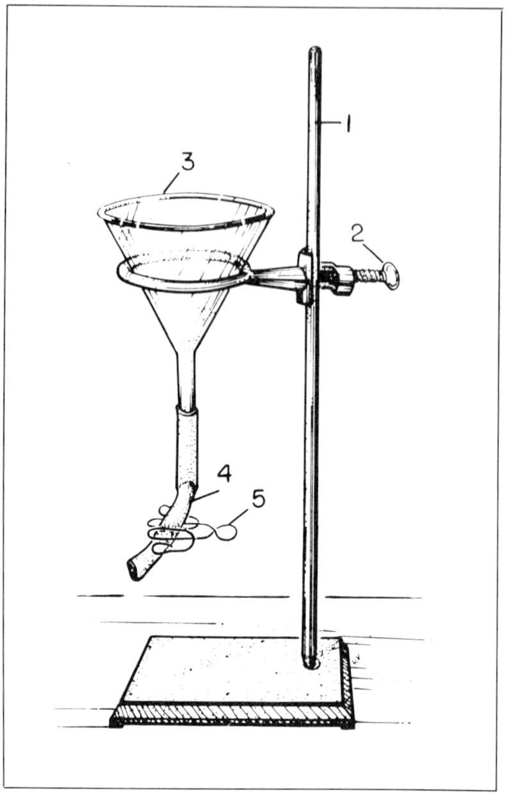

Fig 18. Modified Baermann apparatus: stand (1), support ring (2), funnel (3), rubber tubing (4) and pinch clamp (5).

ples cannot be examined within 2-3 days, they should be placed in 10-15 volumes of 2.5% potassium dichromate solution or in 10% formalin solution.

The method for preparing fecal samples for flotation depends on the equipment available and individual needs. The following methods give good results and can be adapted to suit various circumstances.

One procedure involves (1) placing a sieve (a small tea strainer works well) in a small bowl and putting 5-10 g feces in the sieve, (2) adding about 30 ml water and mixing well with a tongue depressor or spatula so the eggs and feces pass through the strainer, (3) removing the sieve, stirring the suspension and transferring enough to fill a 15-ml centrifuge tube, (4) centrifuging at about 1500 rpm for about 3 minutes, (5) pouring off the supernatant fluid and nearly filling the tube with a flotation solution, (6) mixing the fecal sediment and solution with a wooden applicator stick or small glass rod, (7) placing the tube in a centrifuge and adding flotation solution until the level is slightly above the rim of the tube (a plastic wash bottle is suitable for this), (8) placing a coverslip on the tube and allowing the tube to stand for a few minutes until the coverslip is firmly fixed to it and then centrifuging at 1500 rpm for 3-5 minutes, and (9) removing the coverslip and placing it on a glass slide for examination.

An alternate method that gives equally good results and does not require centrifugation involves (1) performing steps 1 through 3 except using a flotation solution instead of water, (2) placing the tube in a support so it remains vertical and adding flotation solution until its level is slightly above the rim of the tube, (3) placing a coverslip on the tube and allowing it to stand for at least an hour if Sheather's solution is used or for 10 minutes if a concentrated salt solution is used (shorter periods give less reliable results), and (4) removing the coverslip and placing it on a glass slide for examination.

The modified Baermann technic can be used to detect *Strongyloides stercoralis* and *Aelurostrongylus abstrusus* larvae in feces. A small funnel, with a short piece of rubber tubing attached to the end, is placed in a rack (Fig 18). The rubber tubing is closed with a clamp, and the apparatus is filled almost to the top with tap water at a temperature of about 20 C (68 F). From 2-5 g feces are wrapped in porous paper, such as Kimwipes, and placed in the funnel. After the preparation stands for 2-3 hours, about 10 ml fluid are collected from the bottom of the rubber tube by releasing the clamp. The sample should be placed in a small petri dish and examined with a dissecting microscope or low-power objective of a compound microscope. It is essential that fresh fecal samples be used because some parasites pass embryonated or unembryonated eggs from which larvae may hatch in a short time. Difficulty may arise in differentiating these larvae from those of *S stercoralis* and *A abstrusus*.

Vomitus may contain adult parasites of the stomach or upper small intestine. Because of the quantity of mucus present, examination of vomitus by concentration methods is ineffective in detecting parasite eggs or cysts.

Several books contain photomicrographs of the parasite eggs and cysts found in cats.[3,14-16]

Parasites of the Stomach

Nematodes of the genera *Physaloptera* and *Ollulanus* are the only parasites that are usually in the stomachs of cats in North America. *Toxocara mystax* and *Toxascaris leonina* are rarely found there. *Ollulanus tricuspis* is of interest because of its life cycle, but it often has little clinical importance. *Physaloptera* infections are not common in cats, but because of their size and shape, they often are confused with intestinal ascarids.

Ollulanus tricuspis

This trichostrongylid has recently been receiving attention in cats in North America.[17,18] It is more common in cats in Australia and has also been reported in the cat, lion, red fox and pig in Europe.[6,19]

Source of Infection: Infections can be experimentally transmitted by feeding stomach contents or vomitus from infected cats. This may be the normal method of transmission.[20]

Life Cycle: The life cycle of this parasite is unusual in that the females produce third-stage larvae that develop to adults in the stomach.[20] Animals evidently become infected after eating vomitus.

Pathogenesis: The parasite usually is not considered to be highly pathogenic for cats, but it may cause weight loss, gastric irritation and vomiting.[17,18]

Diagnosis: Adults or larvae may be found in vomitus or stomach washings.

Control: Although there is no known treatment, control of this parasite probably can be accomplished by sanitation and preventing ingestion of vomitus from infected cats.

Physaloptera

Three species of *Physaloptera* are found in cats in North America. *Physaloptera praeputialis* is found in the stomach, and *P rara* and *P felidis* in both the stomach and small intestine. Because of their size and shape, these nematodes can be confused with ascarids found in cats (Fig 19).

Source of Infection: The intermediate hosts of *P rara* are cockroaches (*Blatella germanica*), crickets (*Gryllus assimilis*), flour beetles (*Tribolium confusum*) and ground beetles (*Harpalus* spp).[21-22] Intermediate hosts of *P praeputialis* are cockroaches (*B germanica*) and crickets (*G assimilus* and *Centophilus* spp).[22] The intermediate hosts of *P felidis* are unknown but probably are other orthopteran or coleopteran insects.

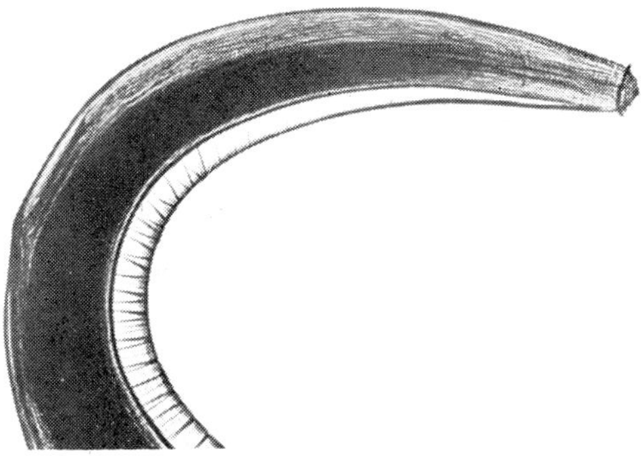

Fig 19. Cranial end of *Physaloptera rara.* (Courtesy of Dr S.M. Gaafar)

Life Cycle: Embryonated eggs are passed in the feces and development to the infective stage occurs after the eggs are ingested by a suitable intermediate host. The eggs of *P praeputialis* may survive 30-40 days at room temperature and up to 60 days at 4 C.[23] The prepatent period of *P rara* is 56-83 days.[21,22]

Pathogenesis: Physaloptera spp attach to the gastric mucosa and feed mostly on blood. They cause erosions and subsequent gastritis, enteritis and increased mucus secretion at the site of attachment.[6]

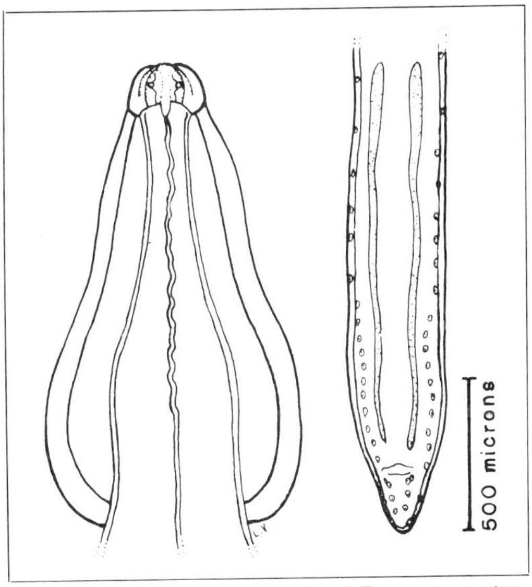

Fig 20. Cranial and caudal ends of *Toxocara mystax.* (Adapted from Morgan and Hawkins: *Veterinary Helminthology,* Burgess Publishing, Minneapolis, 1949)

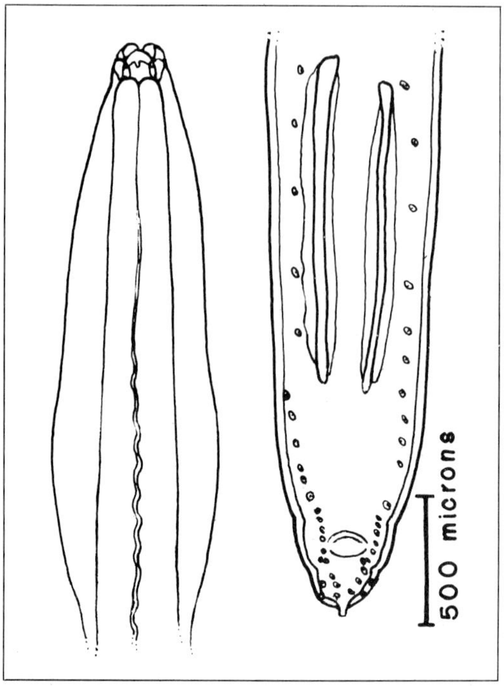

Fig 21. Cranial and caudal ends of *Toxocara canis*. (Adapted from Morgan and Hawkins: *Veterinary Helminthology*, Burgess Publishing, Minneapolis, 1949)

Clinical Signs: P felidis can cause catarrhal gastritis and vomiting, as well as weakness and loss of weight.[6]

Diagnosis: Embryonated eggs may be found in fecal samples. Adult and immature parasites may be present in vomitus from infected cats, but they must be differentiated from intestinal ascarids that may also be in vomitus. At necropsy, *Physaloptera* spp can resemble ascarids; however, ascarids usually are free in the lumen of the intestine or stomach, whereas *Physaloptera* spp usually are attached to the gastric or duodenal mucosa.

Control: There is no known treatment, but infections can be prevented by isolating cats from the intermediate hosts.

Parasites of the Intestine

Ascarids

Three species of ascarids, *Toxocara mystax* (synonym, *Toxocara cati*), *Toxascaris leonina* and *Toxocara canis,* infect the small intestines of cats. They are probably the most common parasites of cats and may also be the most pathogenic. *Toxocara canis* and *T leonina* are also common parasites of dogs and other carnivores. Adult parasites are distinguished by the shape of their cranial and caudal ends (Figs 20-22).

Source of Infection: All 3 species may have a direct life cycle in which infective eggs are ingested. In addition, several species of animals can be transport hosts.[6]

Life Cycle: Unembryonated eggs are passed in the feces. With suitable moisture and temperature, the eggs embryonate and infective larvae are produced; at 25 C the eggs are infective after 9-15 days. At lower temperatures, embryonation requires more time. The eggs do not hatch until ingested.

The life cycles of all 3 species are different. Although the life cycle of *T canis* has not been studied in cats, its life cycle has been well documented in dogs.[6] The following description is based on its life cycle in canine hosts. When eggs are ingested by a susceptible puppy, the larvae hatch in the duodenum, penetrate the intestinal wall and migrate to the liver via the portal circulation. After migration in the liver, they enter the right side of the heart through the venous circulation and reach the capillary beds of the lungs. While in the lungs, the larvae enter al-

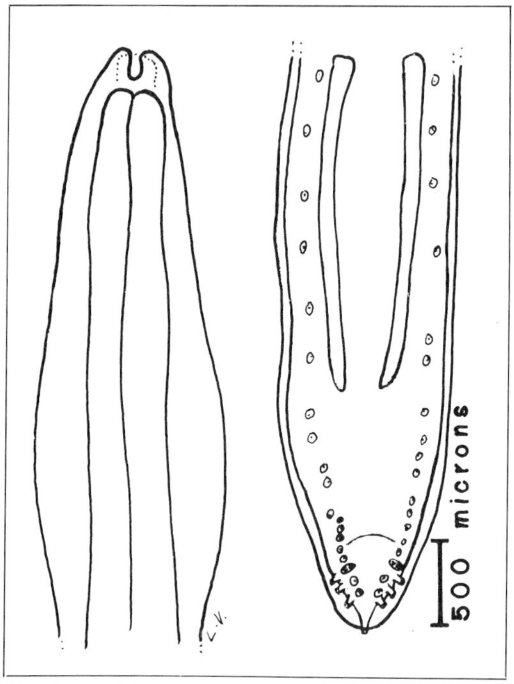

Fig 22. Cranial and caudal ends of *Toxascaris leonina*. (Adapted from Morgan and Hawkins: *Veterinary Helminthology*, Burgess Publishing, Minneapolis, 1949)

veolar lumina, pass up the bronchioles and enter the trachea. After they reach the trachea, the larvae are coughed up and pass via the esophagus to the stomach, where they undergo further development. They then migrate to the small intestine, where they become adults.

Somatic migration of the larvae in bitches and prenatal infection of puppies have been well documented, but nothing is known about this type of life cycle in cats. Many species of animals, including people, may serve as transport hosts for *T canis*. In foreign hosts, the larvae do not develop to adults but remain as second-stage larvae. When a proper definitive host ingests an infected transport host, the larvae are released by digestion and develop to adults in the small intestine.[24]

The life cycle of *T mystax* has been studied in detail.[25-29] If a cat ingests eggs containing infective larvae, the larvae hatch from the eggs and enter the wall of the stomach, from which they migrate to the lungs via the liver. After passing up the trachea, the larvae are swallowed and reenter the stomach wall or burrow into the wall of the small intestine. After a period of development, the larvae return to the lumen of the small intestine, where they develop to adults.

Many species of animals, including mice, can serve as transport hosts. In such animals, infective eggs hatch in the small intestine and migrate to various organs, where they remain alive for several months. When an infected animal is ingested by a cat, the larvae are freed by digestion. Most larvae stay in the digestive tract and develop to adults rather than undergoing tracheal migration. Prenatal infections apparently do not occur but transmammary passage does.[28]

The life cycle of *Toxascaris leonina* has been documented.[29,30] There usually is no larval migration through the lungs and prenatal infections do not occur. After eggs containing infective larvae are ingested, the larvae hatch in the small intestine. They enter the wall of the small intestine and, after a period of development, return to the lumen and become adults. During heavy infections, larvae may migrate to other organs, including the lungs and liver. If the larvae reach the lungs, they may migrate up the trachea, are swallowed and reach the small intestine, where they develop to adults.[29]

Mice may serve as transport hosts for *Toxocara* spp.[25,26] When mice ingest infective eggs, the larvae hatch and migrate to various tissues, where they become encysted. When an infected mouse is ingested, the larvae, released by digestion of surrounding tissues, enter the intestine and develop to adults. The results of one study suggest that cats cannot be infected with eggs of the canine strain of *T leonina*.[30]

Pathogenesis: The pathogenesis of *T canis* in cats is unknown. In dogs larvae migrating through the lungs can cause fatal pneumonia if large numbers are present. Migrating larvae may enter the CNS and cause various disorders. Epileptiform seizures in dogs and cats have been attributed to *T canis* infections.[6]

Larval migration of *T mystax* probably causes most damage when kittens ingest large numbers of eggs containing infective larvae and the larvae migrate through the lungs and liver. Although extensive liver lesions have not been described, experimentally infected kittens may develop medial hyperplasia of the pulmonary arteries identical to that in naturally infected cats.[31] The affected arteries were decreased in diameter and occasionally obliterated.

Because *T leonina* larvae usually do not migrate through the liver or lungs and prenatal infections do not occur, the lesions are confined to the GI tract.

All 3 species can cause digestive disturbances, depending on the severity of the infection.

Diagnosis: Eggs are present in the feces; those of *Toxocara* and *Toxascaris* can be readily differentiated (Fig 23). The eggs of *T canis* resemble those of *T mystax* but the 2 species can be differentiated on the basis of egg size. Eggs of *T canis* are about 85-90 by 75 μ; those of *T mystax* are about 65-75 μ in diameter. The eggs of *T leonina* have a smooth or pitted wall that is thinner than those of the other 2 ascarid species. The egg walls of *T canis* and *T mystax* are rough and thick, and have a darker border than those of *T leonina*. Adults of the 3 species found in vomitus or at necropsy can be differentiated on the basis of size and shape of the cervical alae on the cranial end (Figs 20-22).

Clinical Signs: Gastrointestinal disturbances and loss of condition are common in young cats with heavy intestinal infections. Emaciation, abdominal distention, anemia and listlessness may be apparent. Migrating larvae in the lungs and liver can cause clinical signs related to disease in these organs.

Treatment: Piperazine compounds given at 100 mg/kg (45 mg/lb) have been considered the

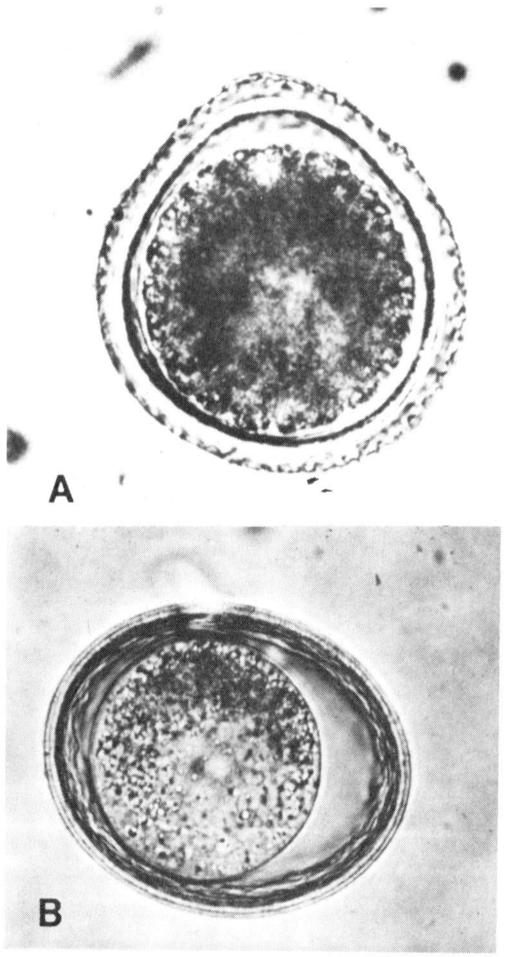

Fig 23. Eggs of *Toxocara* spp (A) and *Toxascaris leonina* (B).

drugs of choice for treatment of ascarids in cats.[32,33] These compounds may be given with or without food.

Dichlorvos (Task Tabs:Squibb), at 11 mg/kg (5 mg/lb), is effective. Pretreatment fasting is not necessary, although feeding simultaneously with treatment may tend to hold the drug in the stomach and reduce its effectiveness in the intestine. Animals under 10 days of age or weighing less than 1 lb should not be treated with Task Tabs.

Diethylcarbamazine, at 55 mg/kg (25 mg/lb), is also effective in removing ascarids. After fasting the animal for 18-24 hours before treatment, administration of the drug resulted in removal of 98% of the ascarids from 11 cats.[34]

Dithiazanine, at 10 mg/kg (4.5 mg/lb) for 4-7 days, has been effective in removing ascarids from cats.[35] Both diethylcarbamazine and dithiazanine may cause vomiting in cats, especially if given when the stomach is empty.

Another effective ascaricide is toluene. When this drug was given at 0.22 ml/kg (0.1 ml/lb), 99% of the ascarids were removed from 25 cats.[36]

None of the compounds mentioned is evidently effective against ascarid larvae during their migration or encystment. Another treatment 2-3 weeks later may be advisable, depending on the age of the animals, whether or not they have had access to transport hosts and the sanitary conditions in the cat's environment.

Control: Good sanitation and preventing contact with intermediate hosts are important in the control of ascarids. This is difficult with unconfined cats. Ascarid eggs are resistant to all of the common disinfectants and also to adverse environmental conditions. Frequent disposal of feces prevents cats and transport hosts from becoming infected. Treatment of queens before breeding and of kittens before the prepatent period aids in preventing eggs from becoming a source of further infections.

Hookworms

Ancylostoma braziliense, A caninum, A tubaeforme and *Uncinaria stenocephala* have been found in cats, but there has only been one report of *A caninum* in cats in North America.[37] *Ancylostoma tubaeforme* is by far the most common. *Uncinaria stenocephala* occurs rarely in cats, although they may serve as accidental hosts.[38] One author considered that the form common in cats and dogs along the Gulf Coast of the US in all probability was *A braziliense*.[6] The following discussion is limited to infections by *A tubaeforme* and *A braziliense*.

Source of Infection: Infective larvae of *A tubaeforme* and *A braziliense* may evidently penetrate the skin or be ingested. Mice are possible transport hosts of *A tubaeforme*.[39]

Life Cycle: The life cycle in cats experimentally infected with *A braziliense* has not been adequately described, but it is likely similar to that of *A caninum* in dogs, which has been well documented.[6] Eggs passed in the feces of infected animals require a favorable temperature and moisture to develop to first-stage larvae. These larvae hatch in 10-12 hours at 30 C, and in 9 hours at 37 C.[40] They feed on bacteria in feces and, after 2 molts, develop to the infective stage (third-stage larvae). Infective larvae may be found in feces 58-66 hours after its elimination when the ambient temperature is 30 C, or in 47 hours when it is 37 C.[40] The infective larvae leave the feces and move onto vegetation.

Larvae may enter a host's body by penetrating the skin or by oral ingestion. After they penetrate the skin, they burrow into blood or lymph vessels, pass to the right side of the heart and enter the lungs. In the lungs, the larvae reach the alveoli and pass up the air spaces of the respiratory tract to the pharynx, where they are swallowed. The larvae move to the small intestine, where they develop to adults.

When larvae are ingested, they may penetrate the intestinal wall and pass in blood vessels to the lungs and back to the intestine. However, most enter gastric gland crypts or crypts of Lieberkühn for a period and then re-enter the lumen to become adults in the small intestine.

The life cycle of *A tubaeforme* has been studied in experimentally infected cats.[41] It is similar to that of *A caninum* in dogs, with infection occurring after cutaneous penetration or ingestion of larvae. Cats were found to be unfavorable hosts of *A caninum* obtained from dogs. They could be more easily infected after 1-2 passages of hookworm in cats.[41]

Prenatal infections of puppies with *A caninum* have been described.[42,43] Infective larvae have been found in colostrum;[44] indeed, transcolostral infections are more common than prenatal ones.[45]

Pathogenesis: Penetration of larvae through the skin may cause a localized dermatitis, but this is not common in naturally acquired infections. Hookworm larvae rarely cause pulmonary lesions during their migration, but such lesions may be found in heavy infections following skin penetration.[6]

Hookworms usually cause their greatest damage by removing blood. When feeding, the adults attach to the intestinal mucosa and erode the surface to start blood flow. They suck blood and frequently move to new sites for feeding. Blood loss is due not only to the parasite's ingestion of blood, but also because the parasites produce an anticoagulant that prevents clotting at the former sites of feeding. The blood loss caused by *A braziliense* in experimentally infected cats is evidently insignificant; clinical signs of parasitism were not observed in kittens harboring 600-800 adult helminths.[46] The pathogensis of *A tubaeforme* in experimentally infected kittens has not been adequately studied.

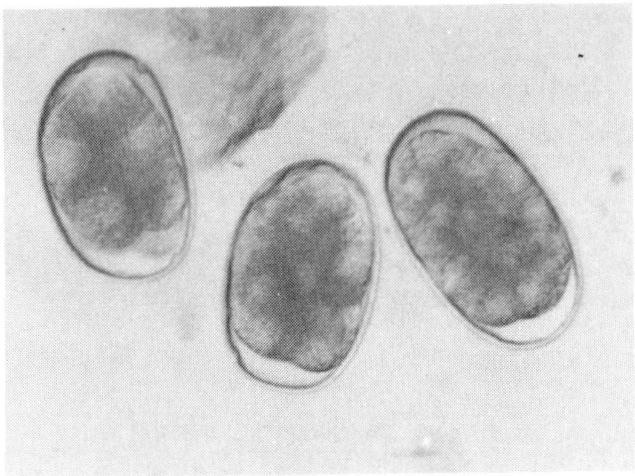

Fig 24. Unembryonated eggs of feline hookworms.

Clinical Signs: Cats with hookworms may have a microcytic hypochromic anemia, appear emaciated and have a rough haircoat.[6] Feces from cats heavily infected with hookworms is often black, and has a tarry consistency and a characteristic putrid odor.

Diagnosis: A presumptive diagnosis of hookworm infection can be confirmed by fecal examination. Because the eggs embryonate and the larvae hatch rapidly at high temperatures, fresh feces should be examined. Unembryonated eggs are shown in Figure 24.

Treatment: Dichlorvos (Task Tabs:Squibb) should be given PO at 11.0 mg/kg (5 mg/lb). Animals under 10 days of age or weighing less than 1 lb should not be treated. Toluene, at 0.22 ml/kg (0.1 ml/lb), has been reported to be 100% effective in removing hookworms from cats.[36] Tetrachloroethylene also is effective in removing hookworms if given at 0.22 ml/kg (0.1 ml/lb).[47] Disophenol injected SC at 9.9 mg/kg (4.5 ml/lb) is effective.

Use of piperazine compounds is not recommended.

A second treatment may be indicated 14-21 days after the first treatment.

Control: Ancylostoma larvae are not resistant to sunlight or drying. By removing feces and cleaning litter pans daily, the main sources of infection can be eliminated. Although it has not been determined whether larvae of *A braziliense* and *A tubaeforme* are transmitted to kittens in colostrum, prebreeding treatment of queens harboring adult hookworms would help prevent such transmission.

Other Intestinal Nematodes

Trichuris campanula

The whipworm, *Trichuris campanula,* has been found in the cecum and colon of cats in various parts of the world, but is rare in the US.[6,48,49] Other species of *Trichuris* have been found in cats but their taxonomic status is uncertain. One author stated that many reports of whipworms in cats were inaccurate because the eggs observed were those of *Capillaria* spp.[50]

Nothing is known about their life cycle, pathogenicity or treatment.

Strongyloides

The taxonomic status of *Strongyloides* species in cats is unclear. Some authors consider *S cati* and *S felis* to be valid species in cats, while others consider them to be the same as *Strongyloides stercoralis. Strongyloides tumefaciens* has also been found in cats in North America and elsewhere.

The following discussion is concerned only with *S stercoralis.* This nematode has been found in the small intestine of cats, dogs, people and other mammals. It can be a serious pathogen in people, and cats and dogs have been considered a source of infection in people.[6] Human infections with *S stercoralis* are rare in the US and are not common in other hosts. Larvae of *S stercoralis* are present in recently passed feces and usually detected by the Baermann technic. If infections with *S stercoralis* are suspected, larvae or fecal samples in 10-15 volumes of 10% formalin or 70% ethanol should be sent to a diagnostic laboratory for identification.

Thiabendazole, given PO at 125 mg daily for 3 days, was effective in clearing *S tumefaciens* from a 1.7-kg cat.[51]

Cestodes

The most common species of tapeworms in cats are *Dipylidium caninum* and *Hydatigera taeniaeformis* (*Taenia taeniaeformis*). *Dipylidium caninum* has fleas as the intermediate hosts and may be found in cats that never leave a human dwelling and also in feral cats. The intermediate hosts of *H taeniaeformis* are rodents, usually mice and rats; consequently, it is more common in free-ranging cats than in those confined. Cats may become infected with *Dibothriocephalus latus* (*Diphyllobothrium latum*) or *Spirometra mansonoides* by ingesting fish or lower vertebrates containing larval stages. Animals that ingest rabbit viscera may become infected with a common dog tapeworm, *Taenia pisiformis.* Cats have been stated to be definitive hosts of *Echinococcus granulosus,* but I have been unable to find any reports in which the cat was confirmed as the definitive host. *Mesocestoides* spp have been found in cats in various parts of the world.

Source of Infection: Cats become infected by eating intermediate hosts containing infective larvae. The intermediate hosts for feline tapeworms are as follows: *Dipylidium caninum:* dog flea (*Ctenocephalides canis*), cat flea (*Ctenocephalides felis*), human flea (*Pulex irritans*) and dog louse (*Trichodectes canis*); *T pisiformis:* rabbits; H taeniaeformis: rodents (usually rats and mice); *S mansonoides:* various vertebrates including frogs and snakes; and *D latus:* several species of fresh-water fish.

Life Cycle of D caninum: Gravid proglottids or egg capsules are passed in the host's feces. For further development, eggs must be ingested by a larval flea or biting louse. The oncosphere is liberated after ingestion and burrows through the gut wall of the intermediate host. In the adult flea or louse, the oncosphere develops to a cysticercoid, which is the infective stage. Cats are infected by ingesting an intermediate host containing a cysticercoid. The cysticercoid evaginates, attaches to the wall of the host's small intestine and develops into a mature tapeworm. The prepatent period is 3-4 weeks.[52]

Life Cycle of T pisiformis and taeniaeformis: Eggs are passed from the host's body in gravid proglottids or occasionally they may be free in the feces. *Taenia pisiformis* eggs are then ingested by a suitable intermediate host, usually a rabbit. The oncospheres are liberated and migrate through the intestinal wall to a blood vessel and are carried to the liver. The larvae migrate through the liver, eventually reach the surface and enter the peritoneal cavity, where they form cysticerci. The definitive host becomes infected by ingesting the viscera of the intermediate host. The cyst is digested except for the scolex, which attaches to the intestinal wall and develops into a mature tapeworm.

The life cycle of *H taeniaeformis* is similar to that of *T pisiformis* except that rodents are the intermediate hosts. The larva, a strobilocercus, is encapsulated in the liver of the intermediate host. The prepatent period of both species is 3-4 weeks.

Life Cycle of D latus and S mansonoides: Eggs of these tapeworms are passed from gravid proglottids and are free in the feces. If the eggs reach water of a suitable temperature, they embryonate and release a ciliated embryo called a coracidium. For the life cycle to continue, the coracidium must be ingested by a copepod crustacean of the genus *Diaptomus* or *Cyclops*.[9] The embryo develops into a procercoid larva in the haemocoel of the copepod. The life cycle of *D latus* continues if infected copepods are ingested by a suitable species of fresh water fish; the procercoid is liberated in the fish's intestinal tract and burrows through the intestinal wall to the musculature, where a plerocercoid larva develops. If an infected fish is eaten by another fish, the plerocercoid burrows through the intestinal wall of the second fish and enters the musculature. The definitive host becomes infected by eating raw or undercooked fish containing plerocercoids. The scolex attaches to the intestinal wall and develops into an adult. Eggs are first passed in the feces 5-6 weeks after ingestion of the plerocercoid.[9]

The life cycle of *S mansonoides* is similar to that of *D latus* except that several different species of vertebrates may serve as the second intermediate host. In the US, the water snake, *Natrix*, is probably the most common second intermediate host.[53]

Pathogenesis: Unless large numbers are present, adult tapeworms in cats cause little harm.

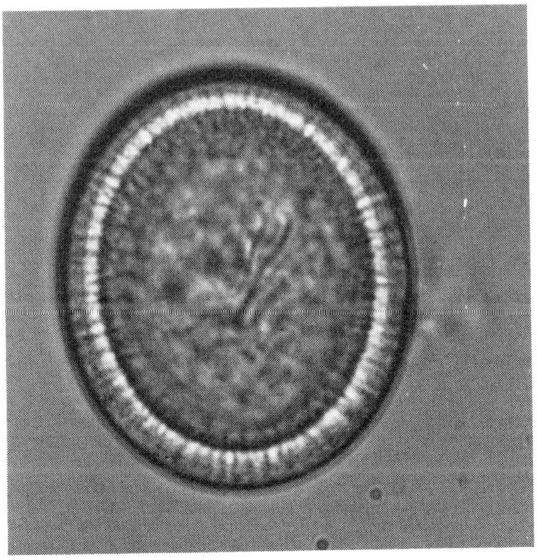

Fig 25. Egg of *Taenia* spp.

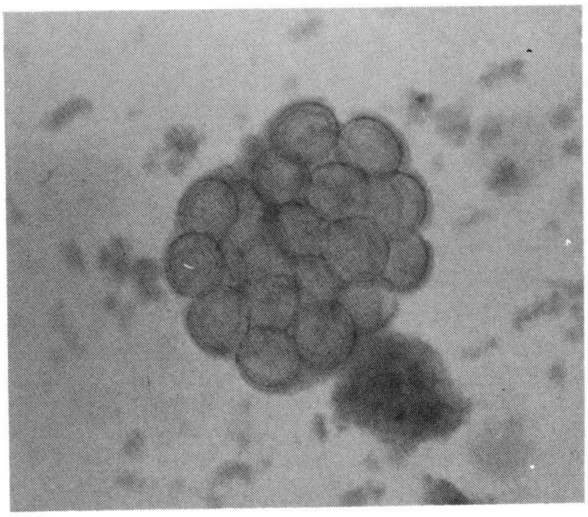

Fig 26. *Dipylidium caninum* egg packet.

It has been stated that tapeworm infection has caused convulsions in cats, but this needs verification.

Clinical Signs: The signs of tapeworm infection in cats are vague. Signs of chronic enteritis and abdominal discomfort, vomiting and diarrhea may occur with heavy infections. The proglottids of *T pisiformis, H taeniaeformis* and *D caninum* are motile when passed and may irritate the perianal region.

Diagnosis: Gravid proglottids of *T pisiformis, H taeniaeformis,* and *D caninum* are found in the perianal region, fecal samples or the animal's bedding (Figs 16, 17). Individual eggs of *T pisiformis* and *H taeniaeformis* and egg packets of *D caninum* occasionally are present in fecal flotations (Figs 25, 26). Eggs of *S mansonoides* and *D latus* are not passed inside gravid proglottids and can be found by fecal flotation (Figs 27, 28).

Treatment: Niclosamide (Yomesan:Haver-Lockhart) is highly effective when given PO at 154 mg/kg (70 mg/lb). An overnight fast is recommended before treatment. Another cesticide, bunamidine hydrochloride (Scolaban:Jen-Sal) is given at 25-50 mg/kg as a single oral dose. This drug is given after withholding food for 3-4 hours; the cat should be fed 3 hours after treatment. Drocarbil (Nemural:Winthrop) has been used to remove tapeworms from cats but is contraindicated in cats less than one year old.

Praziquantel (Droncit:Haver-Lockhart) is an effective cesticide that has recently been approved for use in cats. The tablets may be administered directly or crumbled and mixed with the feed. Fasting is neither necessary nor ad-

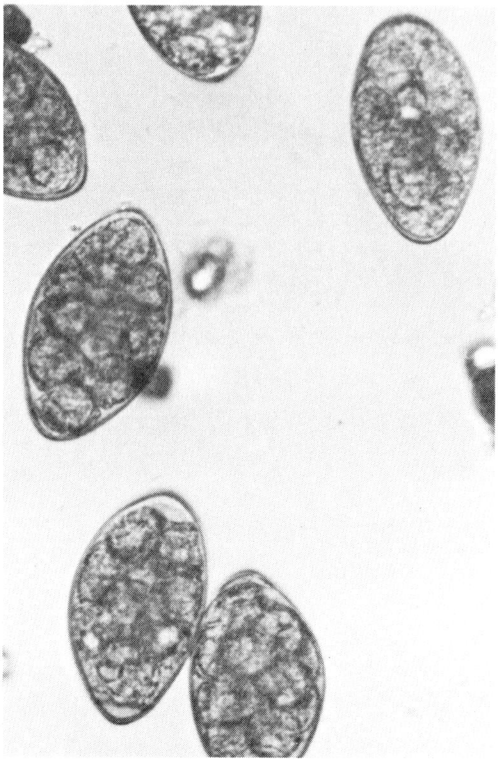

Fig 27. *Spirometra mansonoides* eggs. (Courtesy of Dr J.F. Mueller)

vised. The recommended dosage varies according to body weight. The drug should not be used in kittens less than 6 weeks of age.

Control: Tapeworm infections can be prevented by avoiding contact with intermediate hosts. In cats confined to houses, this is usually accomplished by eliminating fleas. Free-ranging cats may have access to infected vertebrate intermediate hosts. Raw or undercooked fish should not be fed to cats. Animals being added to a cattery should be examined for parasites and treated when indicated.

Trematodes

Trematodes, especially those found in the intestine, are rare in North American cats. All require more than one intermediate host in their life cycle. Little, if anything, is known about their pathogenesis, clinical signs and treatment. Because various species of cold-blooded vertebrates serve as second intermediate hosts, infections can be prevented by not feeding raw or undercooked fish to cats and by preventing them from eating wild vertebrates. The following intestinal trematodes infect cats in North America: *Cryptocotyle lingua, Nanophyetus salmincola, Platynosomum concinnum* and *Alaria marcianae*. Several other species of trematodes in North America have been experimentally transmitted to cats but their natural distribution is unknown.

Cryptocotyle lingua is commonly found in fish-eating birds. Natural infections occur in dogs and the parasite has been transmitted experimentally to cats.[54] The parasite has been found in naturally infected cats in Denmark;[55] its prevalence in cats in North America is unknown. It has been found in dogs in northern Canada.[56] The first intermediate host is the marine snail, *Littorina littorea*.[54] Several species of fish may be the second intermediate hosts.[9,57,58]

Nanophyetus salmincola (*Troglotrema salmincola*) is important because it is the vector of *Neorickettsia helmintheca,* the causative agent of salmon poisoning in dogs. Adult flukes are found in a large number of carnivores, including cats, in the Pacific Northwest region of the US.[59] The first intermediate host is a snail and the second intermediate host may be one of a large number of species of cold-blooded vertebrates, including fish of the salmon family.[60] Infection of the definitive host occurs when intermediate hosts containing metacercariae are ingested. The

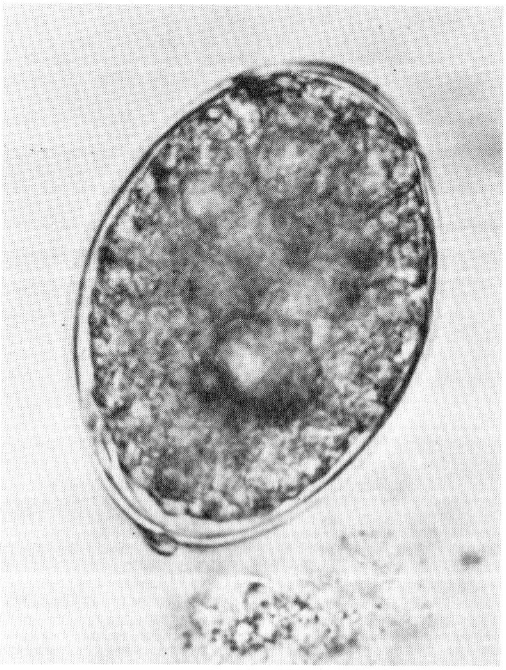

Fig 28. *Dibothriocephalus latus* egg.

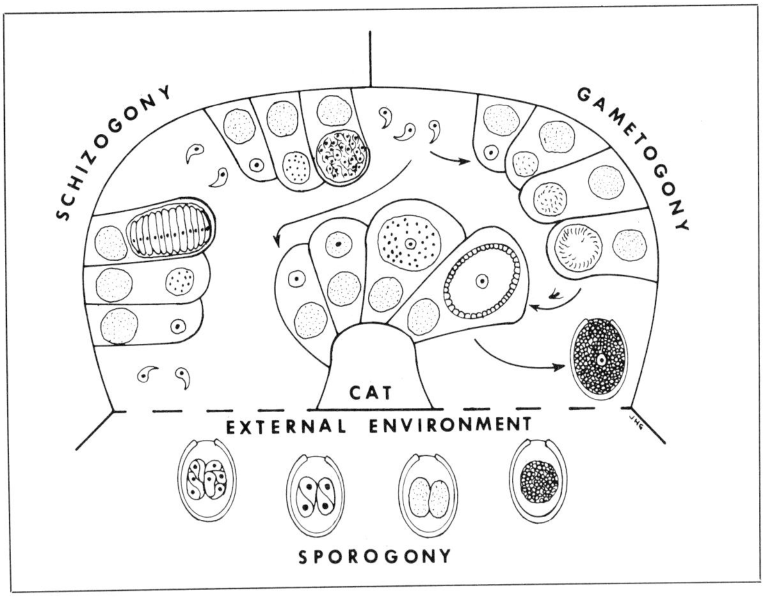

Fig 29. Diagram of the life cycle of isosporan species.

metacercariae develop to adults that become embedded in the mucosa of the small intestine.[61]

Alaria marcinae has been found in the intestine of cats and other carnivores.[58,62] Snails are the first intermediate host and tadpoles of the leopard frog, *Rana pipiens,* are the second intermediate hosts. Mice, rats and chickens may be transport hosts.

Protozoa

All protozoa that normally parasitize cats are found in the alimentary tract. *Toxoplasma gondii* also infects other organs (see Chapter 4).

Five species of *Eimeria* have been found in Felidae. However, no endogenous stages have been described for any of these species nor has experimental transmission been attempted. These may be pseudoparasites of cats.[63]

Until carefully controlled experiments were performed, it was assumed that the same species of *Isospora* infected dogs and cats. Because of negative cross-transmission experiments, it is now known that only *I felis* and *I rivolta* infect cats. *Toxoplasma gondii* and *"Hammondia"* species also produce isosporan oocysts in cats.

Source of Infection: Oocysts from infected cats are passed in the feces. In the presence of O_2, moisture and favorable temperature, they sporulate to an infective stage. Animals become infected by ingesting sporulated oocysts. Under experimental conditions some species of rodents and cattle have been transport hosts for *I felis* and *I rivolta.*[63]

Life Cycle: The *Isospora* species that infect cats are intestinal parasites that undergo intracellular development with both sexual and asexual stages. The life cycles of both species are similar.

After ingestion of a sporulated oocyst, excystation takes place in the small intestine and free-swimming sporozoites are released from the oocysts. The sporozoites enter intestinal epithelial cells and produce meronts (schizonts) containing merozoites. The meronts and host cells rupture and the motile merozoites enter other epithelial cells, where they develop into second-generation meronts. The number of generations depends on the species of coccidium. Merozoites from the last generation of meronts invade new cells and sexual development begins. Some merozoites produce macrogametes and others produce microgametocytes, within which motile microgametes develop. The microgametes leave the host cell and fertilize macrogametes to produce zygotes. A wall forms around each zygote, producing an oocyst that is passed in the feces. A generalized coccidian life cycle is shown in Figure 29. Extraintestinal stages of *I felis* and *I rivolta* have been reported.[63]

Pathogenesis: Coccidiosis usually is a disease of young animals. When the host's intestinal cells are ruptured, loss of the epithelium may result in hemorrhage and anemia. There may be signs of catarrhal enteritis. Many lesions associated with coccidiosis probably are caused by secondary bacterial infection.

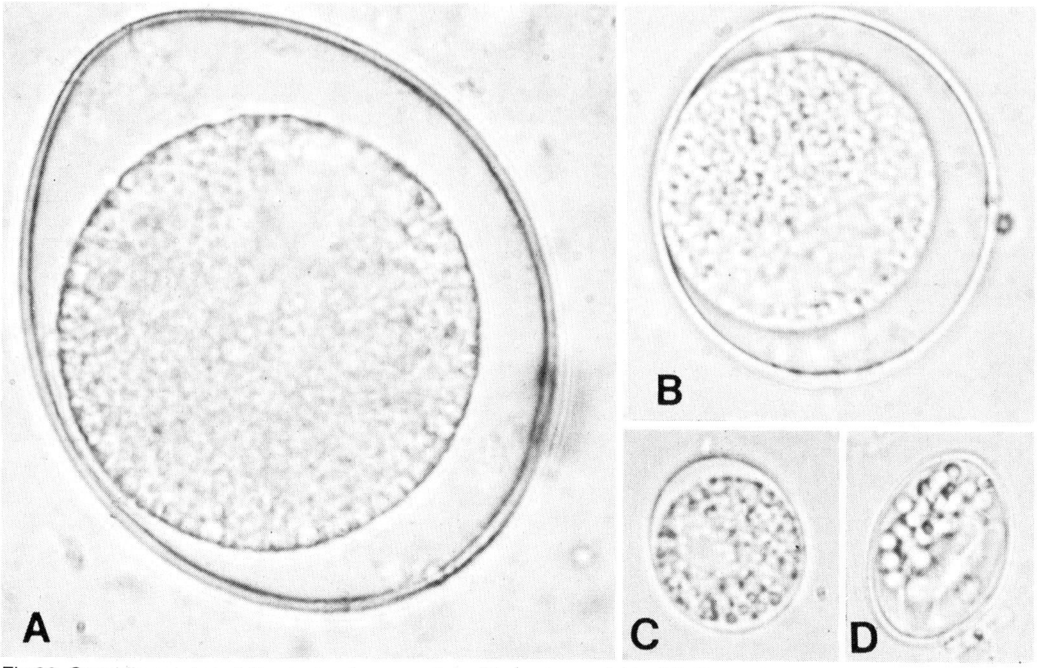

Fig 30. Coccidian cysts in feline feces. *Isospora felis* (A), *Isospora rivolta* (B), *Toxoplasma gondii* (C) and *Isospora bigemina* (sporulated free sporocyst) (D). [From JAVMA 162 (1973) 873]

Clinical Signs: The signs depend on the severity of the infection. Infected cats may be asymptomatic or suffer severe diarrhea that results in death. Clinical signs include anorexia, anemia, emaciation, watery and bloody diarrhea, and fever.[64-66] In kittens experimentally infected with 100,000 oocysts of *I felis,* no clinical signs were observed and infections in kittens given 150,000 oocysts were described as mildly pathogenic.[67,68]

Diagnosis: Oocysts can be found in fecal samples from infected animals after the prepatent period is reached (Fig 30).

Treatment: Several sulfonamides have been used to treat cats with coccidiosis, with varied results. Clinical signs are not observed before oocysts are first seen in the feces. Treatment then includes an attempt to control secondary bacterial infections and support dehydrated animals. This includes administration of antibiotics and/or sulfonamides as well as fluids. Feeding a low-residue diet may be helpful.

Control: As with most parasitic diseases, good sanitation is essential. Because freshly passed oocysts are not infective, removing feces daily prevents new infections. Oocysts are resistant to all disinfectants used commonly but can be killed by heat, sunlight or concentrated ammonia solutions. Care is required if concentrated ammonia solutions are used to disinfect litter pans because of the toxicity of ammonia fumes to people and other animals.

Cats are the definitive hosts for the following species of *Sarcocystis: S hirsuta* of cattle, *S gigantea* of sheep, *S porcifelis* of pigs, *S fusiformis* of water buffalo, *S muris* of mice, *S leporum* of cottontail rabbits, *S cuniculi* of rabbits and *S cymruensiss* of rats.[63] In addition, cats are the intermediate hosts for an unnamed species of *Sarcocystis.*[63]

The life cycle of *Sarcocystis* spp involves a definitive (predator) and intermediate (prey) host, with the asexual cycle taking place in the intermediate host and sexual cycle in the definitive host.

Life Cycle: A generalized life cycle for *Sarcocystis* spp in cats starts with the ingestion of sarcocysts in the muscle of an appropriate intermediate host (Fig 31). The merozoites invade intestinal cells and develop into gamonts that produce macrogametes and microgametocytes. The microgametes fertilize macrogametes to form a zygote, which develops oocysts. The oocysts sporulate in the tissues and sporocysts are passed in the feces. The sporocysts are infectious for the proper intermediate hosts, in which asexual development takes place.

Pathogenesis: Sarcocystis sexual stages apparently are nonpathogenic in cats.[63]

Clinical Signs: Clinical signs of *Sarcocystis* infection are unknown.

Diagnosis: Sporocysts may be found in the feces during the patent period.

Treatment: The treatment for *Sarcocystis* infection is unknown.

Control: Feeding only canned, cooked or dry cat food prevents *Sarcocystis* infection in cats.

Toxoplasma gondii probably has the highest prevalence of any parasite found in people and other mammals. *Toxoplasma gondii* was first described in 1908 but its entire life cycle was not elucidated until 1965, when *T gondii* oocysts were found in the feces of cats that had been fed mice infected with the parasite.[69] It was later postulated that *T gondii* was transmitted in the eggs of the nematode, *Toxocara mystax*.[69] There were subsequent reports about the transmission of *T gondii* to cats in helminth eggs.[70,71] It was then found that *T gondii* could be separated from the eggs and transmitted in the feces of cats not infected with *T mystax*.[72,73] In 1970, it was discovered that *T gondii* produced oocysts in cats and sporozoites developed in tissue cultures.[74-80] This discovery was a landmark in parasitology and it stimulated considerable research and some controversy regarding the role of cats in the transmission of toxoplasmosis. For these reasons, a separate section on the importance of feline infections and human health is included.

Source of Infection: Cats usually become infected by ingesting raw or undercooked meat of intermediate hosts containing extraintestinal forms of *T gondii*. They may also become infected by ingesting infective oocysts of *T gondii* from feces of other cats infected with intestinal stages of the parasite.

Life Cycle: The complex life cycle of *T gondii* cannot be described completely here. Those who desire more information about the life cycle should refer to other sources.[81,82]

The life cycle in cats is summarized in Figure 32. Cats may be infected with enteroepithelial or extraintestinal forms of *T gondii*. Only the intestinal stages are discussed here. Systemic toxoplasmosis is discussed in Chapter 4. A typical coccidian life cycle, such as that for the previously described *Isospora* species, may occur after ingestion of sporulated oocysts from cats infected with the intestinal form of *T gondii*. The parasite undergoes asexual (schizogonic) and sexual (gametogonic) cycles to produce oocysts that are passed in the feces. If the oocysts are in a favorable environment, they sporulate to an infective state. Such oocysts are infective to other cats and may cause extraintestinal toxoplasmosis in cats and other animals. Cats may also become infected by ingesting hosts infected with extraintestinal stages of the organism.

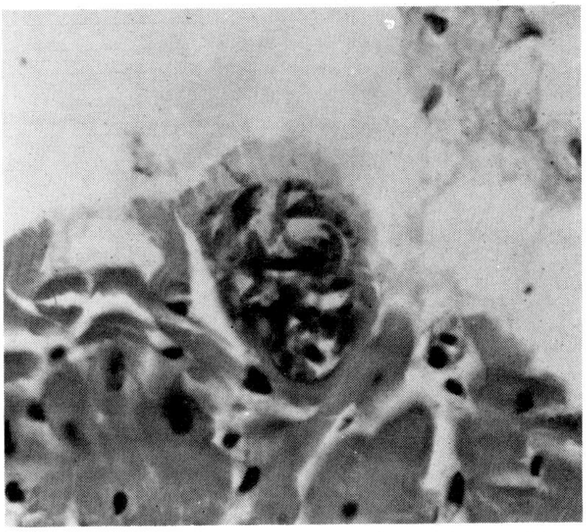

Fig 31. Cyst of *Sarcocystis* spp in bovine myocardium.

Pathogenesis and Clinical Signs: Toxoplasmosis of the CNS and eyes is discussed in Chapters 14 and 17, respectively. Intestinal stages in cats are evidently nonpathogenic.

Diagnosis: Oocysts from enteroepithelial infections may be detected by fecal examination. Because *T gondii* oocysts are of the isosporan type (sporulated oocysts containing 2 sporocysts, with each having 4 sporozoites), they must be distiniguished from those of *Isospora* spp (Fig 30). The largest coccidian oocysts in cat feces are those of *I felis*, ovoid and 35-53 by 26-43 μ. Oocysts of *I rivolta* are ellipsoid and 21-28 by 18-23 μ. Oocysts of *T gondii* are 11-14 by 9-11 μ.

If small oocysts slightly larger than RBC are found in fecal samples, a tentative diagnosis of enteroepithelial toxoplasmosis can be made. Fecal samples should be handled aseptically and sent to a diagnostic laboratory. They should be kept in 10-20 volumes of 2.5% potassium dichromate solution. The sample should be packaged well to avoid breakage in transit and the container should be clearly labeled to indicate the nature of the material.

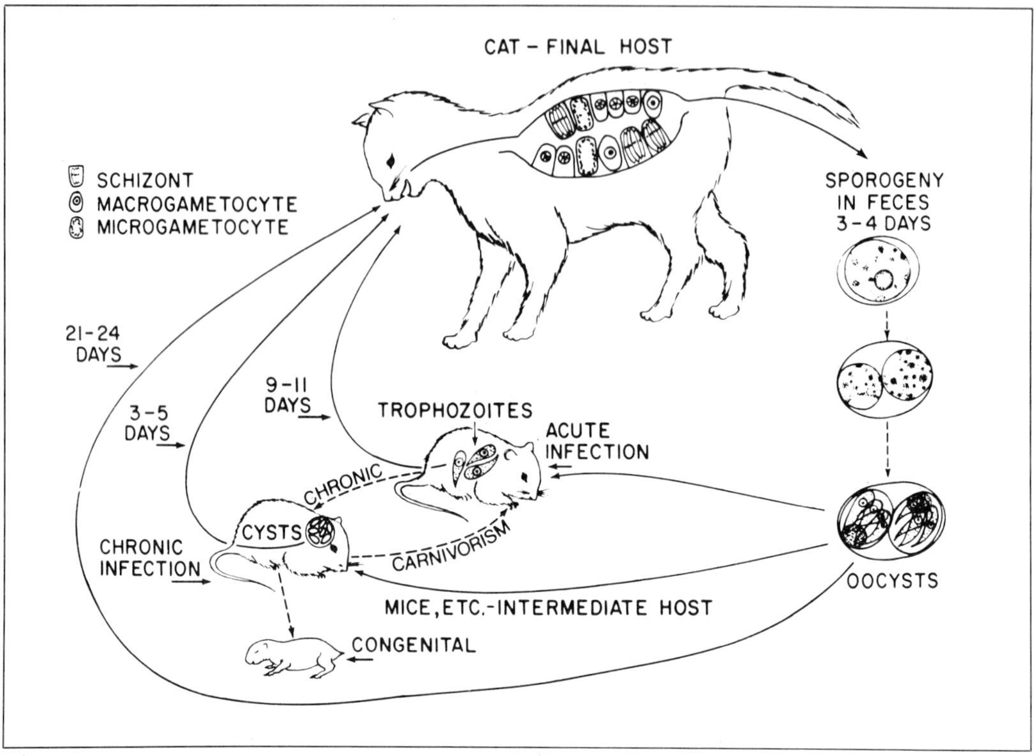

Fig 32. Postulated life cycle of *Toxoplasma* shows transmission by oocysts from cat feces and by ingestion of trophozoites or cysts from intermediate hosts. Days indicated represent time from ingestion of *Toxoplasma* by a cat to excretion of oocysts. Mice represent the many mammals and birds that can serve as facultative intermediate hosts, among which infection can spread, usually by carnivorism. Congenital transmission may occur during chronic infection, as in mice, or during acute infections, as in people. [From *Science* 167 (1970) 893]

Treatment: Kittens can be treated for toxoplasmosis if the disease is diagnosed early. The recommended treatment is sulfadiazine given 4 times daily at 33 mg/kg (15 mg/lb). Addition of pyrimethamine at 2.2 mg/kg (1 mg/lb) improves the therapeutic effect but also increases drug toxicity.[76] Treatment should be continued for 1-2 weeks or for a week after the fever subsides.

Control: Cats should not be allowed to hunt nor should they be fed raw or undercooked meat. With adequate moisture, *T gondii* oocysts in cat feces require 1-5 days to reach the infective stage at temperatures of 15-25 C. Thus, prompt disposal of feces is recommended.[75]

Hazards to Human Health: Toxoplasmosis in people may cause no symptoms or an extremely acute disease. The incidence, pathogenicity and epidemiology of human toxoplasmosis have been summarized.[81,82] Because prenatal infections may be highly pathogenic to the human fetus or neonate, the possibility of transmission to the fetus has received notice in both scientific and popular publications. The postulated transmission of toxoplasmosis is presented in Figure 33. The latest recommendations for preventing toxoplasmosis in humans and cats are as follows: "Avoid contamination with oocysts from cat feces by feeding cats dry, canned or thoroughly cooked food, preventing cats from hunting birds and rodents, emptying litter boxes daily before oocysts sporulate, wearing gloves or thoroughly washing hands after working in the garden or with soil and before eating or touching the face, covering children's sandboxes when not in use, preventing aerosols in the laboratory during centrifugation of potentially infected biologic samples, and boiling drinking water from streams, ponds or lakes frequented by cats.

"Avoid ingestion of tissue cysts by cooking meat to over 66 C and washing hands after handling raw meat.

"The following preventive measures apply to farms and other animal rearing facilities. Avoid contamination of feed or water with oocysts in cat feces by using rodenticides and traps to prevent cats from hunting rodents, covering, closing or locking feed-storage areas to prevent cats from entering and defecating, promptly removing cat feces from buildings, stalls or cages, and flushing, burning or burying it to destroy oocysts, and providing dry, canned or thoroughly cooked food and separate water to prevent cats from sharing facilities used by other animals."[83]

"Hammondia" hammondia and *"Hammondia" pardalis* have been isolated from Felidae. The taxonomic status of *"Hammondia"* is undecided. Some investigators consider *"Hammondia"* the same as *Toxoplasma*.[63] *"Hammondia"* spp are intestinal coccidia of cats. Cats are definitive hosts, and rodents and other mammals serve as experimental intermediate hosts. Unsporulated oocysts are passed in the cat's feces.[63]

Giardia cati (*Giardia felis*) is a protozoan that reportedly occurs in the small and large intestines of cats in North America.[84,85] It is structurally similar to *Giardia canis* and the 2 species may be the same.

Source of Infection: Cysts present in the feces of infected animals are subsequently ingested.

Life Cycle: The life cycle is direct. Trophozoites in the intestinal tract multiply by binary fission.

Pathogenesis: This is unknown but infected cats reportedly showed no signs of enteritis.[85] There is conflicting information about the pathogenicity of *G canis* in dogs. I have seen many cases of enteritis in dogs that have been treated successfully by eliminating *G canis*.

Diagnosis: Infections can be detected by finding cysts in formed feces or trophozoites in diarrheic feces. Trophozoites are found only in feces eliminated recently. Fecal samples can be fixed

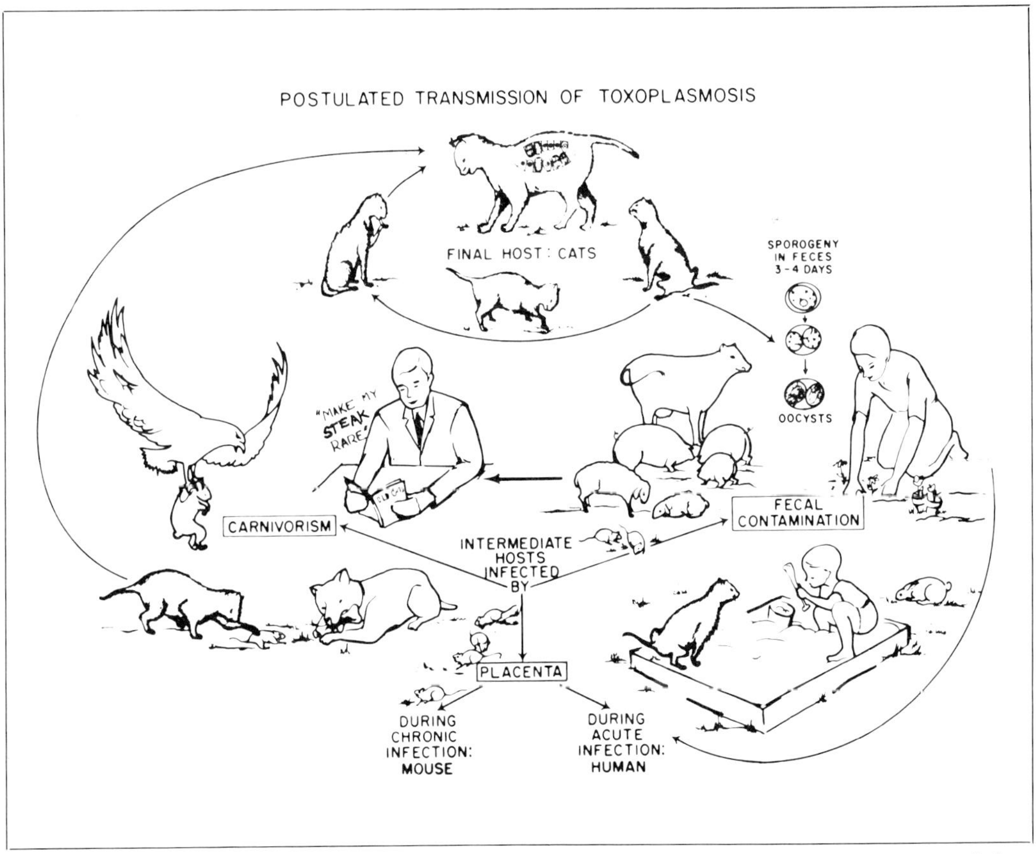

Fig 33. Postulated transmission of toxoplasmosis. Oocysts are shed in the feces of cats and, after sporulation, are infectious to a great variety of hosts by fecal contamination, probably direct, and via transport hosts (right). Carnivorism is the other important means of transmission (left). Cats probably become infected more often by carnivorism than by ingestion of oocysts. Transplacental transmission is indicated at the bottom. (From Frenkel: *Pathology of Protozoal and Helminthic Diseases,* Williams & Wilkins, Baltimore, 1971)

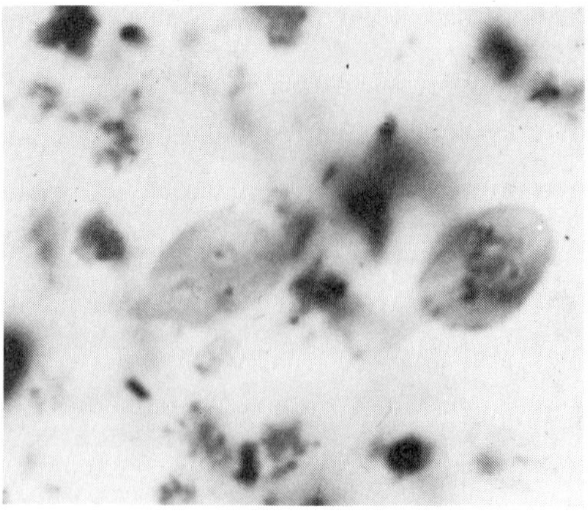

Fig 34. Trophozoites of *Giardia cati* stained with iron hematoxylin.

in 10% formalin and sent to a diagnostic laboratory, where special staining technics are used to identify the parasite (Fig 34). Trophozoites can be stained by adding a drop of Lugol's solution to a fresh fecal smear.

Treatment: One study of the treatment of cats with giardiasis has been reported.[86] Five infected cats were treated with quinacrine PO at 10 mg/kg once daily for 12 days, which resulted in remission of clinical signs. However, 4 of the cats continued to shed cysts after treatment.

Control: Prompt disposal of feces and good sanitation should prevent spread of infection.

Entamoeba histolytica infections of cats are rare. Usually it is found in people and other primates.

Source of Infection: Infective cysts are passed in the feces of infected animals and subsequently ingested.

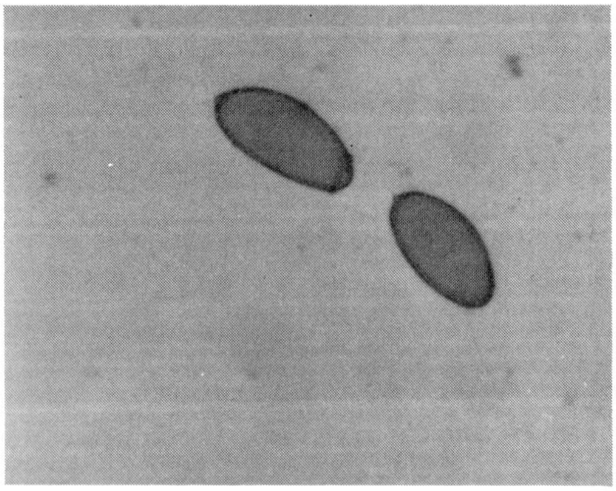

Fig 35. Eggs of *Amphimerus pseudofelineus.*

Life Cycle: Trophozoites reproduce in the intestine by binary fission and may be passed in liquid feces. Cysts are found in formed feces.

Pathogenesis and Clinical Signs: This is unknown in naturally infected cats.

Diagnosis: Cysts and trophozoites may be identified in fecal smears by adding a drop of Lugol's solution. Positive identification of the species usually is made at diagnostic laboratories that use specialized staining methods.

Treatment: Treatment of *E histolytica* in cats is unknown.

Entamoeba gingivalis is found commonly in people and reportedly occurs in cats. Little or nothing is known about its clinical significance in cats.

Parasites of the Liver

Capillaria hepatica

This nematode has rarely been found in the livers of cats. Rodents are the normal definitive hosts and cats are probably accidental hosts. Infections are found infrequently and most cases in cats were discovered at necropsy.

Amphimerus pseudofelineus

This fluke has been found in the livers of cats, coyotes, muskrats and opossums in North America. It has also been found in the larger pancreatic ducts of cats.[87] Because feline infections are rare, cats may be accidental hosts.

Source of Infection: One known second intermediate host is the sucker fish, *Catostomus commersonii.*[88]

Life Cycle: As with other trematodes, the first intermediate host is assumed to be a snail. Fish other than *Catostomus* have not been ruled out as second intermediate hosts.

Clinical Signs and Lesions: Anorexia, emaciation, jaundice, diarrhea, hemoglobinuria, hepatitis and cirrhosis have been observed in infected cats.[87,89-93]

Pathogenesis: The histopathologic lesions caused by the parasite include periportal cirrhosis of the liver, bile duct proliferation and centrilobular fatty degeneration.[87,91,92] Others have found cirrhosis of the pancreas, and chronic inflammation and epithelial proliferation in the larger pancreatic ducts, in which flukes were present.[87]

Diagnosis: Eggs of this parasite may be present in fecal samples (Fig 35).

Treatment: Treatment of *A pseudofelineus* infection has not been reported; infection can be avoided by not feeding raw or undercooked fish.

Platynosomum concinnum

This trematode has been found in the livers and gallbladders of cats in several countries, including the US. It has been considered the most important disease of cats in the Bahamas.[94]

Source of Infection: Cats become infected by ingesting infected lizards, *Anolis cristatellus*, which are the third intermediate hosts.[95]

Pathogenesis: Lesions associated with *P concinnum* infection have been described.[94,96-98] The livers of infected cats are often enlarged, and fatty degeneration, fibrosis and focal necrosis have been observed. Hyperplasia of the biliary epithelium and fibrosis of the bile ducts may cause thickening and distension of the bile ducts. Fatty infiltration of the kidneys, especially of the convoluted tubules, has been associated with infections.

Clinical Signs: The signs vary with the number of parasites present. Cats with slight infections may be asymptomatic. Diarrhea, abdominal distension, anorexia, vomiting and jaundice have been reported in severe cases.[94,97,98]

Diagnosis: Eggs may be present in fecal samples. They are 34-50 by 20-35 μ in size.

Treatment: Although there is no prescribed treatment, this parasitism can be controlled by preventing contact of cats with known intermediate hosts.

Opisthorchis tenuicollis (O felineus)

This parasite occurs in the bile and pancreatic duct of the cat, dog, fox and other animals. It has been reported in various parts of the world, including North America.

Source of Infection: Cats become infected by ingesting infected fish. Known second intermediate hosts are members of the carp family (Cyprinidae).[9]

Life Cycle: Snails are the first intermediate hosts. Fish of the carp family may be infected by cercariae that encyst to form metacercariae. Definitive hosts become infected by ingesting intermediate hosts containing metacercariae. These excyst in the duodenum and migrate up the bile ducts, where they become adults. During heavy infections, the adults may enter the pancreatic ducts or duodenum.[9]

Pathogenesis: The lesions vary with the severity of the infection. Granulomas at the periphery of the hepatic lobes may be minute foci or sizeable consolidated masses. Such lesions can extend up to 2 cm into the liver. The flukes may be encapsulated in calcified cysts.[99]

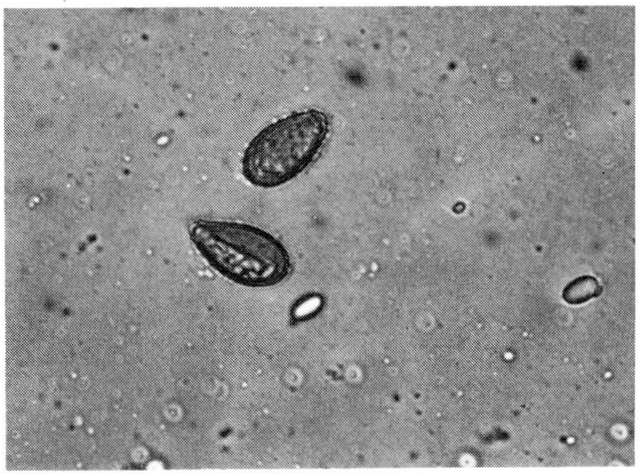

Fig 36. Eggs of *Opisthorchis tenuicollis.*

The parasite can cause catarrhal inflammation and desquamation of the biliary epithelium, which may result in adenomatous thickening. Severe infections can produce marked hepatic cirrhosis and passive venous congestion, leading to ascites and other edematous conditions.[9] Carcinogenic effects have been reported.

Clinical Signs: Although eosinophilia may develop, infected cats usually do not display clinical signs. Vague evidence of liver dysfunction may be confused with other conditions.

Diagnosis: Infections can be detected by finding trematode eggs in feces (Fig 36).

Treatment: Hexachlorophene has been given PO at 20 mg/kg (9 mg/lb) to kill adult trematodes in the liver.[100]

Control: Raw or undercooked fish should not be fed to cats.

Metorchis albidus and *M conjunctus*

These trematodes have been found in the livers of cats and other fish-eating mammals in North America. Both species are found in bile ducts; *M albidus* has also been found in the gallbladder.

Source of Infection: Fresh water fish are the second intermediate hosts.

Life Cycle: Aquatic snails are the first intermediate hosts. The cercariae leave infected snails and encyst in the muscles of fish. When infected fish are ingested, the metacercariae excyst, move up the bile duct to the liver and develop into adults.[9]

Pathogenesis and Clinical Signs: These are similar to those described for *O tenuicollis* infection.

Diagnosis: Operculated eggs may be present in fecal samples.

Treatment: There is none known.

Control: Infections can be avoided by not feeding raw or undercooked fish to cats.

Eurytrema procyonis

Eurytrema procyonis has been found in the gallbladders, pancreatic ducts and bile ducts of cats, raccoons and foxes in North America. The snail, *Nesodon thyroideus,* may serve as the intermediate host. Cats may become infected by ingesting snails containing larval stages of the parasite.[101] Pancreatic ducts containing this trematode have an increased amount of connective tissue due to a slight inflammatory response.[102] Fenbendazole, given PO at 30 mg/kg of body weight once daily for 6 days, eliminated *E procyonis* eggs from the feces of an infected cat.[103]

References

1. Cameron, TWM: The Parasites of Domestic Animals. 2nd ed. JB Lippincott, Philadelphia, 1952.
2. Dunn. AM: Veterinary Helminthology. 2nd ed. W Heinemann Medical Books, London, 1978.
3. Georgi, JR: Parasitology for Veterinarians. 3rd ed. WB Saunders, Philadelphia, 1980.
4. Lapage, G: Veterinary Parasitology. 2nd ed. Charles C Thomas. Springfield, IL, 1968.
5. Levine, ND: Protozoan Parasites of Domestic Animals and of Man. 2nd ed. Burgess Publishing, Minneapolis, 1973.
6. Levine, ND: Nematode Parasites of Domestic Animals and of Man. 3rd ed. Burgess Publishing, Minneapolis, 1980.
7. Levine, ND: Textbook of Veterinary Parasitology. Burgess Publishing, Minneapolis, 1978.
8. Soulsby, EJL: Helminths, Arthropods, and Protozoa of Domesticated Animals. 6th ed. Williams & Wilkins, Baltimore, 1968.
9. Soulsby, EJL: Textbook of Veterinary Clinical Parasitology. Blackwell Scientific Publications, Oxford, 1965.
10. Barriga, OO: The Immunology of Parasitic Infections. Univ Park Press, Baltimore, 1981.
11. Lepp, DL and Todd, KS Jr. Ill Vet **14** (1971) 16.
12. Beaver, PC. Bull Soc Path Exot **55** (1962) 555.
13. Sprent, JFA. Trans Roy Soc Trop Hyg **59** (1965) 365.
14. Sloss, MW and Kemp, RL: Veterinary Clinical Parasitology. 5th ed. Iowa State Univ Press, Ames, 1978.
15. Ivens, VR *et al:* Principal Parasites of Domestic Animals in the United States. Special Publ 52. Coll Ag Vet Med, Univ IL, Urbana, 1978.
16. Thienpont, D *et al:* Diagnosing Helminthiasis Through Coprological Examination. Janssen Research Foundation, Beerse, Belgium, 1979.
17. Greve, JH. Fel Pract **11(4)** (1981) 17.
18. Hargis, AM *et al.* JAVMA **178** (1981) 475.
19. Bearup, AJ. Aust J Sci **21** (1958) 149.
20. Cameron, TWM. J Helminth **5** (1927) 67.
21. Petri, LH. Trans Kansas Acad Sci **53** (1950) 331.
22. Petri, LH and Ameel, DJ. J Parasit **36** (Suppl) (1950) 40.
23. Zago, HF. Rev Brasil Biol **19** (1959) 9.
24. Fulleborn, F. Arch Schiffs Tropenhyg **25** (1921) 367.
25. Lamina, J. Zeitschr Parasitenk **24** (1964) 600.
26. Sprent, JFA. Parasit **49** (1959) 330.
27. Sprent, JFA. Parasit **46** (1956) 54.
28. Swerczek, TW *et al.* Am J Vet Res **32** (1971) 89.
29. Wright, WH. Proc Helm Soc Wash **2** (1935) 56.
30. Okoshi, S and Usui, M. Jap J Vet Sci **30** (1968) 81.
31. Swerczek, TW *et al.* Res Vet Sci **11** (1970) 103.
32. Gibson, TE: Veterinary Anthelmintic Medication. 2nd ed. Commonwealth Ag Bur, Farnham Royal, England, 1965.
33. Sloan, JEN *et al.* J Pharm Pharmacol **6** (1954) 718.
34. Colglazier, ML and Enzie, FD. Proc Helm Soc Wash **18** (1951) 50.
35. McCowen, MC *et al.* Am J Trop Med Hyg **6** (1957) 894.
36. Enzie, FD and Colglazier, ML. J Parasit **39** (Suppl) (1953) 39.
37. Power, LA. J Parasit **57** (1971) 610.
38. Rohde, K. Z Tropenmed Parasit **10** (1959) 402.
39. Miller, TA. J Parasit **56** (Sect II) (1970) 238.
40. McCoy, OR. Am J Hyg **11** (1930) 413.
41. Okoshi, S and Murata, Y. Jap J Vet Sci **29** (1967) 251.
42. Foster, AO. J Parasit **19** (1932) 112.
43. Miller, TA. J Parasit **56** (Sect II) (1970) 239.
44. Stone, WM and Girardeau, MH. Vet Rec **79** (1966) 773.
45. Stone, W and Smith, FW. Exp Parasit **34** (1973) 306.
46. Miller, TA. J Parasit **52** (1966) 856.
47. Link, in Jones: Veterinary Pharmacology and Therapeutics. 3rd ed. Iowa State Press, Ames, 1965.
48. Haas, DK. Fel Pract **8(2)** (1978) 31.
49. Haas, DK and Meisels, LS. Am J Vet Res **39** (1978) 1553.
50. Enzie, FD. JAVMA **119** (1951) 210.
51. Malone, JB *et al.* JAVMA **171** (1977) 278.
52. Olsen, OW: Animal Parasites: Their Life Cycles and Ecology. 3rd ed. Univ Park Press, Baltimore, 1974.
53. Mueller, JF: Host-Parasite Relationships. Oregon State Univ Press, Corvallis, 1966.
54. Stunkard, HW. J Morph **50** (1930) 143.
55. Christensen, NO and Roth, H. Kong Vet Landbohojsk Aarsskr (1946) 114.
56. Cameron, TWM *et al.* Can J Res **18** (1940) 325.

57. Christensen, NO and Roth, H. Kong Vet Landbohojsk Aarsskr (1949) 1.
58. Johnson, AD. J Parasit **54** (1968) 324.
59. Schlegel, MW *et al.* J Parasit **54** (1968) 770.
60. Gebhardt, GA *et al.* J Parasit **52** (1966) 54.
61. Millemann, RE and Knapp, SE. Adv Parasit **8** (1970) 1.
62. Burrows, RB and Lillis, WG. J Parasit **51** (1965) 570.
63. Levine, ND and Ivens, VR. Ill Biol Monogr **51** (1981) 1.
64. Andrews, JM. Am J Hyg **6** (1926) 784.
65. Tomimura, T. Jap J Parasit **6** (1957) 12.
66. Wasielewski, TV: Studien und Mikrophotogramme zur Kenntnis der Pathogenen Protozoen Untersuchungen über den Bau, die Entwichlung und über die pathogene Bedeutung der Coccidien. Johann Ambrosius Barth, Leipzig, 1904.
67. Hitchcock, DJ. J Parasit **41** (1955) 383.
68. Shah, HL. J Protozool **18** (1971) 3.
69. Hutchison, WM. Trans Roy Soc Trop Med Hyg **61** (1967) 80.
70. Dubey, JP. Vet Bull **38** (1968) 495.
71. Rommel, M *et al.* Berl Münch Tierärztl Woch **81** (1968) 309.
72. Frenkel, JK *et al.* Science **164** (1969) 432.
73. Sheffield, HG and Melton, ML. Science **164** (1969) 431.
74. Dubey, JP *et al.* J Parasit **56** (1970) 447.
75. Dubey, JP *et al.* J Exp Med **132** (1970) 636.
76. Dubey, JP *et al.* JAVMA **157** (1970) 1767.
77. Frenkel, JK *et al.* Science **167** (1970) 893.
78. Hutchison, WM *et al.* Br Med J **1** (1970) 142.
79. Overdulve, JP. Koninkel Nederl Akad van Wetenschappen (Amsterdam) Proc Series C **73** (1970) 129.
80. Sheffield, HF and Melton, ML. Science **167** (1970) 892.
81. Frenkel, in Hammond and Long: The Coccidia: *Eimeria, Isospora, Toxoplasma,* and Related Genera. Univ Park Press, Baltimore, 1973.
82. Frenkel, JK: Pathology of Protozoal and Helminthic Diseases. Williams & Wilkins, Baltimore, 1971.
83. Fayer, R. Can Vet J **22** (1980) 344.
84. Burrows, RB and Hunt, GR. JAVMA **157** (1970) 2065.
85. Hitchcock, DJ and Malewitz, TD. J Parasit **42** (1956) 286.
86. Brightman, AH and Slonka, GF. JAAHA **12** (1976) 492.
87. Rothenbacher, H and Lindquist, WD. JAVMA **143** (1963) 1099.
88. Evans, WS. Can J Zool **41** (1963) 649.
89. Essex, HE and Bollman, JL. Am J Trop Med **10** (1930) 65.
90. Koutz, FR. JAVMA **116** (1950) 127.
91. Levine, ND *et al.* Ill Vet **1** (1958) 47.
92. Todd, KS, Jr. *et al.* JAVMA **181** (1982) *In press.*
93. Turk, RD. JAVMA **115** (1949) 23.
94. Leam, G and Walker, IE. Vet Rec **75** (1963) 46.
95. Maldonado, JF. Puerto Rico J Pub Health Trop Med **21** (1945) 17.
96. Levine, ND and Beamer, PD. J Parasit **43** (Suppl) (1957) 29.
97. Retnasabapathy, A and Prathap, K. Vet Rec **88** (1971) 62.
98. Robinson, VB and Ehrenford, FA. Am J Vet Res **23** (1962) 1300.
99. Al-Dabagh, MA *et al.* Vet Rec 76 (1964) 116.
100. Lienert, E. Wien Tierärztl Monatschr **49** (1962) 353.
101. Denton, JF. J Parasit **30** (1944) 277.
102. Sheldon, WG. JAVMA **148** (1966) 251.
103. Roudebush, P and Schmidt, DA. JAVMA **180** (1982) 545.

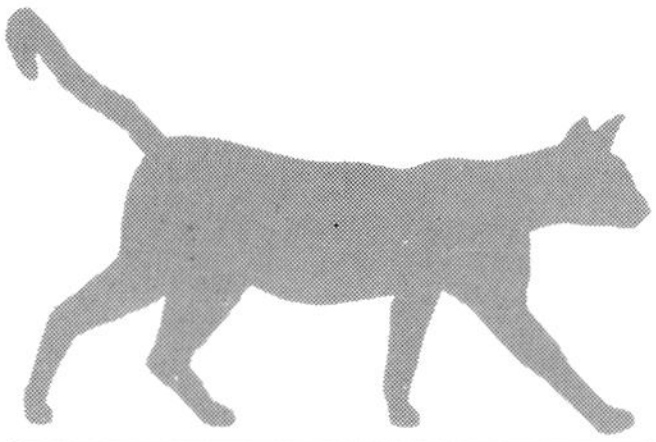

9

the cardiovascular system

P.R. FOX, L.P. TILLEY, AND S.-K. LIU

Feline cardiology is a relatively new field that has developed during the last decade. Competence in this discipline confers the ability to detect symptomatic cardiac abnormalities early through routine physical examination. Criteria for diagnosing heart disease are still being developed in some areas. Electrocardiographic, angiocardiographic and echocardiographic technics continue to define normal values. Many specific cardiac disorders, such as congenital anomalies, lack adequate clinical understanding of their natural history. The causes of cardiomyopathies are still unknown and therapeutic regimens are not well established. Nevertheless, feline cardiology is a rapidly developing specialty in veterinary medicine.

The interest among biomedical researchers in animal models for human disease contributes to the understanding of specific feline cardiac diseases while providing useful information for treatment and control of cardiomyopathy in people. Feline primary myocardial disease (cardiomyopathy) provides an important model for cardiovascular investigators and pathologists since it is similar to hypertrophic and congestive cardiomyopathy in people.[1-3] Naturally occurring aortic thromboembolism in cardiomyopathic cats is also a model for study of thrombolytic and antithrombus drugs.

A significant number of cats are affected with acquired cardiovascular disease. During a 13½-year period, 99,416 cats were examined at the Animal Medical Center in New York City. Acquired heart disease leading to congestive heart failure was diagnosed in 8.5% of 4933 cats necropsied during that period. Congenital cardiac anomalies are much less common. In the same study, cardiac anomalies were clinically diagnosed and confirmed at necropsy in only 1.9% of these cats.[4] Thus, primary myocardial heart disease and congenital cardiac anomalies were present in about 10% of that feline population. It is very likely that the incidence in the general cat population is higher.

EVALUATION OF CARDIAC PATIENTS

An approach to patients with heart disease employs a cardiovascular data base that is part of the general medical examination. Defining heart disease depends upon a logical, methodic approach using the history, physical examination and laboratory tests. Use of a problem-oriented approach provides an organized and efficient system for defining and organizing problems toward a logical solution. Essential components include a defined data base, complete problem list, plan formulation and progress notes (titled and numbered by problem).

The defined data base consists of the history, physical examination and laboratory evaluation. Subjective data include primarily qualitative information comprised of the patient profile and client's history. Objective data is provided by physical examination, and laboratory and diagnostic tests.

History

A thorough and accurate history plays a prominent role in detecting problems and directing the physical and laboratory examination. The patient profile (age, breed, sex) may help suggest or eliminate the likelihood of a disease. For example, a diagnosis of patent ductus arteriosus, aortic stenosis or tetralogy of Fallot is unlikely in a 12-year-old cat. Certain breeds (*eg,* Siamese and Burmese) appear prone to dilated cardiomyopathy. Also, a historical review of other body systems must be performed to detect other diseases and uncover relationships between systemic or metabolic disease and cardiac abnormalities. For example, a history of polyphagia, weight loss, polyuria, voluminous stool, tachypnea and tachycardia in an old cat warrants an evaluation for hyperthyroidism.

Early feline cardiac disease differs markedly in symptomatology from that in dogs and usually is not observed by the client. Coughing is very rare. Exercise intolerance is difficult to appreciate due to the sedentary nature of indoor cats. Hiding and seclusion may be the only abnormalities noted. Anorexia, a common early sign preceding congestive heart failure, may be overlooked in multicat households.

Mild paraparesis that resolves in several days may occur with small distal aortic thromboemboli without total arterial occlusion or severe ischemic neuromyopathy. Acute, severe paraparesis, cool distal extremities, absence of femoral pulses, firm gastrocnemius muscles and cyanotic nail beds indicate a severe distal aortic thrombus secondary to cardiomyopathy or, rarely, vegetative endocarditis.

Decompensated heart disease may be characterized by historical evidence of anorexia and lethargy preceding acute or progressive dyspnea and tachypnea. Abdominal enlargement due to right-sided failure is uncommon even in the presence of severe pulmonary effusion. Stress or excitement can exacerbate a decompensated cardiopulmonary status.

Syncopal episodes may occasionally result from congenital or acquired cardiac disorders. Weakness, loss of consciousness, extensor rigidity and occasionally autonomic release of bladder sphincter tone may occur. Large right-to-left shunts (tetralogy of Fallot, common atrioventricular canal, Eisenmenger's complex) or a fixed outflow obstruction (aortic and pulmonic stenosis) are the congenital diseases usually implicated. Hypertrophic cardiomyopathy, tachyarrhythmias and bradyarrhythmias represent the most commonly acquired cardiac diseases associated with syncope.[5]

Physical Examination

Preliminary inspection begins immediately while the history is obtained. General appearance, posture, behavior and the rate and character of respiration should be noted at this time. Other signs that may be observed include abdominal distension, peripheral edema and discoloration of the tongue or mucous membranes.

Palpation of the thorax and abdomen is best accomplished with the cat resting in sternal recumbency. Palpation of the thorax is often helpful in detecting cardiac disease and is facilitated by the thinness of the feline chest and flexibility of its ribs. The point of maximal cardiac intensity is normally palpated near the cardiac apex beat at the left sternal border or about the fifth to sixth intercostal space. This is best assessed with the palm of the hand held flat against the precordium. Localized movements are often more easily detected with the tips of the fingers. Cats with left ventricular hypertrophy from hypertrophic cardiomyopathy may have an accentuated apex beat. Palpable vibrations (thrills) caused by heart murmurs at their point of maximal intensity may be detected with palpation. The heart rate should be determined and respiratory pattern assessed.

Moving caudad, the abdomen is palpated for hepatosplenomegaly, ascites and integrity of other visceral structures. Femoral arterial pulses should be compared for rate, rhythm and amplitude. Hyperkinetic pulses may occur with hyperthyroidism. A water hammer or rapid, "BB-shot" pulse that rises and falls is associated with rapid diastolic runoff, as in patent ductus arteriosus or aortic insufficiency. A hypokinetic, weak pulse may indicate decreased cardiac output due to primary myocardial disease (especially dilated cardiomyopathy), shock, dehydration, pericardial disease, aortic stenosis or arrhythmias. Cyclic, irregular pulses indicate sinus arrhythmia while noncyclic irregularity suggests arrhythmias. An absence of arterial pulse indicates distal arterial thromboembolism. Venous pulses that are exaggerated in the standing animal are abnormal. Hair over the jugular vein must be clipped to facilitate this observation. Exaggerated venous pulses usually are associated with right-sided failure due to tricuspid insufficiency (usually secondary to tricuspid dysplasia).

Animals in congestive heart failure, especially from dilated or excessive moderator band cardiomyopathy, may be hypothermic. Mild dehydration is common with congestive heart failure.

Auscultation

Auscultation augments inspection and palpation. A quiet room is essential. The cat should be approached gently. The examiner should first palpate the precordium to detect thrills and determine the location of the apex beat. Both femoral arteries are then palpated and compared.

Auscultation is best performed with the animal standing, to facilitate orientation and localization of heart sounds. Purring may interfere with assessment and may be stopped by changing the cat's position or gently palpating the larynx. Shivering, movement, respiration and rubbing the hair can produce artifactual sounds.

The heart should be auscultated at the left apex (mitral valve area over the left fifth to sixth intercostal space at or ventral to the costochondral junction), the left base (aortic and pulmonic valve area over the third to fourth intercostal space dorsal to the costochondral junction), the tricuspid area (right fourth intercostal space dorsal to the costochondral junction), the thoracic inlet, and the mid-sternum (Fig 1).

Initially, the rate and rhythm should be determined with the stethoscope diaphragm placed over the left apex. Thereafter, each of the auscultatory locations described should be examined, focusing attention on heart sounds and murmur detection. Auscultation with the stethoscope diaphragm held snugly against the skin detects high-fequency sounds; the bell is then lightly applied to the chest wall to assess low-frequency sounds.

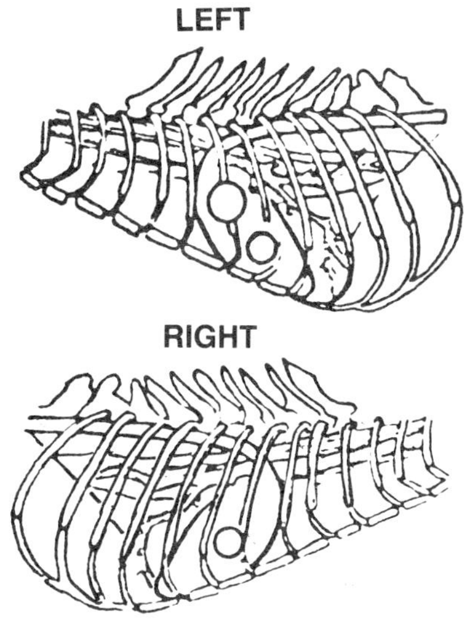

Fig 1. Areas of auscultation are illustrated for the left and right chest wall. The heart should be auscultated at the left apex, left base, tricuspid valve area on the right side, thoracic inlet and mid-sternum.

An understanding of the physiologic origin of normal heart sounds facilitates their identification and clarifies their significance. The first heart sound (S1) occurs at the beginning of the systole. It is related to atrioventricular valve closure, semilunar valve opening, turbulence in the great vessels, and ventricular tension and muscular contraction. It is longer, duller and louder at the apex than the second heart sound. The arterial pulse occurs just after S1.

The second heart sound (S2) is attributed to closure of the aortic and pulmonic semilunar valves and vibrations within the great vessels at the end of systole. The second heart sound can be auscultated by slowly inching the stethoscope from the left apex to left base, where it becomes progressively louder. Splitting of S2 may be difficult to appreciate because of the rapid heart rate in cats. Only S1 and S2 are normally present. A third (S3) or fourth (S4) heart sound usually is abnormal and associated with cardiac disease.

Gallop rhythms occur during ventricular filling. They usually denote myocardial disease, implying abnormal ventricular morphology or function. They usually are a sequence of 3 heart sounds comprised of S1, S2 and either S3 or S4. Gallop rhythms represent a combination of turbulent blood flow, abnormal temporary atrioventricular valve closure and abnormal ventricular motion. They must be differentiated from systolic clicks and murmurs. An S3 heart sound confers a protodiastolic gallop rhythm (S1-S2-S3). Occurring in early diastole, it is most commonly associated with dilated cardiomyopathy. It is lower pitched than S2 and heard best at the left apex, whereas S2 is heard best at the left base. A fourth heart sound (S4) heard at the left base and often at the left apex is termed a presystolic atrial gallop rhythm (S4-S1-S2). It is most frequently associated with hypertrophic cardiomyopathy. A summation gallop rhythm represents merging of S3 and S4. This usually occurs at rapid heart rates. Systolic clicks are higher-frequency sounds. Early systolic clicks are heard best at the left base and occur just after S1. Thus, the click occurs between S1 and S2, preserving the diastolic S2-S1 silent period. This is different from a gallop rhythm, in which S3 is heard in early diastole after S2, with the S1-S2 systolic period preserved, unless a murmur is present.

Phonocardiography may be employed to check, extend and improve auscultation. It transcribes heart sounds and murmurs graphically, describing the timing, frequency and shape (quality) of murmurs. When combined with a simultaneous electrocardiogram (ECG), temporal correlation between heart sounds in the cardiac cycle and cardiac electrical events is facilitated.

Auscultation of a gallop rhythm during physical examination suggests abnormal cardiac function. If the animal is asymptomatic, further diagnostic procedures are warranted to demonstrate and characterize the suspected underlying disease. An ECG is indicated to detect conduction disturbances (*ie,* left anterior fascicular block suggestive of hypertrophic cardiomyopathy), arrhythmias or evidence of cardiac chamber enlargement. A thoracic radiograph is valuable to further assess the cardiovascular system. Radiographic abnormalities are often present with cardiomyopathy, even during the compensated state. Angiocardiography or echocardiography may further define the disease.

Heart murmurs are important indicators of heart disease. When the laminar flow of blood is altered because of cardiovascular disease, turbulence develops. Turbulence or conditions responsible for the turbulent flow, eddies and vortices can cause some murmurs.

Murmurs should be classified according to their timing, intensity, radiation of sound, and quality. Systolic murmurs begin with or after S1 and end with or just before S2. Diastolic murmurs begin with or just after S2 and end before S1. The intensity of murmurs is graded at their point of maximum intensity. A grade-I/VI murmur is the faintest murmur that can be detected, often after minutes of close concentration. Grade-II/VI murmurs are very faint but are heard immediately. Grade-III/VI murmurs are of low intensity to moderately loud. A grade-IV/VI murmur is moderately loud, without a palpable thrill. Grade-V/VI murmurs are loud, with a palpable thrill, but require a stethoscope for detection. Grade-VI/VI murmurs are the loudest murmurs that produce a thrill but are audible without a stethoscope. Certain lesions cause characteristic murmurs and patterns of radiation of sound, although loud murmurs radiate extensively. Therefore, the entire chest should be auscultated. Quality refers to subjective interpretation of the intensity, frequency and nature of the murmur, *ie,* blowing, harsh, musical, rumbling, high pitched or low pitched. Murmurs with mixed high and medium frequencies sound harsh, while those with narrowed frequencies are musical or honking. Thus, interpretation of heart murmurs is based upon their characteristic timing, intensity, duration, location, quality and pitch.

The most common feline systolic murmur is that of mitral regurgitation. Murmurs from tricuspid regurgitation are also common. Most of these are of low intensity and associated with atrioventricular valvular insufficiency due to alteration of the atrioventricular valvular complex in cardiomyopathy. For this reason, detection of a cardiac murmur during physical examination should be followed by additional diagnostic technics similar to those described for gallop rhythms. Murmurs due to intracardiac shunts or semilunar valvular stenosis (pulmonic, aortic) may be encountered less frequently. Diastolic murmurs occur as a component of the continuous "machinery" murmur of patent ductus arteriosus.

Electrocardiography

Indications

Electrocardiography is a well-established and essential tool in clinical evaluation of cats with heart disease. It can also be an important aid in establishing an etiology or diagnosis in certain systemic diseases (pyometra, uremia, neoplasia), toxic myocarditis, electrolyte disturbances (especially K abnormalities), and endocrine diseases (hyperthyroidism). Other indications for obtaining an ECG include tachycardia, bradycardia or arrhythmias detected during auscultation, acute onset of dyspnea or tachypnea, shock, fainting, seizures, monitoring of surgical patients, cardiac murmurs, radiographic abnormalities, cyanosis, evaluating the effects of certain drugs, and serial evaluation for prognosis and diagnosis of cardiac disease. The ECG must be evaluated in conjunction with a complete data base, including a good history, physical examination (inspection, palpation, auscultation, percussion), and laboratory profile (radiographic, echocardiographic, hematologic, serologic and blood chemistry assessment).

Limitations

Certain limitations of electrocardiography should be recognized so the clinician does not read too much into an ECG. The ECG must be interpreted in conjunction with all clinical information. It does not describe the functional status of the heart. For example, animals with congestive heart failure may have a normal ECG and clinically normal animals may have isolated electrocardiographic abnormalities. The ECG may not always suggest a prognosis; however, in general, the more severe the electrocardiographic abnormality, the less favorable the prognosis. The ECG only reflects pathologic changes in the myocardium, not the valves, coronary arteries, endocardium or pericardium. The divisions between normal and abnormal electrocardiographic changes is a continuum and not a sharp, discrete delineation. Finally, every ECG must be recorded properly and consistently.[6] The heart rate of cats is often so rapid that at slow paper speeds of 25 mm/sec, measurements may be difficult to make or impossible to interpret. (All ECGs in this chapter were recorded at a paper speed of 50 mm/sec, 1 cm = 1 mv.)

Use of drugs for restraint during electrocardiography is not advised since possible cardiac actions may alter the ECG. For example, ketamine and diazepam both are antiarrhythmic drugs.[7,8] Tranquilization for restraint, if used judiciously, should not affect P-QRS deflections and electrical axis calculations. However, cardiac rhythm may be affected.

Since the ECG is a mechanical recording, technical or mechanical problems can be superimposed on normal complexes and rhythms. Artifacts may thus interfere with interpretation by simulating tracings of cardiac abnormalities. Electrical interference, muscle tremor, wandering baseline, poorly defined baseline and other artifacts must be identified and distinguished from true cardiac abnormalities.

Technic

The complete ECG should include at least 3-4 complexes of each bipolar standard lead (I, II, III), 3 augmented unipolar limb leads (aVR, aVL, aVF), and at least 15-20 inches of lead II rhythm strip at 50 mm/sec. The unipolar precordial chest leads (CV_5RL, also termed rV_2, CV_6LL or V_2, CV_6LU or V_4, V_{10}) can also be recorded for additional ECG information.

Sternal positioning is used in cats with severe respiratory distress to minimize the stress of restraint, for cats that are difficult to restrain, and when only a rhythm analysis is desired. Right lateral recumbency is used when a complete ECG is recorded for analysis of P-QRS-T and mean electrical axis, when avoiding stress during restraint is not a consideration, and if restraint is reasonably accomplished.

Electrodes of the ECG leads, labeled left arm (LA), right arm (RA), left leg (LL) and right leg (RL), are attached to the cat's skin on the appropriate limbs, just proximal to the olecranon and patella. A fifth lead, the V lead (C), may be attached at various precordial positions according to the intent of the electrocardiographer.

Contact is fostered between the skin and electrodes by moistening them with alcohol or contact gel. An insulated surface is required beneath the cat to avoid electrical artifacts during recording with a standard electrocardiographic machine.[6]

Every ECG should have several features examined systematically. Steps in this analysis include calculation of the heart rate, evaluation of rhythm, measurement of complexes and intervals, assessment of patterns in limb leads I, II, III, aVR, aVL, aVF and V_{10}, and determination of the mean electrical axis.

Measurement of complexes and intervals is completed on the lead II rhythm strip. Figure 2 depicts the P-QRS-T complex with regard to measurements for amplitude and time intervals

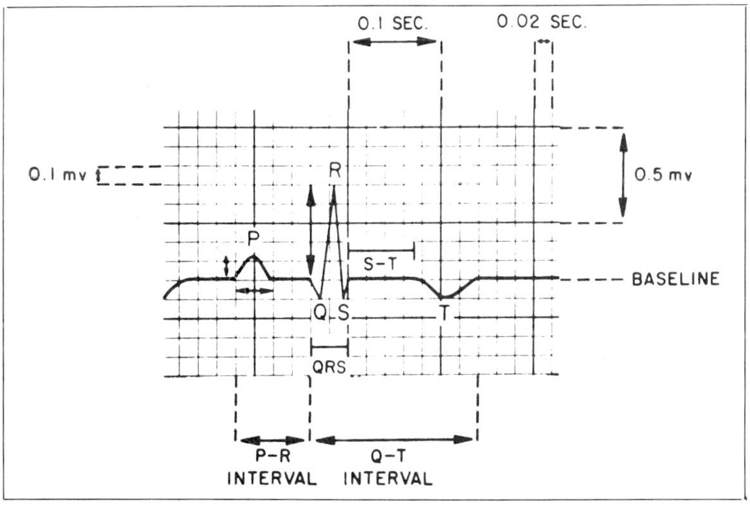

Fig 2. A normal lead-II P-QRS-T complex.[6] (Courtesy of C.V. Mosby)

Table 1. Normal Electrocardiographic Limits in Unanesthetized Cats* [6,9]

Heart rate: 160-240 beats/min (mean 197 beats/min)
Rhythm: normal sinus rhythm or sinus tachycardia (reaction to excitement)
P wave: 0.04 sec max width, 0.02 mv max height
P-R interval: 0.05-0.09 sec
QRS complex: 0.04 sec max width
R wave: 0.9 mv max height
S-T segment: no marked depression or elevation
T wave: positive, negative, biphasic, usually positive; 0.3 mv max height
Q-T interval: 0.12-0.18 sec at normal heart rate (range 0.07-0.20 sec); varies with heart rate (faster rates, shorter interval, slower rates, longer interval)
Electrical axis (frontal plane): 0 to +160°

(Courtesy of C.V. Mosby)

* All measurements at paper speed of 50 mm/sec, 1 cm = 1 mv

as measured in lead II. Calculations include analysis of the P-wave amplitude and width, length of the P-R interval, amplitude and width of the QRS complex, analysis and width of the S-T segment, T wave, and length of the Q-T interval. A summary of the essential criteria for determining normal limits of unanesthetized cats is listed in Table 1.

For sternal recumbency, the values are the same as for right lateral recumbency except that the acceptable height of the P wave is 0.3 mv, the height of the QRS is 1.0 mv, and the axis is −10° to +150°. Sternal recumbency is the position of choice for ease of restraint.[9]

Electrical activity of the heart simultaneously produces potentials in many directions in a 3-dimensional field. The electrical axis refers to the average direction of this activation during the cardiac cycle. The mean electrical axis in the frontal plane can be calculated using 6 limb leads (I, II, III, aVR, aVL, aVF). If the axis shifts to greater than +160°, a right axis is evident. A left axis is represented by a deviation of less than 0° (Fig 3). Even with this broad normal axis, axis calculation can be quite useful, especially when serial ECGs are compared.

Analysis of P-QRS-T Deflections

A normal feline ECG, showing the bipolar standard leads (I, II, III), augmented unipolar limb leads (aVR, aVL, aVF) and unipolar precordial chest leads (CV_5RL, CV_6LL, CV_6LU, V_{10}), is illustrated in Figure 4. Note that the complexes are generally much smaller than those in dogs. The P waves and T waves may be very difficult to observe in some normal cats. It is not

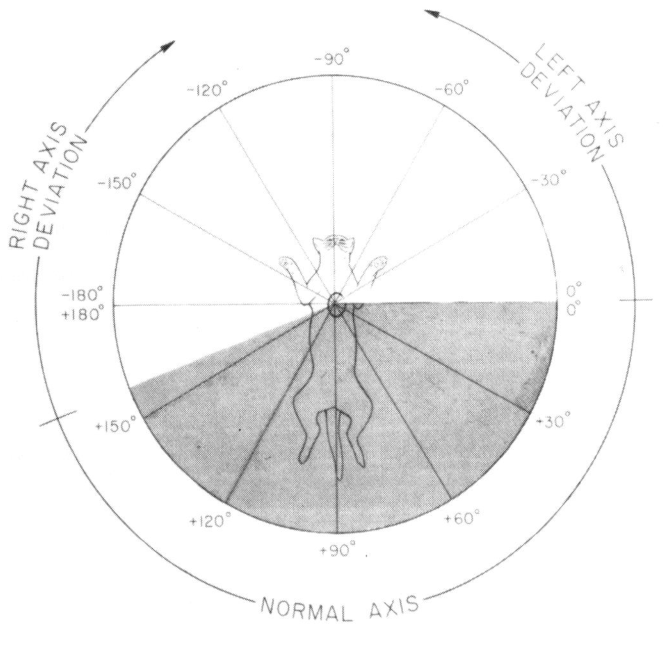

Fig 3. The normal mean electrical axis in the frontal plane is from 0° to +160°. If the axis becomes less than 0°, this is called left axis deviation.[6] (Courtesy of C.V. Mosby)

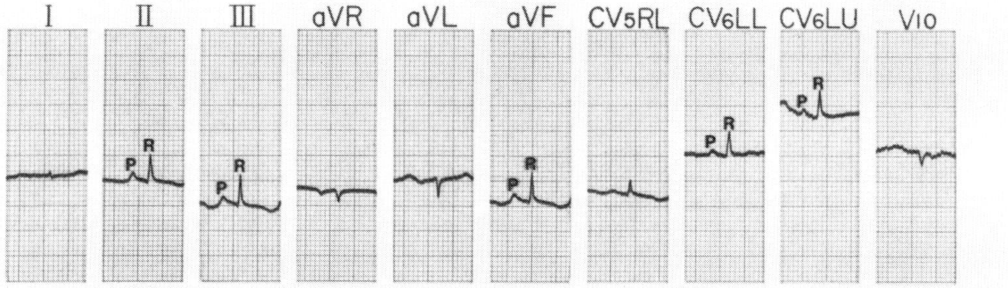

Fig 4. Normal ECG illustrating the bipolar standard leads (I, II, III), augmented unipolar limb leads (aVR, aVL, aVF) and unipolar precordial chest leads (CV_5RL, CV_6LL, CV_6LU, V_{10}). The mean electrical axis is +90°. Note the normal, small amplitudes of complexes in all leads.[6] (Courtesy of C.V. Mosby)

uncommon for complexes to be small and essentially isoelectric in all frontal plane leads. The electrical axis cannot be calculated easily in these situations.

Atrial Enlargement: The P wave represents atrial depolarization. In right atrial enlargement (hypertrophy or dilation), the P wave may be of increased amplitude in leads II, III and aVF. In left atrial enlargement, the P wave is of increased duration and best seen in lead II.

Electrocardiographic diagnosis of atrial enlargement is often inaccurate. Right atrial enlargement can occur with severe chronic respiratory disease, tricuspid dysplasia and occasionally hypertrophic cardiomyopathy. Left atrial enlargement can occur with all forms of cardiomyopathy, some congenital heart defects, and mitral valvular insufficiency. Biatrial enlargement is most often seen with chronic, advanced, hypertrophic cardiomyopathy (Fig 5). Possible mechanisms for P wave abnormalities include elevated end-diastolic pressure with resistance to atrial emptying, distortion of the atrioventricular valves by a hypertrophied ventricular septum, diffuse myocardial fibrosis causing intra-atrial conduction abnormalities, and cardiomyopathies with accompanying atrial enlargement. Electrocardiographic features of atrial enlargement include a P wave with a height greater than 0.2 mv, usually slender and peaked (right atrial enlargement), or a P wave with a width greater than 0.04 sec (left atrial enlargement).

Right Ventricular Enlargement: Right ventricular enlargement often is not evident electrocardiographically unless it is pronounced. Prolongation of the QRS complex does not occur without conduction delay in the right bundle branch. Associated conditions include pulmonic stenosis, tetralogy of Fallot, right-to-left shunts, common atrioventricular canal and heartworm disease. Right ventricular enlargement is uncommon with cardiomyopathy. When it does occur it usually accompanies dilated cardiomyopathy or is secondary to chronic left heart failure associated with hypertrophic or restrictive cardiomyopathies.

Electrocardiographic criteria for right ventricular enlargement have not been well established. The most common signs include S waves

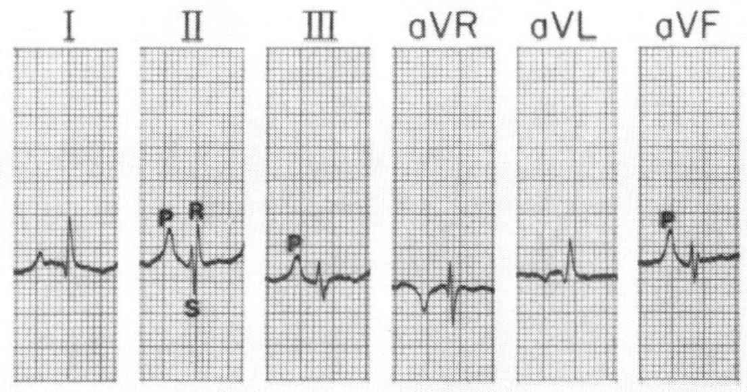

Fig 5. Tracings from a kitten with biatrial enlargement associated with a common atrioventricular canal (septal defect). The P waves are both abnormally wide and abnormally tall in leads II, III and aVF.[6] (Courtesy of C.V Mosby)

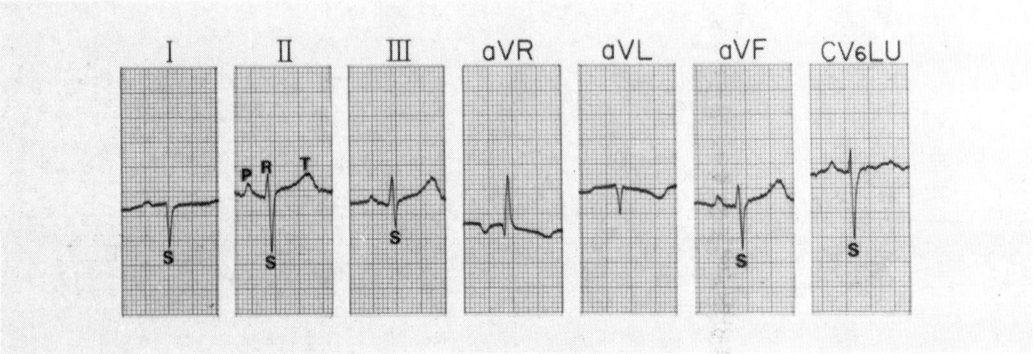

Fig 6. Tracings from a cat with a severe right ventricular enlargement associated with pulmonic stenosis. There is a right axis deviation of about −150°. Note the large S waves in leads I, II, III, aVF and CV_6LU.[6] (Courtesy of C.V. Mosby)

in leads I, II, III and aVF, a clockwise mean electrical axis of the QRS complex in the frontal plane of more than +160°, large S waves in leads CV_6LL and CV_6LU, a positive T wave in lead V_{10}, and right atrial enlargement (Fig 6).[10,11]

Left Ventricular Enlargement: Left ventricular enlargement may indicate dilation or hypertrophy and is common in cardiomyopathic cats, especially the hypertrophic form. Due to the increased muscle mass in hypertrophy, the height of the R wave is increased, the QRS complex is delayed or altered, the S-T segment is depressed, and the T wave or repolarization process is changed (Fig 7). Associated conditions include aortic stenosis, patent ductus arteriosus, ventricular septal defect, hypertrophic and dilated cardiomyopathy, and hyperthyroidism. A positive relationship may exist between renal disease and hypertension with secondary left ventricular hypertrophy. However, this has not been well documented in cats. Electrocardiographic features include an R wave exceeding 0.9 mv in lead II and 1.0 mv in CV_6LU, or QRS complex with a duration greater than 0.04 sec, displacement of the ST segment, repolarization changes causing a T wave with an increased amplitude (greater than 0.3 mv in lead II), and a mean electrical axis deviation in the frontal plane of less than 0°. Other conditions associated with left ventricular enlargement are left or right atrial enlargement and intraventricular conduction defects (left anterior fascicle may be affected from subendocardial fibrosis in left ventricular hypertrophy in hypertrophic cardiomyopathy). Conduction defects may invalidate electrocardiographic features of left ventricular enlargement.

Intraventricular Conduction Defects: An intraventricular conduction defect results from a delay or block in one or more of the conduction

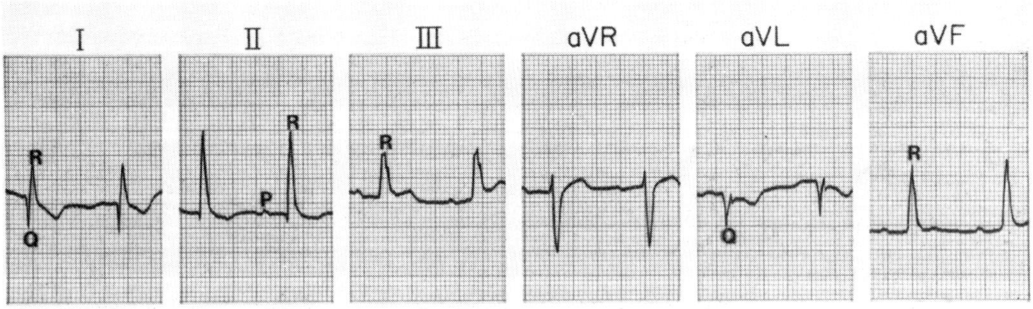

Fig 7. Tracings from a cat with left ventricular enlargement. Note the increased width and amplitude of the QRS complexes in leads II and aVF. Asymmetric septal hypertrophy, with severe obstruction of the left ventricular outflow tract, was found at necropsy.[1] (Courtesy of Am J Path)

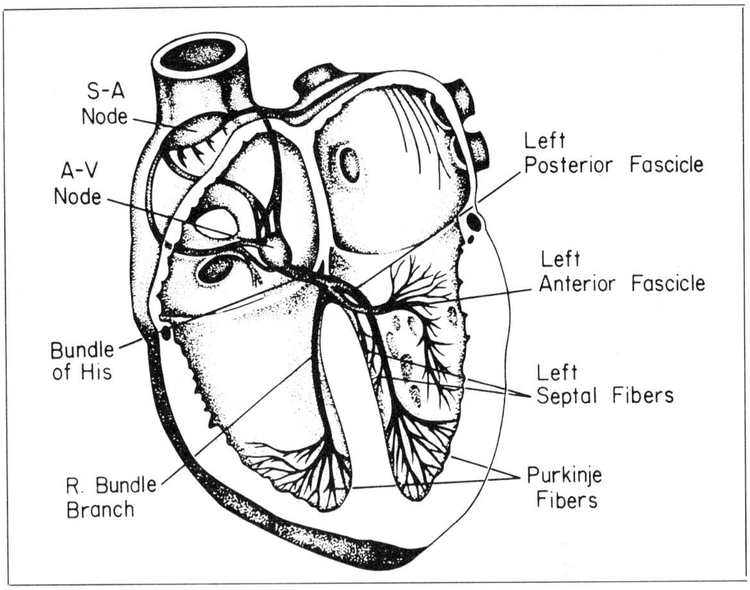

Fig 8. Conduction system of the heart.[11] (Courtesy of W.B. Saunders)

system pathways below the bundle of His. A block can occur in one or all of the 3 major pathways (fascicles) (Fig 8). Intraventricular conduction defects are common in cardiomyopathic cats, especially the hypertrophic form (left anterior fascicular block).

A block or delay in conduction of any of the major pathways causes the affected side to depolarize late. In right or left bundle branch block, the duration of the QRS complex is lengthened. Criteria for diagnosis are extrapolated from those in dogs and people.

Left Bundle Branch Block: Left bundle branch block is a delay or block of conduction in the main left bundle branch or at the level of the anterior and posterior fascicles (Fig 9). These 2 anatomic types cannot be distinguished electrocardiographically.

Electrocardiographic features include a QRS complex with a duration of 0.06 sec or greater, a QRS complex that is wide and positive in leads I, II, III, aVF and leads over the left precordium (CV_6LL, CV_6LU), an inverted QRS complex in leads aVR and CV5RL, and disturbance of the normal initial activation of the septum. Hence, initial activation of the septum is disrupted and the first part of the QRS complex is altered. The Q wave may be absent in leads that record septal activity in the right-to-left axis (leads I, CV_6LU).

Absence of left ventricular enlargement radiographically supports a diagnosis of isolated

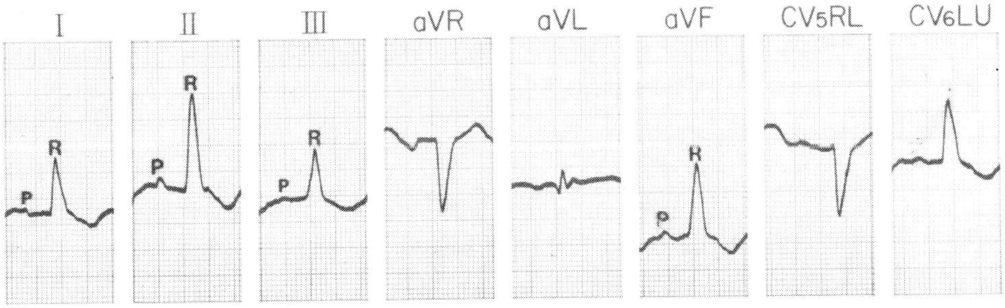

Fig 9. Tracings from a cat with left bundle branch block associated with severe hypertrophic cardiomyopathy. The QRS complex is 0.07 seconds in duration and is positive in leads I, II, III, aVF and CV_6LU. The prolonged P-R interval of 0.12 seconds may indicate involvement of the right bundle branch or the atrioventricular junction.[6] (Courtesy of C.V. Mosby)

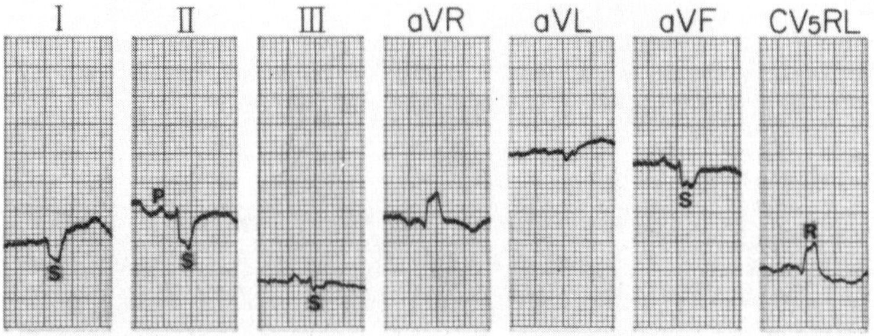

Fig 10. Tracings from a cat with right bundle branch block associated with a common atrioventricular canal. The QRS duration is 0.07 seconds. Large and wide S waves are present in leads I, II, III and aVF. A wide and positive R wave is present in CV_5RL. There is a right axis deviation of −135°.[6] (Courtesy of C.V. Mosby)

left bundle branch block. Left ventricular hypertrophy and left bundle branch block may occur simultaneously.

Left bundle branch block itself does not cause severe hemodynamic abnormalities. However, concurrent right bundle branch block can cause complete heart block, necessitating treatment.

Right Bundle Branch Block: Right bundle branch block refers to a delay or block of conduction in the right bundle branch, causing the terminal QRS complex to become wide and bizarre (Fig 10). It may occur in normal cats or in association with certain congenital defects, such as persistent common atrioventricular canal, cardiac neoplasia, primary myocardial disease (especially cardiomyopathy associated with increased left ventricular moderator bands), and hyperkalemia.

Electrocardiographic features include a QRS complex with a duration of 0.06 sec or greater, right axis deviation, positive QRS complex in a VR and CV_5RL, QRS complex with a wide rsR prime or RSR prime pattern (often M-shaped) in CV_5RL, wide S wave in the QRS complex of leads I, II, III, aVF, CV_6LL and CV_6LU, and an S wave or "W" pattern in lead V_{10}.[11] A diagnosis of isolated right bundle branch block is supported by exclusion of diseases causing severe ventricular enlargement. Thoracic radiographs can be used to evaluate right ventricular enlargement. Intermittent bundle branch block (dependent on tachycardia or bradycardia) may be present in serial tracings or in the same tracing.[12]

Right bundle branch block itself does not cause hemodynamic problems. Therapy should be directed at the primary disease. Complete heart block can result if the 2 fascicles of the left bundle branch are also involved.

Fascicular Block: A block in either the anterior or posterior fascicle of the left bundle causes only slight prolongation of ventricular depolarization. The direction of the depolarization is shifted toward the blocked fascicle. Fascicular blocks are common. Left anterior fascicular block most often is associated with hypertrophic cardiomyopathy.[1] Based on studies in people, the anterior fascicle is more vulnerable because it is longer and thinner, located in the turbulent flow tract of the left ventricle, and has only a single blood supply.[13] Other associated conditions

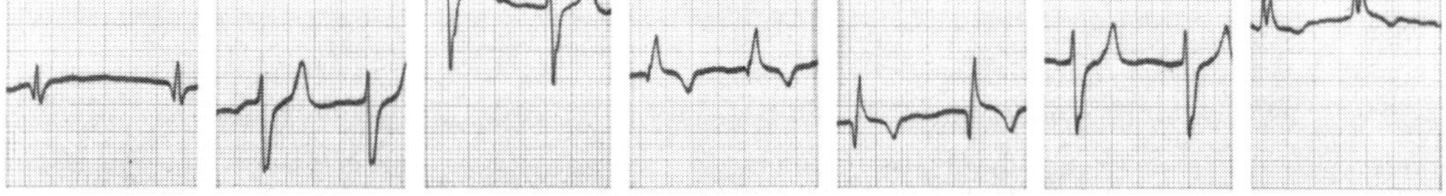

Fig 11. Tracings from a cat with right bundle branch block and left anterior fascicular block associated with hypertrophic cardiomyopathy. Note the wide QRS complex, large S waves in leads I, II, III and aVF, small Q and large R in leads I and aVL, and marked left axis deviation of −90°. Atrial fibrillation is also present, explaining the lack of P waves.[6] (Courtesy of C.V. Mosby)

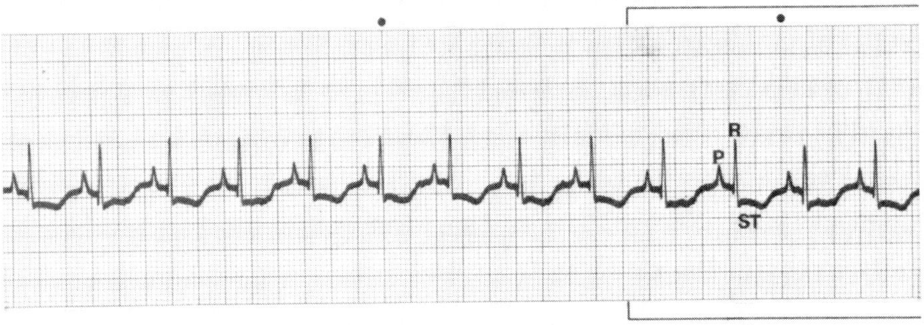

Fig 12. Depression of the S-T segment in a tracing from a cat with hypertrophic obstructive cardiomyopathy. Reduced coronary blood flow can produce myocardial ischemia.[1] (Courtesy of W.B. Saunders)

include causes of left ventricular hypertrophy (aortic stenosis) and hyperkalemia.

Electrocardiographic features include a QRS complex of normal duration or widened to less than 0.06 sec, marked left axis deviation in the frontal plane, a small Q wave and tall R wave in leads I and aVL, and deep S waves in leads II, III and aVF exceeding the small R wave (Fig 11). Other causes of the left anterior fascicular pattern should be excluded, particularly hyperkalemia and left ventricular hypertrophy, before this electrocardiographic diagnosis is made.

Fascicular blocks by themselves do not cause hemodynamic abnormalities. Therapy should be directed at the underlying primary disease, such as hyperkalemia or hypertrophic cardiomyopathy. Right bundle branch block and left anterior fascicular block may lead to second- or third-degree atrioventricular block, making treatment essential.

S-T Segment Abnormalities: The S-T segment, the early phase of ventricular repolarization represented by the end of the QRS interval to the onset of the T wave, may be elevated or depressed in comparison to the baseline (Fig 12). This may be a normal variation in some instances. Depression of the S-T segment in leads II, III, aVF and CV_6LU may occur in myocardial ischemia, hyperkalemia, hypokalemia or digitalis intoxication. Elevation of the S-T segment in leads II, III, aVF and CV_6LU may occur in myocardial infarction, pericarditis or myocardial hypoxia. Treatment should be directed at the underlying disorder.

T-Wave Abnormalities: The T wave represents the recovery period or repolarization of the ventricles. It may be positive, notched, negative or biphasic (Fig 13). Associated conditions include myocardial hypoxia, intraventricular conduction defects, electrolyte imbalances, metabolic

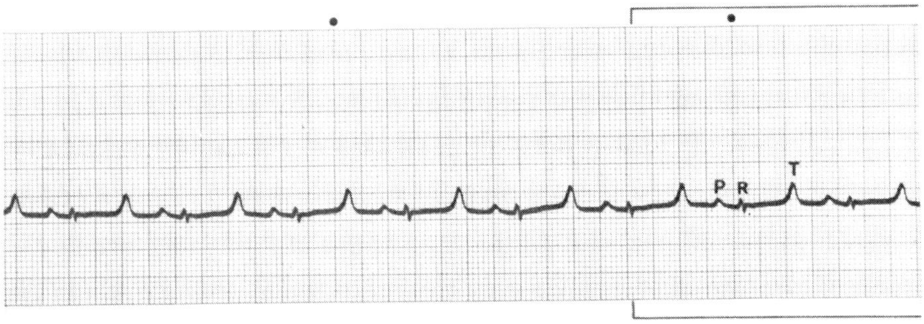

Fig 13. Large and peaked T waves in a tracing from a cat with hyperkalemia. The serum K level was 6.8 mEq/L due to urethral obstruction. The prolonged Q-T interval of 0.23 seconds is also seen with hyperkalemia.[6] (Courtesy of C.V. Mosby)

disease and drug toxicity. Normally the T wave height rarely exceeds 0.3 mv.[9] The T wave is normally slightly asymmetric. Sharply pointed or notched T waves suggest underlying abnormalities. Furthermore, a pronounced change in the morphology of the T wave on serial ECGs usually is abnormal. Although the T wave may be positive or negative, usually it is positive in lead II or in leads with a dominant R wave. Reversal of T-wave polarity on serial ECGs often is abnormal. Treatment is directed toward the underlying cause.

Analysis of Arrhythmias

Arrhythmias include abnormalities in the rate, regularity or origin of impulses and include disturbances in conduction. Anatomic or physiologic abnormalities of impulse formation and conduction (arrhythmias) provide a basis for classification (Table 2).[6]

Table 2. Classification of Arrhythmias[6]

Sinus Rhythm
- normal sinus rhythm
- sinus tachycardia
- sinus bradycardia
- sinus arrhythmia
- wandering sinus pacemaker

Abnormalities of Impulse Formation
- supraventricular
  - sinus arrest
  - atrial premature complexes
  - atrial tachycardia
  - atrial flutter
  - atrial fibrillation
- atrioventricular junction
  - atrioventricular junctional premature complexes
  - atrioventricular junctional escape rhythm
  - atrioventricular junctional tachycardia
- ventricular
  - ventricular premature complexes
  - ventricular tachycardia
  - ventricular flutter or fibrillation
  - ventricular asystole
  - ventricular escape rhythm

Abnormalities of Impulse Conduction
- sinoatrial block
- atrial standstill
- atrioventricular block
  - first degree
  - second degree
  - third degree (complete heart block)

Abnormalities of Impulse Formation and Conduction
- pre-excitation (Wolff-Parkinson-White syndrome, reciprocal rhythm)

(Courtesy of C.V. Mosby)

Knowledge of the anatomy and physiology of the impulse-forming and conducting system of the heart is essential for accurate analysis of cardiac arrythmias. Activation of the myocardium results from spontaneous pacemaker tissue discharge and impulse conduction from cell to cell. The conduction system is composed of the sinoatrial node, internodal tracts, atrioventricular node, the bundle of His and the bundle branches. The sinoatrial node has the highest automaticity and exhibits the fastest inherent discharge rate. Cells from the rest of the conduction system have slower rates of inherent discharge. The normal cardiac rhythm is termed sinoatrial or sinus rhythm because the rate and rhythm are controlled by the sinoatrial node. Pronounced sinus arrhythmia, commonly auscultated in dogs, is rare in cats. Therefore, an irregular cardiac rhythm in a cat generally is considered abnormal. Fright or excitement stimulates the sympathetic nervous system and increases heart rate (may exceed 260 beats/minute) during electrocardiographic examination.

A systematic approach to evaluation of arrhythmias should be developed and followed routinely. General inspection of the ECG is followed by determination of P-QRS-T regularity or irregularity, frequency and repetition of abnormalities. This should help distinguish whether a normal sinus rhythm or an arrhythmia is present. Rhythm strip lead II is used for these analyses. The lead should be scrutinized for discrete P waves, which sometimes may be better visualized in precordial chest leads. The absence of P waves may signify atrial fibrillation, atrial standstill, low-voltage atrial activity, metabolic abnormalities (hyperkalemia) or P waves buried in QRS complexes of atrioventricular junctional rhythms. Alternatively, the P waves may be superimposed on the QRS complex, the S-T segment or T wave of the preceding complex. Recognition of QRS complexes should be made with attention to their morphology, uniformity and regularity. Normal-appearing QRS complexes may be "supraventricular" in origin, whereas wide QRS complexes may suggest ectopic pacemaker activity below the bundle of His ("ventricular") or an intraventricular conduction abnormality. Fusion complexes may occur when one impulse is conducted to the ventricle from the sinoatrial node at the same time an-

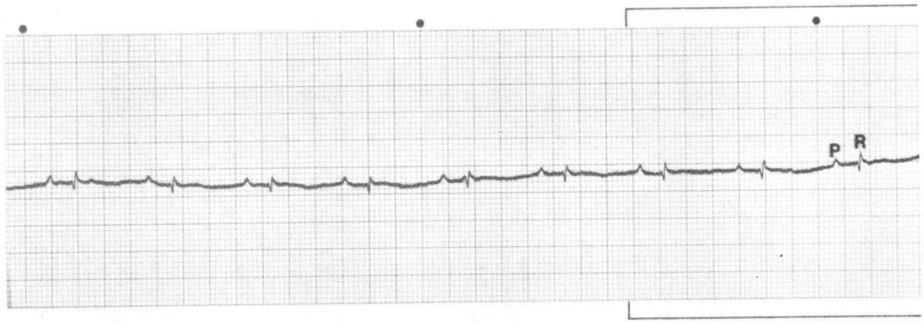

Fig 14. Tracing from a cat with normal sinus rhythm. The heart rate is 160 beats/minute. The rhythm is regular, with no variance in P-P intervals.[6] (Courtesy of C.V. Mosby)

other impulse arrives from a ventricular ectopic pacemaker.

Relationships between P waves and QRS complexes should be scrutinized. The P-R interval is a measure of atrioventricular conduction. Prolonged P-R intervals may indicate a delay in atrioventricular conduction or first-degree heart block. Abnormally short P-R intervals suggest accessory conduction around the atrioventricular node or an atrioventricular junctional rhythm, in which the P wave is situated close to the QRS complex. Second-degree atrioventricular block is present when some P waves are not followed by QRS complexes. Complete (third-degree) heart block may be present when conduction from atrial and ventricular foci occurs independently. Thus, in evaluation of the ECG, the predominant rhythm should be elucidated; it should be determined if the arrhythmia represents an abnormality of impulse formation or impulse conduction. The site of the abnormality should be identified.

Arrhythmias may have variable effects upon normal hemodynamics. Rapid, slow or irregular rhythms can cause cardiac output to decrease, especially when myocardial function is impaired by heart disease. The underlying cause of the arrhythmia should be established since this may affect the clinical approach, interpretation, prognosis and therapy. Arrhythmias may be influenced by the autonomic nervous system (excitement, exercise, pain, fever, respiratory influences on vagal tone, or organic brain disease with sympathetic or vagal stimulation). Cardiac-initiated arrhythmias include those of a hereditary nature, neoplasia and diseases of the atria or ventricles. Noncardiac categories include hypoxia, acid-base disturbances, electrolyte imbalances (especially hyperkalemia), drugs and mechanical stimulation (faulty placement of venous catheter tip in the right atrium or right ventricle).

Normal Sinus Rhythm: The sinoatrial node is the dominant pacemaker and usually depolarizes from 160 to 240 beats/minute in adult cats (Fig 14). During examination the heart rate may increase because of sympathetic stimulation due to excitement. Conversely, increased vagal stimulation may slow the heart rate.

Sinus Arrhythmia: Sinus arrhythmia is an irregular rhythm originating in the sinoatrial node. Manifested by alternating periods of slow and rapid heart rates, it is an uncommon and usually abnormal finding (Fig 15). It may be accompanied by a wandering pacemaker due to a shift in pacemaker activity in the sinoatrial node. The P wave morphology may change but the P-R interval remains basically constant. Vagal stimulation from digitalis toxicity, severe respiratory disease or other influences may cause this arrhythmia. Treatment is directed at the underlying condition.

Sinus Tachycardia and Sinus Bradycardia: A regular sinus rhythm slower than the normal heart rate constitutes sinus bradycardia; that above the normal heart rate represents sinus tachycardia. Sinus tachycardia is the most common arrhythmia in cats and may be related to physiologic causes, such as pain or restraint during examination. Fever, shock, anemia, infection, congestive heart failure, hypoxia and hyperthyroidism may represent pathologic forms of sinus tachycardia. Sinus bradycardia may occur with systemic disease, toxicity (renal failure), hypothermia, dilated cardiomyopathy, general anesthesia, electrolyte disturbances (especially hyperkalemia), and in agonal phases of

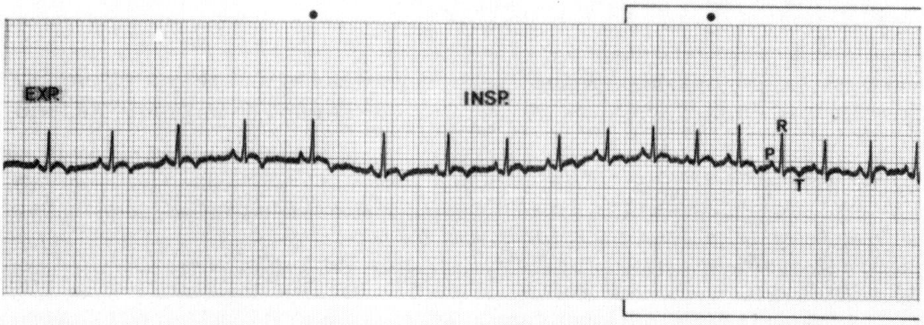

Fig 15. Respiratory sinus arrhythmia in a tracing from a normal cat. The rate increases during inspiration (INSP) and decreases during expiration (EXP). (Paper speed 25 mm/sec.)[6] (Courtesy of C.V. Mosby)

various diseases (Fig 16). Tachycardia can be induced by various drugs, such as atropine, epinephrine or ketamine; bradycardia may result from use of propranolol, digoxin, general anesthetics and lidocaine.

Treatment of sinus tachycardia involves identifying and controlling the underlying cause. Use of propranolol in cats with hypertrophic cardiomyopathy counteracts the effects of stress and the accompanying catecholamine influence on the sinoatrial node. Sinus bradycardia may indicate a serious underlying cardiac or extracardiac disorder and necessitates immediate attention. Atropine may be given IV if life-threatening bradycardia is present.

Atrial Premature Complexes: Atrial premature complexes represent impulses arising from ectopic atrial foci. Also known as atrial extrasystoles and atrial premature contractions, they most commonly occur as a consequence of cardiac disease. Atrial tachycardia, atrial fibrillation or atrial flutter are potential sequelae to atrial premature complexes. Associated conditions include atrial enlargement secondary to dilated, hypertrophic or restrictive cardiomyopathy, congenital cardiac anomalies with atrial enlargement, metastatic tumors, chronic atrioventricular valvular insufficiencies in older cats, digitalis toxicity, general anesthesia and traumatic myocarditis.

Electrocardiographic features usually include a normal heart rate with a disruptive rhythm due to premature P waves. The morphology of the ectopic premature P wave is different from that of the sinus P wave (Fig 17). It may be negative, positive, biphasic or superimposed on the previous T wave. In addition, the QRS complex is premature, although its configuration usually is normal. The QRS complex may be absent if the premature P wave occurs too early during the refractory period of the atrioventricular node, preventing ventricular conduction. With partial recovery of the atrioventricular node or intraventricular conduction system, the

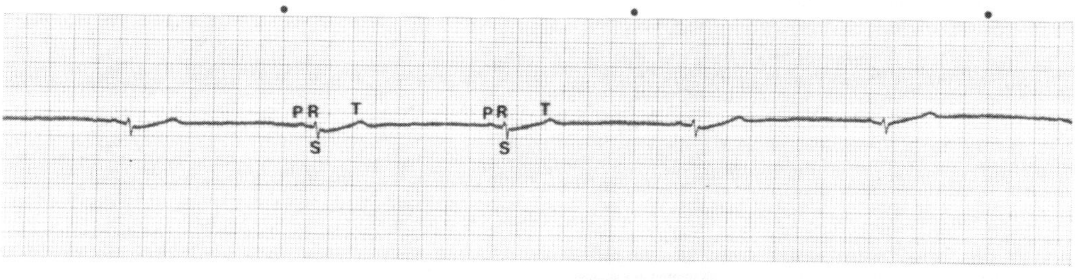

Fig 16. Tracing from a cat with sinus bradycardia due to anesthetic complications during surgery. The heart rate is 75 beats/minute. Termination of anesthesia, administration of 0_2 and atropine, and close monitoring are immediately indicated.[6] (Courtesy of C.V. Mosby)

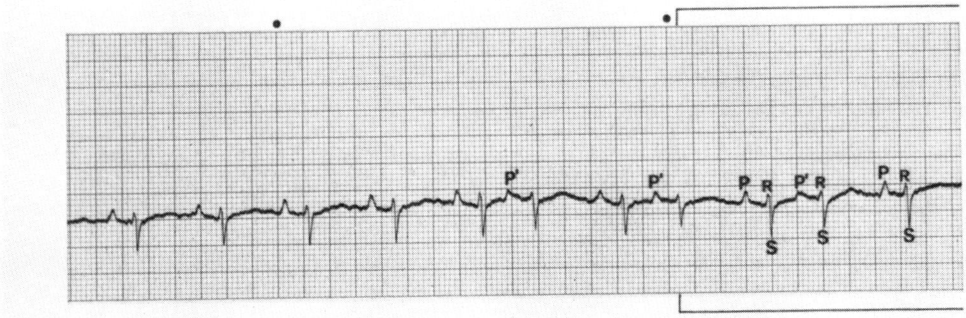

Fig 17. Tracing showing 3 atrial premature complexes in a bigeminal rhythm after the first 5 sinus complexes. The premature P' waves are slightly different from the sinus P waves.[6] (Courtesy of C.V. Mosby)

premature P wave is conducted with a long P-R interval or a change in the normal QRS configuration (aberrant conduction). A noncompensatory pause usually follows an atrial premature complex.

Atrial premature complexes usually decrease in frequency or disappear with rest. Specific antiarrhythmic drugs are rarely needed. Propranolol is beneficial in cats with hypertrophic cardiomyopathy. Treatment is directed toward the underlying condition.

Atrial Tachycardia: Atrial tachycardia is a rapid, regular rhythm originating from a focus in the atria distant from the sinoatrial node (Fig 18). Three or more consecutive atrial premature complexes constitute atrial tachycardia. The term "supraventricular tachycardia" may be used when atrial flutter (atrial rates greater than 300 beats/minute) cannot be differentiated from atrial tachycardia. Associated conditions include diseases causing severe atrial enlargement (most often hypertrophic cardiomyopathy), ventricular pre-excitation (Wolff-Parkinson-White syndrome) and cardiac neoplasia.

Electrocardiographic features include an atrial rhythm in excess of 240 beats/minute, displayed in intermittent paroxysms or as a continuous rhythm. Premature P waves may not be easily seen because of the fast ventricular rate. Configuration of the premature P waves is generally different from that of sinus P waves. The QRS complex configuration is usually normal, although bizarre changes may be due to bundle branch block, aberrant ventricular conduction or ventricular pre-excitation. Varying degrees of atrioventricular block may occur in the presence of a rapid atrial rate, preventing the atrioventricular junction from repolarizing normally. This contributes to lack of conduction of some atrial impulses to the ventricles.

Atrial tachycardia and atrial flutter are usually transient arrhythmias. Although digoxin may be the drug of choice in dogs, it is frequently contraindicated in cats with hypertrophic cardiomyopathy unless the arrhythmia is absolutely uncontrollable and no outflow obstruction is present. Use of propranolol and application of carotid or ocular pressure are often effective in converting the arrhythmia. Propranolol is rel-

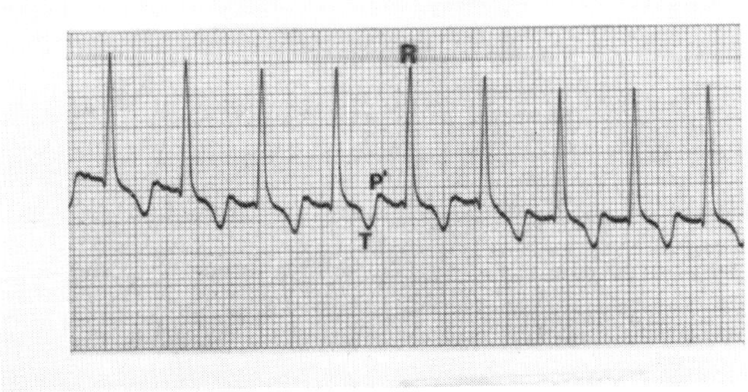

Fig 18. Atrial tachycardia, with a heart rate of 250 beats/minute. This cat had pulmonary carcinoma and secondary cardiac involvement. Note the tall and wide QRS complexes, which indicate left ventricular enlargement.[6] (Courtesy of C.V. Mosby)

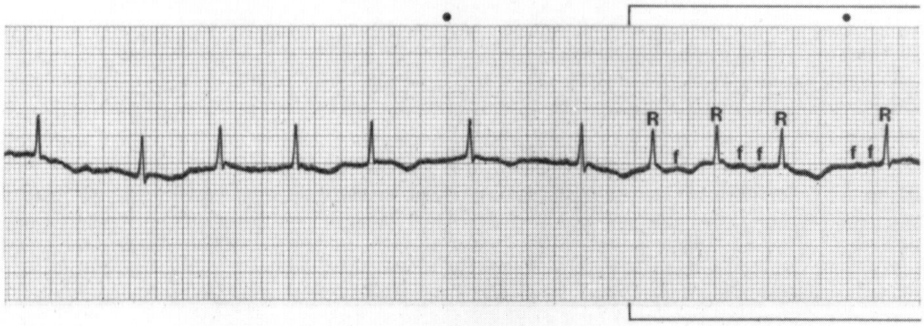

Fig 19. Atrial fibrillation, with an average ventricular rate of 200 beats/minute. This tracing is from a cat with hypertrophic cardiomyopathy. Note the irregularity of the R waves and the absence of P waves, which are replaced by f waves.[6] (Courtesy of C.V. Mosby)

atively contraindicated in the presence of congestive heart failure. However, it may be useful in preventing atrial arrhythmias in hypertrophic cardiomyopathy. Electrical cardioversion or intracardiac pacing may be attempted in the event of uncontrollable, life-threatening arrhythmia.

Atrial Fibrillation: Atrial fibrillation is rare in cats. It is primarily associated with hypertrophic cardiomyopathy, although it has been observed with restrictive and dilated cardiomyopathy. Hypertrophic and restrictive (endocardial fibrosis) cardiomyopathy causes a chronic, increased resistance to left ventricular filling. This results in severe left atrial enlargement and occasionally atrial fibrillation. Electrocardiographic features include a very rapid and irregular heart rate. The normal sinus P wave may be replaced by small, fibrillating ("F") waves (Fig 19). The QRS configuration is normal or wide and bizarre due to intraventricular conduction defects or ventricular pre-excitation.

Digoxin should be administered with caution in cats with hypertrophic cardiomyopathy. However, it is not contraindicated in cats with hypertrophic cardiomyopathy and atrial fibrillation. Propranolol may be added after the cat is adequately digitalized to further slow the ventricular rate.

Escape Rhythms: Escape rhythms occur when the pacemaker with the highest automaticity (usually the sinoatrial node) slows or stops. Slower intrinsic pacemaker activity of lower cardiac regions "rescues" the heart rhythm after a pause in the dominant rhythm. A single, spontaneous impulse from a lower subsidiary pacemaker appearing after a pause is called an escape complex. Escape complexes are most often atrioventricular junctional or ventricular in origin. When ventricular escape impulses con-

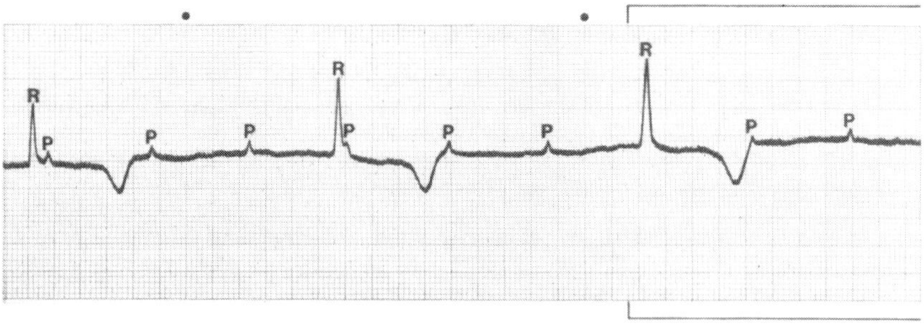

Fig 20. Ventricular escape rhythm in a tracing from a cat with complete atrioventricular block. None of the atrial impulses (P waves) are conducted into the ventricles. The sinoatrial node pacemaker and escape pacemaker fire independently. Some P waves are superimposed on QRS complexes.[6] (Courtesy of C.V. Mosby)

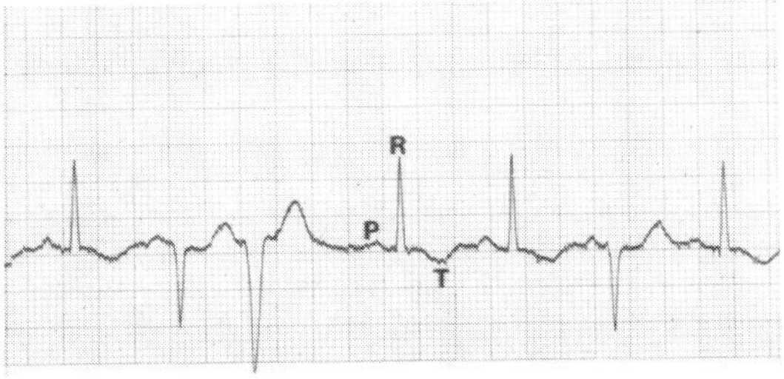

Fig 21. Multiform ventricular ectopic complexes (second, third and sixth complexes) in a tracing from a cat with dilated cardiomyopathy. The second and sixth complexes are shaped differently from the third and follow the simultaneous activation of the ventricles from the sinoatrial node and the ventricular ectopic foci.[6] (Courtesy of C.V. Mosby)

trol the rhythm, the term "idioventricular rhythm" or "idionodal rhythm" is used instead of ventricular escape rhythm. Escape rhythms may occur in association with all causes of sinus bradycardia and atrioventricular block.

The heart rate is slow with junctional escape rhythms. Escape complexes follow a pause that is longer than the normal cycle length (P-P interval). The rhythm is regular when the atrioventricular junction persists as the dominant pacemaker. Here, the P wave usually is negative but the QRS configuration is normal; the P wave may precede, be superimposed on or follow the QRS complex.

Subsidiary pacemakers in cats seem to discharge more rapidly than in dogs. The P waves are not often present unless complete atrioventricular block or high-grade, second-degree atrioventricular block exists. The P waves are then unrelated and precede, are hidden within or follow the ectopic (escape or capture) QRS complexes (Fig 20). The QRS configuration is wide and bizarre (unless a junctional escape rhythm is present), similar to that of ventricular premature complexes. No relationship exists between the P wave and QRS complex.

The escape complex or rhythm should not be treated. It is often the only safety mechanism ensuring and maintaining an adequate cardiac output. The underlying cause of the arrhythmia should be addressed and treated. Use of causative drugs (digoxin, propranolol, anesthetics) should be discontinued. Use of atropine may be indicated.

Ventricular Premature Complexes: Ventricular premature complexes (ventricular premature contractions) are impulses arising from ectopic ventricular foci (Fig 21). Causes include primary myocardial disease (especially dilated cardiomyopathy), infarction, neoplasia, traumatic myocarditis, congestive heart failure, bacterial endomyocarditis, secondary causes (hypoxia, anemia, uremia, pyometra), faulty placement of a venous catheter (into the right ventricle) and use of certain drugs (digitalis, anesthetics, phenytoin).

Electrocardiographic features include premature QRS complexes that disrupt normal sinus rhythm. The QRS complex is premature, bizarre, large and usually followed by a compensatory pause. The T wave is directed opposite the main deflection of the QRS complex. Independent normal P waves may precede, be within or follow the ventricular premature complex.

Treatment should be directed toward the underlying condition. Ventricular premature contractions rarely require aggressive treatment because they tend to disappear spontaneously. Underlying congestive heart failure, acid-base and electrolyte imbalances should be corrected. Propranolol may be cautiously administered IV in small doses in refractory cases.

Ventricular Tachycardia: Ventricular tachycardia implies a series of repetitive ventricular premature contractions, at a rate of 150 beats/minute or more, that are usually of sudden onset (Fig 22). It may be intermittent (3 or more in a row) or persistent. Conversely, an idioventricular escape rhythm is generally less than 100 beats/minute. Ventricular tachycardia usually indicates significant cardiac disease and has been associated with acute myocardial infarction, anesthesia and cardiomyopathy.

Treatment should commence immediately. The underlying disease must be addressed. Supportive measures include correction of acid-base and electrolyte abnormalities and treatment of congestive heart failure, if present. Lidocaine should be used with utmost caution in cats because of their inability to adequately and rapidly

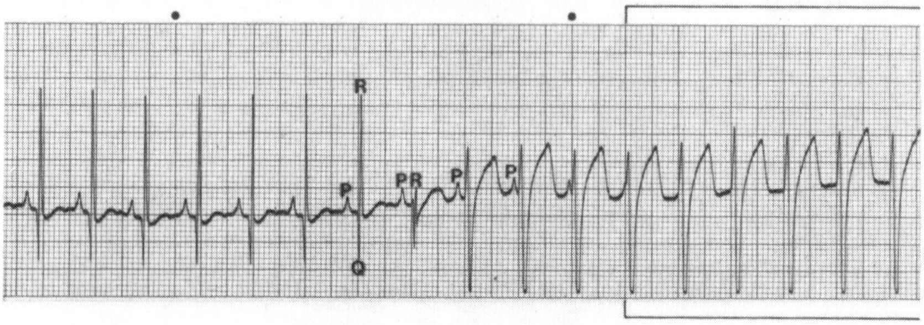

Fig 22. Ventricular tachycardia, with a heart rate of 150 beats/minute, initiated by a ventricular fusion complex in a tracing from a cat with dilated cardiomyopathy and congestive heart failure. The first 7 complexes are all normal sinus complexes. (Paper speed 25 mm/sec.)[6] (Courtesy of C.V. Mosby)

metabolize this drug. Quinidine and procainamide have not been used extensively in cats and should be avoided. A thump on the chest wall over the heart, as a form of cardioversion, may be attempted when other therapeutic regimens are not available.

Ventricular Fibrillation and Asystole: Ventricular fibrillation and ventricular asystole represent cardiac arrest (Fig 23). Irreversible brain damage may occur if the ventricular rhythm is not restored within 3-4 minutes. Cardiac arrest can also be detected if a recordable ECG (P-QRS-T complexes) occurs with absence of palpable femoral pulses. This is termed "electrical-mechanical dissociation." Cardiopulmonary resuscitation should be started immediately in these situations. For ventricular fibrillation, defibrillation with direct current shock may be used. Intracardiac epinephrine and $CaCl_2$ can be given to "coarsen" the fibrillation. For ventricular asystole, epinephrine, $NaHCO_3$, $CaCl_2$, atropine sulfate and IV or intracardiac isoproterenol may be employed in specific instances. The various dosages of these drugs are listed in Table 5.

First-Degree Atrioventricular Block: A delay or interruption in conduction of a supraventricular impulse to the atrioventricular junction and bundle of His is called atrioventricular block. There are 3 types or degrees of atrioventricular block. First-degree block involves a delay in conduction, second-degree block involves intermittent interruptions of conduction, and third-degree block consists of complete or permanent interruption of conduction.

First-degree atrioventricular block may occur in normal cats. Causes include digitalis intoxication, propranolol intoxication, hyperkalemia, hypokalemia and cardiomyopathy (especially dilative).

Electrocardiographic features include a P-R interval longer than 0.09 sec (Fig 24). The P wave and QRS complex are usually of normal configuration. Heart rate and rhythm depend on the presence or absence of other arrhythmias.

Treatment should be directed toward the underlying condition. Consideration should be given to progression to higher degrees of atrioventric-

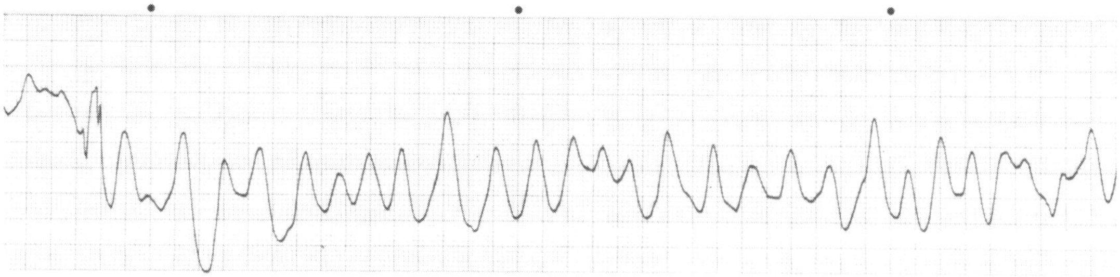

Fig 23. Ventricular flutter-fibrillation in a tracing from a cat with severe myocardial injury from an 11-story fall. The complexes are very wide, bizarre, tall and rapid.[6] (Courtesy of C.V. Mosby)

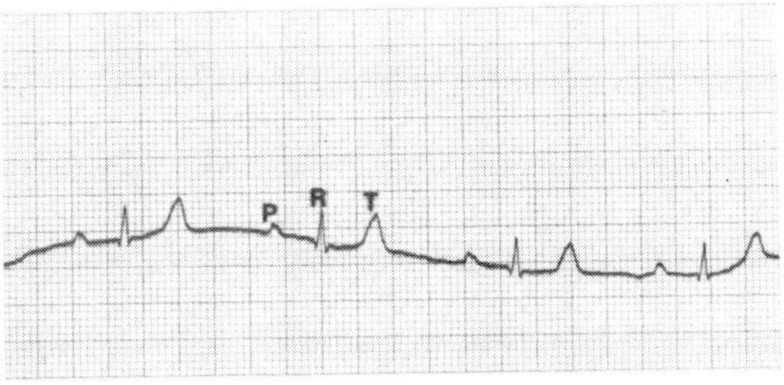

Fig 24. First-degree atrioventricular block in a tracing from a cat with hyperkalemia (serum K level of 7.5 mEq/L). The P-R interval is 0.12 sec. Note the large T waves.[6] (Courtesy of C.V. Mosby)

ular block if an intraventricular conduction defect is also present.

Second-Degree Atrioventricular Block: Second-degree atrioventricular block is characterized by intermittent failure or disturbances of atrioventricular conduction. One or more P waves are not followed by QRS-T complexes (Fig 25). Second-degree atrioventricular block can be classified as Mobitz type I and Mobitz type II. As in dogs, classification can also be based on the QRS duration. A type-A block involves a lesion above the His bundle, with normal QRS complex duration; a type-B block is associated with a lesion below the His bundle, with a wide QRS complex.[14] Conditions associated with second-degree atrioventricular block include supraventricular tachycardia with resultant physiologic block, increased vagal tone, and hypertrophic cardiomyopathy.

In a Mobitz type-I (usually type-A) block, the ventricular rate is slower than the atrial rate because of blocked P waves. The rhythm typically is regular. The P wave and QRS complex usually are of normal configuration. In the typical Mobitz type-I block (Wenkebach phenomenon), progressive prolongation of successive P-R intervals occurs until a P wave is blocked.

In a Mobitz type-II (usually type-B) block, the ventricular rate is also slower than the atrial rate because of blocked P waves. The P waves usually are normal, although the QRS complexes often are abnormal morphologically, exhibiting features of bundle branch block. The P-R interval is always constant. Mobitz type-II (type-B) atrioventricular blocks may progress to higher degrees of atrioventricular block. Two or more consecutively blocked P waves denote advanced atrioventricular block. The presence of ventricular capture complexes indicates that the block is not complete.

Most affected cats usually develop an advanced or complete atrioventricular block. Accompanying clinical signs, such as fainting and weakness, may occur. These cats usually are resistant to medical management; implantation of an artificial pacemaker is the only effective treatment.

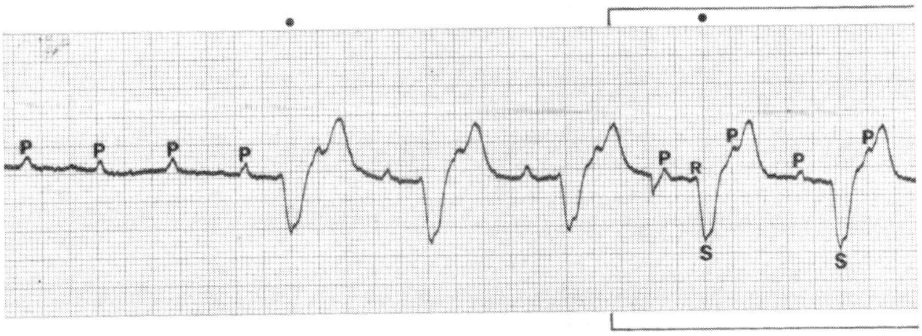

Fig 25. Advanced atrioventricular block (type B), with right bundle branch block, in a tracing from a cat with metastatic lymphosarcoma. Every second P wave is conducted (2:1 block) after the first 3 P waves.[6] (Courtesy of C.V. Mosby)

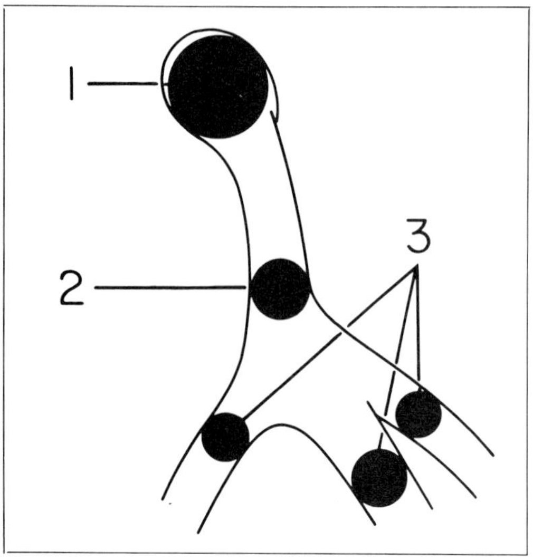

Fig 26. The 3 possible sites of lesions causing complete heart block. 1. atrioventricular node, 2. bundle of His, 3. right bundle branch and left bundle branch (anterior and posterior fascicles).[6] (Courtesy of C.V. Mosby)

Third-Degree Atrioventricular Block: Third-degree (complete) atrioventricular block occurs when atrioventricular conduction is absent and the ventricles are under the influence of subsidiary pacemakers below the area of the block (Figs 26, 27). The atria are thus activated by one pacemaker, usually the sinoatrial node, and the ventricles by another. No relationship between P waves and the QRS complex exists (Fig 27).

Most cases of complete atrioventricular block have been recorded in association with cardiomyopathy.[6] Complete block has also been observed with hypertrophic, dilated and infiltrative cardiomyopathy (with metastatic lymphosarcoma), and in FeLV-positive cats without evidence of lymphosarcoma. Lesions of the atrioventricular node and its bundle branches (degeneration or fibrosis) are commonly associated with endocardial and myocardial fibrosis in cats with cardiomyopathy.[15] Electrocardiographically, however, most cats with cardiomyopathy have normal atrioventricular conduction or first-degree atrioventricular block. Second- and third-degree atrioventricular blocks are rare.

Electrocardiographic features include a ventricular rate that is slower than the atrial rate (more P waves than QRS complexes). The P waves are usually of normal configuration. The QRS complex is wide and bizarre when the pacemaker focus is located in the ventricle but is normal when the escape pacemaker is located in the lower atrioventricular junction (above the His bundle bifurcation). The P waves bear no constant relationship to the QRS complexes. The P-P and R-R intervals are relatively constant.

Ventricular Pre-Excitation: Ventricular pre-excitation is rare in cats and occurs when impulses originating in the sinoatrial node or atrium activate a portion of the ventricles prematurely through an accessory pathway without going through the atrioventricular node. Paroxysmal supraventricular tachycardia with ventricular pre-excitation occurs by the mechanism of re-entry. An impulse traveling to the ventricles through the atrioventricular junction may turn around and re-enter the atria through the accessory pathway. Thus, a reciprocal rhythm or "electrical circuit" is established.[16]

Electrocardiographic features may include a widened QRS complex with slurring or notching of the upstroke of the R wave (delta wave) or a normal configuration of the QRS complexes (Fig

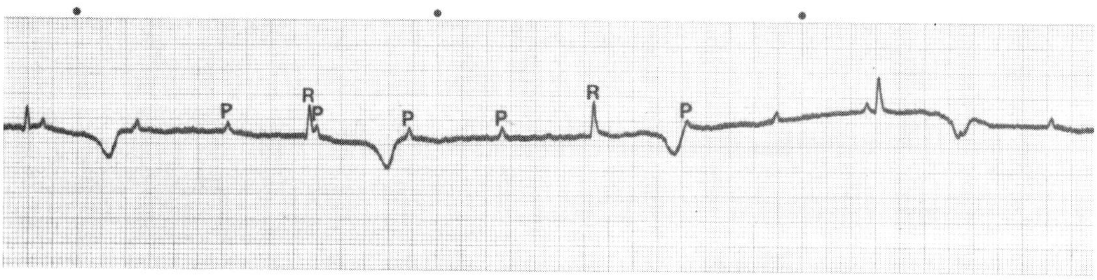

Fig 27. Tracing from a cat with complete heart block. The P waves occur at a rate of 160 beats/minute, independent of the ventricular rate of 50 beats/minute. Because the QRS complex is of normal duration and configuration, the ventricular pacemaker must be above the His bundle bifurcation.[6] (Courtesy of C.V. Mosby)

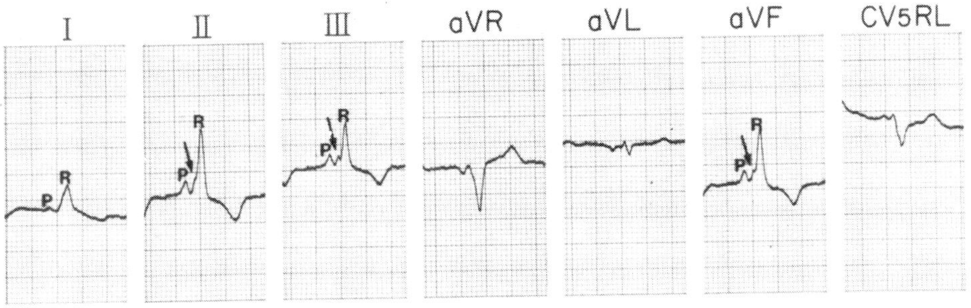

Fig 28. Tracing from a cat with ventricular pre-excitation. Note the short P-R interval in all leads and the easily recognized slur or notch (arrows) in the upstroke of the wide R wave.[6] (Courtesy of C.V. Mosby)

28). The P-R interval in ventricular pre-excitation is short. Sinus P waves may be normal or difficult to recognize.[17,18]

Ventricular pre-excitation without tachycardia does not require therapy. Cats with the Wolff-Parkinson-White syndrome with supraventricular tachycardia may require conversion using propranolol, ocular or carotid sinus pressure, or direct-current shock.

Electrical Alternans: Electrical alternans is manifested as P, QRS or T wave forms (or any combination), originating from the same focus, that alter their configuration in every other complex, every third complex, etc. A 2:1 electrical alternans is the most common alternating ratio (every other complex). The QRS complex alone usually is involved, although various combinations are possible. In dogs, electrical alternans usually is associated with pericardial effusion. Cardiac movement within the pericardial sac is rhythmic and myocardial electrical forces are altered, presumably resulting in electrical alternation.[19] This arrhythmia is rare in cats, having been observed with pericardial effusion (due to septic pericarditis or right-sided heart failure), tetralogy of Fallot, supraventricular tachycardia and cardiomyopathy.

Electrocardiographic features usually include a normal heart rate, with alternating amplitude and configuration of either the P wave or QRS complex. The P wave is always related to the QRS complex. True electrical alternans should not be confused with ventricular bigeminy or a respiratory artifact. Treatment should be directed at the underlying cause. Pericardiocentesis may be indicated if pericardial effusion is severe.

Hyperkalemia: Hyperkalemia is most commonly encountered in cats with feline urethral obstruction. "Blocked" cats may have severely affected cardiac rhythm and conduction, with often lethal consequences if untended. Other conditions, such as renal insufficiency, untreated ketoacidotic diabetes mellitus, iatrogenic K overload or metabolic acidosis, may cause similar consequences.

The electrocardiographic features of hyperkalemia include a spectrum of changes associated with the degree of severity (Fig 29). The earliest alteration is peaking of the T wave, when the serum K level exceeds 5.5 mEq/L. Intraventricular impulse conduction slows with increasing hyperkalemia; prolongation of the P-R interval, QRS complex and Q-T intervals becomes evident. The P wave amplitude decreases progressively and the S-T segment is altered. The P waves disappear (atrial standstill) when the serum K level exceeds 8.5 mEq/L, resulting in a sinoventricular rhythm. A serum K level greater than 10 mEq/L causes pronounced widening of the QRS complex, with eventual replacement by a smooth biphasic curve. Ventricular flutter, ventricular fibrillation or ventricular asystole results if the condition is not resolved.

Treatment is directed toward the cause of hyperkalemia (relieve urethral obstruction). In addition, the serum K level must be lowered. Other causes of electrolyte and acid-base imbalance must be sought and specific therapy instituted. Therapy need not be overzealous when the serum K level is less than 6.5-7.0 mEq/L. However, intensive and prompt attention must be given when serum K concentrations exceed 8.0 mEq/L. Emergency treatment includes IV injection of regular insulin at 0.5-1 unit/kg body weight. This is followed by 2 g dextrose/unit of insulin, half of which is given as an IV bolus and the other half provided in an IV fluid drip. Calcium gluconate (10%) may be added at 0.5-1 ml/kg body weight in life-threatening situations to antagonize the cardiotoxic effects of K. Sodium bicarbonate (1-2 mEq/kg body weight given IV) has been used to promote the transfer of extracellular K to an intracellular location. The ECG should be monitored throughout treatment.[6]

Drug-Induced Arrhythmias: Many drugs affect the cardiovascular system, although a drug-induced arrhythmia often abates after use of the drug is discontinued. For example, administration of inhalant anesthesia should be promptly reduced or stopped if arrhythmias occur intraoperatively. Digitalis may produce virtually any cardiac arrhythmia, although clinical signs (anorexia, vomiting) usually occur before arrhythmias are detected. Propranolol may induce severe sinus bradycardia, atrioventricular block, sinoatrial block or sinus arrest and should be used with extreme caution if congestive heart failure is present. Catecholamines and isoproterenol stimulate beta-1 cardiac receptors; increased excitability (ventricular fibrillation) or increased pacemaker automaticity (atrial or ventricular tachycardia) may result. Beta stimulation influences "irritable" myocardial tissue, which can precipitate arrhythmias in cats with myocardial disease. Lidocaine is not well tolerated by cats. Severe arrhythmias, sinus bradycardia and sinus arrest may result from use of high dosages. Ketamine and atropine may cause tachycardia. Tranquilizers can produce severe bradycardia and depress myocardial contractility and excitability.[6] Profound bradycardia and atrioventricular block may result from overdosage of xylazine.

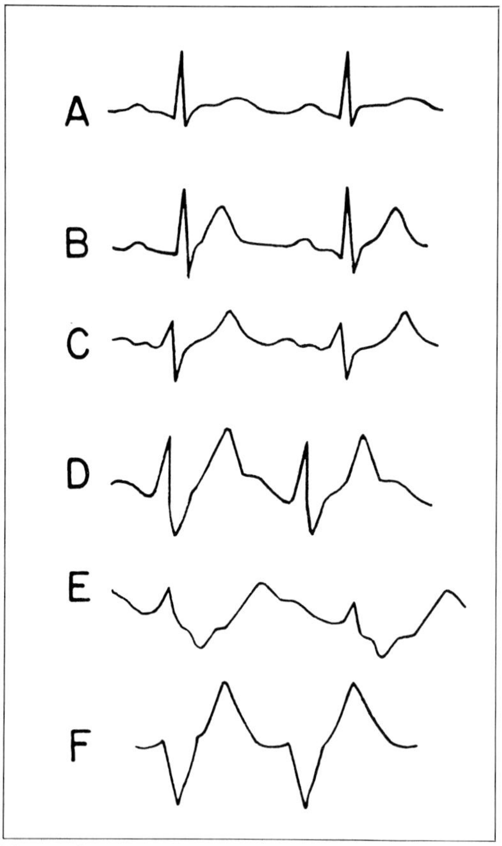

Fig 29. Progressive effects of hyperkalemia on the P-QRS-T complex. A. Normal tracing. B-F. Serial changes in hyperkalemia. [From Vet Clin No Am 7 (1977) 407, courtesy of W.B. Saunders]

Artifacts: Many technical or mechanical factors induce distortions or artifacts during recording of the ECG. When superimposed on a normal cardiac complex or rhythm, artifacts may make measurements and interpretations difficult or impossible. Various arrhythmias or conduction disturbances may be mimicked by artifacts, leading to erroneous conclusions.

Technical recording problems are common. Lead reversal, usually involving the forelimb electrodes, produces negative P waves in leads I and aVL (simulating dextrocardia). In addition, paper speed and standardization often are improperly labeled, causing heart rates and voltages to appear abnormally high or low. Electrical interference (60-cycle artifact) is due to improper grounding. Animal-related factors include muscle tremor and body movements due to struggling, respiration and coughing.

Certain clues can be used to differentiate artifacts from arrhythmias. The rhythm of artifacts is usually irregular and their frequency is variable. Also, artifacts do not interrupt atrial or ventricular rhythms whereas true arrhythmias usually do. This subject has been described and well illustrated elsewhere.[6]

Radiographic Examination

Radiographic examination is essential for a thorough and accurate evaluation of the cardiovascular system. Radiography usually is indicated if auscultation detects a murmur, gallop rhythm, rales or muffled lung and heart sounds, electrocardiographic abnormalities are found, clinical signs compatible with heart failure (dyspnea, cyanosis, hydroperitoneum) are present, acute posterior paresis or paralysis occurs, and for comparison with previous or future radiographs. Radiographs are also indicated if cardiomyopathy or cardiovascular abnormalities are suspected despite the absence of a murmur or electrocardiographic abnormalities, and to discover coexisting or unrelated disease considered in the differential diagnosis.

Information on cardiac size, shape and position, and severity of congestive heart failure can be gained by radiography. However, plain radiographs cannot measure myocardial thickness, chamber volumes or ventricular performance. Certain technical considerations are essential to ensure the diagnostic relevance of the radiographic examination. Accurate positioning is needed for assessment of anatomic abnormalities. This often necessitates tranquilization, especially in an easily stressed, compromised animal. Variations caused by malpositioning of the patient can make interpretation difficult. Exposure at peak inspiration is attempted but may be unobtainable due to rapid rates of respiration. An exposure time of 1/60 second or less is required to reduce motion.

In the lateral view, the normal cardiac silhouette lies between the fourth and sixth intercostal spaces (Fig 30).[20] The apex is at the point of intersection of the right and left ventricular borders and lies immediately above the sternum and cranial to the diaphragm. The right ventricle is cranial to the apex and becomes confluent with the right atrial border, making it nearly impossible to differentiate right atrial from right ventricular enlargement. The left heart border courses dorsad from the apex and is approximately divided from the left atrium by the caudal vena cava.[21] The cardiac base consists of the cranial vena cava, pulmonary arteries and veins, right atrium, ascending aorta, left atrium and caudal vena cava. Normally there is a definable caudal waist. However, the cranial waist may be absent if positional variation of the cardiac vertical axis causes pronounced rostral "tipping." This may confer an accentuated dorsocranial bulge due to a more acute angle between the ascending and descending aorta.

In the dorsoventral view, proper positioning requires superimposition of the sternebrae over the thoracic vertebrae (Fig 30). This is not always attainable in the untranquilized or severely dyspneic cats. The cardiac apex is normally positioned slightly to the right of the midline or occasionally on the midline. The right ventricle and atrium lie to the right of the apex. The aortic arch and descending aorta are visible but superimposed over the heart just to the left of midline. The main pulmonary artery is located in the one o'clock position. The left auricle is at 1-2 o'clock and the left ventricle occupies the rest of the left side up to the apex.

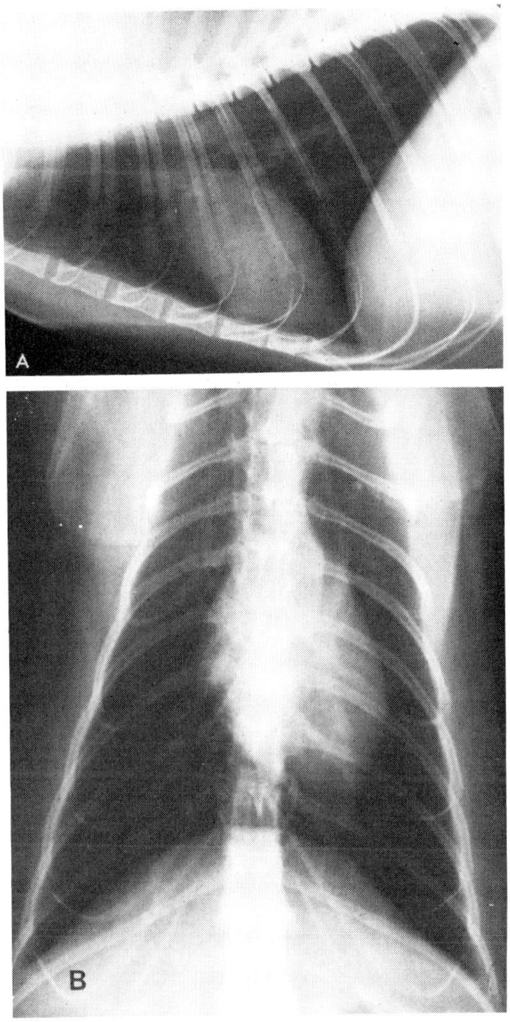

Fig 30. Normal lateral (A) and dorsoventral (B) thoracic radiographs.

Signs of right heart enlargement include increased convexity and more pronounced sternal contact on the lateral view. It causes tracheal elevation in the area of cranial waist and slight elevation of the apex from the sternum on the lateral projection. Displacement of the apex to the left may be present on the dorsoventral view. Loss of the cranial waist on the lateral view may

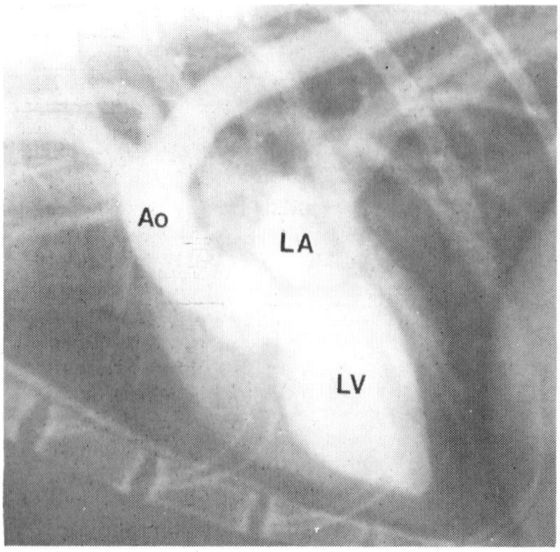

Fig 31. Normal nonselective angiocardiogram obtained about 8 seconds after the injection of contrast medium into the jugular vein. Note the normal size of the left atrium (LA), left ventricle (LV) and aorta (Ao).

occur with enlargement of right atrium (auricle), main pulmonary artery segment or aorta. Isolated right heart enlargement is uncommon but can be associated with pulmonic stenosis, tetralogy of Fallot, tricuspid insufficiency, tricuspid dysplasia, right-to-left shunts (septal defects, patent ductus arteriosus) or heartworm disease. Right heart enlargement may occur with left-sided enlargement in all forms of cardiomyopathy and with hyperthyroidism.

Left ventricular enlargement is associated with left atrial involvement. Left ventricular convexity is increased in both views and the heart is elongated and more upright in the lateral view, causing dorsal elevation of the trachea. Enlargement of the left atrium is seen as a bulge dorsal to the caudal vena cava on a lateral view and as a bulge beyond the left ventrical border (left auricle), with decreased distance between the left heart and thoracic wall, on the dorsoventral view. A prominent "notch" may develop in the caudal cardiac border between the left atrium and ventricle when severe left atrial enlargement is present. This waist is not present with accompanying severe left ventricular enlargement. The apex may be displaced to the right of midline on the dorsoventral view in severe left atrial and ventricular enlargements.[21]

In hypertrophic and restrictive cardiomyopathy, the left auricular bulge may be accompanied by right heart convexity on the dorsoventral view, especially in the 9-12 o'clock position. These changes can confer a valentine-shaped heart appearance. However, this classic cardiac silhouette is only one of many radiographic patterns. Often these cardiomyopathies do not exhibit this classic feature. Left atrial and ventricular enlargements can also be associated with congenital anomalies with left-to-right shunts (patent ductus arteriosus, septal defects), aortic stenosis, mitral insufficiency due to mitral valve complex malformation, and hypertrophic, restrictive, dilated and excessive left ventricular moderator band cardiomyopathies.

Extracardiac radiographic signs caused by the hemodynamic consequences of heart failure may help elucidate the underlying disease and direct a diagnostic and therapeutic regimen. Pleural effusion from right heart failure is much more common than hydroperitoneum or pericardial effusion. These signs may occur occasionally when chronic left heart failure causes pulmonary hypertension and secondary right heart failure. Hepatomegaly and hydroperitoneum may occasionally accompany right heart failure. Left heart failure may cause interstitial or alveolar pulmonary patterns suggestive of pulmonary edema. Classic perihilar edema, as seen in dogs, is less common in cats, in which patchy, focal, peripheral pulmonary edema is usual. Pulmonary undercirculation, characterized by thin vessels and dark lung fields, may occur with pulmonic stenosis and right-to-left shunts (tetralogy of Fallot). Over-circulation is caused by left-to-right shunts (patent ductus arteriosus, septal defects). Prominent pulmonary arteries can occur in heartworm disease.

Sometimes it is impossible to distinguish clearly definable cardiac borders in heart disease, especially if pleural effusion is present. Rather, plain radiographic diagnosis of generalized cardiomegaly, or left or right heart enlargement may have to suffice in many cases. Moderate to severe left atrial enlargement usually is a sequela of primary myocardial disease. When evident radiographically, it strongly suggests cardiomyopathy. Generalized cardiomegaly may occur in all forms of cardiomyopathy. In dilated cardiomyopathy, the apex is often large and globoid on the dorsoventral view, being comprised predominantly of a dilated left ventricle. The left atrium, auricle and ventricle are very enlarged, forming a convex left heart border. In hypertrophic and restrictive cardiomyopathies, the cardiomegaly usually is more associated with severe left atrial enlargement and often right-sided convexity (9-12 o'clock) on the dorsoventral view. The apex is not globiform but rather tapered, and the left ventricle is mildly to moderately enlarged. However, it is not always possible to determine the underlying etiology or distinguish among forms of cardiomyopathy from plain radiographs alone. All available clinical, laboratory and electrocardiographic data must be correlated to facilitate a diagnosis. Nonselective angiocardiography or echocardiography is often necessary to elucidate the underlying disease.

Nonselective Angiocardiography

Angiocardiography permits diagnostic visualization of the cardiac chambers, ventricular and atrial walls, and great vessels (Figs 31, 32). It may be used to support a diagnosis or help elucidate cardiac morphology when clinical data do not indicate the disease.

The technic employs injection of a bolus of contrast medium into a superficial vein, then obtaining one or more sequential radiographs to visualize opacified blood through the heart valves, chambers and great vessels. Although systolic and diastolic phases of the cardiac cycle cannot be assured, both may be represented. Opacification of the right and left heart is often obtained. The technic has been well described and documented elsewhere.[22,23]

Congenital heart defects are best studied with selective catheterization and pressure measurements. However, several anomalies can be adequately diagnosed by nonselective angiocardiography, such as aortic and pulmonic stenosis, patent ductus anteriosus and certain shunts.

Acquired heart disease, on the other hand, can be suitably evaluated nonselectively. Angiocardiography can help differentiate among hypertrophic, dilated and restrictive (due to endomyocardial fibrosis) cardiomyopathies (Figs 44, 49). It does not always clearly distinguish cardiomyopathy associated with excessive left ventricular moderator bands from early dilated or hypertrophic cardiomyopathy. The technic is safe in most cases of hypertrophic and restrictive cardiomyopathy but its use should be avoided when dilated cardiomyopathy is suspected. Examples of angiocardiograms appear in Figures 31, 32, 37-40, 44, 47 and 49.

Clinical Pathologic Examination

Cardiovascular disease and its hemodynamic sequelae may cause abnormalities of the blood, urine or extravascular fluid. To formulate the most accurate conclusions, clinical pathologic data must be interpreted in view of history, clinical examination and other diagnostic tests. Most emphasis in clinical pathology has been

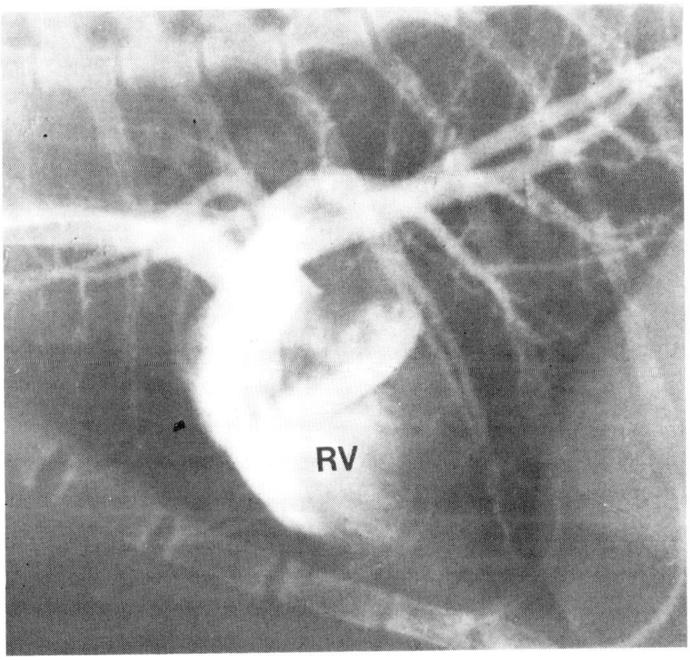

Fig 32. Normal nonselective angiocardiogram obtained about 6 seconds after injection of contrast medium into the jugular vein. Note the normal size of the right ventricle (RV) and pulmonary arteries.

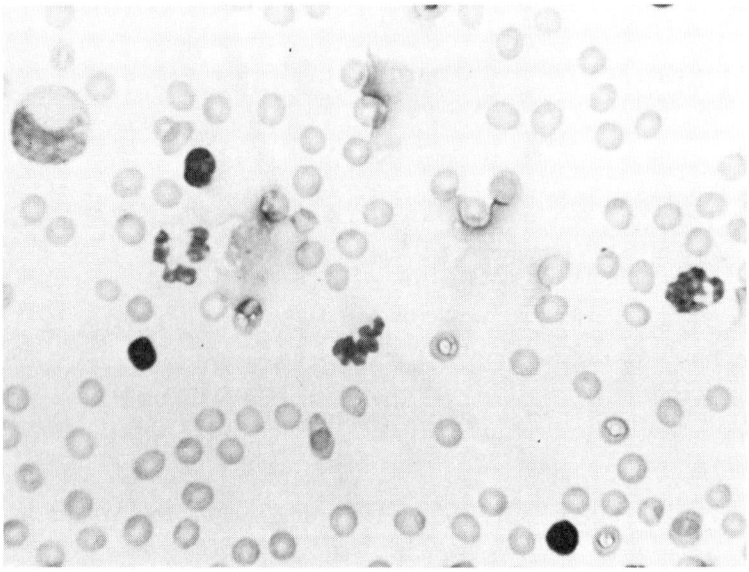

Fig 33. Smear from cell sediment from a sample of thoracic effusion from a cat with cardiomyopathy. Note the mixture of blood cells with normal lymphocytes, occasional macrophages, and smudge fragments. There is minimal evidence of inflammation. (Original magnification 400X)[6] (Courtesy of W.B. Saunders)

placed on assessing primary myocardial disease (cardiomyopathy).[24]

When cardiomyopathy is suspected, a clinical laboratory data base is necessary to reveal underlying complications and formulate a diagnostic and therapeutic plan. Cats with clinically significant cardiomyopathy have usually been anorexic for one to several days. Vomiting sometimes is present. Consequent dehydration causes prerenal azotemia, which is reflected by mild elevations in BUN and serum creatinine levels, and elevation of the PCV and total plasma protein level. Urine specific gravity is usually elevated above 1.025 in the absence of renal dysfunction.

The serum level of lactate dehydrogenase (LDH), an enzyme that catalyzes hydrogen transfer in conversion of lactate to pyruvate, is elevated with cardiomyopathy. Because elevation of the serum LDH level is a nonspecific indication of cell death or hemolysis, isoenzyme electrophoresis can be employed to distinguish individual isoenzymes. In feline serum, 5 isoenzyme bands of activity are recognized. Major isoenzyme fractions in feline cardiac muscle are LD_1 and LD_2; skeletal muscle contains LD_5, and liver contains LD_4 and LD_5. The RBC are the major contributors to elevated serum LDH levels when significant hemolysis is present. Most LDH in normal feline serum is contributed by LD_5 and LD_1 (in hemolyzed samples). Active myocarditis in cardiomyopathic cats may cause increased LD_1 and LD_2 levels in serum. Liver congestion probably causes elevation of serum LD_5 levels secondary to hepatocyte leakage. Elevations of serum alanine aminotransferase (SGPT) levels may accompany this finding.[24] Dramatic increases in total serum LDH, serum aspartate aminotransferase (SGOT) and serum creatine phosphokinase (CPK) levels result from ischemic necrosis secondary to thromboembolism. Such values may remain elevated for 2 weeks or more.

Coagulopathies may accompany thromboembolism with cardiomyopathy. Screening tests for hemostatic disorders may show intrinsic coagulation defects (prolonged activated partial thromboplastin time), extrinsic coagulation defects (prolonged prothrombin time), and hypofibrinogenemia. These abnormalities probably result from consumption of clotting factors and chronic disseminated intravascular coagulation (DIC). Hepatic-mediated coagulopathy may contribute in some cases.[25]

The serum thyroxine (T_4) level, as measured by radioimmunoassay, may be normal or low. However, a TSH-stimulation test results in a normal (elevated) serum T_4 level, suggesting that the depressed pretest serum T_4 level may be due to interference with T_4 binding to plasma proteins as a stress-related phenomenon.

Analysis of pleural and abdominal effusions from cardiomyopathic cats yields characteristic results. Such effusions are sterile and result from increased lymphatic and venous hydrostatic pressure secondary to decreased cardiac output and venous hypertension. Grossly, these obstructive effusions appear serous to serosanguineous in character. Rarely they are chylous. Their composition is a mixture of blood cells and lymphocytes. A nucleated cell to red cell ratio approximates that of blood (Fig 33). Modification of this effusion increases the number of inflammatory cells, resulting in a mixed cellular inflammatory response. Macrophages may display erythrophagia in long-standing effusions.[24] Pleural effusions occur most commonly in dilated cardiomyopathy and often in cardiomyopathy associated with excessive left ventricular moderator bands. Occasionally, cats with hypertrophic cardiomyopathy have pleural effusion.

Echocardiography

Feline cardiovascular assessment has been advanced by the clinical application of echocardiography, a diagnostic technic in which ultrasound is used to visualize cardiac structures and measure heart dimensions. It employs a pulsed ultrasonic beam proportionately reflected from interfaces of differing biologic tissues. This sound wave rebounds as an echo, which is processed into a readable form. The procedure is noninvasive, innocuous and free of the hazards associated with cardiac catheterization and cineangiocardiographic technics.[26]

Ventricular wall thickness and chamber volumes can be measured and correlated with the severity of disease. Valve closure velocity, systolic time intervals and circumferential fiber shortening are reliable indices of ventricular performance.[27]

Echocardiography provides the advantages of directly visualizing motion and measuring dimensions of heart structures as compared to auscultation, which only suggests the nature of lesions and radiography, which does not differentiate hypertrophy, dilatation and pericardial effusion. Additional information can be acquired by combining echocardiography with phonocardiography, pressure recordings and electrocardiography. The capability to differentiate among causes of feline cardiomegaly echocardiographically has been demonstrated.[26] Hypertrophic and dilated (congestive) cardiomyopathic hearts have been differentiated from each other by dimensions of muscle walls and cardiac chambers

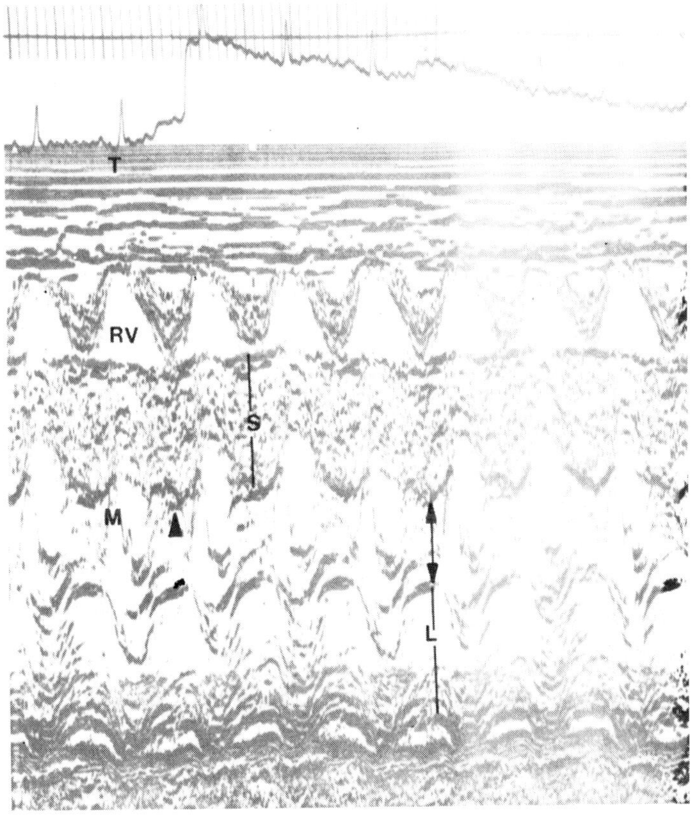

Fig 34. Echocardiogram recorded at the mitral valve level from a male domestic shorthaired cat with hypertrophic cardiomyopathy. The right ventricular free wall demonstrates vigorous systolic motion. The interventricular septum (S) is hypertrophied as compared with normal controls. The left ventricular wall (L) is thickened, with a normal systolic excursion. The left ventricular lumen (arrows) is of normal or decreased diameter. The anterior mitral valve (M) demonstates systolic cranial motion (arrowhead) typical of obstructive cardiomyopathy. The right ventricular lumen (RV) and a transducer artifact (T) are also evident. (Paper speed 50 mm/sec, with 1-cm depth markers every second.) (Courtesy of Dr J.D. Bonagura)

(Figs 34, 35). Pericardial effusion has been identified in cats by the presence of an echo-free space between the ventricular epicardium and pericardial sac.

HEART DISEASE

Congenital Heart Disease

Congenital heart disease is less common in cats than in dogs and is less prevalent than acquired feline heart diseases. In the largest recorded study, 4933 cats were necropsied over a 14-year period. These animals were a subpopulation of 99,416 cats examined during that interval. Necropsy confirmed that 96 animals had congenital heart diseases, totaling 107 anomalies. The most common heart defects included malformation of the mitral valve complex (19), tricuspid valve dysplasia (18), ventricular septal defect (13), aortic stenosis (12), persistent common atrioventricular canal (11), endocardial fibrosis and cardiomegaly (7), patent ductus arteriosus (7) and tetralogy of Fallot (6).[4] Less common defects included incomplete pericardial sac, persistent truncus arteriosus, pulmonary stenosis, atrial septal defect, tricuspid stenosis and right ventricular hypoplasia, double outlet of the right ventricle, patent foramen ovale, right atrial hypoplasia and a caudal vena cava anomaly.

Cats with congenital cardiac abnormalities often die in the first year of life. Moreover, congenital heart defects represent a differential diagnosis when evaluating cats for cardiomyopathy, which may also develop in young cats. No consistent sex or breed predilection has been ade-

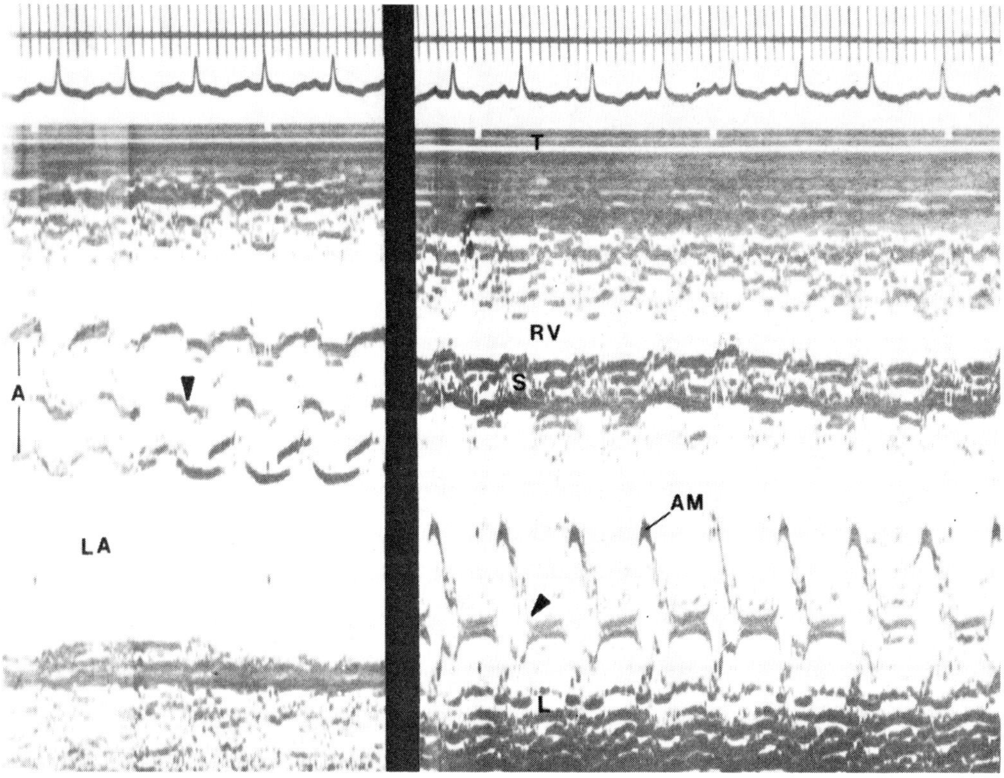

Fig 35. Echocardiograms recorded at the aortic (left) and mitral (right) positions from a male domestic shorthaired cat with dilated cardiomyopathy. The left atrial (LA) to aortic (A) root ratio is increased, suggesting significant left atrial enlargement. Aortic valves are observed in the aortic root in systole and diastole (arrowhead). The echocardiogram at the mitral valve position shows significant left ventricular dilation. The anterior mitral valve (AM) is displaced caudad, suggesting left ventricular dilation. The posterior leaflet is readily seen as it separates and then coapts (arrowhead) with the anterior mitral valve. The pattern is similar to the "double-diamond" mitral configuration observed in people with dilated cardiomyopathy. The left ventricular wall (L) and interventricular septum (S) are of normal thickness and demonstrate marked reductions in systolic motion. (Paper speed 50 mm/sec, with 1-cm depth markers every second.) (Courtesy of Dr J.D. Bonagura)

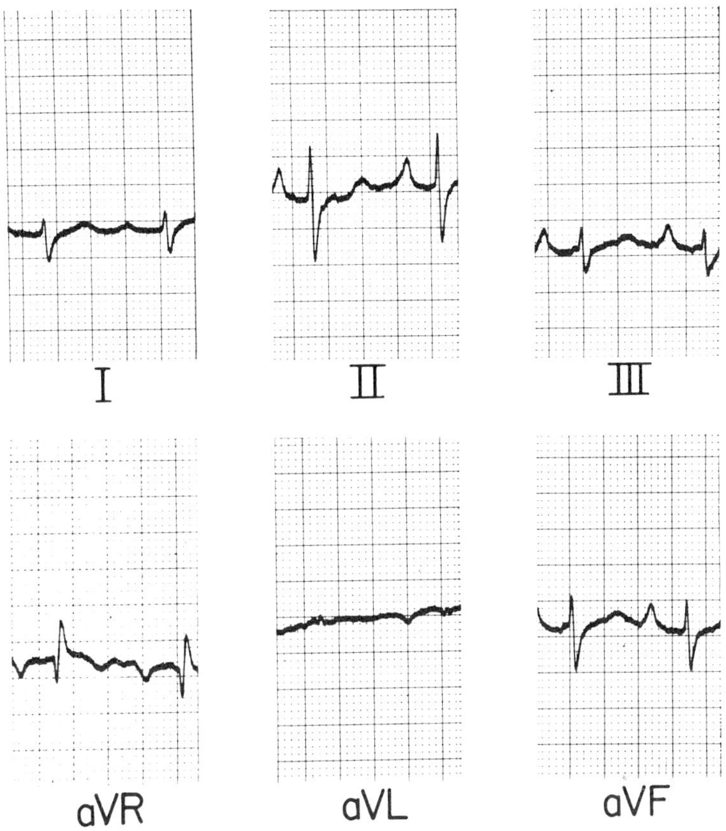

Fig 36. Tracings from a cat with a ventricular septal defect. Right axis deviation (−120°) in the presence of an S wave in leads I, II and III indicate right ventricular enlargement. The tall R waves in lead II may indicate left ventricular enlargement. Biatrial enlargement is indicated by the tall and wide P waves.[29] (Courtesy of W.B. Saunders)

quately demonstrated for congenital feline cardiac anomalies, although familial tendencies have been reported.

Mitral Valve Complex Malformation

The mitral valve complex refers to the mitral valve annulus, mitral leaflets, chordae tendinae, papillary muscles, and associated region of left atrial wall. Malformation of the mitral valve complex is the most common congenital cardiac anomaly in cats. Affected cats usually are young (mean 10 months). Lesions are similar to those in dogs and include annulus enlargement, upward malposition of the atrophic or hypertrophic papillary muscles, abnormal insertion of papillar muscles directly onto valve leaflets, endocardial fibrosis, and left atrial and ventricular enlargement. This anomaly is often accompanied by other congenital heart defects.[4]

Affected cats may be asymptomatic or display variable clinical signs. Lethargy, dyspnea, weight loss and pulmonary edema can occur. Moderate to severe left-sided heart failure, with or without right-sided heart failure, may be present. Radiographic findings may reflect these clinical signs. A holosystolic, mixed-frequency murmur, with the point of maximal intensity at the mitral region or more sternal may be auscultated. Electrocardiographic findings are usually normal or may suggest left ventricular enlargement.

Tricuspid Valve Dysplasia

Tricuspid valve dysplasia is almost as common as malformation of the mitral valve complex.[4] The tricuspid valve complex is similar to the mitral valve complex and gross abnormalities include adherence of the long, thick septal leaflets to the septum, absent or short, thick,

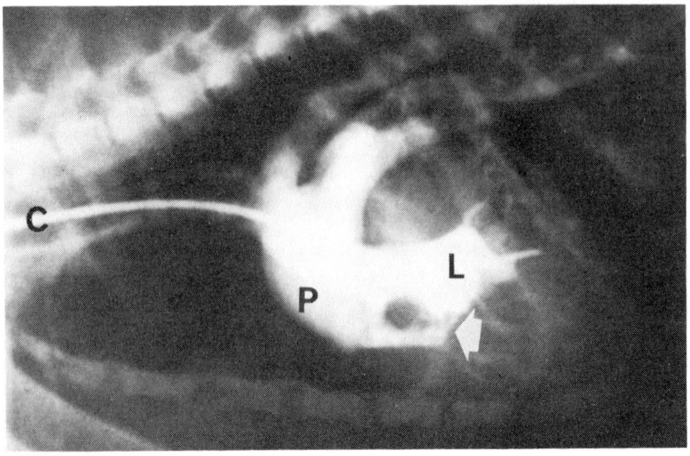

Fig 37. Left ventricular angiocardiogram of a cat with a ventricular septal defect. The catheter (C) passes into the left ventricle (L). Blood flows across the ventricular septal defect (arrow), into the right ventricle, across the pulmonic valve and into the pulmonary artery (P). This causes simultaneous filling of the aorta and pulmonary artery from the left ventricle. [From Vet Clin No Am 6 (1976) 431, courtesy of W.B. Saunders]

fused chordae tendinae, fused, hypertrophic papillary muscles, papillary muscle insertion directly onto lateral leaflets, incomplete development of valves, and enlargement of the right atrium and ventricle.[28] This coexists with malformation of the mitral valve complex in almost half of affected cats and with ventricular septal defect in about 1 in 6 affected cats.

Young cats (mean 9.8 months) usually are affected. Clinical signs may include lethargy, dyspnea, anorexia, weight loss, pleural effusion, ascites and signs of left-sided heart failure. A systolic murmur of tricuspid or mitral insufficiency may be ascultated.

Ventricular Septal Defect

Previously believed to be the most common congenital cardiac anomaly, this defect is reportedly less prevalent than mitral or tricuspid valvular complex malformations. It may occur alone or with other cardiac anomalies. Situated high in the membranous portion of the interventricular septum, this defect usually occurs just below the aortic valve in the left ventricle and beneath the septal cusp of the tricuspid valve of the right ventricle. Rarely the defect occurs in the muscular portion of the septum. Ventricular septal defects and tricuspid valvular dysplasia may coexist in one-third of the cases detected at necropsy.[4]

The functional disturbance from a ventricular septal defect generally depends on the size of the defect and the status of the pulmonary vascular bed. Resistance to left ventricular emptying is an important factor in determining left ventricular pressure and, hence, shunt flow. Such resistance to emptying may occur in hypertrophic obstructive cardiomyopathy. When large quantities of blood are shunted from the left to right ventricle, right ventricular enlargement may occur and pulmonary overcirculation can result. Increased venous return to the left heart may cause left heart enlargement.

Clinical signs may be absent or indicative of heart failure. A systolic murmur may be auscultated over both thoracic walls or loudest at the right fourth to fifth intercostal space near the sternal border. Thoracic radiographs may be normal or reveal biventricular, left atrial and pulmonary artery enlargement. An ECG may be normal or depict biatrial and biventricular enlargement (Fig 36).[29] Selective angiocardiography may be useful to demonstrate the defect (Fig 37). Echocardiography may prove valuable in defining the septal defect by identifying echodense dye bubbles traversing the defect.

Severely affected animals may die within the first days to weeks of life or by one year of age. Medical management is indicated when congestive heart failure is present.[29] Pulmonary artery banding has been used to alleviate clinical signs.[30] This surgical procedure decreases pulmonary artery outflow with the use of constrictive bands. Right ventricular pressure is thereby increased and left-to-right shunting is decreased, thus reducing the volume overload on the left heart. However, if the pulmonary artery occlusion is excessive, pulmonary arterial resistance and right ventricular pressure increase, resulting in an increased potential for a right-to-left shunt.

Aortic Stenosis

Aortic stenosis may be valvular, subvalvular or supravalvular. Supravalvular stenosis involves a fibrous ring encompassing the partial or entire aortic circumference. Subvalvular stenosis, which is more common in dogs, involves formation of a fibrous ring beneath the aortic valve leaflets. In valvular aortic stenosis, there is malformation of the aortic valve. The heart compensates for left ventricular outflow obstruction by concentric left ventricular hypertrophy. Left ventricular compliance becomes diminished and greater intracavitary pressure is required for ventricular filling. Ventricular diastolic filling pressures become elevated. Atrial contraction plays an important role in left ventricular filling with aortic stenosis. Loss of appropriately timed atrial contraction due to arrhythmias may cause rapid deterioration of the patient. Coronary blood flow is impaired by elevated left ventricular end-diastolic pressure and predisposes the heart to ischemia and consequent arrhythmias. Cardiac output may be severely compromised during exertion in animals with significant aortic stenosis.

Clinical signs may occur at a young age and are initially manifested as stunted growth or acute heart failure. A systolic murmur may be present at the aortic-pulmonic area, radiating to the right or craniad up the carotid arteries. The murmur may be loudest at the right sternal border at the third or fourth intercostal space. Decreased femoral pulses may be present but are difficult to appreciate.

Radiographs may be normal or reveal left ventricular and left atrial enlargement, with poststenotic aortic enlargement. Angiocardiography may facilitate diagnosis (Fig 38). Left-axis deviation is usually present on the ECG. Arrhythmias (usually supraventricular) are sometimes encountered.

Surgical correction is not possible. Medical therapy may be attempted using propranolol at 2.5-5 mg 2-3 times daily. The negative inotropic and chronotropic effects of this drug promote ventricular filling and reduce outflow restriction. Coronary perfusion is then enhanced, delaying the onset of ischemia induced arrhythmias. If left-sided congestive heart failure occurs, a low-salt diet and diuretic therapy (furosemide at 5 mg 1-2 times daily) may be used. Digitalis may increase outflow restriction and decrease coronary artery perfusion, making this drug a last choice in the therapeutic regimen.

Persistent Common Atrioventricular Canal

A single defect low in the atrial septum and high in the ventricular septum allows communication of all cardiac chambers through a common atrioventricular canal (Fig 39). Atrioventricular valvular defects and valvular insufficiency may occur as a consequence of their proximity to the septal defect. Shunting of blood from left to right produces volume overload, right atrial and ventricular enlargement, pulmonary artery enlargement and a relative pulmonic stenosis. Increase in venous return to the left heart causes volume overload, left-sided enlargement and failure. Pulmonary hypertension may occasionally develop, causing pressure in the right heart to equal or exceed that of the left and producing a right-to-left shunt and cyanosis. Radiographs are normal or reveal cardiomegaly and occasionally heart failure.[4,29]

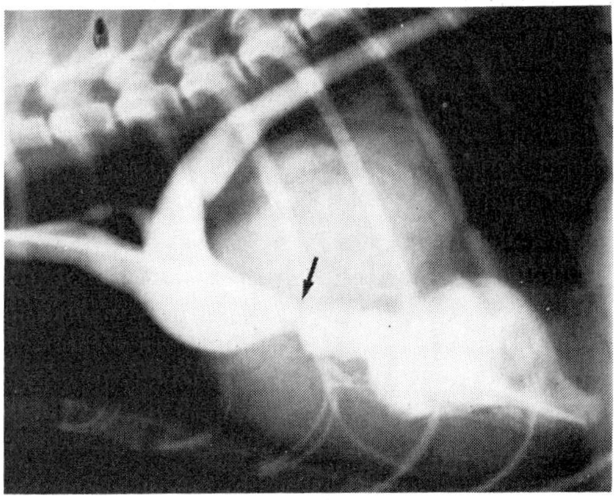

Fig 38. Left ventricular angiocardiogram of a cat with supravalvular aortic stenosis. The stricture (arrow) is in the aorta, above the aortic valve.[29] (Courtesy of W.B. Saunders)

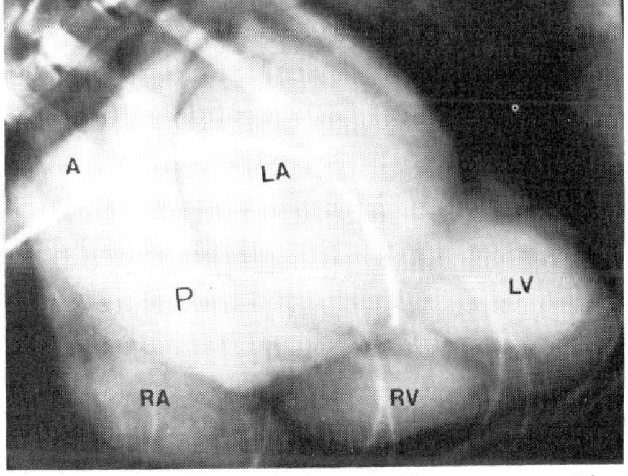

Fig 39. Angiocardiogram of a cat with a common atrioventricular canal. Dye injected into the area of the atrioventricular defect outlines all chambers simultaneously. LA = left atrium, LV = left ventricle, RA = right atrium, RV = right ventricle, A = aorta, P = pulmonary artery.[29] (Courtesy of W.B. Saunders)

Patent Ductus Arteriosus

The ductus arteriosus originates from the distal portion of the left sixth aortic arch. During the fetal period, the ductus is a patent vessel connecting the pulmonary trunk and descending aorta. Most blood from the right ventricle bypasses the unexpanded lungs via the ductus arteriosus and enters the descending aorta. Complete closure of the ductus normally occurs by the end of the second week of life. Mechanisms of closure may include the influences of hemodynamic, neurologic or humoral factors, gas-tension effects initiated by respiration and a drop in pulmonary vascular resistance, or vasoactive substances. When the ductus fails to close, the patent ductus arteriosus allows blood flow from the aorta (high pressure) into the pulmonary artery (low pressure). Shunting usually occurs in systole and diastole, producing a continuous murmur. Pulmonary overcirculation occurs from increased pulmonary artery blood flow. Pulmonary venous return is increased to the left atrium, with resultant volume overload. The left atrium and ventricle enlarge, resulting in biatrial and biventricular enlargement, with aneurysmal dilation of the descending portion of the aortic arch where the ductus arises and the pulmonary artery segments.

Patent ductus arteriosus can occur as an isolated defect or one of a combination of defects. Affected cats may die soon after birth or develop congestive heart failure early in life. Clinical signs in cases of left-to-right shunting include lethargy, anorexia, dyspnea and stunted growth. A systolic-diasystolic "machinery" murmur may be auscultated at the aortic-pulmonic region, with radiation of sound to the right, craniad and ventrad. Radiographic evidence of left atrial and ventricular enlargement may be present. Biventricular enlargement and aortic or pulmonic aneurysmal dilation may be evident or absent. Left ventricular enlargement is often indicated electrocardiographically. Selective catheterization may help define the lesion when nonselective angiocardiography is inconclusive (Fig 40).

In cases of right-to-left shunting associated with pulmonary hypertension, clinical signs differ from those of a typical left-to-right shunt. Cyanosis and syncope may be evident. The heart murmur may be barely audible or conceivably absent if right and left ventricular pressures are equal, eliminating shunting in either direction, or the murmur may be essentially systolic. Radiographic evidence of pulmonary artery tortuosity and attenuation may indicate pulmonary hypertension. Polycythemia can develop secondary to cyanosis. A split second heart sound associated with pulmonary hypertension and delayed closure of the pulmonary valve can occur. Electrocardiographic evidence of a right axis deviation, suggesting right ventricular enlargement, may be present.[31]

Surgery is the treatment of choice in uncomplicated patent ductus arteriosus, but if pulmonary arterial pressures exceed aortic pressures, surgery may cause right-heart failure by eliminating the right-to-left shunt "escape" valve, thus increasing pulmonary hypertension.

Tetralogy of Fallot

Tetralogy of Fallot is a complex congenital heart malformation consisting of a ventricular septal defect high in the septum, just below the origin of the aorta, biventricular origin of the

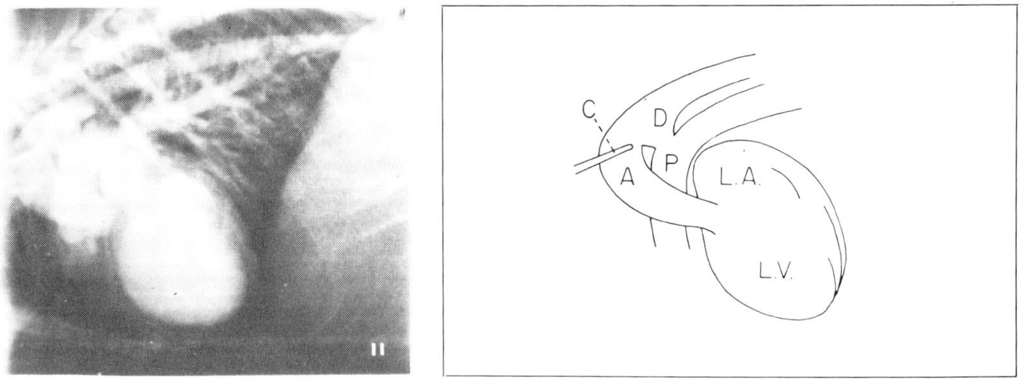

Fig 40. Aortic angiogram of a cat with a patent ductus arteriosus. Dye injected through the catheter (C) into the aorta (A) crosses the patent ductus (D) into the pulmonary artery (P), causing simultaneous filling of both vessels. The left atrium (LA) and left ventricle (LV) are outlined by dye from the lungs via the pulmonary veins. (From JAAHA 11 (1975) 95, courtesy of AAHA)

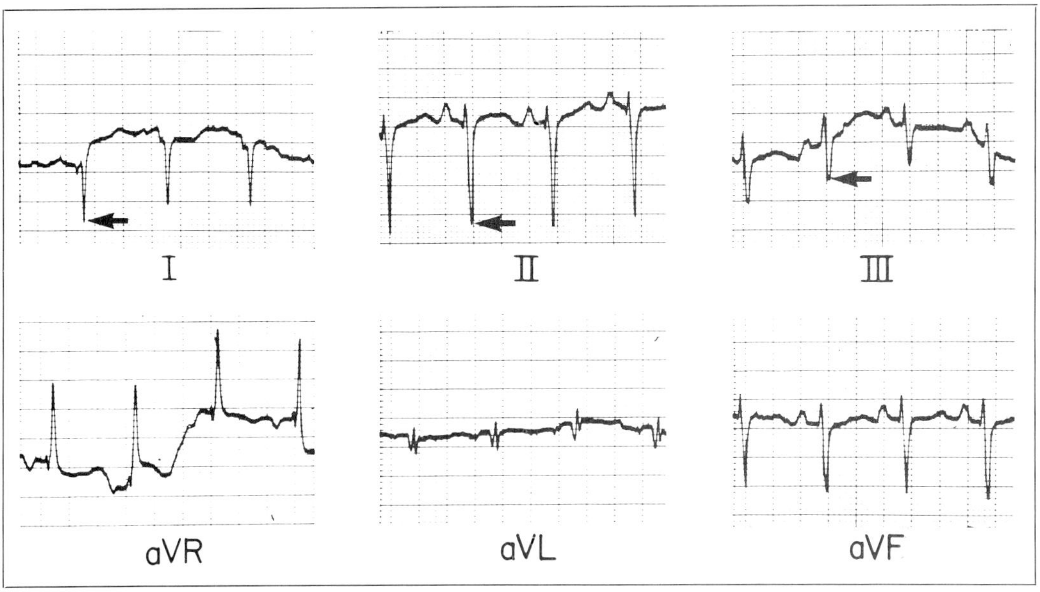

Fig 41. Tracings from a cat with a right-axis deviation (−120°). This indicates right ventricular hypertrophy, typical of tetralogy of Fallot.[29] (Courtesy of W.B. Saunders)

aorta (aorta often originates just dorsal to the ventricular septal defect, readily communicating with both ventricles), pulmonic stenosis (usually subvalvular), and right ventricular hypertrophy (secondary to the fixed outflow obstruction of pulmonic stenosis).

With obstruction to right ventricular outflow, right ventricular pressure becomes elevated until it equals or exceeds left ventricular pressure. Due to the ventricular septal defect, unoxygenated blood is shunted from the right to the left ventricle, a portion of which is ejected through the over-riding aorta into the systemic circulation. This admixture of oxygenated (arterial) and unoxygenated (venous) blood causes cyanosis, which worsens with stress. An elevated PCV (secondary polycythemia) may occur due to secondary hypoxia.

Clinically affected cats may be small and stunted, exhibiting cyanosis, weakness or dyspnea. A holosystolic, mid- to high-frequency murmur associated with the pulmonic stenosis or ventricular septal defect may be present. The murmur may be absent or very soft if pressures of the left and right ventricle are equal and no blood shunts in either direction. The ECG usually displays right axis deviation (Fig 41). Bundle branch block can occur with a bizarre axis shift if bundle branches are interrupted by the ventricular septal defect.[32] Thoracic radiographs may display right ventricular enlargement. If a significant quantity of blood shunts from the right ventricle into the left ventricle (bypassing the lungs), there is decreased pulmonary blood flow, manifested radiographically as hypovascular lung fields.

Selective angiocardiography may be diagnostic. Using right ventricular injection, simultaneous filling of the aorta and pulmonary artery occurs when a right-to-left shunt is present. Nonselective angiocardiography may support a diagnosis of tetralogy of Fallot if the correct phase of the cardiac cycle is delineated by the radiographs.

In milder forms of tetralogy of Fallot, pulmonic stenosis may not be severe. If right ventricular pressure is less than left ventricular pressure, a left-to-right shunt occurs and cyanosis is not manifested. However, some cases may progress to a right-to-left shunt.

Surgical correction of the pulmonic stenosis and ventricular septal defect is the treatment of choice but requires extensive and complex procedures not generally available. An alternate surgical approach is to create a shunt between the aorta or subclavian artery and pulmonary artery, effectively increasing pulmonary blood flow and improving systemic oxygenation.

Propranolol has been used for medical management in dogs.[33] It should be considered for use in cats when surgical intervention is not possible, although its efficacy has not been demonstrated.

Endocardial Fibrosis and Cardiomegaly

Neonatal endocardial fibroelastosis has been observed in kittens 2-6 months of age. Gross and microscopic lesions are not specific but are somewhat similar to those observed in malformation of the mitral valve complex, dysplasia of the tricuspid valve and dilated cardiomyopathy. The true etiology remains obscure and the classification of endocardial fibrosis and cardiomegaly as a distinct congenital cardiac anomaly is doubtful.

Acquired Heart Diseases

Vegetative Endocarditis

Endocarditis is usually bacterial in origin and involves the valvular or mural endocardium. Valvular endocarditis usually occurs in valves experiencing the highest pressure. The mitral valve is most commonly affected, followed by the aortic valve. The tricuspid valve is not often involved and disease of the pulmonic valve is exceedingly rare. Bacterial endocarditis is a sequela to bacteremia. Common causes include wound infections and abscesses. Other predisposing conditions include osteomyelitis, pyelonephritis and dental infections. Pre-existing valvular injury facilitates valvular vegetations, which are composed of fibrin, bacteria and neutrophils. Microabscesses may be present in the myocardium, with ulceration of affected endocardial cells. Nonhemolytic streptococci are commonly responsible for bacterial endocarditis, although hemolytic streptococci, staphylococci, *E coli, Pseudomonas* and *Erysipelothrix rhusiopathiae* have been detected.

Clinical signs usually are obscure. Fevers of unknown origin and acute lameness (paraparesis) may suggest thromboembolism secondary to dislodged valvular vegetations. Bacterial and embolic showers may cause multiple organ involvement and a myriad of signs. Chronic weight loss, anemia, heart murmur, arrhythmia and neutrophilic leukocytosis may be present. Blood cultures usually are negative; samples should be obtained during a febrile period. Nonselective angiocardiography may furnish useful information if selective studies are not available. Echocardiography may demonstrate valvular vegetations.

Positive blood cultures and sensitivity tests identify the infecting bacterium and antibiotic of choice. In absence of positive culture results, intensive IV antibiotic therapy with bactericidal drugs is preferred. Crystalline penicillin, at 1 million IU/kg divided TID, can be used in an IV drip to rapidly attain high blood levels. Treatment may be continued with procaine penicillin at 40,000 IU/kg given IM BID. Oral therapy with ampicillin, at 20 mg TID or QID, should be continued for at least 4 more weeks. Specific therapy also should be directed at particular organ dysfunction if present. Paretic limbs should be given adequate time to regain motor function and for resolution of secondary ischemic neuromyopathy. Use of furosemide and digoxin may be indicated if congestive heart failure develops.

The prognosis must always be guarded. Rapid diagnosis and treatment may facilitate recovery. Unfortunately, the often nonspecific array of signs may preclude early diagnosis. Diffuse embolization and multiple organ dysfunction also dictate the prognosis.

Valvular Heart Disease

Acquired valvular heart disease is uncommon in cats as a distinct entity. Acquired valvular dysfunction usually occurs secondary to cardiomyopathies as a result of distortion of the annulus fibrosus, papillary muscles or myocardium. Mitral and tricuspid valvular insufficiencies are thus encountered.

Clinical signs usually are related to the underlying disease, *ie,* type of cardiomyopathy present. Auscultation usually reveals early to midsystolic murmurs of grades I/VI to III/VI, regurgitant or ejective in quality. They are usually heard best at the mitral valve area and may be loud more ventrad, toward the sternum and occasionally at the tricuspid valve region. Clinical findings depend on the type and stage of underlying disease. Diagnostic procedures include electrocardiography, radiography, angiocardiography, echocardiography and a routine laboratory data base.

Cardiomyopathy

Cardiomyopathy constitutes a major disease in feline cardiology. It represents a significant proportion of the cardiovascular disorders that may lead to cardiac enlargement, congestive heart failure, cardiac arrhythmias and sudden death. Although much progress has been made in clinical recognition of the disease, its etiology is not understood and therapeutic regimens are not well supported with controlled clinical data.

Table 3. Common Clinical Findings in Cats With Dilated and Hypertrophic Cardiomyopathy [35]

Category	Dilated	Hypertrophic
Breed predilection	All breeds, especially Siamese and Burmese	All breeds
Sex predilection	Male	Male
Clinical signs	Shock, hypothermia, anorexia, lethargy, dyspnea, thromboembolism	Dyspnea, thromboembolism, sudden death
Electrocardiographic signs	Ventricular premature complexes, left ventricular enlargement, sinus bradycardia, primary atrioventricular block	Atrial and ventricular arrhythmias, intraventricular conduction disturbances (left anterior fascicular block pattern), left ventricular and atrial enlargement
Radiographic signs	Severe generalized cardiomegaly, pulmonary edema (uncommonly), pleural effusion	Left atrial enlargement, cardiomegaly, pulmonary edema, pleural effusion (rarely significant in early stages)

The various forms of cardiomyopathy are designations that may be appropriate only at a given time. For example, a cat with a specific type of myocarditis may develop chronic cardiac dilation (dilated cardiomyopathy) or possibly restrictive cardiomyopathy. The very early stages of myocardial disease are often unclear. Moreover, a designated form may reflect only the stage at which the animal is examined. Similarly, treatment is based on the clinical stage and form of cardiomyopathy (Table 3).

Primary myocardial disease (cardiomyopathy) is the term applied to an abnormality of the heart muscle of unknown or obscure etiology. Cardiomyopathy is most often classified as primary, *ie,* of unknown etiology, and secondary, *ie,* stemming from systemic disease or other known insult. Primary cardiomyopathy is the most common form of the disease in cats and dogs.

A second method of classification can be developed by separating cardiomyopathy into distinctive patterns according to the nature of the clinical features, hemodynamic alteration and accompanying pathologic changes, *ie,* dilated, hypertrophic, restrictive or excessive left ventricular moderator band cardiomyopathy (Fig 42). In dilated (congestive) cardiomyopathy, dilation of the left and right ventricles occurs with "pump failure," a systolic dysfunction. With hypertrophic cardiomyopathy, left ventricular hypertrophy causes resistance to left ventricular filling, a diastolic dysfunction; the aortic outflow tract also may be obstructed in asymmetric septal hypertrophy. Restrictive cardiomyopathy due to endocardial fibrosis is characterized by a rigid, poorly distensible left ventricular wall that causes greatly diminished compliance. A newly described form of cardiomyopathy due to the presence of excessive left ventricular moderator bands is not yet well characterized hemodynamically.[34] Table 3 lists some of the common clinical findings in cats with the dilated and hypertrophic forms of cardiomyopathy.[35] Clinical findings for restrictive cardiomyopathy are not well established.

A third mode of classification, etiologic, is based on identification of the pathologic process responsible for myocardial damage. Although the specific etiology underlying the functional impairment may be found in some cases, this is not true in most, even after complete evaluation. The term "idiopathic" or primary cardiomyopathy is then applied. Table 4 outlines forms of secondary cardiomyopathy for which an etiologic factor is suspected. These include infections (viral, bacterial, fungal, algal), metabolic disorders (uremia, thyrotoxicosis), infiltrative conditions (neoplasia), parasitism (toxoplasmosis), nutritional disorders, chemicals and drugs.[36]

Hypertrophic Cardiomyopathy

Cats may have either symmetric hypertrophic (most common) or asymmetric septal hypertrophic cardiomyopathy. In asymmetric hyper-

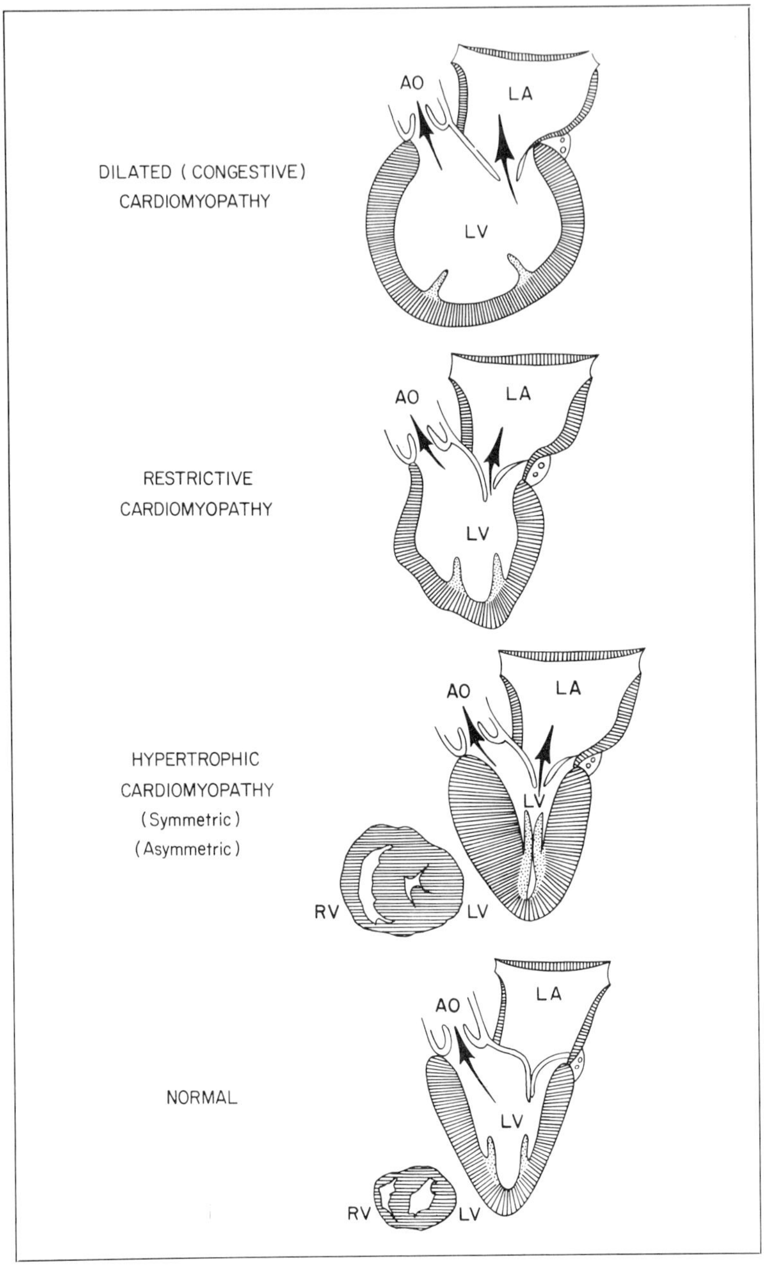

Fig 42. Classification of cardiomyopathy according to the nature of the clinical features, hemodynamic fault and accompanying pathologic changes.

trophy, the septum is thicker than the left ventricular free wall. The cause of hypertrophic cardiomyopathy in cats is unknown but clinical evidence suggests a hereditary component. The disease has been found in related cats. In people a large number of hypertrophic cardiomyopathy cases have a familial incidence.

Clinical Signs: Cats can be affected at any age but hypertrophic cardiomyopathy is most common in middle-aged cats. More males than females are affected. Clinical signs often include acute onset of dyspnea, pulmonary edema, lethargy, anorexia, posterior paresis from aortic thromboembolism, and sudden death.[1,2,35] Moist rales, cardiac murmurs, gallop rhythms (especially S4) and arrhythmias are common. On palpation of the thorax, the point of maximal intensity over the cardiac apex is often exaggerated because of severe left ventricular hypertrophy. If aortic thromboembolism is present, the femoral pulses are absent and the hindlimbs are cool.[37]

Diagnosis: Electrocardiographic abnormalities in hypertrophic cardiomyopathy include atrial and ventricular arrhythmias, intraventricular conduction disturbances, and increased duration and amplitude of P waves and QRS complexes (Fig 7). A left anterior fascicular block pattern is often present and is compatible with an actual conduction defect or left ventricular hypertrophy.[1] Absence of electrocardiographic abnormalities is not uncommon.[37]

Cardiomegaly is almost always evident on thoracic radiographs, with severe left atrial enlargement on the dorsoventral view (Fig 43). Pulmonary edema, identified by generalized fluffy alveolar densities, is common during congestive heart failure. Pleural effusion, a sign of right heart failure, may be present (Table 3).

Nonselective angiocardiograms are indicated when all clinical values are analyzed and the diagnosis is still questionable. Ideally, both the systolic and diastolic phases of the cardiac cycle should be represented, but this is not always possible with nonselective studies. Changes seen include left ventricular thickening, enlarged papillary muscles, decreased ventricular volume and an enlarged left atrium (Fig 44).[23]

Lesions: Necropsy reveals hypertrophy of the left ventricular wall, papillary muscles and septum. Enlargement and hypertrophy of the left atrium is also a consistent finding. In asymmetric septal hypertrophy, the septum is thicker than the left ventricular free wall and impinges on the left ventricular outflow tract (Fig 45). Histologic sections of the ventricular septum in 27% of the cats with hypertrophic cardiomyopathy reveal marked cellular disorganization.

The principal defect is pathologic hypertrophy of the left ventricle, which confers poor distensibility during diastole. Accompanying high left atrial end-diastolic pressure results from greater pressures needed to fill the noncompliant left ventricle. Outflow obstruction in asymmetric septal hypertrophy occurs in some cases. The increased left ventricular mass causes increased 0_2 requirements that eventually cannot be provided by existing coronary blood flow. Stress and tachycardia are precipitating factors in producing dyspnea and pulmonary edema. Tachycardia further shortens diastolic filling time. If the disease progresses gradually, the left atrium enlarges to increase its reservoir capacity. Decompensation occurs eventually. It is not clear if the hypertrophic form progresses to the dilated form of cardiomyopathy.

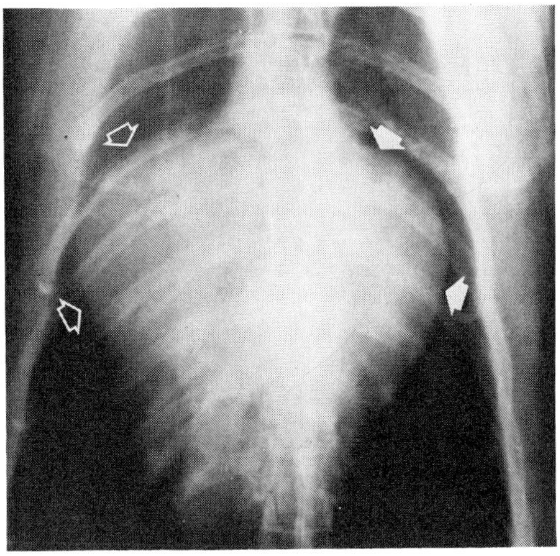

Fig 43. Dorsoventral radiograph of a 2-year-old Persian cat with hypertrophic cardiomyopathy. Enlargement of the right atrium and ventricle (open arrows) and left atrium (solid arrows) give the appearance of a valentine-shaped heart. [From VM/SAC 70 (1975) 313, courtesy of Veterinary Medicine Publishing]

Treatment: Propranolol (Inderal:Ayerst) works primarily by blocking beta-adrenergic receptors. In doing so, it may counteract the effects of stress-related catecholamine release. This drug is intended to reduce the left ventricular diastolic impediment, protect against catechola-

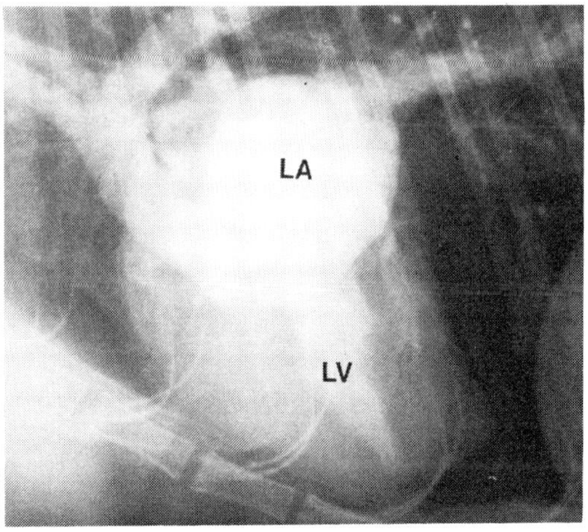

Fig 44. Nonselective left-sided angiocardiogram of a cat with hypertrophic cardiomyopathy. Left ventricular (LV) hypertrophy and left atrial (LA) dilation are seen.

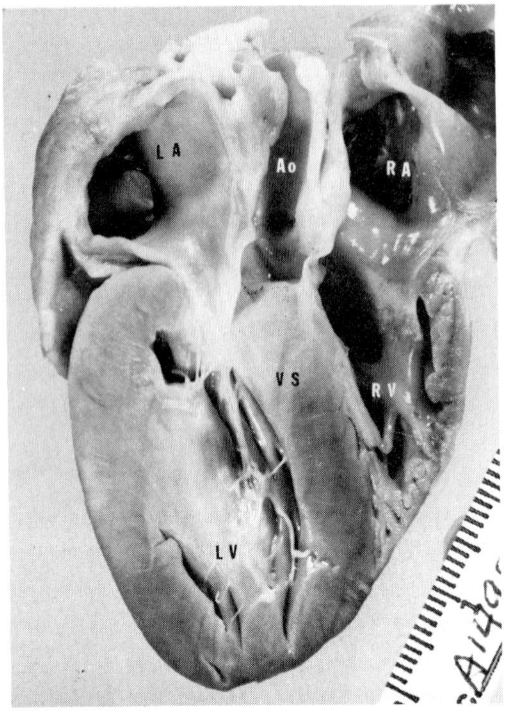

Fig 45. Longitudinal section of a heart from a 3-year-old male Persian cat with hypertrophic cardiomyopathy. The heart has been sectioned at the point where the posterior mitral valve leaflet is not shown. The ventricular septum (VS) is thicker than the left ventricular free wall (LV). The anterior portion of the hypertrophied ventricular septum bulges into and obstructs the lumen of the left ventricular outflow tract. Hypertrophy of the left ventricular free wall, papillary muscles, and ventricular septum causes narrowing of the left ventricular cavity. LA = left atrium, Ao = aorta, RV = right ventricle, RA = right atrium.[1] (Courtesy of Am J Path)

mine-induced arrhythmias and improve ventricular filling. The latter should enhance ventricular performance via the Frank-Starling mechanism.

Propranolol is dosed at 2.5-5.0 mg every 8-12 hours for a 5-kg cat. Therapy must be individualized to achieve a clinical endpoint. Propranolol should be used in cats with hypertrophic cardiomyopathy only after pulmonary edema and other signs of congestive heart failure have been resolved. The drug can depress myocardial performance and thereby accentuate cardiac failure. Therefore, the cat should be closely observed for signs of heart failure during administration of propranolol. Use of the drug should be temporarily discontinued if such signs occur. Untoward effects, such as GI disturbances, weakness and thrombocytopenia, are rare.

Diuretic therapy promotes diuresis, and reduces blood volume and pulmonary capillary pressure, thereby diminishing pulmonary edema. Care must be taken to avoid overuse of diuretics in cats since they seem to be more sensitive and more prone to dehydration and hypokalemia than are dogs.

The 2 major diuretic agents commonly used are furosemide (Lasix:Hoechst-Roussel) and the thiazides. Furosemide is more effective because of its rapid onset of action and is useful when fluid overload is present or imminent. In cats with acute left ventricular failure from hypertrophic or restrictive cardiomyopathy, pulmonary edema and tachycardia require immediate therapy. Furosemide is given IV in these situations. A bolus of 1-2 mg/kg is followed by 1 mg/kg given IV or IM twice or 3 times daily. The dosage is gradually reduced to the smallest effective dose, ideally 1 mg/kg every second or third day.[37]

Dilated Cardiomyopathy

Clinical Signs: Dilated cardiomyopathy is manifested by dilation of the left ventricle, with poor myocardial contractility (Fig 42). Cats with dilated cardiomyopathy sometimes are presented for sudden or gradual onset of lethargy and anorexia as the only clinical signs. Usually they are brought in by the client after these signs have rapidly progressed to depression, dehydration, hypothermia, dyspnea or shock. Some cats have aortic thromboemboli. Affected cats are usually middle-aged and more males than females are affected. Auscultation may reveal a murmur or gallop rhythm but heart and lung

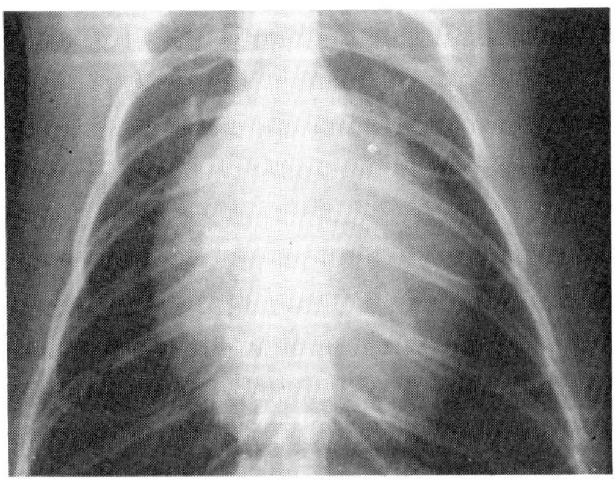

Fig 46. Dorsoventral radiograph of a 10-year-old domestic shorthaired cat with dilated cardiomyopathy. Enlargement of all chambers is evident.[6] (Courtesy of Am J Path)

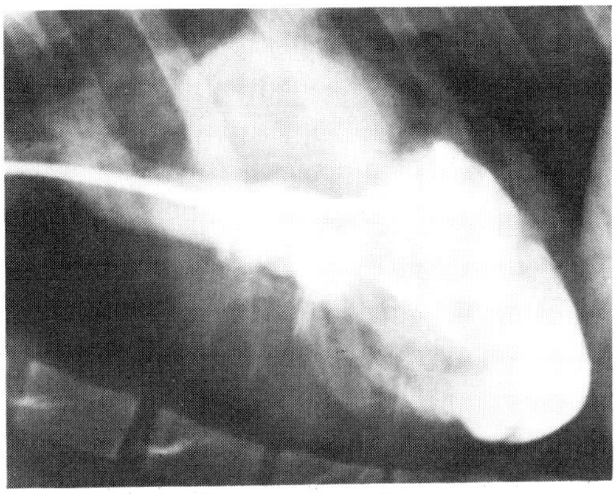

Fig 47. Left ventricular angiocardiogram of a 5-year-old domestic shorthaired cat with dilated cardiomyopathy. Left atrial enlargement is present. The left ventricle is severely dilated.[1] (Courtesy of Am J Path)

sounds may be muffled by pleural effusion. Prerenal azotemia is usually present.

Diagnosis: Common electrocardiographic abnormalities include ventricular premature complexes, tall and wide QRS complexes, first-degree atrioventricular block and sinus bradycardia (Fig 21). Radiographically, pleural effusion often obscures the cardiac silhouette. On dorsoventral thoracic radiographs, all chambers are enlarged (Fig 46). This may be especially evident after thoracocentesis or diuretic therapy. Ascites, a common sequela of right heart failure in dogs, is rare in cats (Table 3).

Because of the critical condition of most cats with dilated cardiomyopathy, discretion must be used in selecting cases for angiocardiography. Angiocardiographic characteristics include dilation of all cardiac chambers, atrophied papillary muscles, a poorly opacified aorta and slow circulation time (Fig 47).

Lesions: At necropsy, the heart is enlarged and globular because of extreme ventricular dilation. The left and right atria are moderately enlarged. The papillary muscles and trabeculae in the ventricles are flattened and atrophic (Fig 48).

Treatment: Dilated cardiomyopathy causes gross left and right ventricular dilation and subsequent impaired systolic function. The large ventricular volume results in increased wall tension that cannot be met by adequate contractile force. The coronary blood supply cannot meet the 0_2 demand required by this increased wall tension. Almost all affected cats develop progressive right heart failure with severe pleural effusion. Mild to moderate left heart failure may occasionally occur simultaneously. Because concurrent shock (a low-output heart failure state) and dehydration are common, it usually is advisable to insert an IV catheter and administer half-strength mixed electrolyte solution and 2.5% dextrose in water, taking care to avoid iatrogenic fluid overload. Very dyspneic cats are placed in an 0_2 cage. Thoracentesis may relieve external pressure on the heart and lungs.

Therapeutic objectives for congestive heart failure associated with dilated cardiomyopathy are to strengthen the heart as a pump, to spare the pump by reducing workload, while still meeting the need for blood flow and perfusion pressure, to prevent secondary damage to the myocardium and other organs, and to promote rapid recovery of myocardial function.

Cats in critical condition are given digoxin IV at 0.002 mg/kg body weight divided into 4 doses given over 4 hours or to effect. The average daily maintenance dosage is 0.005-0.01 mg/kg body weight (*eg*, one-quarter of a 0.125-mg tablet once daily for a 4.5-kg cat or every other day for a 2.5-kg cat). Furosemide is also given IV to cats in critical condition. Vasodilators, such as nitroglycerin ointment (Nitrol:Kremers-Urban, Nitro-Bid:Marion) at 1/4 inch/4-8 kg applied topically TID or QID, may be an effective adjunct in treatment of acute congestive heart failure in some cats. This is a clinical impression, however, and

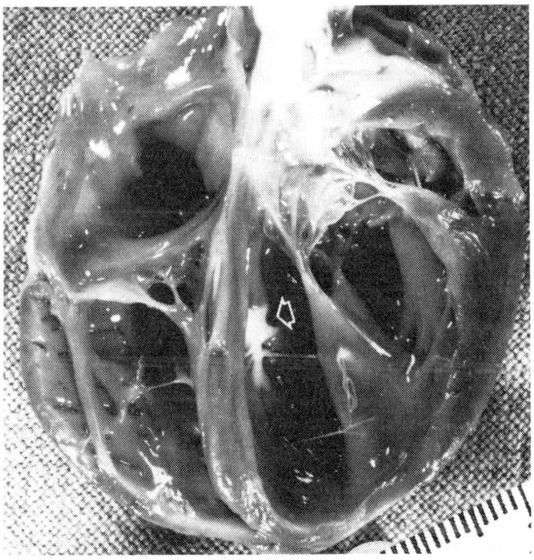

Fig 48. Heart from a 7-year-old male domestic shorthaired cat with dilated cardiomyopathy. All 4 chambers are dilated. Focal endocardial fibrosis (arrow) was found in the left ventricular septum.[1] (Courtesy of Am J Path)

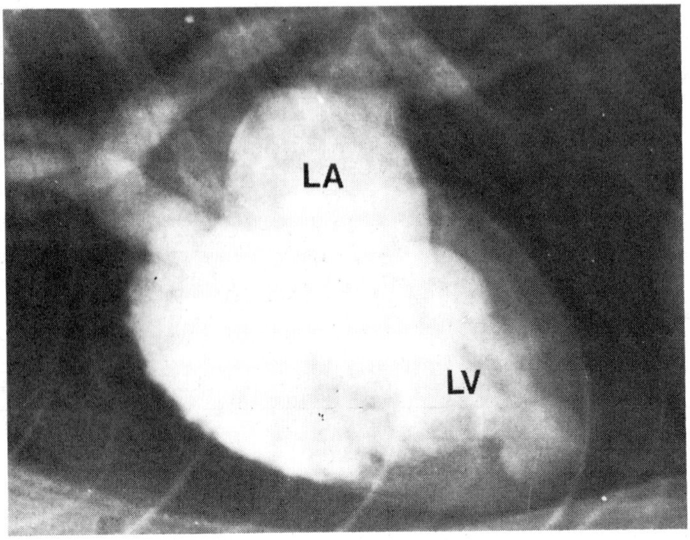

Fig 49. Nonselective angiocardiogram of a cat with restrictive cardiomyopathy. Left ventricular hypertrophy and marked endocardial fibrosis have produced an irregular left ventricular (LV) cavity. The left atrium (LA) is markedly enlarged.

controlled experiments in naturally occurring disease are lacking.

The prognosis for cats presenting with acute dilated cardiomyopathy is grave; they may die within 24-48 hours of presentation. Those surviving long enough to be sent home should be given maintenance digoxin (0.005-0.01 mg/kg) and maintenance furosemide (0.17-0.25 mg/kg 1-3 times daily). Exercise restriction and a low-Na diet should be instituted whenever possible. The long-term use of vasodilators has not been evaluated. Use of beta-adrenergic blockers, such as propranolol, is controversial. Re-examination in 7-10 days is advisable to monitor the efficacy of therapy.

The long term prognosis for cats with dilated cardiomyopathy is poor. Average survival time is often less than one month from onset of clinical signs. Animals may occasionally survive 6 months or more with vigorous and judicious therapy.

Kitten Mortality Complex

The kitten mortality complex is a newly described syndrome associated with an unusually high kitten mortality rate in catteries. Acute dilated cardiomyopathy associated with the kitten mortality complex has been described in adults and kittens in several catteries. Although the cause has not been determined, a viral etiology is suspected. Feline infectious peritonitis has been implicated by virtue of its prevalence in affected colonies. However, the true identity of the underlying factor(s) and the significance of FIP, if any, remain to be demonstrated.[38]

Restrictive Cardiomyopathy

Of the 4 major functional categories of cardiomyopathy (dilated, hypertrophic, restrictive, excessive left ventricular moderator bands), restrictive is the least common (Fig 42). Diastolic dysfunction caused by impaired ventricular filling is the principal hemodynamic abnormality. Various specific pathologic processes can be the cause. Endomyocardial fibrosis results but the etiology usually is unknown.

Most affected cats are mature males (range 1-15 years, average 6.8 years). Clinical signs include dyspnea, lethargy and anorexia. Aortic thromboembolism is common. Conduction and rhythm disturbances, including ventricular premature contractions and atrial fibrillation, are sometimes found. Left atrial enlargement often is observed on radiographs. Pleural effusion and especially pulmonary edema are sometimes present. Angiocardiography may reveal left ventricular apical dilation or irregular filling defects (Fig 49). Gross pathologic changes include severe endocardial thickening, especially of the left ventricular outflow and inflow tracts, extreme left atrial enlargement, and dilation of the right atrium and ventricle. Severe endocardial fibrosis is characteristic histologically.

Only a limited number of cats have undergone treatment, with disappointing results. Digitalis glycosides are indicated in cases of atrial fibrillation to control the ventricular rate. Diuretics help reduce pulmonary edema and effusion, and result in improvement in some cases. However, progression of the disease usually is so advanced by the time of diagnosis that therapy may be of little benefit.[37]

Cardiomyopathy Due to Excessive Left Ventricular Moderator Bands

Another form of cardiomyopathy is associated with excessive numbers of moderator bands bridging the left ventricular septum and free wall, and entangling papillary muscles (Fig 50). Ages of affected animals ranged from 1½ to 13 years (mean 6.5 years); 62% were male. Domestic shorthaired cats comprised 91% of the cases.[34]

Clinical findings included anorexia, lethargy, dyspnea, pleural effusion, pulmonary edema, cardiomegaly, heart murmurs, gallop rhythms, aortic thromboemboli and hypothermia. Electrocardiographic abnormalities, especially conduction disturbances, were observed. Angiocardiographic evidence of irregular or linear left ventricular filling defects were occasionally present. Limited pressure studies revealed evidence of elevated left ventricular end-diastolic pressures. Although pathologic changes are characteristic of this syndrome grossly and histologically, clinical findings often overlapped those of other forms of cardiomyopathy.

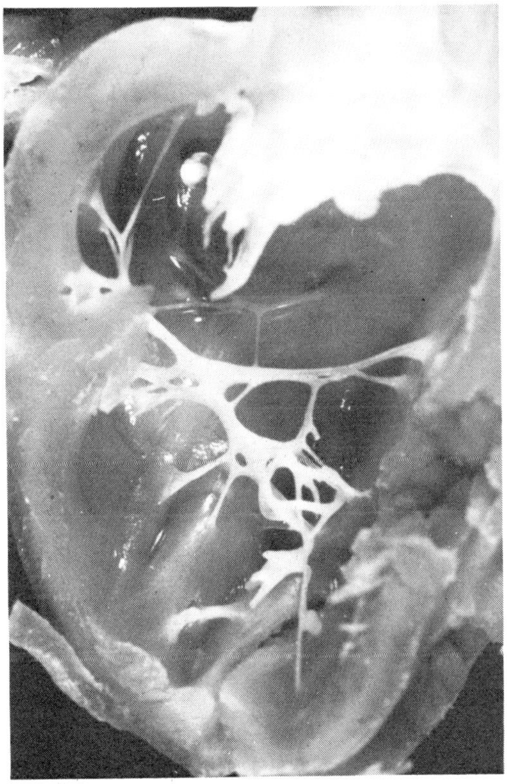

Fig 50. Left ventricle of a 7-year-old spayed female domestic shorthaired cat with excessive numbers of moderator bands bridging the left ventricular septum and free wall. This cat had congestive heart failure, with pleural effusion and severe pulmonary edema.[1] (Courtesy of Am J Path)

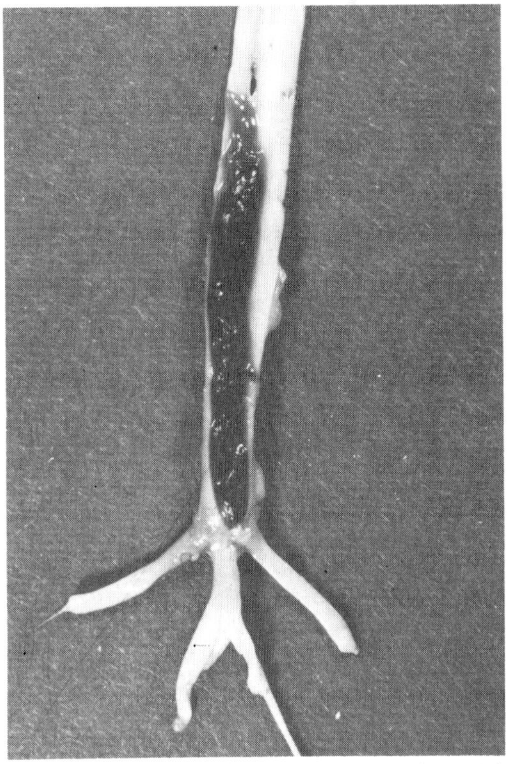

Fig 51. Fresh thromboembolus in the terminal aorta of a 4-year-old domestic shorthaired cat with hypertrophic cardiomyopathy.[1] (Courtesy of Am J Path)

A number of affected cats have successfully responded to diuretics and digitalis. However, clinical and hemodynamic characterization, as well as therapy, have yet to be well defined.[37]

Arterial Thromboembolism

Cause: Arterial thromboembolism is most commonly associated with cardiomyopathy. All forms contribute to spontaneous thromboembolism.[2] Thrombi may originate from the left atrium, from arterial lesions or from hemodynamic aberrations associated with cardiomyopathy. Less often, thromboemboli may originate from vegetative valvular lesions.

The most common location of lodgment of arterial thromboemboli is the terminal aorta at the iliac artery bifurcation (Fig 51). Less com-

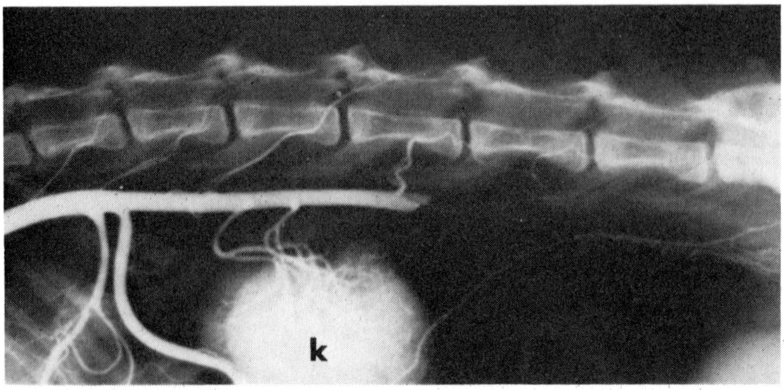

Fig 52. Aortogram of a 4-year-old cat with dyspnea and sudden onset of hindleg lameness. A large thromboembolus in the abdominal aorta, cranial to the iliac bifurcation, blocks the flow of the contrast medium. K=kidney. Hypertrophic cardiomyopathy was evident at necropsy.[1] (Courtesy of Am J Path)

monly, thromboemboli lodge in a front leg or the pulmonary arteries.

The arterial thrombus and not the mechanical occlusion alone contributes to reduced circulation by affecting collateral circulation. Moreover, vasoactive compounds, such as 5-hydroxytryptamine, from degranulated platelets, may be involved in this syndrome.[39] Some degree of collateral circulation persists in most cases, although animals have been observed with gangrenous necrosis of the distal limbs before development of adequate collateral circulation.

Clinical Signs: Distal aortic thromboembolism classically causes acute paraparesis or paraplegia. The distal hindlimbs are cold, the nail beds are cyanotic, and sensory awareness and femoral arterial pulses may be absent. Neurologic examination may reveal flaccid (lower motor neuron) paralysis. Motor function distal to the stifle is most severely affected. Often the lesion is lateralized, with one leg affected more profoundly than the other. This is evidenced by one leg being slightly warmer than the other, with pinker nail beds and pads, weak femoral pulses and greater motor function. Initially, the condition is extremely painful and the limb muscles are soft. A short time later, the limb muscles become very firm or hard, especially the anterior tibial group and gastrocnemius. Serum LDH, CPK and SGOT levels may be greatly elevated. Congestive heart failure and renal, pulmonary, intestinal or myocardial infarction may occur concomitantly.

The effects of ischemia associated with aortic thromboembolism on muscles and peripheral nerves (ischemic neuromyopathy) have been described.[40] The initial ischemic insult usually is of adequate duration to cause posterior paresis. Return of some motor function is common within 2-3 weeks. Recanalization or lysis of the distal aortic thrombus and improved collateral circulation have been demonstrated angiographically 2-4 days after clinical presentation in some cases. Return of femoral pulses, pink nail beds and warm limb extremities may be noted in 2-3 days. Improved motor function is most noticeable initially as an increased ability to flex and extend the hip muscles. At this stage, affected cats drag their rear legs without flexing the tarsus and only minimally flex the stifle. It may take 4-6 weeks to gain full recovery. In some animals, death due to heart disease occurs 1-14 days after thromboembolism. Necropsy of these animals may reveal a large aortic saddle thrombus that has undergone little to no resolution when compared with angiograms taken during onset of signs. Recovery generally is more rapid in cases of forelimb thromboembolism.[37]

Selective arterial or nonselective venous angiography are useful to locate the sites of thromboembolism (Fig 52).

Treatment: Arterial thromboembolism may be managed medically or surgically. Surgical intervention is no longer advocated since ischemic neuromyopathy has usually occurred before surgery and the underlying disease (usually cardiomyopathy and congestive heart failure) makes the animal a poor surgical candidate. Supportive measures are used with primary care directed toward the cardiac abnormality.

There are basic differences between thrombi forming in the arterial system and those in the venous system. Intra-arterial thrombosis is initiated by platelet aggregation, with secondary fibrin deposits, whereas intravenous thrombosis consists primarily of fibrin clots. As a consequence, rational treatment must include use of appropriate agents specific for each type of thrombosis.[41]

Drugs used to treat intravenous thrombi (rare in cats) include heparin and coumarin. Spontaneous recanalization of the thrombus may occur without drug therapy.

Platelet antiaggregates are drugs that theoretically can be considered effective against arterial thrombosis. These drugs include aspirin, dipyridamole, sulfinpyrazone and propranolol.[41]

A quarter of a 5-gr tablet (1.25 gr) of aspirin with an antacid (Ascriptin:Rorer) may be given every second or third day to an average-sized (3-kg) cat.

Other drugs that may be used to treat aortic thrombi include antiserotonergic drugs (cyproheptadine), nonspecific activators of thrombolysis (streptokinase, urokinase) or prostacyclines. These compounds are not yet widely used and have not been clinically tested.

Myocarditis

Myocarditis refers to inflammation of the myocardium, although the term is often used loosely to include degenerative as well as inflammatory myocardial disease. Myocarditis usually is not a singular event but rather occurs in a variety of systemic diseases. Histologic characterization depends in part upon the inciting cause. The true histologic incidence of myocarditis is difficult to determine since most cases probably are subclinical, go unnoticed or resolve spontaneously.

Diseases of diverse etiologies may affect the heart muscle primarily or secondarily, resulting in myocarditis (Table 4). If signs of systemic illness overshadow cardiac signs, the presence of heart disease may be overlooked. Comprehensive patient evaluation may suggest the underlying cause and disease process; however, often the etiology of myocarditis remains obscure.

Clinical signs of myocarditis range from none to fulminant congestive failure. Infectious myocarditis may produce clinical abnormalities during the early convalescent phase of an acute infectious disease. Onset and progression of myocardial inflammation may parallel recovery from the initial signs of the infection.[42] Myocarditis may be a chronic process from the onset or can become chronic after an acute induction. Even when inflammation resolves, lesions may persist to influence myocardial function.

It is difficult to determine if myocarditis is attributable to direct tissue invasion and cellular damage by an infectious agent or if a toxic, allergic or hypersensitivity response to the organism induced the clinical, electrocardiographic and pathologic abnormalities.[42] Electrocardiographic alterations with myocarditis are nonspecific and usually transient. Abnormalities of the S-T segment and T wave have been reported. Atrioventricular and intraventricular conduction defects may be observed, as well as atrial and ventricular arrhythmias.

Treatment is supportive and tailored toward the more dominant disease and its systemic manifestations. Congestive heart failure or arrhythmias are treated with regard to the underlying cause.

Classification of myocarditis may be based on involvement only of the heart (primary myocarditis) or involvement of the heart as part of a generalized multisystemic process (secondary

Table 4. Causes or Possible Associations of Secondary Cardiomyopathy

Type	Cause/Association
Infectious (myocarditis)	Viral (suspected), bacterial, fungal, algal, protozoal
Metabolic	Chronic electrolyte disturbances (hyperkalemia, hypokalemia), uremia
Infiltrative	Neoplasia, amyloidosis
Endocrine	Hyperthyroidism, hyperadrenocorticism, pheochromocytoma
Genetic (unproven)	Hypertrophic cardiomyopathy
Idiopathic	Idiopathic dilated cardiomyopathy, idiopathic restrictive cardiomyopathy, idiopathic hypertrophic cardiomyopathy, idiopathic excessive left ventricular moderator band cardiomyopathy
Toxic	Doxorubicin, others
Inflammatory	Infectious agents, toxins, immune reactions
Other	Heatstroke, hypothermia, malnutrition

myocarditis). Alternatively, an etiologic scheme of classification depends upon identifying a specific pathologic process causing myocardial injury. The designation "idiopathic" is applied when the cause cannot be elucidated.

Inflammatory Myocarditis: Myocarditis occurs when the heart is affected by an inflammatory process, usually an infection. The myocardial cells, interstitium or vessels may be involved. Myocardial injury may occur by direct myocardial invasion of an infectious agent, myocardial toxin production by an infectious agent, or via an immune-mediated reaction. In addition to infectious causes, inflammatory myocarditis can result from radiation, chemicals (lead), drugs (doxorubicin) and metabolic abnormalities (uremia). Histopathologically, lesions are usually focal or diffuse. Clinical cardiac signs depend upon the size, number and location of lesions.[36]

Bacterial Myocarditis: Pyogenic bacteria originating from septicemia or suppurative foci can produce acute, focal myocarditis. Bacterial emboli sometimes can be demonstrated. Myocardial septic embolization secondary to vegetative endocarditis can occur.[43] Clinical signs range from subclinical to nonspecific (lethargy, weight loss), varying with the chronicity and severity of the disease. Fever is not a consistent feature. Heart murmurs usually are absent unless underlying lesions of bacterial endocarditis, concurrent cardiomyopathy or congenital cardiac anomalies or systemic disease (anemia) are present. Arrhythmias may be detected in some cases.

Blood chemistries, hemograms and blood cultures are recommended to facilitate diagnosis. The sudden onset of dysrhythmia accompanying a bacterial infectious disease that has not responded to therapy should prompt consideration of myocarditis as a diagnosis.

Viral Myocarditis: Clinical signs of myocarditis have been associated with systemic viral infections in dogs but are not well documented in cats. Myocardial susceptibility may be enhanced by use of immunosuppressive drugs, malnutrition and previous myocardial disease. Because viral replication in the heart may occur without clinical abnormalities or light microscopic lesions, the diagnosis of viral myocarditis is difficult.[44]

Fungal and Algal Myocarditis: Myocardial involvement in mycotic infections is usually a secondary manifestation of disseminated disease. Systemic fungal infections often occur in conjunction with reduced host defense due to infectious, metabolic or neoplastic disease, or as a result of immunosuppressive therapy. Isolated cases are occasionally encountered. Diagnosis of myocardial involvement may be difficult and is usually of secondary importance in comparison to the generalized systemic disease process.

Parasitic Myocarditis: Toxoplasmosis is caused by the obligate intracellular coccidian parasite, *Toxoplasma gondii.* This zoonotic infectious agent of many birds and mammals is enzootic to a wide geographic area. Cats are the only definitive hosts and may serve as intermediate hosts for infection of other animals.

Acute clinical disease in cats with manifestations of parasitic myocarditis is rare. As immunity to *T gondii* develops, the organisms encyst in various tissues, including the heart. These slowly dividing bradyzoites involved in chronic infection are long-lived. They may rupture (excyst) periodically, causing a hypersensitivity reaction and tissue necrosis. Immune suppression from drugs or disease (FeLV infection) may cause released bradyzoites to rapidly proliferate, with consequent myocarditis.[45]

Clinical signs of toxoplasmosis vary. Diagnosis may be facilitated by histologic identification of organisms in host tissue, animal inoculation, identification of oocysts in cat feces, or by rising serum antibody titers. Arrhythmias detected in conjunction with clinical signs compatible with toxoplasmosis (chorioretinitis, anterior uveitis, encephalitis, granulomatous pneumonia, hepatitis) should increase the suspicion of toxoplasmal myocarditis and generalized toxoplasmosis.

Chapter 4 contains a more detailed discussion of toxoplasmosis.

Noninfectious Myocardial Injury: Many noninfectious agents (toxins, chemicals, drugs) may induce myocardial injury in an acute or chronic process. Myocardial response is often related to the dose and length of exposure. Heatstroke, hypothermia and myocardial allergic reactions to various drugs may produce myocardial injury. Involvement of multiple organ systems often dominates the clinical presentation and obscures myocardial involvement.[36]

Dirofilariasis

Dirofilariasis (heartworm disease) is caused by *Dirofilaria immitis,* a filarial nematode transmitted by mosquitoes. It is prevalent in most mosquito-infested regions and has become an enzootic canine parasite. The dog is the definitive host but many other species have been parasitized, including cats. Although adult filariae are usually confined to the right ventricle and pulmonary arteries, they have been found in the CNS (lateral ventricles, spinal canal, cerebral vessels), bronchioles, eye, vomitus, feces, cysts, abdominal cavity and abscesses.[46] While many cases are discovered at necropsy, there are increasing numbers of reports of feline heartworm disease and accounts of successful therapy, some with IV thiacetarsamide (Caparsolate:Abbott). Extensive reviews of feline dirofilariasis have been published.[47-49]

Feline dirofilariasis may occur either as a patent infection (infective larvae maturing to adults that produce microfilaremia) or as an occult infection (dirofilariasis without circulating microfilariae). Lack of microfilaremia may be due to immune-mediated removal of microfilariae, or the presence of adults of only one sex or only immature adults.

The ages of affected cats reportedly ranges from 9 months to 17 years. Males are affected about 3 times as commonly as females.

Clinical Signs: Presenting complaints include acute respiratory distress and occasionally neurologic signs. Dirofilariasis may be suspected when clinical findings parallel alterations of canine heartworm disease involving the pulmonary, cardiovascular, hepatic, renal and hemopoietic systems. Concurrent radiographic, electrocardiographic, blood chemistry and hematologic changes are related to such alterations. In experimentally infected cats, right heart enlargement, pulmonary artery enlargement and pulmonary parenchymal densities were noted.[50] Right heart enlargement on plain radiographs and adult heartworms in the cranial vena cava, defined by angiocardiography, have been observed in naturally occurring occult dirofilariasis. Adult heartworms have been visualized in pulmonary vasculature with nonselective angiocardiography. Electrocardiographic changes compatible with right ventricular enlargement may be present.

Diagnosis: Diagnosis is based upon the history (dyspnea, coughing or rarely neurologic abnormalities), physical examination, electrocardiographic findings (right heart enlargement pattern) and radiographic signs (right ventricular and pulmonary artery enlargement, pulmonary parenchymal densities). Angiocardiography may provide visualization of adult heartworms in the vena cava, right heart and pulmonary arteries, and defines cardiac changes (right ventricular and pulmonary artery enlargement). Microfilaremia, if present, is diagnostic. In cases of occult dirofilariasis, immunologic testing is essential. The indirect fluorescent antibody technic is used to test for antibodies against microfilarial antigens. The enzyme-linked immunosorbent assay (ELISA) can detect specific antibodies to adult filariae.

The incidence of feline dirofilariasis is low, but heartworm disease or aberrant migration of adult filariae must be considered in differential diagnosis of respiratory disease or unexplained clinical signs associated with the cardiovascular, respiratory, GI or neurologic systems.

Treatment: Treatment of confirmed cases in clinically affected cats may be undertaken. Adult heartworms have been destroyed with IV injections of 1% thiacetarsamide sodium at 0.45 mg/kg every 12 hours for 4 treatments. A complete blood chemistry profile and hemogram should be performed 4-6 weeks later. Cardiopulmonary disease may resolve after successful therapy, but too few cases have been reported for adequate evaluation.

Hyperthyroidism

Hyperthyroidism (thyrotoxicosis) resulting from a hyperfunctioning thyroid adenoma (adenomatous hyperplasia) can produce dyspnea and cardiovascular abnormalities, including cardiomegaly, tachycardia and electrocardiographic changes. [51,52]

Clinical Signs: Clinical signs include hyperactivity, weight loss despite polyphagia, frequent defecation of bulky stools, polyuria, polydipsia, tachycardia, cardiomegaly, murmurs, arrhythmias and palpable enlargement of one or both thyroid lobes.[51] The SGPT, SGOT and SAP levels may be elevated.

Tachycardia ($\geq$240 beats/minute) and increased R-wave amplitude in lead II ($>$0.9 mv) were the most frequently reported electrocardiographic abnormalities. Other changes included atrial premature complexes, atrial tachycardia, ventricular premature complexes, ventricular tachycardia, ventricular bigeminy, prolonged QRS duration and shortened Q-T interval. Intraventricular conduction disturbances (right bundle branch block and left anterior fascicular block) were rare. Multiple ECG abnormalities were present in more than half of the cats with hyperthyroidism. The ECG was normal in one-fifth of affected animals.[52]

Diagnosis: Diagnosis of hyperthyroidism is based on the history, clinical signs and electrocardiographic findings and is confirmed by evaluating serum T_3 and T_4 levels by radioimmunoassay.

Congestive heart failure may occasionally be the presenting complaint. Many electrocardiographic and radiographic changes accompanying hyperthyroidism are similar to those of primary myocardial disease (cardiomyopathy). Therefore, hyperthyroidism should be a differential diagnosis in mature and old cats with suspected cardiomyopathy.

Treatment: Preoperative, intraoperative and postoperative treatment has been described.[51] Hemithyroidectomy or total thyroidectomy resolved electrocardiographic abnormalities.[52] Hypoparathyroidism is a potential postoperative complication of bilateral thyroidectomy due to removal of the parathyroid glands, which are invested in or around thyroid tissue. Tetany and weakness may result from resultant hypocalcemia. Electrocardiographic signs of hypocalcemia include a prolonged Q-T segment. Elevation of the serum Ca level with IV Ca solutions results in shortening of this interval.

CARDIOVASCULAR PHARMACOLOGY

Treatment of feline heart disease is based upon proper clinical, radiographic and electrocardiographic diagnosis to avoid instituting inappropriate or hazardous therapy. The cause, pathophysiology and history of the cardiac disorder should be understood before selecting the proper therapeutic regimen. Appropriate clinical and laboratory investigations should be made to detect noncardiac causes of rhythm disturbances that are correctible without use of antiarrhythmic agents. Knowledge of available drugs, their modes of action and pharmacodynamics, potential drug interactions and contraindications is a prerequisite to pharmacologic intervention. Drugs should be selected to manage arrhythmias, increase myocardial contractility or modify the hemodynamic abnormalitics caused by a failing heart (Table 5).[6]

Specific drugs are not commonly used to treat arrhythmias in cats. Not only is it better to attempt control by removing specific underlying causes, but use of antiarrhythmic drugs may be dangerous or ineffective unless the underlying disorder is treated. For example, in cases of hyperkalemia caused by urethral obstruction, appropriate medical management eliminates the associated arrhythmia. Bradycardia or ventricular premature complexes during general anesthesia may be resolved by decreasing administration of the anesthetic and increasing oxygenation.

When antiarrhythmic agents are used, propranolol (Inderal:Ayerst) and digoxin (Lanoxin:Wellcome) are the drugs most commonly employed. Drugs used extensively in dogs, such as quinidine, procainamide, lidocaine and phenytoin, are not generally advocated for use in cats since inappropriate doses can easily result in toxicity and death.

Lidocaine

Use of lidocaine is dangerous in cats. It is metabolized by the liver. Cats have deficient amounts of glucuronyl transferase and the rate of glucuronide conjugation of drugs is extremely slow in comparison to that in other species. Adverse reactions to lidocaine given IV in dosages of less than 2 mg/kg body weight have been reported. Convulsions and respiratory depression have been observed. Cardiovascular abnormalities from use of lidocaine include bradyarrhythmias, conduction disturbances and sudden death.[41] Heart failure can influence the pharmacodynamics of lidocaine by reducing its plasma clearance and volume of distribution. When necessary, lidocaine is given by slow IV infusion at 0.11 mg/kg.

Phenytoin

The plasma half-life of phenytoin is much longer in cats than in dogs. This is attributable to the inability of cats to hydroxylate phenolic compounds (the phenyl ring is a moiety of phenytoin). Signs of toxicity include sedation, anorexia and ataxia. Maintenance doses of phenytoin may be achieved with a dosage of 2-3 mg/kg/day or 20 mg/kg/week.[53] However, toxicity may still occur due to the drug's prolonged half-life. Therefore, use of phenytoin is best avoided or reserved for special situations.

Propranolol

Propranolol, because of its broad antiarrhythmic action, is the drug of choice in cats. It is a beta-adrenergic receptor antagonist. Stimulation of beta-adrenergic cardiac receptors increases the heart rate (chronotropy), contractility (inotropy), automaticity and rate of impulse conduction. Beta-receptor blockade thus modifies or prevents these effects. Propranolol may be useful for tachyarrhythmias (ventricular tachycardia, atrial tachycardia, atrial flutter, ventricular pre-excitation). Propranolol may also exert a quinidine-like effect, decreasing automaticity and conductivity in the myocardium and Purkinje system, thereby inhibiting ventricular ectopia.[54] It is used in combination with digitalis to decrease conduction through the atrioventricular node, especially in atrial fibrillation. Therapy must be individualized according to clinical response, such as decreased heart rate, elimination or suppression of arrhythmias, and resolution of clinical signs. Propranolol is also useful in treating hypertrophic cardiomyopathy to reduce left ventricular diastolic impedance and thus promote ventricular filling. Ventricular performance is thus enhanced via the Frank-Starling mechanism and coronary perfusion is increased (coronary blood flow is greatest during diastole). Myocardial consumption of 0_2 is diminished. By decreasing contractility, obstruction of the aortic outflow tract also is decreased in hypertrophic obstructive cardiomyopathy. By blocking the catecholamine effects on the heart, stress-induced sinus tachycardia, which can exacerbate or precipitate a failure state, may be prevented and an "irritable" diseased myocardium is protected from the arrhythmogenic properties of catecholamines.

Propranolol is well absorbed from the intestinal tract and metabolized by the liver. Its half-life when given IV is 35 minutes.[54] Its half-life from oral administration, as extrapolated from studies in people, is 3-6 hours, but this duration may be prolonged at high dosages.

Contraindications for propranolol use include asthma, bradyarrhythmias, first-degree heart block and some types of heart failure. It should not be used in left-sided congestive heart failure until pulmonary edema and other signs of failure have resolved since it decreases cardiac per-

Table 5. Drugs Used To Treat Cardiac Arrhythmias [6]

Drug	Dosage and Route of Administration	Indications
Atropine sulfate, 0.4 mg/ml injectable	SC, IM, IV: 0.04 mg/kg every 4-6 hours	Sinus bradycardia, atrioventricular block
Calcium chloride*	IC, IV: 0.05-0.10 ml 10% solution/kg	Ventricular asystole, electrical-mechanical dissociation
Digoxin, 0.125-mg tablets, 0.25 mg/ml injectable	PO: 0.005-0.01 mg/kg, average daily maintenance IV: 0.002 mg/kg in 4 divided doses over 4 hours or to effect	Congestive heart failure, atrial tachycardia, atrial premature complexes, atrial fibrillation, atrial flutter
Epinephrine HCl*, 1:1000 solution, 1 mg/ml injectable	IC: 6-10 μg/kg IV: 0.05-0.1 mg of 1:10,000 dilution	Ventricular asystole, change of fine ventricular fibrillation to coarse ventricular fibrillation
Isoproterenol, 0.2 mg/ml injectable	IV: 0.5 mg/250 ml 5% dextrose/water and titrate to effect	Sinus bradycardia, complete atrioventricular block
Potassium chloride*	IC: 0.25-0.75 mEq, followed by calcium chloride	Depolarization of the heart, chemical defibrillator
Propranolol, 10-mg tablets, 1 mg/ml injectable	PO: 2.5 mg every 8-12 hours for average 5-kg cat, higher dosages to effect IV: 0.25 mg diluted in 1 ml saline, given as 0.2-ml boluses to effect	Sinus tachycardia, supraventricular tachycardia and ventricular arrhythmias, pre-excitation arrhythmias, and with digoxin for atrial fibrillation

(Courtesy of C.V. Mosby) .
* Drugs for cardiac arrest

formance and exacerbates the failure state. It should be used with caution in diabetic animals since it blocks insulin secretion.

Digoxin

Digitalis is used in atrial fibrillation, atrial tachycardia and atrial flutter to decrease the ventricular rate, and in congestive (dilated) cardiomyopathy to improve cardiac performance. It increases strength of contractility (positive inotropy) and decreases the heart rate (negative chronotropy). The latter is a result of decreased atrioventricular nodal conduction velocity, increased refractory period, decreased reflex sympathetic stimulation during heart failure and increased vagal tone.

Digoxin is the form of digitalis used most commonly in cats. Highest plasma digoxin levels were reported with use of the elixir and the lowest with use of crushed tablets mixed with food. Males had higher plasma digoxin levels than females. Food given within 2-3 hours of oral administration of any form of digoxin decreases absorption of the drug.[55] Delayed gastric emptying subjects digoxin to greater hydrolysis, decreasing the quantity of active digoxin absorbed. Because digoxin is excreted primarily by the kidneys, excretion is delayed in cats with renal impairment, and toxicosis may result.

Despite better absorption and the ability to more accurately measure a dose of the drug in elixir form, digoxin is most commonly administered in whole-tablet form because cats often do not tolerate the elixir. A fraction of Lanoxin (Jen-Sal) tablet (usually one-quarter of a 0.125-mg tablet) is easy to administer without food or coated in a very small quantity of food to facilitate swallowing.

Cats are very sensitive to digoxin. Cats given a single oral dose of digoxin elixir (0.01 mg/kg) for 4 consecutive days had daily increases in peak blood digoxin levels with each successive dose. Average blood concentrations by day 4 were 62% higher than after the first dose, which indicates the potential for toxicosis. A plasma digoxin concentration of 2.3 mg/ml was not toxic but concentrations of 4.45 mg/ml and higher caused depression, vomiting, salivation and anorexia before electrocardiographic changes appeared. Alterations in the ECG were minimal, with a slight increase in the P-Q interval, elevation of S-T segment and decreased heart rate being most important. Intact and neutered males were more susceptible to digoxin toxicosis than were intact queens.[55]

Cats with congestive (dilated) cardiomyopathy and heart failure have a very poor prognosis and rapid IV digitalization has been more effective than oral maintenance digitalization. Cats not in critical condition are given digoxin tablets at 0.005-0.01 mg/kg body weight. However, digoxin may accumulate in the serum with consecutive daily dosage, resulting in digoxin toxicosis, especially if the cat has prerenal azotemia from anorexia due to decompensated heart failure. Alternate-day administration of digoxin for maintenance has been used successfully in many such animals.

If digoxin toxicity occurs, administration of the drug should be stopped for at least 24 and sometimes up to 96 hours. Fluid therapy should be instituted and electrolytes balanced as needed. The animal can be re-evaluated in regard to renal function, electrolyte status and clinical condition. The client should be carefully questioned to ascertain if recommended dosages and administration protocol have been followed; calculation of digoxin dosage should be rechecked. The dosage must be modified if any clinical value has changed to influence digoxin pharmacokinetics. Plasma digoxin levels can be measured if a diagnosis of intoxication cannot be made on the basis of clinical signs and history.[37]

Diuretics

Diuretics are very effective in the management of congestive heart failure, especially when used in conjunction with digoxin or propranolol. By inducing diuresis they reduce blood volume and pulmonary capillary pressure. By promoting renal electrolyte and water loss, they help alleviate the compensatory mechanisms of fluid retention activated by heart failure. Diuretics do not increase cardiac output. However, overzealous or untimely application may decrease blood volume and cardiac output, causing cardiac decompensation or precipitating digoxin toxicity. Dehydration, prerenal azotemia, metabolic alkalosis, hypotension and lethargy may occur. Sick animals often are dehydrated due to anorexia and prerenal azotemia can be exacerbated if vigorous diuresis is induced.

Of the 2 most commonly employed diuretic agents in cats (furosemide and thiazides), furosemide (Lasix:Hoechst) is more effective. A potent loop diuretic, furosemide inhibits active Cl transport and passive Na resorption in the thick ascending limb of the loop of Henle. The onset of effect is more rapid than with the thiazides. Intravenous administration of furosemide may cause maximal diuresis within 30-40 minutes, persisting for 2-3 hours. This rapid onset is especially suited for the acute pulmonary edema of left heart failure in hypertrophic or restrictive cardiomyopathy. Long-term therapy involves reducing the dosage of furosemide to the smallest effective dose, such as giving it every second or third day if possible. However, this is not always possible. Some cats require administration at 2 mg/kg twice daily for long periods with little apparent untoward effects. Administration 3 times daily is occasionally necessary in refractory or terminal patients. The potential for electrolyte imbalance is present when high levels of furosemide are given. The most important principle in the use of all diuretics is to administer the smallest possible effective dose.

Vasodilators

Vasodilator therapy is under clinical investigation as a means to "unload" failing ventricles by decreasing excessive blood volume or pressure. Arterial vasodilators decrease impedance to arterial blood flow, lower systemic vascular resistance and improve cardiac output. Hydralazine (Apresoline:CIBA) has been used orally at up to 2.5 mg BID in this fashion. Venous vasodilators increase venous capacitance, decrease ventricular filling pressures and diminish pulmonary edema. Nitroglycerin ointment (Nitro-Bid:Marion) is used topically for this purpose. Hypotension is the major untoward effect of vasodilator therapy unless blood pressure monitoring, sufficiently low doses or concomitant administration of sympathomimetics or catecholamines is used. Clinical indices of arterial pressure that may help assess the results of therapy include pulse pressure, capillary refill time, level of consciousness, urinary output and indirect blood pressure.

Catecholamines

Catecholamines are being investigated for management of acute and chronic congestive heart failure. Dopamine HCl (Intropin:American Critical Care) and dobutamine (Dobutrex:Lilly) increase myocardial contractility and cardiac performance in acute and refractory heart failure. Beneficial effects may result from combination of catecholamines with vasodilators but clinical guidelines are not available.

CARDIOVASCULAR EMERGENCIES

Cardiac arrest may result from primary myocardial disease (cardiomyopathy) or from systemic alterations influencing the heart. Prompt intervention, using a basic approach of patient evaluation, cardiopulmonary resuscitation, and ventilatory and circulatory support, may reverse or control lethal consequences of cardiopulmonary arrest. Arrest can be associated with a variety of predisposing factors that must be treated after resuscitation. Respiratory arrest may precede or occur simultaneously with cardiac arrest.

Early recognition of a potential cardiopulmonary emergency may depend upon appreciating clinical signs of impending arrest. Weak, thready pulses, poor capillary refill, hypothermia, cyanosis, and a change in mentation and respiratory status may shortly precede arrest. Cardiopulmonary arrest is manifested by lack of respiration, heart beat and pulses, dilated, nonresponsive pupils and lack of bleeding from cut surfaces. Electrocardiographic evidence of asystole (lack of ventricular electrical activity), lethal arrhythmia (ventricular fibrillation or bradycardia) or electrical-mechanical dissociation of cardiac function also is present.

Cardiopulmonary arrest necessitates an organized, efficient initial reaction by the attending medical staff if the patient is to survive. This is only possible if all staff members are familiar with resuscitation and emergency procedures and if a "crash cart" and other necessary equipment are available. In this manner, CNS injury, which becomes severe after 4-6 minutes of arrest, may be minimized.

Once cardiopulmonary arrest is detected, the patient is managed according to an "ABCDE" scheme: A. establish a patent airway, B. breathe for the patient, C. restore circulation, D. administer drugs or defibrillate the heart, and E. evaluate the ECG to direct therapy. A flow chart for cardiopulmonary resuscitation and essential therapeutic management has been published.[56,57]

Respiratory support is initiated first by insertion of a cuffed endotracheal tube (or tracheostomy if intubation is prevented by airway obstruction). Forced ventilation is ideally accomplished with a mechanical respirator and 100% O_2 at a rate of 12-16 breaths/minute. If a respirator is unavailable, an Ambu bag may be used to deliver room air or mouth-to-endotracheal tube resuscitation may suffice. Concurrently, closed chest cardiac chest massage (60-80 times/

minute), coordinated with 1 ventilation/5-6 compressions is instituted.

Administration of IV fluids is initiated and drug therapy is guided by evaluation of the heart rate and rhythm, arterial pulse, respiratory effort, results of closed chest massage and duration of cardiopulmonary arrest. Thoracotomy (left fifth intercostal space) may be undertaken as a last resort if a heart beat or pulse is not restored. Successful therapy is followed by cardiovascular monitoring and support. Inciting causes of cardiopulmonary arrest must be corrected.

References

1. Tilley, LP *et al.* Am J Path **87** (1977) 493.
2. Liu, S-K and Tilley, LP. Yale J Biol Med **53** (1980) 191.
3. Tilley, LP and Liu, S-K. Med Times **106** (1978) 2d.
4. Liu, S-K. Vet Clin No Am **7** (1977) 323.
5. Harpster, NK. Vet Clin No Am **7** (1977) 241.
6. Tilley, LP: Essentials of Canine and Feline Electrocardiography. CV Mosby, St. Louis, 1979.
7. Muir, WW *et al.* Am J Vet Res **36** (1975) 1203.
8. Smith, RD and Pettway, CE. Am J Vet Res **36** (1975) 695.
9. Gompf, RE and Tilley, LP. Am J Vet Res **40** (1979) 1483.
10. Harris and Ogburn, in Catcott: Feline Medicine and Surgery. 2nd ed. American Veterinary Publications, Santa Barbara, 1975.
11. Tilley, LP and Gompf, RE. Vet Clin No Am **7** (1977) 257.
12. Rosenbaum, MB and Elizari, MV. Postgrad Med **53** (1973) 87.
13. Rosenbaum, MB. Mod Concepts Cardiovasc Dis **39** (1970) 141.
14. Wantabe, Y and Dreifus, LS: Cardiac Arrhythmias. Grune & Stratton, New York, 1977.
15. Liu, S-K *et al.* Rec Adv Stud Card Struct Metab **10** (1975) 681.
16. Narula, OS. Circ **47** (1973) 872.
17. Friedman, HH: Diagnostic Electrocardiography and Vectorcardiography. 2nd ed. McGraw-Hill, New York, 1977.
18. Ogburn, PN. JAAHA **13** (1977) 171.
19. Bonagura, JD. JAVMA **178** (1981) 574.
20. Hamlin, RL *et al.* JAVMA **143** (1963) 957.
21. Lord, PF and Zontine, WJ. Vet Clin No Am **7** (1977) 291.
22. Owens, JM and Twedt, DC. Vet Clin No Am **7** (1977) 309.
23. Fox, PR and Bond, BR. Vet Clin No Am. *In press,* 1982.
24. Wilkins, RJ. Vet Clin No Am **7** (1977) 285.
25. Fox, PR and Dodds, WJ. Proc Ann Mtg Am Coll Vet Int Med, 1982.
26. Pipers, FS and Hamlin, RL. JAVMA **176** (1980) 57.
27. Popp and Harrison, in Weissler: Noninvasive Cardiology. Grune & Stratton, New York, 1974.
28. Liu, S-K and Tilley, LP. JAVMA **169** (1976) 623.
29. Bolton, GR *et al.* Vet Clin No Am **7** (1977) 341.
30. Sheridan, JP *et al.* J. Sm Anim Pract **12** (1971) 45.
31. Karim, J *et al.* JAVMA **172** (1978) 1432.
32. Bolton, GR *et al.* JAVMA **160** (1972) 1622.
33. Eyster, GE *et al.* JAVMA **169** (1976) 637.
34. Liu, S-K *et al.* JAVMA **180** (1982) 1215.
35. Bond and Tilley, in Kirk: Current Veterinary Therapy VII. WB Saunders, Philadelphia, 1980.
36. Wynne and Braunwald, in Braunwald: Heart Disease. WB Saunders, Philadelphia, 1980.
37. Fox, in Kirk: Current Veterinary Therapy VIII. WB Saunders, Philadelphia, 1983.
38. Scott, in Kirk: Current Veterinary Therapy VII. WB Saunders, Philadelphia, 1980.
39. Bulter, HC. J Sm Anim Pract **12** (1971) 141.
40. Griffiths, IR and Duncan, ID. Vet Rec **104** (1979) 578.
41. Tilley, LP and Weitz, J. Vet Clin No Am **7** (1977) 423.
42. Weneger, in Burch: Cardiomyopathy. FA Davis, Philadelphia, 1972.
43. Knauer, in Kirk: Current Veterinary Therapy VII. WB Saunders, Philadelphia, 1980.
44. Abelmann, WH. Circulation **44** (1971) 950.
45. Jacobson, in Kirk: Current Veterinary Therapy VII. WB Saunders, Philadelphia, 1980.
46. Otto, in Morgan *et al:* Proceedings of the Heartworm Symposium. Veterinary Medicine Publishing, Bonner Springs, 1974.
47. Hawe, RS. JAAHA **15** (1979) 577.
48. Ader, P. Calif Vet **33(11)** (1979) 23.
49. Calvert, CA and Mandell, CP. JAVMA **180** (1982) 550.
50. Donahoe, JM. J Am Vet Rad Soc **17** (1976) 147.
51. Holzworth, J *et al.* JAVMA **176** (1980) 345.
52. Peterson, ME *et al.* JAVMA **180** (1982) 934.
53. Roye, DB *et al.* Am J Vet Res **34** (1973) 947.
54. Weidler, DJ *et al.* Res Commun Chem Path Pharm **26** (1979) 105.
55. Erichsen, DF *et al.* JAAHA **14** (1978) 734.
56. Bonagura, JD. Vet Clin No Am **7** (1977) 385.
57. Adams, HR. Vet Clin No Am **11** (1981) 77.

10

the respiratory system

R.B. FORD

Diseases affecting the upper and lower respiratory tract are among the most diagnostically complex disorders of domestic animals. The variation in clinical signs of respiratory disease, the broad spectrum of etiologic agents capable of causing respiratory disease and the paucity of definitive diagnostic tests explain why the treatment of respiratory disorders is routinely predicated on unconfirmed diagnoses. Discussions in this chapter focus on the clinical orientation of feline respiratory disease. Emphasis is placed on interpreting clinical signs, current diagnostic tests, treatment and prognosis.

Discrete anatomic boundaries separating the upper respiratory tract from the lower respiratory tract have not been defined. However, clinicians attempting to diagnose a specific respiratory disease should initially classify the clinical signs as originating from either the upper or lower respiratory tract. For purposes of this chapter, the upper respiratory tract includes the rhinarium, paranasal sinuses, pharynx and larynx. The lower respiratory tract includes the trachea and associated airways and the lungs. Discussions of diseases of the mediastinum and pleural space are included in the section on lower respiratory tract disease.

To effectively establish a diagnosis, the clinician must properly interpret the clinical signs and localize the respiratory tract segment involved. Once the affected segment has been identified, appropriate diagnostic procedures may be pursued. Obviously, clinical signs of respiratory disease may be caused by primary disorders of the respiratory tract or the clinical signs may be secondary to some underlying problem involving an organ system other than the respiratory tract. Secondary respiratory disorders are discussed in more detail in other chapters.

HISTORY AND PHYSICAL EXAMINATION

Interpretation of the history of cats presented for respiratory disease can be particularly challenging. The owner often is an unreliable source of historical information. Although there is no substitute for actually observing the clinical signs for which an animal is presented, there is no guarantee that the clinical signs will be manifested at the time of examination.

The clinician should at least try to determine the duration and frequency of the clinical signs, the impact of the clinical signs on the cat's general behavior, and the activity level and character of respiration of the cat in its home environment.

Knowledge of the environment in which an animal is maintained can be particularly important in assessing feline respiratory disease. It should be determined whether or not the cat is allowed to roam outside, confined to the house, or caged. In addition, recent known contacts with other cats, ill or healthy, should be determined. The health history of all of the cats in a multiple-cat household should be reviewed when one or more cats are presented.

During the physical examination, the clinician should establish whether the clinical signs are characteristic of upper or lower respiratory tract disease. When clinical signs are evident at presentation, localizing the respiratory tract segment involved generally is not difficult (Table 1). When clinical signs are not evident, the clinician must rely on the owner's ability to describe the signs. This is a considerably less reliable means of determining which respiratory tract segment, if any, is involved.

Table 1. Localization of Clinical Signs

Sign	Respiratory Tract Segment	History/Supporting Signs
Sneezing	Rhinarium	May be acute or chronic; signs are usually paroxysmal; nasal discharge may or may not be present; frontal sinuses may or may not be involved.
Stertor	Pharynx	Snoring sound, loudest during inspiration; may be associated with increased inspiratory effort or open-mouth breathing.
Stridor	Larynx	Wheezing; usually continuous but may be paroxysmal; most evident during expiration.
Cough	Larynx, trachea, bronchi, mediastinum, lungs, heart	Is not a discrete localizing sign; usually intermittent when reported; thorough diagnostic exam is justified.
Dyspnea	Larynx, lower airways, mediastinum, pleura, pleural space, lungs, heart	May be seen at rest or only during exertion; is an emergency situation until proven otherwise; may be associated with orthopnea, tachypnea, open-mouth breathing or cyanosis.

DIAGNOSIS OF RESPIRATORY DISEASE

In addition to a thorough history and physical examination, specific diagnostic procedures may be necessary to confirm a diagnosis.

Auscultation

Although normally part of the routine physical examination, 2 factors significantly compromise the value of thoracic auscultation as a diagnostic procedure in cats with respiratory disease. First, purring completely obliterates any significant lung sounds. Even extremely ill cats may purr despite their poor physical condition. Secondly, the small tidal volume of resting cats is seldom sufficient to enable the clinician to arrive at diagnostic conclusions. Lung sounds described as rhonchi or rales are seldom detected in cats with lower respiratory tract disease. The clinician should develop experience distinguishing normal lung sounds from attenuated or "muffled" lung sounds. This is important in cats suspected of having intrathoracic masses, accumulations of fluid in the pleural space, or diaphragmatic hernias.

Auscultation of the trachea and lungs in cats with upper respiratory disease may be beneficial in cats with laryngeal disorders. Stridor (wheezing) from laryngeal disease may be referred down the trachea and auscultated at the thoracic inlet or over the thorax. The clinician should avoid auscultating the larynx when laryngeal disease is suspected; even slight displacement of the larynx by stethoscope placement may create abnormal sounds.

Radiography

Radiography is a key diagnostic tool in both upper and lower respiratory tract disease.[1]

Upper Respiratory Tract: Plain radiographic studies of the nasal cavity, sinuses and pharynx are indicated when clinical signs of upper respiratory tract disease are evident. A minimum of 2 views, a lateral and an open-mouth ventrodorsal, should be obtained. Frontal radiographs should also be obtained in cats with suspected frontal sinus disease.

Contrast rhinography is accomplished by infusing a water-soluble contrast medium into the rhinarium through the external nares. Radiolucent foreign bodies or soft tissue masses appear as a filling defect in the nasal cavity. The diagnostic value of rhinograms is, however, limited by the absence of published normal rhinograms.

General anesthesia is recommended for all patients subjected to skull radiography. Since lesions of the upper respiratory tract may be subtle, proper positioning and eliminating movement are critical in obtaining diagnostic films. The feasibililty of anesthetizing a patient with upper respiratory disease always depends upon the animal's physical condition.

Lower Respiratory Tract: Lateral and ventrodorsal views of the lung fields are essential components of the diagnostic evaluation of cats with lower respiratory tract disease. In contrast to the technic recommended for upper respiratory tract radiography, cats should not be anesthetized during thoracic radiography. An anesthetized cat is less likely to have normal lung expansion; this may give a false impression of increased interstitial densities.

Contrast studies of the trachea and lower airways are indicated in cats with suspected localized or generalized airway disease. Contrast bronchography is of little diagnostic value in cats with diseases of the lung parenchyma.

Contrast bronchography is performed in the anesthetized patient. Approximately 1 g metrizamide powder (Amipaque:Winthrop) is blown into the lower airways through a catheter placed in the trachea. The contrast material is absorbed within 20 minutes and metabolized by the liver. The diagnostic value of contrast bronchography is limited to structural changes in the lower airways, as from tracheal foreign bodies, tumors, parasitic granulomas, airway collapse and consolidation of a lung lobe.

Endoscopy

Although endoscopic equipment used to diagnose upper and lower respiratory tract diseases in dogs is available, the feasibility of purchasing endoscopic equipment for rhinoscopy and bronchoscopy in cats is limited by the size of their upper and lower airways, and the type and cost of available equipment.

Cultures

Obtaining specimens for bacterial or fungal isolation is indicated in both upper and lower respiratory tract diseases, particularly when mucopurulent nasal/ocular discharges are evident. Collecting samples for bacterial or fungal isolation is most effectively accomplished in an anesthesized cat. Inserting the tip of a nasogastric catheter into the nose permits aspiration of intranasal contents (Fig 1). If nasal secretions are excessively tenacious, 1 ml sterile saline may be infused into the nostril to enhance collection.

The material collected may be placed directly on suitable culture medium or submitted to a laboratory for isolation of a pathogenic organism. Topical anesthetics are bacteriostatic and should not be used to anesthetize the nasal mucosa before collecting bacterial cultures.

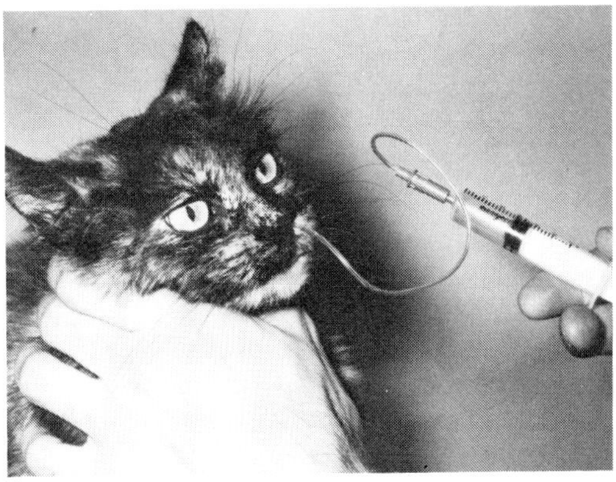

Fig 1. A polyethylene catheter is used to collect intranasal specimens for culture and cytologic examination.

Submission of nasal exudate collected from the external nares is a less reliable technic for recovering pathogenic organisms. This technic should be reserved for cats that should not be subjected to general anesthesia.

Direct microscopic examination of any material collected from the nasal cavity is essential. A small amount of the sample is placed on a clean microscope slide, smeared and allowed to air dry. Slides stained with Wright's stain, Gram stain or new methylene blue are examined for bacteria or fungal hyphae. Specimens from cats with suspected cryptococcosis should be prepared with India ink. It is not unusual to identify fungi on direct microscopic examination while cultures from the same sample are negative.

Tracheal Washings

Pathogenic bacteria may be recovered from the lungs by tracheal washings. The technic used for this procedure in dogs is not well adapted to cats. Instead of passing the catheter through the cricothyroid membrane, it is recommended to pass a sterile polyethylene tube into the trachea directly through the larynx or the endotracheal tube (Fig 2). Volumes of up to 10 ml sterile saline may be infused in 2- to 3-ml aliquots. A rapid injection-aspiration cycle is used to collect samples. The total yield of fluid may be less than 1 ml recovered per 10 ml sterile saline infused. Saline not aspirated is rapidly absorbed and does not cause complications. This procedure may be repeated 2-3 times. Material collected should be submitted for bacterial isolation. A small amount of the sample collected should be stained and examined directly.

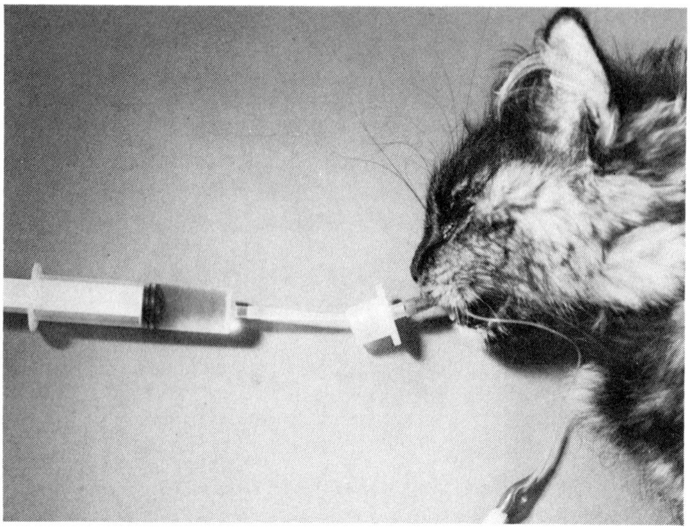

Fig 2. Tracheal washing in an anesthetized cat permits collection of material from the lower airways. Specimens are submitted for culture and cytologic examination.

Table 2 lists the types of bacteria normally found in the upper and lower respiratory tract of cats.

Cytologic Examination

Examination of material collected from the nasal cavity or lower airways may help confirm a diagnosis. Portions of the same material obtained for culture and sensitivity testing can be stained and examined for abnormal cell types. Nasal exudates collected from the external nares should not be used for cytologic examination. Exfoliative cytology should be restricted to material collected during nasal or tracheal washings. Most neoplastic processes have an inflammatory, and possibly bacterial, component associated with the invading tissue. Examination of nasal exudate expelled from the rhinarium is likely to reveal nondiagnostic inflammatory cells. Fine-needle aspiration (1½-inch, 22-ga spinal needle) of obvious masses in the nasal cavity or sinuses or nasal washings are more likely to yield diagnostic cells from cats with nasal tumors.

Table 2. Normal Bacterial Flora of the Upper and Lower Respiratory Tract

Upper Respiratory Tract:
Alpha-hemolytic streptococci
Nonhemolytic streptococci
Staphylococci
Micrococcus sp
Bacillus sp
Moraxella
Coliforms
Pasteurella multocida
Lower Respiratory Tract:
Colonization of bacteria beyond the larynx is unlikely in normal cats. Only light contamination with pharyngeal bacteria should be expected in the trachea and mainstem bronchi.

Biopsy

Collection of tissue samples from the nasal cavity, pharynx or larynx is indicated when a neoplastic process is suspected. Biopsies of pharyngeal and laryngeal tissue may be obtained at the time of visual examination of the oral cavity in an anesthetized cat. In addition to fine-needle aspiration, biopsies of intranasal masses may be obtained with a 21-ga polyethylene IV catheter or modified male urinary catheter. Three factors must be considered when obtaining biopsy samples from the upper respiratory tract: since hemorrhage is common after biopsy of the nasal turbinates, an activated clotting time should be determined before biopsy; the catheter used to obtain the biopsy must be of proper length to avoid penetration of the cribriform plate or calvaria; and the cat must be anesthetized.

Fine-Needle Aspiration of Lung Tissue

Lung tissue may be obtained for cytologic examination by fine-needle aspiration. The technic is indicated in cats with diffuse parenchymal

Table 3. Differential Diagnosis of Pleural Effusions

Gross Appearance	Consistency	Microscopic Appearance	Predominant Cell Type	Laboratory	Differential Diagnoses
A. Turbid: floccular, purulent or opaque; white, cream yellow, grey or lt. green; may be blood-tinged	Thick, tenacious	Bacteria and WBC	Gram + cocci, gram + and − rods, gram + filaments; degenerative neutrophils, macrophages, monocytes ≥100,000/mm^3; many intracellular and extracellular bacteria	Culture may be negative; if culture positive: *Bacteroides*, *Actinomyces*, *Staphylococcus*, *Streptococcus;* protein >3.0 g/dl; may be FeLV positive; may be FIP virus postive	Pyrothrorax: bacterial or mycotic; mixed populations not uncommon
B. Clear, colorless or straw-colored: may be blood-tinged	Serous	Acellular	—	Transudate: protein <3.0 g/dl	Hydrothorax: cardiomyopathy, diaphragmatic hernia, hypoproteinemia from the nephrotic syndrome, protein-losing enteropathy or hepatopathy
	Viscous, tenacious, some particulate matter, fibrinous, may clot on exposure to air	Low cellularity, no bacteria	Occasional neutrophils	Exudate: protein ≥3.0 g/dl	Effusive FIP, subsequent to thoracic surgery or thoracentesis, diaphragmatic hernia
	Slightly viscous	Leukocytosis, no bacteria	Lymphocytes (atypical) w/ lymphoblasts	Modified transudate: protein >3.0 g/dl; FeLV positive	Neoplasia (thymic lymphosarcoma)
C. Turbid: white, peach or pink (blood-tinged);	Slightly viscous	High cellularity, WBC, no bacteria	Lymphocytes, may be atypical lymphocytes	FeLV positive	Chylothorax: thymic lymphosarcoma or traumatic rupture of thoracic duct
opaque: "cream layer" may torm on standing			Lymphoblasts may predominate (>5000/mm^3)		
D. Red, opaque	Hemorrhagic	RBC and WBC, similar to peripheral blood, no bacteria		Hematocrit ≥ that of peripheral blood; exudate: protein >3.0 g/dl	Hemothorax: trauma, inadvertent cardiocentesis, neoplasia (esp. cardiac hemangiosarcoma) or coagulopathy

lung disease. The procedure is not innocuous; complications include pneumothorax and pulmonary hemorrhage. Samples should be obtained from the seventh or eight intercostal space or cranial to the heart. General anesthesia is not a prerequisite for the procedure.

A 1½-inch, 22-ga spinal needle, with stylet in place, is inserted through the thoracic wall and into the lung. The stylet is removed and a 5-ml syringe is used to aspirate. The collected sample is placed on a microscope slide, allowed to air dry and stained with Wright's stain. For at least

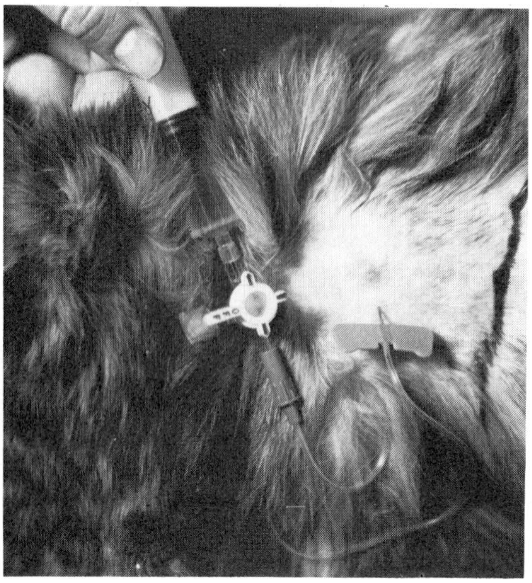

Fig 3. Thoracentesis.

2 hours after the procedure, the patient should be monitored for evidence of dyspnea. Complications are more likely to occur in cats that struggle during or shortly after aspiration.

This procedure is not recommended for routine use. Rather, it is intended for animals with severe, progressive parenchymal lung disease.

Thoracentesis

Pleural effusions are common in cats and can be readily detected by routine radiography. The cause, however, is not usually established by radiography alone. Removal of the fluid is important because fluid in the pleural space may severely compromise respirations, and the fluid removed from the chest has diagnostic importance. Table 3 summarizes the different types of fluid that may be found in the pleural space.

Although cats have a complete mediastinum, this fragile barrier is easily disrupted by intrathoracic disease. Consequently, fluid routinely accumulates in the right and left pleural spaces despite the unilaterality of the primary disease. This is particularly true in cases of pyothorax. Long-standing mediastinal disease may effectively compartmentalize the left thorax from the right thorax.

Thoracentesis is accomplished with a 19- or 20-ga butterfly catheter (Abbott), attached to a 3-way stopcock, inserted at the seventh or eighth intercostal space. The needle should be inserted at the middle or ventral portion of the thorax (Fig 3). The cat is allowed to stand or rest in sternal recumbency during thoracentesis.

Fluid collected during thoracentesis should be examined for bacteria or neoplastic cells. In addition, the specific gravity should be determined if the fluid is clear.

Use of a needle to remove fluid from the pleural space is best reserved for collection of samples for diagnostic studies. This technic is not a substitute for therapeutic drainage through a chest tube.

Blood Gases

Arterial blood-gas determinations are of value in assessing the status of patients with pulmonary disease. Cats with disease severe enough to compromise O_2 exchange at the level of the pulmonary capillaries usually have an abnormally low PaO_2. Venous blood-gas determinations are considerably less reliable in cats. Since arterial blood-gas samples are most reliably collected from anesthetized cats, this procedure is not routinely performed.

DISEASES OF THE UPPER RESPIRATORY TRACT

Of the clincial signs referable to the upper respiratory tract, sneezing is the most common clinical sign for which cats are presented to veterinarians. Sneezing is most commonly caused by disease of the rhinarium. Cats with primary sinus disease and secondary extension to the nasal cavity may also sneeze.

Rhinitis describes any inflammatory process within the nasal cavity. Infectious diseases, neoplasia and foreign bodies are the most common causes of rhinitis in cats. Sneezing may result from generalized, localized, unilateral or bilateral rhinitis.

Cats with chronic, generalized rhinitis may experience loss of olfaction, which may result in anorexia and consequent weight loss. Behavioral changes, such as failure to urinate and defecate in the litter box, have been reported in cats recovering from severe rhinitis. Experimental studies have not confirmed this as a consistent finding after the loss of olfaction.

Acute Sneezing

Physiologic Sneezing

Sneezing is a normal, protective reflex intended to displace foreign material contacting the nasal epithelium. Therefore, cats not affected by rhinitis may sneeze. Whether or not disease exists in a cat presented with the complaint of sneezing may only be determined from a thorough clinical history and physical examination.

Viral Respiratory Disease

Viral upper respiratory disease is perhaps the most common cause of sneezing in cats. Most cases are caused by herpesvirus (feline viral rhinotracheitis) or calicivirus. Clinical signs include severe, paroxysmal sneezing episodes associated with a bilateral, generalized rhinitis. As secondary bacterial infection ensues, any nasal discharge may change from serous to mucopurulent.

Further discussion on the diagnosis, treatment and prognosis of feline viral respiratory disease is in Chapter 4.

Feline Pneumonitis[2]

Feline pneumonitis is caused by the organism *Chlamydia psittaci* and is characterized by mild rhinitis, occasional sneezing and serous conjunctivitis. The term "pneumonitis" is probably inappropriate for this condition since cats rarely develop pulmonary changes associated with the clinical form of this disease.

Clinical Signs: Chlamydia psittaci usually is associated with mild rhinitis, sneezing and serous conjunctivitis. Other findings on physical examination may be normal. The cat may eat well and have normal activity. Secondary bacterial infections and purulent nasal discharges are uncommon in this condition.

Diagnosis: Confirmation of *C psittaci* infection is based on isolation of the organism. Swabs of the conjunctival cul-de-sac and the oral cavity may be inoculated into tissue culture medium. When conjunctival cells are treated with Giemsa stain, this intracellular organism stains red but is small and difficult to identify. Diagnosis is often based on the response to treatment.

Treatment: Chlamydia psittaci is susceptible to many antibiotics. For mild infections of the conjunctiva and nasal epithelium, topical therapy with tetracycline ophthalmic ointment may be the only treatment necessary. Treatment is continued for a minimum of 14 days.

In some cases, the organism may be found in the lower respiratory tract. Cats suspected or known to have *C psittaci* may therefore be treated with systemic tetracycline.

Human psittacosis is caused by infections with an avian strain of *C psittaci*. Human conjunctival infections with feline *C psittaci* have been reported. Considering the zoonotic potential of feline pneumonitis, any cat with a confirmed *C psittaci* infection should be treated.

Prevention: Chlamydia psittaci may be transmitted from one cat to another by direct contact with infective secretions or by airborne fomites. Recurrent infections may be particularly common in catteries. Although vaccines are available, the low incidence of feline pneumonitis and the inability of available vaccines to prevent infection and shedding justify the fact that vaccines are not in widespread use at this time.

Cuterebra Infection

Cats can become infected with larvae of the bot fly, *Cuterebra*. Larvae may hatch and penetrate the skin of a susceptible host. They usually develop in subcutaneous cysts around the head and neck. *Cuterebra* larvae have also been recovered from the nasal cavity of kittens.

Clinical Signs: Cats presented for paroxysmal sneezing associated with a unilateral serous nasal discharge should be examined for the presence of a *Cuterebra* larva within the rostral portion of the nasal cavity. Episodes of sneezing occasionally are accompanied by a serosanguineous nasal discharge. The history is otherwise unremarkable. The findings on physical examination often are normal.

Diagnosis: The presence of a *Cuterebra* larva in the rhinarium is confirmed by visualizing the larva at the nasal orifice. Plain radiography of the nasal cavity is not diagnostic. Contrast rhinography may demonstrate a filling defect on the affected side.

Treatment: Under topical or general anesthesia, the *Cuterebra* larva may be extracted using small forceps. Further treatment is generally not necessary. Left untreated, the larva typically migrates out of the nostril to pupate. Spontaneous remission of clinical signs follows. On the other hand, *Cuterebra* larvae have been suspected of migrating from the nasal cavity through the cribriform plate of the ethmoid bone.

Dental Disease

Chronic dental and periodontal disease can cause sneezing episodes. During visual examination of the oral cavity, particular attention should be paid to the upper dental arcade for the presence of fractured teeth and evidence of oronasal fistulae. These conditions can cause a localized unilateral rhinitis associated with paroxysmal sneezing and a serous nasal discharge. Occasionally the discharge may be serosanguineous.

Diagnosis: The condition may be confirmed by high-quality radiographs of the rhinarium. Increased radiolucency of the tissue around the alveolus of affected teeth may be evident.

Treatment: Fractured teeth, particularly those fractured at the level of the gingiva, are best treated by extraction. Oral antibiotics (hetacillin or amoxicillin) should be given 2 days before and 5 days after extraction.

Foreign Bodies

Although rare, foreign bodies may become lodged in the nasal cavity of cats. Any foreign object contacting the nasal epithelium can elicit a sneezing reflex. A cat presented for recurrent sneezing episodes should be examined for a foreign body. Examination should include a visual examination of the external nares and oropharynx. Radiographs of the rhinarium may be helpful if the foreign object is radiopaque.

Nasal foreign bodies, such as foxtails, can migrate through the tissue surrounding the rhinarium, thereby precluding simple extraction of the foreign body. Objects that migrate through surrounding tissue may cause extensive tissue damage. Surgical exploration of the nasal cavity may be necessary for effective treatment.

Chronic Sneezing

Chronic Rhinitis

The clinical management of viral upper respiratory infections may go beyond supportive therapy and management of the acute disease. Although exact figures are not available, about 80% or more cats that recover from feline viral rhinotracheitis become chronic carriers of virulent herpesvirus. In addition, cats that recover from feline calicivirus infection shed the virus from the oral cavity for at least 2 years. Chronic bacterial rhinitis may also occur in virus-negative cats that have recovered from feline viral rhinotracheitis or calicivirus infection.[2]

Clinical Signs: Rhinitis may be considered chronic when sneezing and nasal discharge persist for more than 2-4 weeks. Although many virus-positive carrier cats manifest no clinical signs, sneezing, a persistent mucopurulent nasal discharge and sonorous breathing are the most common presenting complaints. Some carriers may have chronic periodontal disease or persistent, mild conjunctivitis. Carriers of feline viral rhinotracheitis sneeze and have a nasal discharge subsequent to stress. Surgery, anesthesia, transit to cat shows and corticosteroid therapy are representative sources of stress known to exacerbate clinical signs of rhinotracheitis. Virulent virus may be shed during these episodes. Consequently, clinical signs may be intermittent in some cats.

Diagnosis: Although the clinical signs of chronic rhinitis are readily recognized, defining the exact etiology and prescribing appropriate treatment is less simple. Oral or conjunctival swabs of cats showing clinical signs may be obtained for bacterial or virus isolation. Swabs should be submitted in a small amount of sterile saline or a suitable virus transport medium. Direct microscopic examination of nasal exudates may be helpful in recognizing neoplastic cells stained with Wright's stain or *Cryptococcus* organisms stained with India ink.

Radiography of the rhinarium is indicated to rule out the presence of a space-occupying mass or foreign body. However, chronic rhinitis of viral or bacterial origin is unlikely to be associated with radiographic changes.

Bacterial cultures from material collected from the nasal cavity reveal a variety of common contaminants. In most cases, these are secondary invaders and should not be considered the primary cause.

Treatment: Cats with a significant mucopurulent nasal exudate generally respond dramatically to oral antibiotic therapy. However, discontinuation of medication usually results in reappearance of clinical signs within 2-3 days.

Various treatments have been employed in the management of chronic rhinitis, including topical instillation of antibiotics and corticosteroids, flushing with sterile saline or astringents, infusion of hydrogen peroxide, instillation of enzymes, and topical application of DMSO, alone or combined with antibacterial agents, decongestants, vitamin C and orgotein given IM. These treatment regimens are, at best, palliative. There have been no published studies that conclusively show one regimen to be significantly better than another.

Excluding chronic rhinitis caused by neoplasia or mycotic infection, long-term resolution of clinical signs has been accomplished using a long-acting nasal decongestant and oral ampicillin. One drop of nasal decongestant is instilled into one nostril once daily for 5 days, and in the opposite nostril for the next 5 days. Oral ampicillin therapy is continued for 10-14 days.

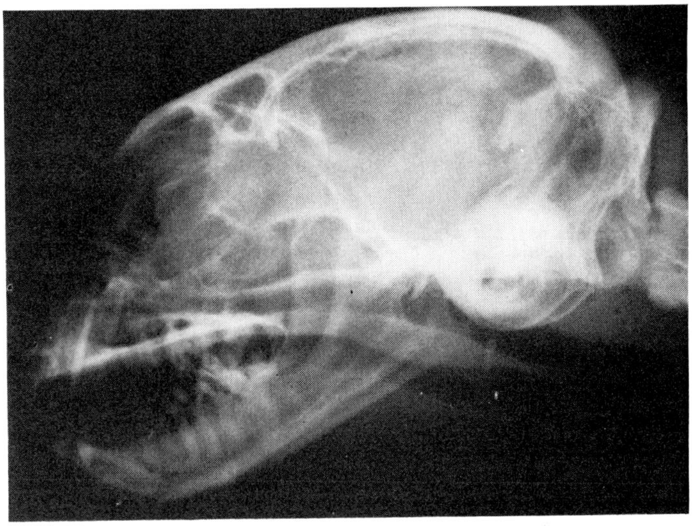

Fig 4. Lateral radiograph of the skull of a cat with chronic sinusitis and otitis media.

Cats followed for over a year have shown gradual spontaneous remission. Upper respiratory infections have been treated with aerosol therapy; conclusive studies on the efficacy of this type of treatment have not been published.

Sinusitis

Infection of the frontal sinuses is a well-recognized chronic disorder. Sinusitis may develop subsequent to direct injury of the frontal sinus (*eg*, penetrating bite wound), neoplasia, or ascending bacterial or fungal infections of the nasal cavity. In addition, cats that have recovered from acute viral upper respiratory infections may develop a secondary bacterial sinusitis.

Clinical Signs: Intermittent sneezing associated with a mucoid or purulent nasal discharge is the most common presenting sign in cats with chronic sinusitis. Owners may observe streaks of blood in the nasal discharge. Duration of clinical signs may be from weeks to years.

Penetrating injuries of the frontal sinus usually are unilateral. Cats so affected may have a unilateral nasal discharge most evident during sneezing. A draining tract may be evident in the skin over the affected sinus.

Other findings of the physical examination generally are normal. Cats with chronic sinusitis, even with secondary bacterial involvement, have normal activity and appetite. Hematologic and blood chemistry profiles usually are normal.

Diagnosis: Lateral and frontal radiographs of the skull are necessary to confirm a diagnosis of sinusitis (Fig 4). Increased radiodensity within the frontal sinus indicates sinusitis. Treatment should be based on radiographic findings rather than clinical signs. Whereas the clinical signs of rhinitis and sinusitis are similar, the treatment is not.

Treatment: Cats with radiographic evidence of a penetrating injury to the frontal sinus should be treated surgically and medically.[3] The penetrating wound should be exposed and debrided as necessary. The infected sinus may be treated by flushing the sinus with sterile saline or 1% Lugol's iodine. In some cases, placement of a tube drain may facilitate repeated flushings. Fractures of the frontal bone seldom require surgical repair. The owner should be warned that a permanent, but usually slight, deformation of the frontal bone may result after healing of frontal bone fractures.

Drugs used to treat sinusitis include antibiotics (including amphotericin B), antihistamines, coricosteroids and enzymes. Surgical therapy is advocated when medical therapy is not successful. Obliteration of the affected frontal sinus is the most commonly used technic. The success of this technic is predicated on complete removal of the sinus mucous membrane, removing the periosteum of the frontal sinus and obstructing the nasal frontal duct (autogenous fat implantation). However, this procedure may not result in complete elimination of clinical signs since involvement of the rhinarium may occur concomitantly.

Surgical treatment usually is supplemented with administration of oral antibiotics, such as ampicillin, hetacillin and amoxicillin, for at least 14 days. Extended treatment periods of up to one month are not uncommon.

Although sinus neoplasia is rare in cats, squamous-cell carcinomas and sarcomas of the frontal sinuses have been reported. Bone destruction usually is evident radiographically.

Cryptococcosis

The respiratory tract is a common site of entry for *Cryptococcus neoformans*. Many, but not all, cats with cryptococcosis have clinical signs referable to the upper respiratory tract. Sneezing, with an associated mucopurulent nasal discharge, is a common presenting complaint. The diagnosis of cryptococcosis is confirmed by identification of the organism in exudates. The reader is referred to Chapter 5 for additional discussions on cryptococcosis.

Reverse Sneezing

The term "reverse sneeze" has been used to describe the rapid inspiratory effort made by an animal attempting to displace material (foreign body or mucus) from the caudal nasal cavity or nasopharynx into the oropharynx. Although more commonly described in dogs, reverse sneezing can occur in cats. Owners may describe reverse sneezing as rapid snorting or gagging. This clinical sign is referable to the nasopharynx.

Clinical Signs: Physical examination of cats with pharyngeal disease may reveal no abnormalities. Often a reverse sneeze cannot be elicited during the examination. Careful interpretation of the clinical history may suggest if the pharynx is involved and if reverse sneezing has actually occurred.

Diagnosis: Cats with suspected pharyngeal disease should be examined under general anesthesia. In addition to the larynx, epiglottis and oropharynx, the soft palate should be pulled rostrad to examine the nasopharynx. Skull radiographs may reveal a radiopaque foreign body imbedded in the retropharyngeal tissues.

Treatment: The treatment of pharyngeal disease is determined by the diagnosis. The most common pharyngeal disorders in cats are foreign bodies and neoplasia. Nasal polyps extending caudad into the nasopharynx have been reported. Surgical removal of these polyps is indicated but frequently not practical. The cause of nasopharyngeal polyps is not known.

Stertor

Comparable to snoring, stertorous breathing suggests a disorder of the soft palate or oropharynx. Unlike reverse sneezing, stertor usually is not intermittent. Stertor is most noticeable on inspiration.

Stertor is generally associated with pharyngeal or soft palate foreign body. Neoplasia, causing significant displacement of the soft palate, pharynx or larynx, may compromise movement of air through the glottis, resulting in stertor.

The diagnosis is based on visual examination of the oropharynx and routine radiography in the anesthetized patient.

The treatment of oropharyngeal and soft palate lesions depends on the diagnosis. The most common tumor of the soft palate and pharynx is squamous-cell carcinoma, which warrants a poor prognosis.

Stridor

Characterized by wheezing, stridor may be intermittent or continuous and may be heard on inspiration or expiration. Occasionally a cat is presented with stridor as the primary clinical complaint. In other cases, stridor may be detected only on auscultation of the cervical trachea. In any event, stridor must be considered a manifestation of laryngeal/tracheal disease.

Laryngitis

Laryngitis may be acute or chronic and is not common in cats. It seldom occurs without concomitant clinical signs of other upper respiratory tract disease, such as feline viral rhinotracheitis.

Clinical Signs: Inflammation of the larynx usually is manifested by stridor. Episodes usually are paroxysmal. Vocalization may be difficult or impossible despite repeated attempts. Manipulation of the larynx and cranial trachea may elicit coughing. Other signs may be evident, depending on the severity of the disease associated with the laryngitis. The inflammatory response, regardless of the cause, may result in significant swelling of the laryngeal and epiglottal epithelium. Consequently, the presenting clinical sign may be dyspnea.

Diagnosis: The diagnosis of laryngitis is confirmed on the basis of the visual examination of the larynx. However, the severity of disease associated with laryngitis may preclude thorough visual examination of the oral cavity under anesthesia. Cats with clinical signs of laryngitis but no additional signs of upper respiratory disease should be examined under anesthesia.

In addition to viral rhinotracheitis, squamous-cell carcinoma of the larynx may result in laryngitis. Exfoliative cytology or biopsy of the affected tissue is used to confirm such a diagnosis.

Treatment: The treatment of laryngitis is determined by the cause. The clinician is cautioned against prescribing arbitrary supportive medication without determining the actual cause.

Of primary importance in the management of laryngitis is to ensure patency of the glottis to air but not to food and saliva. Cats with viral rhinotracheitis may have varying degrees of laryngitis characterized by swelling, ulceration and secondary bacterial colonization. Ampicillin or hetacillin is given IM or SC at 5-10 mg/kg TID for at least 10 days. If laryngeal swelling causes dyspnea, it may be necessary to anesthetize and intubate the cat. Topical application of a 1:10,000 solution of epinephrine may reduce the swelling.

Laryngeal neoplasia in a cat is most likely to be malignant. Surgical debulking of obstructive tumors can help but is unlikely to be curative. Complete laryngectomy is not recommended. Systemic chemotherapy can be attempted in cats with inoperable laryngeal tumors; however, there is no information to support the efficacy of chemotherapy in such cases.

DISEASES OF THE LOWER RESPIRATORY TRACT

The airways of the lower respiratory tract are those extending from the trachea to the alveoli. Lower respiratory disease, however, is not restricted to these anatomic areas. In addition to the airways, lower respiratory disease includes disorders of the thoracic wall, diaphragm, pleura, pleural space, mediastinum, pulmonary vasculature and the supporting interstitial structures (lymphatics and nerves). While most respiratory diseases are the result of changes in the pulmonary-cardiovascular system, secondary respiratory diseases may result from changes in the nervous, endocrine, renal and/or GI systems.

The pulmonary system is a complex system with 2 critical functions. It is necessary for respiration and is a highly integrated defense system that protects the gas-exchange surfaces against potentially harmful biologic and nonbiologic agents. Pulmonary defense mechanisms are outlined in Table 4.[4]

Coughing and dyspnea are the clinical signs most often associated with lower respiratory tract disease. Coughing may result from disorders of the larynx, tracheobronchial tree and lung. Coughing is described as intermittent or paroxysmal and may be acute in onset or chronic. Dyspnea should be considered an emergency until proven otherwise.

Table 4. Major Pulmonary Defense Mechanisms

IMMUNOLOGIC
Secretory IgA
IgG
T-Lymphocyte activation, lymphokine release
Alveolar macrophages
NEUROLOGIC
Cough reflex
Sneeze reflex
PHYSICAL BARRIERS
Mucociliary blanket
Aerodynamic filtration (90% of inhaled particles impact proximal to the carina)
Branching of lower airways
INACTIVATION
Interferon
Lysozyme

Dyspnea, the hallmark of respiratory distress, is characterized by an increased ventilatory effort. Most often associated with lower respiratory tract disease, dyspnea is not a localizing clinical sign. Disorders of the upper and lower respiratory tract, mediastinum, pleural space, thoracic cage and heart can cause dyspnea.

Cough

Mediated by receptors in the pharynx, larynx and tracheobronchial tree, the cough reflex is an important defense mechanism that results in expulsion of inhaled irritant particles, foreign bodies or aspirated food. As in people, this defense mechanism may be attenuated by certain drugs or diseases. The cough reflex, in addition to the other airway clearance mechanisms, is an important physiologic reflex.

Coughing is an important clinical sign of respiratory disease. However, coughing can result from disorders of organ systems other than the respiratory system. Diagnostic evaluation of a cat with a primary complaint of coughing should include the cardiovascular system as well as the respiratory system.

Tracheobronchial Causes of Coughing

Feline Viral Rhinotracheitis

Feline viral rhinotracheitis is associated with frequent and often paroxysmal coughing. However, coughing is seldom the only presenting clinical sign. A more complete description of feline viral rhinotracheitis is found in Chapter 4.

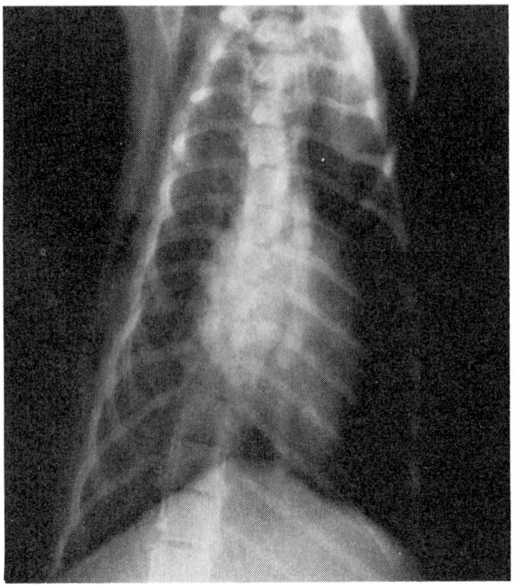

Fig 5. Ventrodorsal radiograph of a cat with subcutaneous emphysema resulting from a cervical bite wound.

Tracheal Trauma

Direct injury to the trachea can result in paroxysmal coughing episodes. Penetrating wounds to the trachea sustained during fights may result in episodic coughing. The onset is acute and may progress rapidly to dyspnea. Cats with bite wounds of the trachea may develop subcutaneous emphysema. Also, penetrating injuries of the trachea may lead to contamination of the subcutaneous tissues. Antibiotic therapy is indicated when the trachea has been penetrated.

Subcutaneous emphysema is a potentially fatal consequence of tracheal penetration or rupture. The condition may develop subsequent to penetration of the cervical trachea (bite wound) or intrathoracic trachea (foreign body penetration from the esophagus). Air in the subcutaneous tissues creates an audible, crackling sound during manipulation of the skin. Radiographs confirm the presence of air in the subcutaneous tissues (Fig 5). Affected cats must be handled with extreme caution. Unnecessary or excessive restraint may worsen the condition. Since hospitalization may be stressful for some cats, patients should be monitored closely for signs of respiratory distress.

Animals with tracheal injury, particularly when penetration of the trachea is suspected, should be treated with oral antibiotics for 7-10 days. The cat should be watched for 24-48 hours for signs of subcutaneous emphysema and respiratory distress.

If subcutaneous emphysema does develop, the cat should be handled carefully to avoid potentially stressful situations, such as restraint for radiography. Some clinicians wrap the cat's thorax in an elastic bandage in an attempt to prevent complications stemming from extension of the emphysema. Extrapulmonic restrictive lung disease, pneumothorax and infection are the major complications of subcutaneous emphysema. In many cases, subcutaneous emphysema subsequent to tracheal injury resolves without complications. Surgical intervention should not be attempted in cats with subcutaneous emphysema unless the site of penetration can be identified.

Bronchial Asthma

Spontaneous asthma-like conditions have been observed in cats. Similar to bronchial asthma in people, feline asthma is characterized by recurrent attacks of coughing, presumably associated with acute bronchoconstriction. However, the immunologic mechanisms involved in feline asthma have not been shown to be the same mechanisms involved in human asthma.[5]

Clinical Signs: Feline asthma is characterized by sudden onset of paroxysmal coughing, which may be mild to severe. The cough is "dry" and nonproductive. Stridor is less commonly associated with the condition. Observation of respiratory patterns may reveal an accentuated expiratory phase. Respiratory rate and depth may be normal. In severe cases, respiratory effort may be significantly increased. Dyspnea is characterized by short inspiratory efforts followed by forceful and prolonged expiratory efforts. Affected cats may become cyanotic.

Since clinical signs may be intermittent, the findings on physical examination of affected cats may be unremarkable. Ocular and nasal discharges are consistently absent in cats with feline asthma. Severe cases may present significant clinical signs. Tachypnea and dyspnea may be apparent. Increased exertion on expiration has been reported. Increased lung sounds or wheezing may be evident on auscultation. This is particularly true during expiration.

Diagnosis: Radiographic findings may be diagnostic. Associated with an increased resistance during expiration, thoracic radiographs may reveal increased density of the lung field, increased thoracic size, and a straight diaphragm. In addition, a prominent interstitial density suggests significant bronchovesicular changes.

About 75% of cats with bronchial asthma have an absolute eosinophilia. In uncomplicated cases, the remainder of the hemogram is normal. Cytologic examination of tracheobronchial washings may contain numerous eosinophils. Standard biochemical profiles are normal in cats with feline asthma.

Treatment: Use of corticosteroids is recommended for treatment of cats with bronchial asthma. A single IM injection of prednisolone, at 0.5-1.0 mg/lb body weight, is followed by prednisolone given PO at 0.5 mg/lb twice daily as needed to control clinical signs. In severely dyspneic cats, hydrocortisone sodium succinate can be given IV at 1.0 mg/lb. Continuation of corticosteroid therapy is based on the clinical response. Aminophylline is an effective bronchodilator and may be used in conjunction with corticosteroids. Aminophylline is administered PO at 10 mg/kg every 8 hours.

Oxygen therapy is indicated in severely dyspneic animals. Morphine sulfate (without atropine) may significantly improve the efficiency of respiration in anxious, asthmatic cats. Morphine should be given at 0.05-0.10 mg/kg divided between the IV and IM routes.

Diuretics, antihistamines and anticholinergics (atropine) are not indicated in the treatment of asthma.

Prognosis: Recurrent attacks can be expected in asthmatic cats if the bronchoconstriction associated with this condition is, in fact, caused by reaginic allergy. However, no such cases have been reported. Identification and removal of the allergen is the preferred treatment in such cases.

Parasitic Pulmonary Causes of Coughing

Considering the size of the pulmonary capillary bed, many types of parasites, or one of their developmental stages, probably pass through the lungs. While some parasites or parasitic larvae are only present temporarily, such as *Toxocara cati,* others, such as *Paragonimus kellicotti,* mature and reproduce in the airways or lung parenchyma. Presumably, most cats with parasites in the lungs or airways never manifest clinical signs; in a few, signs range from a mild, transient cough to bronchopneumonia, dyspnea and death.

Lungworm and Lung Fluke Infection

Among the most common parasites that infect the lower respiratory tract of cats are the lungworms *Aelurostrongylus abstrusus* and *Capillaria aerophila* and the lung fluke *Paragonimus kellicotti.* A chronic, intermittent cough is the most common reason for presentation.[6,7]

Clinical Signs: Although most cats with parasitic lung disease are young, cats of all ages are susceptible. The onset of clinical signs usually is gradual, requiring weeks to months to develop. Coughing is the predominant clinical sign. Other signs include exercise intolerance, gradual weight loss, fever and, in severe cases, dyspnea. Bacterial bronchopneumonia may be a complicating factor. Attenuated lung sounds may be evident over consolidated lobes. Some affected cats manifest no clinical signs.

Diagnosis: Thoracic radiographs, fecal flotation and tracheobronchial washings are used to confirm a diagnosis of lungworm or lung fluke infection. While thoracic radiographs may suggest parasitic lung disease caused by lungworms or lung flukes, they are not diagnostic. Radiographic changes range from a mild, diffuse interstitial density to consolidation of lung lobes and bronchopneumonia. Granulomas may be detected in cats with lung flukes. However, the interstitial densities associated with pneumonia or pulmonary edema may mask the discrete granulomas associated with paragonimiasis.

Both lungworm and lung fluke infections can be diagnosed by identification of first-stage larvae (*A abstrusus*) or ova (*C aerophila* and *P kellicotti*) in feces. *Aelurostrongylus abstrusus* larvae may be concentrated by a fecal flotation method using a sodium dichromate solution with a specific gravity of 1.350 (790 g technical grade sodium dichromate added to 1 L water). Routine sugar or salt flotation solutions have a specific gravity lower than that required to float *A abstrusus* larvae. The ova of *C aerophila* and *P kellicotti* can be identified using routine flotation technics.

Microscopic examination of fluid and mucus from tracheal washings of infected cats may reveal the active larvae of *A abstrusus* or the ova of *C aerophila* and *P kellicotti.*

Peripheral eosinophilia is an inconsistent finding in cats with parasitic lung disease and should not be used in making a diagnosis.

Treatment: Drugs used to treat parasitic lung disease include sodium iodide, diethylcarbamazine citrate, thiabendazole, dichlorvos and levamisole. Levamisole HCl, at 15-20 mg/lb PO every other day for 5-6 treatments, has been used effectively against *A abstrusus*. A similar treatment has been recommended against *C aerophila*. However, conclusive studies of this treatment are not available.

Side effects of levamisole include salivation, vomiting and ataxia. Although levamisole is not an organophosphate nor a cholinesterase inhibitor, atropine sulfate (0.05 mg/lb) given SC 15 minutes before administration of levamisole may prevent salivation and vomiting.

Fenbendazole (Panacur:Hoechst), a broad-spectrum anthelmintic for horses, is effective against *Paragonimus* infection in dogs at 25-50 mg/kg PO given BID for 10-14 days. This same regimen has been used successfully for treating *Paragonimus* infections in cats.

Supplemental antibiotic therapy is recommended for any cat developing signs of bacterial pneumonia.

Prognosis: Most cats with lungworm do not develop significant clinical signs. Many that develop clinical signs recover spontaneously. Aleurostrongylosis is often regarded as a self-limiting disease. Clinical signs and fecal larvae may disappear in 2-3 months without treatment.

Toxoplasmosis

Although most cats with active *Toxoplasma gondii* infection are asymptomatic, the most common clinical manifestation of toxoplasmosis is pneumonitis.

Clinical Signs: Coughing, fever, anorexia and weight loss are seen in cats with *Toxoplasma* pneumonia. Respiratory distress may develop in advanced cases. However, the distribution of *Toxoplasma* organisms is not restricted to the respiratory tract. Cats with toxoplasmosis may develop other clinical signs as well. The reader is referred to Chapter 4 for further discussion.

Diagnosis: Radiographically, ill-defined and patchy densities may be seen throughout the lungs of cats with *Toxoplasma* pneumonia. Air bronchograms become evident as alveoli become filled with exudative fluids.[8] However, thoracic radiographs are not diagnostic of toxoplasmosis. Parasitologic and serologic tests are the most valuable technics in diagnosing toxoplasmosis (see Chapter 4). Oocysts occasionally are identified in the feces of infected cats. *Toxoplasma gondii* may be recovered from tissue biopsies or exudates. Indirect hemagglutination tests and the Sabin-Feldman dye test are the most commonly used serologic tests. Identification of oocysts or the *Toxoplasma* organism is confirmatory. The presence of *T gondii* antibodies, however, indicates previous exposure but does not confirm active infection.

Treatment: The combination of sulfadiazine and pyrimethamine is still recommended for the treatment of toxoplasmosis in cats. These drugs act synergistically to inhibit the biosynthesis of folinic acid required by *T gondii*. Use of sulfadiazine, given PO at 100 mg/kg divided into 4 daily doses with pyrimethamine at 1 mg/kg/day, is recommended. These drugs should be administered for 1-2 weeks.

Pyrimethamine is unpalatable and toxic to cats in addition to being available only in 25-mg tablets that cannot be accurately divided. That, combined with the fact that toxoplasmosis is an important zoonotic disease, should be taken into account before initiating therapy.

Ascarid Migration

Transient coughing may be associated with the tracheal migration of *Toxocara cati* larvae. Second-stage larvae may penetrate the bowel wall, enter the portal vein, liver, postcava and eventually the pulmonary capillaries. Larvae that penetrate the capillary wall and enter the alveoli migrate up the bronchial tree and trachea. The parasite completes its life cycle after being expelled from the trachea and swallowed.

Heavily infected cats may develop a mild, usually transient cough as larvae migrate through the airways. A clinical diagnosis of ascarid migration may be based on the clinical signs, the presence of *T cati* ova in the feces and the exclusion of other diseases known to cause similar signs. Thoracic radiographs of affected cats may demonstrate a generalized interstitial pattern, but may also be normal. Specific respiratory therapy usually is not necessary. Elimination of the adult roundworms from the intestine results in resolution of the respiratory disease.

Dyspnea

Dyspnea represents difficult or painful respiration associated with increased ventilatory effort. It may be characterized as acute respiratory distress associated with tachypnea, open-mouth breathing, orthopnea, cyanosis and increased respiratory effort on inspiration and/or expiration (Fig 6).

While the diagnostic evaluation of dyspnea is not dissimilar to that employed in any lower respiratory disease, the clinical evaluation should not be postponed. Dyspnea is an emergency until proven otherwise.

Table 5 summarizes the common radiographic signs associated with various causes of dyspnea. Since the cause of the dyspnea may not be apparent immediately, the clinician should take prompt, appropriate action to improve ventilation. Use of the following emergency procedures is recommended when confronted with a dyspneic cat. Initial efforts to control dyspnea should include administration of supplemental O_2, and parenteral administration of morphine sulfate at 0.05-0.10 mg/kg.

Morphine sulfate has the advantage of decreasing the anxiety associated with dyspnea, resulting in improved ventilation and O_2 exchange. Oxygen therapy is best administered directly by face mask or O_2 chamber, such as that used to induce general anesthesia. Unconscious cats should be intubated if time permits. Artificial respiration, if necessary, may be administered via face mask.

An attempt to place an indwelling IV catheter should be made at the earliest possible time. Failure to do so may result in delayed administration of a potentially life-saving drug.

Survey radiographs of the thorax and neck should be obtained once it has been determined that the patient can withstand the restraint necessary to obtain good radiographs.

Dyspnea from Diseases of the Larynx and Trachea

Infections

Viral respiratory disease is the most common cause of dyspnea associated with the larynx and trachea. Feline herpesvirus or, particularly, calicivirus infection may be associated with secondary bacterial infections that extend from the rhinarium and pharynx into the trachea and ultimately the lungs. Accumulations of tenacious, purulent secretions may impair normal ventilation.

Once the cat's condition is stabilized, systemic antibiotic therapy should be initiated. This may be combined with aerosol therapy using sterile saline to enhance expulsion of secretions. Antibiotic therapy should be continued for at least 10 days. Aerosol therapy may be administered 3-4 times daily as necessary to decrease the ventilatory effort.

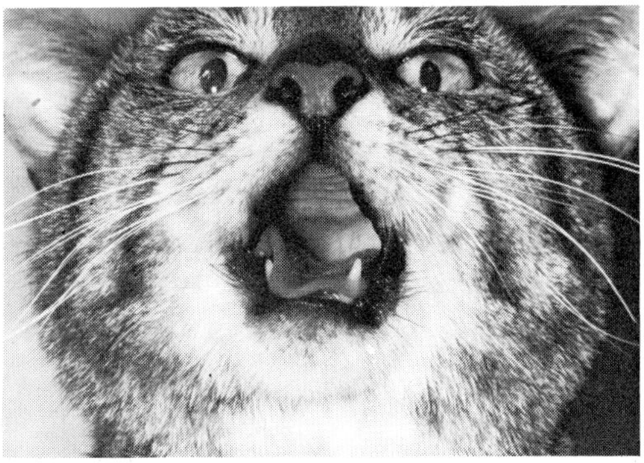

Fig 6. Open-mouth breathing indicates dyspnea.

Trauma

Direct injury to the larynx and trachea may result in acute dyspnea. Tracheal trauma often is complicated by pneumothorax, pneumomediastinum or subcutaneous emphysema. Immediate treatment of dyspneic cats with tracheal injuries is outlined above. Follow-up therapy is determined on the basis of the extent of injury. Often the precise location of penetration or injury cannot be established. In these cases, supportive therapy only is indicated. Cats that do not develop complications within 48 hours have a good prognosis for recovery. Cats that develop pneumothorax and/or subcutaneous emphysema have a guarded prognosis.

Laryngospasm

Clinical Signs: Cats may be presented to a veterinarian with a history of intermittent paroxysms of coughing, wheezing and respiratory distress. The owner usually describes the episodes as occuring sporadically during the day or night. The frequency of episodes may range from once a week to several times a day. Episodes generally last less than 2 minutes. During an episode, the cat is positioned in sternal recumbency with its head extended and low to the ground. These intense episodes of apparent respiratory distress cease as abruptly as they begin. Typically the cat resumes normal activity and eating habits between episodes.

Clinical signs are attributed to laryngospasm that develops subsequent to contact of saliva, hair or mucus with the epithelial surfaces of the larynx. The pathogenesis of this condition is not definitively known. Since clinical signs usually are not evident during physical examination, the diagnosis must be based on the history and owner's interpretation of clinical signs.

Table 5. Radiographic Signs in Dyspneic Cats

A. Normal →

- Cardiac Disease
  1. Cardiomyopathy: ECG, nonselective angiogram
  2. Arrhythmia: ECG
- Upper Airway Obstruction
  1. Neoplasia: examine under anesthesia
  2. Infectious disease: referable to clinical signs
  3. Foreign body: examine under anesthesia
- Drug Toxicity
  1. Acetaminophen toxicosis: cyanosis

B. Hyperlucent Lung Fields →

- Upper Airway Obstruction
  1. Neoplasia: examine under anesthesia
  2. Foreign body: examine under anesthesia

C. Interstitial Alveolar Pattern →

- Pneumonia
  1. Bacterial (usually secondary): tracheal wash, culture and sensitivity, response to antibiotics
  2. Fungal: titers, fine-needle aspirate of lung
  3. Viral: signs of upper respiratory disease
  4. Verminous: fecal flotation, trachael wash
  5. Aspiration: oral exam (cleft palate)
- Pulmonary Edema
  1. Cardiogenic:
     a. Cardiomyopathy: ECG, nonselective angiogram
     b. Left heart failure
     c. Tachyarrhythmia (hyperthyroidism): ECG, serum T3 and T4
     d. Electrocution
  2. Noncardiogenic:
     a. Fluid overload (iatrogenic)
     b. Hypoalbuminemia (<1.0 g/dl)
     c. Allergic
     d. Toxic
- Neoplasia
  1. Metastatic
  2. Primary

Treatment: Treatment has included antibiotics and corticosteroids. Since the exact etiology is unknown, it is difficult to associate any improvement in the clinical signs with response to treatment. The episodes of paroxysmal respiratory distress may be stopped simply by initiating a swallowing reflex by forced administration of liquid. Oral administration of 2-3 ml water usually is adequate.

The prognosis is excellent for control and response to forced feeding of liquid or food. Recurrence of clinical signs is likely in all cats. Owners are informed that the paroxysms are not life-threatening.

Dyspnea from Diseases of the Lung

Pneumonia

There are many causes of pneumonia in cats. Of primary importance are parasitic, bacterial, viral and mycotic pneumonias. Any one or a combination of causes may exist in an individual cat. The existence of bacterial pneumonia, be it primary or secondary, should be determined when the diagnosis of pneumonia has been established. Primary bacterial pneumonia is unlikely to occur in healthy adult cats. More commonly, secondary bacterial pneumonia develops in debilitated cats and can be associated with conditions that alter or impair one or more

Table 5 (continued)

- D. Pleural Space
  - Fluid Density: Thoracentesis (see Fig 6)
  - Air Density (Pneumothorax)
    - Traumatic Pneumothorax
    - Extension of Cervical Emphysema
  - Fluid and Air Density
    - Trauma
      1. Diaphragmatic hernia
      2. Lung trauma
- E. Mediastinum
  - Fluid Density
    - Neoplasia
      1. Lymphosarcoma (FeLV +)
    - Cardiomegaly
      1. Cardiomyopathy
    - Miscellaneous
      1. Hemomediastinum
      2. Abscess
      3. Mediastinal diaphragmatic hernia
  - Air Density (Pneumomediastinum)
    - Trauma
      1. Tracheal laceration
      2. Esophageal laceration
      3. Extension of cervical emphysema
  - Fluid and Air Density
    - Trauma
    - Neoplasia

of the pulmonary defense mechanisms. Bacterial pneumonia can be life-threatening; prompt, vigorous treatment is justified in such cases. The following discussion is limited to the diagnosis and treatment of bacterial pneumonia.

Clinical Signs: Dyspnea is often present in cats with advanced bacterial pneumonia. Depending on the cause, coughing may or may not be present. Once the cat's condition is stabilized, further diagnostic procedures must include survey radiographs of the thorax, careful auscultation of the lungs, routine hematologic examination and a blood chemistry profile. While a diagnosis of pneumonia may be based on clinical signs and thoracic radiographs, it is unlikely that the cause can be determined from this information alone.

The clinician should attempt to determine if the pneumonia has a bacterial component. Anorexia, leukocytosis with lymphopenia, and fever may be the principal clinical features in cats with bacterial pneumonia. As respiratory secretions become tenacious and exudative, moist rales may be auscultated.

Since it is not always apparent whether bacterial pneumonia is primary or secondary, the clinician should attempt to rule out other causes once the bacterial component of the disease is under control. The diagnosis and treatment of parasitic, viral and mycotic pneumonia are discussed elsewhere in this text.

Diagnosis: In addition to clinical signs and laboratory data, thoracic radiographs should be obtained in all cases of suspected pneumonia. Patchy interstitial to alveolar opacities may be

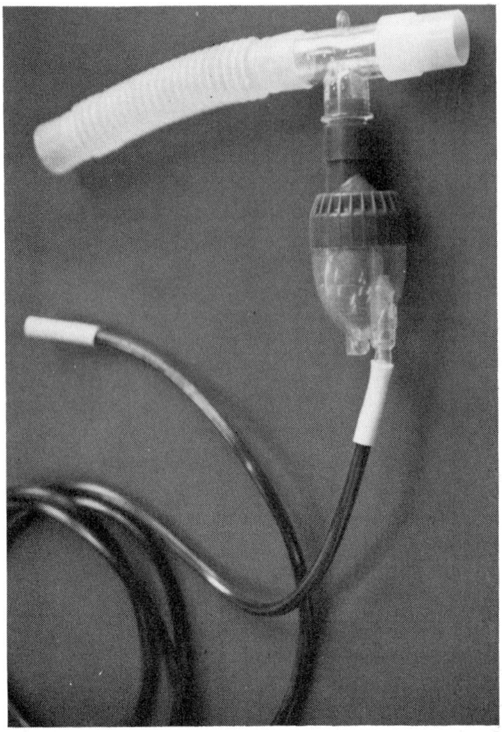

Fig 7. Pneumatic nebulizer used in the treatment of lower respiratory infections.

seen throughout the lung field. Consolidation of one or more lung lobes occasionally is seen.[5]

A diagnosis of bacterial pneumonia may be confirmed by recovery of organisms during tracheal washings. Although most bacterial pneumonias in dogs and cats are caused by gram-negative organisms, culture and sensitivity testing can be important in determining successful treatment of the condition.

Treatment: Successful treatment of bacterial pneumonia hinges on antibiotic therapy. Drug choice, dosage and duration of administration are 3 critical considerations of antibiotic therapy. Systemic therapy with Na or K penicillin G, ampicillin, chloramphenicol or a cephalosporin should be considered. In critically ill patients, parenteral administration of antibiotics should be considered over oral administration. Table 6 lists current recommendations for treating bacterial pneumonia in cats.

The value of fluid therapy in the treatment of bacterial lung disease should not be overlooked. Normal respiratory secretions become tenacious in dehydrated patients. Thickened, tenacious secretions are difficult to expel and may lead to serious ventilation-perfusion abnormalities.

The role of aerosol therapy in treating cats with bacterial pneumonia has not been fully explored. Nebulization therapy decreases respiratory effort. If included as part of the daily treatment regimen, nebulization therapy may actually decrease recovery time. Pneumatic nebulizers are readily available, inexpensive and easily adapted for use in cats (Fig 7). Nebulized sterile normal saline can be delivered into an anesthetic induction chamber (Fig 8). Therapy should be administered for 15-20 minutes 3-4 times daily until improvement in clinical signs is observed. Improvement should be noted in 3-5 days. At this time, there is no known advantage of addition of antibiotics, mucolytics or other drugs to nebulization solutions in the treatment of bacterial pneumonia.[9]

Prognosis: The response to treatment is generally dictated by the cause of the bacterial pneumonia. The hemogram and clinical signs may be monitored to evaluate the response to treatment. The respiratory effort should decrease while appetite and activity increase. Documentation of improvement may be accomplished through serial thoracic radiographs taken at 3- to 5-day intervals during therapy.

Pulmonary Edema

Pulmonary edema is characterized by the accumulation of excess fluid in the interstitial tissues of the lung, alveoli and airways. It must be regarded as a serious complication of a disease rather than a primary disease entity. Pulmonary edema occurs in diseases that increase the permeability of the alveolar epithelium and capillary endothelium, obstruct pulmonary lymphatics or alter the balance between oncotic and hydrostatic pressure in the pulmonary circulation and interstitial tissues of the lung.

Pulmonary edema may develop gradually since compensatory mechanisms that mobilize excess fluid from the lung prevent rapid accumulations of interstitial and alveolar fluid. In the early stages of pulmonary edema, fluid is removed by the lymphatics. Fluid accumulates in the interstitial tissues as the lymphatics become saturated. Alveolar flooding occurs once the compensatory volume of the interstitium has been exceeded. Clinical signs may not be evident until fluid accumulates in the alveoli and distal airways. Despite the fact that pulmonary edema

Table 6. Recommended Protocol for the Treatment of Bacterial Pneumonia

A. Fluid Therapy
see Chapter 2

B. Antibacterial Therapy
1. Ampicillin: 10-20 mg/kg q6h (oral)
   5-10 mg/kg q6h (parenteral)
2. Chloramphenicol: 50 mg/kg q12h (oral or parenteral)
3. Gentamicin: 4 mg/kg (IM, SC) q12h, 1st day only, then 4 mg/kg (IM,SC) daily

C. Aerosol Therapy
3 ml sterile saline nebulized 1-3 times daily.

usually develops gradually, the onset of clinical signs may appear acutely.

Clinical Signs: Dyspnea, characterized by tachypnea, wheezing, orthopnea and open-mouth breathing, is a manifestation of pulmonary edema in cats. Moist rales may or may not be evident. Cats may manifest orthopnea by their unwillingness to assume any position other than sternal recumbency. Dyspnea at rest suggests severe and advanced disease. As fluid enters the alveoli and terminal airways, clinical signs become considerably more dramatic. The oral mucous membranes may be pale grey or light blue.

The increased body temperature associated with stress and respiratory effort should not be interpreted as being associated with an infectious disease.

While it is desirable to distinguish between cardiogenic and noncardiogenic pulmonary edema, harsh lung sounds may preclude cardiac auscultation. Radiographic evaluation and electrocardiography are clearly indicated.

Diagnosis: Thoracic radiographs reveal pulmonary edema. Interstitial edema is recognized as diminished pulmonary radiolucency and loss of contrast of the pulmonary vessels. Interstitial edema may be hilar or generalized. Alveolar edema is recognized by air bronchograms and a mottled appearance of the lung field. Generalized cardiomegaly, associated with congestive cardiomyopathy, supports a diagnosis of cardiogenic pulmonary edema.

Treatment: The principal objective in the treatment of pulmonary edema is to improve the quality of ventilation by mobilizing excess fluid from the alveoli and interstitium of the lung. The cause of pulmonary edema must still be determined and treatment initiated if recurrence of pulmonary edema is to be prevented.

Furosemide, given parenterally or orally at 2-3 mg/kg BID or TID, is the drug of choice in the treatment of pulmonary edema. Cats receiving repeated doses of furosemide should be monitored for hypokalemia. Morphine sulfate (without atropine), at 0.05-0.10 mg/kg divided between the IV and IM routes, reduces anxiety, decreases respiratory effort and improves the quality of ventilation. The dose may be repeated as necessary. Dosages in excess of 0.10 mg/kg may cause excitement.

Bronchodilators are frequently used in the clinical management of pulmonary edema. Aminophylline, at 10 mg/kg every 8 hours, may be given parenterally or orally. In addition to the bronchodilating effect of aminophylline, this drug enchances diuresis, increases heart rate and strengthens myocardial contraction.

In the face of respiratory failure, artificial ventilation must be begun immediately. Using a sterile, cuffed endotracheal tube, 100% O_2 should be given using positive-pressure ventilation.[10]

Prognosis: In the immediate clinical management of pulmonary edema, the response of the patient to therapy should be closely monitored during the first 4-6 hours after the onset of treatment. Thoracic radiographs and clinical signs provide the best means of evaluating patient response. Failure to respond to therapy and persistent dyspnea, cyanosis and tachypnea indicate that therapy must be repeated, intensified or re-evaluated. The ultimate prognosis depends on the clinician's ability to identify and treat the underlying cause of the pulmonary edema.

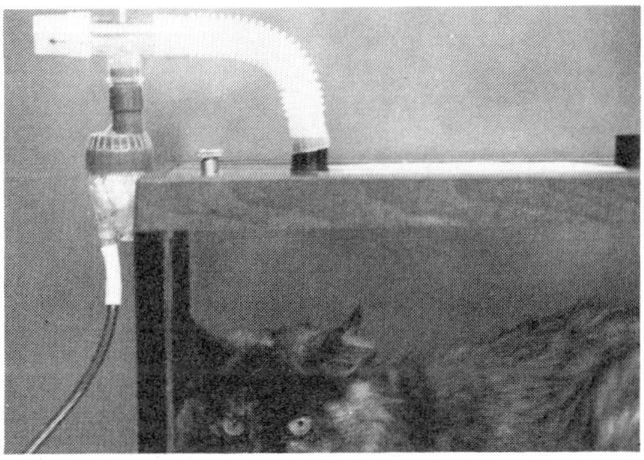

Fig 8. Anesthetic induction chamber used as a nebulization chamber.

Dyspnea from Disease of the Pleural Space

The pleural cavity is best described as a potential space between the parietal and visceral pleurae. The pleural space in normal cats is filled with a thin film of fluid that moistens the mesothelial cells of the pleura. The parietal pleura includes the mediastinal pleura and the pleural lining of the thoracic wall and diaphragm. The visceral pleura covers the lungs. The mediastinal pleura normally completely separates the right and left hemithorax. Due to the delicate nature of this structure, many diseases involving one side of the pleural space extend to the opposite side.

Clinical Signs: Dyspnea at rest is a common presenting sign in cats with pleural space disease. Respiration is rapid and shallow. Unfortunately, early signs of lower respiratory tract disease, such as exercise intolerance, are unlikely to be recognized since cats with lower respiratory disease are reluctant to play or move at all. Attenuated heart and lung sounds may be auscultated over the right or left hemithorax or over the entire thorax. Rales are not evident unless concomitant airway disease exists. Mucous membranes usually are normal in color unless the pleural space disease has resulted in significant atelectasis.

Diagnosis: Fluid in the pleural space is the most common type of pleural space disease in cats. While large volumes of pleural fluid are readily detected radiographically, identification of small volumes of fluid in the pleural space requires high-quality radiographs. As the interlobar fissures fill with fluid, fissure lines may be evident radiographically.[11] This is particularly true on ventrodorsal thoracic radiographs. As the fluid accumulates in the pleural space, the contour of the cardiac and diaphragmatic lung lobes may become obscured and the costophrenic angles become blunted. Since fluid in the pleural space may obscure soft tissue masses in the pleural space of the lung parenchyma, horizontal-beam radiography is useful if an intrathoracic mass is suspected. However, it may be necessary to remove most of the fluid to evaluate the entire thorax. A collapsed or atelectic lung lobe may resemble a soft tissue mass in the thorax.

The presence of fluid in the pleural space justifies thoracentesis. This technic may be used to obtain a specimen for diagnostic studies as well as to relieve the restrictive lung disease caused by the presence of fluid in the pleural space. Table 3 lists the differential diagnoses of pleural effusions.[11-14]

Pneumothorax, the presence of air in the pleural space, is the second most common pleural space disease in cats. Gas in the pleural space precludes complete lung expansion. Therefore, the lungs are displaced from the interior margin of the thoracic wall, resulting in increased radiographic density of the pulmonary parenchyma. Additionally, the cardiac silhouette on lateral radiographs does not contact the sternum. Horizontal-beam radiographs of the lateral thorax confirm the presence of pneumothorax if this cannot be accomplished with routine survey thoracic radiographs. The contrast between pleural air and the compressed lung is accentuated.[1]

Radiographically, soft tissue masses of the pleural space are unilateral and usually associated with displacement of normal thoracic structures. The diagnosis of pleural space masses is best accomplished with selective thoracentesis, using fluoroscopy, or at surgery.

Combinations of soft tissue densities and gas densities in the pleural space occur infrequently. Diaphragmatic hernia is perhaps the most common cause of this radiographic finding. Radiographic changes include obscurity of the cranial margin of the diaphragm, displacement of lung lobes and obliteration of the cardiac silhouette. Fluid may accumulate in longstanding diaphragmatic hernias. In such cases, positive-contrast studies of the upper GI tract may be helpful.

Treatment: The treatment of pleural space disease depends on the specific cause. Obviously, a diagnosis should be made before initiating any treatment. Oxygen therapy and sedation are unlikely to aid in the treatment of pleural space disease.

Pneumothorax should be immediately treated by aspirating air from the pleural space. A butterfly catheter (Abbott), attached to a 3-way stopcock and a 10-ml syringe, is placed into the pleural space at the level of the seventh or eighth intercostal space. Aspiration is continued until moderate resistance develops. Most cases of pneumothorax may be stabilized by removing air from a single site. Occasionally it may be necessary to aspirate air from both the right and left thorax. An attempt should be made to identify the exact cause of the pneumothorax. The cat should be observed for at least 48 hours to determine if air continues to accumulate within the pleural space.

Pyothorax*

Pyothorax refers to the presence of pus in the thoracic cavity. It is the result of infection with a pyogenic organism. Pyothorax is said to be 10 times more common in cats than in dogs. The purulent exudate varies from a creamy yellow and inspissated to a malodorous reddish brown.

Clinical Signs: The condition may be so acute that there is no warning and the cat is found *in extremis* or dead. The exudate puts pressure on the lungs, causing their collapse and progressive dyspnea. Cyanosis may develop; it will be more severe if the animal is placed on its back. The body temperature rises to 39.5-40.0 C (103-104 F), but drops suddenly to a subnormal level just before death. Affected cats are depressed and anorectic, remain in sternal recumbency, and drink considerable water though they remain dehydrated.

Diagnosis: The aforementioned signs suggest the presence of fluid in the thoracic cavity. Standing lateral radiographs of the cat reveal a fluid line within the chest; a dorsoventral radiograph discloses whether both sides of the thorax are involved. The mediastinum usually does not permit passage of inspissated fluid from one side of the chest to the other.

Percussion produces dull sounds, particularly over the ventral thorax, and the heart sounds become muffled due to the intrathoracic fluid. Thoracentesis and aspiration of the typical purulent exudate confirm the diagnosis. The organisms found include *Pasteurella* spp, staphylococci, coliforms, *Nocardia* spp and *Mycobacterium tuberculosis*. Pyothorax must be differentiated from feline infectious peritonitis, in which coughing, dyspnea and pleural effusion also occur.

Treatment: Unless the cat is handled carefully, it may suffer a fatal circulatory collapse.

Draining the pleural cavity with an 18-ga needle at the eighth intercostal space rapidly alleviates the dyspnea. A plastic indwelling catheter or polyethylene tube may be introduced through the needle and, in conjunction with a 2-way stopcock or clamp, used to drain the chest daily for 4-5 days. A stockinette can be used to hold the tube against the cat's body and prevent the animal from dislodging it.

Antibiotics can be administered through the drainage tube, as may proteolytic enzymes. The choice of antibiotic should be based on a sensitivity test after a culture of the aspirated exudate. Treatment should be continued until the signs subside. When *Nocardia* is involved, the treatment should be continued for 4-5 days after the cat is asymptomatic.

Due to the severe dehydration, fluid replacement is important. Severely affected, dyspneic animals should be placed in an oxygen cage.

Chylothorax*

Although chylothorax usually is the result of a crushing force over the abdomen, it may occur spontaneously. Rupture of the thoracic duct may also be related to thoracic infections or neoplasms.

Clinical Signs: Dyspnea consistently accompanies chylothorax, and visible mucosae become pale or cyanotic. In chronic cases, the signs develop over several months and include anorexia, malaise and weakness. Fever is not common.

Diagnosis: Radiographs disclose the presence of fluid in the thoracic cavity and permit differentiation from diaphragmatic hernia. The fluid should be aspirated to determine its character. Chyle has a milky appearance, although it is occasionally bloodstained as a result of the original injury. As a diagnostic test, the fat droplets in the chyle may be stained with Sudan III.

Treatment: The thoracic duct is ligated with nonabsorbable sutures placed caudal to the rupture. The thoracotomy can be performed on either the left or right side. The duct may be very difficult to find, and it has been reported that its ligation at the diaphragm "obviates looking for the duct."[16] If a fatty meal or milk is given 2 hours before the surgery is performed, the thoracic duct may become visible.

Dyspnea from Diseases of the Mediastinal Space

Similar to disease of the pleural space, mediastinal disease is caused by the presence of gas, fluid, or a combination of these in the mediastinal space. Unlike the pleural space, the mediastinal space of normal cats contains several organs, vessels, lymph nodes and nerves. Radiographically, however, only the trachea, aorta, caudal vena cava, thymus (in cats less

*by G. Sumner-Smith and C. Eger

than one year of age) and heart can be seen in the mediastinal space of normal cats. Knowledge of the location of these structures is important if abnormalities are to be detected.

The mediastinal pleura comprises the lateral boundaries of the mediastinal space and separates the left hemithorax from the right. However, diseases of the mediastinum may readily and easily extend through the mediastinal pleura into the pleural space.

Clinical Signs: Dyspnea is a common presenting complaint in cats with mediastinal disease. The character of respirations is not dissimilar to that noted in cats with disease of the pleural space. However, mediastinal disease does not attenuate heart and lung sounds unless significant amounts of fluid accumulate secondarily within the pleural space. Auscultation of the heart and lungs usually is normal if the pleural space is not involved.

Dyspnea associated with mediastinal disease may be caused by tracheal or bronchial compression, restriction of lung expansion, extension of disease into the pulmonary parenchyma or the pleural space. Table 5 lists some causes of mediastinal disease.[15]

Diagnosis: Both lateral and ventrodorsal survey radiographs of the thorax are necessary to confirm mediastinal disease. Soft tissue densities or fluid within the mediastinal space are recognized by an increased opacity and size of the mediastinum. Displacement of the lungs, heart and/or trachea may be evident. By virtue of their position, enlarged mediastinal lymph nodes displace the trachea dorsad. Cats with evidence of mediastinal lymph node enlargement or cranial mediastinal masses should be tested for FeLV. Ventral displacement of the trachea is likely to be associated with an esophageal mass or mediastinal abscess rather than a lymphoid mass. Fluid in the mediastinal space may obliterate visualization of a soft tissue mass. Horizontal-beam radiographs of the lateral thorax may provide additional information. Positive-contrast esophagrams may reveal a soft tissue mass within the mediastinum. However, these procedures may not yield a definitive diagnosis. Thoracotomy may be the only means available to diagnose mediastinal masses.

The presence of free gas in the mediastinum is called pneumomediastinum. Radiographically, pneumomediastinum is readily identified by enhanced visualization of mediastinal structures. The azygos vein and cranial vena cava, not normally seen on lateral thoracic radiographs, may be evident in cats with pneumomediastinum. In addition, the adventitial surface of the trachea is also evident, indicating the presence of air around the trachea.

Although dyspnea is not usually caused by pneumomediastinum, it is likely to be associated with the source of the mediastinal air. Tracheal or pulmonary lacerations are common causes of pneumomediastinum. Since the cranial mediastinum communicates with the fascial planes of the cervical region via the thoracic inlet, traumatic cervical emphysema may extend into the mediastinum.

Treatment and Prognosis: Although cardiomegaly and lymphosarcoma are the most common abnormalities of the feline mediastinum, the specific diagnosis must be established if treatment is to be pursued and a prognosis made. Treatment of these entities is discussed elsewhere in this text.

References

1. Kealy, JK: Diagnostic Radiology of the Dog and Cat. WB Saunders, Philadelphia, 1979.
2. Ford, RB. Compend Cont Ed Pract Vet **1** (1979) 337.
3. Bright, in Bojrab: Pathophysiology in Small Animal Surgery. Lea & Febiger, Philadelphia, 1981.
4. Hjerpe, CA. Proc Ann Mtg Am Coll Vet Int Med, 1973.
5. Suter, in Ettinger: Textbook of Veterinary Internal Medicine. WB Saunders, Philadelphia, 1975.
6. Georgi, JR: Parasitology for Veterinarians. WB Saunders, Philadelphia, 1969.
7. Dubey, JP *et al.* JAVMA **174** (1979) 835.
8. Bartels, JE. Feline Pract **2(3)** (1972) 11.
9. McKiernan, B. Proc III Vet Resp Symp, 1978.
10. Bonagura, in Kirk: Current Veterinary Therapy VII. WB Saunders, Philadelphia, 1980.
11. Gruffydd-Jones, TJ and Flecknell, PA. J Sm Anim Pract **19** (1978) 315.
12. Losonsky, JM *et al.* Feline Pract **8(4)** (1978) 35.
13. Tomlinson, J. Feline Pract **10(6)** (1980) 26.
14. Schalm, OW *et al.* Feline Pract **4(6)** (1974) 41.
15. Thrall, DE and Losonsky, JM. Feline Pract **8(6)** (1978) 47.
16. Garber, ER. JAVMA **146** (1965) 242.

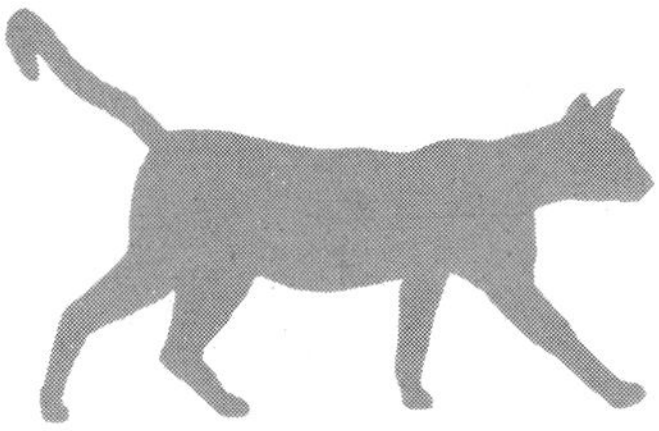

11
the endocrine system

S.L. MARTIN AND C.C. CAPEN

Disorders of endocrine glands occur less frequently in cats than in dogs and people. Diabetes mellitus, hyperthyroidism and secondary hyperparathyroidism associated with dietary imbalances of calcium (Ca) and phosphorus (P) or long-term renal failure are the major endocrine diseases encountered in cats. Since recent scientific advances have greatly expanded our understanding of metabolic skeletal disorders, a section has been included on the hormonal control of Ca metabolism. Less frequently encountered diseases of endocrine glands discussed in this chapter include pituitary neoplasms, hypopituitarism, disturbances of growth in the thyroid gland, and diseases of the adrenal cortex.

THE PITUITARY GLAND

Syndromes associated with pituitary neoplasms occur infrequently in cats as compared with dogs. Nearly all of the pituitary adenomas reported in the literature and studied at Ohio State University have been endocrinologically inactive but resulted in functional disturbances by virtue of compression atrophy of the pituitary gland and extension into the brain.

Anatomy and Physiology

The pituitary is a complex endocrine gland of dual ectodermal origin. The adenohypophysis develops from an outpouching of oral ectoderm (Rathke's pouch) and the neurohypophysis develops from downgrowth of diencephalic neuroectoderm. Close apposition of these 2 primordia is necessary for differentiation of the pars intermedia from the wall of Rathke's pouch. The pituitary gland in adults is completely separated from the oral cavity. It is situated in the sella turcica, a concavity of the sphenoid bone, and enveloped by an extension of dura mater.

The pituitary (hypophysis) is subdivided anatomically into the adenohypophysis (anterior lobe) and neurohypophysis (posterior lobe). In the cat the adenohypophysis completely surrounds the pars nervosa of the neurohypophyseal system.

A specific population of endocrine cells in the pars distalis synthesizes and secretes each of the pituitary tropic hormones.[1] Secretory cells in the adenohypophysis are subdivided into acidophils, basophils and chromophobes, based on interaction of the secretory granules with pH-dependent histochemical stains. Acidophils are further subdivided into either somatotrophs that secrete growth hormone (GH, somatotropin) and luteotrophs that secrete luteotropic hormones (LTH, prolactin).[2,3] Basophils include gonadotrophs that secrete luteinizing hormones (LH) and follicle-stimulating hormone (FSH), and thyrotrophs that secrete thyrotropic hormone (TTH).[4,5] Chromophobes are pituitary cells that do not have obvious cytoplasmic secretory granules by light microscopy. They include the endocrine cells concerned with the synthesis of adrenocorticotropic hormone (ACTH) and melanocyte-stimulating hormone (MSH), nonsecretory follicular cells, and undifferentiated stem cells.

Each population of endocrine cells in the adenohypophysis is under the control of a corresponding releasing hormone (factor) from the hypothalamus (Fig 1). These releasing hormones are small peptides synthesized by neurosecretion by neurons in the hypothalamus.[6] They are transported by axonal processes to the median eminence, where they are released into capillaries and conveyed by the hypophyseal portal system to specific endocrine cells in the adenohypophysis. There they stimulate the rapid release of preformed tropic hormones (Fig 2).

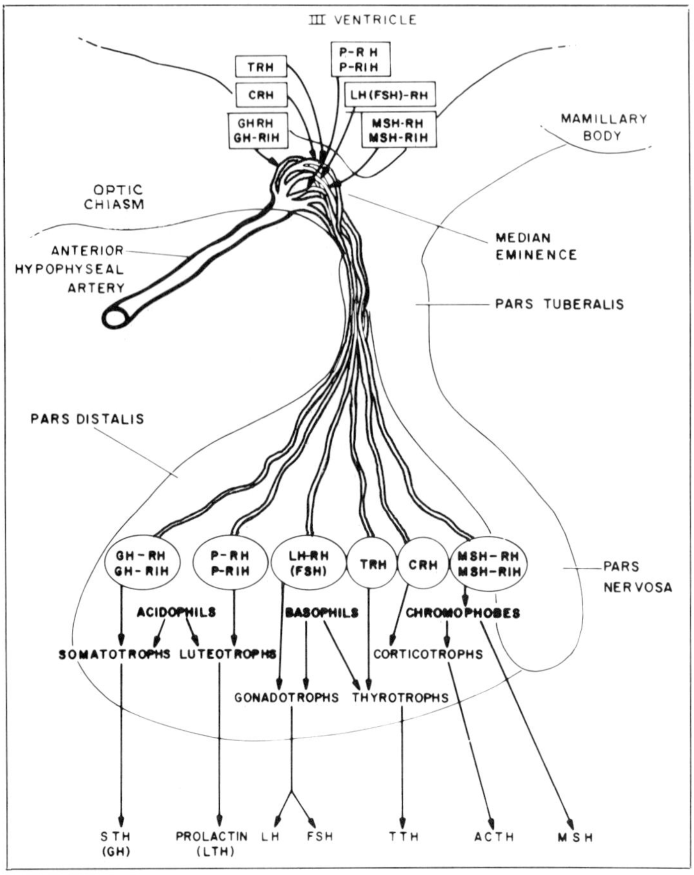

Fig 1. Control of tropic hormone secretion from the adenohypophysis by hypothalamic-releasing hormones (RH) and release-inhibiting hormones (R-IH). The releasing and release-inhibiting hormones are synthesized by neurons in the hypothalamus, transported by axonal processes, and released into capillary plexuses in the median eminence. They are transported to the adenohypophysis by the hypothalamic-hypophyseal portal system, where they interact with specific populations of tropic hormone-secreting cells to govern the rate of release of preformed hormones, such as somatotropin (GH, STH), prolactin (LTH), luteinizing hormone (LH), follicle-stimulating hormone (FSH), thyrotropin (TTH), adrenocorticotropin (ACTH) and melanocyte-stimulating hormone (MSH).

There appear to be 7 different hypothalamic releasing hormones that regulate the rate of secretion of each tropic hormone secreted by the adenohypophysis. For most pituitary tropic hormones, negative-feedback control is accomplished by the blood concentration of the hormone produced by the target endocrine gland (*eg*, thyroid gland, adrenal cortex, ovary, testis). The hormone produced by the endocrine glands exerts negative-feedback control on the neurosecretory neurons in the hypothalamus that synthesize the corresponding releasing hormone; however, GH, prolactin and MSH do not act on target endocrine organs to stimulate secretion of a hormone. Negative-feedback control of these last 3 pituitary hormones is effected by production of a corresponding release-inhibiting hormone (factor) by neurons in the hypothalamus. The relative local concentrations of the specific releasing hormone and release-inhibiting hormone appear to govern the rate of release of GH, LTH and MSH from the adenohypophysis.

The neurohypophysis consists of 3 anatomic subdivisions. The pars nervosa (posterior lobe) represents the distal component of the neurohypophyseal system. It is composed of numerous capillaries supported by modified glial cells (pituicytes). The capillaries in the pars nervosa are termination sites for the nonmyelinated axonal processes of neurosecretory neurons in the hypothalamus. Secretion granules that contain the neurohypophyseal hormones, *ie*, oxytocin and antidiuretic hormone (vasopressin), are synthesized in hypothalamic neurons but are released into the blood in the pars nervosa. The infundibular stalk joins the pars nervosa to the overlying hypothalamus and is composed of unmyelinated axonal processes from neurosecretory neurons. Neurosecretory neurons in the hypothalamus receive impulses from higher centers and translate these into endocrine output in the form of hormonal secretion. In addition to the usual structural features of neurons, they contain prominent arrays of rough endoplasmic re-

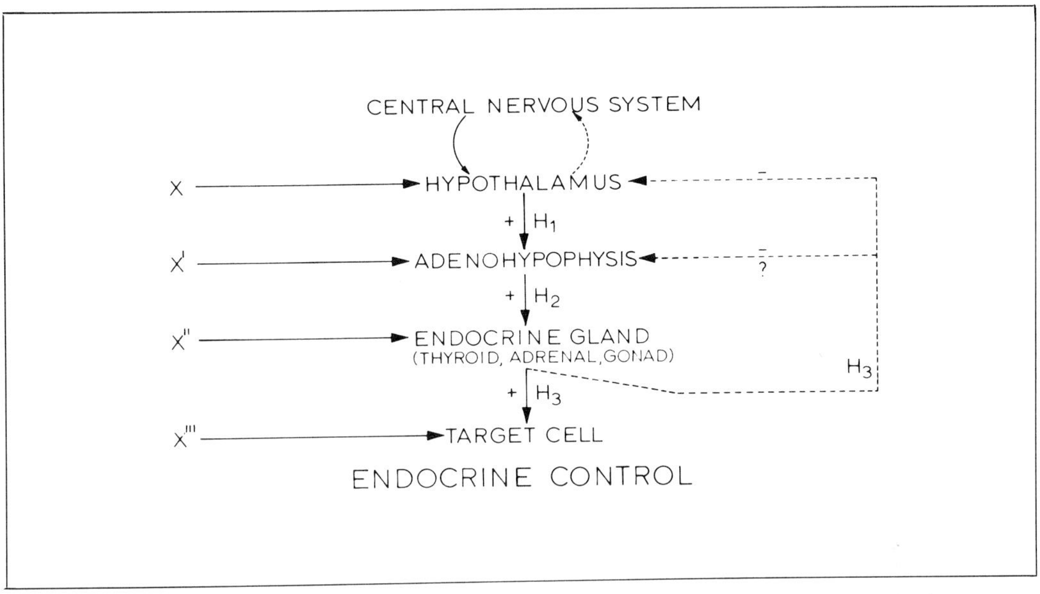

Fig 2. Highest order of endocrine control involving interrelationship with the CNS. Receptors in the nervous system detect changes in the internal or external environment and convey this information through neural impulses to neurosecretory neurons in the hypothalamus. Releasing hormones (H_1) produced in response to the neural input stimulate rapid release of corresponding tropic hormone (H_2) from the adenohypophysis. Tropic hormones influence the rates of existing reactions in the corresponding endocrine gland (thyroid, adrenal cortex, gonad) and increase secretion of hormones (H_3) from target endocrine organs, which are carried by the bloodstream to specific target cells to elicit a biologic response. Negative-feedback control is effected by the blood concentration of the final endocrine product (H_3), primarily on target cells in the hypothalamus. Local autoregulatory mechanisms (X) at each level influence the functional activity of components of this endocrine control system.

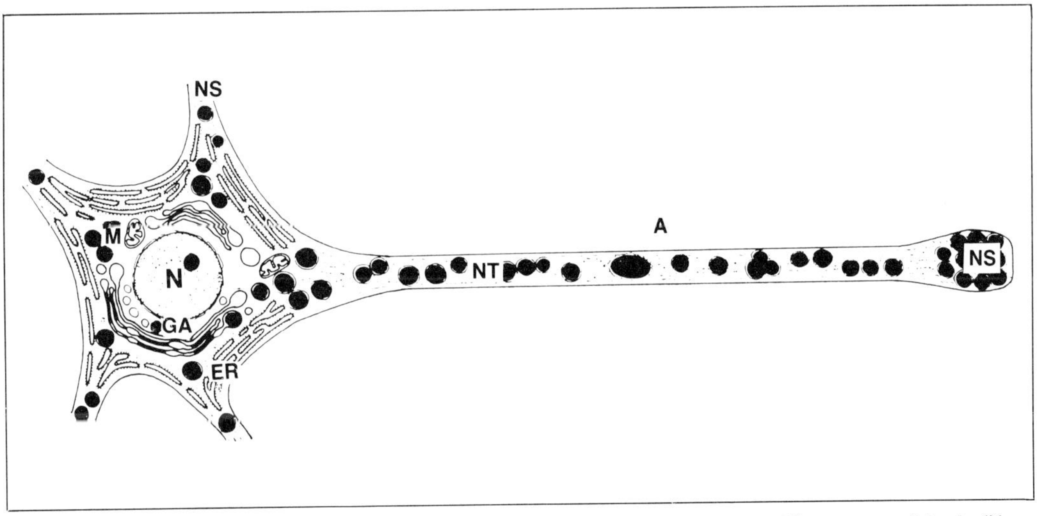

Fig 3. Structural characteristics of a neurosecretory neuron in the hypothalamus. The nerve cell body (N = nucleus) has dendritic and axonal (A) processes with arrays of rough endoplasmic reticulum (ER), large mitochondria (M), and a prominent Golgi apparatus (GA). Hormone-containing, membrane-limited neurosecretory granules (NS) are formed in the Golgi apparatus and transported along the axon to the site of release at the termination on capillaries. Neurosecretory neurons synthesize the releasing and release-inhibiting hormones of the adenohypophysis and the hormones of the neurohypophysis (oxytocin, antidiuretic hormone). NT = neurotubules.

ticulum, large Golgi apparatuses, and numerous membrane-limited secretory granules in the nerve cell body and axonal process (Fig 3). The neurosecretory neurons concerned with hormone synthesis are segregated into anatomically defined regions, called nuclei, in the hypothalamus. The supraoptic nucleus is concerned primarily with the synthesis of antidiuretic hormone, whereas oxytocin is produced predominantly by neurons in the paraventricular nucleus.

The neurohypophysis in most animals is supplied directly by the posterior (inferior) hypophyseal arteries that branch from the internal carotid arteries. Branches of the anterior (superior) hypophyseal arteries originate from the internal carotid arteries and from the posterior communicating arteries of the circle of Willis. Arteriolar branches penetrate the pars tuberalis, lose their muscular coat, and form a capillary plexus near the median eminence. These vessels subsequently drain into hypophyseal portal veins that supply the pars distalis. There also may be a small direct arterial supply to the adenohypophysis of minor importance that arises from the posterior hypophyseal arteries.

Diseases of the Pituitary Gland

Pituitary Adenoma and Hypopituitarism

Clinical Signs: Cats with pituitary adenomas are presented with functional disturbances related to CNS dysfunction or lack of secretion of pituitary tropic hormones and diminished end-organ function.[7-9] The history often includes complaints of depression, weakness, collapse with exercise, marked personality changes, incoordination and other disturbances of balance. The cat may become unresponsive to its owners and develop a tendency to hide at the slightest provocation.[8] In long-standing cases the cats often are blind, with dilated and fixed pupils. The body condition may vary from progressive cachexia to obvious obesity. The cat may appear dehydrated, as evidenced by a dry, lusterless haircoat, and the owners may notice increased water consumption and frequency of urination. Occasionally a cat that is housebroken begins to urinate on furniture and defecate outside of its litterbox.

Lesions: Pituitary adenomas usually grow to considerable size before they cause obvious clinical signs or result in death. The proliferating tumor cells incorporate the remaining structures of the adenohypophysis and infundibular stalk (Fig 4). The neoplasms are firmly attached to the base of the sella turcica but there is no evidence of erosion of the sphenoid bone. Because the diaphragma sellae is incomplete in cats, the line of least resistance favors dorsal expansion of the progressively enlarging adenoma, resulting either in a broad-based indentation or extension into the overlying brain. The entire hypothalamus may be compressed and replaced by the tumor, which extends through the thalamus and protrudes into the lateral ventricles. The optic nerves are compressed and incorporated within the large neoplastic mass on the ventral aspect of the brain, accounting for the blindness observed clinically.

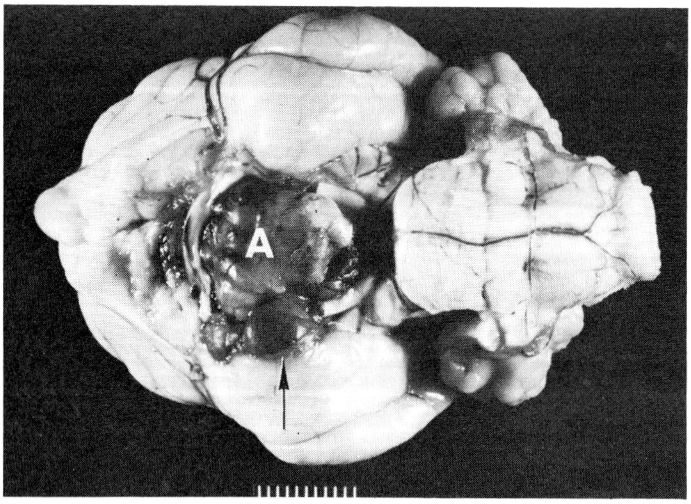

Fig 4. Ventral view of the brain of a 4-year-old male Siamese, illustrating a large chromophobe adenoma (A) in the pituitary gland. The neoplasm has completely incorporated the pituitary, extended into the brain and destroyed the optic nerves. An arrow marks the junction of the neoplastic tissue and brain parenchyma. (scale = 1 cm)

Microscopically the tumor cells are polyhedral and subdivided into small pockets by fine connective tissue septa with prominent capillaries. Special histochemical technics for pituitary cytologic examination either have failed to demonstrate secretory granules or have demonstrated numerous acidophilic granules within the cytoplasm of the tumor cells.

The adrenal glands of cats with pituitary adenomas are often small and difficult to find at necropsy. The adrenals consist primarily of medullary tissue surrounded by a narrow band of atrophic cortex (Fig 5). The adrenal cortex appears as a thin, yellow-brown rim composed of a moderately thickened capsule and secretory cells of the zona glomerulosa. The zonae fasciculata and reticularis are severely atrophied as compared with those in the adrenal glands of normal cats. Thyroid glands of cats with large pituitary neoplasms may be smaller than normal but the reduction in size is to a lesser degree than in the adrenal cortex. Most follicles are large, lined by flattened cuboidal epithelium and filled with densely stained colloid. The seminiferous tubules of males are small, with little evidence of active spermatogenesis.

Treatment: Since pituitary tumors in cats are endocrinologically inactive, their presence is not recognized until the masses grow large enough to produce neurologic signs and surgical removal is not feasible (Fig 5). Secondary signs of hypopituitarism, such as hypothyroidism and corticosteroid deficiency, can be alleviated with oral thyroxine and prednisolone.

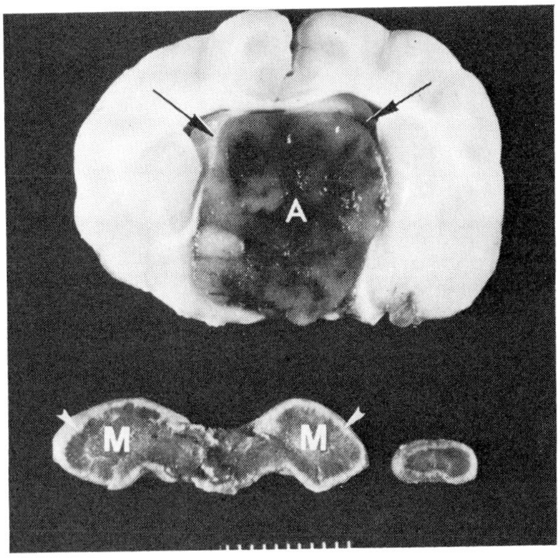

Fig 5. Pituitary chromophobe adenoma of the cat in Figure 4. Cross-section of the brain reveals massive extension of the adenoma (A) into the hypothalamus and thalamus, with protrusion into the lateral ventricle (arrows). The junctions between the adenoma and brain parenchyma are sharply defined. The adrenal glands are small and consist primarily of medullary tissue (M) surrounded by an atrophied layer of cortex (white arrowheads). (scale = 1 cm)

Diabetes Insipidus

Diabetes insipidus is a disorder in which inadequate antidiuretic hormone (ADH) is produced or target cells in the kidney lack the biochemical systems to respond to secretion of normal or elevated circulating levels of hormones. The hypophyseal form of diabetes insipidus develops from compression and destruction of the pars nervosa, infundibular stalk or supraoptic nucleus in the hypothalamus. The lesions responsible for this disruption of ADH synthesis or secretion include large pituitary neoplasms, a dorsally expanding cyst or inflammatory granuloma, and trauma to the skull, with hemorrhage and glial proliferation in the neurohypophyseal system. Sporadic cases of hypophyseal diabetes insipidus may be the result of an inherited biochemical defect in the synthesis of ADH and its corresponding neurophysin I, as has been well characterized in the Brattleboro strain of rats.[10]

In the nephrogenic form of diabetes insipidus, blood levels of ADH are normal or elevated but target cells in the distal nephron and collecting ducts cannot respond due to a lack of adenylate cyclase in the plasma membrane.

Diabetes insipidus has been observed infrequently in cats.[11,13] One case occurred after trauma and involved an apparent partial deficiency of ADH.[13] The marked polydipsia and polyuria decreased after administration of vasopressin, hypertonic saline or chlorpropamide. The response to hypertonic saline and chlorpropamide injection indicated that ADH was released from the neurohypophysis. The cat died suddenly after treatment for 7½ months with chlorpropamide. At necropsy the pituitary gland was half the normal size and there was caudal displacement of the pituitary stalk and optic chiasma. The hypothalamus appeared normal.

Cats with diabetes insipidus excrete large volumes of hypotonic urine, which in turn necessitates the intake of equally large amounts of water to prevent dehydration and hyperosmolality of body fluids. Urine osmolality is decreased below normal plasma osmolality (about 300 mOsm/kg) in both hypophyseal and nephrogenic forms of diabetes insipidus. In response to water deprivation, urine osmolality remains below that of plasma in both forms of diabetes insipidus, in contrast to that observed in normal animals. The elevation of urine osmolality above that of plasma in response to exogenous ADH in the hypophyseal form but not in the nephrogenic form of diabetes insipidus is useful in the clinical separation of these 2 forms of the disease.

THE THYROID GLAND

Anatomy and Physiology

The thyroid originates as a thickened plate of epithelium in the floor of the pharynx. Branched cell cords develop from the pharyngeal plate and migrate dorsolaterad, but remain attached to the pharyngeal area by the narrow thyroglossal duct. A portion of the thyroglossal duct may persist postnatally and form a cyst due to accumulation of proteinic material secreted by the lining epithelium.

The 2 thyroid lobes in cats are located on the lateral surfaces of the trachea. The principal blood supply to each lobe is the cranial thyroid artery, a branch of the common carotid artery.

The thyroid gland is the largest of the endocrine organs that function exclusively as an endocrine gland. The basic histologic structure of the thyroid is unique for endocrine glands, consisting of follicles of varying size that contain colloid produced by the follicular cells. The follicular cells are cuboidal to columnar and their secretory polarity is directed toward the lumen of the follicles. An extensive network of inter- and intrafollicular capillaries provides the follicular cells with an abundant blood supply. Follicular cells have long profiles of rough endoplasmic reticulum and a large Golgi apparatus in their cytoplasm for synthesis and packaging of substantial amounts of thyroglobulin, a protein that is transported into the follicular lumen. The interface between the luminal side of follicular cells and the colloid is modified by numerous microvillar projections.

The biosynthesis of thyroid hormones is unique among endocrine glands because the final assembly of hormones occurs extracellularly, within the follicular lumen. Essential raw materials, such as iodide, are trapped efficiently by follicular cells from plasma, transported rapidly against a concentration gradient into the follicular lumen, and oxidized by a peroxidase in microvillar membranes to iodine. The assembly of thyroid hormones within the follicular lumen is made possible by a unique protein (thyroglobulin) synthesized by follicular cells.

Thyroglobulin is a high molecular-weight glycoprotein synthesized in successive subunits on ribosomes of the rough endoplasmic reticulum in follicular cells. The constituent amino acids (tyrosine and others) and carbohydrates (mannose, fructose, galactose) are derived from the circulation. Recently synthesized thyroglobulin leaving the Golgi apparatus is packaged into apical vesicles and extruded into the follicular lumen.[14,15] The amino acid tyrosine, an essential component of thyroid hormones, is incorporated within the molecular structure of thyroglobulin. Iodine is bound to tyrosyl residues in thyroglobulin at the apical surface of follicular cells to form successively monoiodotyrosine and diiodotyrosine (Fig 6).[16] The resulting monoiodotyrosine and diiodotyrosine combine to form the 2 biologically active iodothyronines (thyroxine, triiodothyronine) secreted by the thyroid gland.

The secretion of thyroid hormones from stores within the luminal colloid is initiated by elongation of microvilli on follicular cells and formation of pseudopods. The length of these elongated cytoplasmic projections is increased by pituitary thyrotropin. They extend into the follicular lumen, and indiscriminately phagocytize a portion of adjacent colloid. Colloid droplets in follicular cells fuse with numerous lysosomal bodies that contain proteolytic enzymes.

Triiodothyronine (T_3) and thyroxine (T_4) are released from the thyroglobulin molecule and secreted into adjacent capillaries. The iodinated tyrosines (monoiodotyrosine, diiodotyrosine) released from the colloid droplets are deiodinated enzymatically and the iodide generated under normal conditions is either recycled to the lumen to iodinate new tyrosyl residues or released into the circulation. These unique structural and functional characteristics of the phylogenetically oldest endocrine gland suggest the thyroid may have evolved toward a more "ideal" structure to perform its vital metabolic functions.

Negative-feedback control of thyroid hormone secretion is accomplished by the coordinated response of the adenohypophysis and certain hypothalamic nuclei to circulating levels of T_3 and T_4. A decrease in thyroid hormone concentration

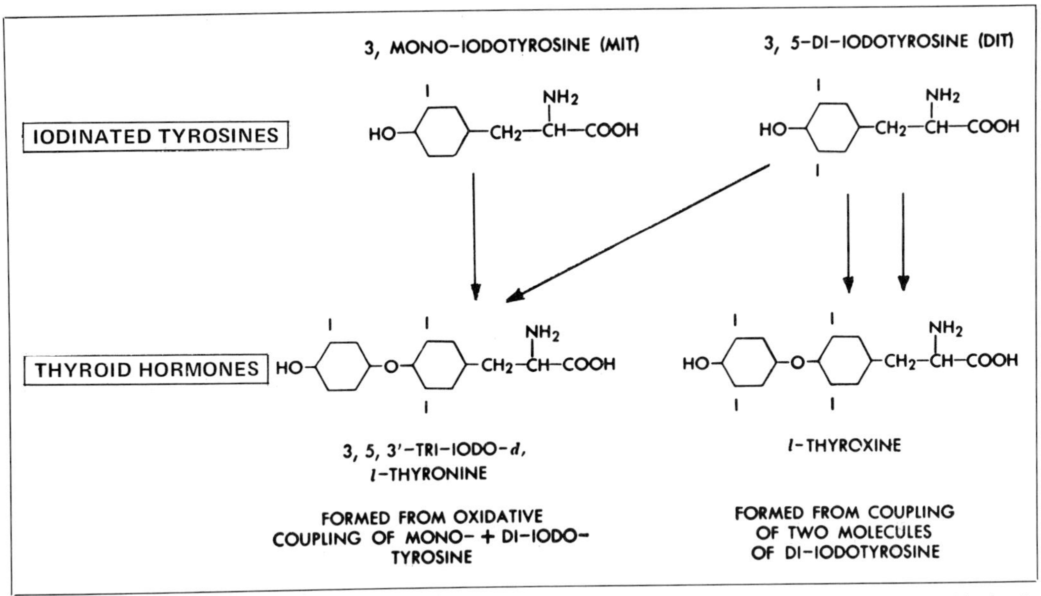

Fig 6. Formation of thyroid hormones from iodinated tyrosines within the follicular lumen of the thyroid gland. (Courtesy of R.W. Rawson and Clinical Symposia)

in plasma is sensed by groups of neurosecretory neurons in the hypothalamus that synthesize and secrete a small peptide into the hypophyseal portal circulation.[17] Thyrotropin-releasing hormone (TRH) binds to isoreceptors on the plasma membrane of thyrotropic basophils in the adenohypophysis and activates adenyl cyclase, resulting in the formation of 3′5′ cyclic adenosine monophosphate (cyclic AMP). The intracellular accumulation of cyclic AMP in thyrotropic basophils results in contraction of microfilaments and the peripheral movement and discharge of thyrotropin containing secretion granules into pituitary capillaries. Thyrotropin is conveyed by the blood to thyroid follicular cells, where it binds to the basilar aspect of the cell, activates adenyl cyclase, and increases the rate of most biochemical reactions concerned with the biosynthesis and secretion of thyroid hormones. An initial response by follicular cells to thyrotropin is the formation of numerous cytoplasmic pseudopodia, resulting in increased endocytosis of colloid and release of preformed hormone stored in the follicular lumen. The converse of what has just been described occurs in response to an increased level in circulating thyroid hormone.

Once T_4 and T_3 are released into the circulation, they act on many different target cells in the body. The overall function of T_4 and T_3 is similar, although much of the biologic activity may be the result of monodeiodination of T_4 to T_3 before interacting with receptors in target cells.[18] The subcellular mechanism of action of thyroid hormones appears to resemble that of steroids in that free hormone enters into target cells and binds to a cytosol-binding protein.[19] Free T_3 either binds to receptors on the inner mitochondrial membrane to activate mitochondrial energy metabolism or binds to a nuclear receptor and increases transcription of the genetic message to facilitate new protein synthesis.[20] The overall effects of thyroid hormones are to: increase the basal metabolic rate; make more glucose available to meet the elevated metabolic demands by increasing glycolysis, gluconeogenesis and glucose absorption from the intestine; stimulate new protein synthesis; increase lipid metabolism, conversion of cholesterol into bile acids and other substances, activation of protein lipase, and sensitivity of adipose tissue to lypolysis by other hormones; stimulate the heart rate, cardiac output and blood flow; and increase neurotransmission, cerebration and neuronal development in young animals.

Diseases of the Thyroid Gland

Disturbances of Growth

Disturbances of growth involving the thyroid gland are not uncommon in cats. The literature

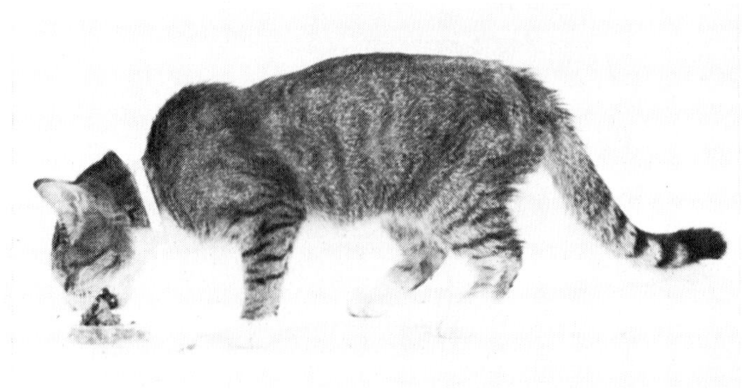

Fig 7. Hyperthyroid cat with a functional adenoma derived from follicular cells. The cat had lost a considerable amount of body weight despite its ravenous appetite.

and our experience suggest that adenomas and "multinodular goiters" are encountered more commonly than thyroid carcinomas.[21-31] Adenomas and carcinomas are most likely to be encountered in aged cats, whereas goiters can occur at any age. The mean age of cats with benign tumors was reported as 12.4 years and thyroid carcinomas as 15.8 years.[27]

Clinical Signs: Until recently, most proliferative lesions encountered in the feline thyroid gland were found incidentally at necropsy and were not recognized as being associated with obvious clinical disturbances. Recent reports have described a syndrome in aged cats of hyperthyroidism usually associated with multinodular goiter, adenomas and occasionally adenocarcinomas derived from follicular cells of the thyroid.[24,26,30] Large adenomas and carcinomas may be detected by palpation of swelling in the cranioventral cervical region. Arterial thrombosis has been observed in a cat with a bilateral thyroid carcinoma.[23] The cat was unable to use the left front leg, which was cool to the touch as a result of a tumor cell embolus occluding the left brachial artery. Dyspnea and dysphagia were reported in a cat with a rapidly growing anaplastic giant-cell adenocarcinoma of the left thyroid.[31] The mass had partially enclosed the trachea and esophagus.

Lesions: Thyroid adenomas usually appear as solitary, soft nodules that enlarge and distort the contour of the affected lobe. A thin, fibrous connective tissue capsule separates the adenoma from the adjacent, often compressed, thyroid parenchyma. The neoplastic cells tend to form irregularly shaped follicles, with occasional papillary infoldings of epithelium and variable amounts of colloid. Focal areas of necrosis, mineralization and cystic degeneration are present in larger adenomas. Multiple sections of adenomas fail to reveal histologic evidence of either vascular or capsular invasion by tumor cells. Certain atypical thyroid adenomas are composed of poorly differentiated follicular cells arranged into compact cellular foci and small, closely packed follicles either devoid of colloid or with many endocytotic vacuoles at the interface with the follicular cells. They are differentiated from thyroid carcinomas by the lack of vascular and/or capsular invasion and absence of metastases in regional lymph nodes and lung.[27]

Thyroid adenomas also must be differentiated from multinodular adenomatous hyperplasia ("goiter") that occurs in old cats. These multiple areas of thyroid hyperplasia usually are microscopic and do not enlarge the affected lobe of thyroid. In contrast to adenomas, the areas of nodular hyperplasia are not encapsulated and adjacent thyroid parenchyma is not compressed. Histopathologically, these hyperplastic nodules are composed of irregularly shaped, colloid-filled follicles lined by cuboidal follicular cells.

Thyroid carcinomas occur less frequently than either adenomas or multinodular hyperplasia in cats. They often result in considerable enlargement of one or both thyroid lobes and may invade adjacent structures. Carcinomas are characterized by the invasion of vessels and the connective tissue capsule by neoplastic cells. Metastases to regional lymph nodes (retropharyngeal, mandibular, deep cervical) and distant sites have been reported in less than 50% of thyroid carcinomas in cats.[27] The more well-differentiated thyroid carcinomas are relatively solid and composed of a uniform pattern of small follicles containing little colloid and occasional compact cellular areas. Strands of dense connective tissue, with an abundant capillary network and

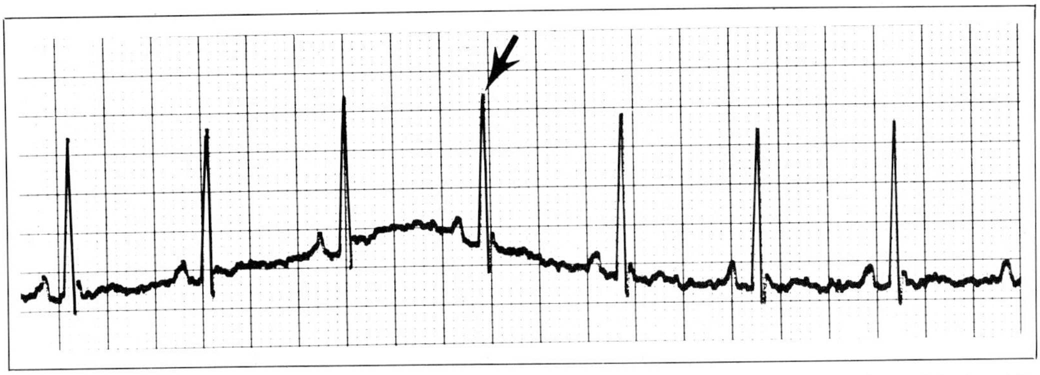

Fig 8. Electrocardiogram from a cat with hyperthyroidism, illustrating high-voltage R waves (arrow) in Lead II. Heart rate, 210 bpm; calibration, 1 cm = 1 mV; paper speed, 50 mm/sec.

foci of lymphocytes, subdivide the neoplastic cells into small lobules. Other follicular carcinomas are composed of large, cystic spaces lined by pleomorphic tumor cells arranged into irregular follicles or compact groups. Papillary carcinomas of the thyroid are rare in cats and are composed of projections of neoplastic cells on a fibrous vascular core that extend into fluid-filled cystic spaces.

Hyperthyroidism

In a report of 26 cases of hyperthyroidism in aged cats, all affected cats were short- or long-haired crossbreeds ranging in age from 9 to 22 years.[24] Both sexes were equally represented.

Clinical Signs: The most common clinical sign reported was weight loss in spite of a normal or increased appetite (Fig 7). Polydipsia and polyuria occurred in some cats. Increased frequency of defecation and increased volume of stools were observed in about half of affected cats. Restlessness and increased activity occurred in some previously quiet cats.

A common clinical finding in hyperthyroidism is tachycardia accompanied by premature beats and/or a systolic murmur.[32] Electrocardiographic changes observed in cats with hyperthyroidism are sinus tachycardia, often with heart rates greater than 240 beats/minute, and increased R wave voltages in lead II, indicative of left ventricular enlargement (Fig 8). Cardiomegaly may be evident on radiographs (Fig 9). The changes usually regress after treatment.

Lesions: One or both thyroid lobes are enlarged in hyperthyroid cats. Solitary adenomas derived from thyroid follicular cells, in our experience, are the most common lesion associated with hyperthyroidism in cats. The affected thyroid lobe is partially or completely incorporated by the adenoma (Fig 10). Functional thyroid adenomas are composed of cuboidal to columnar follicular cells that form follicles of varying size and shape. Usually the follicles are partially collapsed and contain little colloid due to the intense endocytotic activity of neoplastic follicular

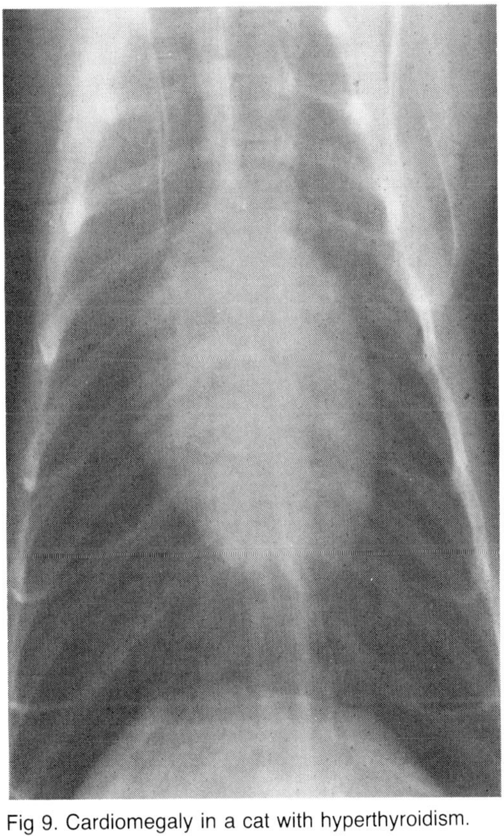

Fig 9. Cardiomegaly in a cat with hyperthyroidism.

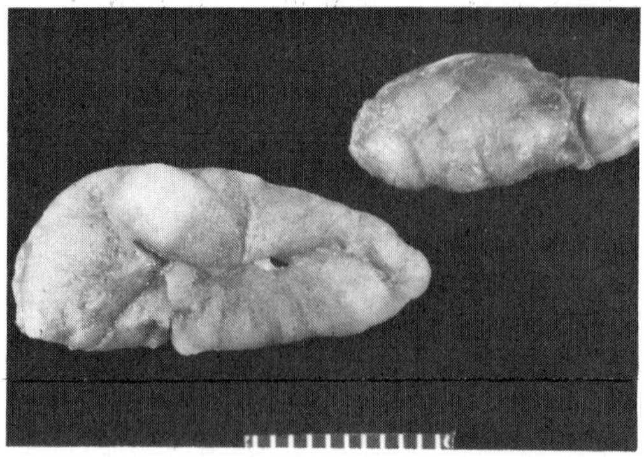

Fig. 10. Functional thyroid adenoma excised from a hyperthyroid cat, illustrating cut (bottom) and external (top) surfaces. The adenoma was coarsely nodular and firm in consistency. (scale = 1 cm)

cells. Long cytoplasmic projections often extend from the follicular cells into the lumen to phagocytize colloid. As a result of the marked endocytotic activity, numerous colloid droplets are present in the apical cytoplasm of follicular cells in close proximity to the many electron-dense lysosomal bodies.

Functional thyroid adenomas are partially or completely separated from remnants of the adjacent "normal" thyroid by a fine connective tissue capsule. Follicles in the rim of "normal" thyroid around a functional adenoma are markedly enlarged and distended by accumulation of colloid. The follicular cells are low cuboidal and atrophied, with little evidence of endocytotic activity in response to the elevated levels of thyroid hormones.

The opposite thyroid lobe should be carefully evaluated in cats with solitary adenomas for evidence of focal hyperplasia or "microadenomas." In our experience, the opposite thyroid lobe in cats with unilateral functional adenomas often has discrete, small areas of multinodular hyperplasia of follicular cells that cause recurrence of hyperthyroidism several months to a year or more after surgical removal of the tumor.

Diagnosis: Cats with hyperthyroidism usually have markedly elevated serum T_4 and T_3 levels. Normal serum levels of T_4 by radioimmunoassay are 1.5-5 μg/dl.[24] Normal serum T_3 levels by radioimmunoassay are 60-200 ng/dl. The serum T_4 levels in 7 cats with hyperthyroidism ranged from 3.4 to 30 μg/dl and serum T_3 levels ranged from 179 to 470 ng/dl.[24] Increased serum enzyme levels, including SGPT, SGOT and serum alkaline phosphatase, occur in hyperthyroid cats.

Treatment: Surgical excision of affected thyroid lobe(s) is the treatment of choice for cats with hyperthyroidism (Fig 11). Bilateral thyroidectomy should be performed if both glands are abnormal in appearance at surgery. At least one parathyroid gland should be left with an intact blood supply if bilateral thyroidectomy is performed. A thyroid-blocking agent, such as propylthiouracil, can be used for several days before surgery to alleviate some of the clinical effects of hyperthyroidism. A dose of 50 mg BID or TID has been used.[24]

Preoperative stabilization of cardiac function with a beta-adrenergic-blocking agent, such as propranolol, is indicated in cats with marked cardiac dysfunction.

When bilateral thyroidectomy has been performed, careful monitoring of the serum Ca level is indicated to detect hypocalcemia secondary to hypoparathyroidism. If the serum Ca level drops below 8 mg/dl, supplementation with Ca and vitamin D should be given until the Ca level is stabilized. After bilateral thyroidectomy, replacement therapy with thyroxine is also required to maintain a euthyroid state. Sodium levothyroxine at 0.05-0.1 mg given SID, starting 5-7 days after surgery, is adequate to maintain normal serum T_4 and T_3 levels in most cats.

Hypothyroidism

Well-documented cases of hypothyroidism are uncommon. Hypothyroid cats are obese and lethargic, and may not groom themselves (Fig 12).

A poorly defined clinical entity attributed to a hypofunction of the thyroid gland by some clinicians has been designated as feline endocrine alopecia (see Chapter 16). However, hypothyroidism has not been confirmed in these cats by evaluation of serum T_4 levels or thyroid biopsy.

Diagnosis: Cats with hypothyroidism have low serum T_4 and T_3 levels. A serum T_4 level below 1μg/dl and a T_3 level below 60 ng/dl supports a clinical diagnosis of hypothyroidism.

Treatment: The response of a hypothyroid cat to replacement of T_4 is dramatic. Sodium levothyroxine, at 0.05-0.1 mg SID, is adequate therapy for most affected cats.

THE PARATHYROID GLANDS

Anatomy and Physiology

Both the external and internal pairs of parathyroid glands of cats are in close proximity to

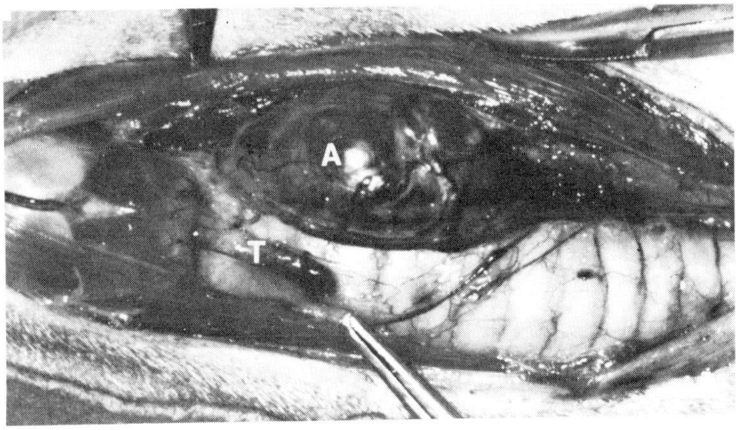

Fig 11. Surgical dissection of the ventral cervical region of the cat illustrated in Figure 7. Note the large unilateral thyroid adenoma (A) and small thyroid (T) gland on the opposite side.

the thyroid gland. The larger external parathyroid gland is situated near the cranial pole of each thyroid lobe and outside of the thyroid capsule. The internal parathyroid gland is smaller and situated near the dorsomedial aspect of each thyroid lobe and may be located within the thyroid capsule.

The parathyroid glands contain a single basic type of secretory cell concerned with elaboration of one hormone.[33] The parathyroid glands are composed of chief cells in different stages of secretory activity and in transition to oxyphil cells.[34] In most species chief cells interpreted to be an inactive (resting or involuted) stage of their secretory cycle predominate in the parathyroid glands. Active chief cells have an increased cytoplasmic density due to the close proximity of secretory organelles and numerous secretion granules.[35]

Oxyphil cells are not present in the parathyroid glands of young animals. They first appear at puberty and increase in number with advancing age, often forming nodules in the parathyroids of old animals. They occur singly or in small groups interspersed among chief cells in parathyroid glands. They are larger than chief cells and their abundant cytoplasmic area is filled with numerous, large, often bizarre-shaped mitochondria. Glycogen particles and free ribosomes are interspersed among the mitochondria.

Granular endoplasmic reticulum, Golgi apparatuses and parathyroid hormone-containing secretory granules are poorly developed in oxyphil cells of normal animals, suggesting that they do not have an active function in the biosynthesis of parathyroid hormone. Associated with the marked increase in mitochondria, oxyphil cells have a higher oxidative and hydrolytic enzyme activity than do chief cells.[36-38]

Cells are observed in parathyroid glands with cytoplasmic characteristics intermediate between those of chief and oxyphil cells. These transitional oxyphil cells have numerous mitochondria but secretory organelles also are present. The significance of oxyphil cells in the pathophysiology of parathyroid disease has not been elucidated; however, they are not altered in response to either short-term hypocalcemia or hypercalcemia in animals. Present evidence suggests that oxyphil cells do not appear to be degenerated chief cells as previously thought but rather are derived from chief cells as a result of aging or some metabolic derangement.

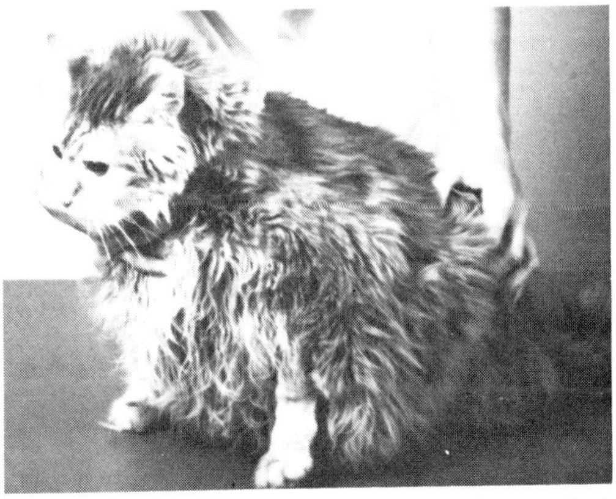

Fig 12. Hypothyroidism in a cat, illustrating marked obesity and poor grooming. The serum T_4 and T_3 levels were markedly reduced.

Parathyroid Hormone

The biosynthetic precursor of parathyroid hormone (PTH), pre-proparathyroid hormone, is synthesized on ribosomes of the rough endoplasmic reticulum in chief cells.[39-47] Pre-proparathyroid hormone is rapidly converted to proparathyroid hormone (proPTH), which moves within membranous channels of the endoplasmic reticulum to the Golgi apparatus.[48] Within the membranes of the Golgi apparatus, proPTH is converted enzymatically to biologically active PTH (Fig 13).[49-51] Active PTH is packaged into membrane-limited, macromolecular aggregates in the Golgi apparatus for subsequent storage in chief cells. Under certain conditions of increased demand, PTH may bypass this packaging phase and be released directly from chief cells. Low serum Ca levels increase the rate of PTH secretion and decrease the resting phase of chief cells; conversely, high serum Ca levels suppress the rate of PTH secretion and increase the resting phase of the secretory cycle.

Molecular fragments of PTH are formed in the liver, kidney, at target cells of the hormone,and possibly within chief cells. The immunoheterogeneity created by the multiple circulating fragments of PTH has caused significant problems in the development and application of highly specific radioimmunoassays for PTH to clinical diagnostic problems.[52]

The chief cells in the parathyroid glands secrete PTH continuously and store relatively small amounts of PTH in secretory granules. They can respond to minor fluctuations in serum Ca concentration by rapidly altering the rate of PTH secretion and more slowly by altering the rate of PTH synthesis.[53,54] In contrast to most endocrine organs, which are under complex controls involving both long- and short-feedback loops, the parathyroids have a unique feedback control via the serum Ca level.[55]

The serum P concentration has no direct regulatory influence on the synthesis and excretion of PTH; however, certain conditions in animals with hyperphosphatemia (chronic renal failure, excess dietary P) are associated with hyperparathyroidism. An elevated serum P level may lead indirectly to parathyroid stimulation by virtue of its ability to lower the serum Ca level when the serum is saturated with these 2 ions.[56]

The magnesium (Mg) ion has an effect on parathyroid gland secretory rate similar to that of Ca but is not equipotent.[57-59] The more potent effects of the Ca ion in the control of PTH secretion, together with its preponderance over Mg in the extracellular fluid, suggest a secondary role for Mg in control of PTH secretion.

Parathyroid hormone is the principal hormone involved in the minute-to-minute regulation of the serum Ca level. It directly influences the function of target cells, primarily in bone, kidney and intestine, to maintain serum Ca levels sufficient to ensure the optimal functioning of a wide variety of body cells. The overall action of PTH on bone is to mobilize Ca from skeletal reserves into extracellular fluids (Fig 14). Administration of PTH causes an initial decline, followed by a sustained increase, in circulating levels of Ca. This transitory decrease in serum Ca level is considered the result of sequestration

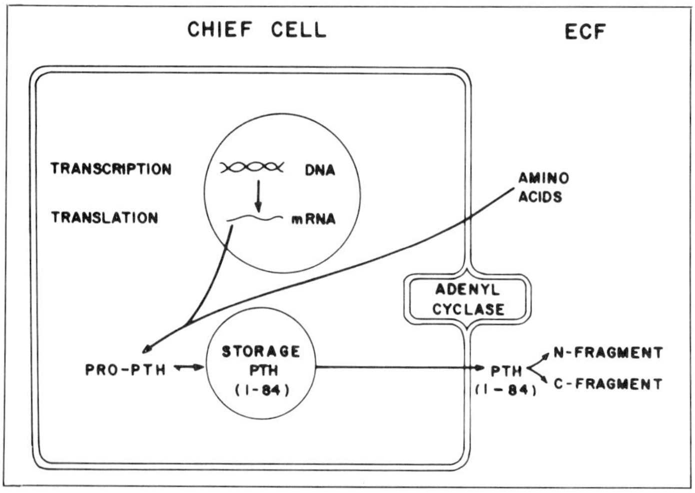

Fig 13. Biosynthesis of pro-parathyroid hormone (pro-PTH) in chief cells and conversion to biologically active PTH (1-84) prior to storage in secretory granules. PTH is converted to amino-terminal (N-) and carboxy-terminal (C-) fragments by peripheral tissues and possibly within chief cells before secretion.

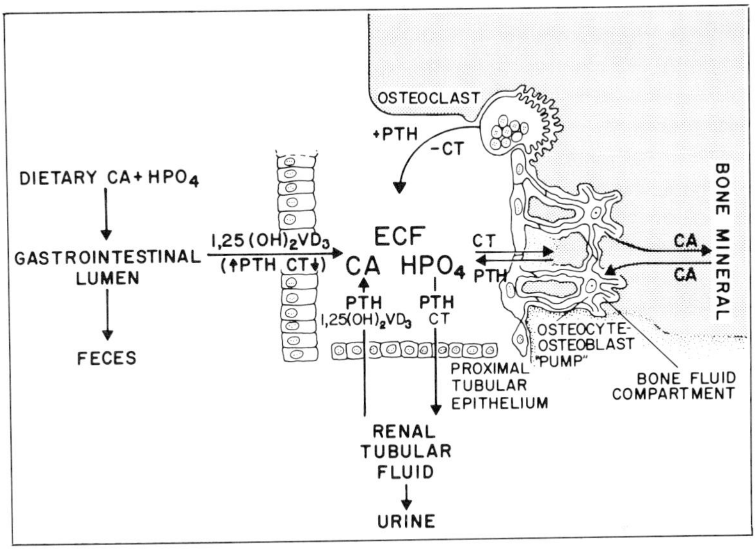

Fig 14. Interrelation of parathyroid hormone (PTH), calcitonin (CT) and 1,25-dihydroxycholecalciferol (1,25-$(OH)_2VD_3$) in the hormonal regulation of Ca and P in extracellular fluids.

of calcium phosphate in bone and soft tissues.[60] The subsequent increase in the serum Ca level results from interaction of PTH with osteoclasts and osteocytes in bone.

The response of bone to PTH is biphasic. The immediate effects are the result of increased activity of existing osteocytes and osteoclasts present in bone. This immediate effect depends upon the continuous presence of PTH and results in an increased flow of Ca from deep in bone to bone surfaces. Later effects of PTH are potentially of greater magnitude and not dependent

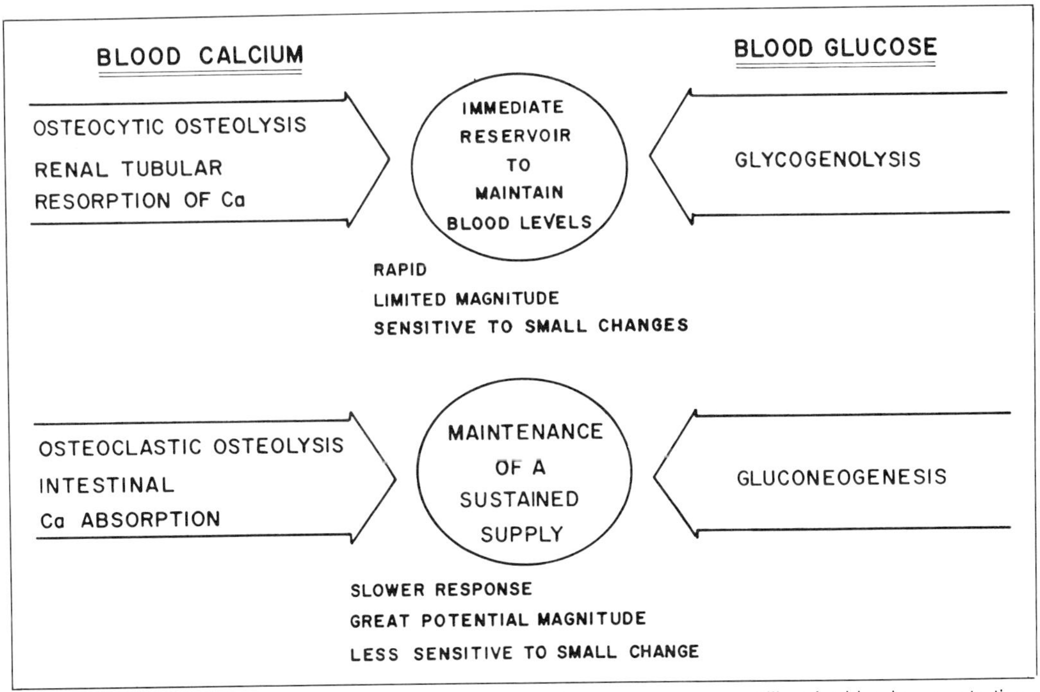

Fig 15. Comparison of immediate and long-term homeostatic mechanisms controlling the blood concentrations of Ca and glucose.

upon the continuous presence of PTH. Osteoclasts appear to be primarily responsible for the long-term action of PTH on increasing bone resorption and overall bone remodeling. If the increase in PTH secretion is sustained, the active osteoclast pool in bone is increased by activation of osteoprogenitor cells in the endosteal and other bone-cell envelopes.[61] A long-term increase in PTH secretion may also result in formation of greater numbers of osteoblasts, with a resultant increase in bone formation as well as resorption; however, resorption is usually greater than formation, leading to a net negative skeletal balance.

Renal tubular function is affected directly within 5-10 minutes by PTH, resulting in decreased resorption of P in the proximal tubule and consequent phosphaturia (Fig 14). Additionally, PTH leads to increased urinary excretion of K, Na, bicarbonate, cyclic adenosine monophosphate and amino acids.

Parathyroid hormone also enhances renal resorption of Ca in the distal tubules and is of considerable importance in the maintenance of Ca homeostasis (Fig 14). The urinary excretion of Mg, ammonia and titratable acids also is decreased by PTH. The other important effect of PTH on the kidney is enhanced conversion of 25-hydroxycholecalciferol to 1,25-dihydroxycholecalciferol and other vitamin D metabolites.

Parathyroid hormone promotes the absorption of Ca from the GI tract. This effect is not as rapid as the action on the kidney and is not observed in vitamin D-deficient animals. It is uncertain if this increased intestinal Ca transport is a direct effect of PTH on absorptive cells or rather an indirect effect of PTH by its action of stimulating renal synthesis of the biologically active metabolite of vitamin D.

Osteocytic osteolysis and the renal conservation of Ca function as an immediate reservoir to maintain the serum levels of Ca within narrow limits (Fig 15). Osteoclastic osteolysis and increased intestinal absorption of Ca respond more slowly to slight changes in serum Ca concentration and maintain the supply of Ca in the extracellular fluid (Fig 15).

Hormonal Control of Calcium Metabolism

The normal serum concentration of Ca in cats is approximately 8.5-10.5 mg/dl. The Ca in serum is composed of protein-bound and diffusible fractions. The diffusible fraction consists of biologically active or free (ionic) Ca and Ca that has formed complexes with anions, such as phosphate and citrate. Because the Ca ion plays a key role in many fundamental biologic processes, including muscle contraction, blood coagulation, enzyme activity, neural excitation, hormone release and membrane permeability, precise control of the concentration of this ion in extracellular fluids is vital. The endocrine control mechanisms that maintain a constant serum concentration of Ca despite marked variations in intake and excretion primarily consist of the interactions of PTH, calcitonin and vitamin D (Fig 14). Other hormones, such as adrenal corticosteroids, estrogen, thyroxine, somatotrophin and glucagon, also may contribute to Ca homeostasis under certain conditions.

Calcitonin: Calcitonin is secreted by a second endocrine cell population in the thyroid gland, the parafollicular or C-cells. They are distinct from the thyroid follicular cells, which secrete T_4 and T_3.[62] They are situated either within the follicular wall or as small groups of cells among follicles (Fig 16). The C-cells do not border the follicular colloid directly and their secretory polarity is oriented toward the interfollicular capillaries. The distinctive feature of C-cells is the presence of numerous small, membrane-limited secretory granules in the cytoplasm.

The concentration of Ca ion in serum and extracellular fluid is the principal physiologic stimulus for secretion of calcitonin by C-cells.[63] Calcitonin is secreted continuously under conditions of normocalcemia but the rate of secretion is increased greatly in response to elevation of the serum Ca level.

The C-cells store substantial amounts of calcitonin in secretory granules in their cytoplasm, in contrast to parathyroid cells, which store relatively small amounts of preformed hormone. In response to hypercalcemia, there is a rapid discharge of stored hormone from C-cells into interfollicular capillaries (Fig 17).[64] If the hypercalcemic stimulus is sustained, this is followed by an increased development of cytoplasmic organelles concerned with synthesis and secretion of calcitonin. Hyperplasia of C-cells occurs in response to long-term hypercalcemia.[65,66] When the serum Ca level is lowered, the stimulus for calcitonin secretion is diminished and numerous secretory granules accumulate in the cytoplasm of C-cells (Fig 17).

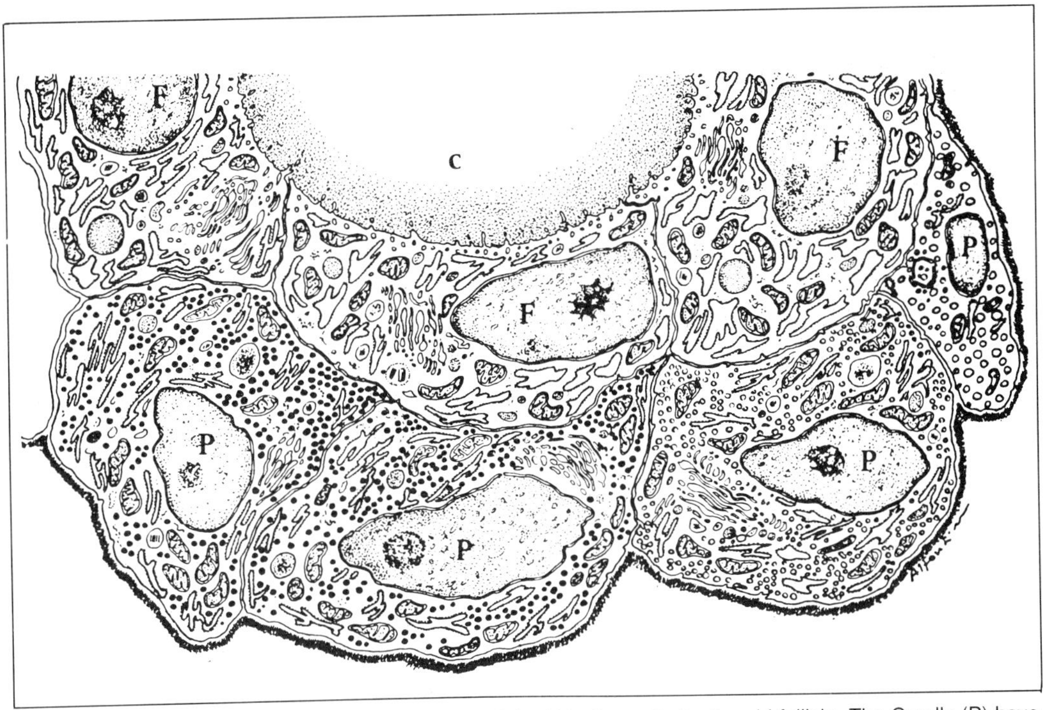

Fig 16. Calcitonin-secreting C-cells (parafollicular cells) within the wall of a thyroid follicle. The C-cells (P) have many small secretory granules in their cytoplasm. Thyroxine-secreting follicular cells (F) directly line the lumen and extend microvilli into the colloid (C). (From Proc Symp Thyrocalcitonin and C-cells. W. Heineman, London, 1968)

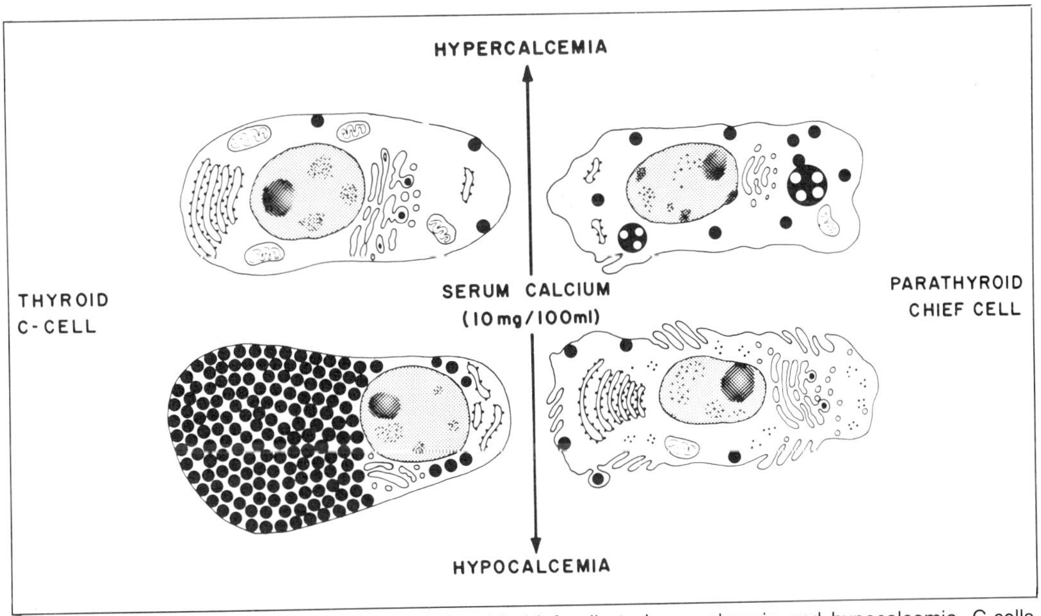

Fig 17. Response of thyroid C-cells and parathyroid chief cells to hypercalcemia and hypocalcemia. C-cells accumulate hormone-containing secretory granules in response to hypocalcemia, whereas chief cells are nearly degranulated but have a greater development of synthetic and secretory organelles. In response to hypercalcemia, C-cells are degranulated and chief cells are predominantly in the inactive stage of the secretory cycle.

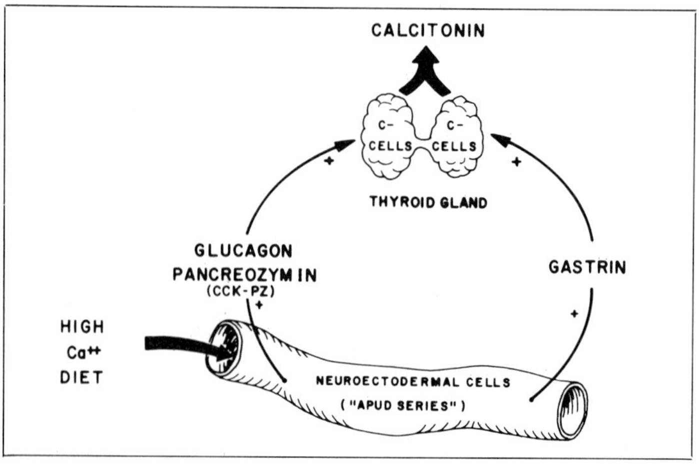

Fig 18. Gastrointestinal hormone-thyroid C-cell axis provides a mechanism for rapid release of calcitonin from the thyroid in response to a high-Ca diet before a significant elevation in blood Ca levels.

Calcitonin secretion is increased in response to a high-Ca meal, often before a significant rise in serum Ca level can be detected. The cause of this increase in calcitonin secretion may be due either to a small undetectible rise in the level of ionized Ca in the serum or a direct stimulation of certain GI hormones by the oral Ca load, which in turn stimulate secretion of calcitonin from the thyroid gland.[67] Gastrin, pancreozymin and glucagon stimulate calcitonin release under experimental conditions in animals.[68] These findings suggest that GI hormones may be important in triggering the early release of calcitonin to prevent hypercalcemia after ingestion of a high-Ca meal (Fig 18).[69]

The Mg ion has an effect on calcitonin secretion similar to that of Ca but only under experimental conditions when it is present in nonphysiologic amounts.

Administration of calcitonin or stimulation of endogenous secretion results in varying degrees of hypocalcemia and hypophosphatemia. These effects of calcitonin on serum Ca and P levels are most evident in young animals or adult animals with increased rates of skeletal remodeling. Calcitonin exerts its function by interacting with target cells, primarily in bone, kidney and, to a much lesser extent, the intestine. The action of PTH and calcitonin are antagonistic on bone resorption but synergistic on decreasing renal tubular resorption of P. The hypocalcemic effects of calcitonin are primarily the result of decreased entry of Ca from the skeleton into plasma due to temporary inhibition of PTH-stimulated bone resorption.[70,71] Hypophosphatemia develops from calcitonin's increasing the rate of movement of P out of plasma into soft tissue and bone, as well as from inhibition of bone resorption.[72] The action of calcitonin is not dependent on vitamin D since it acts both in vitamin D-deficient animals and after administration of large doses of vitamin D.

Inhibition by calcitonin of bone resorption stimulated by PTH and other factors results from blockage of both osteocytic and osteoclastic osteolysis (Fig 14). Specific structural alterations are produced in osteoclasts by calcitonin. Osteoclasts withdraw from resorptive surfaces, and the brush border and transitional zone become atrophied.[73,74] There also is a decrease in the rate of activation of osteoprogenitor cells to preosteoclasts and osteoclasts, resulting in fewer osteoclasts in bone. Although calcitonin can block bone resorption completely, the inhibition is transitory. Continuous administration of calcitonin in the presence of PTH leads to an "escape phenomenon," whereby the effects of PTH on increasing bone resorption are manifested in the presence in calcitonin.[71]

Calcitonin and PTH both decrease renal tubular resorption of P, leading to phosphaturia; however, the adenylate cyclase-linked receptors for calcitonin are found in the ascending loop of Henle and distal convoluted tubule. Calcitonin also causes diuresis of Na, Cl and Ca, whereas PTH infusion leads to renal retention of Ca and hydrogen ions.[75]

Calcitonin and PTH, acting in concert, provide a dual negative-feedback mechanism to maintain the concentration of Ca in extracellular fluids. Parathyroid hormone is the major factor concerned with minute-to-minute regulation of serum Ca levels under normal conditions. Calcitonin appears to function more as an "emergency" hormone to prevent development of hypercalcemia during the rapid postprandial absorption of Ca and to protect against excessive loss of Ca and P from the maternal skeleton during pregnancy.

Cholecalciferol: The third major hormone involved in regulation of Ca metabolism and skeletal remodeling is cholecalciferol or vitamin D_3. Although this compound has been considered a vitamin for a long time, recent evidence suggests it can equally be considered a steroid hormone.[76] Cholecalciferol is ingested in small amounts in the diet and can be synthesized in the epidermis through a pre-vitamin D_3 intermediate form.[77] This reaction is catalyzed by ultraviolet irradiation from the sun. A high-affinity, vitamin D-binding protein transports cholecalciferol from the skin into the blood.[78,79]

Vitamin D must be metabolically activated before it can interact with target cells, primarily in the small intestines and bone.[80-82] Vitamin D_3 from dietary sources is absorbed by facilitated diffusion and bound to an alpha-2 globulin in the blood for transport. Endogenous cholecalciferol synthesized in the skin from 7-dehydrocholesterol also is bound to an alpha-2 globulin for transport to the liver (Fig 19).

The first step in the metabolic activation of vitamin D is conversion of cholecalciferol to its first metabolite in the liver.[83] This metabolite is transported to the kidney, where it undergoes further transformation to a more polar and active metabolite (Fig 20).[84] The final step in the metabolic activation of vitamin D is complex and regulated in part by the serum Ca concentration and its influence on the rates of secretion of PTH and calcitonin.[85-87] Parathyroid hormone and conditions that stimulate its secretion increase production of the hormonal form of vitamin D_3. High serum P levels suppress and low serum P levels stimulate formation of the active metabolite of vitamin D in the kidney.

The active metabolite of vitamin D increases absorption of Ca and P from the intestine, thereby maintaining adequate levels of these electrolytes in the extracellular fluid and permitting mineralization of bone matrix and function of a wide variety of tissues. From a functional view, vitamin D causes retention of sufficient mineral ions to ensure mineralization of bone, whereas PTH maintains the proper ratio of Ca to P in extracellular fluid.[88]

The major target tissue for the active metabolite of cholecalciferol is the mucosa of the small intestine, where it increases active transcellular transport of Ca out of the proximal small intestine and P out of the distal small intestine into the blood.

The active metabolite of cholecalciferol also acts on bone (Fig 20).[89] In young animals it is required for the orderly growth and mineralization of cartilage in the growth plate. Young animals fed diets deficient in vitamin D and housed indoors without exposure to ultraviolet irradiation develop rickets. In the absence of vitamin D, the cartilaginous matrix fails to mineralize

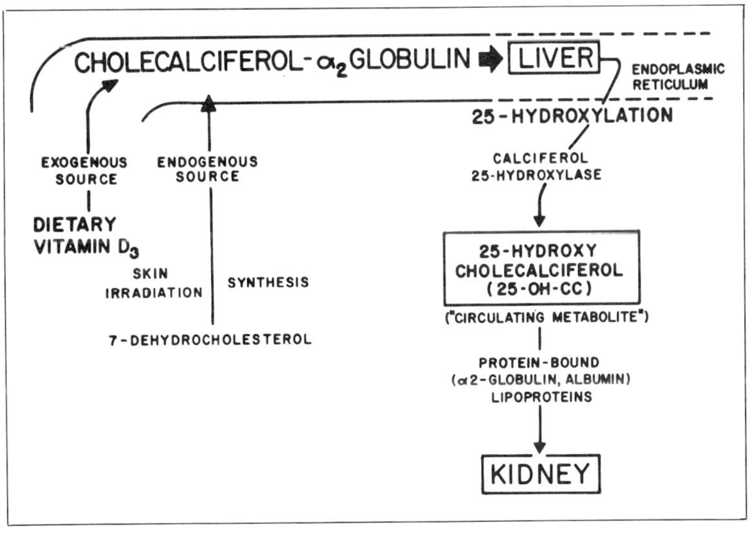

Fig 19. Metabolism of vitamin D_3. The initial step in the metabolic activation of Vitamin D_3 from endogenous and dietary sources is in the liver to form 25-hydroxycholecalciferol.

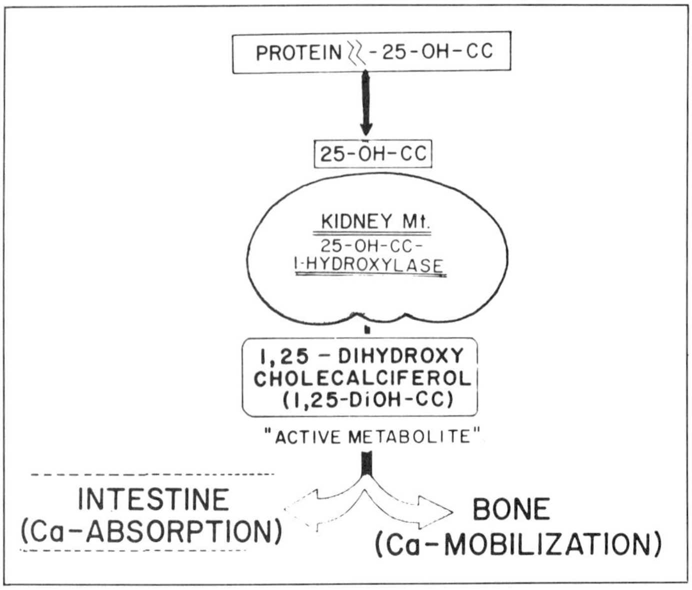

Fig 20. Metabolism of vitamin D_3. The final step in the metabolic activation of vitamin D_3 is in the kidney, where 25-hydroxycholecalciferol (25-OH-CC) is converted to 1,25-dihydroxycholecalciferol (1,25-DiOH-CC). 1,25-dihydroxycholecalciferol acts on target cells, primarily in the intestine and bone.

and the formation of woven bone on spicules of cartilage and subsequent remodeling to lamellar bone are blocked. The epiphyseal plate is irregularly thickened as progressively more primordial cartilaginous matrix accumulates and fails to mineralize.

In addition to this effect on mineralization of bone matrix in young animals, vitamin D is necessary for osteoclastic resorption and Ca mobilization from bone in adults. Small amounts of the active metabolite of vitamin D permit osteolytic cells to respond to PTH ("permissive effect") under physiologic conditions.

Considerably less is known regarding the action of cholecalciferol and its active metabolites on the kidney. The active metabolite of vitamin D stimulates Ca retention by increasing distal renal tubular resorption. The active metabolite of vitamin D may have a direct suppressive effect on secretion of PTH by the parathyroid gland in addition to its well-characterized action on intestine and bone.[90-92]

Disorders of Calcium Metabolism

Primary Hyperparathyroidism

Cause: Hyperparathyroidism is a rare metabolic disorder in which excessive amounts of PTH are secreted by the parathyroid glands, resulting in disturbances of mineral and/or skeletal homeostasis. In primary hyperparathyroidism, excess PTH is produced by a functional lesion in the parathyroid glands. Primary hyperparathyroidism does not appear to be a sequela of long-standing secondary hyperparathyroidism in animals.

Pathophysiology: The normal control mechanisms for PTH secretion by the serum level of Ca are lost in primary hyperparathyroidism. Hormone secretion is autonomous and the parathyroid glands produce excess hormone in spite of the increased serum Ca level.[93] Parathyroid hormone acts on cells of the renal tubules initially to promote the excretion of P and retention of Ca. Prolonged increased secretion of PTH results in accelerated osteocytic and osteoclastic bone resorption. Mineral is removed from the skeleton and replaced by immature fibrous connective tissue. The bone lesion of fibrous osteodystrophy is generalized throughout the skeleton but is accentuated in local areas such as in the cancellous bone of the skull.

Clinical Signs: Hypercalcemia results in anorexia, vomiting, constipation and generalized muscular weakness due to decreased neuromuscular excitability. Other functional disturbances result from weakening of bones by excessive osteoclastic resorption. Lameness or fractures of long bones due to severe demineralization occur after relatively minor trauma. Compression fractures of weakened vertebral bodies may exert pressure on the spinal cord and nerves,

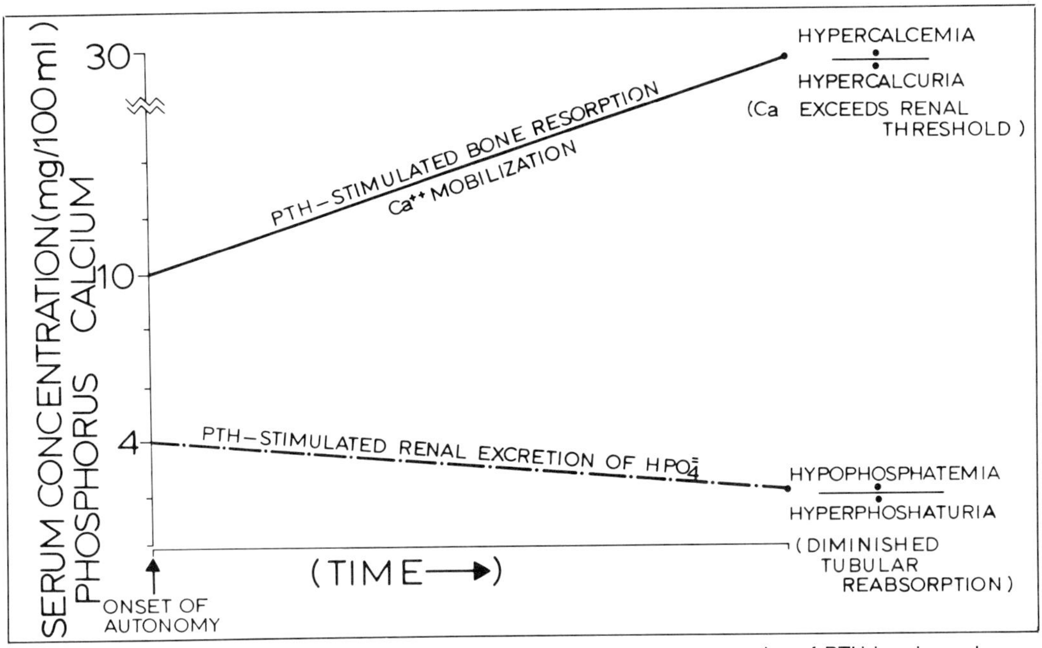

Fig 21. Alterations in serum Ca and P levels in response to autonomous secretion of PTH in primary hyperparathyroidism.

resulting in motor and/or sensory dysfunction. Bones of the skull are markedly thin from increased osteoclastic resorption and have a characteristic "moth-eaten" appearance on radiographs.

Diagnosis: Primary hyperparathyroidism should be included in the differential diagnosis of older cats with a history of severe, generalized skeletal demineralization and normal renal function. Radiographic evaluation reveals areas of subperiosteal cortical resorption, loss of lamina dura, soft tissue mineralization, bone cysts and a generalized decrease in bone density and fractures in advanced cases.

The most important and practical laboratory test used to establish the diagnosis of primary hyperparathyroidism is measurement of the total blood Ca level. Although other laboratory findings may be variable, hypercalcemia is a consistent finding and results from accelerated release of Ca from bone (Fig 21). Serum Ca values consistently above 12 mg/dl should be considered as hypercalcemic and cats with primary hyperparathyroidism usually have a greatly elevated serum Ca level (12-20 mg/dl or above). The blood P level is low or low-normal because of inhibition of renal tubular resorption of P by excess PTH (Fig 21). The activity of alkaline phosphatase may be elevated in the serum of cats with overt bone disease. Increased activity of this enzyme is thought to result from a compensatory increase in osteoblastic activity along trabeculae in response to mechanical stress of bones weakened by excessive resorption.

The urinary excretion of P, and often Ca, is increased and may result in nephrocalcinosis and urolithiasis. Accelerated bone matrix catabolism is reflected by an increased excretion of hydroxyproline in urine. Detection of elevated circulating levels of PTH by radioimmunoassay in people has greatly facilitated diagnosis of hyperparathyroidism in its early stage.

Other causes of hypercalcemia that must be considered in the diagnosis of primary hyperparathyroidism are vitamin D intoxication, malignancies with osseous metastases, secretion of hormones with PTH-like activity or other bone-resorbing substances by malignancies of nonparathyroid origin without metastases to bone, multifocal osteolytic lesions associated with septic emboli, complete immobilization, osteosarcoma, hypoadrenocorticism (Addison's-like disease, and chronic renal disease.[94-96]

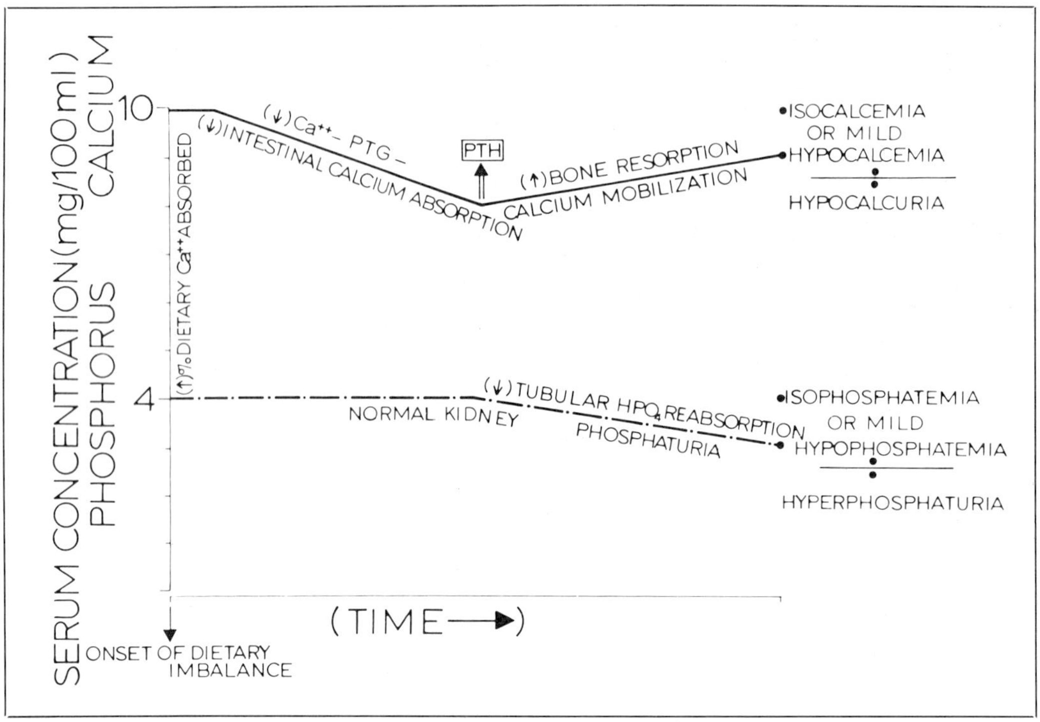

Fig 22. Alterations in serum Ca and P levels during nutritional secondary hyperparathyroidism caused by a low- Ca diet.

Treatment: The aim of treatment is to eliminate the source of excessive PTH production. An attempt should be made to identify all 4 parathyroid glands before excising any tissue. Parathyroid adenomas appear as light brown-red, encapsulated nodules, usually many times the size of normal glands. Successful removal of a functional parathyroid tumor results in rapid decrease in circulating PTH levels because the half-life of PTH in plasma is about 20 minutes. Plasma Ca levels in patients with overt bone disease may decrease rapidly and be subnormal within 12-24 hours after surgery, resulting in severe hypocalcemic tetany. Postoperative hypocalcemia (5 mg/dl and lower) can be the result of depressed secretory activity of chief cells due to long-term suppression by chronic hypercalcemia or injury to the remaining parathyroid tissue during surgery, abruptly decreased bone resorption due to lowered PTH levels, and accelerated mineralization of osteoid matrix that has previously been prevented from undergoing mineralization by elevated PTH levels. Infusions of Ca gluconate to maintain the serum Ca level at 7.5-9.0 mg/dl, plus feeding high-Ca diets and supplemental vitamin D, correct this postoperative complication.

Nutritional Secondary Hyperparathyroidism

The increased secretion of PTH in this metabolic disorder is a compensatory mechanism directed against a disturbance in mineral homeostasis, induced by nutritional imbalances. The disease occurs in both domestic cats and wild felidae kept as pets. Hyperparathyroidism has been observed most often in Siamese and Burmese kittens but skeletal lesions can be induced readily in other breeds. The indulgence of fussy eating habits with undesirable diets, rather than a genetic predisposition, probably accounts for the higher incidence in these breeds. A wide variety of synonyms have been used to describe this metabolic disorder in cats, including osteogenesis imperfecta, juvenile osteoporosis, paper-bone disease and Siamese cat disease.

Cause: Dietary mineral imbalances of etiologic importance in the pathogenesis of nutritional secondary hyperparathyroidism include a low Ca content, excess P with normal or low Ca, and inadequate amounts of vitamin D. The

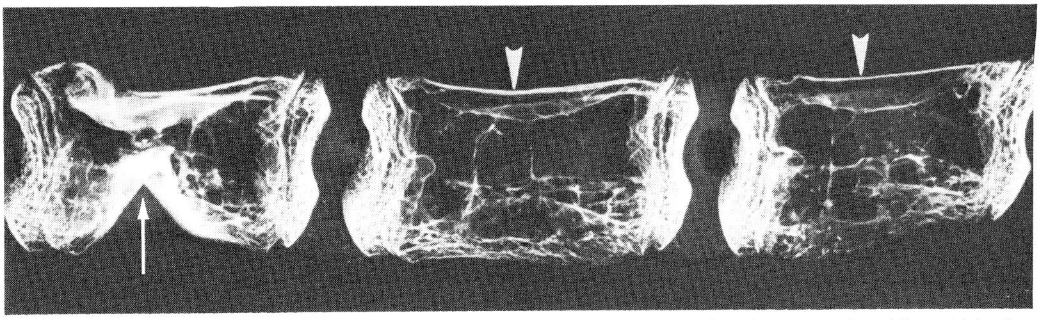

Fig 23. Radiograph of lumbar vertebrae from a kitten with nutritional secondary hyperparathyroidism. Note the loss of trabecular bone, thinning of the cortex (arrowheads), and cavitation of the vertebral body (arrow).

result is hypocalcemia, which causes parathyroid stimulation (Fig 22). The most common cause is a low-Ca diet that fails to supply the daily Ca requirement even though a greater proportion of ingested Ca is absorbed from the intestines and hypocalcemia develops.[97,98] Ingestion of excess P results in increased intestinal absorption and elevation of serum P levels. Hyperphosphatemia does not stimulate the parathyroid gland directly but does so indirectly by virtue of its ability to lower the serum Ca level.

The disease develops most commonly in young cats fed a predominantly meat diet. For example, beef heart or liver contains minimal amounts of Ca (7-9 mg/100 g) and has a markedly imbalanced Ca to P ratio (1:20-1:50). The diet of kittens up to 6 months of age should supply 200-400 mg Ca and about 200 μg iodine daily, and 10,000-15,000 IU vitamin A weekly.[98] Addition of iodine to all-meat diets prevents thyroid hyperplasia but not the skeletal disease.

Pathophysiology: In response to the nutritionally induced hypocalcemia, the parathyroid glands undergo hypertrophy and hyperplasia. Since kidney function is normal, the increased levels of PTH result in diminished renal tubular resorption of P and increased resorption of Ca, returning blood levels toward normal (Fig 22). In addition, osteoclastic bone resorption is accelerated and release of Ca elevates serum Ca levels to the low-normal range. Continued ingestion of the unbalanced diet sustains the state of compensatory hyperparathyroidism, leading to progressive metabolic bone disease.

In general, kittens are more susceptible and develop more severe skeletal lesions than adult cats fed a similar diet. Adult cats fed a beef heart diet develop osteoporosis slowly after a period of months in response to increased PTH secretion, whereas kittens develop severe generalized osteitis fibrosa within a few weeks.[97] The disease develops rapidly because the dietary imbalance is wide and the skeletal metabolic rate of kittens is high. Resorption proceeds faster than repair by fibrous connective tissue proliferation, resulting in decreased bone volume (hypostotic fibrous osteodystrophy). Vertebral fractures, with compression of the spinal cord and paralysis, are common in kittens but rare in adults (Fig 23).

Clinical Signs: Kittens fed only beef heart develop functional disturbances within 4 weeks. Clinical signs are dominated by disturbances in locomotion, manifested by a reluctance to move, rear-leg lameness, and an uncoordinated gait. The kittens often assume a standing position with characteristic medial deviation of the paws. The skeletal disease becomes progressively more

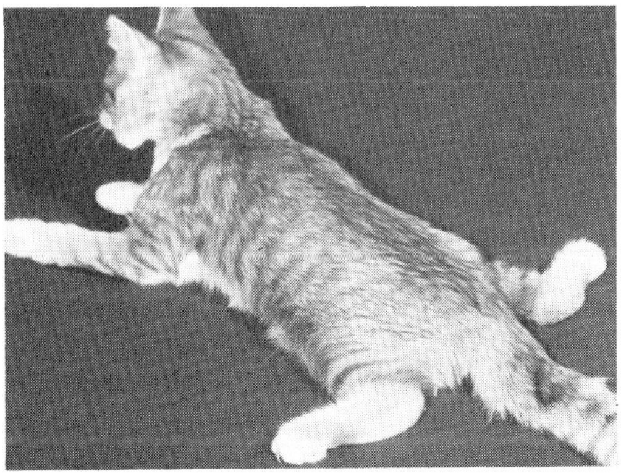

Fig 24. Nutritional hyperparathyroidism of 7 weeks' duration in a kitten. The kitten was in sternal recumbency, with its hindlegs abducted at the pelvis, due to extensive demineralization, and had difficulty supporting its weight.

severe after 5-14 weeks and the weakened skeleton is unable to support the body weight (Fig 24). The cortex of long bones is greatly thinned due to increased bone resorption and the medullary cavity is widened (Fig 25). The long-term increase in PTH secretion results in formation of numerous large, multinucleated osteoclasts on trabecular surfaces, with resorption of underlying bone. Haversian canals in cortical bone are widened and filled by a layer of hyperplastic osteoblasts and proliferating fibroblasts.

As the disease progresses the kittens become quiet and reluctant to play. They assume a sitting position or are in sternal recumbency, with the rear legs abducted (Fig 24). Normal activities may result in sudden onset of severe lameness due to incomplete or folding fractures of one or more long bones and vertebral bodies (Fig 23). The ends of fractured long bones often are joined by a poorly mineralized fibrous callus (Fig 26). The high content of digestible protein (over 50% on a wet basis) and fat promotes rapid growth in kittens fed beef heart. They appear well nourished, with a lustrous haircoat (Fig 24).

A severe osteoporotic bone disease has been recognized in adult cats 2-5 years of age and fed primarily beef liver for long intervals.[99] There is no history of previous traumatic injury or secondary hyperparathyroidism. Although the pathogenesis is not entirely clear, etiologic factors of importance appear to be the low Ca content of the beef liver diet, with a widely imbalanced Ca:P ratio (1:50), the high vitamin A content of liver, and restricted exercise. The disease is characterized by subperiosteal and medullary new bone formation, increased cortical resorption, and abnormal marrow fat. Although all bones may be affected, the cervical vertebrae and bones of the forelegs often are more severely involved. Lesions may cause impaired movement and fusion of adjacent joints, resulting in deforming ankylosis.

Diagnosis: The diet of all cats with skeletal disease, particularly young and rapidly growing kittens, should be evaluated for Ca and P content. In nutritional secondary hyperparathyroidism, there is radiographic evidence of generalized skeletal demineralization, loss of the dental lamina, subperiosteal cortical bone resorption, bowing deformities, and multiple fractures of long bones, with poorly mineralized calluses (Fig 27). Values of laboratory tests, used to assess renal function are normal in patients with this metabolic disease.

Analysis of the serum for Ca, P and alkaline phosphatase should be undertaken with an appreciation that one determination may be of limited diagnostic value. Since the body's complex compensatory mechanisms with this disease are operating when the animal is first presented, results of a single determination must be evaluated as one would a single frame from a long motion picture. When the dietary imbalance is a deficiency of Ca, with adequate P, patients have either mild hypocalcemia or isocalcemia, and a normal or slightly reduced serum P level (Fig 22). Serum alkaline phosphatase activity may be elevated in animals with overt bone disease. The increased secretion of PTH acts on the normal kidneys to increase P and decrease Ca excretion in the urine.

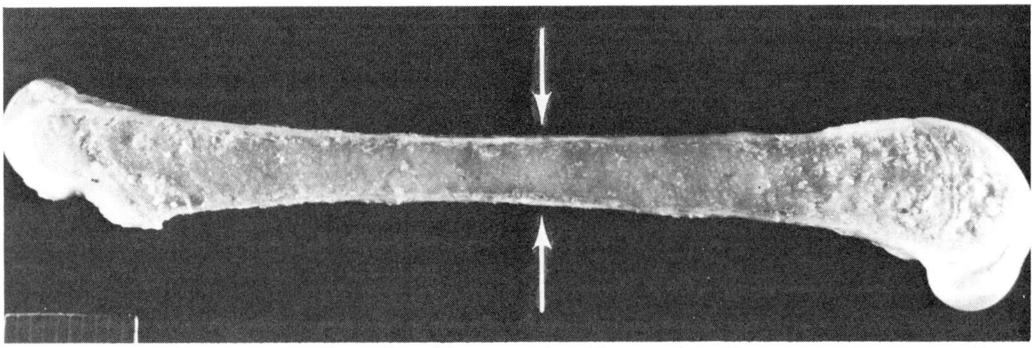

Fig 25. Femur from a young cat with nutritional hyperparathyroidism produced by consumption of a beef heart diet for 13 weeks. The cortex of the femur is extremely thin (arrows) due to excessive resorption stimulated by PTH and the marrow cavity is widened. (scale = 1 cm)

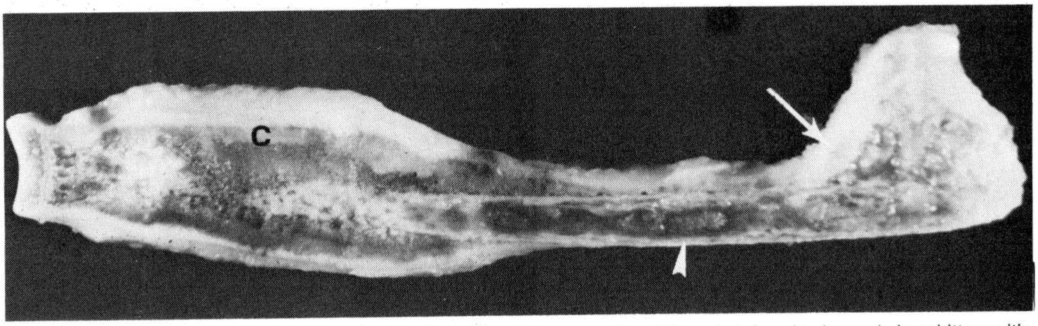

Fig 26. Fracture of the radius, with a poorly mineralized fibrous callus (C) and deformity (arrow), in a kitten with nutritional hyperparathyroidism. The cortex (arrowhead) was thin and had undergone extensive resorption stimulated by PTH.

Treatment: The aim of treatment is to decrease PTH secretion by correcting the dietary mineral imbalance. The diet should be balanced and provide the recommended total daily requirements of Ca and P. Initially more Ca than P (2:1) should be fed to increase intestinal absorption and elevate the serum Ca level. Hypercalcemia suppresses secretion of PTH, decreases bone turnover rate, and increases bone accretion, possibly by stimulating release of calcitonin from the thyroid gland. Feeding excess Ca for prolonged periods should be avoided since it may retard growth and bone remodeling in young cats.

Affected kittens should be fed a diet that fulfills their high demand for animal protein and meets the daily requirements for Ca (200-400 mg) and P (150-200 mg). Calcium gluconate, lactate or carbonate alone or in combination should be used as a dietary supplement to achieve a 2:1 Ca to P ratio during the healing phase in cats with severe bone disease. Additional vitamin D usually is not necessary since the requirements of cats are low (50-100 IU vitamin D_3 daily) but may be indicated in severely affected cats to increase intestinal absorption of Ca. The addition of potassium iodide to meat diets to supply 150-200 g iodine daily reverses thyroid hyperplasia. Calcium gluconate should be given parenterally if the appetite is depressed.

The SC administration of 22 ml 10% Ca gluconate provides 200 mg Ca daily. This should be given in divided doses and discontinued when a balanced Ca:P supplement is accepted by the kitten.

Affected cats must be closely confined in flat-bottom cages for at least 3 weeks after initiation of feeding the corrected diet (2:1 Ca to P ratio). The response to therapy is rapid and within a week the kittens become more active and their attitude improves. Jumping or climbing must be prevented since the skeleton is still susceptible to fractures. The restrictions need to be less rigid after 3 weeks but confinement with limited movement is indicated until the skeleton returns

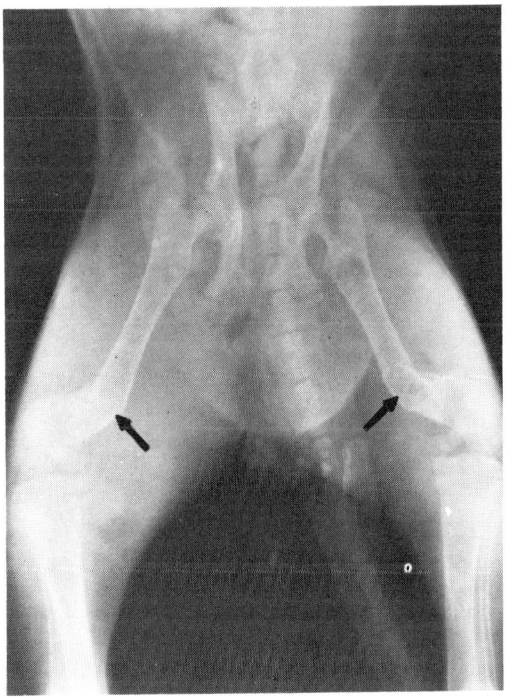

Fig 27. Radiograph of a kitten with nutritional hyperparathyroidism, illustrating generalized skeletal demineralization with bilateral folding fractures of the femur (arrows), thin cortices of long bones, and fracture of the pelvis near the acetabulum.

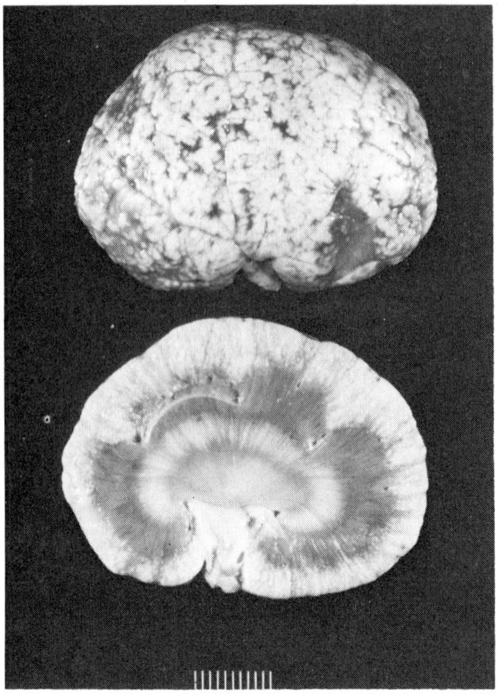

Fig 28. Malignant lymphoma of the kidney, resulting in long-standing renal failure and secondary hyperparathyroidism. (scale = 1 cm)

to normal. Improvement of the skeleton during dietary supplementation can be followed radiographically. Fracture calluses become radiodense and the overall mineral density and cortical bone thickness increase progressively with treatment. The skeleton usually is healed after feeding the corrected diet for 8-9 weeks. Subsequently the diet should supply the total daily requirements of Ca and P and be balanced at about 1.2:1.

The prognosis for recovery is good unless vertebral fractures have resulted in injury to the spinal cord and posterior paralysis. Even advanced cases respond favorably to dietary supplementation. Good nursing care is essential to prevent complications, such as decubital ulcers, constipation and additional fractures. Healed pelvic fractures may predispose to dystocia and obstipation.

Prevention: The disease can be prevented by feeding commercial cat food supplemented with table scraps, cottage cheese and skim milk.

Renal Secondary Hyperparathyroidism

Secondary hyperparathyroidism, as a complication of chronic renal failure, is a metabolic state characterized by an excess, but not autonomous, rate of PTH secretion. Secretion of PTH by the hyperplastic parathyroid glands in cats with renal disease usually remains responsive to fluctuations in serum Ca levels.

Cause: The primary etiologic mechanism in this disorder is long-standing, progressive renal disease. Chronic renal insufficiency in cats results from interstitial nephritis, glomerulonephritis, nephrosclerosis, amyloidosis and malignant lymphoma (Fig 28). Several congenital anomalies, such as polycystic kidneys and bilateral hydronephrosis, may result in renal insufficiency in younger cats (Fig 29).

Pathophysiology: When the renal disease progresses to the point at which there is significant reduction in the glomerular filtration rate, P is retained and progressive hyperphosphatemia develops (Fig 30). Although the serum concentration of P has no direct regulatory influence on the synthesis and secretion of PTH, it may, if elevated, contribute to parathyroid gland stimulation by virtue of its ability to lower the serum Ca level. Parathyroid stimulation in patients with chronic renal disease can be attributable directly to the hypocalcemia.

Recent evidence suggests that impaired intestinal absorption of Ca due to an acquired defect in vitamin D metabolism plays a significant role in development of hypocalcemia in chronic renal insufficiency and uremia.[100,101] Chronic renal disease interferes with production of 1,25-dihydroxycholecalciferol by the kidney, thereby diminishing intestinal Ca transport and causing hypocalcemia.

The parathyroid glands of affected cats are considerably enlarged due to hypertrophy of chief cells initially, and subsequently by hyperplasia, as compensatory mechanisms to increase PTH secretion in response to the hypocalcemic stimulus. Although the parathyroid glands are not autonomous, the concentration of PTH in the peripheral blood in people with chronic renal failure may exceed that in people with primary hyperparathyroidism. Parathyroid hormone increases osteoclastic resorption and bone remodeling, resulting in release of stored Ca from bone.[102-105] The long-standing increase in bone resorption that attempts to return the serum Ca level to normal eventually results in the metabolic bone disease associated with chronic renal insufficiency. Progressive glomerular and tubular dysfunction, with loss of target cells, interferes with an expression of the phosphaturic response by the increased circulating PTH in renal disease. Phosphate is retained and the serum P level continues to rise in spite of the secondary hyperparathyroidism (Fig 31).

Clinical Signs: The clinical signs of vomiting, dehydration, polydipsia, depression and ammoniacal odor to the breath are related to the progressive renal insufficiency and uremia. A spectrum of skeletal lesions of secondary hyperparathyroidism may be present, from minor changes in early or mild renal disease to the severe fibrous osteodystrophy of advanced renal failure. The volume of affected bones usually is normal (isostotic fibrous osteodystrophy), particularly in older cats, due to the slow onset of renal failure and lower metabolic activity of bones.

Although skeletal involvement is generalized in renal secondary hyperparathyroidism, it does not affect all parts uniformly. Lesions become apparent earlier and reach a more advanced degree in certain areas. Resorption of alveolar socket bone and loss of the dental lamina occur early and result in loose teeth, which may be dislodged easily and interfere with mastication. Cancellous bone of the maxillae and mandible also is a site of predilection in hyperparathyroidism. Due to accelerated resorption, the bones become soft and pliable, and the mouth may fail to close properly. Fractures after relatively mi-

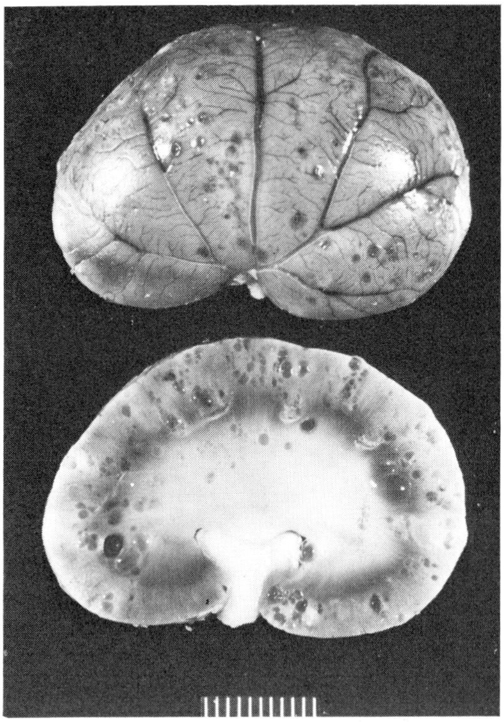

Fig 29. Congenital polycystic kidney, with numerous fluid-filled cysts in the cortex, from a cat with renal secondary hyperparathyroidism. (scale = 1 cm)

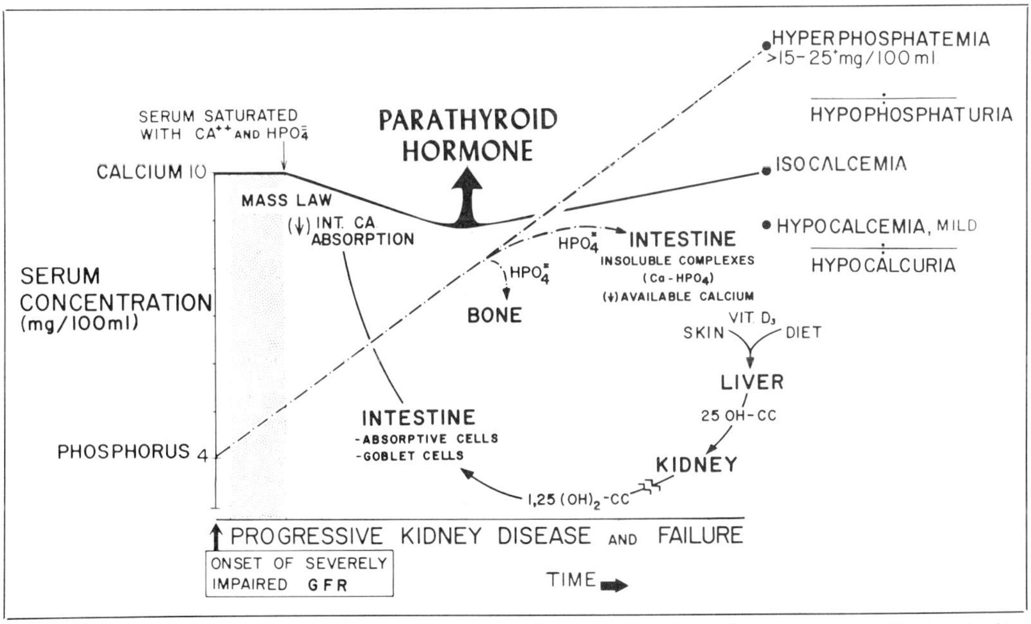

Fig 30. Alterations in serum Ca and P levels during secondary hyperparathyroidism associated with progressive renal failure.

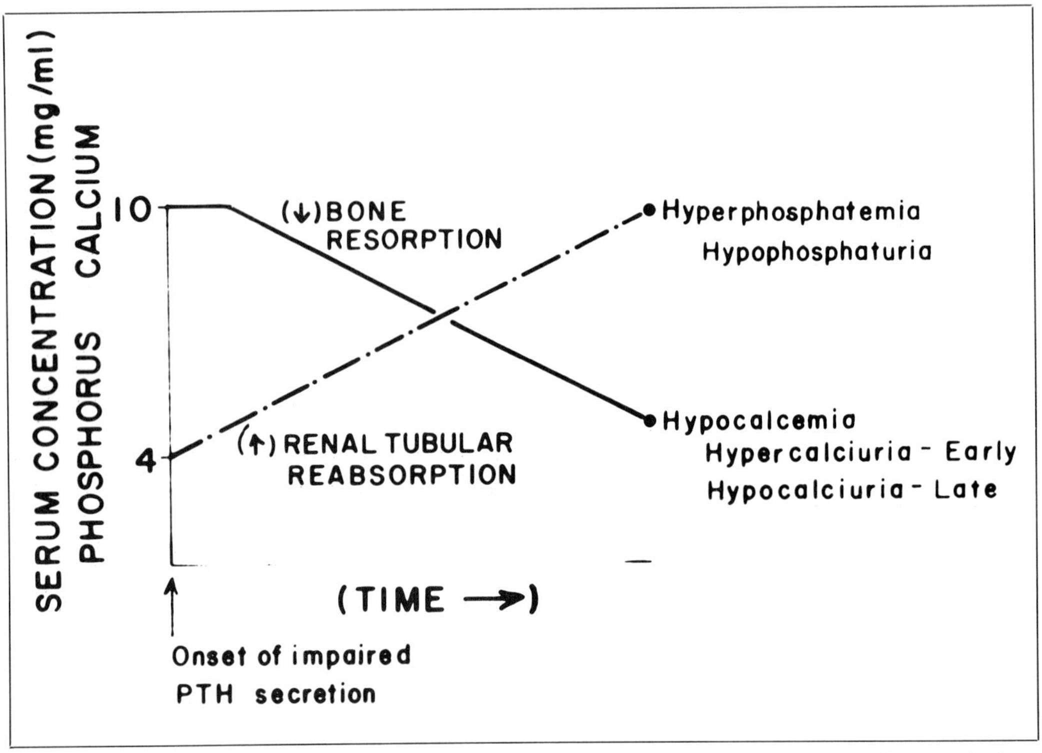

Fig 31. Alterations in serum Ca and P levels in response to inadequate secretion of PTH. This results in a progressive increase of serum P levels and a marked decline in serum Ca levels to the point of increased neuromuscular excitability and tetany.

nor trauma, lameness and a stiff gait may result from increased bone resorption. Areas of subperiosteal resorption by numerous osteoclasts may disrupt the osseous attachment of tendons, leading to elevation and stretching of the periosteum, bone pain and inability to support the body's weight.

Diagnosis: A combination of laboratory and radiographic evaluation aids in diagnosis of secondary hyperparathyroidism in patients with chronic renal insufficiency. There is radiographic evidence of generalized skeletal demineralization in advanced cases, with localized areas of accentuation and loss of the dental lamina. Several laboratory procedures are useful to assess the extent of renal disease. The BUN and serum creatinine levels are elevated consistently, whereas the glomerular filtration rate and effective renal blood flow are decreased. Dilute urine in the presence of clinical dehydration, proteinuria and/or large numbers of casts in the urine suggests a diagnosis of renal disease.

Serum should be analyzed for Ca, P and alkaline phosphatase. Results of a single determination must be interpreted with an appreciation that considerable variation exists, depending upon the stage of the disease, due to the body's compensatory mechanisms (Fig 30). Hyperphosphatemia of 6 mg/dl and above is a consistent finding and results from retention of P by the damaged kidney. The serum Ca level is considerably more variable but is usually near normal (10 mg/dl) or low-normal due to mobilization of skeletal Ca reserves by increased PTH secretion. Alkaline phosphatase activity may be elevated in cats with overt bone disease. Urinary excretion of Ca and P is decreased.

Treatment: The aim of treatment with this metabolic disorder ideally would be to interrupt the progression of kidney disease and restore renal function to normal. However, due to the late stage at which the disease often is diagnosed and the progressive nature of the renal lesions, treatment realistically is directed toward reducing the renal excretory load and replacing substances (Na, water, etc) the failing kidney cannot conserve. Feeding a prescription diet, with supplemental Ca (gluconate or lactate) and vitamin

D, may diminish the severity of hyperparathyroidism and accompanying bone lesions.

Pseudohyperparathyroidism

Cause: Pseudohyperparathyroidism ("hypercalcemia of malignancy") is a metabolic disorder in which substances that induce bone resorption are secreted in excessive amounts by malignant tumors of nonparathyroid origin. Prostaglandins, PTH-like polypeptides, vitamin D sterols and osteoclast-activating factor can be produced by tumor cells and induce Ca mobilization from bone.[106-113]

Hypercalcemia and hypophosphatemia develop in cats, dogs and people affected by various malignant neoplasms in the absence of bone metastases and functional lesions in the parathyroid glands. The hypercalcemia is the result of ectopic secretion of bone-resorbing substances by anaplastic tumor cells, most likely by the mechanism of genetic derepression.[114,115]

Lymphosarcoma is the most common neoplasm associated with hypercalcemia in cats.[116] It is uncertain if the hypercalcemia develops from the production of humoral substances by neoplastic cells and/or from physical disruption of trabecular bone due to frequent bone marrow involvement. Serum immunoreactive PTH levels were subnormal in hypercalcemic dogs with lymphosarcoma and plasma immunoreactive prostaglandin E_2M levels did not differ from those in controls.[117] Studies involving radiolabeled Ca suggested that local production of factors that induce bone resorption is important in stimulating Ca release from bone in some dogs with lymphosarcoma and hypercalcemia.[118]

Clinical Signs: Clinical signs in cats with pseudohyperparathyroidism include generalized muscular weakness, anorexia, vomiting, bradycardia, depression, polyuria and polydipsia.[116] These signs are primarily the result of severe hypercalcemia and complicate the problems associated with the malignant neoplasm.

Diagnosis: Criteria for diagnosis of pseudohyperparathyroidism include persistent hypercalcemia and hypophosphatemia, absence of radiographic or pathologic evidence of metastases in bone, atrophy of parathyroid glands and C-cell hyperplasia in the thyroid gland, remission of hypercalcemia when the tumor is destroyed or excised, demonstration of active PTH-like polypeptides or other substances that induce bone resorption in tumor tissue, and exacerbation of hypercalcemia if the tumor recurs after therapy.

Treatment: Since many of the effects of hypercalcemia associated with malignancy are accentuated by dehydration, disturbances in fluid balance should be corrected. Replacement fluids, such as isotonic solutions, lactated Ringer's solution or 0.9% saline, should be administered IV. Calciuresis may be enhanced by administering 0.9% saline IV because the additional Na presented to the renal tubules diminishes Ca resorption. If the serum concentration of Ca is only moderately increased (12-14 mg/dl), these therapeutic measures alone may result in adequate lowering of the serum Ca level.

Additional measures to combat hypercalcemia may be necessary when the elevation of the serum Ca level (15 mg/dl or more) and clinical signs are more severe. Furosemide, ethacrynic acid and sodium sulfate are calciuretic agents that may be used. It is important to maintain adequate extracellular fluid volume by proper administration of IV fluids while using these diuretics. Furosemide, given IV to dogs with experimental hypercalcemia at 5 mg/kg, reduces the serum Ca concentration. Thiazide diuretics reduce the urinary excretion of Ca and, therefore, are contraindicated in cases of hypercalcemia. Peritoneal dialysis is an effective alternative method of removing Ca from the body, particularly in uremic animals.

Corticosteroids sometimes are effective in lowering the serum Ca concentration. Their effects are thought to be mediated by inhibiting intestinal absorption of Ca and increasing urinary Ca excretion. In addition, direct antitumor activity may be responsible for a reduction of the serum Ca concentration, most notably in cases of lymphosarcoma. Mithramycin and calcitonin are agents sometimes used in the therapy of hypercalcemia in people but clinical experience in dogs, cats and other animals with hypercalcemia is lacking.

In hypercalcemic crises, IV administration of $NaHCO_3$ may be of value to temporarily reduce toxic effects of elevated ionizing Ca concentration. The beneficial effect is related to diminution of the level of ionized Ca associated with alkalosis induced by $NaHCO_3$ administration.

Since prerenal factors are commonly associated with hypercalcemia, proper attention to fluid therapy helps maintain renal perfusion, thereby minimizing progressive ischemic damage to nephrons. If the hypercalcemia can be controlled and the patient kept alive long enough, tubular lesions may be repaired by regeneration and functional adaptations. Dissolution of mineral deposits in the kidney also may occur, although this is a slow process.

Since neoplasia is commonly found to be the underlying cause of hypercalcemia, total surgical extirpation of the tumor is indicated. When this is not possible because malignant neoplasms have infiltrated locally or metastasized, radiotherapy in combination with chemotherapy and immunotherapy may be of value in reducing tumor mass and concomitant hypercalcemia. Remission of the tumor usually is accompanied by remission of hypercalcemia.

Hypoparathyroidism

In hypoparathyroidism, subnormal amounts of PTH are secreted by the diseased parathyroid glands or the PTH secreted is unable to interact normally with target cells. Hypoparathyroidism is rare in cats and occurs much less frequently than hyperparathyroidism.

Cause: Several pathogenic mechanisms can cause inadequate secretion of PTH. The parathyroid glands may be damaged or inadvertently removed during surgery on the thyroid gland, such as removal of a functional thyroid adenoma. If the glands or their vascular supply have only been damaged and not removed, there often is regeneration of adequate functional parenchyma and subsequent disappearance of clinical manifestations.

Agenesis of both pairs of parathyroid glands is a rare cause of congenital hypoparathyroidism. Idiopathic hypoparathyroidism associated with progressive lymphocytic parathyroiditis and extensive degeneration of chief cells, probably an autoimmune phenomenon, may cause hypoparathyroidism. Another possible cause of hypoparathyroidism is invasion and destruction of the parathyroid glands by primary or metastatic neoplasms in the cranial cervical area. Diffuse atrophy of the parathyroid glands has occurred in cats with severe hypercalcemia from vitamin D intoxication or with multifocal osteolytic lesions, in which release of Ca is caused by tumor metastases.

Clinical Signs: The clinical manifestations of hypoparathyroidism primarily are the result of increased neuromuscular excitability and tetany. Due to the lack of PTH, bone resorption is decreased and serum Ca levels diminish progressively (to 4-6 mg/dl (Fig 31). Affected animals are restless and ataxic, and have intermittent tremors of individual muscle groups that progress to generalized tetany and convulsive seizures. Concurrently, serum P levels are substantially elevated due to increased renal tubular resorption of P.

Treatment: Serum Ca levels should be returned to near normal by slow IV administration of Ca solution to stop the tetany. Long-term maintenance of normal serum Ca levels in the absence of normal PTH can be attempted by feeding diets high in Ca and low in P, supplemented with large amounts of vitamin D_3 (10,000 IU or more daily). The dose of vitamin D should be adjusted after determining the effect on serum Ca levels to protect against development of hypercalcemia and extensive soft tissue mineralization. After the dose of vitamin D is adjusted, a 5-day interval should precede the next serum Ca determination to fully assess the effects of changes in vitamin D dose. Once serum Ca levels return to normal, substantially smaller doses of vitamin D usually are required for long-term maintenance of serum electrolyte levels. Replacement therapy with parathyroid extract or PTH derived from other species is expensive and ineffective on a long-term basis due to development of antibodies. Synthetic PTH and the more potent active metabolites of vitamin D (1,25-dihydroxycholecalciferol and 1,alpha-hydroxycholecalciferol) may become useful in treatment of hypoparathyroidism.

Puerperal Tetany

Considerably less is known about the pathogenesis of hypocalcemic syndromes in dogs and cats than is known about their development in cattle. Puerperal tetany, or eclampsia, is encountered occasionally in cats.[119,120] Severe hypocalcemia may develop in queens during the nursing period, from several days to several weeks portpartum.

Pathophysiology: There is little evidence to suggest that puerperal tetany in queens is the result of interference in PTH secretion. Severe hypocalcemia and often hypophosphatemia develop near the time of peak lactation, probably from an imbalance between the rates of inflow and outflow from the extracellular Ca pool (Fig 32). Feeding high-Ca diets to dairy cows in the prepartum period has a provocative effect on development of hypocalcemic disorders after parturition because of diminished responsiveness of PTH-mediated bone resorption.[121-123] The

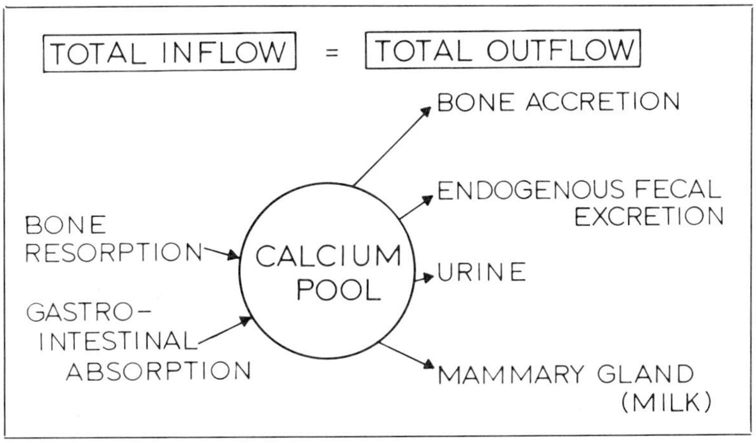

Fig 32. Homeostasis of Ca in extracellular fluids, illustrating dependency upon the balance between inflow and outflow from the Ca pool. Puerperal tetany and hypocalcemia appear to be related to an imbalance between these rates of movements of Ca, favoring outflow from the Ca pool into the milk.

reduced availability of Ca from skeletal sources leads to an excessive reliance on intestinal Ca absorption.

Clinical Signs: Puerperal tetany is characterized by nervousness, anxiety, intermittent muscular spasms, and incoordination. In advanced stages of the disease, affected queens often have dilated pupils, elevated or subnormal body temperature, vomiting and coma.

Diagnosis: Diagnosis of puerperal tetany usually is based on history, clinical signs and response to IV administration of Ca solution. If laboratory facilities are readily available, demonstration of hypocalcemia, with serum Ca levels less than 7 mg/dl, confirms the diagnosis. The serum P level often is lowered to a comparable degree. The blood glucose level is in the low-normal range or decreased from the intense muscular activity associated with tetany.

Treatment: Slow IV administration of about 5 ml of an organic Ca solution, such as 10% Ca gluconate, to effect usually results in rapid improvement and cessation of tetanic spasms within 15 minutes. Intravenous administration of Ca solution should proceed slowly to avoid inducing ventricular fibrillation and cardiac arrest.

Kittens should be removed from the queen for 24 hours to reduce lactational drain of Ca. During this period kittens should be fed a milk substitute or other appropriate diet (see Chapter 1). If the kittens are mature enough, they should be weaned; otherwise they should be returned to the queen after the 24-hour period.

Prevention: During gestation, feeding a good-quality balanced diet with a Ca to P ratio of 1:1 or less that provides the required (but not excessive) amounts of Ca may result in a more responsive Ca homeostatic mechanism to meet the markedly increased demands of lactation. Calcium homeostasis in animals fed balanced or relatively low-Ca diets during part of gestation is apparently under better control by PTH secretion with the approach of parturition and the initiation of lactational drain. The higher levels of PTH secreted during the prepartum period by an expanded population of actively synthesizing chief cells apparently results in a larger pool of active bone-resorbing cells to fulfill the increased needs for Ca mobilization at the critical time near parturition and during lactation. Queens so fed appear less susceptible to the influence of decreased Ca absorption and flow into the extracellular pool, which can occur in the immediate postpartum period during peak lactation.

Hypercalcitoninism

Syndromes associated with abnormalities in secretion of calcitonin are recognized much less often than disorders of PTH secretion. Hypersecretion of calcitonin is well characterized in people and bulls with medullary (ultimobranchial) thyroid neoplasms derived from C-cells but incompletely studied in other species.[124-127] In people the syndrome often is familial. Chronic stimulation of ultimobranchial derivatives in the thyroid by high-Ca diets may be related to the pathogenesis of the neoplasm in bulls. Cows do not develop ultimobranchial lesions under similar dietary conditions, probably because of the high physiologic requirements for Ca imposed by pregnancy and lactation.

Clinical Signs: The prevalence of C-cell tumors in cats is uncertain but they appear to be uncommon. These neoplasms often are firm on palpation due to the presence of large amounts of amyloid in the stroma. The C-cell tumors in people and bulls often are associated with concurrent pheochromocytomas and neoplasms in other endocrine organs.[125,128]

Diagnosis: Serum Ca and P levels in adult people with a chronic excessive secretion of calcitonin usually remain in the low-normal range due to the relatively low turnover rate of bone.

Hypocalcitoninism

Specific syndromes caused by a lack of calcitonin secretion have not been recognized in any species. However, experimentally thyroidectomized animals are less able than normal to metabolize a Ca load and may develop hypercalcemia.[129]

THE ENDOCRINE PANCREAS

Anatomy and Physiology

The pancreas of cats usually is subdivided into the right (duodenal) lobe, angle of the pancreatic body, and the left (splenic) lobe. The endocrine function of the pancreas is performed by small groups of islets of cells (islets of Langerhans) surrounded by acinar (exocrine) cells that produce digestive enzymes.

The pancreatic islets of normal cats contain 3 types of cells.[130] Beta cells are the predominant secretory cells and synthesize insulin. Alpha cells are less numerous and secrete glucagon. Delta cells are found near the periphery of pancreatic islets and secrete somatostatin.

Secretory granules are stored in the cytoplasm of beta cells until there is an appropriate stimulus for insulin secretion. Although changes in the concentration of glucose in extracellular fluid are the principal physiologic stimuli for insulin release, other sugars (fructose, mannose, ribose), amino acids (leucine, arginine), hormones (glucagon, secretin), drugs (sulforylureas, cAMP, theophylline), fatty acids and ketone bodies may also stimulate insulin secretion under certain conditions.[131] Endocrine cells, such as pancreatic beta cells, have the unique ability to respond to a specific physiologic stimulus with release of stored hormone in a modulated fashion rather than releasing all of the hormone at once. If the latter were to occur in the case of insulin, the animal would die from hypoglycemia.

The secretory response of endocrine cells involves not only the immediate release of hormone but also a series of intracellular events that control the rate of release. For example, insulin secretion in response to elevation of blood glucose concentration proceeds in a biphasic pattern (Fig 33). The rate of insulin release increases immediately after the blood glucose level is above 100 mg/dl and reaches a maximum 4-5 minutes after stimulation. This initial phase of insulin secretion apparently is associated with release of preformed insulin in peripherally situated storage granules in contact with the mi-

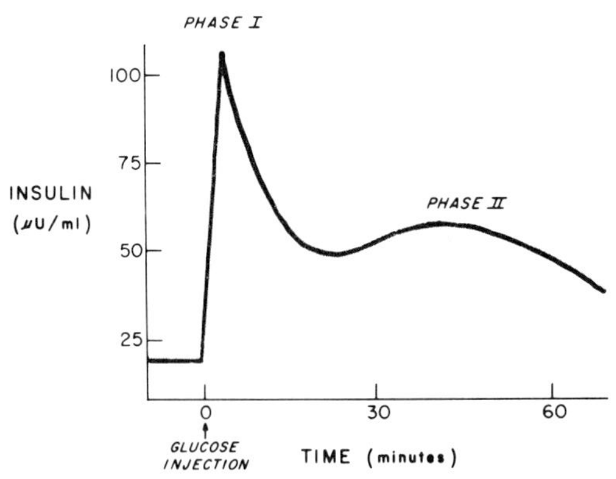

Fig 33. Biphasic insulin secretory response to glucose injection and hyperglycemia. The initial phase (I) of insulin release consists of secretion of storage granules from a rapidly mobilized pool. These granules appear to be peripherally situated in beta cells and associated with the microtubular-microfilamentous system. The second (II) phase of insulin secretion is delayed for 30-40 minutes and results from peripheral movement of additional storage granules, plus secretion of newly synthesized insulin. [From Levine, R. N Engl J Med 283 (1970) 522]

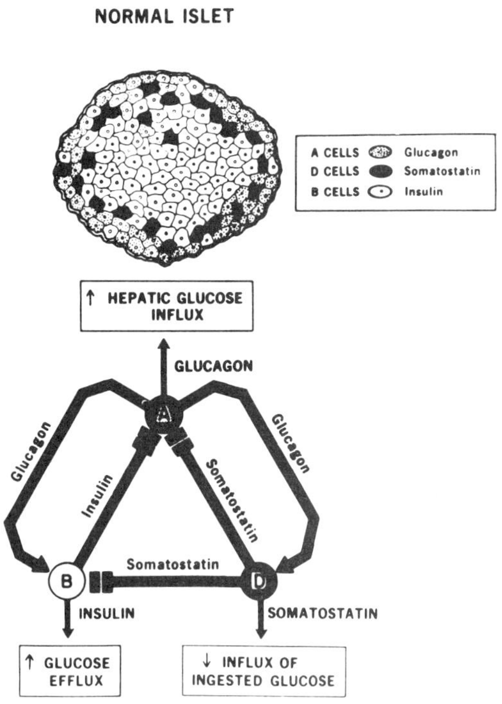

Fig 34. Schematic representation of an islet of Langerhans reveals the characteristic relationship of the 3 major cell types, the postulated "paracrine" (direct hormone-cell interactions), and the endocrine functions of the 3 hormones. Glucagon stimulates secretion of both insulin and somatostatin, whereas insulin inhibits secretion of glucagon from alpha cells. Somatostatin inhibits secretion of both glucagon and insulin. The overall effect of glucagon is to increase the influx of glucose from the liver into extracellular fluids. Insulin increases the efflux of glucose from extracellular fluids into insulin-sensitive tissues. [From Unger, RH and Orci, L. Arch Int Med 137 (1977) 482]

crotubular-microfilamentous system in beta cells. The second phase of insulin release occurs 30-60 minutes after a hyperglycemic stimulus and is maintained until the blood glucose level returns to normal. It apparently is associated with the peripheral movement of additional storage granules containing preformed insulin, plus the secretion of newly synthesized insulin.

Insulin is a powerful hormone with broad biologic influences on every organ in the body. Tissues especially responsive to insulin include skeletal and cardiac muscle, adipose tissue, fibroblasts, liver, WBC, mammary glands, cartilage, bone, skin, aorta, pituitary gland and peripheral nerves.

The main function of insulin is to stimulate anabolic reactions involving carbohydrates, fats, proteins and nucleic acids. It catalyzes the formation of macromolecules used in cell structure, energy stores and regulation of many cell functions. Insulin also stimulates synthesis of protein from amino acids, nucleic acids from mononucleotides, polysaccharides from monosaccharides, and lipids from fatty acids.

Liver, adipose cells and muscle are 3 principal target sites for insulin. Insulin generally increases the transfer of glucose and certain other monosaccharides, some amino acids and fatty acids, and K and Mg ions across the plasma membrane of target cells, enhances glucose oxidation and glycogenesis, and stimulates lipogenesis, protein synthesis and the formation of ATP, DNA and RNA. It also decreases the rate of lipolysis, proteolysis, ketogenesis and gluconeogenesis. Some of insulin's actions result from its inhibition of the supply of cAMP in target cells, causing diminished activity of protein kinases. This is associated with less phosphorylation of enzymes but an increase in activity of some nonphosphorylated enzymes that promote anabolic reactions. Insulin does not promote glucose transport in RBC or neurons, nor does it stimulate renal tubular resorption of glucose or intestinal absorption of glucose.

Glucagon is the second major hormone secreted by the pancreatic islets. It is secreted by alpha cells situated at the more peripheral parts of the islet in an external mantle (Fig 34). It is a single, long-chain polypeptide with a different amino acid composition and sequence than that of insulin.

Glucagon secreted in response to a reduced blood glucose level is a hormone of energy release from target cells. It mobilizes stores of energy-yielding nutrients by increasing glycogenolysis, gluconeogenesis and lipolysis, thereby elevating the blood glucose level.

Glucagon and insulin, acting in concert through a "push-pull" system, maintain the concentration of glucose in extracellular fluids within relatively narrow limits. A "glucosensor" in the peripheral tricellular region of the pancreatic islets controls the relative mixture of these 2 biologic antagonists secreted from the microendocrine organ (Fig 34). Glucagon controls glucose influx from the liver into the extracellular space and insulin controls glucose efflux from the extracellular space into such insulin-sensitive tissues as fat, muscles and liver.

The delta cells that secrete somatostatin are interspersed among the outer layer of alpha cells and inner core of beta cells (Fig 34). In this peripheral tricellular region afferent vessels and nerves enter the islet. Somatostatin inhibits the secretion of glucagon and insulin (Fig 34).

Diseases of the Endocrine Pancreas

Diabetes Mellitus

Incidence: Since the first report of diabetes mellitus in a cat in 1928, there have been a number of case reports of this endocrinopathy in the literature.[132-143] A suggested incidence of diabetes mellitus in cats of about 1 in 800 was lower than the incidence in dogs (1 in 200).[144] The incidence of diabetes mellitus was 1 in 484 in cats admitted to the Animal Medical Center in New York.[143]

Diabetes mellitus occurs most commonly in middle-aged or older cats. A review of cases treated in our hospital and those reported in the literature suggests that the mean age of onset of clinical signs is 9 years, with a range of 3.5 to 17 years. Male cats apparently are more often affected than females, although one study indicated this difference is not statistically significant.[143] Most affected cats in the Veterinary Teaching Hospital at Ohio State University have been domestic shorthairs.

Clinical Signs: Polyuria and polydipsia are the clinical signs most often associated with diabetes mellitus in cats. Because many cats use indoor litterpans, the increased volume of urine becomes readily apparent to observant owners. Loss of weight, polyphagia or partial to complete anorexia, depression, lethargy, weakness and icterus also have been observed in cats with diabetes mellitus. Enlargement of the liver, from fatty infiltration and/or cirrhosis, is apparent on abdominal palpation of most diabetic cats (Fig 35). Cystitis may be a complication and radiographic evidence of emphysematous cystitis is strongly suggestive of diabetes mellitus.[144] Catheterization of the bladder should be performed with caution because of the danger of introducing infection. Diabetic cats have a diminished resistance to bacterial infection and may develop suppurative cystitis, as well as dermatitis and bronchopneumonia.

Lesions: Cats with diabetes mellitus usually have specific degenerative lesions localized selectively in the islets of Langerhans, whereas the remainder of the pancreas appears to be normal. This is in contrast to dogs, in which the pancreatic islets usually are destroyed secondary to pancreatitis, with associated hemorrhage or fibrosis.[145,146] The selective deposition of amyloid in islets, with degenerative changes in alpha and beta cells, is the most common pancreatic lesion in cats with diabetes; however, amyloid deposits in the pancreatic islets occur in many cats without development of overt diabetes mellitus.[147-152] A study of the relationship of pancreatic cells with early development of amyloid deposits in cats demonstrated that amyloid is formed initially in nonendocrine perivascular cells in the islets.[153]

Another common islet lesion in cats with diabetes mellitus is hydropic (vacuolar) degeneration of the beta and alpha cells.[154,155] The cytoplasmic area of beta cells is expanded by massive accumulation of glycogen particles. Secretory organelles, such as the rough endoplasmic reticulum, Golgi apparatus, mitochondria and insulin-containing secretory granules, are displaced to the periphery of the beta cell by the glycogen accumulation. This selective islet lesion has been observed in cats that were resistant to large doses of exogenous insulin. Vacuolar degeneration with glycogen accumulation in cats appeared to develop in beta cells as a response to long-term overstimulation ("exhaustion") because of insulin resistance.

Other pancreatic lesions observed include preferential inflammatory cell infiltration of islets, decreased numbers and granularity of beta cells, and chronic pancreatitis, with fibrosis leading to secondary destruction of islets. Primary or metastatic neoplasms of the pancreas with destruction of islets are an infrequent cause of diabetes in older cats.

Diagnosis: Diabetes mellitus is diagnosed primarily by demonstration of persistent glucosuria and fasting hyperglycemia. A diagnosis of diabetes mellitus should not be made on the basis of detection of glucose in the urine without determining the blood glucose level since transitory glucosuria, with a normal blood glucose level, has been observed in cats with cystitis and renal disease. A consistent fasting blood glucose level of more than 120 mg/dl is suggestive of diabetes mellitus. An IV or oral glucose-tolerance test should be performed when the blood glucose determination is equivocal.

The urine of diabetic cats is more viscid than normal and often has a sweet odor. Urine specific gravity is elevated when the blood glucose level exceeds the renal threshold and large amounts of glucose are excreted in the urine. Ketonuria often indicates an advanced clinical stage of the disease and necessitates immediate therapy. Serum immunoreactive insulin levels, both before and after glucose administration, are reportedly low or undetectable in cats with diabetes mellitus and amyloidosis of the pancreatic islets as compared with normal cats.[146]

Treatment: The primary objectives of therapy in nonketoacidotic diabetic cats are reduction of the blood glucose level by administration of insulin and correction of complicating factors, such as dehydration, concomitant infections and hepatic lipidosis. Diabetic cats should be hospitalized until the dosage of insulin is established. An insulin preparation with intermediate activity, such as NPH insulin, is injected SC once daily with a tuberculin or insulin syringe. An initial dosage of 0.25 units/lb body weight is administered, and the blood and urine glucose levels are monitored 8-10 hours postinjection. Cats may be quite sensitive to insulin and the dosage should be adjusted by 0.5-unit increments until a blood glucose level between 150 and 200 mg/dl is obtained and there is only a trace of glucose in the urine.[143]

The cat should be fed high-protein, low-carbohydrate cat food twice daily. Use of canned foods is preferred over other types for cats with diabetes mellitus. If the cat is dehydrated, IV lactated Ringer's solution should be administered to effect.

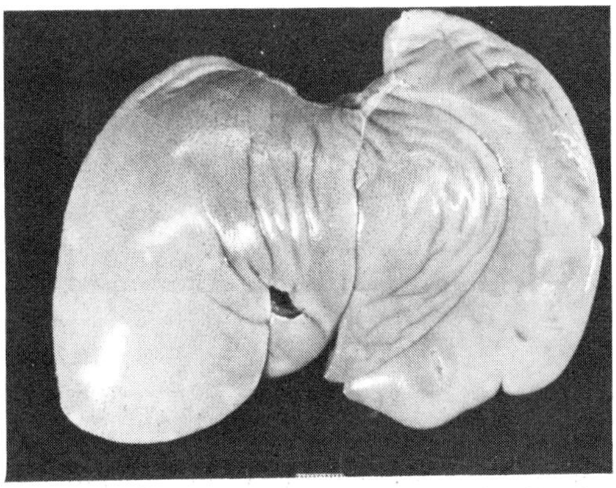

Fig 35. Hepatomegaly due to marked fatty infiltration in a cat with long-standing diabetes mellitus associated with resistance to insulin.

The owner should be informed that certain cats may develop hypoglycemia with insulin therapy and be advised of the early clinical signs, such as weakness and fatigue after exercise, generalized muscular weakness, mental confusion and ataxia leading to periodic tonic-clonic convulsions. Karo syrup (2-3 tbsp) should be given immediately by the owner. If signs of hypoglycemia persist after an hour, the cat should be returned to the hospital. Glucose is administered IV to effect and the dosage of insulin is reduced in 0.5-unit increments.

Ketoacidosis is a serious complication of diabetes mellitus and must be regarded as a true medical emergency. Ketoacidotic diabetic cats should be hospitalized under close supervision to monitor the response to therapy. The principles of therapy of ketoacidotic cats include correction of dehydration and electrolyte imbalances by IV administration of appropriate fluids, and reduction of ketonuria, acidosis and hyperglycemia with crystalline insulin. Correction of metabolic acidosis with $NaHCO_3$ may be indicated in critical cases but the danger of causing paradoxic acidosis of the CSF should be recognized as a possible complication of such therapy.

An initial blood sample should be drawn for glucose, BUN, creatinine and, if possible, blood-gas and electrolyte determinations. A urine sample should be collected by gentle manual expression of the bladder for evaluation of glucose and ketone content. Insertion of an indwelling IV catheter facilitates therapy. The amount of fluid required to rehydrate the cat, plus that required for daily maintenance, should be calculated and administered via the catheter.

In severe dehydration associated with diabetic ketoacidosis, about half the calculated daily fluid requirement can be administered in 4-6 hours (see Chapter 2). Physiologic saline has been recommended as the fluid of choice for correction of the dehydration. Once the severe dehydration and circulatory collapse are corrected, lactated Ringer's solution can be used for maintenance.

The amount of $NaHCO_3$ required to correct acidosis can be estimated by multiplying the bicarbonate deficit (normal serum level minus the measured level) times one-half the body weight in kilograms. This calculated dose should be given over a 48-hour period to avoid paradoxic acidosis in the CSF.[156] Chapter 2 contains more information on this topic.

Although ketoacidosis may increase the resistance to insulin, care should be observed when treating cats with insulin because of their sensitivity to this hormone. An initial crystalline insulin dosage of 0.25 units/lb body weight is given SC or IV if the cat is comatose. Urinary glucose and ketone levels should be carefully monitored about every 4 hours and the dose of insulin varied by 1-2 units, depending on laboratory findings. If the levels of urine glucose and ketone bodies remain high, the insulin dose should be increased by 2 units. When the urine becomes negative for both glucose and ketones, blood for a glucose determination should be drawn. If hypoglycemia develops during insulin therapy for diabetic ketoacidosis, judicious addition of glucose to the IV fluids is indicated.

Once the condition of a cat with diabetic ketoacidosis is stabilized with the IV fluid and crystalline insulin therapy, the type of insulin used can be changed to NPH insulin, used at about the same dosage as for crystalline insulin. For long-term maintenance the dosage of NPH insulin can be adjusted as for cats with uncomplicated diabetes mellitus.

THE ADRENAL GLANDS

Anatomy and Physiology

The adrenal glands in the cat are flattened organs situated cranial and slightly medial to the kidneys. The adrenal glands are enclosed in a fibrous capsule and surrounded by fat. The cortex and medulla can be distinguished grossly by their color and consistency. The adrenal cortex is firm, yellow and nearly of uniform thickness. The medulla is soft, brown and surrounded by cortex on all sides.

The adrenal glands are richly vascularized. The arteries form a vascular plexus in the capsule that eventually supplies the entire adrenal gland through separate channels to the capsule, cortex and medulla. A capillary network formed about the cell columns of the adrenal cortex empties into the venous tree at the periphery of the medulla. The larger branches of the venous tree empty into the adrenal vein.

Adrenal Function

The adrenal cortex is subdivided into 3 layers or zones, although the demarcation between zones often is not distinct. The zona glomerulosa is composed of columns of cells next to the capsule. This peripheral zone is responsible for secretion of mineralocorticoid hormones. The secretory cells of the zona fasciculata are arranged in long anastomosing cords separated by numerous small capillaries. This middle zone is composed of cells that contain abundant cytoplasmic lipid and is responsible for the secretion of glucocorticoid hormones. The zona reticularis accounts for the remainder of the adrenal cortex. The secretory cells are arranged in small groups surrounded by capillaries. This inner layer is responsible for secretion of sex steroids. The corticomedullary junction often is irregular and groups of cortical cells may project for a short distance into the medulla.

Glucocorticoids: Glucocorticoids secreted by the adrenal cortex are concerned with the intermediary metabolism of glucose. Cortisol and lesser amounts of corticosterone are the most important glucocorticoids secreted by the adrenal gland. In general, the actions of glucocorticoids on carbohydrate, protein and lipid metabolism result in decreased glucose use and increased glucose production.[157] Glucocorticoids decrease the uptake of glucose in adipose tissue, skin, fibroblasts and lymphoid tissue, followed shortly by increased catabolism of these tissues and muscles. This provides amino acids for increased gluconeogenesis, mainly in the liver. In addition, glucocorticoids decrease lipogenesis and increase lipolysis in adipose tissue, which results in release of glycerol and free fatty acids.

Glucocorticoids also suppress both inflammatory and immunologic responses and thereby attenuate associated tissue destruction and fibroplasia. Under the influence of high levels of glucocorticoids, there is an enhancement of the spread of infections and reduced resistance to a number of bacterial, viral and fungal diseases. Glucocorticoids may impair the immunologic response at any stage, from the initial interaction and processing of antigens by cells of the reticuloendothelial system through the induction and proliferation of immunocompetent lymphocytes and subsequent antibody production. Inhibition by glucocorticoids of a number of lymphoid cell functions forms part of the basis for suppression of the immunologic response. Although all lymphoid tissues can be depleted by glucocorticoid treatment, some populations of lymphocytes are steroid-resistant.

Glucocorticoids also decrease the initial inflammatory reaction and its classic manifestations of heat, swelling and pain. The degree of hyperemia, extravasation, cellular migration and infiltration at the site of injury is decreased. Especially important are the effects on the usual vascular responses of increased permeability, diapedesis and extravasation. In addition, a number of phagocytic mechanisms are inhibited by glucocorticoids and clearance is impaired of particulate substances by the reticuloendothelial system. Accumulation of engulfed antigens in macrophages probably is related in part to the enhanced stability of lysosomal membranes induced by glucocorticoids.[158]

Glucocorticoids exert a profound negative effect on wound healing. Animals receiving high therapeutic levels of glucocorticoids may have postoperative wound dehiscence. The basic mechanism involved is inhibition of fibroblast proliferation and collagen synthesis, leading to a decrease in scar tissue formation.

Mineralocorticoids: Mineralocorticoids are adrenal steroids that have their principal effects on ion transport by epithelial cells, resulting in a loss of K and conservation of Na. The most potent and important natural mineralocorticoid is aldosterone. The enzymatically controlled electrolyte "pumps" in epithelial cells of the renal tubule and sweat glands respond to mineralocorticoids by conserving Na and Cl, and by excreting K.[159] In the distal convoluted tubule of the nephron, a cationic exchange mechanism exists for resorption of Na from the glomerular filtrate and secretion of K into the tubular lumen (Fig 36). These reactions are accelerated by mineralocorticoids but move much more slowly in their absence.[160] A lack of secretion of mineralocorticoids, as in Addison's-like disease, may result in lethal retention of K and loss of Na.

Sex Steroids

Secretion of sex steroids by cells of the zona reticularis occurs under normal conditions but in minute amounts that probably are of little

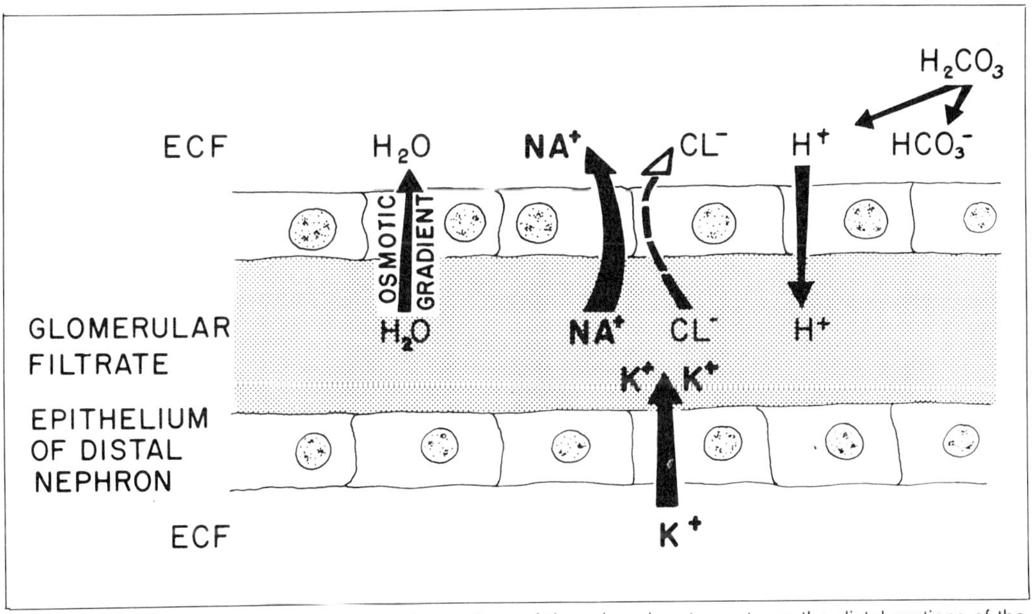

Fig 36. Aldosterone secreted by the zona glomerulosa of the adrenal cortex acts on the distal portions of the nephron to increase tubular excretion of K and increase resorption of Na (and secondarily Cl). The osmotic gradient created facilitates movement of water from the glomerular filtrate into the extracellular fluid.

physiologic significance. Progesterone, estrogens and androgens are synthesized by secretory cells of the inner zone of the cortex.

Control of Adrenal Function

Adrenocorticotropic hormone (ACTH) secreted by the adenohypophysis is the principal regulator of adrenal cortical growth and secretory activity, particularly cells in the zona fasciculata and zona reticularis. The adrenal cortex secretes significant quantities of cortisol only in response to ACTH stimulation. Cyclic adenosine monophosphate serves as the intracellular mediator of ACTH action by stimulating certain key enzymes (*eg*, protein kinases) to initiate the biochemical events leading to biosynthesis of corticosteroid hormones.[161]

Control of ACTH secretion by the adenohypophysis is governed largely by the overlying hypothalamus through secretion of corticotropin-releasing hormone (CRH). This peptide is secreted by neurons of the hypothalamus into capillaries that form the hypothalamic-pituitary portal system and convey CRH to the corticotropic cells of the adenohypophysis. Negative-feedback control of ACTH secretion is exerted mainly by the circulating level of cortisol acting on secretory cells in the hypothalamus.

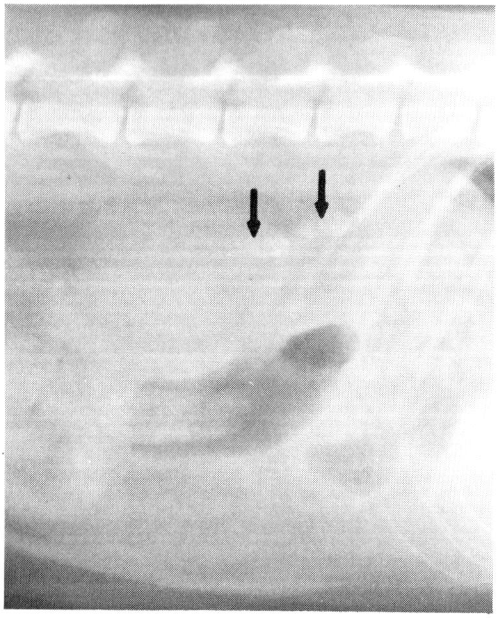

Fig 37. Radiodense adrenal glands, with extensive mineralization, situated cranial to the kidneys and ventral to the lumbar vertebrae.

The renin-angiotensin system is the major regulator of aldosterone production by the zona glomerulosa of the adrenal cortex.[162] Renin is an enzyme released into the circulation by cells of the juxtaglomerular apparatus in the kidney. It acts to cleave the plasma globulin, angiotensinogen, to form angiotensin I. This decapeptide is further hydrolyzed to angiotensin II by a converting enzyme. Angiotensin II is both a potent vasoconstrictor and a tropic hormone that stimulates synthesis and secretion of aldosterone. It is a very labile peptide that is quickly inactivated in plasma and tissues by angiotensinases.

A number of factors are reportedly concerned with the regulation of renin secretion by the kidney. The "short loop" of negative-feedback control is the direct inhibition exerted by circulating levels of angiotensin II. The "long loop" of this servomechanism is exerted by an indirect feedback-inhibition on renin secretion by aldosterone. Renin release and eventually aldosterone secretion are increased by conditions that compromise bloodflow and pressure to the kidney, severe dehydration that results in decreased intravascular blood volume, and Na depletion.

Diseases of the Adrenal Glands

Mineralization of the Adrenal Glands

Extensive deposits of minerals in the adrenal glands of adult cats occur frequently. A 30% incidence was reported for cats, vs only 5.7% for dogs.[163] The cause is unknown. The mineral deposits, although often bilateral and extensive, usually are not associated with clinical signs attributable to hypoadrenocorticism in cats.

Occasionally a dog with extensive mineralization and degeneration of the adrenal glands dies suddenly after relatively minor stress.[164] The mineralized adrenals may be detected at necropsy or during routine radiographic evaluation of the abdomen as 2 radiopaque bodies situated ventral to the cranial lumbar vertebrae (Fig 37).

Extensively mineralized adrenal glands are coarsely nodular, firm and mottled with multiple yellow-white foci throughout the cortex and extending into the medulla (Fig 38). They are difficult to incise and gritty.

The clinical significance of adrenal gland mineralization is unclear.

Hyperadrenocorticism

Cause: Inadequate numbers of cases have been studied or reported to determine which of

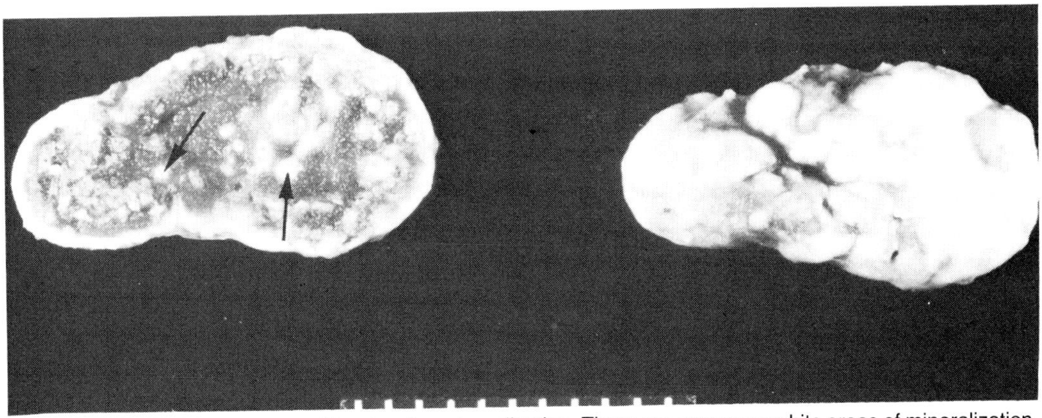

Fig 38. Adrenal gland from a cat with extensive mineralization. There are numerous white areas of mineralization throughout the cortex and medulla (arrows). The surface is coarsely nodular (right) due to regenerative hyperplasia of the remaining viable cortical cells. (scale = 1 cm)

the several potential pathogenic mechanisms is most important in development of hyperadrenocorticism in cats. Based on our experience, the syndrome of cortisol-excess in cats has been observed most often after long-term, high-level administration of potent, synthetic corticosteroids in the treatment of a variety of corticosteroid-responsive conditions.

Clinical Signs: Animals with hyperadrenocorticism usually have a distinctive appearance. The catabolic effects of cortisol on protein metabolism result in gradual wasting of skeletal muscles. The cat may not be as active as normal and exhibits muscular trembling. Limb muscles atrophy and abdominal muscles also are weakened, resulting in a pendulous abdomen. Accumulation of fat in the abdomen and liver, resulting in hepatomegaly, contribute to the "pot-bellied" appearance of affected animals.

The skin becomes progressively thinned and more fragile in cats with naturally occurring and iatrogenic cortisol-excess. The epidermis and dermis atrophy and the skin becomes extremely thin and tears or hematomas develop after minor trauma (Fig 39). Excessive cortisol favors prolongation of the telogen or resting phase of the growth cycle of hair follicles. As a consequence, the hairs are less firmly attached to the base of the hair follicle and tend to be dislodged by accumulations of keratin.

Animals with hyperadrenocorticism are more susceptible to infection. Chronic pyoderma, with focal epidermal ulceration, and cystitis are common sequelae. Hospitalized animals are more susceptible to respiratory infections that may progress to suppurative bronchopneumonia. Because affected animals spend more time recumbent, pressure necrosis of skin overlying bony prominences, such as the elbows and tuber ischii, is common. Fibroblastic proliferation and synthesis of collagen are inhibited by elevated serum cortisol levels. Therefore, areas of necrosis are slow to heal and susceptible to infection.

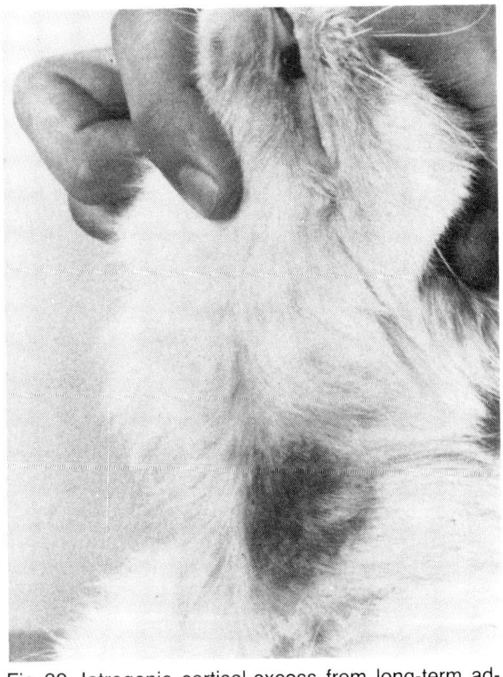

Fig 39. Iatrogenic cortisol-excess from long-term administration of glucocorticoids resulted in a large hematoma after jugular venipuncture.

Increased serum cortisol levels antagonize the action of antidiuretic hormone on the renal tubules. Therefore, most animals with hyperadrenocorticism have varying degrees of polyuria and polydipsia.

Affected animals often have a ravenous appetite. The increased hunger appears to be the result of a direct effect of glucocorticoids on the appetite center in the brain.

Diagnosis: Cortisol-excess consistently affects the hematopoietic system. There is intravascular destruction of eosinophils or sequestration of circulating eosinophils in the lung and spleen, with resulting eosinopenia. Involution of lymphoid tissues occurs in response to increased secretion of cortisol, resulting in lymphopenia. Corticosteroids stimulate the formation of neutrophils in bone marrow and decrease the migration of these cells into areas of infection. Animals with the syndrome of cortisol-excess often have a neutrophilia that is great enough to cause leukocytosis. Because the neutrophils remain in circulation for longer than normal periods, an increased number of hypersegmented neutrophils may be present.

Hyperadrenocorticism also affects glucose metabolism and affected animals may have moderately elevated blood glucose concentrations and an abnormal response to exogenous administration of glucose. Such serum electrolytes as Na, K and Cl usually are within normal limits. Because animals with the syndrome of cortisol-excess usually produce large volumes of dilute urine, a urinalysis should be performed to assist in establishing the diagnosis. A specific gravity of less than 1.015 has been present in most dogs with the syndrome of cortisol-excess evaluated in our hospital.

A definitive diagnosis of hyperadrenocorticism should not be based solely on laboratory tests that indirectly evaluate the metabolic effects of excessive cortisol secretion. The most precise assessment is obtained by measuring blood levels of corticosteroids under specific conditions compared with age-matched, clinically normal animals. Satisfactory measurement of cortisol levels may be obtained by a number of methods, including fluorometric, competitive protein-binding, and radioimmunoassay.

Too few cats with hyperadrenocorticism have been evaluated in our hospital at present to determine if blood cortisol levels are consistently elevated above normal. Plasma cortisol levels in dogs with hyperadrenocorticism overlap the range established for clinically normal dogs and a resting plasma cortisol level by itself often does not identify a dog with hyperadrenocorticism. Therefore, monitoring changes in plasma cortisol levels after stimulation of the adrenal cortex with exogenous ACTH and suppression with dexamethasone is necessary to establish the diagnosis and determine the most likely pathogenic mechanism for the cortisol excess.

Treatment: Treatment of animals with proven hyperadrenocorticism can be medical or surgical. Oral use of mitotane (o,p'DDD) (Lysodren: Bristol) has been the most common medical method of therapy since 1973.[165] This drug is an isomer of the insecticide DDD and is selectively cytotoxic for the zonae fasciculata and reticularis of the adrenal cortex in dogs. Since a dosage schedule and the toxicity of mitotane have not been determined in cats, its use would appear contraindicated due to known susceptibility of cats to insecticides of this group.

Since experience with hyperadrenocorticism in cats is very limited, the best approach to recommend at this time for treatment would be either unilateral (functional adenoma or carcinoma) or bilateral (adrenal cortical hyperplasia) adrenalectomy. It should be emphasized that the surgery is demanding and postoperative care is critical, time-consuming and expensive. The adrenal glands can be approached surgically through a ventral midline or bilateral paracostal incisions. Medical management of the patient before, during and after surgery has been described in detail for dogs and is of major importance in the animal's survival.[166] These experiences should serve as a guideline in establishing a similar course of pre- and postoperative therapy in cats.

Hypoadrenocorticism

Chronic adrenocortical insufficiency in people was first described by Thomas Addison in 1855 and was the first recognized endocrine disease. Although hyperadrenocorticism is a common endocrinopathy in dogs, it is encountered infrequently in cats.

Cause: Lesions in the adrenal cortex responsible for a deficient production of all 3 classes of corticosteroids (mineralocorticoids, glucocorticoids, adrenal sex steroids) and development of hyperadrenocorticism include bilateral adrenocortical atrophy, granulomatous adrenalitis, thrombosis of adrenal vessels with infarction of the gland associated with disseminated intravascular coagulopathies, invasion and destruction by metastatic neoplasms, hemorrhage and necrosis with subsequent replacement by fibrous connective tissue, and extensive amyloid deposition along adrenal sinusoids.

In idiopathic adrenocortical atrophy, all layers of the cortex are markedly reduced in thickness. Although the pathogenesis of idiopathic atrophy is unknown, an immune-mediated process may be responsible.[167] No pituitary lesions have been observed and all 3 zones are severely atrophied, including the zona glomerulosa, which is not under ACTH control. Granulomatous adrenalitis, with necrosis of cortical parenchyma caused by *Histoplasma capsulatum, Blastomyces dermatitidis, Mycobacterium tuberculosis* or *Toxoplasma gondii,* may be related to suppression of the inflammatory response and local cell-mediated immunity by the high levels of glucocorticoids in the adrenal cortex.[168]

Large neoplasms of the anterior pituitary gland may result in decreased blood levels of ACTH and subsequent tropic atrophy of the adrenal cortex but do not lead to hypoadrenocorticism (Fig 5). Although there is severe atrophy of the zona fasciculata and zona reticularis, the aldosterone-secreting zona glomerulosa remains essentially normal.

Clinical Signs: A variety of signs is observed in animals with hypoadrenocorticism, including recurrent gastroenteritis, a slowly progressive loss of body condition, and failure to respond appropriately in stressful situations, such as hospitalization, minor illnesses or surgery. Less commonly, the animal is presented in a shock-like coma with no history of previous illness.

A reduction in the synthesis and secretion of mineralocorticoids, primarily aldosterone, results in marked alterations of serum K, Na and Cl levels (Fig 36). Less K is excreted by the kidney, resulting in a progressive rise in serum K levels. Less Na and Cl are resorbed from the glomerular filtrate in renal tubules, leading to varying degrees of natriuresis and hyperchloruria, with a corresponding decline in blood levels. The severe hyperkalemia often produces marked cardiovascular disturbances reflected by changes in the EGC.[169]

A progressive decrease in blood volume contributes to hypotension, weakness and microcardia that is apparent on radiographs. Peripheral circulatory collapse may result from the progressive hemoconcentration. Emesis, diarrhea and anorexia also occur in animals with hypoadrenocorticism and contribute to the patient's deterioration. Weight loss often is severe. Although development of clinical signs often is insidious and not readily apparent to the owner, affected cats often are presented with acute circulatory collapse and evidence of renal failure.

Diagnosis: Hematologic alterations that occur with hypoadrenocorticism include an increase in the PCV and hemoglobin level due to dehydration and loss of intravascular fluid volume. Changes in the WBC count vary considerably, but eosinophilia and lymphocytosis often are observed. Since recently administered glucocorticoids can rapidly affect the WBC count, this should be taken into account in interpreting the hematologic data. The hyponatremia, hypochloremia and hyperkalemia that occur with hypoadrenocorticism may vary from slight to severe, depending upon the stage and severity of the disease. Determination of the Na:K ratio may be helpful in evaluating electrolyte values in animals with suspected adrenal cortical insufficiency. The BUN and serum creatinine levels begin to rise as renal perfusion and urine output decrease. The serum glucose level ranges from low-normal to moderately subnormal in animals with hypoadrenocorticism.

Treatment: Adrenal cortical insufficiency should be regarded as a medical emergency that requires intensive therapy to correct associated shock, dehydration and electrolyte imbalances. The reduced blood volume and dehydration should be corrected initially with IV fluid replacement. Physiologic saline or 5% dextrose in physiologic saline solution is the preferred replacement fluid. A corticosteroid with marked mineralocorticoid activity, such as desoxycorticosterone acetate (Percorten:Ciba), is administered IM at a total dose of 1-2 mg. Injections are repeated at 24-hour intervals and adjusted as needed to return Na and K levels to their normal ranges. Soluble glucocorticoids are administered IV to reverse circulatory collapse and shock. When the animal is rehydrated and has normal blood electrolyte levels, supportive therapy can be reduced gradually. Fluids and electrolytes can be replaced PO if the animal is not vomiting. A maintenance dose for desoxycorticosterone acetate should be established by frequent monitoring of serum Na, K and Cl levels.

References

1. Ricci, V and Russolo, M. Acta Anat **84** (1973) 10.
2. Wilhelmi, AE. Yale J Biol Med **41** (1968) 199.
3. Papkoff, H. Proc Soc Exp Biol Med **153** (1976) 498.
4. El Etreby, MF and Fath El Bab, MR. Cell Tissue Res **193** (1978) 211.
5. El Etreby, MF and Fath El Bab, MR. Cell Tissue Res **186** (1978) 399.
6. Schally, AV. Science **202** (1978) 18.
7. Capen, in Moulton: Tumors in Domestic Animals. 2nd ed. Univ Calif Press, Berkeley, 1978.
8. Zaki, FA and Liu, S-K. Vet Path **10** (1973) 232.
9. Zaki, F *et al.* J Comp Path **85** (1975) 467.
10. Sokol, HW and Valtin, H. Endocrin **77** (1965) 692.
11. Green, RA and Farrow, CS. JAVMA **164** (1974) 524.
12. Grieg, WA. Proc 17th World Vet Cong, 1963.
13. Rogers, WA *et al.* JAVMA **170** (1977) 545.
14. Pelletier, G. *et al.* Endocrin **98** (1976) 1253.
15. Ekholm, R *et al.* Endocrin **97** (1975) 337.
16. Ekholm, R and Wollman, SH. Endocrin **97** (1975) 1432.
17. Guillemin, R. Science **202** (1978) 390.
18. Chopra, IJ *et al.* Clin Endocrin Metab **36** (1973) 1050.
19. Oppenheimer, JH *et al.* Recent Prog Horm Res **32** (1976) 529.
20. Hammarström, S *et al.* Science **197** (1977) 996.
21. Brodey, RS. Adv Vet Sci Comp Med **14** (1970) 309.
22. Clark, ST and Neier, H. Zbl Vet Med **5** (1958) 17.
23. Holzworth, J *et al.* Cornell Vet **45** (1955) 487.
24. Holzworth, J *et al.* JAVMA **176** (1980) 345.
25. Johnson, KH and Osborne, CA. JAVMA **156** (1970) 906.
26. Jones, BR and Johnstone, AC. N Zeal Vet J **29** (1981) 70.
27. Leav, I *et al.* Am J Path **83** (1976) 61.
28. Lucke, VM. J Sm Anim Pract **5** (1964) 351.
29. Whitehead, JE. VM/SAC **62** (1967) 357.
30. O'Brien, SE *et al.* Vet Rec **107** (1980) 199.
31. Patnaik, AK and Lieberman, PH. Vet Path **16** (1979) 687.
32. Peterson, ME *et al.* JAVMA *In press*, 1982.
33. Capen and Roth, in Iaochim: Pathobiology Ann. Vol 3. Appleton-Century-Crofts, New York, 1973.
34. Capen, in Branley and Cornelius: Advances in Veterinary Sciences and Comparative Medicine. Academic Press, New York, 1975.
35. Capen, CC and Rowland, GN. Anat Rec **162** (1968) 327.
36. Balogh, K and Cohen, RB. Lab Invest **10** (1961) 354.
37. Harcourt-Webster, JN and Truman, RF. J Path **97** (1969) 687.
38. Tremblay, G and Pearse, AGE. Br J Exp Path **40** (1959) 66.
39. Arnaud, CD *et al.* Am J Med **40** (1971) 630.
40. Cohn DV *et al.* Am J Med **56** (1975) 767.
41. Habener JF *et al.* Proc Nat Acad Sci **68** (1971) 2986.
42. Kemper, B *et al.* Proc Nat Acad Sci **69** (1972) 643.
43. MacGregor RR *et al.* Endocrin **93** (1973) 1387.
44. Potts, JT, Jr *et al.* Clin Endocrin **5** (Suppl) (1976) 307.
45. Sherwood, LM *et al.* Proc Nat Acad Sci **67** (1970) 1631.
46. Habener, JF and Kronenberg, HM. Fed Proc **37** (1978) 2561.
47. Habener, JF and Potts, JT, Jr. N Engl J Med **299** (1978) 580.
48. Habener, JF and Potts, JT, Jr. Endocrin **104** (1979) 265.
49. Habener, JF *et al.* Biochem **16** (1977) 3910.
50. Habener and Potts, in: Handbook of Physiology, Endocrinology. Vol VII Am Physiol Soc, Washington, DC, 1976.
51. MacGregor, RR *et al.* J Biol Chem **253** (1978) 2012.
52. Arnaud, CD. Am J Med **55** (1973) 577.
53. Pott JT, Jr *et al.* Am J Med **50** (1971) 639.
54. Roth, SI and Raisz, LG. Lab Invest **13** (1964) 331.
55. Targovnik, JH *et al.* Endocrin **88** (1976) 1477.
56. Krook, L and Lowe, JE. Path Vet **1** (Suppl 1) (1964) 1.
57. Mayer, GP. Abstr 56th Ann Mtg Endocrin Soc, 1974. No A181.
58. Mayer, GP and Hurst, JG. Endocrin **102** (1978) 1803.
59. Morrisey, JJ and Cohn, DV. Endocrin **103** (1978) 2081.
60. Parsons, JA and Robinson, CJ. Nature (London) **230** (1971) 581.
61. Rasmussen, H and Bordier, P: The Physiological and Cellular Basis of Metabolic Bone Disease. Williams & Wilkins, Baltimore, 1974.
62. Kalina, M and Pearse, AGE. Histochemie **26** (1971) 1.
63. Copp, DH. Ann Rev Physiol **32** (1970) 61.
64. Capen, CC and Young DM. Am J Path **57** (1969) 365.
65. Collins, WT Jr, *et al.* Am J Path **87** (1977) 603.
66. Nunez EA *et al.* Lab Invest **31** (1974) 96.
67. Cooper, CW *et al.* Endocrin **91** (1972) 1079.
68. Care, AD *et al.* J Endocrin **48** (1970) 667.
69. Gray TK and Ontjes DA. Clin Orthop **111** (1975) 238.
70. Aliapoulious, MA *et al.* Science **151** (1966) 330.
71. Friedman, J *et al.* Endocrin **82** (1968) 149.
72. Talmadge, RV *et al.* Endocrin **90** (1972) 1185.
73. Kallio, DM *et al.* J Ultrastruct Res **39** (1972) 205.
74. Weisbrode, SE and Capen, CC. Am J Path **77** (1974) 395.
75. Rasmussen, in Williams: Textbook of Endocrinology. WB Saunders, Philadelphia, 1973.
76. Kodicek, E: Lancet **2** (1974) 325.
77. Holick, MF *et al.* Science **210** (1980) 203.

78. Holick, MF and Clark, MB. Fed Proc **37** (1978) 2567.
79. Holick, MF *et al.* Biochem Biophys Res Commun **76** (1977) 107.
80. DeLuca, HF. N Engl J Med **289** (1973) 359.
81. DeLuca, HF. Biochem Pharm **26** (1977) 563.
82. Kodicek, E *et al.* Nature (London) **228** (1970) 763.
83. Haussler, MR and McCain, TA. N Engl J Med **297** (1977) 974.
84. Haussler, MR *et al.* Proc Nat Acad Sci **68** (1971) 177.
85. Fraser, DR and Kodicek, E. Nature (London) **241** (1973) 163.
86. Garabedian, M *et al.* Proc Nat Acad Sci **69** (1972) 1673.
87. Rasmussen, H *et al.* J Clin Invest **51** (1972) 2502.
88. Capen, in McDonald: Veterinary Endocrinology and Reproduction. Lea & Febiger, Philadelphia, 1980.
89. DeLuca, HF. Am J Med **56** (1974) 871.
90. Hughes, MR and Haussler, MR. J Biol Chem **253** (1978) 1065.
91. Wecksler, WR *et al.* Arch Biochem Biophys **183** (1977) 168.
92. Capen, CC *et al.* Abstr 6th Parathyroid Conference, 1978. p 48.
93. Arnaud, CD. Fed Proc **37** (1978) 2557.
94. Olson, H and Capen, CC. Am J Path **86** (1977) 437.
95. Walser, M *et al.* J Clin Invest **42** (1963) 456.
96. Musselman EE. VM/SAC **70** (1975) 1433.
97. Rowland, GN *et al.* Path Vet **5** (1968) 504.
98. Scott, PP. Symp Zool Soc (London) **21** (1968) 21.
99. Riser, WM *et al.* J Am Rad Soc **9** (1968) 37.
100. Avioli, LV and Haddad, JG. Metabolism **22** (1973) 507.
101. Brickman, AS *et al.* Ann Int Med **80** (1974) 161.
102. Weisbrode, SE *et al.* Lab Invest **30** (1974) 786.
103. Norrdin, RW *et al.* Virchows Arch (A) Path Anat Hist **375** (1977) 169.
104. Norrdin, RW *et al.* Calcif Tiss Res **24** (1977) 99.
105. Villafane, F *et al.* Calcif Tiss Res **23** (1977) 171.
106. Galaska, CSB and Bennett, A. Nature **263** (1976) 508.
107. Seyberth, HW *et al.* N Engl J Med **293** (1975) 1278.
108. Tashjian, AH Jr. Cancer Res **38** (1978) 4138.
109. Voelkel, EF *et al.* Metabolism **24** (1975) 973.
110. Powell, D *et al.* N Engl J Med **289** (1973) 176.
111. Singer, FE *et al.* Ann Int Med **78** (1973) 365.
112. Mundy, GR *et al.* N Engl J Med **291** (1974) 1041.
113. Mundy, GR *et al.* N Engl J Med **290** (1974) 867.
114.Stewart, AF *et al.* N Engl J Med **303** (1980) 1377.
115. Omen, in Ioachim: Pathobiology Annual. Vol 3. Appleton-Century-Crofts, New York, 1973.
116. Chew, DJ *et al.* JAAHA **11** (1975) 46.
117. Meuten, DJ *et al.* Lab Invest *In press*, 1982.
118. Heath, H *et al.* Calcif Tiss Int **30** (1980) 127.
119. Edney, ATB. J Sm Anim Pract **10** (1969) 231.
120. Bjerkas, E. J Sm Anim Pract **15** (1974) 411.
121. Black, HE *et al.* Lab Invest **29** (1973) 437.
122. Capen, CC and Black, HE. Am J Path **74** (1974) 377.
123. Capen *et al*, in Arceneaux: 31st Ann Proc Electron Microsc Soc Am. Claitor's Publishing, Baton Baton Rouge, 1973.
124. Hazard, JB. Am J Path **88** (1977) 214.
125. Sipple, JH. Am J Med **31** (1961) 163.
126. Black, HE *et al.* Cancer **32** (1973) 865.
127. Capen, CC and Black HE. Am J Path **74** (1974) 377.
128. Yarrington, JT and Capen, CC. Vet Path **18** (1981) 316.
129. Swaninathan, R *et al.* J Endocrin **54** (1972) 525.
130. Legg, PG. Z Zellforsch **80** (1967) 307.
131. Williams, RH and Ensinck, JW. Diabetes **15** (1966) 623.
132. Hjärre, A. Arch Wiss Prakt Tierheilk **57** (1928) 1.
133. Rubarth, S. No Am Vet **17** (1936) 49.
134. Bloom, F. N Engl J Med **217** (1937) 395.
135. Lande, KE. Am J Clin Path **14** (1944) 590.
136. McEvoy, JP. No Am Vet **30** (1949) 449.
137. Schlotthauer, CF and Miller, JAS. JAVMA **118** (1951) 31.
138. Dlugach, J. JAVMA **123** (1953) 118.
139. Holzworth, J and Coffin, DL. Cornell Vet **43** (1953) 502.
140. Keep, JM. Aust Vet J **30** (1954) 347.
141. Joshua, JO. J Small Anim Pract **4** (1963) 275.
142. Gepta, W and Toussaint D. Diabetologia **3** (1967) 249.
143. Schaer, M. JAAHA **9** (1973) 548.
144. Root, CR and Scott, RC. JAVMA **158** (1971) 721.
145. Meier, H. Diabetes **9** (1960) 485.
146. Coffin, DL and Thordal-Christensen, A. Vet Med **48** (1953) 193.
147. Finn, JP *et al.* J Sm Anim Prac **11** (1970) 607.
148. Johnson, KH and Stevens, JB. Diabetes **22** (1973) 81.
149. Rubarth, S. Scand Vet-tidskrift **25** (1935) 750.
150. Yano, BL *et al.* Vet Path **18** (1981) 621.
151. Johnson, KH *et al.* Path Vet **7** (1970) 153.
152. Yano, BL *et al.* Vet Path **18** (1981) 310.
153. Yano, BL *et al.* Lab Invest **45** (1981) 149.
154. Williamson, JR and Lacy, PE. Arch Path **72** (1961) 637.
155. Dohan, FC and Lukens, FDW. Endocrin **42** (1948) 244.
156. Schall, WD and Cornelius, LM. Vet Clin No Am **7** (1977) 613.
157. Baxter, JD and Forsham, PH. Am J Med **53** (1972) 573.

158. Thompson, EB and Lippman ME. Metabolism **23** (1974) 159.

159. Pelletier, M *et al.* Arch Int Med **129** (1972) 248.

160. Horton, R. Metabolism **22** (1973) 1525.

161. Liddle, in Williams: Textbook of Endocrinology. WB Saunders, Philadelphia, 1974.

162. Williams, GH and Dluhy, RG. Am J Med **53** (1972) 595.

163. Howell, JM and Ormrod, AN. J Comp Path **74** (1964) 280.

164. Howell, JM and Ormrod, AN. Vet Rec **74** (1962) 469.

165. Schechter, RD *et al.* JAVMA **162** (1973) 629.

166. Siegel, ET *et al.* JAVMA **157** (1970) 2081.

167. Blizzard, RM and Kyle, M. J Clin Invest **42** (1963) 1653.

168. Frenkel, JK. Am J Path **86** (1977) 749.

169. Mulnix, JA. JAAHA **7** (1971) 220.

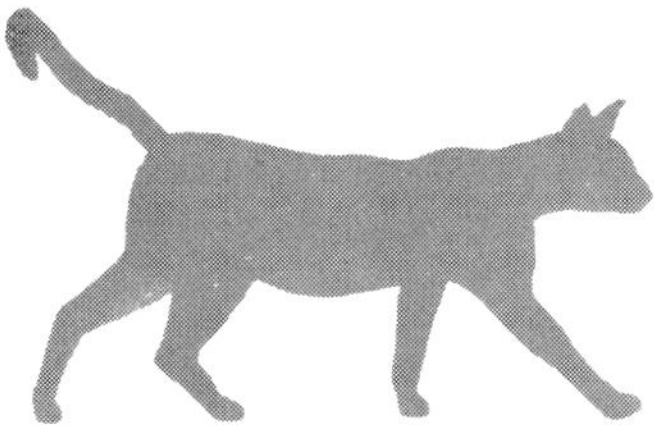

12

the urinary system

D.R. FINCO, J.A. BARSANTI, AND W.A. CROWELL

Cat owners frequently consult veterinarians because of urinary tract disorders in their pets. This chapter summarizes current knowledge of these disorders. Emphasis has been placed on mechanisms of disease so that rational diagnostic and therapeutic procedures can be established. Because of the prevalence of feline urologic syndrome, this disease has been given special attention.

ANATOMY AND PHYSIOLOGY

A thorough knowledge of anatomy and physiology is a prerequisite to the successful clinical management of feline urologic problems. Textbooks of anatomy and physiology should be consulted for comprehensive reviews of mammalian, and specifically of feline, urinary tract structure and function.[1-4] Of particular relevance is a knowledge of gross and microscopic renal anatomy and knowledge of physiologic concepts, such as renal blood flow, glomerular filtration, tubular resorption and secretion, and the countercurrent mechanism of urine concentration. Several distinctive features of the urinary tract of the cat are not discussed or are inadequately discussed, however, in standard texts. The following features have immediate or potential clinical significance.

Renal Lipids

The kidney of the cat has more lipid than that of any other common domestic species. The lipid is located in the proximal tubule, with an abrupt transition between the fat-free and fat-laden portions.[5-7] Age, sex and sexual activity appear to be significant factors regarding the quantity of fat present. Kittens and immature cats have less fat and finer fat globules than adults.[5,8,9] Only moderate amounts of fat are in the kidneys of sexually active males, but sexually inactive males have heavy lipid deposits. Castration of males causes an increase in renal lipid content within 3 weeks.[7] In the queen, only small amounts of renal lipid are found during anestrus, a moderate amount during proestrus or estrus, and increased amounts during the luteal phase. The kidneys of pregnant females are heavily laden with fat.[5,7] No correlation appears to exist between the amount of fat in the kidney and in the liver, and body weight is not related to the amount of renal fat.[5]

The relationship of fat deposition to sexual activity has resulted in the theory that renal lipids might be sex steroids. Semiquantitative thin-layer chromatography has revealed, however, that the principal component is triglycerides. Cholesterol and phospholipids are present in smaller quantities, but no estrogen has been detected.[10] The high fat content of the cat's kidney and alterations in quantity dependent on age, sex and sexual activity should be considered when evaluating the morphology of the kidneys of the cat.

Vitamin A has been found in cat kidneys at a concentration far in excess of that in other species.[11] No consistent correlation has been found, however, between the concentrations of fat and vitamin A in the kidney. Vitamin A is particularly prevalent in the medullary rays, which does not coincide with the predominant location of fat. The possible role of vitamin A in amyloidosis in the cat will be discussed later.

Renal Vascular System and Blood Flow

In the cat, the main segmental arteries of the kidney have branches that supply the outer cortex, and a subcapsular network of veins drains directly into the renal vein at the hilus.[12,13] There is evidence that the subcapsular veins provide exclusive drainage of the superficial renal cortex under normal venous pressure. On this basis, the function of the superficial cortical area was compared with the combined deep cortical and medullary areas by separate sampling of the subcapsular and the remaining venous effluent.[14-18] The findings indicated differences in function of superficial and deep nephrons in the mammalian kidney. These differences may aid in explaining renal dysfunction as more data become available.

Total blood flow to the cat's kidney was measured with a flow meter implanted around a renal artery and other abdominal arteries.[19] This facilitated blood-flow measurements during normal activity. Considerable renal vasodilation occurred during sleep, and vasoconstriction occurred both in preparing for and during fighting. Alterations in renal blood flow paralleled the direction of alteration of arteries to the gut, but were variable in direction compared with arteries to the hindlimb.

In the cat, halothane anesthesia causes a reduction in renal vascular resistance. A decrease in systemic blood pressure has been associated with anesthesia, and renal blood flow was decreased to about 74% of control values.[20] This anesthetic has the same effect in the dog, although there is some evidence that renal cortical blood flow increases when halothane is given to a dog with preexisting hypotension.[21] The reduction in renal blood flow with halothane should be considered when giving this anesthetic to cats.

Renin, a renal hormone that converts a plasma globulin to angiotensin I, has been isolated from the cat's kidney.[22,23] Most renin is localized in the afferent arterioles. Cats have a higher renin activity per gram of kidney tissue than dogs or people, but a lower serum concentration of angiotensinogen.[24,25] The clinical significance of the renin system in hypertension in cats is unknown since blood pressure determinations are not commonly performed.

Kidney Size

Kidney size is determined routinely during physical examination to aid in evaluating the urinary system. Studies have revealed that no significant difference in weight exists between the right and left kidneys in normal cats.[26,27] The formula (total kidney weight in g = 9.825 x body weight^{71} − 1.09) was reported to provide a satisfactory estimate of normal kidney weight in kittens and adult females.[26] Adult males weighing more than 3 kg apparently have larger kidneys than females of the same weight.[27] Consequently, the formula is less accurate for heavy male cats. The quantity of protein in the diet may influence kidney size in mammals, whereas body fat depots probably do not.[28] These factors should be considered when using body weight to predict whether the kidney weight is normal or abnormal.

Renal Tubular Function

Analysis of fluid from renal tubules obtained by micropuncture of superficial nephrons has been valuable in studying renal function. From such analyses, it is possible to determine tubular cell function at various levels of the nephron. Extensive use of this and other technics has resulted in generalizations concerning mammalian tubular function that may or may not apply to cats. Although it is likely that most mammals share common mechanisms of renal function, some variation has been documented. Micropuncture studies of distal tubules reveal that, in dogs, luminal fluid was markedly hypotonic to plasma along the entire length of the distal tubule. In cats, fluid is initially hypotonic but becomes isotonic as it progresses along the distal tubule due to passage of water from the tubule.[29]

Differences in renal handling of certain solutes in cats have also been reported. In dogs and people, essentially all filtered glucose is resorbed until a maximum tubular capacity for resorption is reached. All glucose filtered in excess of this quantity is eliminated in the urine. In cats, no maximum resorption rate was established. Resorption was practically complete up to 230 mg/dl glomerular filtrate, but resorption continued thereafter at a slower rate.[30] In contrast to some other species, no maximum resorption rate for P has been found for cats, and P resorption by the tubule seems to be enhanced by high plasma glucose concentration.[30] If these observations were correct, they may be relevant in the feline patient with diabetes mellitus if urine glucose concentration is used exclusively in determining insulin dosage.

Species differences exist in the ability to concentrate urine; the cat has exceptional ability in this regard. Specific gravity values greater than 1.070 and urine osmolality of greater than 1900 mOsm/kg urine have been found.[31,32] This may be related to the large amount of medullary versus cortical tissue in this and other species with exceptional concentrating ability. All of the cat's nephrons have long loops of Henle that course deeply into the medulla, and thus the countercurrent system may be more efficient in this species.[15] Because of this concentrating ability, cats can survive without detriment if maintained solely on rations containing 75% water.[32]

Bladder and Urethral Structure and Function

The anatomy of the male urethra is of interest because of the common occurrence of urethral obstruction. The portion between the bladder and prostate gland (abdominal portion) is thin-walled and contains only smooth muscle fibers. The portion from the prostate gland to the bulbourethral glands (pelvic portion) has smooth muscle covered by a layer of striated muscle fibers. The urethra between the bulbourethral glands and the tip of the penis (penile portion) has thick walls, forming the corpus cavernosum urethrae, and is covered by a strong tunica albuginea.[33,34] The lumen of the penile urethra is smaller than the remaining urethra.[33-35] The lining is predominantly stratified columnar epithelium in the penile urethra, mixed columnar and transitional epithelium in the pelvic urethra, and transitional epithelium in the abdominal urethra.[36]

Trauma and urethral obstruction may cause micturition defects in cats, and mechanical urethral obstruction may be complicated by urethral spasm. The cat has been used extensively for experimental investigation of urinary bladder and urethral structure and function.[37-56] Recently, clinical evaluation of bladder and urethral function with use of cystometrograms to evaluate the micturition reflex, urethral pressure profiles to evaluate urethral muscle tone, and electromyography to evaluate sphincter muscle activity have been studied.

EVALUATION OF THE URINARY SYSTEM

Clinical Examination

Principles of history-taking and physical examination are similar for most species and essential for accurate diagnosis. Reviews of physical diagnosis should be consulted.[57-59] Even when the history strongly suggests urinary tract disease, a complete physical examination should be performed. Diseases of the urinary tract can cause secondary changes in other body systems, and concurrent unrelated diseases of other systems may be present.

The cat lends itself to thorough physical examination of the urinary tract. Both kidneys are usually palpable and should be examined for location, size, shape, character of the surface, and presence or absence of pain. The urinary bladder is usually palpable and should be examined for shape, position, character of the wall, and intraluminal abnormalities. The pelvic urethra can be examined by rectal examination, and the penis and vulva can be inspected directly.

Collection and Evaluation of Urine

Urinalysis is of value in diagnosis of both urinary and extraurinary diseases. Textbooks of veterinary clinical pathology can be consulted for standard procedures of urinalysis and their interpretation.[60-63] This discussion is restricted to points that deserve special emphasis because of their importance.

Urinalysis specimens are obtained by collecting urine voided naturally, by manual compression of the urinary bladder, by catheterization, or by cystocentesis. Technics for collection of urine have been described.[63] The choice of the method of collection should take into account both the welfare of the patient and the likelihood of success of obtaining a specimen.

Collection of a naturally voided specimen is least traumatic to cats but difficult to accomplish. With hospitalized patients the litter pan and cage paper may be removed and replaced after several hours with a clean, chemical-free pan. Urine often can be obtained when the cat subsequently voids.

If the urinary bladder is moderately distended at the time of examination, cystocentesis is probably the easiest way to obtain urine. Such a sample is superior for both urinalysis and urinary culture since debris and bacteria normally found in the urethra and genital tract do not contaminate the specimen. If performed properly, cystocentesis entails little risk to the patient (Fig 1). One disadvantage of a cystocentesis sample is that RBC may be present because of iatrogenic trauma. For this reason, a naturally voided specimen is preferable in instances when the purpose of urinalysis is to establish if hematuria exists.

Urine may also be obtained by manually expressing it from the bladder. Pressure should be applied with the hand enveloping the bladder as completely as possible; pressure on the bladder should be increased slowly. If moderate pressure does not result in micturition, the cat

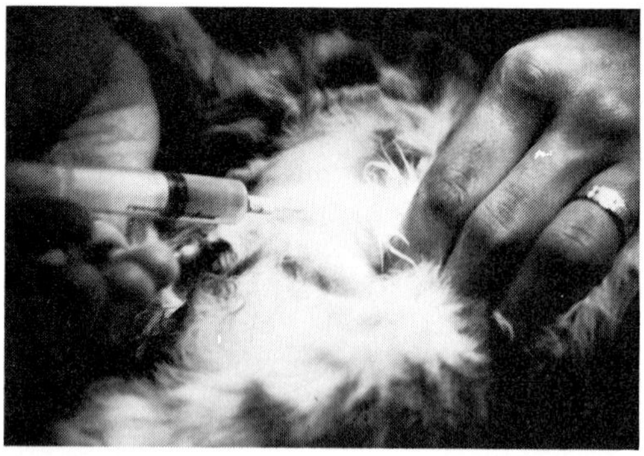

Fig 1. Cystocentesis being performed to obtain urine from a cat. A 22-ga needle is inserted through the cleansed abdominal wall into the bladder as the latter is immobilized by the operator's left hand. The penis is visible just beneath the syringe on the left.

should be returned to the cage; spontaneous micturition often occurs in the next few minutes.

Catheterization of male cats for the sole purpose of obtaining urine is generally inadvisable because it is difficult to perform aseptically unless chemical restraint is provided, and the penis and urethra may be injured. Females can be catheterized using a "blind" technic. A local anesthetic is instilled into the vagina and the rigid catheter is inserted along the ventral floor of the vagina into the urethra. Several attempts may be required for success. There is a greater chance of carrying microorganisms into the bladder using the blind technic than when catheterization is performed by direct visualization of the urethral orifice. A sterile otoscope cone can be used as a vaginal speculum to visualize the urethral orifice for catheterization of females.

When dysuria results in voiding of small quantities of urine at frequent intervals, the bladder may never attain a size sufficient to either manually express it or perform cystocentesis. In such instances it may be necessary to use a spontaneously voided specimen obtained by confining the cat to a metabolism cage or a cage with a dry, chemical-free litter pan.

Interpretation of the urinalysis must be related to the method of urine collection. Occult blood, increased RBC numbers, and proteinuria may be caused iatrogenically by manual compression of the bladder, catheterization or cystocentesis. This hematuria is transient and usually not detectible in urine obtained without trauma on the following day.

If WBC and bacteria are present in a sample obtained during spontaneous voiding, the possibility of contamination from the lower urinary or genital tract must be considered.

The specific gravity of the urine should be considered when interpreting all aspects of urinalysis. Urinary components are likely to be concentrated in urine samples of high specific gravity and diluted with low specific gravity.

Protein determinations with the dipstick method are often slightly to moderately positive for feline urine. The same specimen may be negative for protein, however, when the nitric acid or sulfasalicylic acid test for protein is used. The dipstick method may be overly sensitive for protein. In addition, immersion of the stick in urine for too long washes buffer from the strip and yields positive results. Higher urine pH values also increase the probability of false-positive results with dipsticks.[64] For these reasons, positive results for protein with dipsticks should be confirmed by other methods before proteinuria is diagnosed.

Although the pH of feline urine is usually acid, the diet may result in slightly alkaline urine.[65,66] Regardless of the composition of the diet, alkaline urine may be produced by cats for several hours after a meal. This is believed to be due to removal of hydrogen ions from blood during gastric secretion of HCl, mild alkalemia, and renal excretion of bicarbonate. Urine pH values above 8.0 may occur in normal cats because of this phenomenon. For these reasons, it should not be assumed that the presence of alkaline urine denotes infection.

Glucosuria is normally detected either by highly specific methods that use the enzyme glucose oxidase for part of the reaction or by nonspecific methods that measure any reducing substance. Vitamin C, when used as a urinary acidifier, can affect the detection of glucose. It inhibits the glucose oxidase reaction, which may produce negative results with dipsticks or tapes when glucose is actually present. With nonspecific reducing methods (boiling tablets), vitamin C may produce a positive reaction when glucose is absent.[67] Consequently, in patients that have received vitamin C, a urine glucose test that is negative is accurate when a nonspecific reducing method is used, and a positive result is accurate when the glucose oxidase reaction is used.

Microscopic examination of urine sediment is essential and should be performed even if dipstick tests are negative. The urinalysis is not complete if microscopic examination of sediment is not performed. Most components of feline urine sediment are similar to those in canine urine. Fat in feline urine may be related to the high fat content of the kidney and is considered a normal urine constituent. A combination of factors is responsible for phosphate crystals in urine. The pH is one; it is common to find crystals during microscopic examination of urine sediment from specimens with a pH above 6.8. Phosphates are normal constituents of urine and the presence of phosphate crystals simply denotes that the character of the urine has changed.

Evaluation of Renal Function

The levels of urea or creatinine in serum or plasma are routinely measured as screening tests for evaluation of renal function. Since both urea and creatinine diffuse into RBC, levels are nearly the same in serum, plasma and whole blood. Thus the term blood urea nitrogen (BUN) is used, although whole blood is rarely analyzed. As in other species, BUN and serum creatinine levels rise in cats only after considerable renal dysfunction; the measurements can only be expected to detect severe levels of abnormality. Normal values in cats are 15-35 mg/dl for BUN and 0.7-1.5 mg/dl for serum creatinine. Because of minor interlaboratory differences, normal values should be defined for each laboratory. Advantages and limitations of BUN and serum creatinine values for domestic species have been reviewed.[60] Although the BUN level may be slightly altered by diet or tissue catabolism, there is no evidence that one of these tests has a significant advantage over the other. Elevation of the BUN or serum creatinine level is not pathognomonic for renal disease because impaired renal perfusion or interference with urine outflow may cause abnormally high values when the kidneys are normal.

Urine concentration has been used in other domestic species to aid in detecting renal dysfunction, but it is of less value in cats. Impaired ability to concentrate urine precedes development of azotemia (*ie*, elevation of BUN or serum creatinine level) in dogs with chronic renal failure. However, cats with renal dysfunction may develop azotemia while considerable concentrating ability is retained.[68] Specific gravity readings above 1.030 may exist with azotemia due to primary renal failure. This finding creates a dilemma for the clinician since urine specific gravity readings may not distinguish prerenal and primary renal failure.

Since BUN and serum creatinine levels are crude indices of renal function, normal values may exist in cats with considerably impaired renal function. When it is necessary to document renal dysfunction not detectible by BUN and serum creatinine assay, other tests have been employed. The rate of disappearance of a compound from the blood following IV injection measures renal function if the compound is not metabolized and is excreted exclusively by the kidney. Studies of sodium sulfanilate and phenosulfonphthalein (PSP) indicated that sulfanilate is an acceptable compound for measuring renal function in cats, while PSP was less sensitive.[68] Para-aminohippurate has also been claimed to be of value.[69] The methods of performing these tests are described elsewhere.[63,68,69]

Radiography

The technics for diagnosing urinary tract disorders in cats are similar to those used in dogs; textbooks of radiology can be consulted for details. The following comments are directed at specific points that deserve emphasis.

For all radiographic procedures, the patient should be fasted for 24 hours. Warm-water enemas should be administered about 6 hours prior to radiography to avoid difficulties in interpretation due to the presence of feces.

Survey Radiographs: These are generally indicated when signs referable to the urinary tract are present and the patient cannot be adequately palpated because of obesity. The kidneys of cats are usually more visible than those of dogs on survey radiographs. Standard technics are used to obtain 2 views.

Excretory Urography: This technic is generally indicated when abnormalities in renal size or shape are present; it also aids in confirming and differentiating other suspected abnormalities. It is of particular value in differentiating hydronephrosis from a uniform increase in kidney size due to other causes. Although not a sensitive indicator of renal function, the excretory urogram may reveal differences in the 2 kidneys' ability to excrete contrast medium. Renal blood flow, glomerular filtration rate, ability to concentrate urine, and diameter of the collecting system are the significant factors in determining the radiopacity of the kidneys and collecting system. The excretory urogram also can provide information regarding the urinary

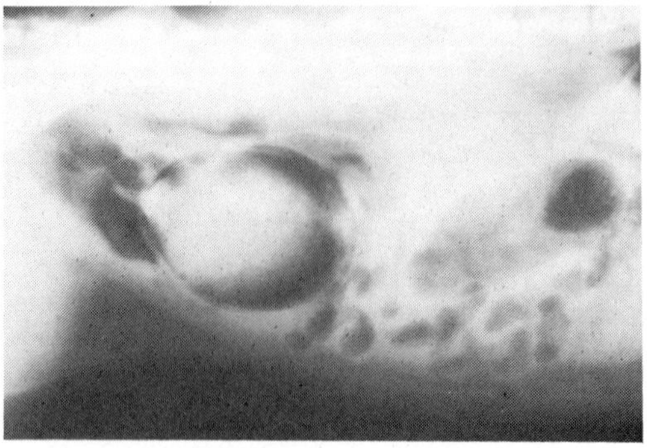

Fig 2. Lateral radiograph with double-contrast cystography. The CO_2 is located between layers of the bladder wall, having penetrated via mucosal lesions. The potential for gas embolism exists in such instances.

bladder. It is probably inferior to procedures in which contrast medium is injected via a urethral catheter because the bladder can be distended more with the latter.

Excretory urography usually can be performed without inducing general anesthesia; use of a tranquilizer may facilitate the procedure in some patients. Several organic iodine compounds are available (*eg*, Conray 400: Mallinckrodt), and a 50-70% solution seems to provide good results.[70] After survey radiographs are obtained, an indwelling catheter is placed in a cephalic vein and the contrast medium is administered at 2.2 ml/kg body weight by rapid injection. Generally the injection can be completed within a few seconds. A ventrodorsal radiograph is obtained 10-12 seconds after the injection and a lateral view is obtained immediately afterward. These exposures enable visualization of the kidneys because the medium is in the renal vasculature and tubules. Additional radiographs are obtained 5 minutes later to visualize the pelves and ureters, and 5-10 minutes later to visualize the ureters and bladder. Subsequent exposures may be needed.

Use of larger volumes of diluted contrast medium may improve visualization of structures.[71] There is no advantage in administering the contrast medium slowly (drip infusion) because concentration rather than volume is the significant factor in visualization. Increased volumes of fluid may increase urine output and further distend the urinary bladder. Although compression of the abdomen with a band has been advocated to compress the ureters, this procedure appears to add little to visualization of the ureters and it distorts the normal anatomic relationship of abdominal structures.[72] Through excretory urography, the kidney length in 30 normal cats was found to be best predicted by the following formula: kidney length = 23.45 mm + (1.045 x L_2 vertebra length in mm).[73]

Cystography: This technic may aid in defining acquired or congenital bladder defects. The patient is usually sedated to facilitate both catheterization and radiography. For positive-contrast studies, 1 part of 50% organic iodine solution (Conray 400:Mallinckrodt) is diluted with 9 parts of sterile water. Sufficient volume is injected via a urethral catheter to distend the bladder prior to radiography. For negative-contrast studies, CO_2 is used as the contrast agent. Either positive- or negative-contrast agents may be forced into bladder wall blood vessels after intravesicular injection of patients with eroded bladder epithelium. While positive-contrast agents generally cause no problem, embolism may occur when air is used as a negative-contrast agent.[74] CO_2 is more soluble than air in blood and reduces risk of embolism.

Double-contrast cystography may be performed by instilling about 10 ml diluted positive-contrast agent in the bladder, rolling the cat to disperse the agent in the bladder, and then distending the bladder with CO_2 (Fig 2).

Urethrography: This procedure is of value in assessing the urethra whenever lesions altering normal urethral outflow are suspected. Medium diluted with 3 parts of sterile water is injected via a catheter positioned just within the tip of the urethra. Small balloon-type catheters, such as the Swan Ganz type, are valuable for this procedure since retrograde flow of contrast medium from the urethra is prevented when the balloon tip of the catheter is inflated. Radiographs are obtained as the medium is injected. Repeated injections of 5-10 ml of medium are made with the cat in lateral and oblique positions for maximum visualization of urethra. Air urethrography should be avoided because of the risk of embolism.

When interpreting the radiograph, one should recall that a cat's bladder is normally more cranial than a dog's, and that a tapered, long abdominal urethra is normal (Fig 3).

Arteriography: This technic has occasional application in cases of renal masses and trauma. In people, the diagnostic information obtained may aid in localizing and identifying renal masses, and in evaluating the extent of renal injury after trauma. The technic may also be used to visualize the renal vasculature and kidney outline in patients with severe azotemia and in which the kidneys are not visualized by excretory urography.

Although aortography has been used under experimental conditions, its clinical application has been limited.[75,76] After inducing general anesthesia, the femoral triangle area is surgically prepared and the femoral artery is exposed. A 4- or 5-Fr, sterilized, radiopaque catheter is attached to a syringe containing saline-heparin solution. The lumen of the catheter is filled with the solution and the barrel is secured to the syringe to prevent reflux of blood. Between 2 loosely applied ligatures, held taut to avoid blood loss, the artery is incised sufficiently to allow insertion of the catheter. The catheter is passed proximad in the aorta to the level of the junction of the first and second lumbar vertebrae.[77] Fluoroscopy or radiography can aid positioning of the catheter. The ligatures around the femoral artery are tied to avoid blood loss. With the cat in ventrodorsal recumbency, 6 ml organic iodine contrast agent are injected into the catheter as quickly as possible and a radiograph is obtained immediately after the injection. The injection may be repeated if necessary. When radiography is completed, the arterial incision may be sutured. If difficulty is encountered, the artery may be ligated since collateral circulation to the hindlimb is sufficient to allow the femoral artery to be sacrificed.

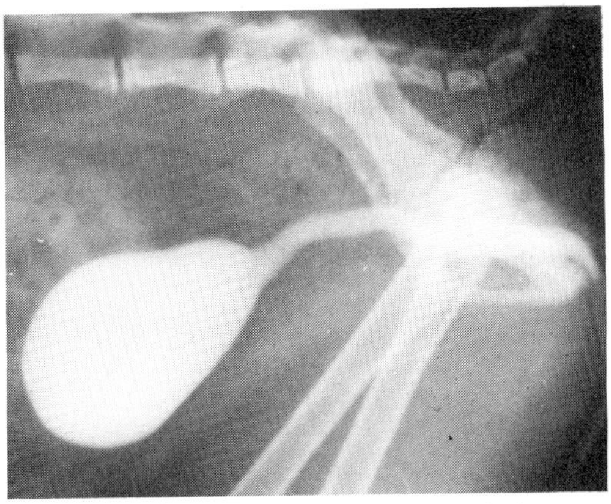

Fig 3. Retrograde cystogram of a cat with contrast medium in the urinary bladder and urethra. The feline bladder is situated cranial to the pelvic brim. The long, wide pelvic and abdominal urethra is seen tapering caudad.

Renal Biopsy

Biopsy of the kidney is a valuable technic for the nephrologist. Useful information concerning cause, pathogenesis, prognosis and therapy can be obtained in this way. Although the procedure is not innocuous, hundreds of renal biopsies have been performed on dogs and cats at the University of Georgia Veterinary Hospital without a fatality.[78] The technic can be performed more quickly and with greater ease in cats than in dogs because both kidneys can be immobilized in most cats by abdominal palpation.[79]

Biopsy of a kidney may be indicated for a variety of reasons. It has most value in assessment of renal disease that has not progressed to the stage at which the kidneys are small and shrunken (end stage). Biopsy of end-stage kidneys currently has limited value because examination of tissue usually does not reveal the cause and the lesions are so advanced that they are irreversible. When it is questionable whether kidneys are shrunken or when renal disease is present and the kidneys are normal or increased in size, biopsy should be considered.

The cat's blood-clotting ability should be evaluated preoperatively with a few simple procedures. The PCV should be determined and a blood smear examined for platelets. The number of platelets can be quickly estimated by examining a blood smear on which a drop of new methylene blue stain has been placed. The clotting properties of the blood and tendency to hemorrhage can be evaluated at the time blood is drawn for the PCV determination and blood smear. If available, an activated coagulation time determination may be used to evaluate intrinsic clotting mechanisms.

An ultrashort-acting general anesthetic agent is most convenient for the biopsy procedure. With all equipment available and the biopsy site prepared for surgery, a bolus IV injection of thiamylal sodium allows sufficient time for the biopsy and allows recovery of the cat from anesthesia within 10-15 minutes. Biopsy may be conducted in patients that are poor anesthetic risks with sedation and infiltration of the abdominal wall with local anesthetic. Ketamine should be used cautiously in an azotemic patient because it is excreted via the urine and narcolepsis may be prolonged.

Either aspiration or punch biopsy can be performed. An aspiration biopsy is easier to perform and may be advantageous when a renal cyst,

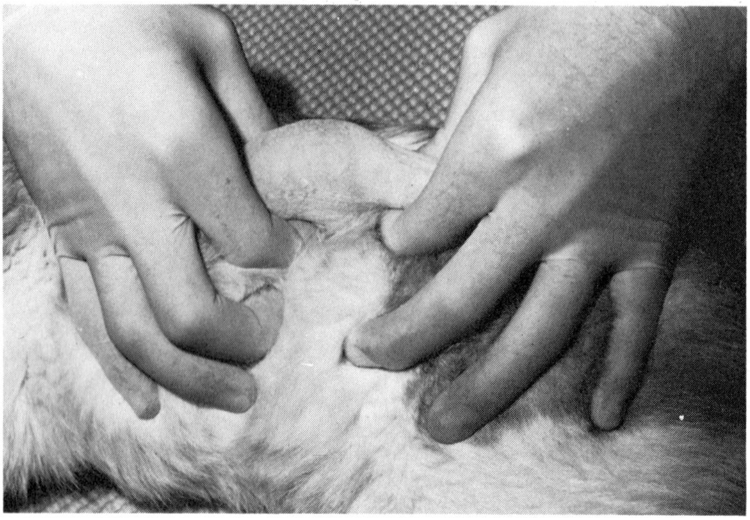

Fig 4. Immobilizing the left kidney of a cat. For biopsy, the kidney must be firmly immobilized to procure an adequate specimen and to avoid unnecessary trauma.

abscess, diffuse infection or metastatic neoplasm is suspected. The small-gauge needle used for aspiration biopsy minimizes the chance for dissemination of infectious agents and production of hemorrhage. However, samples obtained by aspiration biopsy are inferior to those obtained by punch biopsy because the architecture of the renal parenchyma cannot be evaluated.

A specimen can be aspirated with a 6-ml disposable syringe and 1½ inch, 22-gauge disposable spinal needle. After preparing the surgical site, the kidney is grasped and brought to a position just beneath the skin (Fig 4). Reliable immobilization of the kidney is imperative for all biopsy procedures and biopsy should not be attempted without it. A 2-mm incision in the overlying skin facilitates insertion of the spinal needle and helps avoid sudden overpenetration of the needle into the kidney. After the needle has been inserted into the kidney, an assistant removes the needle stylus, attaches the syringe, and slowly aspirates a specimen. The needle is then withdrawn and digital pressure is maintained on the biopsy site for 3 minutes to control hemorrhage. The material obtained is examined with conventional cytologic and laboratory tech-

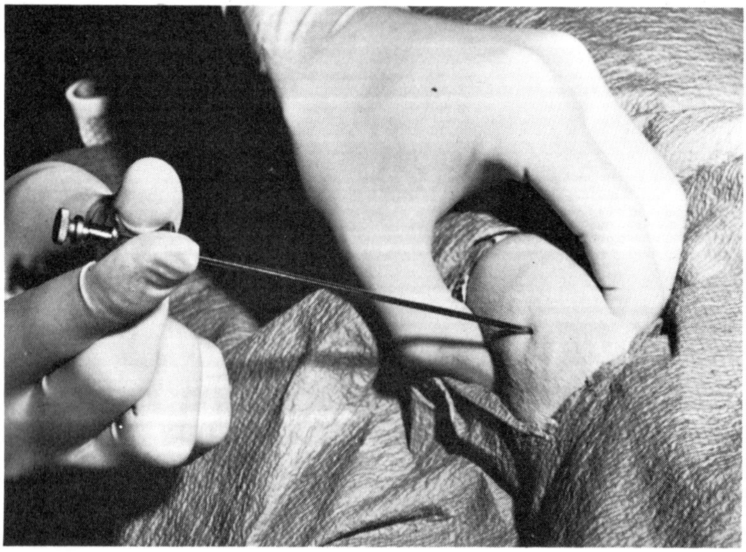

Fig 5. The biopsy needle is inserted through the abdominal wall and the kidney is grasped and positioned for the biopsy procedure.

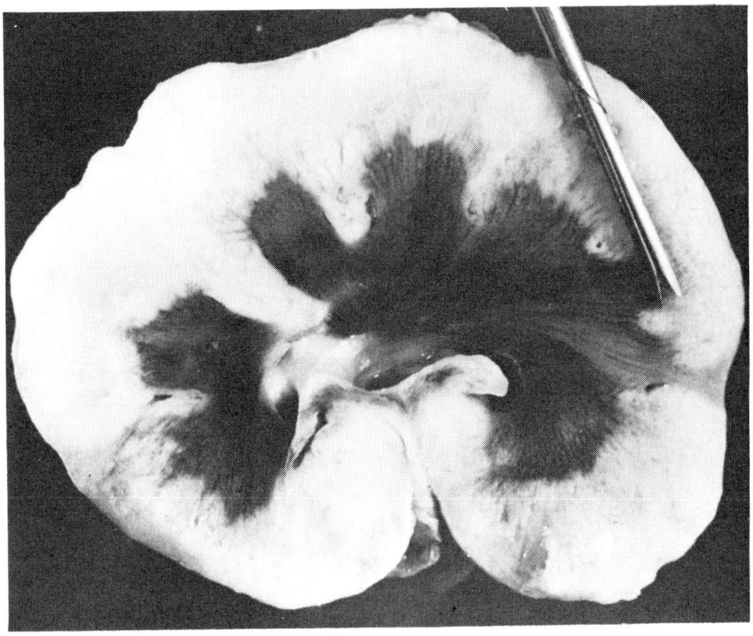

Fig 6. Acceptable position of the biopsy needle. Notice that the cortex has not been overpenetrated and that the needle is directed away from the renal pelvis and vessels.

nics. Pieces of parenchyma large enough for histologic examination are usually not obtained by aspiration.

The punch biopsy provides a superior specimen for examination and an effort should be made to use this method whenever possible. We have used both the Franklin-modified Vim-Silverman needle (Mueller) and the Travenol Tru-Cut needle (Baxter Laboratories) for biopsy of cat kidneys. The latter is manufactured as a disposable instrument but may be used up to 6 times if handled carefully and sterilized with ethylene oxide. To perform the biopsy, the kidney is grasped through the abdominal wall and immobilized. The biopsy site within the kidney can be selected through detection of focal abnormalities by palpation or radiography. If no specific location for biopsy can be determined, the specimen should be taken from either pole rather than the middle of the kidney to avoid the pelvis and renal vessels. A small nick is made in the skin overlying the area of the kidney selected for biopsy. The kidney is released and the biopsy needle is inserted through the abdominal wall. The kidney is again grasped and brought into position under the needle (Fig 5). A common error in biopsy is to overpenetrate the kidney with the needle. If this occurs, the specimen may consist of only medullary tissue. If it is not imperative to have medullary tissue, the needle can be directed so it courses parallel to the kidney surface within the cortex (Fig 6).

With both types of needles, the cutting portion is quickly thrust into the kidney while the kidney and outer cannula remain stationary. It is usually most convenient for the clinician to immobilize the kidney and place the outer cannula in position, and to have an assistant thrust the cutting prongs into the kidney. Once the cutting thrust has been made, the assistant holds the cutting portion stationary while the clinician brings the outer cannula over the cutting prongs (Fig 7). The assistant must be careful that the cutting prongs do not move in or out of the kidney during this procedure. If the Vim-Silverman needle is used, the cutting prongs can be marked to indicate when the needle has been advanced enough to free the specimen, and thus avoid overpenetration.[80]

The specimen should be gently removed from the needle and fixed in 10% buffered formalin in preparation for histologic examination. If neoplasia is suspected, impression smears may be made by touching the specimen to a glass slide prior to formalin fixation. The slide can be examined after staining it with new methylene blue. After removing the biopsy specimen aseptically, the needle is swirled in liquid culture medium if a culture is desired.

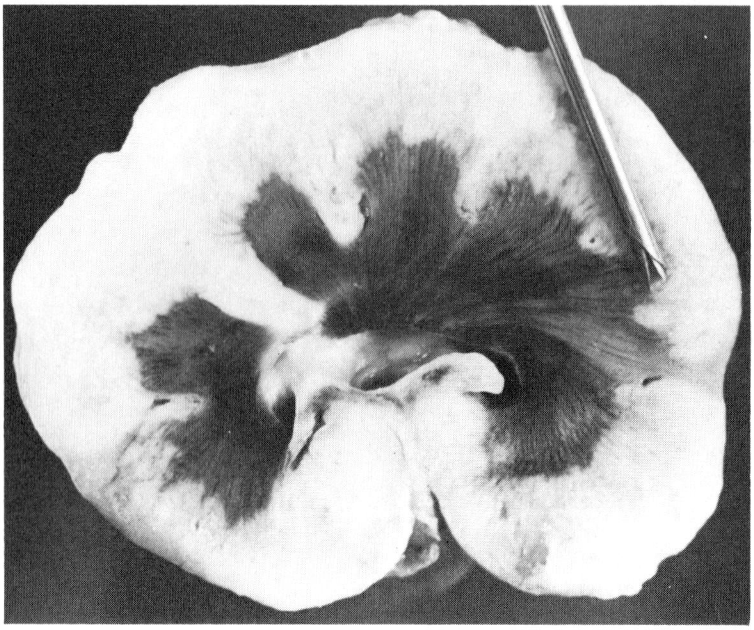

Fig 7. The cutting prongs have been thrust into the kidney. The outer cannula and kidney must remain immobilized when the prongs are inserted.

After the biopsy instrument has been removed, the kidney is grasped and digital pressure is applied over the renal biopsy site for 3 minutes to control hemorrhage. The vital signs are monitored for 2 hours postoperatively because the most common complication of biopsy is hemorrhage. Microscopic hematuria for 1-3 days is common, but gross hematuria is infrequent. In one series, 6 of 10 biopsy specimens from cats contained transitional epithelium, indicating penetration of the renal pelvis; one cat developed a degree of hydronephrosis due to a blood clot in the renal pelvis.[81] Diuresis is therefore recommended after renal biopsy to increase urine flow and minimize the chance of clot formation in the renal pelvis. In 13 consecutive biopsies on 10 cats at the University of Georgia, complications were restricted to the presence of transitional epithelium in one specimen.

Complications in biopsy are usually due to inexperience of the surgeon. Therefore, the technic should be practiced on cadavers prior to use on live animals.

A limitation of all biopsy procedures is the small size of the specimen obtained. In diffuse disease, adequate tissue is usually obtained; however, if the lesion is localized, it may not be included in the biopsy sample. This limitation is minor because renal disease is frequently generalized prior to its recognition.

RENAL DISEASE AND RENAL FAILURE

Pathophysiology

An understanding of renal pathophysiology is essential for clinical management of renal dysfunction. Unfortunately, few studies have been conducted in cats to determine if renal response to injury in this species is the same as in people and dogs. Some of the following discussion is an extrapolation of information obtained from studies of other species and may require modification as more data are accumulated. This subject has been reviewed in recent publications; only clinically significant points are discussed.[63,82,83]

Disease vs Failure: Renal disease is a general term used to indicate deviations of renal function from normal. The disease may or may not be of significance because a renal reserve capacity exists, and a nonprogressive lesion affecting a minority of nephrons may not adversely affect the patient.

Renal disease may be detected during necropsy. Although this information is valuable in documenting the incidence and types of spontaneous diseases, observations at necropsy cannot be interpreted as an indication of the incidence of clinically significant renal disease in the same proportion of living cats of that age. The statement that "most old cats have renal disease" may be true on a histologic basis but is usually not true in terms of clinical relevance.

Renal failure and uremia refer to clinical signs caused by inadequate renal function. In this discussion, the term renal failure is used to encompass signs from the earliest (polydipsia, polyuria) until death. The term uremia is reserved for cases in which the more profound signs (vomiting, depression, anorexia, weight loss) are present. Signs due to renal failure do not occur until two-thirds of renal tissue or more are nonfunctional. Therefore, in slowly developing abnormalities, a cat may have renal lesions for a prolonged period prior to the onset of signs.

Pathogenesis of Uremia: Uremia may be induced by any cause of impaired renal function. The kidneys may or may not be primarily involved because they depend on adequate perfusion to perform their functions and they also depend on adequate urine outflow to eliminate nitrogenous waste from the body. When uremia or azotemia is present, it is imperative that causes of impaired renal perfusion (prerenal) and causes of urine outflow impairment (postrenal) be considered, as well as primary renal disease.

A common cause of prerenal azotemia is severe dehydration. Cardiovascular abnormalities, leading to decreased renal blood flow, may also cause prerenal azotemia. Causes of marked protein catabolism may elevate BUN levels because of increased generation of urea.

Common causes of postrenal azotemia are urethral obstruction and rupture of the urinary bladder. If prerenal and postrenal causes of azotemia are quickly corrected, normal renal function ensues. More prolonged impairment can cause irreversible kidney damage. Renal ischemia induced by clamping the renal artery for 4 hours results in irreversible ischemic nephrosis. Unilateral complete ureteral obstruction results in hydronephrosis. If the obstruction is removed within 4 weeks, sufficient renal function is salvaged to sustain life if the contralateral kidney is removed. After 4 weeks of obstruction, insufficient tissue remains to sustain life after contralateral nephrectomy.

Acute vs Chronic Disease: In this discussion, acute renal disease refers to that present for days to a few weeks, and chronic disease to that present for months to years. This is related to the duration of time subsequent to renal insult; it cannot invariably be related to the duration implied by the owner because renal disease can be insidious and undetected for long periods.

It is important to establish whether the renal impairment is acute or chronic to provide a prognosis. A patient with acute renal disease may be presented with azotemia prior to onset of any morphologic compensatory mechanisms and prior to the time that damage to nephrons has been repaired. In cats with acute renal disease, a potential exists for repair and resumption of normal or nearly normal renal function. As compensatory mechanisms have not been mobilized, some improvement can be anticipated with their advent in uninjured nephrons, even if injured nephrons cannot be repaired.

In contrast, a cat with chronic renal disease has had time for compensatory mechanisms to operate before signs of uremia appear. In fact, the patient with chronic irreversible renal failure has exhausted its compensatory mechanisms by the time uremia develops.[84] Any improvement in clinical status thereafter reflects an effect of extrarenal factors rather than parenchymal rejuvenation.

The course of chronic renal failure in cats is usually characterized by a progressive decrease in functional renal mass, manifested clinically by polydipsia, azotemia and then uremia. Exacerbation of signs does not imply sudden destruction of parenchyma, nor does remission of signs imply renal parenchymal hypertrophy or repair. Exacerbation of signs usually is associated with extrarenal factors (water deprivation leading to dehydration and poor renal perfusion, tissue catabolism associated with stress, slowly developing acid-base and electrolyte deviations), and remission of signs accompanies correction of these extrarenal factors. The terms "uncompensated" and "compensated" chronic renal failure are erroneous if used to imply that the appearance or disappearance of clinical signs is due to alterations in renal function that are primarily renal in origin.

Response to Injury: The kidney has limited ability to respond to injury. Some functional responses are observed within hours of injury, but most morphologic responses require weeks. Therefore, as a generality, response to injury (*ie,* compensatory hypertrophy) is associated more with chronic renal failure than with acute failure. The subsequent discussion applies predominantly to chronic failure.

Since the number of nephrons is fixed with maturation of the kidney during the first few

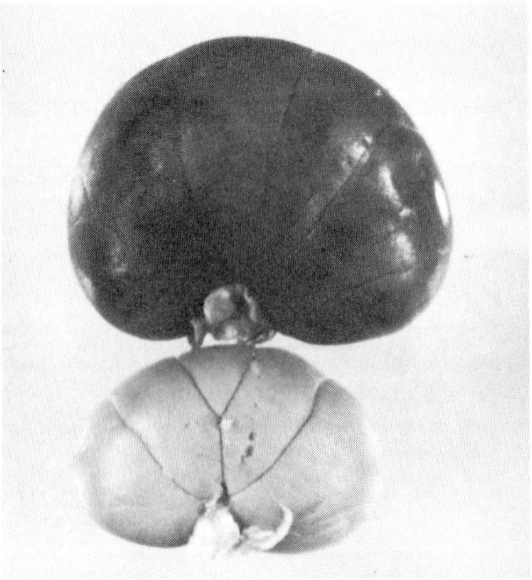

Fig 8. Renal compensatory hypertrophy. The smaller kidney, removed from a normal cat, was histologically normal. The larger kidney, also histologically normal, was obtained at necropsy of the same cat 3 months later.

weeks of life, compensatory mechanisms involve increased activity of existing nephrons rather than formation of new ones. Damage to tubules may be repaired if the tubular basement membrane remains intact. If some nephrons are lost because of disease, residual nephrons respond by hypertrophy and altered activity. The glomerular filtration rate of individual residual nephrons increases so that the whole-organ glomerular filtration rate, although subnormal, is greater than before hypertrophy. The tubular activity of residual nephrons is likewise altered so that body content of water and electrolytes remains normal until the late stages of renal failure. For example, tubules of residual nephrons resorb less Na, Cl and P but secrete more K and hydrogen ions than they did when a normal complement of nephrons existed.

Kidney size is variably altered by injury and response to injury. Depending on the degree of injury (*ie,* the number of nephrons destroyed) and its type, kidney size may increase, remain the same or decrease. A normal kidney increases in size when the opposite one has undergone severe damage (Fig 8). In injured kidneys, size is often determined by the balance between contraction associated with fibrosis and the increase in size associated with hypertrophy of residual nephrons.

Signs of Renal Disease

Renal disease usually escapes detection until signs of failure appear. Exceptions to this generalization may occur when increase in kidney size may be noticed by the owner or detected during physical examination, or when such abnormalities as gross hematuria are noted. Although urinalysis may reveal WBC, blood or protein that may be of renal origin, the lower urinary and genital tracts must be considered potential sources because they are more frequently responsible for these findings than are renal diseases. The persistent presence of urinary casts is reliable evidence of renal disease. Pain referable to the kidneys or ureters may occur with stretching of the renal capsule or distension of a ureter. Pain should be considered of renal origin only when manifested as the kidneys are palpated. Pain elicited by palpation of the vertebral column is usually not renal in origin. Chronic renal disease is not accompanied by evidence of renal pain. The BUN or serum creatinine levels may be elevated in the absence of clinical signs. One must rule out prerenal and postrenal causes of azotemia in such patients before diagnosing primary renal disease.

Signs of Renal Failure

Renal failure is characterized by a predictable group of signs that occur regardless of cause of failure. These signs include depression, anorexia and vomiting. Polyuria may be present with acute or chronic primary renal failure; oliguria or anuria may exist with acute failure, terminal chronic failure, prerenal azotemia or outflow obstruction. "Uremic breath" has been described in people and probably occurs in cats; it is associated with respiratory excretion of dimethyl and trimethyl amines.[85] Chronic renal failure may be associated with mucosal pallor due to nonregenerative anemia; decreased bone density may be associated with renal secondary hyperparathyroidism. The presence and duration of certain findings are helpful in assessing the duration of the disease and may aid in categorizing the disease as acute or chronic (Table 1).

Contrary to some old ideas, the specific gravity of urine is not a valid criterion for differentiating acute and chronic renal disease. Urine may be of low specific gravity in either acute or chronic disease. In addition, the urine can be moderately

Table 1. Observations That May Aid in Differentiating Acute and Chronic Renal Failure*

Observation	Acute	Chronic
History of chronic weight loss	No	Frequent
History of chronic polydipsia, polyuria	No	Frequent
Nonregenerative anemia	No	Frequent
Renal secondary hyperparathyroidism (clinical)	No	Occasional
Decrease in kidney size	No	Frequent
Increase in kidney size	Variable	Unusual
Low specific gravity of urine	Frequent	Frequent
Renal casts	Variable	Variable
WBC in urine	Variable	Variable

* Signs described may have causes other than renal failure; the clinician must consider the possibility of coexisting unrelated diseases.

concentrated in chronic failure, making differentiation of the latter from prerenal azotemia difficult.

Progression of Renal Failure

Renal failure is often progressive, even when known causes have been removed or when no cause is apparent. Studies in rats suggested that progression of renal failure depended on mineral imbalances associated with the disease.[86] Renal mineralization was responsible for deterioration of renal function and restricting P intake prevented progression of renal failure. It is not clear if these phenomena are related to renal secondary hyperparathyroidism since renal tissue content of minerals during uremia does not seem related to parathormone levels in dogs.[87] Some experimental studies in cats made azotemic by reduction of renal mass suggested that renal mineralization occurred when dietary P levels were not restricted.[88] Cats on a P-restricted diet had minor changes in plasma parathormone levels, while cats on a higher-P diet had marked increases in plasma parathormone levels.[78] The implications of these findings in the conservative management of renal failure in the cat are subsequently discussed.

Causes of Renal Disease

Several causes of renal disease are known but it is likely that a greater number have yet to be found. The clinician frequently deals with cats with chronic renal failure in which the cause cannot be determined despite exhaustive diagnostic efforts. In those instances, therapy is symptomatic. Although such therapy may be beneficial, a more logical and effective treatment includes elimination of the underlying cause. Knowledge of the cause also aids in prognosis and provides the opportunity to establish prophylactic procedures.

Congenital Defects

Renal agenesis, polycystic kidneys, fused (horseshoe) kidneys, and dystopia have been reported, and there are textbook references to renal hypoplasia and vascular anomalies. The causes of these abnormalities have not been elucidated. Although there is evidence of inherited renal disease in people and dogs, only in the case of polycystic disease is an inherited or familial tendency described in cats. In addition to inherited factors, renal development in other species has been affected by prenatal infection, drugs and chemicals.

The clinical detection and significance of developmental renal disease depend on several factors. Unilateral disease may be undetected or an incidental finding. With severe unilateral disease, the contralateral kidney may undergo compensatory hypertrophy, which should not be confused with disease.

Agenesis: Renal agenesis (aplasia) in cats has been reported.[89-106] Although there are insufficient data to indicate whether a sex difference in prevalence exists, most reported cases have been in females. Other developmental defects in the urogenital tract often accompany renal agenesis because the urinary and genital tracts have common or adjacent embryologic origins. The presence of multiple abnormalities suggests that the defect may have been initiated early in

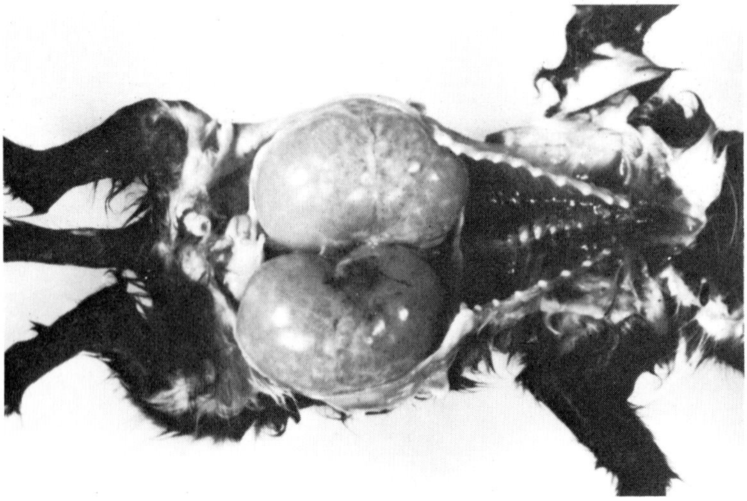

Fig 9. Enlarged polycystic kidneys from a young cat with familial polycystic disease.

embryologic development, prior to differentiation of tissues.

The most common defect associated with renal aplasia is abnormal development of the uterus or ductus deferens. For inapparent reasons, about 3 times as many abnormalities have been found on the right side as on the left. The adrenal gland and gonad on the affected side have been missing in a few cats. Although the adrenals and gonads develop independently from the kidney, ureter and genital ductal system, the origin of all these structures is contiguous.

A study of developmental renal abnormalities in Beagles indicated that complete absence due to agenesis was erroneously assumed, when in fact careful examination revealed the presence of remnants of renal tissue.[107] The presence of renal tissue remnants is called dysgenesis. Not all cats with presumed renal agenesis have been examined in sufficient detail to exclude the possibility of dysgeneses.

Although bilateral renal agenesis in cats has not been reported, some neonatal mortalities may result from this condition. Unilateral agenesis is compatible with life as long as adequate functional tissue is present in the remaining kidney. Hypertrophy of the remaining kidney usually occurs as a compensatory mechanism. Unilateral agenesis may be discovered in cats with renal failure due to disease of the remaining kidney. When uterine dysplasia is found during ovariohysterectomy, the patient should be examined for renal aplasia or dysgenesis.

Cysts: Isolated cases of polycystic kidneys in cats have been reported;[108-114] a familial episode also was documented.[115] Renal cysts in the young or newborn, or cysts in kidney and other parenchymal structures, such as the liver, are highly suggestive of developmental anomalies.

In this juvenile form of disease, extreme abdominal enlargement because of increased kidney size may be a prominent sign, while in adult cats only moderate kidney enlargement has been reported (Fig 9).

Histologic studies in human cases do not support the theory that cysts are due to a simple failure of fusion of the metanephric ductal system with the nephrogenic mass.[116] The pathogenesis of congenital cyst formation remains controversial.[117]

Acquired cysts probably develop from obstruction of tubules with exudate or obstruction associated with interstitial inflammation or connective tissue deposition. Differentiation of acquired and hereditary renal cystic disease may be difficult or impossible in individual patients because genealogic studies are required. Polycystic disease with a known hereditary basis occurs in children as an autosomal recessive trait and in adult people as an autosomal dominant. The disease is usually bilateral but may develop at different rates in each kidney.[117]

The clinical significance of renal cysts depends on the degree of parenchymal damage associated with the disease. With generalized involvement, the decrease in function may result in uremia; a few small cysts may cause no clinical signs. Kidneys that are markedly enlarged because of cysts can be palpated. Massive cysts or infection associated with cysts may require surgical re-

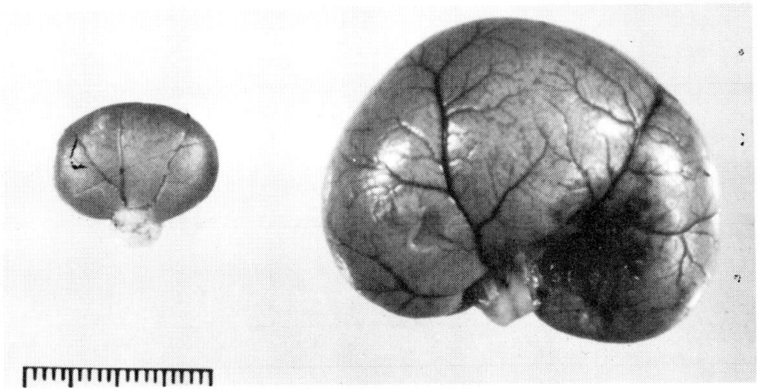

Fig 10. Two kidneys from the same cat. The small kidney could have shrunken due to disease. However, the cortex was smooth and uniform, the capsule was nonadherent and histologic changes were minimal. This kidney may have been hypoplastic. The opposite kidney was histologically normal and enlarged due to compensatory hypertrophy.

moval of the kidney but the primary concern of the clinician should be preservation of functional renal tissue. Unilateral nephrectomy should be performed only after careful evaluation of the other kidney's function and exhaustion of more conservative forms of therapy.

Capsular or capsulogenic cysts in cats have also been described.[118-121] Technically these structures are pseudocysts since epithelial lining is absent. Affected animals had massive abdominal enlargement and the cyst enveloped the kidney. Although the pathogenesis of these cysts is unknown, acquired or congenital obstruction of the capsular veins or lymphatics, or urine leakage may be involved. The kidney may be otherwise normal or abnormal. The cyst and involved kidney were excised in one cat, which became uremic 3 months later and was euthanized. If it is not infected, the cyst should be incised widely and sutured to the abdominal wall to establish constant drainage of fluid into the abdominal cavity. This procedure may prevent pressure necrosis of the kidney by the surrounding cyst and preserve renal function.

Fusion: Fusion of the kidneys is presumed to be due to compression of primitive tissues by the umbilical arteries during ascent of the kidneys from the pelvis;[122] it occurs occasionally in cats.[123-125] The fusion in cats usually occurs caudad, with a band of renal parenchyma or fibrous connective tissue connecting the kidneys. Fused kidneys may not ascend from the pelvis to the normal abdominal location, they may not rotate normally (the convex surface is dorsal initially but rotates to become lateral in the newborn), they may retain fetal lobulation, and they may be displaced to one side of the abdominal cavity.[122] No data are available concerning the clinical significance of fused kidneys in cats. About 40% of affected people eventually have complications; external trauma, ureteral obstruction associated with angulation of the ureters as they leave the kidney, abdominal pain, and pyelonephritis have been reported.[121]

Other Defects: Other defects in other species have been reported less frequently or have not been reported in cats. A singular pelvic kidney in a cat has been reported.[126] This defect apparently results from failure of cranial migration. Congenital renal ectopia (abnormal location) in people is thought to be due to anomalous vascular attachment.[122]

Renal hypoplasia has been considered a congenital anomaly in cats, but documentation of this abnormality is difficult because of confusion with unilateral or bilateral end-stage renal disease. Merely finding small kidneys is not justification for a diagnosis of congenital renal hypoplasia inasmuch as acquired unilateral or bilateral renal disease is known to cause "shrunken kidneys" (Fig 10). In hypoplasia, the kidney is small but has essentially normal parenchyma and a patent ureter; the cells may be smaller than normal, with a greatly reduced number of nephrons.[122] Hypoplastic kidneys in people are reported to be subject to secondary infection, and differentiation from atrophic pyelonephritis is difficult.

Vascular anomalies of the kidney are apparently rare in cats. There is less variation in renal vasculature in cats than in dogs.

Renal and Ureteral Trauma

The kidneys of the cat may be injured by blunt trauma and occasionally by penetrating wounds.[127,128] Multiple injuries may accompany renal trauma. The superficial capsular vessels of the feline kidney may enhance the chances

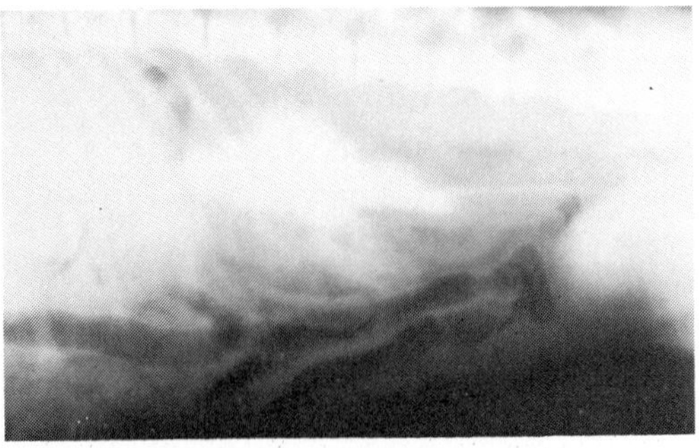

Fig 11. Lateral radiograph taken after IV injection of radiopaque contrast material. Material has accumulated in the abdominal cavity because of ureteral rupture.

of subcapsular hematoma in this species, and the loose attachment of the kidneys to the body wall makes retroperitoneal hemorrhage less likely than in dogs. This mobility of the cat's kidneys may reduce the chance of injury.

The degree of renal trauma and signs referable to trauma are variable. Rupture of major vessels leads to death in minutes by exsanguination. Rupture of the renal capsule may result in hemorrhage into the abdominal cavity. Abdominocentesis should be performed when traumatized patients are in shock; aspiration of blood in patients unresponsive to fluid replacement indicates the need for immediate laparotomy. Damage to the kidney without capsular rupture may result in restriction of the hemorrhage to the subcapsular site or infiltration of blood around the renal pedicle and into the retroperitoneal area. Such hematomas may be palpable; their size should be evaluated periodically to aid in determining if hemorrhage is continuing. Depending on the severity of injury, hematuria may be present.

Damage to the renal pelvis or ureter may result in escape of urine into the abdominal cavity or retroperitoneal area. Hypertonic urine can cause a tissue reaction, leading to gradual increase in the size of a retroperitoneal mass over a period of days.

Diagnosis of urine leakage frequently requires a radiographic examination (Fig 11). An excretory urogram can confirm the presence of leakage and aid in its location.[129,130] Angiograms may be helpful in assessing the effects of trauma on renal vasculature and the parenchyma.

Subcapsular hematoma generally is not an indication for surgical intervention because resolution usually occurs, with good preservation of renal function. With capsular rupture and lacerations and contusions of the kidney, the degree dictates the need for materials to aid hemostasis (oxidized regenerated cellulose, Gelfoam), partial nephrectomy or nephrectomy. Before nephrectomy is performed, the contralateral kidney should be examined for assurance of adequate functional renal parenchyma.

Sequelae to renal trauma include hydronephrosis due to outflow blockage by blood clots or strictures, renal infarction and atrophy due to impairment of circulation, and perirenal abscesses and fistulas associated with leakage of urine. Serial radiographic examinations may aid in evaluating the patient.[129]

Primary Renal Neoplasia

Primary neoplasms of the feline kidney are rare. A recent literature review of 43 cases included 19 carcinomas, 9 nephroblastomas, 8 sarcomas, 2 undifferentiated neoplasms, 3 transitional-cell carcinomas and 2 adenomas.[131]

Until more data are accumulated, conclusions concerning the biologic behavior of primary renal neoplasms in cats are tentative. Metastases have been reported.[132,133]

A primary neoplasm should be considered when an enlarged kidney is palpable. However, the much higher incidence of metastatic neoplasms and hydronephrosis as a cause of kidney enlargement should be kept in mind.

In view of the potential for metastasis of primary renal neoplasms, a thorough physical examination and radiography of the thorax should be performed prior to surgical intervention. The abdominal organs should be examined carefully during laparotomy.

For renal carcinoma in people, radical excision of the tumor offers the best hope for cure. Chemotherapy has not been highly rewarding, although testosterone and progesterone reportedly cause tumor regression. Treatment of nephroblastomas in people by combining nephrectomy, postoperative radiation and use of actinomycin D has been fairly successful. The prognosis is apparently better if the neoplasm is more highly differentiated.

Removal of a nephroblastoma in a cat was complicated by postcaval occlusion.[134] In this patient and in 4 normal cats, however, there was immediate adaptation to sudden total occlusion of the postcava between the renal veins and the liver. The vertebral veins apparently provide adequate collateral circulation. This suggests that more radical surgical procedures may be possible with renal vein involvement inasmuch

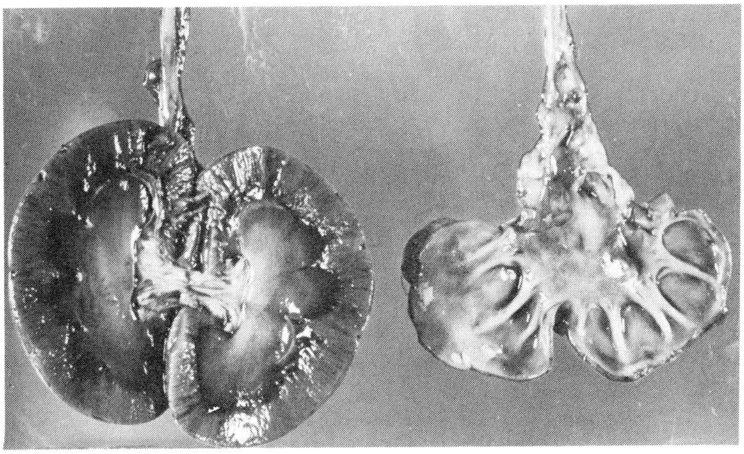

Fig 12. Unilateral hydronephrosis in a cat. Life was sustained by the normal kidney (left), while massive parenchymal destruction occurred in the affected kidney.

as postcaval patency in this area need not be maintained.

Hydronephrosis

Hydronephrosis refers to dilation of renal pelves subsequent to impairment of urine outflow from the kidneys. Depending on the duration and severity of outflow impairment, the kidney may undergo mild reversible pelvic dilation, enlargement of the collecting system and permanent destruction of variable quantities of renal parenchyma, or renal atrophy that could be mistaken for hypoplasia.[135,136]

When the involvement is bilateral, the degree of hydronephrosis is limited because uremia develops and death occurs before parenchymal destruction is severe. When the obstruction is unilateral, hydronephrosis may progress to the point where functional parenchyma cannot be found in the affected kidney (Fig 12).

Impaired urine outflow is usually due to partial or total mechanical obstruction. Congenital abnormalities that are obstructive include torsion, kinking, stenosis or atresia of the ureters or urethra and aberrant renal vessels that constrict the ureters.[63] Acquired causes of hydronephrosis include ureteral and urethral masses (neoplastic or non-neoplastic), calculi, and iatrogenic complications of ovariohysterectomy.[63] Besides mechanical obstruction, ureteral aperistalsis should be considered a cause of hydroureter and hydronephrosis.

In the reported cases of hydronephrosis in cats, the cause was not always apparent.[137-146] Enlargement of the abdomen was a consistent sign. Fever, leukocytosis and pyuria occasionally were present, indicating coexistent bacterial infection. Abdominal radiographs frequently reveal a cranial abdominal mass. Excretory urograms may fail to reveal excretion of contrast media in kidneys with minimal perfusion but disclose dilated collecting systems in cases of lesser impairment (Fig 13). When the diagnosis is in doubt, aspiration biopsy can be performed.

Treatment of hydronephrosis is directed at removing the underlying cause. Depending on the duration and degree of obstruction, functional renal tissue may or may not be salvaged. In experimental dogs subjected to unilateral total ureteral obstruction for as long as 4 weeks, there was resumption of some ipsilateral renal

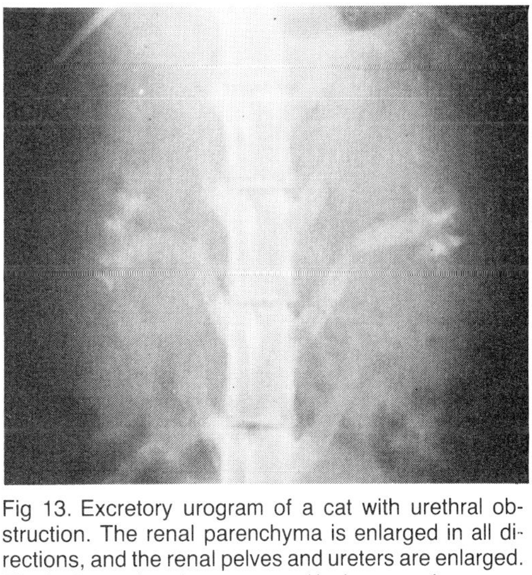

Fig 13. Excretory urogram of a cat with urethral obstruction. The renal parenchyma is enlarged in all directions, and the renal pelves and ureters are enlarged. The hydronephrosis was caused by increased pressure following urethral obstruction.

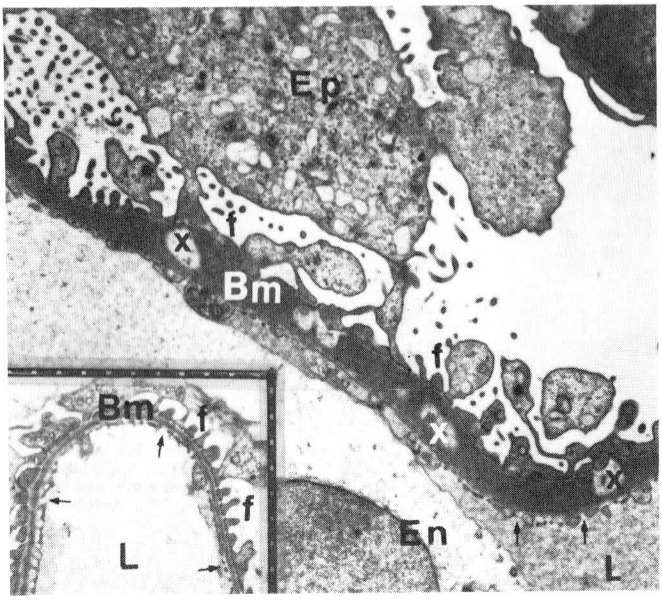

Fig 14. Electron micrographs of glomerular capillaries of a normal cat (insert) and of a cat with glomerulonephritis, taken at the same magnification. Portions of an epithelial cell (Ep) and its foot processes (f), an endothelial cell (En), pores in the endothelial cell cytoplasm (arrows), the basement membrane (Bm) and capillary lumen (L) are visualized. Note that the basement membrane in the diseased glomerulus is thickened and has holes associated with dense deposits (x). Foot processes are altered over some parts of the diseased glomerulus.

function; in one experiment it was sufficient to sustain life when the contralateral kidney was removed.[147-150] This suggests that moderate hydronephrosis does not necessarily mean that the kidney can no longer function; efforts should be made to salvage the organ. In severe hydronephrosis, when only a shell of nonfunctional tissue remains, nephrectomy may be indicated to relieve associated signs. It is imperative, however, to evaluate the contralateral kidney first. Compensatory hypertrophy of the opposite kidney should not be confused with disease.

Secondary bacterial infection may be associated with hydronephrosis. General principles of antibacterial therapy should be employed and long-term or continuous therapy may be required if the underlying cause of hydronephrosis is not corrected.

Bone has been found in the kidneys of cats with hydronephrosis.[141] This is apparently associated with the ability of transitional epithelium to initiate osteogenesis, and is observed both in other spontaneous diseases and in experimental animals in which transitional epithelium is transplanted to other body sites.[63]

Glomerulonephritis

Spontaneous glomerulonephritis in cats has been reported.[151-162] In other species, glomerulonephritis can be caused by immunologic mechanisms and 2 distinct forms of immunologic disease occur. In one type, antibody is produced against antigens present in glomerular basement membrane (anti-GBM glomerulonephritis). This antibody becomes attached to the basement membrane in a linear, diffuse pattern. The characteristic pattern can be detected by immunofluorescent and electron microscopy.

In the other type, circulating antigen-antibody complexes are deposited within glomerular capillaries, and are particularly prevalent in the basement membrane of the capillary (immune-complex glomerulonephritis). The deposition of these complexes is not related to the antigenicity of the renal tissue, but appears to be a nonspecific entrapment by the basement membrane of the glomerular capillary. Immune complexes are distributed in aggregates (lumpy, bumpy deposits) rather than in a diffuse, linear pattern. These deposits may be visualized in thin section by light microscopy but are more reliably detected by immunofluorescent studies and electron microscopy (Fig 14).

Both types of immune processes stimulate an inflammatory response that is detrimental to the host. Glomerular damage results in marked protein leakage into the glomerular filtrate and urine. Both types of glomerulonephritis occur spontaneously in people but the immune-complex disease is far more prevalent.[157] Only immune-complex glomerulonephritis has been observed in cats, but this may be due to lack of

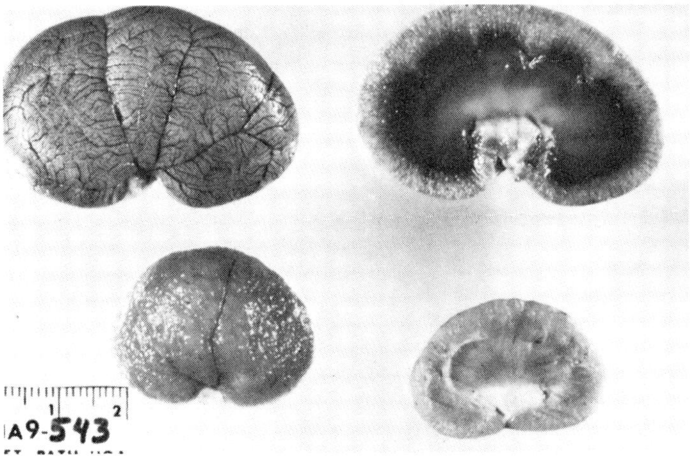

Fig 15. A kidney from a cat with chronic glomerulonephritis (lower) and a kidney from a normal cat of the same size. Contraction and pitting are apparent in the diseased kidney.

comprehensive studies of glomerulonephritis in this species.

Information on the causes of glomerulonephritis is incomplete. Although an immunologic basis exists for both types, the causes of anti-GBM antibody production are speculative. The reason that antigen-antibody reactions cause disease in some patients and not in others may be related to differences in host response to antigen, and to the relative quantities of antigen and antibody. Glomerulonephritis in cats has been reported in association with porphyria, malignant lymphoma and myeloid leukemia, and has been described in cases in which the antigenic stimulus was unknown.[156,160,162] Glomerulonephritis has also accompanied lupus erythematosus in cats.[154,161]

A diagnosis of glomerular disease should be considered if severe proteinuria exists in the absence of WBC, RBC or cellular debris in the urine. Clinical signs may be absent until uremia or the nephrotic syndrome develops. Kidney size varies, depending on the stage of disease (Fig 15). The diagnosis is usually confirmed through light microscopy of renal biopsy specimens.

Treatment of glomerulonephritis is directed toward controlling or removing the primary cause, and providing symptomatic therapy as described in later sections of this chapter.

In some cases in other species, removal of the antigen source causes remission. Glomerulonephritis secondary to lupus erythematosus may subside with suppression of the immunologic reaction with corticosteroids or antimetabolites. However, the benefit of corticosteroids in treatment of other causes of glomerulonephritis is controversial. Inadequate data are available for evaluating treatment of cats with glomerulonephritis because of the low numbers of cases and lack of controlled studies. Two cats with glomerulonephritis survived without treatment, with very slow progression of azotemia and without development of uremia for over a year.[153,154]

Nephrotic Syndrome

The nephrotic syndrome is a combination of alterations caused by proteinuria and hypoproteinemia. The prominent clinical sign is generalized edema (Fig 16). The edema is due to the decrease in colloid osmotic pressure of plasma caused by hypoproteinemia. A plasma albumin concentration of about 1 g/dl is usually associ-

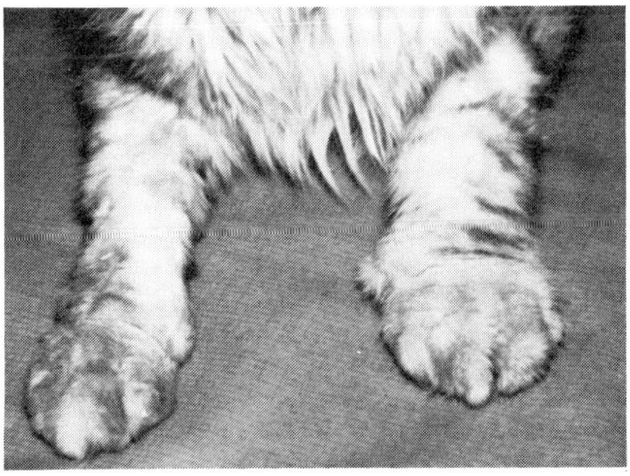

Fig 16. Edema in the left foreleg of a cat with the nephrotic syndrome. Edema is usually symmetric in dependent portions of the body but may be altered by position or other local hemodynamic factors.

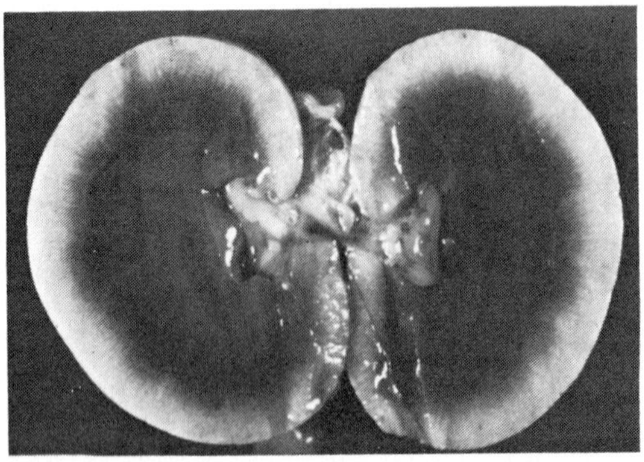

Fig 17. Kidney from a cat that died from ethylene glycol toxicosis. The only gross lesion was pallor of the renal cortex.

ated with edema. For reasons not apparent, the serum cholesterol concentration is markedly elevated. The nephrotic syndrome has occurred in cats with glomerulonephritis.[152,155,158] Several drugs cause profuse proteinuria in people; salicylamide has caused it in cats.[163]

The nephrotic syndrome must be differentiated from other causes of hypoproteinemia, including protein-losing enteropathies and hepatic failure. Proteinuria is absent in the nonrenal diseases.

Cats with the nephrotic syndrome have been treated with corticosteroids and antimetabolites. The efficacy of these drugs varies and probably depends on the underlying cause of the glomerular lesion. Low-Na diets and diuretics (furosemide) aid in controlling the edema. High-protein diets are indicated in the absence of azotemia. In azotemic nephrotic cats, attention must be directed toward alleviating the signs that appear most life-threatening (*ie,* edema vs azotemia).

Chemical and Ischemic Nephrosis

Nephrosis is a degenerative lesion of the renal tubules. Occasional cases of chemical nephrosis in cats have been reported.[153,154] Although ischemic nephrosis has not been documented in cats, clinical impressions suggest that it occurs.

Most nephrotoxic chemicals cause proximal tubular necrosis due to the direct effects of the material's high concentration in the intratubular fluid at that site. Ischemic nephrosis is most likely related to vasospasm and causes patchy lesions throughout the tubules.[63] Numerous causes of renal ischemia (hemorrhage, trauma, anesthesia, profound dehydration, shock, major vascular surgery) are identified in people. Chemical nephrosis due to bismuth, mercury and arsenic may occur iatrogenically, and other heavy metals (lead, thallium, uranium) and glycols have potential nephrotoxicity (Fig 17).[164,165] Several drugs, particularly neomycin, polymyxin B, gentamicin, amphotericin B and kanamycin, have the potential for nephrotoxicity and should be used with caution in azotemic patients.

The history may reveal the likelihood of exposure to a chemical agent. Depending on the severity of injury, anuria or polyuria may be present. In addition to signs of uremia, evidence of neurologic disorder can occur with glycol toxicity; signs of gastroenteritis and hepatic dysfunction may accompany heavy-metal toxicity.[63] The kidneys may be normal in size or enlarged on palpation. Oxalate crystals may or may not be in the urine of cats suffering glycol poisoning. Casts, WBC, RBC and tubular epithelial cells may be in the urine of cats with chemical poisoning. Chemical tests for heavy metals in blood or urine may confirm the diagnosis; renal biopsy may aid in diagnosing glycol poisoning.

Treatment of chemical nephrosis should be primarily directed toward the cause, with secondary consideration given to symptomatic therapy. Textbooks of toxicology should be consulted for antidotes and dosage (also see Chapter 3).

Patients with ischemic nephrosis are treated symptomatically for renal failure. Osmotic diuresis has been helpful in preventing ischemic nephrosis in people undergoing prolonged surgical procedures.

Multisystemic Diseases

In a significant number of diseases that affect the kidneys, disease also occurs in other body systems. In the subsequent discussion, emphasis is placed on those conditions in which renal dysfunction may be sufficiently severe to cause significant clinical signs. Additional information appears in other chapters about these diseases.

Lymphosarcoma: Lymphosarcoma accounts for a third of all feline neoplasms, and the annual incidence was reported as 41.6 cases per 100,000 cats at risk.[166] In one study, the kidney was affected in 31 of 78 cases of lymphosarcoma.[167] In another, renal involvement produced the most prominent clinical signs in 20% of cats with lymphosarcoma.[168,169] Although uremia may not be the cause of death in most cats with lymphosarcoma, mild to moderate azotemia may be present and the signs may be referable to kidney disease. Alterations in the size and shape of the kidneys are frequently detected by physical or radiographic examination.[170-172]

Feline lymphosarcoma is caused by an RNA virus transmitted horizontally and possibly vertically. The mean age of involvement is about 5 years, but over 40% of affected cats are under 3 years. Although lymphatic tissue anywhere in the body may be involved, the neoplasms are frequently predominantly in one of the body cavities. Peripheral lymph node enlargement occurs in only 10-20% of affected cats, and leukemia is not usually present. The signs are referable to organs of major involvement and may vary considerably.

Renal involvement with lymphosarcoma may be either diffuse or focal (Figs 18, 19). Although survey radiographs and excretory urography have been used to delineate the lesions and identify renal masses, similar information often is obtained by abdominal palpation.[170,171] Renal angiography may provide information concerning vascularization of the kidney. Stretching of vessels without neovascularity has been observed after neoplastic infiltration.[172]

Needle aspiration or punch biopsy of the kidney may confirm the diagnosis.[63] Renal biopsy is not contraindicated in lymphosarcoma because neoplastic cells usually are already widely disseminated. Although hypercalcemic nephropathy has been associated with canine lymphosarcoma, it has not been observed in cats.

Amyloidosis: Amyloidosis refers to abnormal deposition of a glycoprotein in several tissues throughout the body. In cats with amyloidosis, renal dysfunction can occur but signs referable to failure of multiple organs may be more significant. In contrast, signs of renal dysfunction predominate in dogs.

Amyloid formation is thought to result from stimulation of reticuloendothelial cells and numerous agents are known to induce amyloidosis.[173] Hypervitaminosis A has been incriminated as a cause of amyloidosis in cats, and their kidneys appear to have a high concentration of vitamin A.[11,174] However, amyloidosis seems more closely associated with alteration of normal immunoglobulin production. A few cases have been diagnosed in cats, but the disease may be overlooked.[173-180]

Renal amyloid deposition is mainly in the renal papilla and outer medulla, but there may be sufficient glomerular involvement to cause proteinuria.[181]

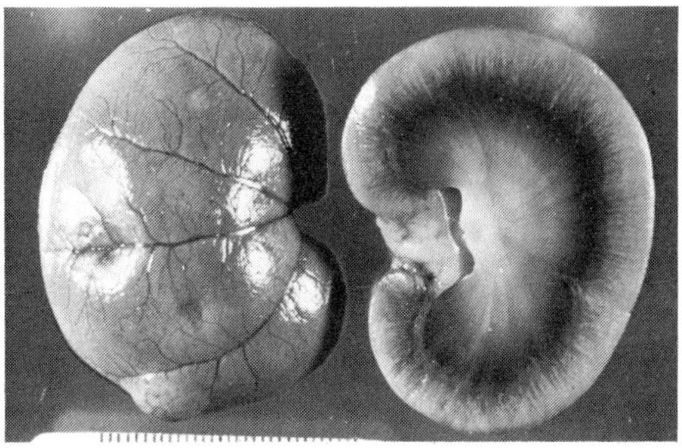

Fig 18. Histologic examination of this kidney revealed diffuse involvement with lymphosarcoma. Direct observation revealed only a circumscribed elevated area at the caudal pole (lower left).

Amyloidosis should be considered if splenomegaly, hepatomegaly, anemia and proteinuria are present. An organ biopsy is helpful in confirming the diagnosis. Unfortunately, other than removal of agents responsible for immunologic stimulation, the treatment is symptomatic.

Polyarteritis Nodosa: This disease has been observed infrequently in cats.[182,183] The disease is characterized by necrotizing arteritis affecting small- and medium-sized arterioles of numerous organs. Fever, anorexia, muscle spasm, stiffness of the extremities, and leukocytosis were observed. In human patients, improvement may occur with corticosteroid therapy.

Feline Infectious Peritonitis: Feline infectious peritonitis is of viral origin and may be accom-

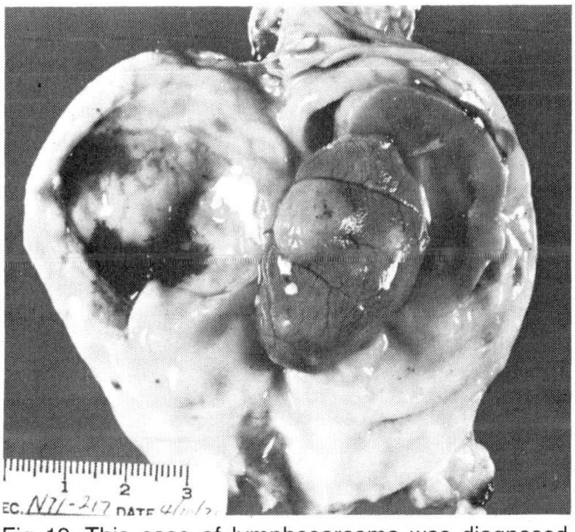

Fig 19. This case of lymphosarcoma was diagnosed histologically. The preponderance of the mass is extrarenal.

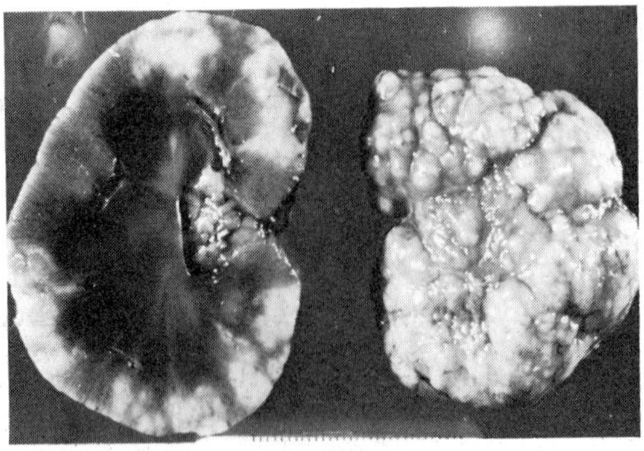

Fig 20. Kidneys from a cat with FIP. Gross inspection cannot distinguish FIP from lymphosarcoma.

panied by a wide variety of signs. Persistent or sporadic fever, weight loss, anemia and ascites are common. Granulomatous reactions may occur in several organs of the body and occasionally there is irregular enlargement of one or both kidneys (Fig 20). Renal biopsy has been performed to help diagnose the condition in cases without typical abdominal effusion. No unique changes have been present in the urine of a limited number of affected cats. The condition seems to occur frequently with lymphosarcoma.

Systemic Lupus Erythematosus: This disease may be associated with immune-complex glomerulonephritis in cats. In dogs, renal failure is frequently responsible for death.[184] Inadequate data are available to evaluate the significance of renal lesions in this disease in cats.

Pyometra: Inability to concentrate urine and morphologic evidence of glomerulonephritis are present in dogs with pyometra.[63] Although unproved, clinical impressions suggest that the same alterations occur in cats. Evidence in dogs indicates that the glomerulonephritis is of the immune-complex type. Although the cause of the urine-concentrating defect has not been definitely established, large doses of *E coli* endotoxin given to experimental dogs caused transient concentrating defects. The disturbance could not be attributed to ADH deficiency, progesterone excess, K depletion, or disturbances in Ca metabolism.[185] The renal lesions of pyometra may heal if ovariohysterectomy is performed and immediate postoperative care is successful.

Diabetes Mellitus: Little information is available concerning renal lesions associated with diabetes mellitus in cats. Amyloid or amyloid-like material has been found in the pancreas and kidneys of affected cats and has been incriminated as the cause of the diabetes.[186,187] Proteinuria was present in one case but absent in others. Nephrosclerosis was present in one affected cat.[186] Glomerulosclerosis, which is characteristic of diabetes in people, has been observed in dogs but has not been documented in cats.[63] Renal disease apparently is not a common complication of diabetes mellitus in cats.

Systemic Mycoses: The kidneys of the cat are occasionally involved in systemic mycoses. Renal failure generally is not a significant aspect of these infections. The nephrotoxic potential of amphotericin B should be considered if it is used for treatment of patients with renal lesions.

Multiple Myeloma: Multiple myeloma is rare in cats.[188,189] It may be accompanied by proteinuria due to permeability of the renal glomeruli to immunoglobulin fragments of low molecular weight. Plasma-cell infiltration of several tissues may occur, but the prevailing view is that renal failure associated with multiple myeloma in people is due to ancillary aspects of the disease, including obstruction of tubules with protein casts and subsequent tubular atrophy, decreased renal blood flow, increased blood viscosity, and hypercalcemia.[190] Because proteinuria is not invariably detected by common laboratory methods in patients with multiple myeloma, its absence does not exclude the disease as a differential diagnosis.

Leptospirosis: In several serologic surveys there have been positive reactions to leptospiral antigens in a small percentage of cats.[191-193] Clinical signs of leptospirosis have not been reported, however. Experimental infection of cats resulted in microscopic renal lesions consistent with acute interstitial nephritis in people and dogs with leptospirosis.[194] In dogs and people, the acute nephritis subsides if the patient survives.[195] Leptospirosis in these species is no longer considered an important cause of chronic renal disease in most parts of the world.[63] There is no evidence that leptospirosis is a cause of chronic renal disease in cats.[196,197]

Chronic Interstitial Nephritis

Renal disease characterized by interstitial connective tissue proliferation and mononuclear cell infiltration occurs in cats.[198-204] Necropsies of cats that died from causes other than renal failure revealed that these changes were present in kidneys in which disease was not markedly advanced. In earlier stages of the disease, glomerular changes were minimal or absent.

The descriptive pathologic term chronic interstitial nephritis has been applied to this renal disease in cats. Use of this term is justified when morphologic evidence of the disease process is obtained, but it has no application in clinical medicine until biopsy or necropsy histologic studies have been performed. Chronic nephritis or end-stage kidney is a more appropriate clinical term.

Although many theories have been proposed for causes of chronic interstitial nephritis in cats, none has been proven. Infection (pyelonephritis, bacterial endocarditis, respiratory infection), renal ischemia, and autoimmune mechanisms have been postulated.[198-204]

End-Stage Kidney

This term refers to kidneys that have undergone fibrosis and decrease in size as a consequence of damage and efforts at repair. At this stage the renal morphology is so distorted that it usually is impossible to accurately assess the pathogenesis of the disease. Essentially all nonneoplastic diseases discussed previously can produce end-stage kidneys. It is likely that causes of renal disease not yet identified or proven are responsible for other cases of end-stage kidney. Renal disease in cats has frequently progressed to the end stage by the time uremia occurs. Because elaborate studies at this point shed no light on the cause or pathogenesis, end-stage kidney is the best description.

Prognosis of Renal Failure

With regard to renal failure, it may be helpful to make a short-term and long-term prognosis. The short-term prognosis is based on the clinician's ability to combat the signs of renal failure during the first several days or weeks of illness, regardless of the underlying cause. The long-term prognosis refers to the potential for eliminating or controlling the underlying morphologic and functional disturbances.

The prognosis of renal failure should not be based on a single observation or a single laboratory determination. Such an approach ignores significant data that may be easily obtainable.

A far more logical approach for establishing a prognosis of renal failure involves accumulating as much information as possible and formulating a prognosis on the basis of all the data. This data can be evaluated by attempting to answer the following questions. What is the cause of the renal failure? What is the degree of renal dysfunction? What is the potential for reversing the lesions and achieving permanent improvement in renal function?

Causes of Failure

Knowledge of the way in which renal failure develops is helpful in establishing a prognosis because the effect of specific injuries to the kidney and its response to these injuries are known.

Prerenal failure may be caused by cardiovascular impairment due to any cause of heart disease, hypovolemia, shock and adrenocortical insufficiency. If prerenal failure is quickly and adequately treated, the prognosis is excellent because there is no renal damage. More prolonged or extensive renal ischemia may result in secondary kidney damage.

In some cases, prerenal failure may be differentiated from primary renal and postrenal causes of failure on the basis of clinical signs referable to cardiovascular involvement. In other instances, the clinical signs are not helpful and additional diagnostic tools must be used. Renal biopsy is probably the best of the other available methods for making the differentiation.

Postrenal failure is commonly caused by urethral obstruction, or rupture of the urinary bladder or proximal urethra. If the cause of postrenal failure is obstruction and is corrected within a few days, the prognosis is good because there is no secondary damage to the kidney. More prolonged obstruction can result in hydronephrosis, which may be reversible or irreversible. In contrast to postrenal failure associated with obstruction, rupture of a segment of the urinary tract is not accompanied by backup of urine, so renal damage does not occur. In these cases, the prognosis depends on successful repair of the leak and treatment of renal failure (short-term factors).

The prognosis of primary renal failure varies and cannot be based only on the knowledge that renal failure is due to primary kidney disease. When available, knowledge of the action of a specific microbial or chemical agent provides the clinician with information that can be of value in establishing the prognosis. For example, chemical toxins usually cause acute nephrosis. This enables one to give a good long-term prognosis, although the short-term prognosis depends on the severity of damage and response to therapy. Renal amyloidosis is a slowly progressive and ultimately fatal disease. Therefore, knowledge that a patient has this condition warrants a poor long-term prognosis. The short-term prognosis depends on the stage of the disease. Unfortunately, the specific cause of primary renal disease is not always known. In these cases, the clinician must use other information to give a reasonable prognosis.

Degree of Renal Dysfunction

The degree of renal dysfunction can be estimated by common laboratory procedures, such as determination of the BUN or serum creatinine concentration. Both the BUN and serum creatinine determinations are adequate for evaluating the degree of dysfunction in renal failure inasmuch as values for both are elevated by the time renal failure occurs. Serum creatinine concentration has the advantage of being affected by fewer extrarenal factors than is the BUN level. For example, dietary protein intake affects the BUN level but not that of serum creatinine; the rate of protein catabolism may affect the BUN level but does not affect serum creatinine concentration. For these reasons, serum creatinine determination is superior to measurement of BUN level for prognosis of renal failure. While serum creatinine concentration is more likely to reflect the actual degree of renal function than BUN level, neither test taken alone provides an adequate basis for prognosis. The ratio of BUN to creatinine values provides no information about the cause of the disease. The failure could be prerenal or postrenal. Likewise, no information is obtained concerning the potential reversibility of the lesions in primary renal failure.

Intensive supportive and symptomatic treatments make it possible to sustain life for short periods despite severe renal dysfunction. Because the short-term prognosis is thus improved, the long-term prognosis assumes more importance in the overall prediction of the outcome. Long-term prognosis is more dependent on knowledge of the cause and morphologic status of the kidney than on a single assessment of renal function.

Whereas basing prognosis on a single determination of the BUN or serum creatinine level has no logical or theoretic basis, serial determinations of renal function may provide additional information. This helps the clinician judge the kidneys' response to therapy and their ability to compensate and regenerate.

Reversibility of Renal Lesions

Reversibility of renal disease depends on the extent and severity of the lesions, and on the kidneys' ability to repair the injury. Generally there is potential reversibility of kidney lesions and improvement in function in patients with acute renal failure. In acute disease, compensatory methods have not been exhausted and parenchymal regeneration has not started. In contrast, the potential for reversibility of lesions in chronic renal failure is poor because compensatory mechanisms have been exhausted and parenchymal regeneration has not had an opportunity to occur.

Although the long-term prognosis with chronic renal failure is poor, vigorous therapeutic measures may reverse the signs so that a patient with chronic renal failure may live comfortably for several months to years despite progressive renal disease. This reversal of uremic signs in chronic renal failure is due to correction of prerenal factors that were superimposed on the degree of dysfunction due to primary renal disease. The clinician should use all available information to differentiate acute from chronic disease because these terms may be considered synonymous with reversible and irreversible renal disease. Information helpful in making this differentiation follows.

The duration of clinical signs may aid in differentiating acute from chronic renal disease. When signs referable to renal failure have been present for several weeks or more, the condition generally can be considered chronic. The clinician should hesitate to distinguish acute from chronic renal disease on the basis of an acute onset of signs, however. In many instances, signs of uremia may appear to occur abruptly during chronic disease because of the owner's casual attention to the animal or because of the insidious onset of chronic renal failure.

Acute and chronic renal failure share many common signs, including depression, anorexia, vomiting, diarrhea, polydipsia, polyuria, oliguria and dehydration. Some signs usually are restricted to chronic renal failure, including weight loss, mucosal pallor due to anemia, and skeletal changes caused by renal secondary hyperparathyroidism.

An effort should be made to palpate the kidneys because knowing something about their size may aid in differentiating acute from chronic renal failure. Knowing that the kidney size is normal is not informative because this is possible with either acute or chronic disease. Increased kidney size may occur with acute renal disease but can also accompany hydronephrosis, compensatory hypertrophy, amyloidosis or neoplasia. Decreased kidney size is usually associated with chronic, generalized renal disease.

Radiographs may aid in differentiating acute from chronic disease inasmuch as kidney size may be difficult to ascertain by physical examination in obese or uncooperative cats. In some instances, kidney size can be determined from survey radiographs. In others, excretory urography may aid in evaluating kidney size. It is unfortunate that, in azotemic cats, visualization of the kidneys with contrast agents is impaired due to decrease in renal blood flow and impaired ability of the kidneys to concentrate the contrast medium. In addition to providing information about kidney size, radiographs may be of value in assessing skeletal decalcification due to renal secondary hyperparathyroidism. Decalcification is not detectible in acute renal failure but may be observed with chronic renal failure.

No test that measures renal function enables differentiation of acute from chronic renal disease. Contrary to other reports, determination of serum creatinine, BUN or serum P levels has not been of value for this differentiation in cats. Urinalysis data are of limited value in differentiating acute from chronic disease. Likewise, proteinuria is an unreliable indication of whether a process is acute or chronic. Examination of urine sediment may help determine if renal failure is associated with an inflammatory process; however, the inflammation may be acute or chronic. Casts may be in the urine in both acute and chronic renal disease.

Renal biopsy provides the only method of establishing the morphologic status of the kidney in the living patient. This procedure provides a basis for determining the reversibility of kidney lesions. Correlation of biopsy results with history, physical examination, radiography and laboratory tests enables the most precise prognosis of renal disease.

Management of Primary Renal Failure

Specific therapeutic measures should be employed when the cause of renal failure can be identified and a specific regimen of therapy is available for the cause. Unfortunately, the cause often cannot be identified and specific therapeutic agents are frequently not available. Under these circumstances, symptomatic therapy may alleviate some of the signs associated with renal failure and may prolong life.

Despite the multiplicity of causes of uremia, the signs of renal failure are the same, being more dependent on the quantity of functional tissue remaining than on the cause. Even with an impaired glomerular filtration rate, sufficient nephron mass may be present so that polyuria occurs spontaneously or can be induced with diuretics. This phase of renal failure is thus called polyuric renal failure. When the glomerular filtration rate is further reduced, oliguria or anuria may occur. The imbalances and approach to therapy with oliguria are significantly different than in polyuric failure, even though the cause of the renal failure may be the same.

Polyuric Primary Renal Failure

Patients with polydipsia and polyuria may remain otherwise asymptomatic for months or years. Polydipsia and polyuria without azotemia may or may not indicate primary renal disease, and consideration should be given to other diagnostic possibilities.

When polyuria is due to renal disease and azotemia is absent, symptomatic therapy includes providing access to water, dietary supplementation with a multiple B-vitamin preparation, and efforts to avoid stress of the animal.

When polyuria and azotemia are the only signs present, other therapeutic measures in addition to those previously listed should be employed. These measures are directed toward minimizing the level of BUN, preventing volume contraction and poor renal perfusion, preventing acidosis, preventing renal mineralization, and minimizing erythron depression.

The BUN levels should be minimized because signs of uremia are clinically related to elevation of the BUN level. Although urea itself is relatively nontoxic, other catabolites of protein apparently contribute to uremia. Ideally, only the amounts and types of amino acids required for protein anabolism should be given. Amino acids not used for protein synthesis are metabolized to such products as urea and elevate the BUN level. If inadequate amounts of amino acids are ingested, body proteins may be catabolized to provide amino acids needed for new protein synthesis. Proteins may also be catabolized if the total caloric intake via fats or carbohydrates is inadequate. Unfortunately, the appropriate quality and quantity of protein to be fed to the azotemic cat has not been established. Cats normally have a higher requirement for dietary protein than dogs, and may require larger quantities of protein during azotemia as well (see Chapter 1).

Until experimental data are available, specific feeding recommendations for azotemic cats cannot be made. Tentative recommendations are diets that provide 70-80 cal/kg body weight, with a maximum of 20% of the dietary calories supplied as high-quality protein. This is equivalent to about 8% protein for canned food and 20-22% for dried food.[205] One prescription diet for cats (c/d:Hill's) approximates this composition. Alternately, nonglandular animal proteins may be fed to supply 50% of total caloric needs, and the remainder can be provided as fat and carbohydrates. High levels of dietary fat are tolerated by normal cats and increase the palatability of food. Animal and vegetable fats should be provided to assure a supply of arachidonic acid. A tentative recommendation of a dietary fat level sufficient to supply 25-40% of its total caloric requirements is suggested, with the remaining 10-25% made up of carbohydrates.

Individual cats should be monitored for response to the dietary regimen. Body weight should be maintained and plasma protein levels should remain normal. The BUN levels should remain proportionately lower than serum creatinine levels.

Volume contraction is to be avoided to prevent prerenal factors from being superimposed on the primary renal failure. Free access to fresh water is essential and close monitoring of the cat is essential to detect a negative water balance soon after its onset. In dogs and people, high Na intake leads to volume expansion and increased glomerular filtration rate when compared to low Na intake. Water turnover rate in normal cats is enhanced by salt ingestion.[206,207] Because these factors may aid azotemic cats by improving renal function, oral administration of salt may have therapeutic value. On the other hand, a high-salt diet could accentuate any hypertension in cats with azotemia. Clinical trials are needed to determine if alteration of dietary salt levels is beneficial for azotemic cats. We will continue to advocate its use until proved ineffective or harmful. A dose of 0.5-2.0 g salt is recommended daily for an adult cat.

Acidosis of varying degrees may exist in cats with azotemia. Oral administration of $NaHCO_3$ is beneficial for correction of acidosis. Precise maintenance dosages have not been established. Ideally, an initial dosage is selected and serial evaluations of blood pH and plasma bicarbonate concentration are used to adjust the dosage. An empiric dose of 5-10 gr daily may be used in adult cats.

As discussed previously, altered mineral metabolism associated with uremia may cause renal mineralization and progression of renal failure. Phosphate restriction appeared to benefit cats with experimentally induced azotemia. Although not proved to be effective in the naturally occurring disease, it seems prudent to recommend phosphorus restriction in these cases. Diets low in P may be employed and oral P-binding agents, such as aluminum hydroxide gel, may be beneficial. No standard dose can be recommended because of variation among cats. Although definitive studies have not been conducted to prove reliability in preventing calcification, the serum P concentration should be kept below 6.0 mg/dl.

Steroids related to testosterone have anabolic effects that may help azotemic cats. Anabolic steroids stimulate protein synthesis when adequate calories and protein are ingested. This effect is general, but it may be particularly advantageous for specific tissues adversely affected during azotemia. Testosterone can stimulate RBC production in anemic azotemic patients and may be administered as a reposital injection of 15-25 mg once monthly.

Residual renal tissue is apparently required for stimulation of erythropoiesis by anabolic steroids inasmuch as anephric people maintained by dialysis may not respond to testosterone.[208] Anabolic steroids may be beneficial in instances of acute failure when kidney regenerative processes are active. In chronic failure, regenerative processes are already exhausted and anabolic steroids probably have no direct effect on the kidney. They may be beneficial, however, to other body tissues. In contrast to the anabolic steroids, glucocorticoids are contraindicated in uremic patients because of their catabolic effects.

When a uremic crisis (depression, anorexia, vomiting, diarrhea, dehydration) occurs, the oral route of therapy cannot be used. Parenteral therapy must be initiated to correct imbalances of water, electrolytes, acid-base and calories. With chronic disease, there may be a remission of signs for weeks or months. For acute cases, there is hope of repair and resumption of normal function. In addition to parenteral fluid therapy during the uremic crisis, B vitamins and anabolic steroids should be given parenterally.

Each patient in uremic crisis should be thoroughly evaluated to determine the fluid requirements. Whereas certain trends in alterations can generally be anticipated in cats with polyuric renal failure, marked individual differences may exist in the degree of abnormality. The duration and severity of diarrhea, vomiting or anorexia contribute to these differences, in addition to the alterations caused by the underlying renal disease. Evaluation of the individual patient involves consideration of the history, physical examination and laboratory tests. When planning therapy, it is helpful to consider specific types of abnormalities, such as water deficit, electrolyte deficits or excesses, acid-base status and nutritional derangements.

Water Balance: Patients with polyuric renal failure are frequently dehydrated. The magnitude of the deficit can be estimated by physical examination and determination of the PCV and total plasma protein level. Changes in body weight reflect changes in body water content if excessive tissue catabolism is not occurring.

Clinical signs of dehydration occur only when water constituting about 5% of body weight has been lost. At the other extreme, life is usually incompatible with a loss of body water in excess of 15% of body weight. Consequently, when estimating the water deficit in an obviously dehydrated cat, the clinician knows that an amount of water equal to 5-15% of the body weight has been lost.

When the cat is about 5% dehydrated, the skin has a slightly doughy, inelastic consistency. This is the only clinical sign apparent at this stage of dehydration. When evaluating dehydration, the skin covering the cervical area should not be assessed because it does not immediately return to the usual position, even in normal patients. With 7% dehydration, the skin assumes the position to which it is pulled. At this stage of dehydration, the eyeballs are slightly depressed in the orbit. When dehydration is 10-12% of body weight, the aforementioned signs are more severe. Shock may occur in debilitated animals and involuntary muscle twitching may be apparent. At 12-15% dehydration, shock occurs and death is imminent.

As normal values for the PCV and total plasma protein have a relatively broad range, this information is initially used only to confirm the degree of dehydration, and not for quantitative calculations. Once therapy has been initiated, the PCV and total plasma protein values can be used to monitor day-by-day variation in the state of hydration.

Once percent of dehydration has been estimated, water deficit can quickly be calculated. For example, a 3-kg cat that is 10% dehydrated has a fluid deficit of 0.3 kg or 300 ml.

Electrolyte Balance: Patients with polyuric renal failure may have deficits of Na, K and Cl ions because of renal loss associated with polyuria and volume contraction. Associated signs, such as vomiting and diarrhea, may contribute to loss of these ions. Although body deficits of these ions may exist, the serum electrolyte concentrations may be normal, suggesting proportionate loss of both water and electrolytes (isotonic dehydration). Cats with polyuric renal failure usually do not have elevated concentrations of serum K. When renal function is more severely impaired and oliguria or anuria ensues, the serum concentration of K may increase. With chronic renal failure, there is a negative body balance of Ca; however, the serum concentration of Ca remains normal until late in the course of disease. Hypocalcemic tetany is rare in patients with chronic renal failure. Administration of Ca is probably not of prolonged benefit to cats with renal failure, except when tetany occurs, because hyperphosphatemia can result in deposition of Ca in soft tissues.

In planning electrolyte therapy for cats with polyuric renal failure, knowledge of the serum concentration of Na, K and Cl is helpful. With this information, attention can be directed to specific electrolyte deficits or excesses. Accurate determination of the total quantity of electrolyte deficit or excess cannot be deduced from the plasma concentration, however, and repeated serum determinations after therapy are required to assess the efficacy of therapy. In the absence of specific electrolyte data, it is logical to administer fluids with a composition similar to extracellular fluid, such as lactated Ringer's solution.

Acid-Base Balance: Alterations in acid-base balance associated with renal failure are usually in the direction of acidosis, even in vomiting patients, as a result of impaired ability of the kidney to excrete hydrogen ions. Unfortunately, physical examination of the patient is not a reliable method of evaluating acid-base balance. Although compensatory hyperpnea or polypnea should occur with acidosis, severe acidosis has occurred in cats with renal failure in which no alteration in respiratory function was detectible. Determination of urine pH may give some information concerning acid-base status inasmuch as a urine pH below 5.5 suggests increased excretion of hydrogen ions. With a normal urine pH, acidosis is still possible because, with renal failure, the kidneys may have impaired ability to excrete hydrogen ions. Determination of plasma bicarbonate concentration provides information that can be used to estimate the total bicarbonate deficit with the following formula: deficit (mEq) = body weight (kg) x 0.6 x (25 minus patient's plasma bicarbonate concentration). A 3-kg cat with a plasma bicarbonate concentration of 14 mEq/L would require 20 mEq bicarbonate according to the following calculations: 3 x 0.6 x (25-14) = 20 mEq.[209]

When the plasma bicarbonate concentration is unknown, there is little to guide the clinician in estimating the magnitude of the bicarbonate deficit. Because renal failure is associated with metabolic acidosis and the severity of renal failure can be evaluated by clinical signs and BUN or serum creatinine determination, patients can be assessed on the assumption that a parallel exists between the severity of the disease and severity of the acidosis. Table 2 provides guidelines for therapy based on this assumption. When $NaHCO_3$ is given IV, the rate of administration should be slow so that sudden changes in blood pH do not occur. Small doses over 48 hours are preferable to a single large dose.

Table 2. Estimation of Bicarbonate Deficit in Patients with Renal Failure

Severity of Signs	Estimated Bicarbonate Deficit (mEq/L)	Bicarbonate Required to Alleviate the Deficit (mEq/kg)
Mild	5	3
Moderate	10	6
Severe	15	9

Caloric Balance: As patients with renal failure frequently are anorectic, a negative caloric balance is often present. Carbohydrate stores are soon depleted, and body fats and proteins are used as sources of calories. Protein catabolism is particularly harmful because the resulting nitrogenous wastes cannot be readily excreted by the kidneys. Unfortunately, it is difficult to provide adequate calories by parenteral routes to fulfill maintenance requirements. For example, to provide the maintenance requirements for a 3-kg cat, more than a liter of 5% dextrose is required every 24 hours. To avoid spillover of dextrose in the urine, the dextrose should be administered over a 15-hour period.[209]

In polyuric renal failure, however, there is an advantage in inducing diuresis by maintaining hyperglycemia. For this reason, administering 20% dextrose may serve not only to provide calories but also to induce diuresis. The induction of osmotic diuresis is discussed subsequently.

It may seem advantageous to administer amino acid solutions with protein catabolism and tissue wasting that may be observed in polyuric renal failure. Unless adequate calories are provided, amino acids are not used for tissue synthesis but are deaminated and used as a source of calories. For this reason, amino acid solutions are not indicated in renal failure prior to adequate caloric replacement. Parenteral hyperalimentation has promise in improving survival rate in people with acute renal failure.[210] In this procedure, adequate carbohydrate and amino acids are provided so that caloric requirements are met and tissue anabolism occurs. A solution of 25% dextrose and 5% amino acids is constantly infused into a large vein. Results of using this technic in cats have not been reported.

Fluid therapy is discussed in Chapter 2.

Consideration of these 4 aspects of therapy (water, electrolytes, acid-base, calories) is followed by developing a plan of action. In summary, a specific estimate of water deficit can be made. Electrolyte deficits are difficult to quantify, but a fluid with the electrolyte composition of extracellular water is usually adequate. For this purpose, lactated Ringer's solution is preferred. Severe acidosis may not be alleviated with lactated Ringer's solution, however, because it contains only 27 mEq lactate per liter. It may be necessary to administer additional base as sodium lactate or $NaHCO_3$. As nutritional needs are difficult to meet, one should attempt to provide calories in the next phase of therapy.

If dehydration is severe, fluid should be replaced IV through an indwelling catheter. To facilitate initiation of the next phase of therapy, the entire deficit may be administered in 3-6 hours. The patient should be monitored closely during rehydration for evidence of cardiovascular overload.

After the patient is rehydrated, an effort is made to increase the rate of body fluid turnover by inducing osmotic diuresis. This facilitates excretion of metabolic wastes but has no specific beneficial effect on the underlying renal disease. The predominant effect is achieved by inhibiting tubular resorption of solute and subsequent inhibition of passive diffusion of water from the tubular lumen back into tubular cells. In addition, osmotic diuresis with glucose moderately increases the glomerular filtration rate.[39] If it is questionable that the patient can excrete large volumes of urine, one must proceed cautiously to avoid overhydration. Osmotic diuresis has been induced with mannitol, but there are distinct advantages in using 20% dextrose in cats. Not only is dextrose cheaper but a considerable quantity of it can be used to partially alleviate the caloric deficit. The following is a step-by-step procedure for osmotic diuresis:[211]

1. After deficit therapy, the animal is weighed. This is the baseline weight to be used to assess underhydration or overhydration during subsequent therapy.
2. Then 20% dextrose is given IV in the amount of 25-65 ml/kg and at a rate of 2 ml/minute for 10-15 minutes. The infusion rate is then reduced to 1 ml/minute.
3. The patient's bladder is catheterized when the infusion of glucose is begun and the bladder is emptied.
4. Newly formed urine (if any) is tested for glucose.
5. If the test is positive, sufficient glucose to exceed the renal threshold has been administered and anuria does not exist. Urine volume should increase if the procedure can safely be continued. The urine volume should be 1-2 ml/minute.
6. If adequate urine flow is not seen by the time half the glucose is given, the procedure must be discontinued because of possible overhydration and hyperosmolality.
7. If adequate urine flow is obtained, all of the osmotic agent may be given. Administration of lactated Ringer's solution, in an amount equivalent to 3-5% of body weight, and glucose is then repeated. Fluid input and urine output are measured to maintain a reasonable balance. Every 24 hours, 2-3 cycles of dextrose and lactated Ringer's solution are administered.
8. After 24 hours, the patient is re-evaluated by a physical examination, determining body weight and measuring the BUN level.
9. The entire procedure is repeated if necessary. A gain in weight indicates fluid retention and contraindicates the administration of lactated Ringer's solution prior to administration of the osmotic agent. Loss of weight reflects a fluid deficit and lactated Ringer's solution should be given in sufficient quantity to rectify the deficit.
10. Extreme weakness suggests K deficiency. If the serum K concentration is less than 3.0 mEq/L, solutions containing K at 25-35 mEq/L should be administered at a rate of 0.5 mEq/kg/hour.
11. Initially all fluids should be given IV. Lactated Ringer's solution given to maintain hydration can be administered SC if it is absorbed well. A favorable response to therapy, as indicated by a decrease in BUN level, generally occurs within 2-4 days. Good nursing care by the owner may result in dramatic clinical improvement. Failure to respond indicates severe functional impairment and dictates the use of supplementary measures, such as peritoneal dialysis.

If diuresis with dextrose fails, furosemide may be given at the recommended dosage to attempt to induce diuresis. If no urine forms after an hour, the dosage can be doubled. If this is not successful in inducing urine output, it usually can be assumed that the patient must be treated for anuria.

When there is a favorable response to therapy, oral alimentation and medication are gradually resumed as parenteral therapy is discontinued. Oral administration of salt, bicarbonate, anabolic steroids and B vitamins is continued indefinitely in chronic disease or until renal function has improved to the point of resolution of azotemia.

Anuric Primary Renal Failure

Oliguria or apparent anuria may be observed in dehydrated cats with normal renal function as a consequence of efforts to conserve water. It may also be observed in a cat with renal failure because the combination of dehydration and renal failure markedly reduces the glomerular filtration rate. In both instances, restoration of circulatory volume may increase the urine flow rate. For this reason, a cat with suspected anuric renal failure must be challenged appropriately to produce urine before anuric renal failure is diagnosed. The challenge imposed is the procedure for osmotic diuresis previously described. This is superior to volume expansion with isotonic fluids since osmotic diuresis may overcome renal effects of antidiuretic hormone while isotonic volume expansion may not. Fear, pain and vomiting stimulate release of antidiuretic hormone. Alternatively, volume expansion with isotonic fluids and furosemide administration may be used to differentiate anuric from nonanuric conditions. If the cat fails to produce urine after these maneuvers, anuric primary renal failure or outflow tract obstruction or rupture should be suspected.

In our experience, the prognosis of anuric primary renal failure is extremely poor. The only chance for survival is apparently to maintain the cat until renal dysfunction improves sufficiently to sustain life. Hemodialysis and renal transplantation have not been developed for clinical use in cats, but peritoneal dialysis is feasible. Even with the use of this technic, the prognosis is poor because of mechanical difficulties with fluid exchange. The technic for peritoneal dialysis as described for dogs may be applied to cats.[63,212]

Ancillary Considerations in Chronic Renal Failure

Nonregenerative anemia due to depression of bone marrow is common in chronic failure. Anabolic steroids may help to maintain the PCV within satisfactory limits. Blood transfusions generally are of value only when anemia is severe enough to cause clinical signs. Although there may be variation among cats, little benefit can be anticipated unless the Hb concentration is below 6 g/dl. Other than increasing the circulating red cell mass, transfusion has no known benefit for uremic patients.

Vomiting and diarrhea are sometimes associated with renal failure. Gastroenteritis has been attributed to ammonia that is produced by bacterial degradation of urea. Vomiting may also occur because of stimulation of the chemoreceptor trigger zone.[213,214] Phenothiazine tranquilizers and GI protectives may be helpful, but they rarely eliminate all of the signs.

Pruritus and neurologic signs other than depression are rarely associated with renal failure. Their presence should focus attention on abnormalities of body systems other than the urinary tract.

Bacterial Infection of the Urinary Tract

Pathogenesis

All body orifices have exposure to microbial agents and have protective mechanisms that usually prevent systemic infection. Defense mechanisms of the urinary tract include the flushing action associated with micturition, anatomic barriers (mucosal lining, urethral length, ureterovesical flap valves) and antibacterial properties of urinary tract components (prostatic fluid, urine, local antibody production).

Specific studies have not been conducted to examine the role of all of these factors in cats, but some properties of cat urine may be particularly valuable for antibacterial defense. Specifically, low urine pH and high urine osmolality are detrimental to growth of most bacteria considered to be common urinary pathogens. The high osmolality of cat urine may act as a significant factor in prevention of urinary tract infection in this species.[215]

Clinical impression suggests that urinary infection is more common in dogs than in cats. Nevertheless, urinary tract infections occur naturally in cats.[216,217]

Urinary infections are presumed to develop because of failure of defense mechanisms previously described. Ascent of organisms from the periurethral area via the lower urinary tract is believed to occur, although hematogenous infection is also possible.

The spectrum of organisms is similar to that in dogs except for the higher incidence of *Pasteurella* spp urinary infection in cats.[218]

Bacterial Pyelonephritis

The term pyelonephritis is often used to describe inflammatory lesions of the renal pelvis and medulla. Unfortunately, the term implies a bacterial origin to lesions from which bacteria were not isolated. The term bacterial pyelonephritis is used in this discussion with specific reference to kidneys and renal pelves from which bacteria are isolated.

Ascent of bacteria from the bladder to the kidneys may be aided by bacterial motility and by ureteral aperistalsis induced by endotoxin. The renal medulla is vulnerable to infection because

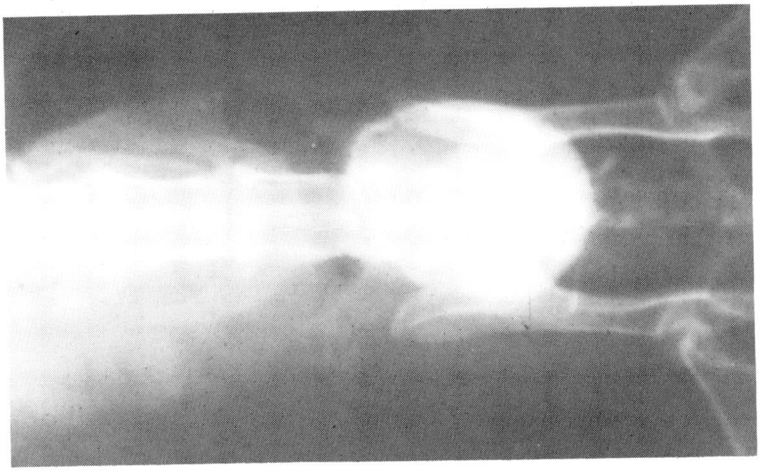

Fig 21. Excretory urogram from a cat with suspected pyelonephritis. The cat had significant bacteriuria and bilateral dilation of the ureters and renal pelves.

the hyperosmolality results in impaired WBC and complement activity.[219]

Acute pyelonephritis in people is apparently associated with sufficiently distinct signs (fever, renal pain, leukocytosis) to enable a reasonably accurate diagnosis.[219,220] Chronic pyelonephritis presents a diagnostic challenge in that pyuria is the only sign, and differentiation from lower tract disease is extremely difficult. Collecting urine by ureteral catheterization is considered to be the only accurate method of diagnosis.[219]

Pyelonephritis in cats has been diagnosed in isolated cases (Fig 21).[221] It is not known whether many asymptomatic infections are present in cats that eventually are presented with end-stage disease.

Factors that may predispose to pyelonephritis include any cause of urine retention within the collecting system. Nephrolithiasis is frequently associated wtih bacterial infection in other species. Vesicoureteral reflux has been incriminated as a cause of ascending infection in people. Although vesicoureteral reflux sometimes can be demonstrated radiographically in cats, its significance is unknown (Fig 22).

Bacterial Cystitis

Bacterial cystitis is assumed to exist in cats inasmuch as signs of lower urinary tract infec-

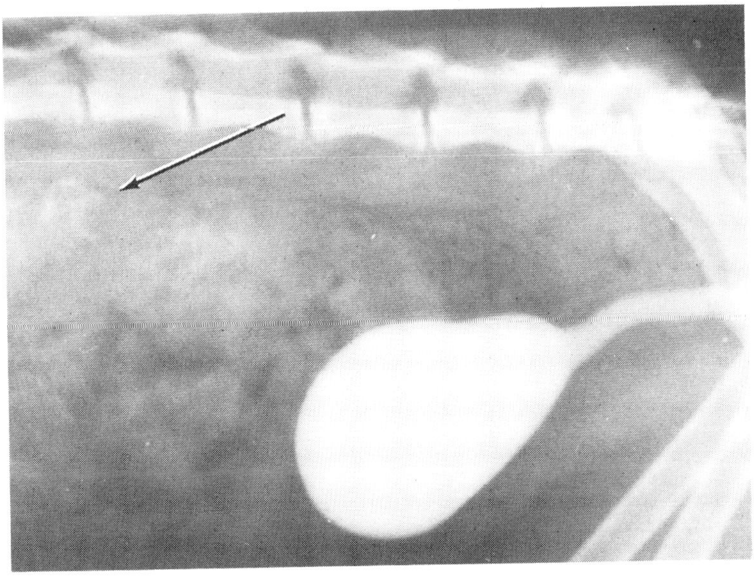

Fig 22. Cystogram revealing reflux of contrast medium into the renal pelvis (arrow).

tion (dysuria, hematuria) may be accompanied by numerous bacteria in urine obtained by cystocentesis. The role of bacteria in the feline urologic syndrome is discussed subsequently. In addition to dysuria and hematuria, thickening of the bladder wall may be palpable or visualized radiographically. This observation is consistent with but not diagnostic of bacterial cystitis. Patients with bacterial cystitis are usually afebrile and do not have leukocytosis.

The presence of lower urinary tract (urethra, bladder) signs does not preclude the simultaneous existence of upper urinary tract infection. Likewise, the absence of lower urinary tract signs does not eliminate the bladder as the source of infection since chronic or mild infections of the lower urinary tract may not produce clinical signs.

Bacterial infection of the lower urinary tract is assumed to be caused by ascending infection in most instances. Persistent or recurrent bacterial cystitis may be related to resistant microorganisms, urolithiasis or an anatomic defect in the bladder wall or urethra resulting in urine retention.

Diagnosis of Bacterial Infections

The history and clinical signs may aid diagnosis of bacterial infection. Because of the prevalence of lower urinary tract signs in feline urologic syndrome of nonbacterial origin, however, a diagnosis of bacterial infection must be proven by laboratory procedures. For these procedures, it is essential to obtain a urine sample without bacterial contamination from the genital tract, to collect the specimen in a sterilized container, and to process the sample immediately to avoid multiplication of bacteria prior to their enumeration. A sample obtained by cystocentesis is ideal and is sterile in normal animals if aseptic technic is used for its procurement. A specimen obtained after careful cleaning of the external genitalia and manual expression of the bladder is usually satisfactory if midstream urine is obtained, but some bacterial contamination is likely even with the best technic.

Quantitative bacterial culture has been used to differentiate infection from contamination on the assumption that large numbers of organisms indicate urinary tract infection, whereas small numbers represent contamination. Counts of greater than 1×10^5 organisms have been considered indicative of infection in dogs and people.[220,222] Although data are not available for the cat at present, this value is probably equally valid in this species. The number of bacteria in urine can easily be estimated with commercially available culture tubes. Alternatively, a drop of fresh uncentrifuged urine can be examined under the microscope (440X). Visualizing bacteria in the urine correlates fairly well with colony counts of 1×10^5 or greater, but an inexperienced individual may make serious errors in interpretation.[220,223]

Counts greater than 1×10^5 organisms/ml should be considered indicative of bacterial infection in a properly collected specimen, but counts of less than 1×10^5 organisms/ml should not be ignored. Patients with relatively high counts should be observed and re-evaluated.

Particularly with chronic or recurring infections, it is advisable to perform antibiotic sensitivity tests and identify the organism in addition to quantitative culture.

Treatment of Bacterial Infections

Antibacterial therapy of urinary tract infection should be chosen on the basis of the drug's known effectiveness against the microorganism, ability to achieve adequate urine and blood levels, side effects and cost. Urinary acidifiers and antiseptics are inferior to antibiotics, sulfonamides and nitrofurantoins in the treatment of bacterial infections and should generally be used as adjuncts to other therapeutic agents. They may be used as the exclusive treatment when prolonged or life-long therapy is required, or when organisms are resistant to all other antibacterial drugs.

With acute onset of lower urinary tract signs, parenteral therapy should be continued for 10-14 days, regardless of earlier remission of signs. If infection persists or recurs, the patient should be thoroughly re-examined for evidence of factors that predispose to urinary infection, such as urine retention, resistant microorganisms or calculi.

Antibacterial therapy is needed for at least 4 weeks in chronic infections. The cat should be evaluated at intervals after suspending therapy to determine whether the infection has definitely been eradicated.

Infusion of antibiotics into the urinary bladder is usually a poor method of therapy. Therapeutic levels of antibiotics are obtained in both blood and urine by parenteral administration, whereas therapeutic levels are obtained only in urine by bladder infusion. Also, the frequent urination characteristic of cats with lower urinary tract infection usually results in voiding of instilled drugs soon after their administration.

Urolithiasis

In this discussion, urolithiasis refers to solid uroliths composed of layers of mucoprotein and mineral. This description is consistent with definitions in other species and differentiates this condition from feline urethral obstruction due to unorganized crystals, mucus and debris. Other authors have made a distinction between uroliths and urethral debris.

Although sufficient information on etiology is not available to draw definite conclusions, the causes of the 2 conditions probably are different. The frequent occurrence of urethral obstruction in males and its counterpart of dysuria and hematuria in females, along with the infrequent occurrence of uroliths in both sexes, seems incompatible with a common cause.

Although cases of urolithiasis in cats have been described, the condition is far less common in cats than in dogs (Fig 23).[171,224-231] Oxalate, ammonium urate and phosphate calculi have been identified, with the last being most common. They are usually found in the urinary bladder, but nephrolithiasis has been reported.

In a survey of 16 intact female, 63 spayed female, 14 intact male and 38 castrated male cats with cystic calculi, a peak incidence at 2-5 years of age was noted, with no apparent breed predisposition.[231] Qualitative analysis of calculi revealed phosphate in 124 of 128. Urine culture of 86 cases was positive in 28, with *Staphylococcus* spp isolated from 14 cats. This study raises the question of whether phosphate calculi in cats are caused by infection with urea-splitting bacteria as described in dogs. Further study is required to establish this point since negative urine cultures at the time of examination do not rule out the possibility that the infection that initiated stone formation was later resolved spontaneously. In the absence of urine infection, it may be helpful to culture the calculi themselves as previously described.[232] Positive calculus cultures are consistent with a bacterial etiology. Negative urine and calculus cultures suggest a dietary etiology or a metabolic defect in urinary mineral excretion.

The uroliths should be removed unless circumstances contraindicate surgery. Calculi should be analyzed to determine their mineral composition because this knowledge provides the only rational basis for therapy. Kits are available for qualitative analysis; quantitative analysis is performed by the Urolithiasis Laboratory, PO Box 25375, Houston, TX 77005. Prophylactic therapy, as used in dogs, should be done until other data dictate a different approach.[233]

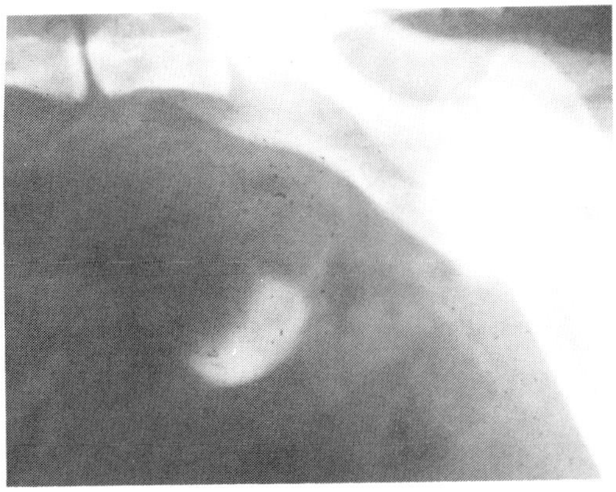

Fig 23. Radiopaque objects in the urinary bladder. Calculi were removed surgically.

Diseases of the Ureters

Diseases of the cat's ureters are rare. Abnormalities leading to obstruction and hydronephrosis were mentioned previously. Trauma to ureters is uncommon, but they may be injured in association with other abdominal injuries. Ectopic ureter has not been observed in cats and vesicoureteral reflux has not been studied sufficiently to establish its incidence or significance in this species. Primary neoplasms of the ureter of the cat have not been reported.

Feline Urologic Syndrome

A syndrome characterized by urethral obstruction in the male and dysuria with or without hematuria in both sexes has been given various names in the veterinary literature, including cystitis-urethral obstruction complex, feline urethral obstruction, feline urolithiasis, feline urolithiasis syndrome, urethroadenocystitis, feline urinary retention and retention cystitis. We will use the term feline urologic syndrome (FUS) since it describes the condition at the present level of its comprehension.

Incidence: This syndrome is the most common urologic disease for which cats are presented to veterinarians and is one of the most common of all cat diseases for which veterinarians' services are sought. Surveys in the US and England indicate the incidence in any one year is about 0.6% of the total cat population.[234,235]

A definite age predisposition for FUS occurs, with young adults chiefly affected.[236-239] The disease is infrequent in cats under 1 year, has a high incidence in males 1-3 years of age, and then diminishes in frequency. Its relationship to age in females appears to parallel that in males. Although one epidemiologic study suggested a predisposition of the Persian breed to the disease, other studies have not demonstrated a breed susceptibility.[240,241] Data are not clear concerning the sex distribution of cases of FUS. Some studies report a greater frequency in the male, but this may be related to anatomic factors predisposing the male to outflow obstruction. The effect of neutering on the incidence of the disease is discussed subsequently. Some reports of seasonal variation in incidence occur, but this point is controversial.[241-244]

Clinical Signs: Cats with FUS use their litter pans frequently; the owner may erroneously interpret this as a sign of constipation. It is also common for the history to include the voiding of small quantities of bloody urine in bathtubs or sinks. In the absence of urethral obstruction or in its early stages, the cat remains alert and the appetite is reported to be normal. The owner may note that the obstructed male licks its penis.

Findings are normal on physical examination of nonobstructed cats. The urinary bladder is usually empty because of dysuria. Depending on several variables, including duration of obstruction, urine concentration, bladder epithelium integrity and bladder volume, obstructed cats may be alert or depressed to the point of being moribund. Body temperature is normal to subnormal, and cats may be dehydrated if adipsia and vomiting have occurred. Abdominal palpation reveals a large, turgid urinary bladder. Bradycardia or an irregular heart rhythm may be encountered in cats with hyperkalemia.

Laboratory Data: Hemograms usually are normal in cats with FUS unless massive hemorrhage or severe bladder necrosis has occurred. The stress response (mild mature leukocytosis, lymphopenia, eosinopenia) may be observed.[245]

On urinalysis, evaluation of sediment reveals few WBC, but an increased number of RBC is common.[246] Phosphate crystalluria is often present, but it is important to recognize that these crystals are commonly present in the urine of normal cats. Urine pH is sometimes elevated. The role of urine pH in etiology will be discussed subsequently. Positive glucose reactions have frequently been associated with FUS.[245,247,248] It has been proposed that the positive reaction is due to glucose loss through hemorrhage into the urinary system or that it is due to tubular leak of glucose due to renal damage.[245,248] However, hyperglycemia of undetermined origin was present in cats with both naturally occurring and induced obstruction; this could explain glucosuria in some cases. Other positive reactions may be due to nonglucose-oxidizing substances.[248] Proteinuria may be present in cats with FUS. This is most likely due to hemorrhage and plasma extravasation and should not be attributed to glomerular leakage. Urine specific gravity is high unless obstruction has caused impairment of concentrating ability or postobstruction diuresis is occurring.

Blood chemical changes in obstructed cats include metabolic acidosis, mild hyponatremia, hyperkalemia, hypermagnesemia, hypocalcemia, hyperphosphatemia, hyperglycemia, hyperproteinemia and azotemia. In experimentally obstructed cats, blood chemical changes were minimal during the first 48 hours but developed rapidly between 48 and 72 hours after obstruction.[249] Clinical observations suggest that mentally alert cats have minor blood chemical changes but lethargic or depressed cats have an increased likelihood of blood abnormalities. Of the abnormalities noted, dehydration, hyperkalemia and acidosis are most life-threatening; therapy described later is directed toward correcting these imbalances.

Electrocardiograms obtained from cats with hyperkalemia reveal changes similar to those associated wtih hyperkalemia in other species.[250] These changes include depression in amplitude of P waves, spiked T waves, and prolongation of the QRS complex.

Obstructing Material: Material retrieved from cats with signs of FUS has been analyzed by x-ray diffraction.[236,251] The mineral component usually was struvite (magnesium ammonium phosphate). Other components found occasionally include newberyite (magnesium phosphate), calcium oxalate, ammonium urate brushite (calcium phosphate), and calcium carbonate. The mineral material is present as an unorganized aggregate of crystals rather than an orderly composition, as in uroliths (Fig 24). As previously indicated, the term urolith is not descriptive of the debris usually present in cats. In some debris, the quantity of mineral is low or absent, as indicated by absence of a mineral diffraction pattern or by gross inspection.[236,251]

The nonmineral component has not been studied in detail. In one study it was found to contain antigen unique to cats with obstruction.[252] It migrated on electrophoresis with serum globulins but was antigenically distinct from them. In another study, differences in physiochemical properties of proteins and mucoproteins from obstructed cats and normal cats were found but it was not established if this was a cause or effect of obstruction.[253]

Cause: Numerous causes or contributing factors have been proposed for FUS, including infectious agents (bacteria, virus), changes in character of urine as a consequence of diet (crystalluria, high pH, high urine mineral content, concentrated urine due to oliguria, high mineral content of water, vitamin A deficiency), changes in character of urine independent of diet (unique matrix protein, lack of protective colloids, limited exercise and infrequent urinations) castration, heredity, stress, anatomic bladder defects and hyperparathyroidism.[236,239,243,247,252,254-260]

The involvement of some of these factors has been disproven with considerable certainty. Others seem unlikely to be involved in view of present opinions but have not been excluded for certain. Still other factors seem to be involved but do not have universal support. One school of thought is that the syndrome is multifactorial, with synergism between several factors being required for disease.

One factor that infrequently causes signs of FUS is bacterial infection. Several studies have documented a lack of significant bacteriuria in cases of FUS when common methods of aerobic bacterial culture are used.[241,246,261] Attempts to isolate anaerobes, mycoplasma, spirochetes and fastidious organisms have failed, even when special media supplemented with feline urine, feline serum or extracts of feline renal tissues have been used.[261] Scanning electron microscopy on urinary sediment from cats with FUS has also been negative for bacterial agents.[261] Occasional cases of bacterial urinary infection occur in cats and these animals may have clinical signs identical to FUS. We prefer to exclude these cases from the definition of FUS, since their etiology and management is unique to that generally encountered with the syndrome.

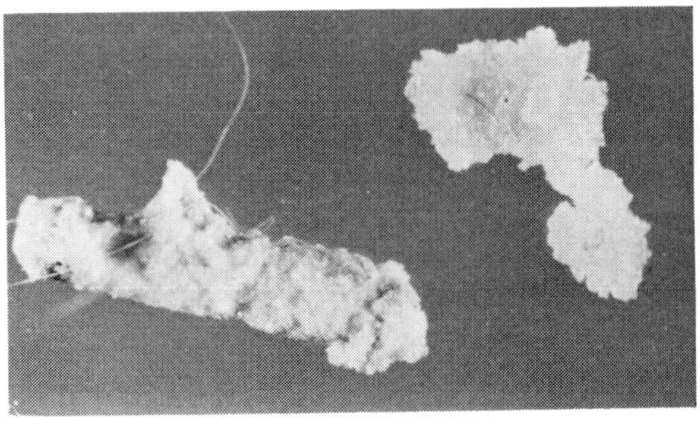

Fig 24. Debris removed from a male cat with an obstructed urethra. Notice that the debris has conformed to the shape of the urethra and is not organized as are urinary calculi.

Although not studied thoroughly, such factors as stress, vitamin A deficiency, mineral content of water, hyperparathyroidism and bladder trauma are not considered significant in FUS.

Factors that have more support, albeit sometimes undocumented, for contributing to FUS include the remainder of those previously itemized. Several of these factors share a common theory of pathogenesis of obstruction. This theory presumes that obstructing crystalline debris forms as a consequence of alteration of the physicochemical properties of urine. The amount of solute normally in urine is in excess of that which can be explained on the basis of simple solubility. Consequently, urine has been described as a stable colloid from which solute might aggregate if conditions are altered. The conditions of change considered most relevant to FUS are the volume of fluid (urine water) in which urinary solutes are suspended and the pH of urine. The relationship between amount of solute and solvent can be varied by either excreting less urine or by excreting more minerals in a "normal" urine volume.

In regard to diet, ingestion of dry food is thought to lead to oliguria in cats. Some studies in England indicated less urine output by cats eating dry food than by cats fed canned food, but studies in the US indicate no difference.[262,263] This difference may be related to differences in the composition of canned food in the 2 countries.[206] Epidemiologic studies have been done to define the role of dry foods in FUS but conflicting results have been obtained. Some studies have incriminated them in the genesis of FUS but others have found them not at fault for recurrence.[240,264,265] Epidemiologic studies, in addition to giving inconsistent results, by their nature fail to pinpoint any characteristics of dry foods that may cause the problem.

Studies have been conducted with canned and dry foods to evaluate the role of Mg, Ca and P intake in FUS. Cats given diets high in Mg alone or in combination with Ca or P have developed urethral obstruction.[266,267] Of these minerals, Mg was fed at the levels most atypical of commercial foods (0.4-1.0% Mg experimental diets vs 0.08-0.25 in commercial foods). Question exists concerning the relationship of this experimental disease of FUS since the levels of minerals were much higher than cats normally encounter and since mineral composition of the obstructing material was different than FUS. Ammonium was almost absent from the experimental disease but is usually present in naturally occurring cases of obstruction. More conclusive evidence must be presented before this model of experimental urethral obstruction can be accepted as a valid representation of FUS. Based on these data, it does not seem appropriate to claim that a high level of dietary minerals causes FUS.

One factor relevant to the dietary theory of FUS is the distinction between percent of various minerals in the diet and the urinary levels of minerals of cats fed those diets. Total mineral intake depends on the amount in the food and the amount of food ingested. If 2 foods have identical percentages of minerals but differ in caloric density, cats ingest more of the lower caloric density food and thus ingest more minerals. Intestinal absorption of minerals by the cat is also poorly defined at present. Absorption of ingested minerals may depend on their form in the food and their relative proportions to one another in the diet. Thus the influence of diet on urinary mineral content is best determined by analysis of urine rather than by analysis of the diet. Such analyses should be performed in cats known to be at risk for FUS rather than in normal cats since there is no assurance that cats with FUS respond the same as normal cats to the diets available. Hyperabsorption states and urinary mineral "leaks" in people may predispose to calculi formation because of a metabolic abnormality of the gut or the kidney.[268]

Another popular theory of the cause of FUS is viral infection. This theory has received support from one laboratory but has not been supported by others.[255,261,269,270] Advocates of the viral theory have incriminated 3 different viruses at various phases of the investigation. A cell-associated herpesvirus presently is favored as the cause. Signs of FUS have been produced in cats inoculated with one or more of the viruses but skepticism persists regarding these findings. Inconsistencies in results sometimes are attributed to accidental infections, and sham-operated control cats apparently were not used to rule out obstruction following mechanical manipulations. Isolation procedures and transmission trials from 3 other laboratories have failed to incriminate a virus. The latter findings have been criticized since urine that was used for transmission and isolation studies may inactivate the cell-associated herpesvirus.

On the other hand, intact cells frequently are sloughed into the urine with FUS, so shedding of viable virus via these cells could be expected. Yet 58 of 59 urine samples from cats with FUS were negative for viral culture in one study, as was one bladder tissue explant.[261] Ironically, some of the early studies reported by proponents of the virus theory reported induction of FUS by urine transmission.[271] It will be necessary for the positive results of viral studies to be duplicated in more than one laboratory before the viral theory achieves scientific credibility.

Conflicting findings have been reported concerning the role of castration in FUS. Some epidemiologic studies suggested that castration predisposed cats to FUS while others found no association.[240,264] An anatomic study revealed no difference in penile urethral diameter between castrates and noncastrates.[272] The tip of the penis in castrates contained slightly more fibrous tissue, however, and the author emphasized that the study was an anatomic rather than a physiologic one.[272] Whether the increase in connective tissue would reduce maximal dilation of the castrate's urethra compared to that of the noncastrates has not been established. As the role of castration in FUS has been attributed to urethral diameter, smaller cats or those with a smaller penis should have a predisposition for FUS. No data indicate this is so. In summary, no clear-cut data exist to condemn or refute a role for castration in FUS. The common occurrence of the syndrome in intact cats suggests that if it plays a role, it is a subtle factor.

High urine pH has been incriminated in FUS as it is known that struvite is more soluble in acid solution. Urine pH is influenced by the type of metabolic wastes that must be excreted. Diets containing protein of animal origin usually cause production of acid urine and diets containing vegetable proteins cause production of

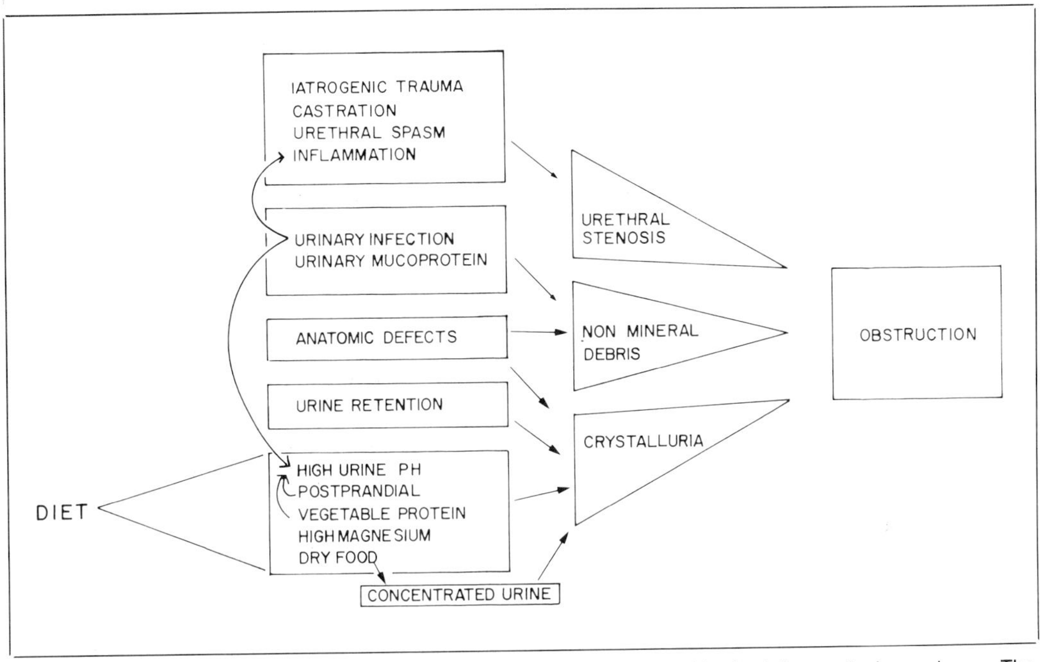

Fig 25. Schematic representation of the multiplicity of factors incriminated in the feline urologic syndrome. The role of specific factors and interrelationship of factors are unproved in many instances.

alkaline urine. However, existing commercial diets of the canned and dry types cause little difference in urine pH.[206]

Regardless of the type of diet, consumption of foodstuff may cause transient production of alkaline urine in association with secretion of HCl by the stomach. This secretion causes alkalemia, which results in bicarbonate secretion by the kidney. Studies in normal cats have shown that alkaline urine exists in the bladder at least between 2 and 6 hours after eating.[273,274] The role of this postprandial phenomenon in FUS has not been studied.

Urine pH may also be modified by bacterial infection in that the metabolic products of urea-splitting organisms may cause alkaline urine. The infrequent presence of bacteriuria in cats with urinary disease makes this an unlikely factor in most cases of FUS.

Such factors as urinary protective colloids, protein matrix, frequency of urinating, heredity and anatomic defects have been nearly untouched in terms of investigative work. One report indicated a high incidence of urachal remnants in cats with FUS and improvement when the remnants were surgically excised.[259]

Postmortem investigations have added little to the knowledge concerning the cause of FUS. These studies revealed changes that would be expected subsequent to outflow obstruction. In some cases the abnormalities have been restricted to the lower urinary tract and in others changes in the kidneys have been found.[236,275,276] While it is tempting to relate renal changes to the cause of FUS, mechanical obstruction could also cause the abnormalities observed.

The previous discussion indicates that the cause(s) of FUS is not established at present. Until more data are accumulated, many of the causes that have been proposed should be regarded as predisposing factors. Several of them may be responsible for FUS because of their simultaneous occurrence or interrelationships. This multicausation concept is illustrated in Figure 25.

Pathophysiology: Obstruction of the urethra may occur at any point along its course but is most common in the penile urethra due to its smaller diameter. The diameter of the penile urethra was estimated to be about 1.0 mm. Cylindric implants 3 mm in diameter placed in the bladder lodged in the bulbourethral area.[55]

Azotemia occurs after obstruction due to accumulation of urine in the bladder and subsequent suppression of renal function. The integrity of the bladder mucosa may be a factor in determining the onset of azotemia since experimental obstruction without bladder scarification caused azotemia after 4-5 days, but azotemia occurred in 3 days or less with bladder scarification.[276] The BUN and serum creatinine concentrations increased at a similar rate in these experiments. Renal function is suppressed because back-pressure of urine in the ureter counters the blood pressure, which is responsible for glomerular filtration. Although some glomerular filtration occurs, tubular resorption results in minimal urine formation. Nonmechanical factors may also play a role in impaired renal function. Experiments in dogs disclosed that maintaining distension of the urinary bladder while alleviating back-pressure on the kidneys by transection of the ureters still resulted in impaired renal function.[277]

A transient minor increase in blood pressure is associated with distension of the urinary bladder of cats but this is probably not of clinical significance. Blood pressure returns to normal when the obstruction is removed.[278]

Anuria results in retention of normal urine constituents. As a result, several blood biochemical alterations previously listed may occur, with dehydration, hypercalcemia and acidosis being the most relevant.

Dehydration is commonly associated with obstruction despite the anuria. Although not proven, this is probably due to continued loss of water through the respiratory tract and skin, and by vomiting without replacement by oral intake.

To avoid imbalances that may occur during this period, it is important to recognize some aspects of the postobstruction state. Diuresis occurs in some patients during the acute postobstructive period in association with elimination of urea and other urine components that accumulated during anuria. This diuresis may be considered physiologic and may occur in the absence of renal damage.[279] Diuresis may also occur because of direct effects of renal obstruction. Impairment of the renal concentrating mechanism is one of the earliest manifestations of obstructive nephropathy, and may be due to defects in proximal and distal tubular transport of Na.[280]

The following events have been demonstrated in other species and probably occur in cats. Due to hyperosmolality associated with retention of solutes in the extracellular compartment during obstruction, there is a shift of water from the intracellular compartment to the extracellular compartment. This helps maintain plasma volume in dehydrated patients.[279] With removal of obstruction, the expanded hyperosmolar extracellular fluid provides adequate renal perfusion to result in marked osmotic diuresis. All extracellular components (urea, Na, K, etc) are lost. If water losses and original water deficit are not replaced, however, hypovolemia, poor renal perfusion and prerenal uremia can occur.

If renal damage associated with obstruction is superimposed on this situation, the potential for morbidity is greater. The hypovolemia that follows initial diuresis is not accompanied by the kidney's ability to concentrate urine, resulting in further loss of water and solute. The end result may be severe dehydration and excessive loss of such electrolytes as Na, K and bicarbonate. Affected cats must receive adequate fluid therapy until renal function is restored.

Some observations have suggested that the urine's specific gravity was related to duration of obstruction and thus to prognosis.[238] Unfortunately, these observations are not consistent with specific gravity determinations made by others nor do they consider the physiologic osmotic diuresis that occurs after removal of obstruction.[236]

Treatment: The best treatment for any disease is to remove the underlying cause. As the cause of FUS is not known, the treatment is symptomatic. As a consequence, there is a wide variety of treatments.

Males and females that do not have urethral obstruction but have dysuria and perhaps hematuria should have a urinalysis and/or urine culture to determine if bacterial cystitis exists. In the absence of bacteria, antibacterial therapy is of questionable value. Response to chloramphenicol therapy was no better than response to a wheat flour placebo, raising serious question to the testimonials that antibiotics are of value in a disease of nonbacterial origin.[261] Parasympathomimetic drugs, such as homatropine methylbromide or propantheline, may be given to relieve spasm of bladder musculature. Other treatments that may be appropriate for unobstructed cats are listed subsequently in a discussion of prophylaxis.

Patients with urethral obstruction should be considered an emergency and should receive immediate attention. The approach to therapy is dictated by the cat's clinical condition. Those that are normothermic, alert and euhydrated are not in imminent danger. Removal of outflow obstruction has first priority and can be conducted in a more leisurely fashion, although it should be done immediately. On the other hand, moribund obstructed cats must be treated immediately and intensively if recovery is to be achieved.

The objectives are to reduce hyperkalemia, restore fluid and acid-base balance and correct hypothermia. The following are logical approaches to achieving these goals and are listed in the order in which they should be performed.

(1) An indwelling catheter is placed in a peripheral vein and a warmed alkalizing solution is infused. A blood sample may be obtained at the time of venous catheterization if pretreatment laboratory values are desired. Fluids are administered at a rate of 90 ml/kg/hr until a volume equal to the fluid deficit is administered. The deficit is calculated by multiplying body weight (kg) by percent dehydration. Thus, a 3-kg cat with 7% dehydration would require 210 ml of fluid. Since the maximal rate of administration recommended is 90 ml/kg/hr, the entire deficit in this case could be given in 50 minutes.

(2) When administration of fluids has been started, the cat's rectal temperature is determined and the cat is placed on a heating pad if hypothermia exists or develops.

(3) Bladder back-pressure is relieved so that urine formation resumes. Removal of the urethral obstruction is the preferred method. If this cannot be achieved within a few minutes, cystocentesis should be performed. Obstructing material may often be removed by decompression of the urinary bladder by cystocentesis.

(4) An indwelling catheter is placed in the urinary bladder once the obstruction has been removed.

As previously indicated, the primary objective of therapy is to correct dehydration, acidosis and hyperkalemia that are likely to exist. The regimen of therapy described above is successful in achieving these goals because:

(1) Rapid correction of dehydration restores circulatory volume. Thus, renal perfusion should be adequate so that renal excretion of wastes can resume once the bladder is emptied.

(2) Administration of alkalizing agents corrects the acidosis. This treatment not only has general beneficial effects on cell metabolism but also specifically causes cell uptake of K to aid in alleviation of hyperkalemia.

(3) Emptying of the bladder removes renal back-pressure and facilitates resumption of urine flow. The kidney is able to resume its homeostatic role with regard to body water and electrolyte balance. Studies in obstructed cats demonstrated a marked increase in urinary potassium excretion after removal of obstruction.[249]

The type of fluid initially used for therapy in obstructed cats is probably not too relevant except that it should be alkalizing and should decrease hyperkalemia by dilution. Several preparations can be used with equal efficacy. For example, lactated Ringer's solution, with $NaHCO_3$ added at 25 mEq/L or saline with $NaHCO_3$ added at 50 mEq/L, could be used. The K content of some solutions may seem to contraindicate their use but this should be kept in perspective. Administration of solutions containing K at 4.0 mEq/L, when compared with the elevated blood K levels in obstructed cats, still causes a decrease in serum K levels. The decrease could be expected to be less rapid, however, than when saline with $NaHCO_3$ added at 50 mEq/L is used.

The cat's urine production should be monitored. Renal excretion of K occurs once flow is resumed. For maintenance and contemporary loss therapy, a balanced electrolyte solution (lactated Ringer's or Multisol-R) should be used.

Glucose and insulin have been used for treatment of hyperkalemia in other species since these compounds are associated with cellular uptake of K. Although these compounds have been advocated for use in cats, they have been used only in combination with fluid therapy and relief of obstruction. Thus, proof of efficacy for the dose of insulin-glucose recommended for cats has not been reported. In view of the success of removal of obstruction and fluid therapy alone, glucose-insulin use does not seem to be indicated or required for the postrenal failure associated with FUS.[249,281]

The actual procedure for removal of urethral debris is important. The approach to be outlined embodies our own ideas and those of other clinicians. A cardinal rule in all procedures involving manipulation of the penis, sheath or urinary bladder is to be extremely gentle to minimize iatrogenic trauma. Repeated manipulation of the penis or manual compression of the urinary bladder can only accentuate existing damage. Sedation or anesthesia is induced as required to handle the patient but not if moderate manual restraint suffices. Although sedatives or anesthetics are considered by some clinicians to facilitate removal of debris, no objective studies have been performed to evaluate their efficacy in this regard. Phenothiazine tran-

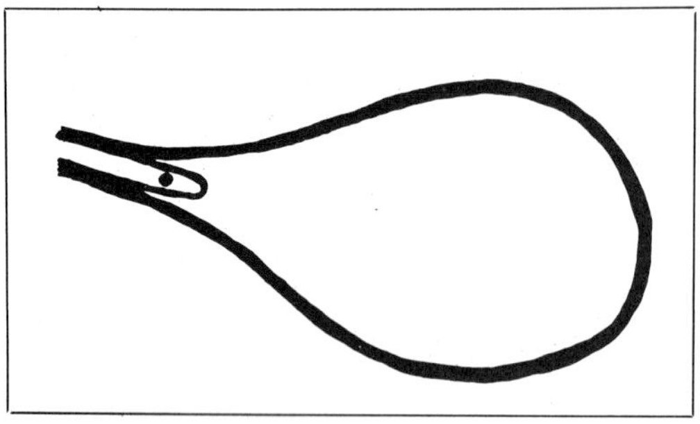

Fig 26. Schematic representation of an indwelling urinary catheter properly placed in the urinary bladder. Notice that the catheter barely protrudes into the bladder lumen. This placement assists in preventing extrusion of the catheter as the bladder contracts.

quilizers and thiamylal sodium are generally used for pharmacologic restraint. Although ketamine is popular for this purpose, the drug is excreted via the urine, and its effect may be prolonged in animals with renal dysfunction. Epidural anesthesia has been induced with 1-1.5 ml of 2% lidocaine injected at the lumbosacral junction.[275] This provides many of the advantages of general anesthesia without the risk.

To remove the obstruction, the cat is placed in lateral recumbency and the penis is gently extruded from the sheath. The urethral orifice is inspected for obstructing debris. The penis is gently massaged to mechanically express debris. If this fails, efforts are made to remove the obstruction by backflushing. After gently washing the penis and prepuce with a mild soap, an open-ended polyethylene catheter (Sherwood Medical) is coated with sterilized lubricant and gently inserted into the urethra while the penis is grasped and gently extended toward the tail. After the obstruction is encountered, sterile saline solution is injected. Initially the solution is allowed to flow back around the catheter to the outside in the hope of flushing the obstructing material out via the external urethral orifice. If this is not successful, the penis is grasped more tightly to prevent reflux of the saline solution. Subsequent injection of saline solution exerts pressure on the obstructing debris.

If the material is forced from the urethra back into the urinary bladder, the resistance on the syringe decreases as the saline enters the bladder. The catheter is then removed, and urine may be voided spontaneously or micturition may be induced by gentle compression of the bladder through the body wall. If the size of the stream is large, the urine is not grossly bloody, bladder emptying is complete as determined by palpation, and the cat was not severely depressed when admitted, use of an indwelling catheter may be avoided. However, the cat should be hospitalized for 24 hours and palpated to determine if spontaneous micturition results in complete emptying of the bladder.

In instances of a small urinary stream, bloody urine, difficulty in emptying the bladder or severe depression, we prefer the use of an indwelling urinary catheter. A soft rubber 3.5-Fr catheter (Sherwood Medical) is used for indwelling purposes because it is less traumatic than a polyethylene catheter.[282] The penis is cleansed, and the lubricated catheter is inserted and advanced as saline solution is injected. The solution probably dilates the urethra and facilitates the passage of both debris and catheter into the bladder. Once the catheter's tip is near the bladder, aspiration is performed. When urine can be aspirated, insertion of the catheter is discontinued. This assures correct placement of the catheter in the bladder so that the tip does not protrude into the bladder to cause trauma (Fig 26). The extruding end of the catheter is dried and wrapped with a strip of ¼-inch adhesive tape. Two sutures are placed through the tape and prepuce to secure the catheter, and the excess length of catheter is cut (Fig 27). The bladder usually empties spontaneously and manual compression is unnecessary unless atony has occurred. Vacuum decompression has been described but seems unnecessary.[283] An Elizabethan collar is placed around the cat's neck to prevent it from removing the catheter. The catheter is left in place until the urine is no longer grossly bloody, usually for 2-4 days. During this time, the bladder is palpated gently a few times daily to determine if outflow is occurring. Blockage of an indwelling catheter is rare, but if it occurs the catheter can be flushed *in situ*. After the catheter is removed, the cat is kept in the hospital for 24 hours to determine if spontaneous micturition occurs.

The use of indwelling urinary catheters in cats is controversial. Long-term use of such catheters in people is accompanied by a high rate of urinary tract infection. One study in cats indicated that indwelling catheters were associated with urinary infection, particularly if dilute urine was formed as a consequence of concomitant parenteral fluid therapy.[284] Morphologic lesions of the urethra and bladder were noticed with use of indwelling catheters, particularly in cats with infection. Although these studies did not establish if infection persisted beyond the period of catheterization, even its temporary presence is undesirable since urethral inflammation and increased debris in the urine may increase the likelihood of reobstruction. Ampicillin administration decreased the incidence of infection but did not prevent its occurrence in all cats.[284] It is obvious that the clinician must weigh the disadvantages and advantages of indwelling catheters in deciding on their use. The possibility of urinary infection in catheterized cats cannot be ignored.

On the other hand, the advantages of an indwelling catheter are considerable. Prior to their use, relief of obstruction by backflushing often was followed by repeated obstruction on the same or subsequent days. Efforts to relieve repeated obstructions have resulted in severe trauma to the urethra and penis. The diuresis frequently associated with removal of an obstruction results in large volumes of urine, and repeated efforts to express urine from the bladder by manual compression have accentuated existing injury and hemorrhage. Use of indwelling catheters eliminates such added trauma. In our opinion, the advantages of short-term indwelling catheters greatly outweigh their disadvantages, if the patient is monitored for bacterial infection.

Occasionally it is not possible to relieve obstruction by back-flushing. Cystocentesis, followed by back-flushing, may be successful in these cases. Although there is controversy about the role of cystocentesis for an obstructed cat, there are few alternatives if the obstruction cannot be removed. To perform cystocentesis, the abdominal area overlying the bladder is prepared as for surgery. A 22-ga, 1½-inch needle is attached to a 3-way valve and a 20-ml syringe. The needle is inserted as the bladder is palpated. Care should be taken to prevent movement by the patient during the procedure, to minimize the risk of lacerating the bladder. This can occur when the bladder is friable or necrotic but it is uncommon when the tissue is viable. Although leakage from the puncture site is a potential complication, it usually does not seem to be clinically significant. If the obstruction cannot be relieved, cystocentesis may be required at intervals indicated by distension of the bladder. When supportive therapy results in improvement in the cat's condition, surgical intervention may be considered. Although their use in cats has not been reported, indwelling prepubic catheters have been used in people for temporary alleviation of urine retention.[285]

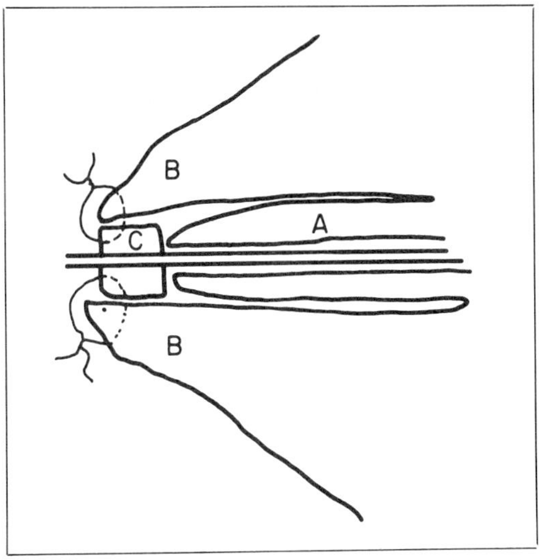

Fig 27. Schematic representation of an indwelling catheter properly placed and immobilized in the male cat. A. penis. B. prepuce. C. adhesive tape wrapped around catheter. The distal edge of the tape is sutured to the prepuce so that only the tip of the catheter protrudes from the urethral orifice.

Various solutions have been advocated for back-flushing obstructed cats to dissolve crystals and mechanically remove them, including $\frac{1}{12}$ N sulfuric acid, tap water, 2% lidocaine, 0.2% acetic acid, 0.5% dyclonine, proparacaine and sodium EDTA solution.[53,54,254,286-289] No objective comparisons have been made concerning the relative efficacy of these solutions. Studies of the acetic acid-acetate buffer indicated that it dissolved macroscopic struvite crystals in 4 minutes and microcalculi weighing 5 mg in 4 hours.[286] Using a buffered solution is more rational than a strong acid for dissolving calculi inasmuch as an extreme pH is avoided; a buffer probably better maintains a pH near the desired level. The acetate-acetic acid buffered solution may support bacterial growth *in vitro,* and it must be sterilized and stored where it can be kept sterile.

Use of anesthetic solutions has been advocated for back-flushing on the theory that local anesthesia may relieve urethrospasm. No objective studies have been performed to confirm this theory nor has the potential toxicity of these agents on inflamed or eroded urinary tract epithelium been investigated.

Use of smooth muscle relaxants has also been advocated for relief of urinary tract obstruction. Statements testifying to their efficacy and lack of it exist but there have been no objective studies of these products.[63,236,289] The use of smooth muscle relaxants is not a part of our therapeutic regimen because to us they seem ineffective.

Use of other technics and instruments has been advocated to facilitate removal of urethral debris. Their efficacy is probably related to the clinician's familiarity with a particular technic. Any procedure that quickly relieves obstruction and maintains urethral patency with minimal trauma to the urinary tract fulfills the requirements of this aspect of therapy.

Other treatments advocated during the early phase of therapy include corticosteroids for reduction of inflammation, testosterone, castor oil, progesterone, vitamin A and hyaluronidase.[290-293] We do not recommend use of any of these drugs since rationale for their use frequently is lacking and their efficacy is unproven.

Once outflow obstruction has been rectified, attention should be directed to other aspects of FUS. Studies in experimental cats indicated that urethral obstruction caused a severe catabolic state.[249] Force-feeding and gavage should be initiated after the initial 24 hours of therapy and should be continued unless voluntary eating or vomiting occurs.

Postobstruction diuresis, as previously discussed, is not uncommon, although it does not occur in all cats. Diuresis may be associated with water and electrolyte loss. Oral administration is the best approach to providing water and electrolytes but parenteral fluid therapy, using lactated Ringer's solution, may be required to supplement fluid needs.

The azotemia of urethral obstruction resolves in about 72 hours if renal damage has not occurred secondary to the obstruction.

Prophylaxis: Long-term prophylactic therapy is a highly controversial aspect of FUS because of the lack of information concerning the underlying cause of the disease. Few, if any, of the procedures that have been advocated have been evaluated objectively. Among the suggested measures are use of a high salt intake to stimulate polyuria, urinary acidifiers, low-mineral diets, avoidance of dry foods, oral sodium EDTA and oral sodium polyphosphate.[53,63,252,289,294-298]

Until better data are available, personal opinion dictates what is considered appropriate prophylactic therapy. On the premise that certain treatment will not harm the cat and may or may not help it, we institute the following measures. An attempt to increase the rate of urine formation is considered the single most important procedure. This dilutes solutes and minimizes urine stagnation in the bladder. Sodium chloride is administered orally as tablets (0.25-1.0 g/day) or by salting the food fairly heavily. Free access to fresh water is essential.

Use of urinary acidifiers is recommended after the uremic phase of disease because they may decrease the quantity of struvite crystals in the urine, even in cats that already have an acid pH.[66] As osmotic agents, they may also increase the volume of urine formed. Several urinary acidifiers are available and their advantages and disadvantages have been reviewed.[299] Some urinary acidifiers are of questionable efficacy in reducing urine pH in cats. These include dl-methionine, ascorbic acid and ethylenediamine dihydrochloride.[273,274] Ammonium chloride appeared more effective and may be used at a dose of 15 gr daily for a 3- to 4-kg cat. Urine pH should be checked at intervals to assure adequate dosage. Methenamine has been mentioned for use in cats but we know of no reports that assure its safety in this species.

Methylene blue and products containing methylene blue are contraindicated because they induce Heinz body formation and hemolytic anemia in cats.[300,301]

On the basis of data previously presented, low-mineral moist food probably can be fed without harm to the patient or serious inconvenience to the client. It is our impression, however, that diet is not a significant factor as long as salt is given PO. Therefore, no specific dietary recommendations are made for our patients.

Treatment of Complications: Complications of urethral obstruction include urethral fistula, bladder atony and urethral stricture (Fig 28). Initially a ruptured urethra is treated with an indwelling urinary catheter, to enable urine outflow while providing the opportunity for spontaneous healing. If this is unsuccessful, surgical repair may be attempted.

Following atony, bladder musculature usually regains tone after a catheter is left in the urethra for several days. Bethanicol (1-2 mg TID) may be used if the outflow tract is patent.[287]

Urethral stricture may be a problem subsequent to the acute phase of FUS. Dilating the urethra with a urinary catheter may be helpful.

Several surgical procedures have been developed for correction of obstruction associated with FUS, including amputating the tip of the penis, splitting the penis, ureterocolostomy, cystocolostomy, urethrocolostomy, antepubic urethrostomy, preputial urethrostomy and technics for perineal urethrostomy. Details concerning some of these procedures can be found in surgery texts.

Wilson's perineal urethrostomy procedure is presently favored as the operation of choice. In a report on 128 cases, a 9% incidence of stricture occurred, requiring a second surgical procedure.[302] Since the recurrence rate for FUS is lower in cats over 4 years of age, we do not recommend surgery in these cats with the first obstructive episode.[265] In younger cats, opinion is divided concerning the recommendation for surgery with the first or later obstructions. Available data indicate that some cats, regardless of age, do not have recurrences after a single episode of obstruction that is managed by nonsurgical means.

Although various prosthetic devices have been developed for facilitating long-term urine outflow in cats, none has gained acceptance.

Congenital Bladder Anomalies

Urachal remnants have been observed in cats.[258,303-305] Three abnormalities have been reported: persistent patent urachus, through which urine passes out via the umbilicus; persistent urachus that is confluent with the bladder but ends blindly in the abdominal cavity; and persistent urachus with leakage of urine or secretion of urachal epithelium into the abdominal cavity.[304]

Treatment of persistent urachus entails surgical extirpation of the urachal stalk. Pre-existing urinary tract infection should be controlled prior to surgery. The theory of urachal remnants leading to FUS was previously mentioned.

Bladder Neoplasia

Primary neoplasms of the bladder are uncommon in cats.[63,306-310] None was found at the necropsy of 2019 cats, whereas 36 were found at the necropsy of 12,030 dogs.[310] This has been attributed to the fact that cats do not metabolize the amino acid tryptophan in the same way as other common species. Cats excrete minimal quantities of carcinogenic orthaminophenols in the urine as products of tryptophan metabolism.[311]

Of the primary neoplasms reported, most have been malignant (carcinomas). Benign tumors (papillomas) have also been observed.

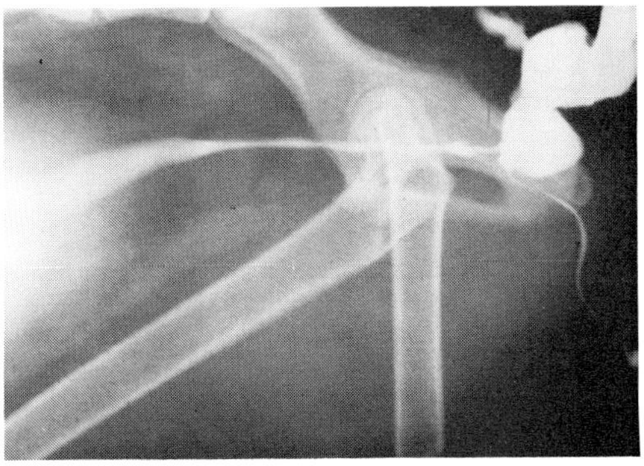

Fig 28. Lateral radiograph of a male cat presented with urine draining from a lesion lateral to the base of the tail. Contrast medium injected into this lesion is seen filling the urethra, which deposits the medium into the urinary bladder and to the external urethral orifice.

Metastatic neoplasms of the cat's bladder are rare but have been reported. Two metastatic lymphoid tumors were found during the necropsies of 2019 cats.[310]

Clinical signs of bladder neoplasia are indistinguishable from those of cystitis in the earlier stages. Dysuria and hematuria are observed. When the neoplasm is larger, diffuse or focal abnormalities in the bladder wall may be palpable; these lesions may also be demonstrated radiographically.

Neoplasms must be differentiated from diffuse or polypoid cystitis and from blood clots in the bladder (Fig 29). As these lesions cannot be dif-

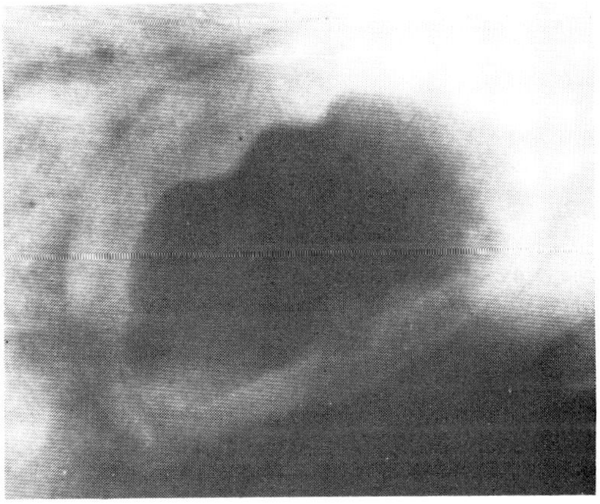

Fig 29. Pneumocystogram of a cat with a bladder wall that is thickened and contains nodular irregularities. At surgery, organized blood clots were found lining the bladder wall.

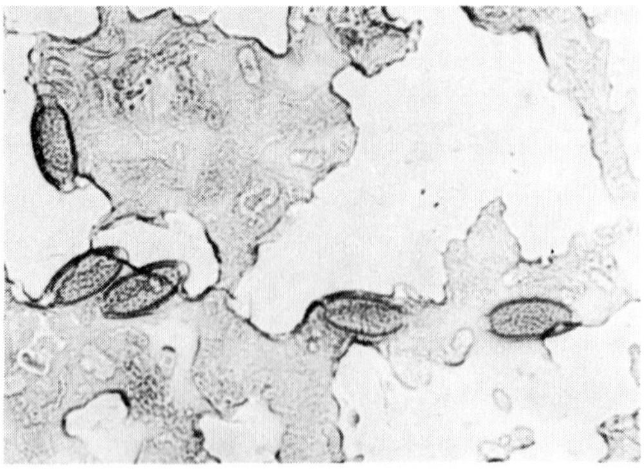

Fig 30. Urine sediment from a cat infected with *Capillaria feliscati*. Five ova appear in the field (original magnification 440X).

ferentiated radiologically, other examinations must be performed. Urine sediment should be examined by a cytologist to determine if neoplastic cells are present. A positive finding confirms the diagnosis but negative results do not exclude neoplasia. Blood clots may be lysed over a period of several days. Exploratory laparotomy may be required for a definitive diagnosis. The lesion and regional lymph nodes may be biopsied and the lesion extirpated by partial cystectomy if possible. The abdomen should be examined for evidence of metastasis.

Chemotherapy and radiation therapy of bladder malignancies in other species have not been highly effective. There have been no reports of such therapy in cats.

Bladder Parasites

The urinary bladder parasite *Capillaria feliscati* has been reported in cats in Australia and Egypt but it is rare in the US.[63,312,313] Diagnosis is by identifying eggs in the urine (Fig 30). Both direct and indirect life cycles involving the earthworm have been postulated. Most cats with the parasite demonstrate no clinical signs, but dysuria and hematuria may occur since occasionally dogs with *Capillaria plica* have these signs. A safe, effective treatment is not known.

Bladder and Urethral Trauma

Trauma to the bladder and urethra occasionally is associated with severe blunt trauma as well as penetrating wounds.[314,315] Rupture of the outflow path can cause signs of uremia and peritonitis due to urine leakage into the abdominal cavity. Hemoconcentration may be severe because of shifts of fluid into the abdominal cavity as a result of leakage of hypertonic urine. Survey radiographs using a horizontal beam, excretory urography and a urethrogram are helpful in diagnosis. Abdominocentesis may yield a fluid with a higher creatinine concentration than in peripheral blood. Therapy includes parenteral fluids and peritoneal dialysis. The defect is usually repaired surgically.

Trauma resulting in urethral edema and diffuse intrapelvic urine leakage may not be apparent in radiographs because of the small or diffuse lesion. If the bladder is intact, an indwelling catheter may be inserted in hope that the defect will heal spontaneously. The patient must be carefully examined when the catheter is indwelling so that laparotomy and surgical repair can be attempted if leakage persists.

Urinary Incontinence

Urinary incontinence is rarer in cats than in dogs. Ectopic ureters and incontinence following ovariohysterectomy have not been reported.

Urinary incontinence of neurogenic origin has been observed in cats after spinal cord and pelvic trauma, and with diffuse inflammatory disease of the urinary bladder. Hereditary vertebral disease of Manx cats caused urinary and fecal incontinence.[316] Incontinence has also been associated with bladder, bladder neck and urethral masses of debris.

Treatment of urinary incontinence is directed at correcting the underlying cause. When overflow incontinence occurs, the potential exists for secondary bacterial infection because of urinary stasis.

References

1. Crouch, JE: Atlas of Cat Anatomy. Lea & Febiger, Philadelphia, 1969.
2. Gilbert, SG: Pictorial Anatomy of the Cat. Univ Washington Press, Seattle, 1971.
3. Pitts, FR: Physiology of the Kidney and Body Fluids. Yearbook Medical Publishers, Chicago, 1968.
4. Swenson, MJ: Dukes' Physiology of Domestic Animals. Cornell Univ Press, Ithaca, 1977.
5. Modell, W. Anat Rec **57** (1933) 13.
6. Foote, JJ and Graffin, AL. Anat Rec **72** (1938) 169.
7. Lobban, MC. J Anat **89** (1955) 92.
8. Gairns, FW and Morrison, SD. J Physiol **110** (1949) 17.
9. Smith, C and Freeman, BL. Proc Soc Exp Biol Med **86** (1954) 775.
10. Helmy, FM and Longley, JB. Acta Histochem **25** (1966) 300.
11. Moore, T *et al.* Res Vet Sci **4** (1963) 397.
12. Fuller, PM and Huelke, DG. Acta Anat **84** (1973) 516.

13. Simic, V and Popvic, S. Anat Anz **113** (1963) 224.
14. Nissen, OI and Galskov, A. Circ Res **30** (1972) 82.
15. Nissen, OI. Acta Physiol Scand **68** (1966) 286.
16. Nissen, OI. Acta Physiol Scand **73** (1968) 329
17. Nissen, OI. Acta Physiol Scand **73** (1968) 320.
18. Galskov, A and Nissen, OI. Circ Res **30** (1972) 97.
19. Baccelli, G. Europ J Clin Invest **1** (1970) 125.
20. Westermark, L and Wahlin, A. Acta Anaesth Scand **13** (1969) 185.
21. MacDonald, AG. Br J Anaesth **41** (1969) 644.
22. Faarup, P. Acta Path Microbiol Scand **71** (1967) 509.
23. Faarup, P. Acta Path Microbiol Scand **72** (1968) 109.
24. Schaffenberg, CA *et al.* Am J Physiol **199** (1960) 788.
25. Coote, JD *et al.* J Physiol **226** (1972) 15.
26. Latimer, H. Growth **3** (1939) 89.
27. Hall, VE and MacGregor, WW. Anat Rec **69** (1937) 319.
28. Smith, HW: The Kidney, Structure and Function in Health and Disease. Oxford Univ Press, New York, 1951.
29. Suzuki, A. Jap J Pharm **21** (1971) 75.
30. Eggleton, MG and Shuster, S. J Physiol **124** (1954) 613.
31. Wolf, AV *et al.* Am J Physiol **196** (1959) 633.
32. Prentice, PG *et al.* Am J Physiol **196** (1959) 626.
33. Carbone, MG. Vet Clin No Am **1** (1971) 281.
34. Meier, RW. JAVMA **137** (1960) 67.
35. Jackson, OF. J Physiol **201** (1969) 97.
36. Bharadwaj, MB and Calhoun, ML. Am J Vet Res **20** (1959) 841.
37. McPherson, A. J Physiol **185** (1966) 185.
38. Garry, RC and Garven, HSD. J Physiol **139** (1957) 1P
39. Garry, RC *et al.* J Physiol **149** (1959) 653.
40. Fletcher, TF *et al.* J Comp Neur **136** (1969) 1.
41. Fletcher, TF and Bradley, WE. Am J Anat **128** (1970) 145.
42. Evans, JP. J Physiol **86** (1936) 396.
43. Elbadawi, A and Schenk, EA. Am J Anat **126** (1969) 107.
44. Edvardsen, P. Acta Physiol Scand **72** (1968) 157, 172, 183, 234.
45. Bowen, JM *et al.* Invest Urol **13** (1976) 327.
46. Domer, FR *et al.* Invest Urol **15** (1978) 404.
47. Sjostran, SE *et al.* Acta Pharm Tox **31** (1972) 241
48. DeGroat, WC and Ryall, RW. J Physiol **200** (1968) 87.
49. DeGroat, WC and Saum, WR. J Physiol **220** (1972) 297.
50. Uemura, E *et al.* Am J Anat **136** (1973) 305.
51. Alexander, RS. Am J Physiol **220** (1971) 1413.
52. Fletcher, TF and Bradley, WF. Am J Vet Res **30** (1969) 1655.
53. Weiss, RM *et al.* Am J Physiol **222** (1972) 378.
54. Edge, ND J Physiol **127** (1955) 54.
55. Shehata, R. Acta Anat **77** (1970) 139.
56. Arlhac, A. C R Soc Biol **165** (1971) 616.
57. Bovee, KC. Vet Clin No Am **1** (1971) 119.
58. Custer, in Catcott: Feline Medicine and Surgery. American Veterinary Publications, Santa Barbara, 1964.
59. Low, DG *et al:* Internal Medical Disorders of the Dog and Cat. WB Saunders, Philadelphia, 1974.
60. Finco, DR: Clinical Biochemistry of Domestic Animals. Academic Press, New York, 1980.
61. Benjamin, M: An Outline of Veterinary Clinical Pathology. Iowa State Univ Press, Ames, IA, 1967.
62. Medway, W *et al:* A Textbook of Veterinary Clinical Pathology. Williams & Wilkins, Baltimore, 1969.
63. Osborne, CA *et al:* Canine and Feline Urology. WB Saunders, Philadelphia, 1972.
64. Thysell, H. Acta Med Scand **185** (1969) 401.
65. Worden, AN. J Sm Anim Pract **1** (1960) 11.
66. Rich, LJ and Kirk, RW. Am J Vet Res **29** (1968) 2149.
67. Mayson, JS. Am J Clin Path **58** (1972) 297.
68. Ross, LA and Finco, DR. Am J Vet Res *In press,* 1981.
69. Bieri, P. Zbl Vet Med A **24** (1977) 642.
70. Borthwick, R and Robbie, B. J Sm Anim Pract **13** (1971) 579.
71. Dure-Smith, P. Am J Roent, Rad Therap, Nuc Med **108** (1970) 691.
72. Zeskov, B. Vet Archiv **27** (1957) 171.
73. Barrett, RB and Kneller, SK. Acta Radiol **(Suppl) 319** (1972) 279.
74. Thayer, GW *et al.* JAVMA **176** (1980) 643.
75. Kneller, SK *et al.* Am J Vet Res **33** (1972) 2111.
76. Smallwood, JE and Sis, RF. Am J Vet Res **34** (1973) 955.
77 . Kneller, SK *et al.* J Am Vet Rad Soc **12** (1971) 65.
78. Finco, DR, Univ Georgia: Unpublished data, 1981.
79. Osborne, CA *et al.* JAVMA **151** (1967) 1474.
80. Osborne, CA. J Urol **107** (1972) 358.
81. Osborne, CA. JAVMA **158** (1971) 1213.
82. Bricker, NS. Am J Med **46** (1969) 1.
83. Finco, DR *et al:* Internal Medical Disorders of the Dog and Cat. WB Saunders, Philadelphia, 1974.
84. Bernstein, LM: Renal Function and Renal Failure. Waverly Press, Baltimore, 1967.
85. Simmenhoff, ML *et al.* N Engl J Med **297** (1977) 132.
86. Ibels, L *et al.* N Engl J Med **298** (1978) 122.
87. Arieff, A *et al.* J Clin Invest **53** (1974) 387.
88. Ross, LA and Finco, DR, Univ Georgia: Unpublished data, 1981.
89. Brouwers, L and Dewaele, A. Ann Med Vet **104** (1960) 229.
90. Berg, R. Anat Anz **109** (1961) 36.
91. Riedel, W. Berl Munch Tierarztl Wschr **81** (1968) 159.
92. Ball. Arch Vet Wissensch (1898) 430.
93. Pierson, DL and Grollman, SS. Acta Anat **40** (1960) 385.
94. Radasch, HE. Am J Med Sci **136** (1908) 111.
95. Potter, GC. Turtox News **32** (1954) 228.
96. Hunt, HR. Anat Rec **15** (1918) 221.
97. Robinson, GW. JAVMA **147** (1965) 516.

98. Verstraete, A *et al.* Vlaams Diergenesk Tijdschr **37** (1968) 81.
99. Ekman, G. Ann Sec Fenn Vanamo **4** (1926) 213.
100. Ekman, G. Ann Sec Zool-bot fenn **14** (1934) 136.
101. Tannreuter, GW. Anat Rec **25** (1923) 59.
102. Mack, CO and McGlothlin, JH. Anat Rec **105** (1949) 445.
103. Hill, KJ. Vet Rec **66** (1954) 107.
104. Lombard, CH. Rev Med Vet **6** (1934) 206.
105. Lombard, CH and Florio, R. Rev Med Vet **9** (1937) 707.
106. Henschen, in Joest: Spezielle Pathologische Anatomie der Haustiere. III Band 206 Richard Scholtz, Berlin, 1923.
107. Merti, GS. JAVMA **146** (1965) 1120.
108. Harzti, J. Mag Allator Lapja **9** (1954) 350.
109. Silverstro, D. Acta Med Vet Napoli **13** (1967) 349.
110. Battershell, D and Garcia, JP. JAVMA **154** (1969) 665.
111. Sehic, M and Bauer, M. Vet Arhiv **49** (1970) 152.
112. Lettow, E and Dammrich, K. Kleintier-Prax **12** (1967) 35.
113. Northington, JW and Juliana, MM. J Sm Anim Pract **18** (1977) 663.
114. Rendano, VT and Parker, RB. J Sm Anim Pract **17** (1976) 479.
115. Crowell, WA *et al.* JAVMA **175** (1979) 286.
116. Osathanondh, V and Potter, EL. Arch Path **77** (1964) 459.
117. Dalgaard, OZ: Diseases of the Kidney. Little, Brown and Co, Boston, 1971.
118. Ticer JW. JAVMA **143** (1963) 613.
119. Kraft, AM and Kraft CG. VM/SAC **65** (1970) 692.
120. Mitten, RA. Iowa State Vet **40** (1978) 65.
121. Chastain, CB and Grier, RL. Feline Pract **5 (4)** (1975) 51.
122. Hayman, JM: Diseases of the Kidney. Little, Brown and Co, Boston, 1971.
123. Johnson, CE. Anat Anz **46** (1914) 69.
124. Ekman, G. Ann Soc Zool Bot Fenn **6** (1928) 37.
125. Meyer, AW. J Anat Physiol **48** (1914) 172.
126. Johnson, CA. JAAHA **15** (1979) 599.
127. Osborne, CA and Finco, DR. Vet Clin No Am **2** (1972) 259.
128. Borthwick, R. J Sm Anim Pract **12** (1971) 623.
129. Kleine, LJ and Thornton, GW. JAAHA **7** (1971) 318.
130. Burt, JK and Root, CR. JAAHA **7** (1971) 328.
131. Caywood *et al*, in Kirk: Current Vet Therapy VII. WB Saunders, Philadelphia, 1980.
132. Collet, R *et al.* Bull Soc Sci Vet Lyon **53** (1952) 47.
133. Montoro, L and Botija, CS. Trab Inst Biol Anim Madr **3** (1935) 121.
134. Potkay, S and Garman, R. J Sm Anim Pract **10** (1969) 345.
135. Craven, JD and Leeky, JW. Rad **101** (1971) 555.
136. Friedland, GW and Dale, RL: Rad **99** (1971) 273.
137. Lucam, F and Brion, A. Bull Acad Vet Fr **15** (1942) 74.
138. Northway, RB. Sm Anim Clin **2** (1962) 526.
139. Imhoff, RK. JAVMA **145** (1964) 123.
140. Rex, MAE. N Zeal Vet J **14** (1966) 94.
141. Hall, MA *et al.* JAVMA **160** (1972) 857.
142. Schneck, G. Dtsch Tierarztl Wschr **80** (1973) 541.
143. Hayes, J. Mod Vet Pract **60** (1979) 827.
144. Weller, RE *et al.* VM/SAC **6** (1979) 1109.
145. Robotham, GR. Feline Pract **8(3)** (1978) 23.
146. North, DC. J Sm Anim Pract **19** (1978) 237.
147. Finkle, AL and Smith, DR. Invest Urol **8** (1970) 299.
148. Steckler, JF and Gillenwater, JY. Invest Urol **8** (1971) 377.
149. Pridgen, WR *et al.* JAVMA **178** (1961) 149.
150. Kerr, WS. Am J Physiol **184** (1956) 521.
151. Bown, P. Vet Rec **89** (1971) 557.
152. Farrow, BRH *et al.* Path **1** (1969) 67.
153. Crowell, WA, Univ Georgia: Unpublished data, 1981.
154. Slauson, DO *et al.* J Path **103** (1971) 131.
155. Farrow, BRH and Hustable, ERR. J Comp Path **81** (1971) 463.
156. Anderson, LJ and Jarrett, WFH. Res Vet Sci **12** (1971) 179.
157. Osborne, CA and Vernier, RL. JAAHA **9** (1973) 101.
158. Nash, AS *et al.* Vet Rec **63** (1979) 71.
159. Scott, RC *et al.* JAAHA **11** (1975) 53.
160. Glick, DW *et al.* Am J Path **92** (1978) 321.
161. Scott, DW *et al.* JAAHA **9** (1973) 530.
162. Ward, JM *et al.* JAVMA **155** (1969) 879.
163. Bekemeier, H and Mendler, E. Acta Biol Med **16** (1966) 79.
164. Kelly, DF *et al.* JAVMA **149** (1971) 413.
165. Jonsson, L and Rubarth, S. Nord Vet Med **19** (1967) 265.
166. Hardy, WD. Proc 40th Ann Mtg AAHA, 1973.
167. Nielsen, in Catcott: Feline Medicine and Surgery. 1st ed. American Veterinary Publications, Santa Barbara, 1964.
168. Willson, JE and Gilmore, DE. JAVMA **140** (1962) 1068.
169. Holzworth, J. JAVMA **136** (1960) 47.
170. Battershall, D and Garcia, JP. Mod Vet Pract **50:9** (1969) 51.
171. Osborne, CA *et al.* JAVMA **158** (1971) 2058.
172. Bush, M *et al.* J Am Vet Radiol Soc **14** (1973) 27.
173. Crowell, WA *et al.* JAVMA **161** (1972) 1127.
174. Clark, L and Seawright, AA. Path Vet **6** (1969) 117.
175. Nakamatsu, M *et al.* Jap J Vet Sci **28** (1966) 259.
176. Hjarre, A. Acta Path Microbiol Scand **Suppl 16** (1933) 132.
177. Clark, L and Seawright, AA. Aust Vet J **44** (1968) 584.
178. Hartigan, PJ *et al.* Irish Vet J **34** (1980) 1.
179. Saegusa, S *et al.* Jap J Exp Med **45** (1975) 403.

180. Saegusa, S *et al.* Arch Path Lab Med **103** (1979) 413.
181. Jubb, KVF and Kennedy, PC: Pathology of Domestic Animals. 2nd ed. Academic Press, New York, 1970.
182. Lucke, VM. Vet Rec **82** (1968) 622.
183. Altera, KP and Bonash, H. JAVMA **149** (1966) 1307.
184. Lewis, in Kirk: Current Veterinary Therapy IV. WB Saunders, Philadelphia, 1971.
185. Asheim, A. JAVMA **147** (1965) 736.
186. Finn, JP *et al.* J Sm Anim Pract **11** (1970) 607.
187. Meier, H. Diabetes **9** (1960) 485.
188. Farrow, BRM and Penny, R. JAVMA **158** (1971) 606.
189. Holzworth, J. Cornell Vet **47** (1957) 302.
190. Walker, WG *et al:* Diseases of the Kidney. Little, Brown and Co, Boston, 1971.
191. Esseveld, H *et al.* Meded Dienst Volksgezondh Ind **29** (1940) 1.
192. Murphy, LC *et al.* Cornell Vet **48** (1958) 3.
193. Hemsley, LA. Vet Rec **68** (1956) 300.
194. Fessler, JF and Mortar, RL. Cornell Vet **54** (1964) 176.
195. Low, DG *et al.* Am J Vet Res **28** (1967) 731.
196. Lucke, VM and Crowther, ST. Vet Rec **77** (1965) 647.
197. Freudiger, U. Kleintier Prax **13** (1968) 153.
198. Bloom, F: Pathology of the Dog and Cat. American Veterinary Publications, Santa Barbara, 1954.
199. Blaehser, S. Rec Med Vet **137** (1961) 589.
200. Hamilton, JM. J Sm Anim Pract **7** (1966) 445.
201. Riedel, W. Berl Munch Tierarzt Wschr **82** (1969) 397.
202. Lucke, VM. Vet Rec **102** (1978) 301.
203. Lucke, VM. J Path Bact **95** (1968) 67.
204. Holzworth, J. Mod Vet Pract **40** (1959) 22.
205. Osborne, CA *et al.* JAAHA. *In press,* 1981.
206. Holme, DW. Proc Kal-Kan Symposium, 1977.
207. Hamar, D *et al.* JAAHA **12** (1976) 514.
208. Fried, W *et al.* Ann Int Med **79** (1973) 823.
209. Finco, DR. JAAHA **8** (1972) 166.
210. Abel, RM *et al.* N Engl J Med **288** (1973) 695.
211. Low, in Kirk: Current Veterinary Therapy IV. WB Saunders, Philadelphia, 1971.
212. Parker, in Kirk: Current Veterinary Therapy VII. WB Saunders, Philadelphia, 1980.
213. Black, DA. Arch Int Med **126** (1970) 906.
214. Borison, HL and Herbertson, LM. Am J Physiol **197** (1959) 850.
215. Lees, GE and Osborne, CA. JAAHA **15** (1979) 135.
216. Finco, DR. Am J Vet Res. *In press,* (1981).
217. Kelly, DF *et al.* J Comp Path **89** (1979) 125.
218. Wooley, RE and Blue, JL. J Clin Microb **4** (1976) 326.
219. Braude, A. Med **52** (1973) 257.
220. Cass, RJ *et al.* J Am Med Assoc **225** (1973) 1509.
221. Brandt, ME. VM/SAC **66** (1971) 123.
222. Kirk, RW. Proc 37th Ann Mtg AAHA, 1970.
223. Robbins, EG *et al.* Lancet **1** (1975) 476.
224. Lawler, DC. Vet Rec **83** (1968) 103.
225. Heller, RA. Southwest Vet **23** (1970) 129.
226. Jackson, OF and Sutor, DJ. Vet Rec **86** (1970) 335.
227. Ryan, CP and Smith, RA. JAVMA **158** (1971) 1946.
228. Fisherman, H and Slatko, L. No Am Vet **34** (1953) 355.
229. Jarvis, J. Vet Rec **72** (1960) 519.
230. Frost, RC. Vet Rec **70** (1958) 765.
231. Bohonowych, RO *et al.* JAVMA **173** (1978) 301.
232. Stamey, TA: Urinary Infections, Williams & Wilkins, Baltimore, 1981.
233. Finco *et al,* in Catcott: Canine Medicine. American Veterinary Publications, Santa Barbara, 1979.
234. Tomey, SL and Follis, TB. Feline Pract **8(1)** (1978) 39.
235. Anonymous. Vet Rec **100** (1977) 208.
236. Osbaldiston, GW and Taussig, RA. VM/SAC **65** (1970) 461.
237. Foster, SJ. J Sm Anim Pract **8** (1967) 207.
238. Jackson, OF. J Sm Anim Pract **12** (1971) 555.
239. Practice Survey. Feline Pract **3(1)** (1973) 9.
240. Willeberg, P. Nord Vet Med **27** (1975) 1.
241. Dorn, CR *et al.* Am J Vet Res **34** (1973) 433.
242. Barker, J and Povey, RC. J Sm Anim Pract **14** (1973) 445.
243. Holzworth, J. Cornell Vet **53** (1963) 157.
244. Brodey, RS. Mod Vet Pract **52:3** (1971) 20.
245. Rich, LJ and Kirk, RW. JAVMA **154** (1969) 153.
246. Schecter, RD. JAVMA **156** (1970) 1567.
247. Carbone, MG. JAVMA **147** (1965) 1195.
248. Loeb, WL and Knipling, GD. Mod Vet Pract **52** (1971) 40.
249. Finco, DR and Cornelius, LC. Am J Vet Res **38** (1977) 823.
250. Parks, J. JAAHA **11** (1975) 102.
251. Sutor, DJ *et al.* Res Vet **11** (1970) 298.
252. Rich, LJ and Norcross, ML. Am J Vet Res **30** (1969) 1001.
253. Duch, DS *et al.* Biochem Med **19** (1978) 236.
254. Meier, RW. JAVMA **151** (1967) 1059.
255. Fabricant, CG. Comp Immun Microb Inf Dis **1** (1979) 121.
256. Armistead, WW. No Am Vet **34** (1953) 276.
257. Gilbride, AP. Norden News, Summer (1970) 6.
258. Livingston, ML. VM/SAC **60** (1965) 705.
259. Hansen, JS. VM/SAC **72** (1977) 1735, 1744.
260. Lyngset, A. Nord Vet Med **24** (1972) 577.
261. Barsanti, J *et al,* Univ Georgia: Unpublished data, 1981.
262. Jackson, OF and Tovey, JD. Feline Pract **7(5)** (1977) 30.
263. Thrall, BE and Miller, LG. Feline Pract **6(1)** (1976) 10.
264. Reif, JS *et al.* JAVMA **170** (1977) 1320.
265. Bovee, KC *et al.* JAVMA **174** (1979) 93.
266. Lewis, LD *et al.* JAVMA **172** (1978) 559.
267. Kallfelz, FA *et al.* Feline Pract **10(4)** (1980) 25.

268. Broadus, AE and Thier, SO. N Engl J Med **300** (1979) 839.
269. Jackson, OF. Vet Rec **96** (1975) 70.
270. Gaskell, RM *et al.* Vet Rec **105** (1979) 243.
271. Fabricant, CG *et al.* Cornell Vet **59** (1969) 667.
272. Herron, MA. JAVMA **160** (1972) 208.
273. Finco, DR. Am J Vet Res **42** (1981) 670.
274. Chow, FHC *et al.* Feline Pract **8(4)** (1978) 29.
275. Rich, LJ. Cornell Vet **61** (1971) 542.
276. Robinette, JD. Master's thesis, Washington St Univ, 1969.
277. Tolls, RE and Dille, JM. J Urol **74** (1955) 197.
278. Watkins, AL. J Physiol **39** (1938) 32.
279. Chandler, M *et al.* Invest Urol **11** (1973) 114.
280. McDougal, WS and Wright, FS. Kidney Int **2** (1972) 304.
281. Burrows, CG and Bovee, KC. JAVMA **172** (1978) 801.
282. Lees and Osborne, in Kirk: Current Veterinary Therapy VII. WB Saunders, Philadelphia, 1980.
283. Frye, FL and Detrick, JF. VM/SAC **68** (1973) 424.
284. Lees, GE *et al.* Am J Vet Res **42** (1981) 825.
285. Jackson, GW. Am J Obstet Gyn **105** (1969) 59.
286. Jackson, OF. Vet Rec **87** (1970) 667.
287. Fishler, J. JAVMA **127** (1955) 121.
288. Damitz, WF. JAVMA **159** (1971) 90.
289. Phillips, LR. Anim Hosp **2** (1966) 15.
290. Kowall, NL. Feline Pract **1(2)** (1971) 9.
291. Sharpnack, in Kirk: Current Veterinary Therapy IV. WB Saunders, Philadelphia, 1971.
292. Lumb, WV. Vet Med **50** (1955) 26.
293. Stallings, EP. Proc 19th World Vet Congr **1** (1971) 300.
294. Osborne and Lees, in Kirk: Current Veterinary Therapy VII. WB Saunders, Philadelphia, 1980.
295. Holmes, JR *et al.* Vet Rec **90** (1972) 578.
296. Bentley, MAW and Waterlow, J. Vet Rec **90** (1972) 612.
297. Jackson, OF. Vet Rec **91** (1972) 292.
298. Burch, GR. Mod Vet Pract **48:3** (1967) 47.
299. Hardy, RM and Osborne, CA. Proc 40th Ann Mtg AAHA, 1973.
300. Spicer, SS and Thompson, EC. J Indust Hyg Tox **31** (1949) 206.
301. Schecter, RD *et al.* JAVMA **162** (1973) 37.
302. Tomchick and Green, in Kirk: Current Veterinary Therapy VII. WB Saunders, Philadelphia, 1980.
303. Scherzo, CS. JAVMA **151** (1967) 1329.
304. Hansen, JS. VM/SAC **67** (1972) 379.
305. Hansen, JS. VM/SAC **67** (1972) 1090.
306. Osborne, CA *et al.* Am J Vet Res **29** (1968) 2041.
307. Wimberly, HC and Lewis, RM. Vet Path **16** (1979) 223.
308. Dorn, AS *et al.* Feline Pract **8(5)** (1978) 14.
309. Dill, GS *et al.* JAVMA **160** (1972) 743.
310. Gruber, R. Inaug Diss Tierarztl Fak Munchen **86** (1970).
311. Brown, RR and Price, JM. J Biol Chem **219** (1956) 985.
312. Waddell, AH. Aust Vet J **43** (1967) 297.
313. Waddell, AH. Aust Vet J **44** (1968) 33.
314. Alcantara, P and Costa, ME. J So Afr Vet Assoc **43** (1972) 409.
315. Andre, PG and Jackson, OF. J Sm Anim Pract **13** (1972) 101.
316. Leopold, HW *et al.* JAVMA **164** (1974) 520.

13

the musculoskeletal system

M.R. HERRON

Although the domestic cat constitutes a high percentage of small animal patients seen by veterinarians, diseases affecting the musculoskeletal system are uncommon. If we exclude those diseases caused by trauma, very few diseases are recorded when compared with muscular and osseous diseases in dogs.[1] Some of the problems to be described are so unusual they are almost items of curiosity rather than of clinical significance. We should not forget, however, that any lesion of the musculoskeletal system is possible in cats, and never rule out a possible diagnosis simply because it has not been reported.

As long as breeders are satisfied with the musculoskeletal conformation of cats, many of the abnormalities found in dogs probably will not occur. With the few obvious exceptions, the anatomy of the cat's locomotor system has changed little if any from that of the domestic cat's ancestors. Some of the obvious skeletal changes that have resulted from breeding practices include brachycephalic conformation in some breeds and lack of a tail in the Manx. Because most of the problems of the musculoskeletal system are traumatic in origin, surgery texts should be consulted for solutions to these problems.

Congenital Disease

Although cats are potentially subject to an unlimited number of congenital diseases, few occur commonly. Some are inherited and others are associated with infection *in utero*. Surviving cats with congenital diseases should not be bred.

Maxillofacial Compression

Shortening of the maxilla and mandible, as in the Persian, Angora and Himalayan breeds, has been exaggerated by inbreeding of lines of breeding cats with brachycephalic traits. The condition predisposes to upper respiratory, pharyngeal and ocular problems related to corrugation of the soft tissues in the facial area.

Amelia and Hemimelia

Amelia, the congenital absence of a limb or limbs, and hemimelia, the congenital absence of the distal part of a limb, occur occasionally in kittens. Radial and ulnar hemimelia are most common.

Congenital lack of a tail, as in Manx cats, can be considered a form of amelia. Extreme shortening of the tail, to include the sacrum, can result in neuromotor deficits, megacolon, urine retention and reproductive failure.

Exostoses

Exostoses are benign outgrowths of the bones, typically occurring near the epiphyses of long bones. Multiple cartilaginous exostoses should be considered hereditary in cats.[2]

Hip Dysplasia

Abnormalities of the coxofemoral joint and associated lameness, characteristic of hip dysplasia in dogs, are rare in cats.[3] The lesions are the same as in dogs (Fig 1). Cats respond well to femoral head and neck ostectomy.

Patellar Luxation

Patellar luxation may be acquired or congenital and is rare in cats.[4] Traumatic luxations may be treated by reduction and immobilization. Congenital patellar luxation can be treated by trochleoplasty, joint capsule imbrication or tibial tubercle transplantation.

Acquired Diseases

Trauma

Myositis, tendinitis and osteitis are most commonly caused by bite wounds. Ritualistic fight-

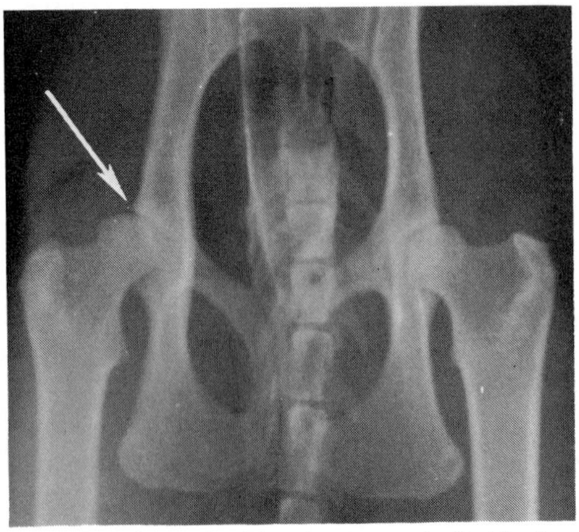
Fig 1. Coxofemoral subluxation in a cat with hip dysplasia.

ing among cats leads to puncture wounds and the associated cellulitis that often follows. The spread of bacterial infection may involve muscles, tendons, bones and joints.

The early, disseminated subcutaneous infections generally are easily controlled with systemic antibiotics. The tendency for cats to form abscesses is well recognized. Once abscessation occurs, use of antibiotics alone seems less than adequate to control the disease. Generally it is necessary to establish drainage, provide some cautery to the abscess directly, and protect the patient with systemic antibiotics.

Some cases of myositis or osteomyelitis may become chronic.[5] Any time an infection becomes chronic and unresponsive to routine therapy, consideration should be given to a few problems that require special attention. When cellulitis begins to form dissecting, unresponsive lesions of the skin and surrounding tissues, consideration should be given to the possibility of *Nocardia* infection, and appropriate diagnostic tests and therapy instituted (see Chapter 5).

If the skeletal system is involved in puncture wounds, thought should be given to osteomyelitis and sequestration of bone. Diagnostic radiographs and therapeutic sequestrectomy usually lead to resolution of the problem.

Foreign bodies, including teeth and claws, occasionally cause chronic unresponsive infections. Surgical exploration and foreign body retrieval are curative.

Trauma by automobiles and blows by objects are the cause of many musculoskeletal diseases in cats. Muscle trauma generally is self-curative, with anti-inflammatory agents and muscle relaxants to provide relief of pain. Muscle tears must be treated with external support or surgical repair.

The most common disease of the feline skeleton is fractures. Fracture repair is beyond the scope of this chapter and specifics should be consulted in surgery texts.[6] Fracture repair in cats is essentially like that in dogs, with minor variations. The size of the cat allows for some technics to work well in the cat that might not in large dogs. Cats are very cooperative orthopedic patients and appropriate orthopedic procedures yield gratifying results.

Figure 2 illustrates a severe example of trauma caused by a shotgun blast. The multiple fractures and joint destruction would lend themselves to amputation of the limb very easily. However, external coaptation was elected. A modified full-pin splint was applied for 6 weeks, and the cat showed normal ambulation 4 weeks after splint removal (Figs 3, 4). This is a rather vivid example of how well cats respond to good orthopedic care.

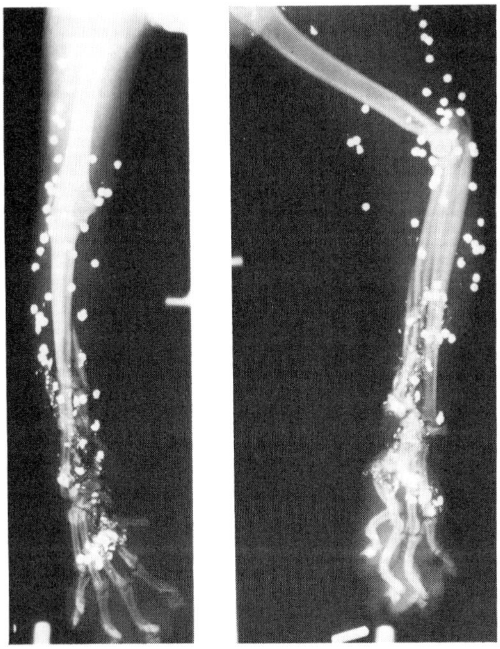
Fig 2. Forelimb of a cat injured by a shotgun blast.

Infection

Other than bacterial osteomyelitis, as caused by puncture wounds described earlier, bone infection usually is related to open fractures or open surgical fracture reduction. Bacterial osteomyelitis generally begins with infection by gram-positive organisms, with the gram-negative bacteria as secondary invaders. Treatment should be directed at antimicrobial therapy and fracture stabilization. Nocardiosis should be considered in unresponsive cases of osteomyelitis.

Brucellar osteomyelitis and anaerobic bacterial infections occur in dogs and both should be considered in chronic, unresponsive feline osteomyelitis. Fungal osteomyelitis should be considered in enzootic areas. Blastomycosis, coccidioidomycosis and histoplasmosis can be manifested as bone infections even though the disease may be systemic (see Chapter 5).

Polyarthritis

Polyarthritic syndromes occur in cats and consideration should be given to all feline patients with multiple joint disease as having some systemic disease. Septicemia may precipitate septic synovitis and usually is seen in kittens.

Therapy involves joint aspiration and intra-articular injections of broad-spectrum antibiotics. Mesenchymal diseases may cause polyarthritis and patients should be evaluated for antinuclear antibody, lupus erythematosus and Rh factors. Infection by FeLV reportedly causes a polyarthritis syndrome.[7,8] Cats with multiple joint involvement should be tested for FeLV.

Osteoarthritis

Arthritis in cats is more common than is generally supposed. Degeneration of articular cartilage is secondary to the same causes as in other species. Some show only subtle lameness when they actually have severe arthritis. Lameness is exaggerated in cold, wet weather and after excessive activity.

The causes of arthritis in cats include sepsis, trauma, articular fractures, luxation and ligamentous injuries. Once the cause is corrected,

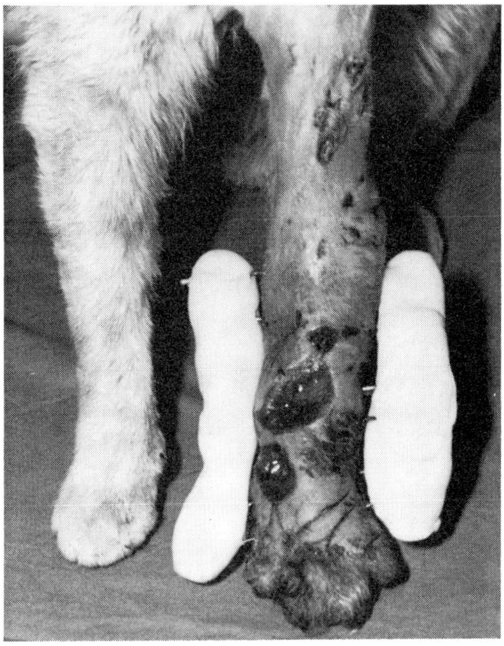

Fig 3. The limb was stabilized with full-pin splintage, K wires and methyl methacrylate.

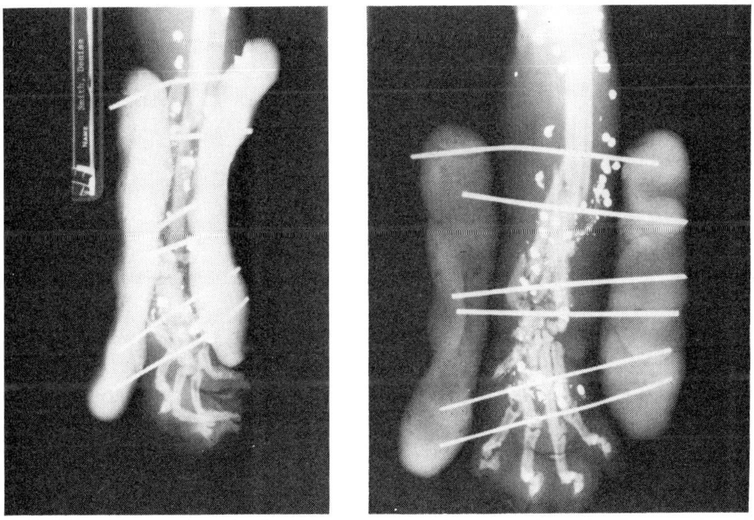

Fig 4. Radiograph of the foreleg of the cat in Figures 2 and 3 after fixation.

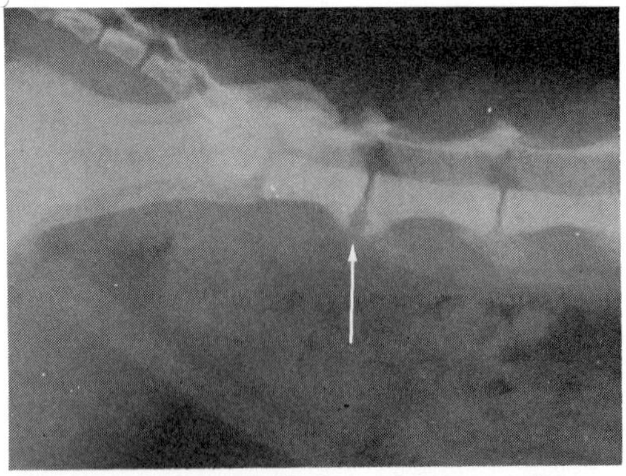

Fig 5. Spondylosis (arrow) of the lumbar vertebrae.

therapy with anti-arthritics works well to ameliorate signs. Ascriptin (Rorer), given PO at 25 mg/kg every third day, works well in minor cases of arthritis. For severe cases of arthritis, oral prednisolone is used at 5 mg BID, with the dosage gradually being reduced to 1.25 mg or less BID and maintained at low levels. Arthrodesis is quite successful in cats, and consideration of the feline crouching position should be given before deciding on the angle of fusion.

Spinal Disc Protrusion

Herniation of intervertebral discs in cats is not as common as in some breeds of dogs. It causes the same signs as in affected dogs (see Chapter 14). The lesion may be more commonly associated with trauma in cats than in dogs. There are signs of posterior paresis, with loss of sensory and motor activity of the rear legs.

The diagnosis is based on clinical signs and confirmed by radiography. Treatment of disc protrusion involves decompression hemilaminectomy. Patients treated early in the course of the disease respond well.

Hypertrophic Osteoarthropathy

Hypertrophic osteoarthropathy is characterized by subperiosteal hypertrophic osteogenesis of the long bones and occasionally the pelvis and vertebrae.[9] The skeletal changes are commonly associated with thoracic lesions, such as tumors, lung disease, heart defects and mediastinal lesions, but have also occurred in cats with abdominal lesions.

The cause is thought to be a circulatory disturbance somehow related to the thoracic or abdominal lesion. Resolution of the thoracic or abdominal lesion results in regression of the periosteal new bone growth.

Spondylosis

Spondylosis, ankylosis of a vertebral joint, is another uncommon lesion in cats. It occurs secondary to vertebral trauma or as a senile change and may be evident radiographically (Fig 5).

Use of analgesics, such as aspirin or prednisolone used as for arthritis, may be necessary if the lesion causes pain. Pain typically ceases after osseous bridging between vertebrae is complete. Cats unresponsive to medical therapy can be treated by vertebral body stabilization.

Metabolic Disease

Dietary Deficiencies

Dietary deficiencies of Ca, P, Se, Cu and vitamins A, D and E may result in musculoskeletal disease.[10] Rickets, a lack of vitamin D, is essentially nonexistent and deficiencies of vitamins A and E are rare.

Nutritional deficiencies are more common in cats fed only one type of food, such as all liver, fish or meat. Such diets may also lead to toxic excesses of vitamins A and D.

Chapter 1 contains more information on nutritional deficiencies.

Hypervitaminosis A

Cats fed an exclusive diet of raw liver are subject to excessive levels of vitamin A. The resultant toxicosis causes hyperostosis and vertebral ankylosis. Other clinical signs include manifestation of pain, abnormal ambulation, depression and muscle wasting.[11]

There is no specific, effective therapy in addition to eliminating the all-liver diet and feeding a balanced diet. Mildly affected cats may recover. High serum levels of vitamin A persist due to continuous release of vitamin A stored in the liver.

Hypervitaminosis D

This condition is rare and causes high serum levels of Ca. Although it may be of no clinical significance, chronic hypervitaminosis D may result in bone resorption. Hypercalcemia also can lead to cardiac abnormalities and metastatic calcification of soft tissues.

Nutritional Hyperparathyroidism

Nutritional hyperparathyroidism, also known as paper-bone disease, osteogenesis imperfecta and juvenile osteoporosis, is a disease of young, confined cats.[12] It is characterized by hypocortical osteodystrophy, with loss of bone minerals.

Owners of catteries have thought this condition was inherited and related to osteogenesis imperfecta. Histologically, it is not similar to osteogenesis imperfecta, however, other than that in both cases the bone cortices lack mineral and the bones are easily fractured.

Cause: Nutritional hyperparathyroidism is directly related to a lack of dietary Ca. The natural diet of cats consists of rodents and birds. In the wild state, cats consume the entire carcass, including bones, intestines and skin. This provides a balanced intake of minerals, proteins, carbohydrates and vitamins. When confined as pets, cats are seldom fortunate enough to receive all of these nutrients in abundance. Furthermore, cats are creatures of habit and, when given certain food, even for a short time, may develop a liking for it and refuse all others.

Household cats, both young and old, often are fed meat exclusively. They drink infrequently and, once they acquire a taste for meat, accept little else even though milk is offered. Even young cats may refuse milk. The usual meat diet consists mostly of muscle or organs, such as heart, kidneys and liver. All meat has a low Ca and high P content. The Ca:P ratio in most meat is 1:20. This means the average cat eating such a restricted diet receives insufficient Ca.

In growing animals, Ca deficiency causes acute, severe metabolic disturbances involving the parathyroid gland, resulting in demineralization of the skeleton. The degree of demineralization depends on the intake. Growing cats should receive food rich in minerals, with a Ca:P ratio of about 1.5:1. During the first 6-8 months of life, while the cat's skeleton is developing, there is a special need for minerals.

The serum Ca level in normal cats is 10-11 mg/gl and the normal serum P level is 4-5 mg/dl, with a normal serum Ca:P ratio of 2:1. A low mineral intake, particularly of Ca, causes hypersecretion of parathormone. This hormone causes minerals to be resorbed from bone if dietary Ca is not readily available (see Chapter 11). Blood levels of Ca and P show little fluctuation of the 2:1 ratio until late in the disease.

Demineralization of young bones occurs very rapidly if the dietary deficiency is great. Resorption is from the diaphyses of bones. Mineral is transferred in the blood to the growth plates, enabling bones to grow at a normal rate.

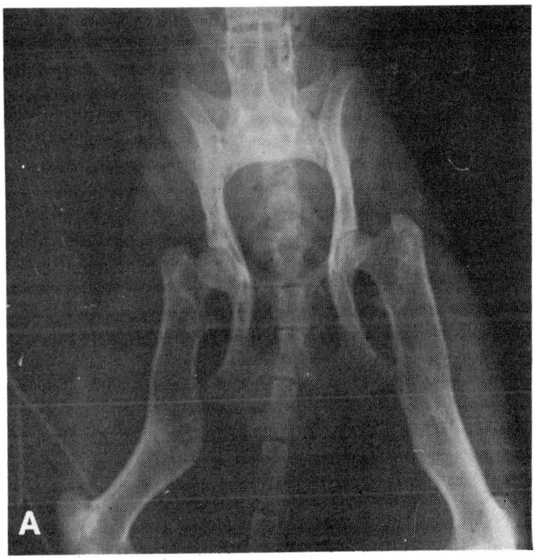

Fig 6. A. Ventrodorsal radiograph of a cat with severe nutritional hyperparathyroidism. Note the old femoral fractures. B. Lateral radiograph of the same cat reveals spinal curvature.

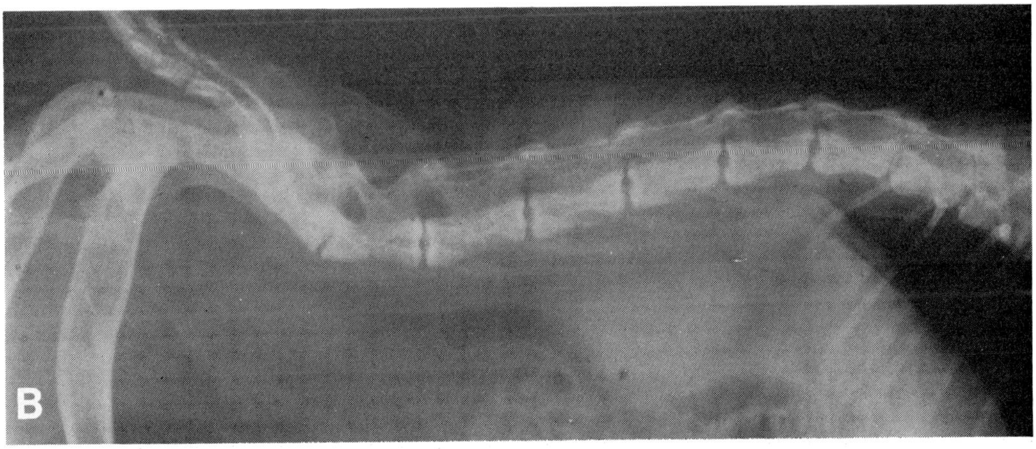

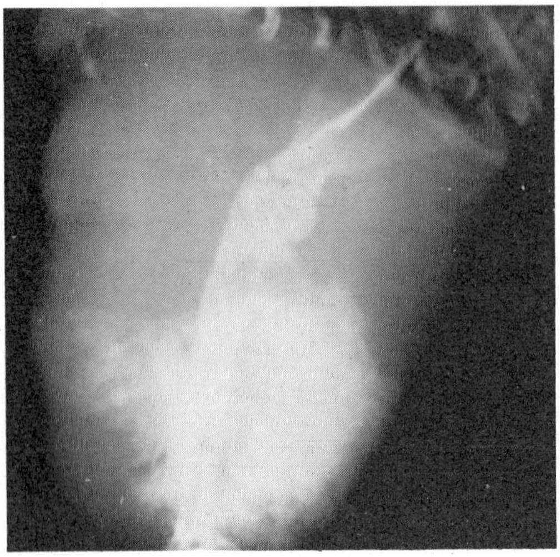

Fig 7. Osteosarcoma of the humerus. The tumor appears to originate at midshaft. There is considerable proliferation of bone as well as lysis.

Clinical Signs: During the peak of the growth period, at 6-14 weeks of age, cats fed distilled water and meat, particularly beef heart exclusively, become demineralized to the extent that fractures of their long bones may occur in as short a time as 2-3 months (Fig 6). It is difficult to determine the amount of mineral present in the skeleton by radiography, but it can decrease 30% before evidence of depletion can be detected radiographically.

When fed a meat diet exclusively, cats maintain body weight and a normal haircoat; however, due to demineralization, the legs become bowed and the spine arched. Spontaneous fractures of the long bones and vertebrae are prominent signs of the disease.

If the condition becomes severe enough, the cat refuses to walk, and as many as 25-50 spontaneous fractures may occur. There also is evidence of muscle soreness and hypersensitivity. Instability of the periosteum around the demineralized bone usually is responsible for the pain. After the condition progresses sufficiently, muscular spasms may be noticed.

Chronic constipation and retention of urine are common. Because of pelvic obstruction, defecation and urination become so painful that the bladder and bowels are not emptied. Death due to uremic poisoning and megacolon occurs in extreme cases.

Treatment: The initial treatment is slow IV administration of 10 ml, in an average-sized cat, of 10% Ca gluconate solution. Considerable improvement usually is evident within 24 hours, after which time large doses of Ca (*eg*, Ca gluconate at 1-2 g/day) should be given PO. The diet should also be corrected to meet the minimum daily requirements for all nutrients.

It sometimes is very difficult to entice a cat to eat a balanced diet. They relish the soft bones of chickens, small birds and rodents, however, and in this form adequate Ca may be ingested.

Renal Hypoplasia and Nephritis

There are 2 other forms of hypocortical osteodystrophy resulting from secondary hyperparathyroidism. One is associated with impaired renal function, which may result from either nephritis or congenital hypocortical renal dystrophy. As in the case of a low-Ca diet, parathyroid activity is increased due to the hyperphosphatemia and hypocalcemia. Increased production of parathormone then causes resorption of bone mineral.

When renal complications exist, there are changes in the skull, particularly the mandible. The resulting condition is very similar to the one in horses known as "bighead" and in dogs as "rubber jaw." The normal architecture of the bones is changed through absorption of mineral. The bony trabeculae are replaced by cancellous bone, which is interspersed with fibroplastic tissue and blood vessels that crowd out the marrow.

Secondary Hyperparathyroidism

A third form of bone demineralization occurs in older, confined cats eating meat diets. The Ca requirements of adult cats normally are lower than for kittens because skeletal growth has stopped. Cats conserve Ca well enough to remain asymptomatic for some time while in a negative Ca balance. However, prolonged Ca deficiency results in resorption of bone mineral, hyperostosis and formation of poor-quality periosteal new bone.

Cats with this condition usually are presented for treatment of chronic constipation. The owner seldom realizes that the trouble is due to a narrowed pelvic opening caused by pelvic collapse when the depleted bones lose their rigidity and ability to support the cat's weight. The diagnosis of such cases is dependent on radiographic examination. The collapsed pelvis, arched back and hyperperiostosis of the long bones are the diagnostic signs.

If the skeletal changes are recognized early enough, the diet can be corrected and the cat's condition improved, provided feces and urine can be eliminated without too much difficulty. Calcium gluconate, fish with bone, and other high-mineral foods should be given.

Neoplasia

Although bone tumors are not common, any cell type is potentially neoplastic. Of primary bone tumors, the origin may be osteogenic, chondrogenic, collagenic or myelogenic.[13-15] In addition to primary bone tumors, soft tissue tumors of any type may directly invade bone or metastasize to bone.[16] A tumor in bone could be of any cell type.

Without attempting to describe all the tumors of bone, suffice it to say that when a neoplasm of bone is suspected, there should be no hesitation to biopsy the growth and confirm clinical and radiographic suspicions of neoplasia. Diagnosis in the absence of histopathologic confirmation is unwarranted.

Osteosarcomas are the most common bony tumor. They tend to become quite large before being noticed and differ from the same tumor in dogs. In cats, osteosarcomas tend to occur at an older age and do not necessarily originate at the metaphyses of long bones (Fig 7). This malignant tumor has developed on the skull and feet of cats. In younger cats, osteosarcomas tend to involve membranous bones and are more lytic than proliferative. In older cats, the long bones are affected and the tumors are proliferative as well as lytic (Fig 7).

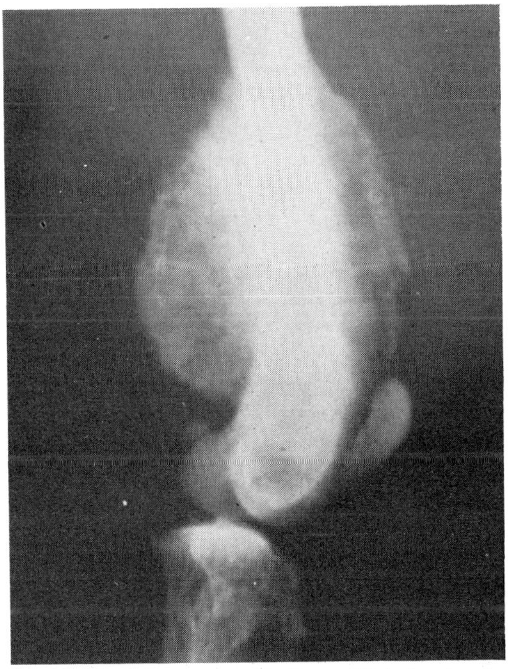

Fig 8. Parosteal sarcoma of the femur. Note the density of this tumor as compared with the more lytic appearance of the osteosarcoma in Figure 7.

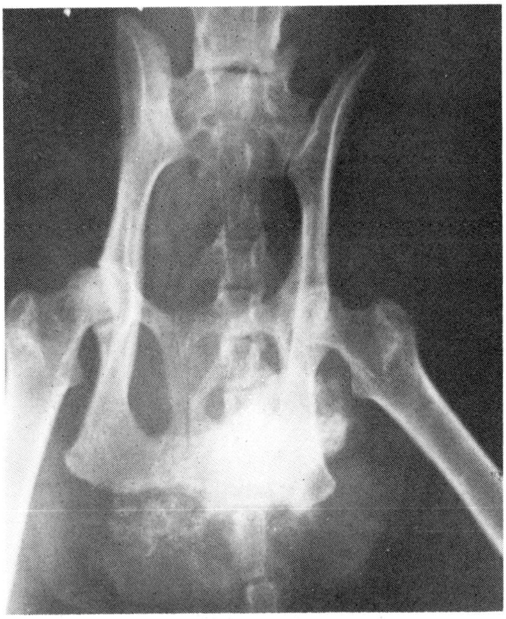

Fig 9. Myxochondrosarcoma in an aged cat.

Parosteal sarcomas are less common bony tumors in cats. They may be mistaken for periosteal fibrosarcomas, but they tend to grow less rapidly and are more dense and slower to metastasize (Fig 8).

Tumors of cartilaginous origin, such as chondrosarcomas or myxochondrosarcomas, occur at the epiphyses and in membranous bone (Fig 9).

Osteomas generally are benign and grow slowly. They occur on the membranous bones of the head, ribs and pelvis.

Once the tumor type has been determined, the proper approach to therapy can be instituted. The tumor type and mitotic index dictate the use of surgical, radiation, chemical or immunologic therapy, or a combination of these.

To illustrate the potential for therapy of skeletal neoplasia, Figure 10 shows a composite radiograph of preoperative and postoperative views of a cat with an osteogenic sarcoma of the femur. Because of the slow metastatic rate of this tumor type in the cat, the distal femur was resected

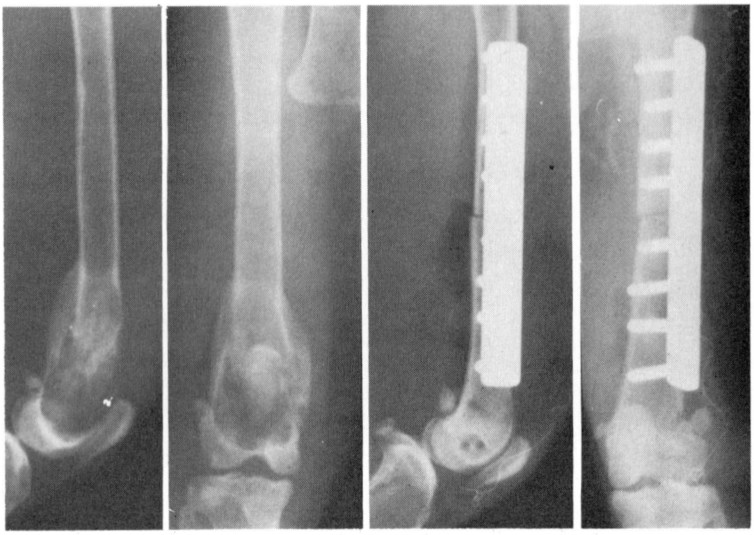

Fig 10. Preoperative (left) and postoperative radiographs of a cat with osteosarcoma of the distal femur. The affected portion was resected and an allograft implanted, with bone plates for stabilization.

and a frozen allograft used to replace the resected bone. Figure 11 shows a sagittal section of the resected distal femur and the tumor destruction. This patient was alive and showing no signs of tumor or lameness one year postoperatively. Although this case illustrated what can be done in some cases of neoplasia, sometimes amputation is the best solution. The key to success is a diagnosis confirmed by biopsy.

Neoplasia of muscle tissue is very uncommon. The same approach to diagnosis and treatment is indicated with muscle tumors as discussed with bony tumors.

Confusing Lesions

Several diseases are easily confused with musculoskeletal conditions but are unrelated.

Saddle Thrombus of the Caudal Aorta

In middle-aged and old cats, paralysis of the hindlimbs may occur following embolism at the bifurcation of the iliac arteries. The blood clot that lodges there assumes the shape of a saddle and is so-named. The lesion may be an extension of endocarditis, but it occasionally occurs after severe vascular trauma.

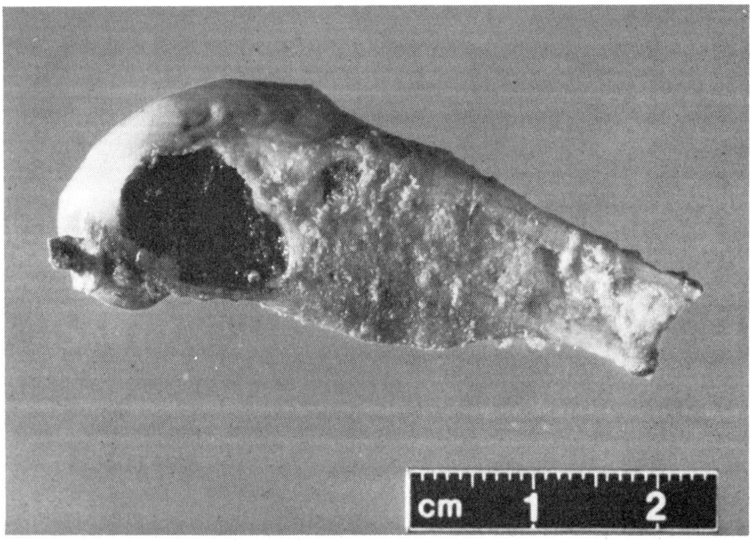

Fig 11. Sagittal section of the resected portion of the femur from the cat in Figure 10.

An affected cat is presented with posterior paralysis, cold rear extremities, and absence of a femoral pulse. The condition is serious and prompt surgical correction is indicated.

Surgery involves temporary ligation of the caudal aorta, incision through the aorta, and removal of the thrombus. After vascular closure, the aortic ligature is removed and the patient is checked for a femoral pulse. If these cases are diagnosed and treated promptly, return of locomotor function is possible. Chapter 9 contains a detailed discussion of thromboembolism.

Cerebellar Hypoplasia

Incomplete development of the cerebellum in kittens was once thought to be inherited but is now known to be caused by *in utero* infection by feline panleukopenia virus. Affected kittens lose their balance and are unable to coordinate head, body and limb movements. Although the condition may be noticed earlier, it generally is not recognized until the kittens are 6-8 weeks old, when they should normally be walking well. Affected animals are not even able to coordinate eating movements and begin to lose weight.

At necropsy, a small underdeveloped cerebellum is found with a normal-sized cerebrum and medulla.

Chapter 4 contains more information on this subject.

Gangliosidosis

Gangliosidosis, an inherited neurologic disease in cats, can easily be confused with a disorder of the musculoskeletal system. The condition is due to a marked accumulation of GM_1 ganglioside in the cerebral cortex. Affected cats show motor disability beginning at 2-3 months of age. There is progressive muscular and neurologic degeneration, causing sudden deterioration and death at about 11 months old.

This disease may be inherited as an autosomal recessive trait and may be analogous to juvenile GM_1 gangliosidosis of children. The condition seems to start after an apparently normal developmental period. The diagnosis can be confirmed by measuring galactosidase activity in the skin of a cat with the suspected disease.[17]

References

1. Rousch, JC. Feline Pract **10(3)** (1980) 10.
2. Pool, RR and Carris, CB. Vet Path **9** (1972) 350.
3. Holt, PE. J Sm Anim Pract **19** (1978) 273.
4. Vaughn, LC. Pedigree Dig **5(1)** (1978) 5.
5. Griffiths, GL and Bellenger, CR. Aust Vet J **55** (1979) 587.
6. Herron, in Catcott: Feline Medicine and Surgery. 2nd ed. American Veterinary Publications, Santa Barbara, 1975.
7. Pedersen, NC *et al.* Am J Vet Res **41** (1980) 522.
8. Wilkinson, GT and Robins, GM. J Sm Anim Pract **20** (1979) 293.
9. Brodey, RS. Vet Annual **19** (1979) 179.
10. Bennett, D. Vet Rec **98** (1976) 313.
11. Seawright, A *et al.* J Comp Path **77** (1967) 29.
12. Watson, ADJ. Aust Vet Pract **5** (1975) 164.
13. Knecht, CD and Greene, JA. JAVMA **171** (1977) 1077.
14. Hinko, PJ *et al.* JAAHA **15** (1979) 737.
15. Thornburg, LP. Vet Path **16** (1979) 255.
16. Madewell, BR *et al.* J Am Vet Rad Soc **17** (1976) 213.
17. Baker, HJ *et al.* Science **174** (1971) 838.

14

the nervous system

A.J. PARKER, D.P. O'BRIEN, AND S.A. SAWCHUK

NEUROLOGIC DIAGNOSIS

Recognizing the Problem

Defining the presenting complaint of the owner or the sign the cat is showing is generally a simple matter; however, signs caused by lesions of the nervous system are often misinterpreted because veterinarians overinterpret. The differential diagnosis tables in this chapter are organized along simple lines to help avoid such mistakes. The clinical signs should be initially defined as simply as possible: paralysis, pain, ataxia, behavior, muscle spasm, seizure, etc. This simple diagnostic approach also applies as the lesion is localized and the differential diagnosis attempted.

Interpreting the Signalment, History and Physical Examination

The significance of the signalment, history and physical examination in neurologic diagnosis is frequently overlooked, especially by generalists. They seem to think that neurologists do not use such mundane information in making a differential diagnosis. Although neurologists use advanced technology, they also make much use of the basic information available to everyone. They are interpreters.

The history, signalment and physical examination are free sources of information that only cost time to obtain. If the information they provide is ignored, it is likely that expensive and possibly unprofitable tests will be substituted. This simple information also plays a major part in selection of treatment and in the prognosis.

The factors to be considered include species, breed (purebred in general, specific combinations of breeds, specific breeds), age, sex (female, estrus, parturition), color (white), size (obese, cachectic), environment (places, people, animals), habits (roams, diet, chews things, annoys neighbors), first sign of the problem, speed of onset, progression/recovery (anatomic spread or degree of severity), presence of pain and its localization, probability of trauma, history of other diseases or treatments (mild or severe, kitten diseases, vaccinations, origin, birth), evidence of current non-neurologic problems (pulse, color, respirations, vomition) and behavior/personality.

Neurologic Examination

The neurologic examination is not an end in itself. In a normal animal it is an extension of a routine physical examination. Most clinicians examine gait, coordination, position sensation of the limbs (conscious proprioception), balance and most cranial nerve functions in their routine examination. Muscle atrophy, skin lesions (self-mutilation) and focal pain are also likely to be detected. The client usually furnishes information about the cat's ability to eat and drink (swallow), smell, hear and see, and about such things as behavior, seizures or episodic weakness.

Probably the only parts of the neurologic examination ignored in the routine physical examination are the segmental spinal reflexes and the placing/hopping (higher) reflexes.

Among the client's complaint, the history and the physical examination, the generalist is not likely to miss the fact that there is a neurologic problem. A neurologic examination is not magic and its results are not difficult to interpret or use in diagnosis, when logic is used.

The tables on differential diagnosis in this chapter are used as the starting point from which neurologic examinations are described and the findings interpreted. There is always a diagnostic reason for examining a neurologic function; it is not done just because a textbook says it should be.

Principles of Neurologic Diagnosis

The 3 classic objectives in neurologic diagnosis are localization of the lesion, determination of the character or type of lesion (irritative or destructive), and determination of the lesion's cause. These objectives readily lend themselves to incorporation into the problem-oriented medical record system. Localization and characterization of the lesion are determined just before the differential diagnosis list ("rule outs") is drawn up.

Most neurologic signs are deficits. The nervous system can cause many signs, but most are deficits that indicate the location of a lesion.

Nervous tissue responds to injury or disease in only 4 ways: deficiency, shock, release and discharge.

Deficiency: Deficiency refers to absence of a function of part of the nervous system. For example, a peripheral nerve may be severed, a vertebral fracture may destroy a lower motor neuron, eliminating a reflex and producing flaccid paralysis, an optic nerve may be compressed, causing loss of vision, or a vestibular lesion may cause loss of balance.

Shock: Shock of the CNS is difficult to diagnose except in retrospect. It has been suggested that shock is a molecular disturbance. Two forms of CNS shock are concussion and spinal shock. Concussion will be discussed later. We have never seen true spinal shock in a feline clinical case. It is a depression of all lower motor neurons and other neuronal activity caudal to a site at which the spinal cord is either anatomically or functionally severed. In experimental cats it lasts only a few minutes.

Release: This term refers to escape of a lower (more primitive) part of the nervous system from higher (more sophisticated) control. The major clinical example is release of lower motor neurons from upper motor neuron inhibition. This results in increased segmental reflex response to a stimulus (*eg,* tapping the straight patellar ligament). Such increased reflex activity is sometimes called hyper-reflexia.

Discharge: Discharge refers to abnormal electrical activity of part of the nervous system. The most common manifestation of discharge is a convulsion. Irritation of lower motor neurons can cause them to discharge, resulting in fasciculations or rigidity in the muscles they supply.

Localization of the Lesion

Neurologic localization frightens many clinicians because they assume one has to be a neuroanatomist to do it. To interpret every possible neurologic sign, this is true; however, it is not true when it comes to making a diagnosis. A diagnosis depends on knowledge of a combination of history (speed of onset of signs), signalment (age, species), signs observed and the examination.

It is initially only necessary to say that the signs are brain, spinal cord, peripheral, non-neurologic or multifocal in origin. Even if some confusion exists it is likely that only 2 of these broad categories are involved.

The next step is to say if the lesion(s) is on the left and/or right, if it is mild or severe, or if it is irritative or obliterative. For brain lesions one can usually say if cranial nerves, the cerebellum, motor, behavioral, visual or balance mechanisms are involved. For spinal lesions one can often identify the level of the lesion (cervical, thoracolumbar or lumbosacral). The exact spinal nerve or spinal segment involved in peripheral or spinal lesions is not usually critical in making a diagnosis but is useful in giving a prognosis and knowing where to radiograph or perform surgery. This is usually adequate information to make up a list of differential diagnoses regardless of where the lesion is.

Efficiency of Diagnosis

A logical and simple approach to neurologic diagnosis is usually an efficient one. Factual knowledge, interpretation skills and understanding how one's mind works in making a diagnosis lead directly to accuracy and profitability.

A clinician is usually solving a problem when making a diagnosis. Clinical knowledge functions at 3 levels when it is used in problem-solving. Level 1 is the recognition of the presenting sign, elicitation of the history, performance of the physical and neurologic examinations, and interpretation of this information. It is important to interpret as much as possible at level 1 before moving to level 2.

Level 2 is the use of level-1 information and its interpretation to produce a limited list of probable diagnoses from comprehensive differential diagnosis lists. One also must select, perform and interpret a number of diagnostic tests so the list can be reduced to conform to the diagnostic objectives of the client or practice. One must decide how far to push diagnosis in many situations. How limited a diagnosis do the clients want or can they afford? Is it reasonable to proceed just until all remaining differential diagnoses on the list are treated the same way or are treated compatibly? Note that to function at level 2, one must do such things as obtain quality radiographs and interpret them. A level-2 diagnosis leads directly to level 3. Excessive activity at level 2 usually results in loss of profit.

Level 3 is simply client education, prognosis and treatment. It also involves performing any surgical treatment. Most sources of information (lectures, books, articles, seminars) are level 3 in nature, and one must virtually know the diagnosis to use them.

The reference sources one uses most often are comprehensive lists of causes of clinical signs, such as the differential diagnosis tables in this chapter, tables of normal results of tests and lists of treatments. One depends heavily on diagnostic skills (facts and interpretation experience) and knowledge about the signs various diseases can cause.

Perspectives on Diseases

The last part of this chapter describes the clinical features of each neurologic disease, using a systematic approach. A clinician cannot make a diagnosis by leafing through such a section, looking for inspiration. The differential diagnosis section is written for that purpose. The disease descriptions are provided to help clinicians get a perspective on what signs any given disease can cause.

Having an accurate perspective on the diseases is important when one reads a differential diagnosis table and selects the likely diseases that could be responsible for the signs in the case at hand. Not knowing that a disease could cause the signs in any given case is a major cause of errors in diagnosis.

Differential Diagnosis of Presenting Signs

The presenting complaint or signs should be interpreted as simply as possible. The signalment and history should be recorded and interpreted with the findings of the physical and neurologic examinations. The lesions should be localized, at least in general terms if not specifically. The appropriate differential diagnosis table(s) should be consulted and the likely diseases selected from it/them.

One must always consider the more common diseases first. Follow the general rules initially and only consider unusual diseases and exceptions to the general rules later. The text accompanying each table helps in further examination of the appropriate part of the nervous system and in the selection of tests. No test should be selected that is likely to make the cat's condition worse than will the possible diseases. Tests, the results of which are unlikely to change the form of therapy or prognosis, must be selected with care. Any deviation from such an attitude to advance knowledge should be justified to the client in light of the expense and the possible needless suffering of the cat. Select and interpret suitable tests at least until the remaining differential diagnoses are all untreatable, are all treated the same way, or can be treated in combinations which are compatible. Do not "wait-and-see" when the remaining differential diagnoses are urgent for therapeutic or public health reasons.

Refer cases promptly if you are unable to perform the required diagnostic tests. Always get a good pathologic study performed whenever the diagnosis is not final or a question of infection/genetic etiology has arisen. Do not ignore the value of repeated neurologic or radiologic examinations in difficult cases. In the tables, each disease is followed by a list of suggested tests. The suggestions often include apparently unnecessary tests, usually because the diagnosis is made by eliminating other diseases or because closely related differential diagnoses would require such a test. The tables tend to be over-inclusive at times because it is easier to ignore a suggestion than to think of it oneself. The tables tend to overlap in places to make up for some misinterpretation of clinical signs. For example, signs of paralysis or weakness (paresis) of cranial nerves can be handled with Table 1 (brain), Table 3 (head tilt) or Table 9 (neuritis). When doubt exists over which table is most applicable, it is wise to consult them all.

Ataxia, Paresis, Paralysis and Pain

These are the major signs of disease of the spinal cord/vertebrae, but they can also be caused by cranial, peripheral and non-neurologic processes.

Some of the data from the basic signalment, history and physical examination could be applied in Table 1 as follows in cases with signs of spinal lesion: pain (trauma, meningitis, tumor of vertebra); no pain (tumor, myelitis, demyelination, spinal vascular accident, CNS degeneration); slow onset (tumor, myelitis, CNS degeneration, inherited diseases); fast onset (trauma); onset over 1-3 days (meningitis, mye-

Table 1. Some Causes of Real or Apparent Ataxia, Paresis and Paralysis

Involving Spinal Cord or Vertebrae	Methods of Diagnosis
Trauma:	
Vertebral fracture or fracture-dislocation	C,H,PR,(CR)
Cord contusion/laceration	C,H,PR,(CR)
Projectile injury	C,H,PR
Hematomyelia or hemorrhagic necrosis of spinal cord	C,H,PR,(CR)
Intervertebral disc, traumatic or spontaneous	C,H,PR,(CR)
Neoplasms and Space-Occupying Lesions:	
Vertebral tumor	C,H,PR
Cord tumor, nerve root tumor	C,H,PR,CR
Spinal cord cyst	C,H,PR,CR
Epidural granuloma or hematoma	C,H,PR,CR
Infection:	
Myelitis/meningomyelitis	
FIP or FeLV	C,H,OP,CP,S,CSF,E
toxoplasmosis	C,H,OP,CP,CSF,E
rabies	Hopefully B
unknown, polioencephalomyelitis, demyelination, vaccinal	C,H,PR,CSF,S,CR,E,B
Vertebral osteomyelitis, spondylitis/discospondylitis/ epidural abscess	C,H,PR,M
Spinal meningitis (fungal, bacterial, algal)	C,H,PR,CSF,M,S
Congenital and Genetic:	
Lysosomal enzyme deficiencies—glycolipid/lipoprotein catabolism disease (leukodystrophy, gangliosidosis, etc)	C,H,OP,PR,CR,CSF,E,B, S
Other inherited CNS degenerations	C,H,OP,PR,CR,CSF,E,B
Spina bifida (occulta, meningo- or meningomyelocele)	E,H,PR,CR,CSF,E
Syringomyelia/spinal dysraphism	E,H,PR,CR,CSF,E
Hemivertebra and other anomalies	C,H,PR,CR
Other:	
Spinal vascular accident	C,H,OP,PR,CSF,CR,E
Migrating parasites or larvae	C,H,PR,CSF,CR,B
Tetanus	C,H,CP,E
Hypervitaminosis A	C,H,PR,CP
Idiopathic	C,H,OP,PR,CP,CSF,CR, S,E,B

CODE: **B**—biopsy, aspiration or necropsy; **C**—clinical signs and examination (includes neurologic examination); **CP**—clinical pathologic examination; **CR**—contrast radiography; **CSF**—cerebrospinal fluid analysis; **E**—electrophysiologic examination (EEG, EMG, ECG, ERG, isotope brain scan, CAT scan); **H**—history; **M**—microbiologic examination; **OP**—ophthalmologic examination; **PR**—plain radiography; **S**—serologic examination, skin tests, FeLV slide test (paired serum samples often needed); **T**—treatment.

litis); young animal (infections, trauma, inherited disease, congenital anomalies); older animal (tumors). Such an approach usually limits the differential diagnoses to relatively few diseases.

Localizing and understanding the effects of spinal lesions requires knowledge of some simple neuroanatomy. Clinically it is important to understand reflex, motor and sensory functions, as well as the clinical signs of spinal cord disease (pain, ataxia, paresis, paralysis).

All fibers leaving (efferent) the CNS are motor, and it is customary to refer to them as lower

Table 1 (continued)

Involving Brain and/or Associated Structures	Methods of Diagnosis
(also see Table 3)	
Encephalitis (FIP, FeLV toxoplasmosis, rabies, CNS reticulosis or granulomatous encephalitis, pseudorabies, polioencephalomyelitis, vaccinal)	C,H,CSF,PR,CR,E
Tumor	C,H,CSF,PR,CR,E
Cerebrovascular accident	C,H,CSF,E
Trauma	C,H,CSF,PR,E
Hydrocephalus	C,H,PR,E,CR
Cerebellar hypoplasia and other cerebellar or cerebellar-tract degenerations or encephalitis	C,H,PR,CSF,E
Intracranial meningitis	C,H,CSF,CP,M,E,S
Epilepsy (see Table 5)	C,H,CP,CSF,E
Hallucinogenic drugs	C,H,CP,CSF,E
Idiopathic feline vestibular syndrome	C,H,PR,CSF,CP,E
Inherited CNS disease (already mentioned)	
Thiaminase toxicity	C,H,CP,CSF,T
Granuloma/migrating larvae	C,H,CP,PR,CR,CSF,E
Involving PNS but May Suggest Spinal Lesions Initially	**Methods of Diagnosis**
(Also see Table 9)	
Trauma ± fracture	C,H,PR,E
Polyradiculoneuritis	C,H,PR,E,B
Immune neuritis of brachial plexus	C,H,PR,E,B
Injection injury	C,H,PR,E
Nerve tumor	C,H,PR,E
Non-PNS tumor pressing on nerve	C,H,PR,E
Toxicity (lead, acrylamide, organophosphate)	C,H,CP,E
Idiopathic	C,H,PR,E,B
Not Directly Involving Nervous System	**Methods of Diagnosis**
Arterial occlusion (aortic or other artery embolus, DIC)	C,H,CR
Cardiac failure	C,H,PR,CP,E
Fractured pelvis or limb	C,H,PR
Arthritis	C,H,PR
Heart blocks (complete or intermittently severe)	C,H,E
Addison's disease, severe hypothyroidism	C,H,CP,PR,E
Polymyopathies	C,H,E,B
Myasthenia gravis	C,H,E,B
Botulism, tick paralysis	C,H,T,E
Hypoglycemia	C,H,CP
Generalized toxicity (thiaminase)	C,H,CP,CSF,S,E
Depression (general disease processes)	C,H,CP,PR
Drugs (eg, phenytoin)	C,H
Sedatives	C,H,E
Obesity	C,H
Anemia	C,H,CP

motor neurons. The cell bodies of the spinal lower motor neurons are in the ventral horn of the spinal cord grey matter (Fig 1). Lower motor neurons innervate both voluntary striated and involuntary (smooth) muscles. The lower motor neurons receive many synapses from afferent (incoming) components of the segmental spinal reflexes and directly or via interneurons from a

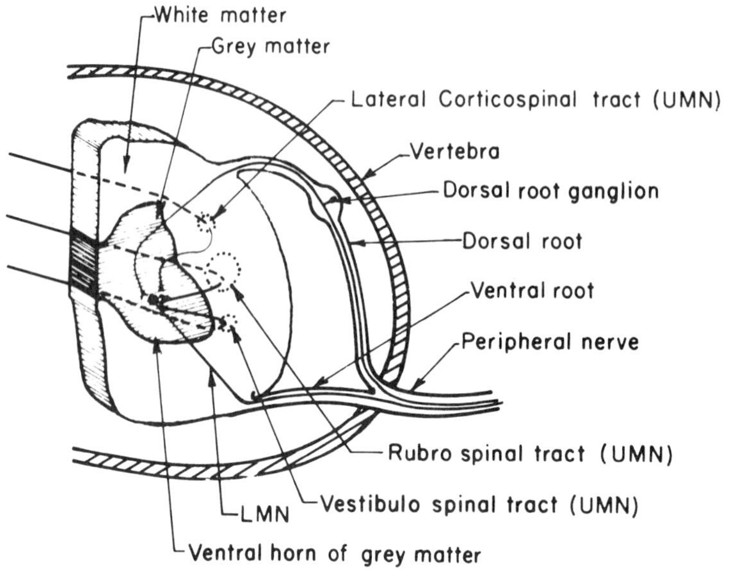

Fig 1. Diagram of half of one spinal cord segment. Ascending sensory spinal cord tracts are not shown.

variety of descending motor tract fibers in the spinal cord. The descending fibers, originating from the cerebral hemispheres, midbrain and brainstem, are called upper motor neurons.

Because the lower motor neurons are the only motor fibers leaving the CNS and because they are the final common fiber through which all upper motor neurons and reflexes must operate, lower motor neurons are often referred to as the final common pathways. The lower motor neurons are neurotrophic to the striated muscles they innervate, *ie,* they supply some of the metabolic needs of muscles and also innervate them. After lower motor neuron injury (within the spinal cord or in the peripheral nerves), the striated muscles atrophy rapidly. Mere electrical stimulation is insufficient to reverse the atrophy, although it slows it. This continued atrophy is in part attributed to loss of lower motor neuron neurotrophic activity.

Upper motor neurons are divided into voluntary and involuntary types. The major voluntary tracts in cats are the rubrospinal tracts and, to a lesser extent, the lateral corticospinal tracts. Upper motor neurons are generally inhibitory to lower motor neurons, whereas the segmental spinal reflex inputs to the lower motor neurons are excitatory. Therefore, the lower motor neurons would respond to a greater extent to afferent reflex information were it not for the inhibitory upper motor neurons. There are a few upper motor neuron tracts that are excitatory to lower motor neurons, *eg,* the involuntary vestibulospinal tract. In cats, upper motor neurons run on the same side (ipsilateral) of the cord as the limbs they supply (Figs 1, 3).

A reflex is a circuit beginning at the sensory organ (*eg,* muscle spindle in knee jerk). This generates an action potential in a sensory (afferent or toward the CNS) nerve fiber. This enters the CNS and may synapse locally (segmental reflex) (Figs 1, 2). The effector (efferent) part of the reflex arc is the lower motor neuron to the muscle. If any part of the reflex arc (sense organ, dorsal root, spinal cord segment, lower motor neuron, peripheral nerve or muscle) is not functional, the reflex is absent. If the reflex extends to or descends from the brain, it is called a higher reflex (Fig 2).

Clinically it is not critical to know exactly where in the cord each motor tract runs, but it is necessary to know which cord segments mediate the major reflexes.

The sensory functions we test in the cat's limbs are of 2 types: conscious proprioception or limb position sense and pain (superficial and deep).

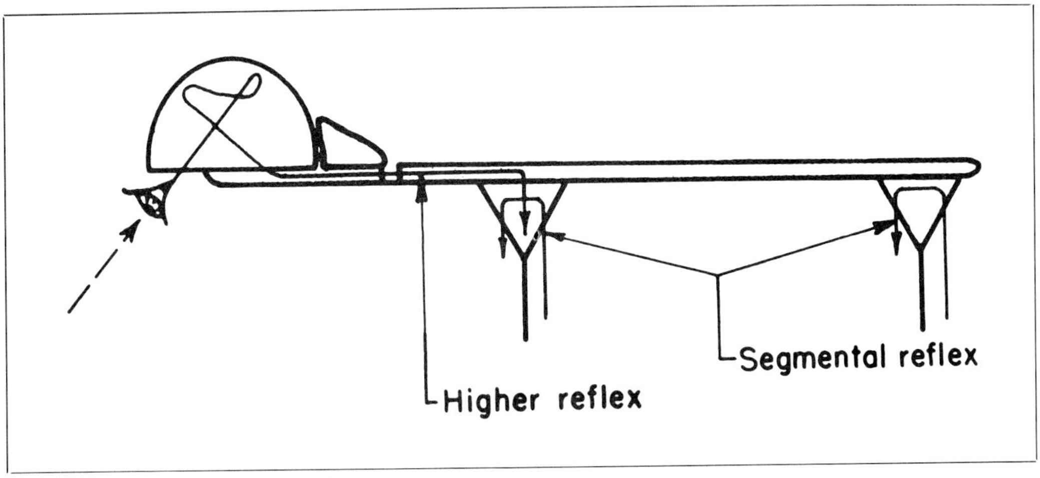

Fig 2. Higher reflex vs a segmental reflex.

Conscious proprioception information travels in the dorsal white columns of the cord ipsilateral to the limb of origin. Pain information apparently is processed similarly but there is disagreement about which tract is involved (Fig 3). The spinocervical tract seems to be a major pathway. The spinothalamic tracts are apparently of less significance in cats as compared to people. Another pathway is the network of short fibers wrapped around the grey matter, called the fasciculus proprius.

Clinically it is not critical to know where each sensory tract runs, but it is essential to know how to test the sensory functions.

Once in the brainstem, most sensory pathways cross over to the opposite (contralateral) side. Most limb functions (except cerebellar) are mediated by the opposite half of the brain. Similarly, the motor pathways (except the vestibular) cross before they leave the brainstem.

Painful foci may be difficult to localize but every attempt should be made to do so by careful manipulation and palpation of the spinal and limb muscles for spasms (Table 2). One can at least usually decide if the pain involves the cervical or lumbar spine as opposed to being in the thorax or abdomen. Palpation dorsal to the transverse processes normally elicits more pain than does abdominal palpation if the source is the spine. Manipulation of the neck slowly, then suddenly laterad and in flexion/extension elicits at least a muscle spasm if not cries of pain with

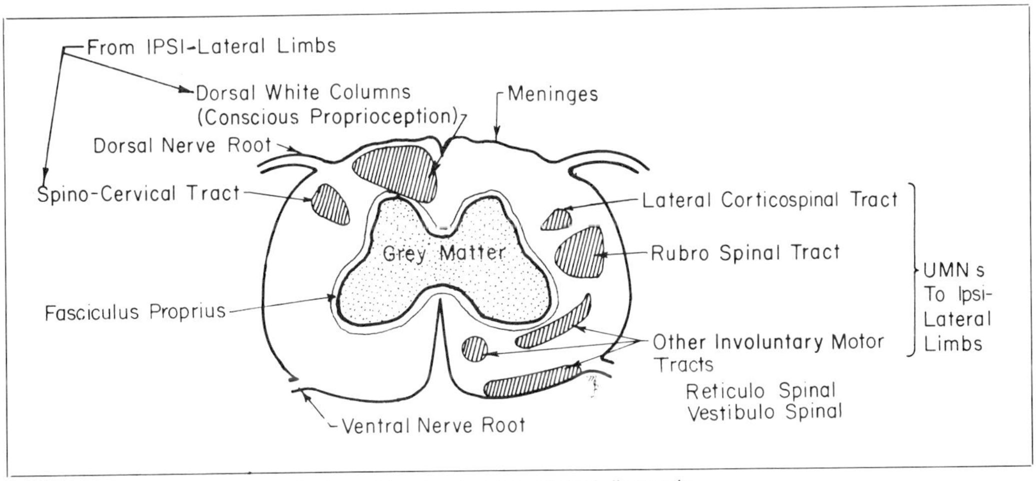

Fig 3. Diagram of the major spinal cord tracts of use in clinical diagnosis.

Table 2. Some Causes of Real or Apparent Pain of Neurogenic Origin

Involving Spinal Cord or Vertebrae	Methods of Diagnosis
Lesions Caused by Trauma:	
Vertebral fracture or fracture-dislocation	C,H,PR
Cord contusion/laceration	C,H,PR
Projectile injury	C,H,PR
Intervertebral disc (traumatic)	C,H,PR
Intervertebral disc (spontaneous)	C,H,PR
Neoplasms:	
Vertebral tumor, metastasis to vertebrae, or local invasion of vertebrae	C,H,PR,CR
Nerve or nerve root tumor	C,H,PR,CR
Cord tumor (unlikely unless rapidly growing and involving meninges or nerve roots)	C,H,PR,CR
Congenital or Genetic Lesions:	
C_1-C_2 subluxation	C,H,PR
Infection-Inflammation:	
Vertebral osteomyelitis or spondylitis	C,H,PR,M,S
Discospondylitis	C,H,PR,M,S
Spinal meningitis or epidural abscess	C,H,PR,CSF,M,S
Myelitis (FIP, pseudorabies)	C,H,OP,CP,PR,CSF, (CR),E
Spinal arthritis	C,H,PR
Other Causes:	
Hypervitaminosis A (multiple exostoses)	C,H,PR,CP
Involving No Direct Damage to Spinal Cord or Vertebrae	**Methods of Diagnosis**
Feline hyperesthesia syndrome	C,H,CP,PR,T
Fractured pelvis or other bones	C,H,PR
Contusion of muscles	C,H,PR,CP
Any cause of pain on opening mouth	C,H,PR
Any cause of thoracic pain	C,H,PR,CP
Any cause of abdominal pain	C,H,CP,PR,CR
Polyarthritis	C,H,CP,PR
Polymyositis	C,H,CP,E,B
Neuritis (see Table 9)	
Lead toxicity neuritis (usually dyesthesia)	C,H,CSF,CP,E
Anal gland impaction/inflammation	C,H
Subcutaneous abscess or cellulitis	C,H,CP,M
Postsurgical scar contraction	C,H
Epilepsy (psychomotor) (see Table 5)	C,H,CSF,E
Hallucinogenic drugs	C,H,CP,CSF,E
Intracranial meningitis	C,H,CSF,E
Intracranial pressure elevated from brain tumor, edema or abscess	C,H,CSF,CP,CR
Myasthenia gravis (stutter steps may mimic painful gait)	C,H,E,B

CODE: **B**—biopsy, aspiration or necropsy; **C**—clinical signs and examination (includes neurologic examination); **CP**—clinical pathologic examination; **CR**—contrast radiography; **CSF**—cerebrospinal fluid analysis; **E**—electrophysiologic examination (EEG, EMG, ECG, ERG, isotope brain scan, CAT scan); **H**—history; **M**—microbiologic examination; **OP**—ophthalmologic examination; **PR**—plain radiography; **S**—serologic examination, skin tests, FeLV slide test (paired serum samples often needed); **T**—treatment.

cervical lesions. Intracranial pain is rarely difficult to separate from cervical pain because lesions that cause intracranial pain also usually cause head pressing and other signs of brain involvement. Pain may be exhibited as favoring one or more limbs or as apparent pain or manipulation of the limb. Although limb pain that causes the cat to hold its leg up is most commonly caused by lesions not involving the nervous system, it can be caused by any lesion compressing or inflaming the spinal cord meninges, vertebrae or peripheral nerves and their roots. Spinal pain may lead to constipation (straining raises CSF pressure in the cord), absence of sudden movements and a careful, deliberate gait.

Ataxia (dysmetria, wobbly gait) and paresis (weak voluntary motor function) are sometimes difficult to separate; however, as both are frequently caused by the same diseases, their separation is often academic. A stiff gait and lack of sophistication in the gait (hopping) may also be caused by several of these same diseases.

Ataxia of spinal origin usually involves depression of conscious proprioception function in the affected limbs. Ataxia of intracranial origin, which may also affect conscious proprioception, is usually accompanied by other signs, such as personality changes, cranial nerve changes, head tilt, circling or seizures. One must not forget that a combination of signs may be seen because some diseases may involve several parts of the nervous system, as in feline infectious peritonitis. If the cerebellum is involved there is usually an intention tremor, which is absent during rest or tight manual restraint and worse when testing the placing reflexes and involves the head, and a hypermetria (goose stepping), with no loss of conscious proprioception.

Ataxia occasionally may be a difficult sign to interpret because even careful observation may fail to localize the lesion and it can be produced by many diseases affecting many sites. Other strange gaits included in Table 1 are hopping and the stilted stiff-limb gait.

Paresis may be confused with ataxia. Paresis is weakness in voluntary motor function and may be considered as a degree of paralysis. Paresis accompanied by deficits in conscious proprioception is strongly suggestive of a neurologic lesion but on occasion a cat may just be too weak to reposition its feet when conscious proprioception is being tested. The presence of normal conscious proprioception with paresis is suggestive of cardiovascular, respiratory, nerve conduction, neuromuscular function or electrolyte problems. When weakness is intermittent, muscles should be palpated at rest and after strenuous exercise (Table 12). Tissue hypoxia usually causes cramping and pain, whereas reduced nerve conduction velocities, electrolyte abnormalities and neuromuscular junction problems do not.

Paralysis indicates loss of motor function to muscles. It may involve visceral structures, such as the esophagus, diaphragm and bladder, or the muscles of the head and limbs. Motor function may be lost due to lesions of the muscles themselves (myositis), the neuromuscular junction (botulism, myasthenia), the peripheral nerve (trauma), the motor nerve root (polyradiculoneuritis), the grey matter of the spinal cord segment to the affected muscle (myelitis, spinal vascular accident), the entire spinal cord (trauma) or many parts of the brain (encephalitis). Paralysis, unlike ataxia, is a sign that permits fairly easy localization of a lesion.

Paralysis can be classified clinically as flaccid, spastic or rigid. Flaccid paralysis arises from lower motor neuron damage, in which affected muscles have no tone or reflexes, and also during the first 12-24 hours of complete upper motor neuron loss, during which affected muscles have no tone on palpation but reflexes are present.

Spastic paralysis is caused by complete upper motor neuron loss. This state is a dynamic one that develops from the initial flaccidity, with intact reflexes in the first few hours, through a gradually increasing palpable tone and hyperreflexia. After 1-2 months the animal can usually support weight on affected limbs and make cyclic reflex leg movements (spinal walking).

Rigid paralysis describes a state of involuntary rigidity due to partial loss of upper motor neuron function, direct lower motor neuron irritation (spasms), loss of lower motor neuron inhibition loops (Renshaw cells), as in strychnine toxicity or tetanus, and as part of the Schiff-Sherrington sign. The Schiff-Sherrington sign is seen with a severe thoracolumbar lesion; the rear legs are paralyzed but the forelegs are rigid (the Schiff-Sherrington sign) when the animal stops making conscious movements with them, *ie,* the front-limb rigidity in this instance is not a paralysis.

If the spinal cord is anatomically severed or has its function totally interrupted, lower motor neurons caudal to that point are released from the normal constant or intermittent upper motor neuron inhibition. The uninhibited lower motor neurons gradually develop more and more independent activity. For example, if the cord is cut at the thoracolumbar junction, immediately thereafter the hindlimbs are flaccid or have a very weak tone (virtual flaccidity), with intact segmental reflexes (knee jerk). The flaccidity of upper motor neuron loss is perhaps better thought of as early spastic paralysis rather than a true flaccid paralysis. After 12-24 hours the tone gradually increases, segmental reflexes become more exaggerated, and abnormal reflexes begin to appear.

Tone and reflex activity continue to increase until, after 1-2 months, the animal is usually capable of spinal walking. Spinal walking is a cyclic repetition of exaggerated segmental reflexes, giving the cat the appearance of walking, especially when its rear end is supported.

If cord damage is partial, with some involuntary motor tracts remaining intact, the limbs caudal to the lesion are usually rigid, even immediately after the injury. This is termed involuntary rigidity to separate it from spastic paralysis. In time there are noticeable changes in cats with spastic paralysis, but animals with involuntary rigidity rarely change until voluntary function begins to return. Involuntary rigidity is rarely confused initially with spastic paralysis because of the severity of the rigidity (capable of supporting the animal's weight) when compared to spastic paralysis of a day's duration.

Deep pain perception is intact in limbs with involuntary rigidity. After about 2-4 weeks, spastic tone may resemble involuntary rigidity. Involuntary rigidity does not prevent abnormal reflexes, such as the crossed extensor reflex, from appearing; however, this reflex rarely develops in cases of involuntary rigidity except in animals in which cervical lesions produce the involuntary rigidity. An animal with involuntary rigidity of the hindlimbs, when supported by its tail and allowed to walk on its forelegs, moves in crude, stiff, jerking steps with its hindlegs, even in cases of a few hours' duration. Involuntary rigidity frequently masks a knee jerk reflex because the limbs are not relaxed.

Many authors do not make a distinction between involuntary rigidity and spastic paralysis, and refer to both states as spasticity. We make the differentiation because of the different prognoses when trauma is the cause; spasticity is from a much more severe injury.

If a lesion directly damages the lower motor neurons within the spinal cord or in the peripheral nerves such that the lower motor neurons are nonfunctional, the muscles innervated by those lower motor neurons are paralyzed and flaccid. Segmental spinal reflexes are also gone. This does not necessarily indicate a worse prognosis; it simply indicates the site of the lesion. Lower motor neurons are, however, sensitive to anoxia and this should be taken into account in such situations. Unless early decompression is performed or inflammation rapidly reduced, significant numbers of lower motor neurons may be irreversibly destroyed.

Lower motor neurons mildly affected by inflammation or hypoxia may become irritated constantly (lower motor neuron rigidity) or intermittently (fasciculations). The latter are visible as twitchings under the skin, in contrast to muscle fibrillations, which are caused by single muscle fibers and cannot be seen through the skin. Fasciculations are produced by whole groups of muscle fibers (motor units) under the control of one lower motor neuron.

The Schiff-Sherrington sign is an extensor rigidity of the forelimbs only apparent when the animal is at rest. The animal retains full voluntary motor function in the forelimbs but has usually lost it in the hindlimbs. The sign occurs when lower motor neurons or more cranial cord segments are released from the inhibitory tone of more caudal spinal cord segments. The Schiff-Sherrington sign is usually associated with thoracic cord injury (never with an injury cranial to T_2) or more rarely with lumbar cord injury. It usually occurs after severe cord injury, but occasionally after only slight injury. It can develop within a few hours after the injury or may be delayed several days.

If a disease involves the spinal cord, the lesion(s) may be at one point in the spinal cord and unilateral or bilateral. Unilateral lesions may affect one leg (front or rear) or may affect both legs on one side. Bilateral lesions ("transverse cord syndrome") may affect both hindlegs only, both front legs only (lower motor neuron lesions only), or all 4 legs.

Lesions may also be diffuse throughout the spinal cord but with signs that appear localized as in singular lesions or with signs that are obviously due to several lesions, such as lower motor neuron lesions in front and rear limbs.

The localization of spinal lesions depends upon the use of the segmental spinal reflexes, whereas

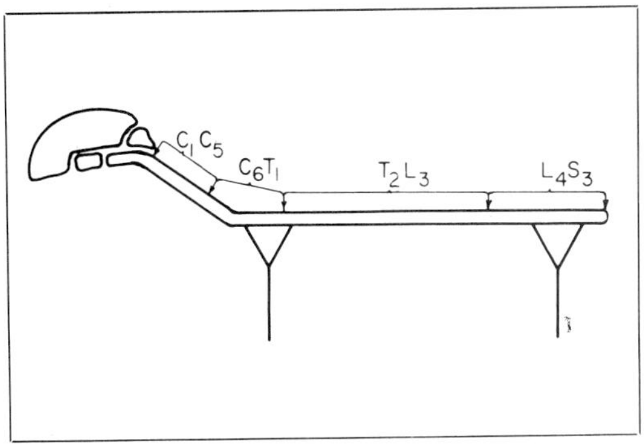

Fig 4. Spinal cord segments of major clinical significance.

the identification of the severity of the lesion (and thus the prognosis) depends on the use of the spinal tracts.

As shown in Figure 4, the spinal cord can be divided into 4 major segments. The segments from C_6 to T_1 contain the lower motor neuron to the forelimbs and thus are the segments mediating flexor withdrawal and the triceps' reflexes to the forelimbs. Segments L_4 to S_3 contain the lower motor neuron to hindlimbs and perineal region, as well as the anal and bladder sphincters. Therefore, this segment mediates the hindlimb flexor withdrawal reflex (L_6-S_2), the knee jerk reflex (L_4-L_6), and the anal reflex (S_1-S_3). Segments T_2 to L_3 contain lower motor neurons to the thoracic and abdominal muscles but not to the limbs. The phrenic nerve usually originates from nerves C_4 to C_7 and innervates the diaphragm. Therefore, any severe spinal cord lesion in segments C_1 and C_5 is fatal because all respiratory movements cease. With diaphragmatic respiration, resulting from a severe lesion somewhere from C_6 to the upper thoracic area, the thorax expands on expiration and not on inspiration as in normal respiration.

There are 8 cervical cord segments and nerves in the cat but only 7 cervical vertebrae (Fig 5). This has little clinical significance but may be confusing when interpreting radiographs, as in a fracture of C_4 that damages cord segment C_5.

Figure 6 shows how the last 4 lumbar and the sacrococcygeal cord segments are telescoped within vertebrae L_3 to L_6. Although the spinal cord ends at about the L_6-L_7 junction in the cat, the spinal nerves still run within the spinal canal and emerge at their respective foramina. The clinical significance of this arrangement is that lesions of vertebrae L_3 to L_6 damage the lower motor neurons of several cord segments caudad. Therefore, the clinician must be careful when translating the vertebral number (from

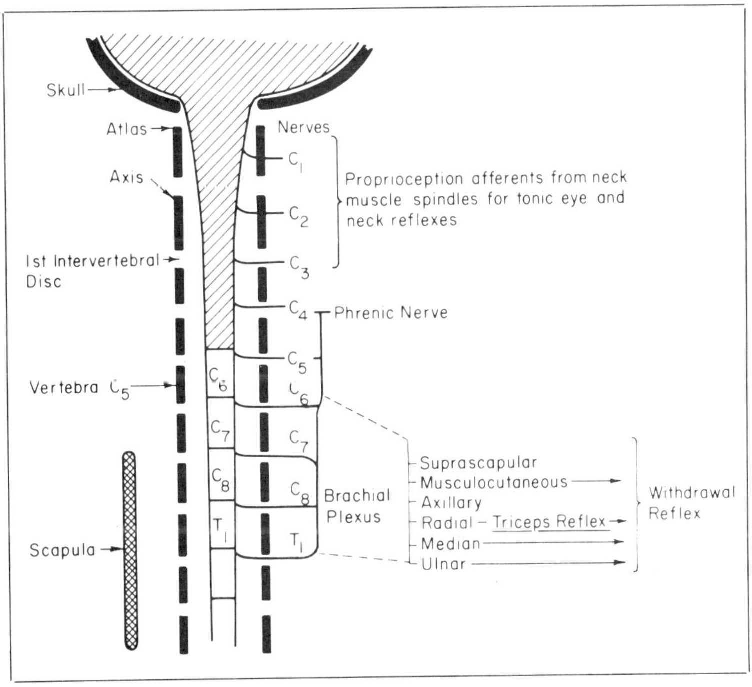

Fig 5. Diagram of the cervical and first thoracic spinal cord segments.

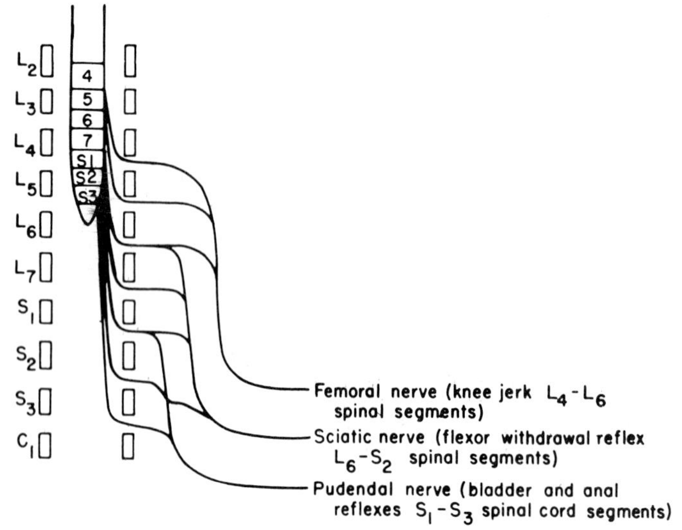

Fig 6. Diagram of the lumbosacral plexus.

radiographs) into the cord segments or spinal nerves it contains.

To accurately assess the degree of functional damage to the spinal cord, the long spinal tracts are used. The larger the diameter of the nerve fiber, the faster pressure or anoxia causes dysfunction. Therefore, the spinal cord tracts containing the widest fibers are the first to be affected by a lesion causing increased pressure on the spinal cord. In descending order of component fiber diameter, the spinal cord functions that can be tested clinically are conscious proprioception (dorsal white columns), voluntary motor (rubrospinal and lateral corticospinal tracts, superficial or skin pain (spinocervical and spinoreticular tracts), involuntary motor (reticulo-, tecto- or vestibulospinal tracts). The approximate positions of some of these tracts within the spinal cord are shown in Figure 3. The only components of the spinal cord more sensitive to pressure or anoxia than the conscious proprioception fibers are the lower motor neurons, the cell bodies of which are approximately 2-5 times the diameter of conscious proprioception fibers and have a high metabolic demand.

By combining the functional degree of cord damage with the information about spinal cord segments, certain dysfunctions can be explained as follows. Clinical signs may affect the limb or limbs on one side of the body only. In some cases this may make the attribution to the spinal cord, rather than to the brain, confusing if other signs (cranial nerve deficits or a head tilt) of brain involvement are absent.

Flaccid paralysis of the hindlimbs with or without the presence of pain in the hindlimbs: This is the result of a lesion affecting cord segments L_4 to S_3, and damaging the lower motor neuron to the hindlimbs. All hindlimb reflexes are abolished. In some cases, the knee jerk (L_4 to L_6), the withdrawal reflex (L_6 to S_2) or the anal reflex (S_1 to S_3) might be spared, with tone being present in some hindlimb muscles if the lesion is more focal than all segments L_4 to S_3.

Hindlimb paralysis, with muscle tone present in the hindlimbs and the forelimbs normal: This is produced by a lesion at some point from segments T_2 to L_3. The panniculus reflex can be used to further localize the lesion if it is moderately severe. In mild lesions, with some voluntary upper motor neuron loss, rear-leg reflexes are exaggerated. If some primitive involuntary motor tracts are intact but all other upper motor neuron function is lost, the hindlimbs may be rigid (involuntary rigidity), pain sensation remains and the reflexes may be hidden by the stiffness. If the cord has no motor tracts intact, muscle tone is weak for the first few days but increases as mentioned earlier. Hindlimb segmental reflexes are exaggerated and abnormal reflexes (*eg*, crossed-extensor) appear.

Forelimb paresis or flaccid paralysis with or without the hindlimbs affected: This is caused by

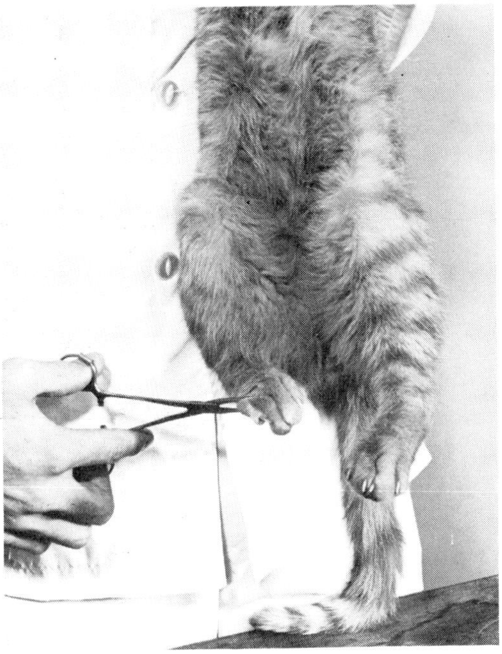

Fig 7. Stimulating the withdrawal reflex.

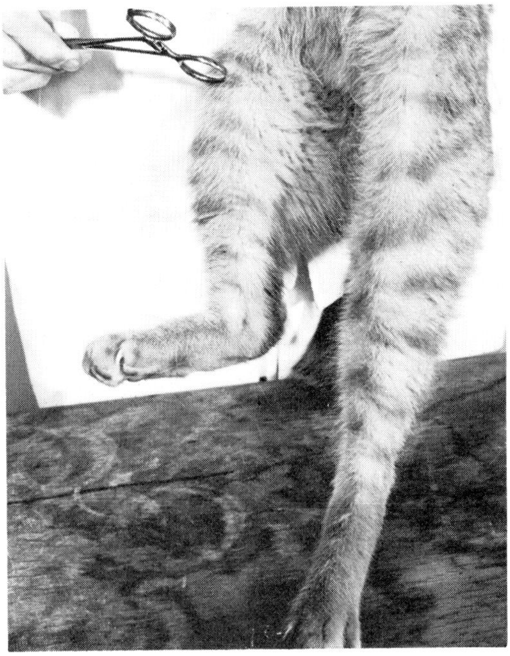

Fig 8. Stimulating the knee jerk reflex.

a lesion in segments C_6 to T_1. With a mild lesion, the hindlimbs are normal or only have conscious proprioception loss, but the front legs collapse. Pain sensation usually is present in all limbs but forelimb sensation may be lost. Forelimb reflexes are depressed or abolished. A moderate lesion produces involuntary rigidity in the hindlimbs; severe lesions produce spastic hindlimbs. In the last 2 cases, the forelimbs are flaccid.

Quadriparesis (voluntary muscle weakness of all 4 limbs) or quadriplegia (paralysis), with all 4 limbs showing similar tone and reflexes: Affected animals have a lesion in or cranial to cord segment C_6. If the lesion is severe and cranial to C_6, the cat dies of respiratory paralysis. It is just possible for a cat to remain alive with a lesion involving segments C_1 to C_5 causing involuntary rigidity (quadriplegia) of all 4 limbs.

Flaccid quadriplegia or quadriparesis, with depressed or absent reflexes in all limbs: This condition is due to a lower motor neuron lesion of all 4 limbs, as in polyradiculoneuritis. Superficial (skin) pain function is usually intact.

To use this knowledge, one must accurately test and interpret all of the reflexes, tracts and signs already discussed.

Tests of spinal segmental reflex and tract function: A segmental reflex can be abolished by a lesion that destroys any part of the reflex arc: the receptor organ, afferent nerve, dorsal nerve root, segment of the spinal cord involved, lower motor neuron, ventral nerve root, efferent nerve or effector organ. The reflex may also be obscured by excessive activity of other reflexes in the same limbs, excessive voluntary movements in progress, involuntary rigidity, or spasms in effector muscles. Higher reflexes can be abolished or masked by any of these factors and by lesions in spinal segments or regions of the brain transmitting or mediating reflex activity. It is important to remember that many different lesions may depress any one reflex.

The flexor withdrawal reflex can be tested in each limb by pinching each foot in turn (Fig 7). The response is withdrawal of the stimulated limb. A conscious response (cry of pain) may not necessarily occur when the reflex is intact. Foreleg reflexes are mediated in cord segments C_6 to T_1 (musculocutaneous, radial, median and ulnar nerves). The hindlimb reflexes are mediated in cord segments L_6 to S_2 (sciatic nerve).

The knee jerk reflex is tested by tapping the straight patellar ligament and observing the kick of the lower leg (Fig 8). A similar reflex can be elicited by tapping most muscles or their tendons of insertion but only the anterior tibial

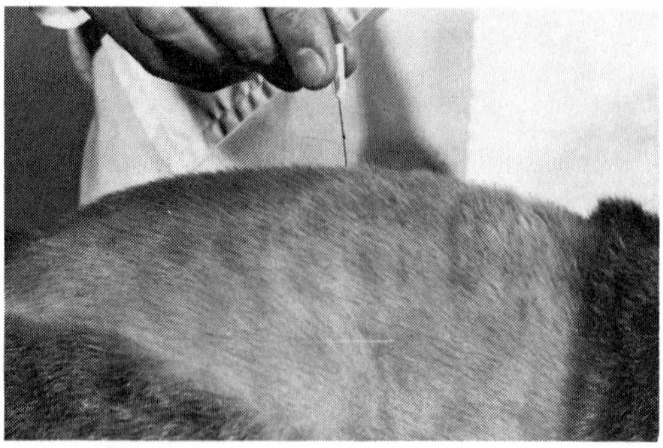

Fig 9. Stimulating the panniculus reflex with a needle.

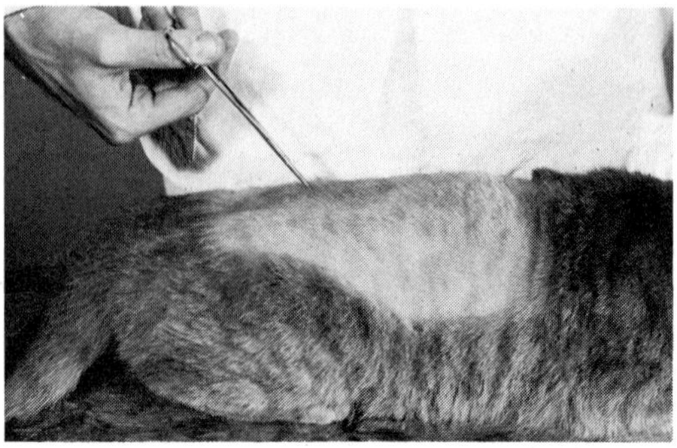

Fig 10. Stimulating panniculus reflex with hemostats.

muscle is as reliable in the normal animal as the knee jerk. The triceps tendon is used in the forelimb; tapping it just proximal to the olecranon usually causes straightening of the lower limb if the animal can be induced to relax its limb. The knee jerk reflex is mediated in cord segments L_4 to L_6 (femoral nerve) and the anterior tibial in L_6 to S_2. The triceps reflex is mediated in cord segments C_7 to T_1 (radial nerve).

The anal reflex is elicited by pinching the skin of the anus and observing constriction of the anal sphincter. It is mediated in cord segments S_1 to S_3 (pudendal nerves).

The panniculus reflex is elicited by pricking or pinching the skin over the back at each vertebra from L_7 to T_2 (Figs 9, 10). The response is a twitch of the skin over the whole back. The afferent components of the reflex are sensory fibers from the skin, with an input to the reflex at each segment. There is only one efferent component of the reflex, from cord segments C_8 to T_1 to the subcutaneous panniculus muscle of the back (Fig 11). The reflex can only be elicited by stimulating the skin innervated by a spinal nerve and cord segment cranial to a severe cord lesion. Stimulating skin innervated by a cord segment caudal to a severe cord lesion does not produce a twitch of the back muscles because there is no intact afferent input to the reflex. Because spinal nerves angle caudad and innervate skin 2-3 vertebral segments caudal to their origin from the cord, it is necessary to count 2-3 segments cranial to the level at which the reflex can first be elicited to find the caudal extent of normal spinal cord. Mild cord lesions have no effect on the reflex. Moderate cord lesions can cause difficulties in interpreting changes in this reflex. When the reflex is elicited, the whole back twitches, even the skin behind the cord lesion. In normal animals the reflex is usually exaggerated if the skin over L_1 is stimulated.

The crossed-extensor reflex can be elicited by pinching one toe and observing withdrawal of that leg (normal flexor withdrawal reflex) and extension of the other limb (Fig 12). The reflex can be produced in the front and rear limbs. It indicates a severe upper motor neuron lesion in the thoracolumbar region (reflex seen only in the hindlimbs) or a mild cervical, midbrain or brainstem lesion (reflex seen in front and/or rear limbs). This reflex does not occur in normal an-

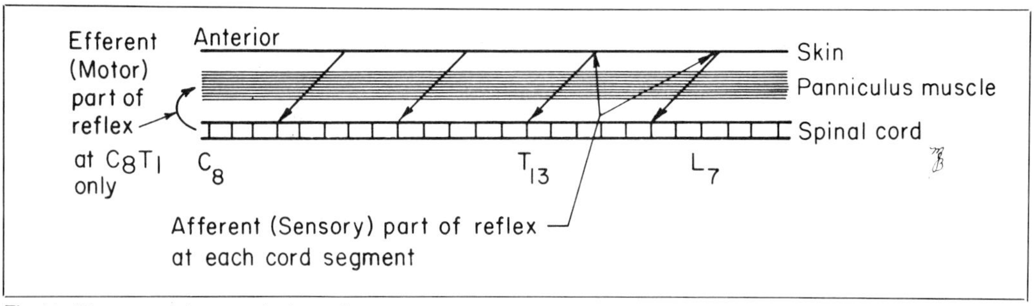

Fig 11. Diagram of the panniculus reflex.

imals. It may appear within hours after the lesion develops but is marked after 2-3 days.

Spinal walking has already been discussed. It can be elicited in the hindlimbs by supporting the cat by the tail and allowing it to walk on its normal forelimbs. Its hindlimbs make rhythmic cyclic withdrawal movements resembling steps as its toes or skin are stimulated by touching the ground. The cat may be able to support its rear end for a few meters when the tail is released. It indicates total functional cord damage of 1-2 months' duration. It is not likely to be confused with involuntary rigidity because of the delay between the injury and its appearance and because of its characteristic cyclic steps.

Conscious proprioception is position sensation, *ie,* the knowledge of how one's limbs are positioned. It is tested by supporting the animal and knuckling over each foot in turn (Fig 13). Normal animals resist attempts to knuckle their feet over and immediately reposition them. If the function is absent, the affected limb(s) remain knuckled over until the animal moves (Fig 14). If the animal is not supported and begins to fall, vestibular mechanisms cause the animal to reposition its legs; that is not a test of conscious proprioception. The function is said to be depressed if the animal takes a few seconds to reposition its foot.

An animal that has totally lost conscious proprioception is usually ataxic, but partial loss may not affect the gait.

Conscious proprioception is mediated in the contralateral cerebral cortex, with impulses reaching there via the ipsilateral spinal cord and brainstem, where they decussate and proceed to the midbrain. Intracranial lesions, as well as spinal lesions, may affect this function. Sciatic or radial nerve lesions may cause knuckling, mimicking loss of conscious proprioception.

Voluntary motor function can only be tested by observing the animal move. If the function is weak, it is called paresis. If the function is

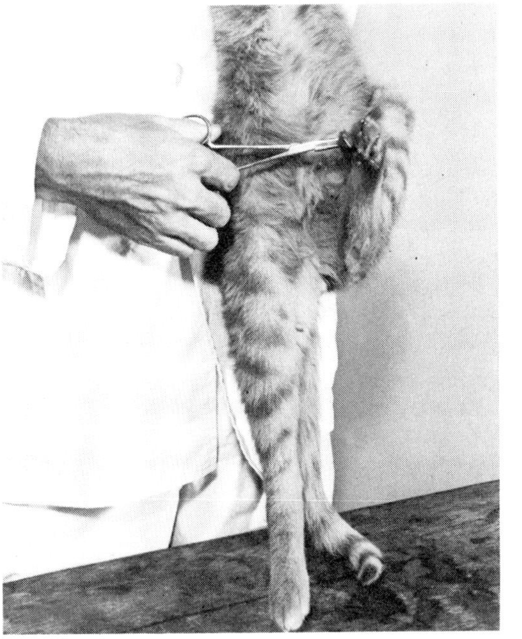

Fig 12. Stimulating the crossed-extensor reflex. Notice the extension of the limb not stimulated.

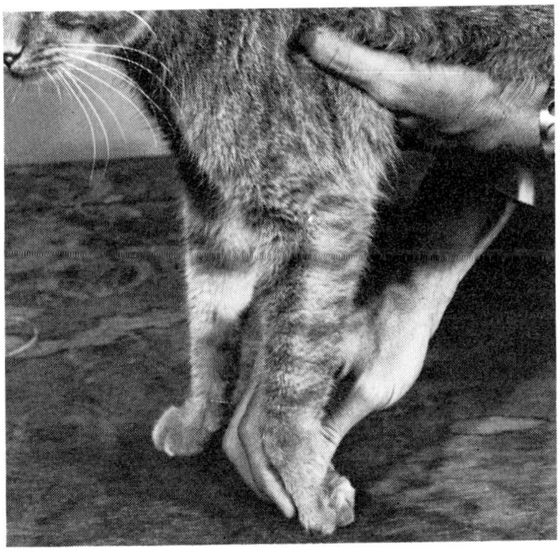

Fig 13. Testing conscious proprioception function.

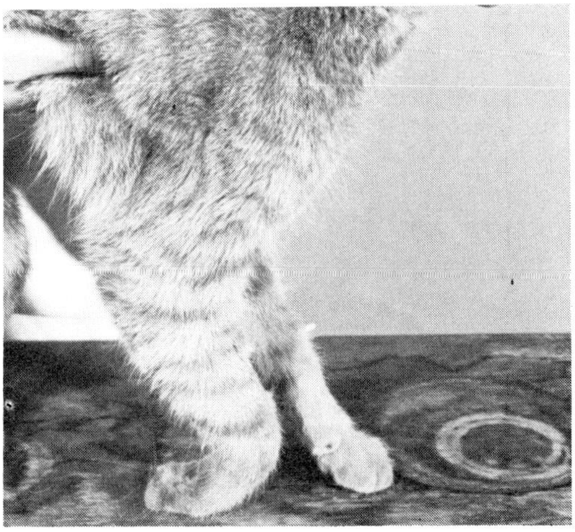

Fig 14. Loss of conscious proprioception in the right front leg.

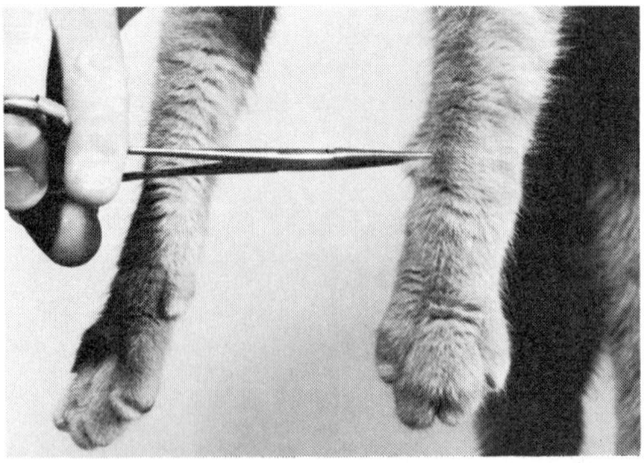

Fig 15. Testing superficial pain function by pinching the skin at points on the limb being tested.

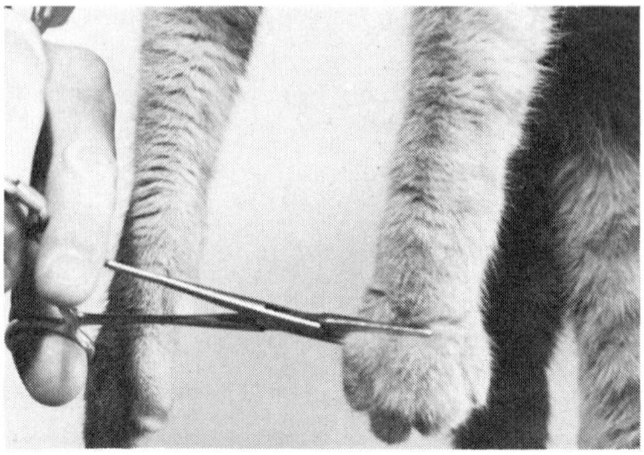

Fig 16. Testing deep pain function by squeezing a digit with hemostats.

absent, it is called paralysis. Different types of paralysis have already been described.

Voluntary motor function is mediated in the contralateral cerebral hemisphere and midbrain. Impulses reach the limbs via the brainstem, where the fibers decussate, and the ipsilateral spinal cord. As with conscious proprioception, intracranial or peripheral nerve lesions, as well as spinal lesions, affect voluntary motor function.

Signs of involuntary rigidity in a limb can only be detected by palpating affected limbs and feeling the rigidity. If the animal is supported, crude, stiff involuntary jerks of affected limbs may be seen as the cat tries to walk. Deep pain sensation is always intact when involuntary rigidity is present.

Response to superficial pain in each limb is tested by pinching the skin of each foot (Fig 15). Deep pain response is tested by squeezing a whole toe or foot pad in forceps (Fig 16). Response to deep pain is the last spinal cord tract function to be lost when the cord comes under increasing pressure or inflammation from a lesion.

The superficial and deep pain responses are conscious reactions (cries or attempts to bite or escape) and are not just a withdrawal of the limb being pinched. The responses are mediated via the ipsilateral and perhaps contralateral spinal cord, brainstem (where the ipsilateral fibers decussate), midbrain, thalamus and cerebrum.

Muscle wasting can indicate lower motor neuron damage if the wasting is localized. Most muscles without their lower motor neurons lose approximately 50% of their bulk in 1-2 weeks, become stringy in 1-2 months, and become fibrotic in 2-6 months. Upper motor neuron damage produces slight wasting that may become moderate (less than 30%) after 2-3 months. The affected muscles have tone and reflexes, whereas those without their lower motor neurons are flaccid and without reflexes at all times.

Information about bladder and anal control is useful in regard to the nursing care required, but it is of little use for diagnosis and prognosis except with lesions of the lumbosacral or sacrococcygeal junctions and pudendal nerves. In such cases, urethroanal electromyography and cystometrography may be necessary to assess the lesion.

The character of respirations should be noted because it may help indicate the area of a spinal lesion. Phrenic (diaphragmatic) respiration has already been discussed and may also be reflected by the cat's inability to mew at normal volume.

Head Tilt, Circling and Nystagmus

Table 3 outlines the differential diagnosis of obvious neurologic signs of intra- or pericranial disease (head tilt, circling, nystagmus). The table is applicable to cases of intracranial causes of ataxia and those with signs of cranial nerve disease (paralysis, twitching, fasciculation, spasm). However, when intracranial diseases cause ataxia, they usually cause other signs, such as seizures, behavioral changes, cranial nerve signs, head tilt, circling or nystagmus. Most diseases causing cranial nerve signs also usually cause other signs of intracranial disease.

In cats with a head tilt, the lower the lesion is in the brain, the more severe is the degree of head tilt. Otitis interna also causes a head tilt.

Table 3. Causes of Head Tilt, Circling, or Nystagmus
(Including Intracranial Causes of Ataxia and Causes of Cranial Nerve Signs)

Cause	Head Tilt	Circling	Nystagmus	Methods of Diagnosis
Encephalitis (FIP, FeLV, toxoplasmosis, rabies, polioencephalomyelitis, pseudorabies, vaccinal reticulosis)	Y	Y	Y	C,H,E,CSF,S,OP
Idiopathic feline vestibular syndrome	Y	Y	Y	C,H,PR,CSF,E,CP
Otitis media/interna	Y	R	Y	C,H,PR,E
Tumor (brain, nerve root, bone, connective tissue)	Y	Y	Y	C,H,PR,E,CSF,CR
Trauma (brain, skull)	Y	Y	Y	C,H,PR,E,CSF
Trauma (middle inner ear)	Y	R	Y	C,H,PR
Cerebrovascular accident (stroke)	Y	Y	Y	C,H,E,CSF
Intracranial meningitis (fungal, bacterial or algal)	Y	Y	Y	C,H,E,CSF,M
Hydrocephalus	R	R	R	C,H,E,PR,CR
Toxicity (thiaminase, streptomycin)	Y	Y	Y	C,H,E
Migrating parasites (heartworm)	Y	Y	Y	C,H,E,B
Congenital blindness	N	N	Y	C,H
Postictal (postseizure)	Y	Y	Y	C,H,CSF,E,CP
Torticollis (not usually an intracranial process but might mimic a head tilt)	Y?	N	N	C,H,PR,CSF,S,E,CR
Siamese cat nystagmus (biphasic fast)	N	N	Y	C,H

Y = seen with this cause; N = not seen with this cause; R = rarely seen with this cause

CODE: **B**—biopsy, aspiration or necropsy; **C**—clinical signs and examination (includes neurologic examination); **CP**—clinical pathologic examination; **CR**—contrast radiography; **CSF**—cerebrospinal fluid analysis; **E**—electrophysiologic examination (EEG, EMG, ECG, ERG, isotope brain scan, CAT scan); **H**—history; **M**—microbiologic examination; **OP**—ophthalmologic examination; **PR**—plain radiography; **S**—serologic examination, skin tests, FeLV slide test (paired serum samples often needed); **T**—treatment.

If there are bilateral lesions, the animal may be spread-eagled flat on the ground and totally disoriented. In severe cases, with brainstem lesions or otitis interna, the animal may roll continuously sideways. The tilt is usually to the same side as the lesion except with a few cortical lesions, in which it may be variable to one side or the other, and with some cerebellopontine angle tumors, in which it may be to the opposite side (paradoxic head tilt). Intracranial lesions (especially cortical ones) may cause the animal to tilt its head and avert its nose up, down or to the side. This is referred to as head aversion rather than head tilt. In head tilt, the nose points rostrad; the head is simply twisted about the longitudinal axis. Similar signs are caused by cervical scoliosis and torticollis, in which the head is twisted to one side or tilted.

Head pressing refers to an animal standing with its head down, leaning it against an obstruction. This is seen frequently in conditions of increased intracranial pressure (brain tumor, encephalitis, toxicity, and trauma). Head pressing is really a form of circling. Constant pacing with or without dummy behavior or dulled personality, may accompany head pressing.

Circling may be associated with brain lesions in any area from the frontal cortex to the brainstem. Generally, the lower the lesion is in the brain, the greater is the tendency to circle and also to circle to the side of the lesion. Cerebral lesions may cause only a tendency to circle, which may be constantly to one side or vary from side to side. Discrete cerebellar lesions do not cause circling. Except in some cases of acute inner ear disease, circling is not caused by extracranial lesions.

Nystagmus refers to constant or variable horizontal, vertical, diagonal or rotatory flicking movements of the eyes. There is usually a slow phase (drifting) and a fast one (flick). Nystagmus may be caused by extracranial lesions of the vestibular apparatus (semicircular canals), intracranial lesions of the vestibular nuclei in the brainstem, or from brain edema or distortion effects of a brain lesion at almost any point. Lesions of the cerebellum usually cause a biphasic fast (intention) tremor type of nystagmus. This type of nystagmus is seen in Siamese cats, especially when they are nervous. Nystagmus can be induced normally by the caloric test, for which we have little practical clinical use in cats (see Chapter 18). By deep flushing the external ear canal with cold water, horizontal nystagmus can be induced if the vestibular system to that ear is intact. Another normal type of nystagmus is the vestibular type (see under testing the eighth cranial nerve).

There are 4 types of pathologic nystagmus of clinical interest. Spontaneous horizontal or rotatory fixed nystagmus is the peripheral, horizontal, constant type not changed by varying head position. This is caused by extracranial lesions (vestibular apparatus). Positional or variable nystagmus is rotatory, vertical, horizontal or diagonal, changes direction with the position of the animal's gaze, and can be induced to change by changing the position of the animal's head. It is caused by intracranial lesions. Fixating or intention nystagmus is only apparent when the animal stares. It is cerebellar in origin and frequently resembles "trembling" of the eyeball because both directional phases are fast. Wandering nystagmus is a form in congenitally or neonatally blind animals in which the eyes drift aimlessly.

Strabismus (squint) may be seen with lesions of the vestibular system (ear, brainstem) or midbrain. It is often difficult to interpret which of the cranial nerves (third, fourth or sixth) to the extraocular muscles is affected because it is not necessarily the nerve or its nucleus that is directly involved, but the vestibular or neck position information to the nerves' nuclei that has been affected.

The vestibular syndrome refers to the signs seen when the vestibular system (vestibular apparatus in the ear, eighth nerve, vestibular nuclei) is affected. Signs include ataxia, head tilt, nystagmus and perhaps strabismus, circling and nausea. Not all signs are present in every case. The character of the nystagmus, the presence of limb proprioception deficits, seventh (facial) nerve changes and evidence of Horner's syndrome (sympathetic ophthalmoplegia) are used to determine if the syndrome is central (in the brain) or peripheral. Such a differentiation radically changes the diagnosis, the tests selected and the possible treatments.

The objectives in the diagnosis of intracranial lesions are to ascertain if the lesion is solitary or if there are multiple foci, thus providing a clue about the possible cause, to decide the severity and if surgery is required and feasible, and to monitor changes in the signs of the lesion.

As pointed out in the previous section on spinal cord lesions, each of the long spinal sensory or motor tracts originates in or ascends to the brain. Each tract may or may not cross from one side of the brain to the other at different levels in the brain. Figure 17 shows how the upper motor neuron tracts are arranged. The rubrospinal (red nucleus, midbrain) tract is the most important voluntary motor tract in the cat. The conscious proprioception tracts (dorsal white columns) are arranged almost parallel to the voluntary motor (corticospinal) tracts from the cerebral cortex. The conscious pain tracts in lower mammals are a topic for much discussion but clinically one can regard the spinocervical tracts as a theoretic base for use. The spinocervical tracts run parallel to the conscious proprioception tracts but ventrolaterad in the spinal cord. Pain fibers are assumed to ascend to the thalamus and cerebral cortex roughly parallel to the conscious proprioception fibers. Other pain fibers ascend the spinal cord in the spinoreticular tracts, which run close to the grey matter of the cord in the fasciculus proprius, to the brainstem reticular formation. Transmission to the thalamus is assumed.

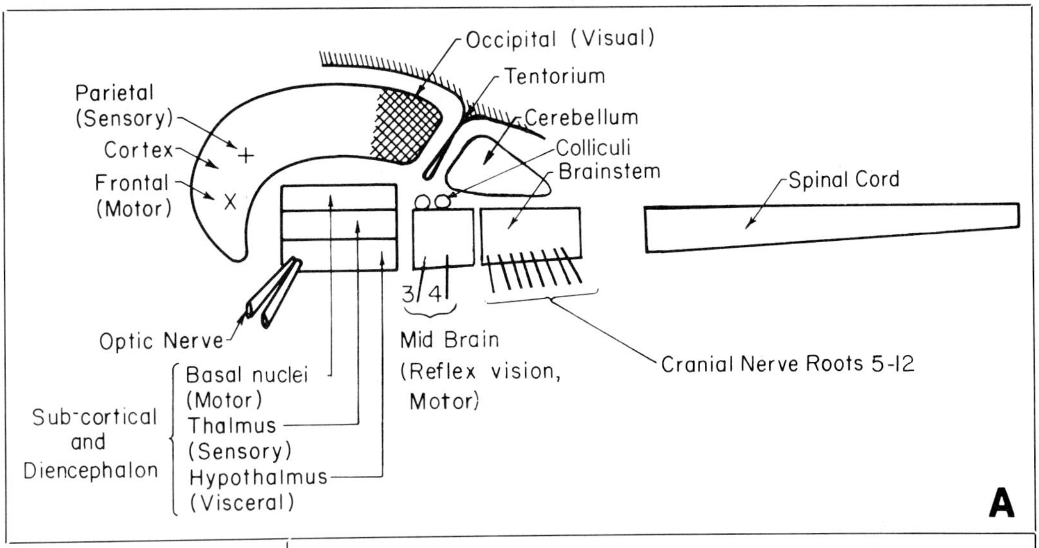

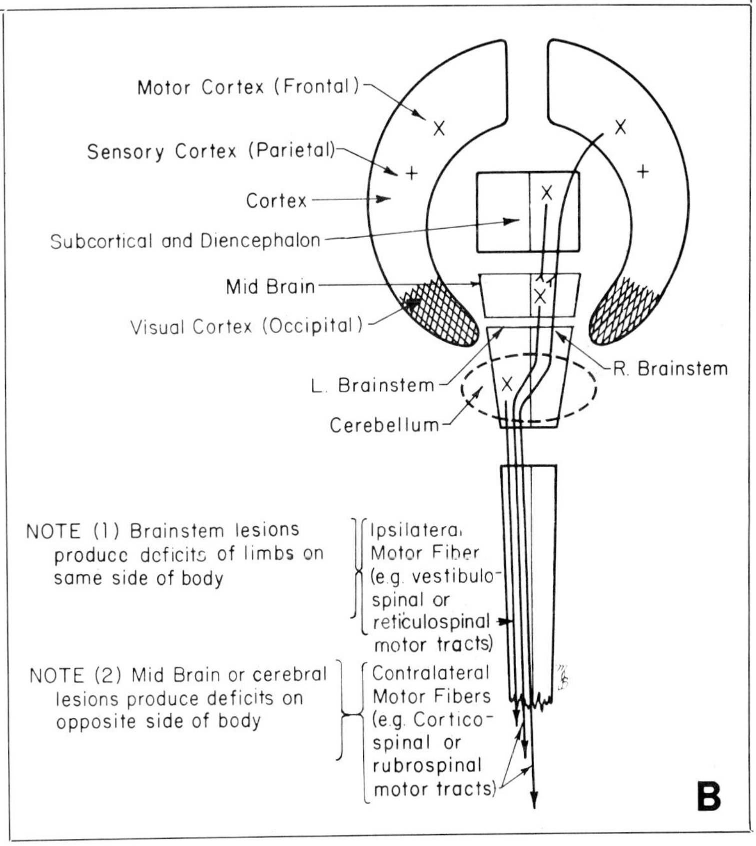

Fig 17. Diagram of the major areas of the brain. A. Lateral. B. Ventrodorsal.

Intracranial lesions may affect any of these tracts (usually only conscious proprioception and upper motor neurons are involved in the clinical deficits) at almost any level in the brain. If the lesion is in the caudal brainstem, all 4 or the 2 ipsilateral limbs may lose conscious proprioception and upper motor neuron function. If the lesion is in the rostral brainstem, midbrain or cerebral cortex, all 4 or the 2 contralateral limbs may be affected. To complicate the clinical pic-

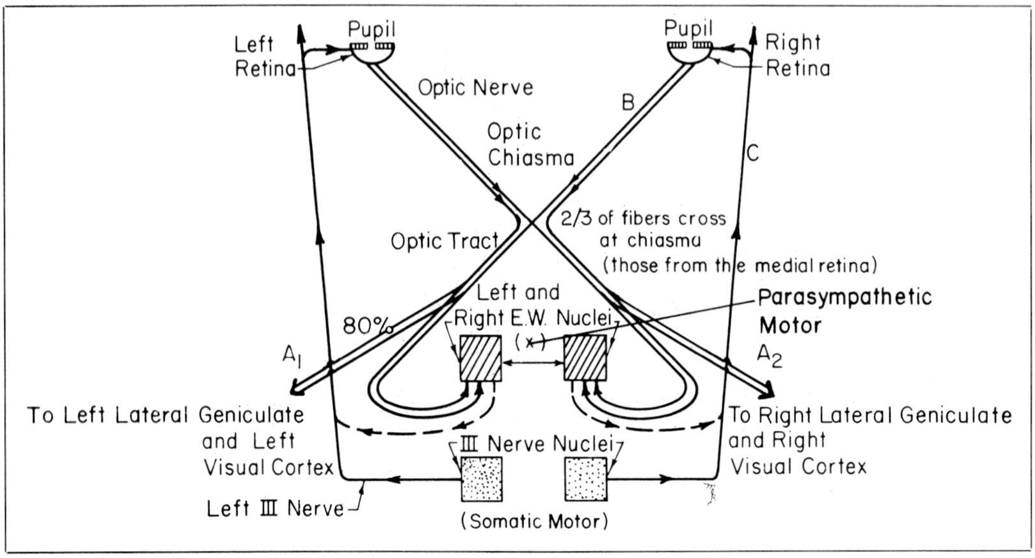

Fig 18. Diagram of the tracts involved in the pupillary reflexes.

ture, one or both hindlimbs may be affected before or more severely than the forelimbs.

Figure 17 also shows the approximate position of the cranial nerves in the brain. Note how they are in the midbrain and brainstem, with the exception of the first 2, which are the olfactory and optic. They are inaccessible surgically. Figure 17 is perhaps an oversimplification of the anatomy of the brain but it has functional value. The brain can be subdivided usefully into 5 areas (cortex, subcortex-diencephalon, midbrain, brainstem, cerebellum). This is an effective base for understanding the important signs of intracranial disease processes.

The tentorium is a shelf of bone and connective tissue that separates the cerebrum from the cerebellum. It creates a narrow ring of bone with the petrous temporal bones at the level of the midbrain and marks the rostral limit of the caudal fossa of the brain. The rostroventral portion of the tentorium extends to the colliculi of the midbrain. Structures in the brain are often referred to as sub- or supratentorial. Subtentorial structures include the fourth ventricle, cerebellum and brainstem; the cerebrum, subcortex and diencephalon are supratentorial structures. This classification is important in intracranial hemorrhage or other space-occupying lesions, such as a tumor. If the lesion is supratentorial, the pressure rise and swelling may produce a pressure cone through the bony ring formed by the tentorium, petrous temporal bones and base of the skull. This pressure cone can produce hemorrhages from small vessels in the midbrain and brainstem, leading to decerebration.

Decerebrate rigidity appears as an extensor rigidity of the limbs and spine, usually with the neck held back in opisthotonus and the toes curled. Mild cases may mimic the involuntary rigidity of all 4 limbs seen with a cord injury at C_1 to C_5; however, decerebrate rigidity is associated with signs of intracranial damage (coma, small pupils).

Pupil changes occur as intracranial pressure rises and the tentorial pressure cone develops. Generally the pupils become smaller, then pinpoint before dilating as brain death approaches. Respiration also changes character. Motor, pupil and conscious state changes are discussed under Brain Trauma.

Cranial nerves may be injured intracranially, as they pass through the skull or extracranially. The signs produced by cranial nerve lesions and the means of testing the cranial nerves are summarized in Table 4. Certain cranial nerves, such as 1, 4, 6 and 11, are difficult to test reliably and lesions involving them can only be detected by gross clinical signs. Others, such as 9 and 10, are difficult to test. The owner's comments about ability to eat and drink are often more informative. There is no way of easily ascertaining if the eleventh cranial nerve is functional, except by electromyography.

The cranial nerves most useful for clinical diagnosis are the optic (2), oculomotor (3), trigeminal (5), facial (7), auditory (8), glossopharyngeal (9), vagus (10) and hypoglossal (12). The optic and oculomotor nerves are tested together by the pupillary reflexes. The trigeminal and facial nerves are also tested together by tapping, pricking or pinching each side of the face (Table 4).

There are 2 pupillary responses to retinal stimulation with light (Fig 18). The first is constriction of the pupil in the eye being stimulated, which is the direct response. The second is constriction of the pupil in the eye that is not being stimulated, which is the consensual or indirect response.

In the cat, two-thirds of the optic nerve fibers cross in the optic chiasma to the opposite side of the brain (optic tract); 80% of the optic tract projects via the lateral geniculate nucleus to the visual cortex of the cerebrum (visual perception) and 20% goes to the midbrain (rostral anterior colliculus and underlying tegmentum). The midbrain structures function in reflex vision (following moving objects, seeing stationary objects, gaze fixation, visual input balance, pupils). The visual cortex also supplies the opposite (contralateral) seventh nerve nucleus with information via the pons and cerebellum that enables a blink response to a menace gesture. Hence, the clinician examines conscious visual perception, pupil reflexes and the menace response. When the fifth and seventh nerves are tested, one uses a facial tap, touch of the cornea, or pinprick of the face out of the visual field to get a blink response; this is not a menace response.

A menace response involves threatening the eye (place a hand over the eye from out of the visual field or open a clenched fist in front of the eye) without causing air currents to stimulate hairs or the cornea. The important fact to note about the menace response is that it can be absent in one eye with ipsilateral cerebellar lesions (or bilaterally with diffuse cerebellar lesions) and the cat need not be blind. One must test "conscious" cortical vision by observing the animal walk in the examination room (maze test), accurately follow a dropped cotton ball, and accurately follow hand movement. Crude appreciation of a doorway or light in a dark room is testing no more than midbrain circuits. "Conscious" vision may be referred to as "central vision" by ophthalmologists who apply either term to a blind animal with normal eyes and intact pupillary reflexes.

Each optic nerve supplies both left and right Edinger-Westphal nuclei (parasympathetic lower motor neuron to the eye) because of the two-thirds decussation at the chiasma. The Edinger-Westphal nuclei supply each other and their iris with fibers that join the third cranial nerve. The third nerve nuclei are close to the Edinger-Westphal nuclei in the midbrain. A light shone into the left eye produces an impulse in the left optic nerve, which activates the left Edinger-Westphal nucleus and produces left pupillary constriction (direct). Many fibers also cross to the right Edinger-Westphal nucleus from the left optic nerve, resulting in right pupillary constriction (consensual).

Lesions at A_1 or A_2 in Figure 18 produce blindness (of one visual field, called hemianopsia) of central origin yet leave optic reflexes normal and crude visual responses (light perception, some ability to follow objects) intact because midbrain circuits are present. A lesion involving the right optic nerve (B) results in complete blindness of the right eye, absence of direct response in the right eye, and absence of consensual reflex to the left eye when the right is stimulated by light. A consensual reflex is present in the right eye when the left is stimulated because the right third nerve is intact. Direct response in the left eye is normal. A lesion at C does not affect sight but abolishes the direct pupillary response in the right eye. It does not prevent the consensual response in the left eye to right eye stimulation. This lesion abolishes the right eye's consensual response to stimulation of the left eye.

Hemianopsia is a term applied to blindness not of one eye but of one visual field. Objects approaching from the left side are perceived by the left medial retina and right lateral retina. Because of the decussation of medial retinal fibers at the chiasma, this left visual field information is transported by the contralateral right optic tract, right lateral geniculate, right visual cortex and right midbrain. Lesions of these structures thus abolish left visual field vision (left hemianopsia). This is hard to appreciate clinically but if one is suspicious of left hemianopsia, one should blindfold the functional (right) eye and note how the cat cannot see an object laterad on its affected left side or may bump into such left lateral objects. Objects to its right or straight ahead are seen by the unaffected right visual field, of which a small part of the visual impulses is processed by the left lateral retina;. One looks for contralateral hem-

Table 4. Methods of Testing the Cranial Nerves

Nerve	Signs of Nerve Destruction	Test	Result of Test if Nerve Damaged
1. Olfactory	Anosmia (inability to smell)	Difficult to test accurately	Observe cat's behavior: normal cats will smell strange objects, such as the exam table
2. Optic	Blindness in one or both eyes, mydriasis if bilateral (pupils dilated)	A. Sudden hand movement over or toward eye (menace) B. Light into each eye in turn (pupil light reflex) C. Maze test, follow hand or cotton ball (central vision)	A. Absence of blink B. Direct pupil constriction response absent in affected eye. Consensual response to other eye also absent. C. Negotiates maze, follows objects
3. Oculomotor	Mydriasis, ptosis, eye deviated laterad and ventrad	A. Light in affected eye B. Light in normal eye	A. Direct response absent, consensual response to other eye is present B. Direct response present, consensual response to other eye is absent
4. Trochlear	Eye may be deviated mediad	It is rarely possible to detect abnormalities in this nerve	Eyes may be unable to move ventrolaterad
5. Trigeminal	A. Motor: inability to close mouth B. Loss of sensation to face and eye	A. Tone in jaw muscles B. Prick, pinch or tap side of face out of visual field (cover eye). Touch cornea with wisp of cotton	A. Reduced or absent muscle tone (temporal, masseter) B. No blink. May be uni- or bilateral, partial or complete, involving one or more branches of the nerve
6. Abducens	Eye deviated mediad	Turn head or move hand for cat to follow	Eye unable to move laterad or to retract

Table 4 (continued)

Nerve	Signs of Nerve Destruction	Test	Result of Test if Nerve Damaged
7. Facial	Facial muscles paralyzed, eyelid, mouth droop, ear motion reduced	Tap face on: A. Affected side (hard) B. Normal side	A. Blink only on normal side B. Blink only on normal side
8. Auditory: Cochlear Branch	Deafness	Make noise behind the animal	No ear prick up or head turn response to the noise
Vestibular Branch	Circling, head tilt, nystagmus	Caloric test	Absence of nystagmus when affected side tested
9. Glossopharyngeal	Difficulty in eating (dysphagia)	Touch base of tongue	No gagging response
10. Vagus	Dysphagia, soft palate sags	A. Pressure on eyes B. Squeeze larynx C. Gag test as for 9	A. No cardiac slowing (difficult to induce) B. No cough C. No response
11. Spinal Accessory	Atrophy of trapezius and sternocephalicus muscles	No accurate test except electro-myography	
12. Hypoglossal	Tongue deviates to unaffected side (after fibrosis has occurred, this is reversed)	Observe tongue movements	Abnormal tongue movements

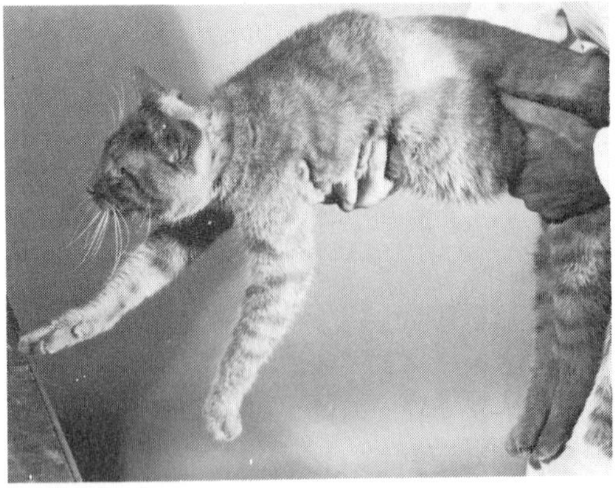

Fig 19. Normal foreleg response during testing of the visual placing reflexes.

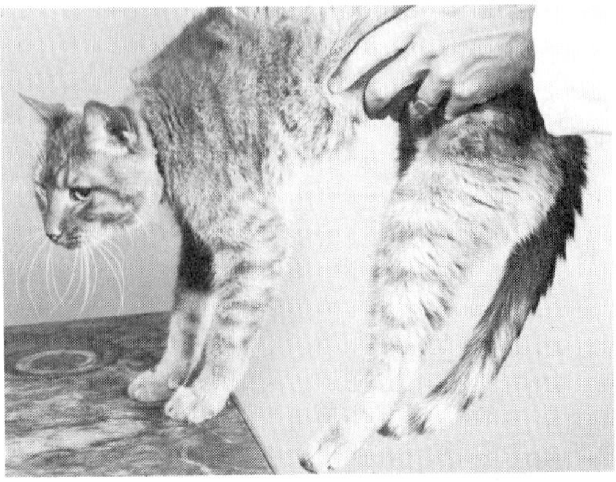

Fig 20. Normal hindleg response during testing of the visual placing reflexes.

ianopsia when evaluating unilateral cerebral or optic tract lesions when pupillary light reflexes are intact.

Conjugate eye movement is the term used to describe the eyes moving simultaneously as a pair. This is tested by moving a hand for the cat to follow and observing the eyes moving as a pair. If they do not, they are called dysconjugate. Lesions in the midbrain and rostral brainstem cause dysconjugate eye movements.

The fifth cranial nerve is sensory in function except for its innervation of the muscles of mastication (part of its mandibular branch). The fifth nerve's sensory function is tested by observing a conscious pain response (cry, avoidance) or a grimace of the facial muscles, which are innervated by the seventh nerve. If the motor branches of both fifth nerves have been damaged, the mandible hangs loosely. Damage of one fifth nerve causes rapid atrophy of the ipsilateral masseter and temporal muscles. If the seventh nerve is damaged, the ipsilateral lips and ear droop, and blinking is absent ipsilaterad, except for eyeball retraction (sixth nerve) causing a third eyelid flick.

The fifth and seventh cranial nerves are tested by tapping, pinching, or pricking each side of the face gently (out of the vision field) and then hard. If there is a fifth nerve lesion on one side, tapping on that side does not stimulate a blink in either eye. A hard tap or prick on the unaffected side produces a blink, even on the side with a fifth lesion. If there is a seventh nerve lesion on one side, apart from its being obvious at first examination, there is no blink on the affected side regardless of how hard either side of the face is tapped.

The third eyelid position is controlled indirectly by the sixth nerve (eyeball retraction) and by sympathetic fibers, the tone of which keeps it retracted. If the animal sees the hand or object, there is an avoidance withdrawal of the eyeball and the third eyelid falls across the eye when the face is tapped; this is not a blink. Because some animals do not acknowledge the pain of pinpricks or pinches on the face, one must be wary of diagnosing fifth nerve sensory deficits. Always test 3 sensory areas corresponding to the 3 branches of the fifth nerve dorsal and caudal to the eye (ophthalmic branch), ventral to the eye, on and in the nose (maxillary branch), and the mandible (mandibular branch).

The auditory branch of the eighth nerve is tested by response to a noise that cannot be transmitted via the floor or table, causes no air turbulence, and is produced by a movement that the animal does not see. The cat turns its ear or looks. Damage to the vestibular branch, its apparatus or the vestibular nuclei may produce the vestibular syndrome (head tilt, nystagmus, ataxia) on the same side. Their function can also be tested by the caloric test or by use of the normal vestibular (optokinetic, doll's eye, or railway) nystagmus. If the head is turned laterad, dorsad or ventrad, the eyes exhibit nystagmus, with the fast phase in the direction of head movement. The vestibular system mediates this nystagmus. Absence of such nystagmus when the head is moved to the left or right suggests a vestibular system lesion on that side.

The pituitary gland is situated close to the optic chiasma and lesions of either often affect the other. The hypothalamus is the highest center of the autonomic nervous system and lesions here produce changes in body temperature, thirst or appetite. The hypothalamus, along with a variety of structures around it (the limbic system), is also involved in behavior. Because the cerebellum controls coordination of movements, lesions of it cause intention tremors (including of the head and eyes), hypermetria (goose-stepping), swaying of the body and ataxia (without conscious proprioception loss). These signs are often more severe in the hindlimbs than the forelimbs. Limb hypermetria is sometimes seen if the spinocerebellar tracts in the spinal cord are selectively injured.

Figure 17 shows the significant areas of the cerebral cortex that the clinician can test: motor and proprioception functions (frontal, parietal) and vision (occipital). Lesions in the prefrontal and temporal (lateral) cortices may cause behavioral changes.

Evidence of nasal, auricular or retrobulbar disease is worth seeking because it often is a clue to the site or cause of neurologic signs.

Multiple Lesions: If deficits in long spinal tracts occur without any head tilt, circling nystagmus, cranial nerve deficits or other signs of intracranial disease, one initially assumes a spinal lesion. If any of these other cranial signs or deficits are present, then one initially assumes an intracranial lesion. However, there are exceptions and both spinal and intracranial may be present simultaneously, as in feline infectious peritonitis.

The postural reflexes or reactions are also used to study intracranial disease but these reflexes also involve the spinal cord, peripheral nerves and muscles. Therefore one must carefully interpret the results of testing these reflexes. When all structures except the brain are normal, the tests are useful. They are especially useful when there are no cranial nerve deficits and cerebral lesions are suspected. They help show which hemisphere is involved by revealing deficits in the contralateral limb or limbs on one side. They may even help distinguish a lesion in the rostral cortex from one in the caudal cortex. For example, the tactile reflex does not require an intact occipital cerebral cortex but the visual placing reflex does.

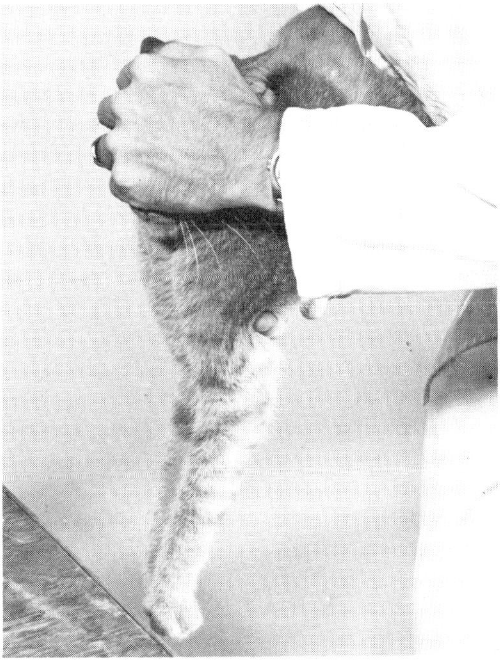

Fig 21. Testing tactile placing reflexes involves covering the cat's eyes and moving it slowly forward until the forelegs touch the edge of the table.

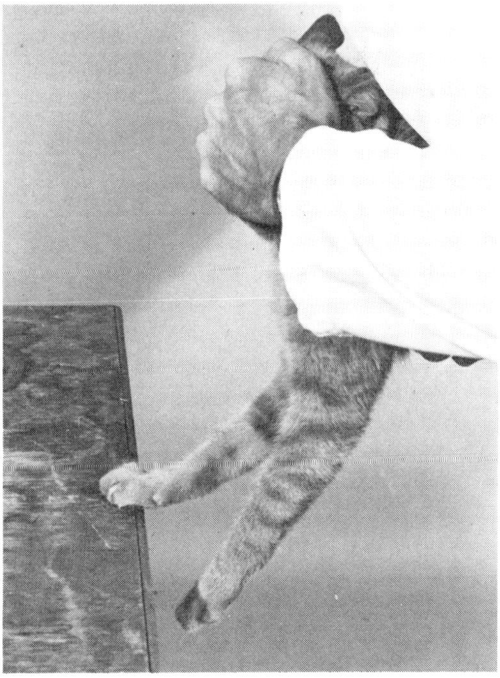

Fig 22. Normal response to the tactile placing reflex test.

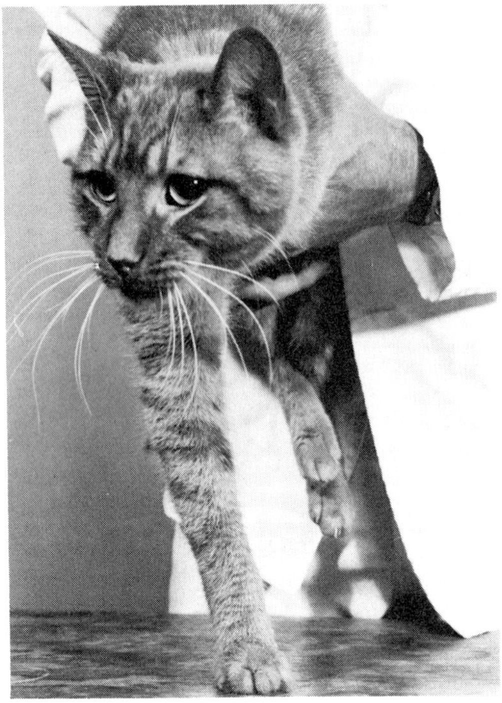

Fig 23. Testing the hopping reflex in the right foreleg.

Conscious proprioception is considered a postural reaction, although we have discussed it mainly as mediated by a long spinal tract.

The tonic neck and eye reflexes are variable in the normal uncooperative cat and have rarely provided us with any useful clinical information we could not have obtained in other ways. Both are tested by standing the animal on all 4 legs and flexing and extending the neck to extremes. As the neck is extended, the eyes maintain their forward gaze but the forelegs extend and the hindlegs flex. The reverse happens when the neck is flexed. These reflexes maintain the original direction of vision and head position. They are mediated in the brainstem and their sensory components are in the first 3 cervical nerves (from muscle spindles and tendon organs in the cervical muscles). In our experience, brainstem and midbrain lesions provide more striking evidence of CNS disease than does simple abolition of these reflexes.

To test the visual placing reflex, the animal is brought to the edge of a table. It normally reaches out with its front legs, places them on the table and swings its back legs up (Figs 19, 20). Each foreleg can be tested separately by restraining one leg at a time.

To test the tactile placing reflex, the same procedure is followed except that the animals' eyes are covered and the animal is moved slowly toward the table until the paws just touch it (Fig 21). This prompts the animal to put its front and then back feet on the table (Fig 22). If the animal remembers and reaches to where the table is in relation to its position, then one rotates oneself and the animal 360° on the spot to disorientate the animal after first covering its eyes. The animal's feet should not be brought up to the table too fast because the vestibular system detects the forward acceleration and may cause the animal's legs to reach out without mediation by the cerebral cortex.

The hopping reflex is tested by restraining 3 limbs and standing the cat on the fourth (Fig 23). All 4 limbs are tested in turn. If the animal is moved in any direction (except mediad), it should hop on the free leg. Many normal animals have difficulty hopping mediad. This reflex is mediated in a way similar to the placing reflex except that the vestibular system is involved. The hopping reflex is used mainly to test the

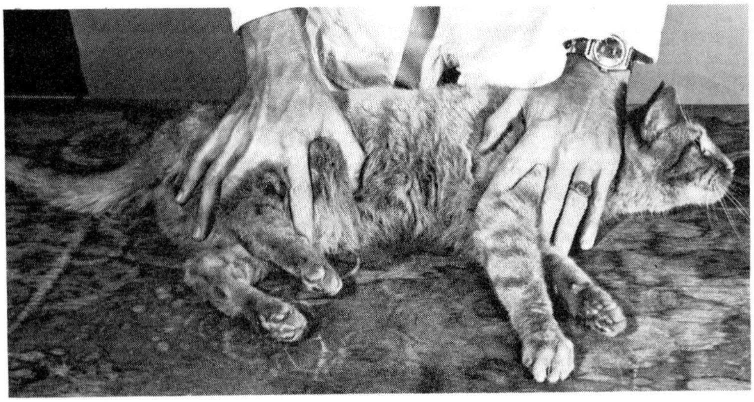

Fig 24. Correct way to test the righting reflex.

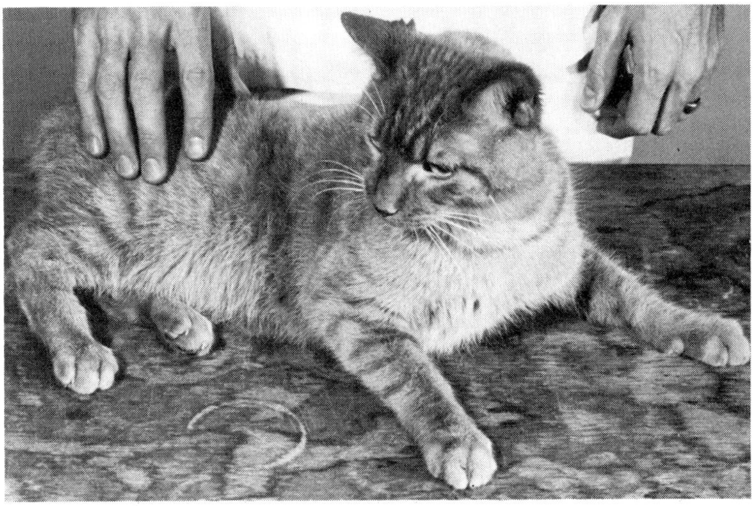

Fig 25. Normal response to the righting reflex test.

mediation of contralateral parietal cortex to the limb being tested.

The cat can be tested further by standing it on the 2 limbs on one side of the body and forcing it to walk (hemiwalking) forward or hop hemi-hopping) sideways. This helps confirm any suspicions aroused by an abnormal hop in one leg.

The extensor postural thrust reflex is tested by lowering the animal's rear paws until they just touch the ground, upon which the cat shuffles its feet to adjust its position. Any loss of proprioception in the hindlegs affects this reflex. It is used to test the contralateral parietal cortex's effect on the limb involved. This reflex should not be confused with the extensor thrust reflex, which is an unreliable segmental reflex of the limbs for which we find little practical use because the other segmental spinal reflexes serve equally well.

The righting reflex should be tested by placing the blindfolded animal on its side and releasing it (Figs 24, 25). The animal should sit up. This is repeated by placing the animal on its other side. This reflex is mediated via the vestibular systems and their motor tracts. A weak or depressed cat may remain laterally recumbent, and this should not be confused with loss of the righting reflex. The cat should not be tested as

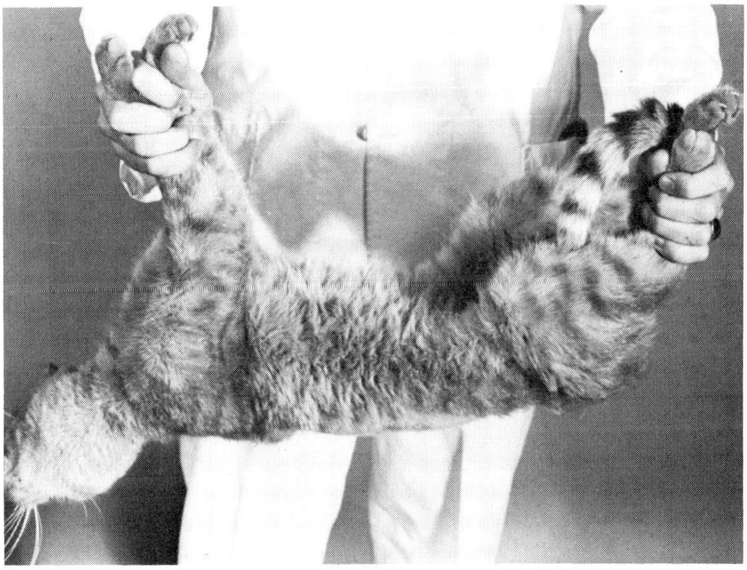

Fig 26. Wrong way to test the righting reflex.

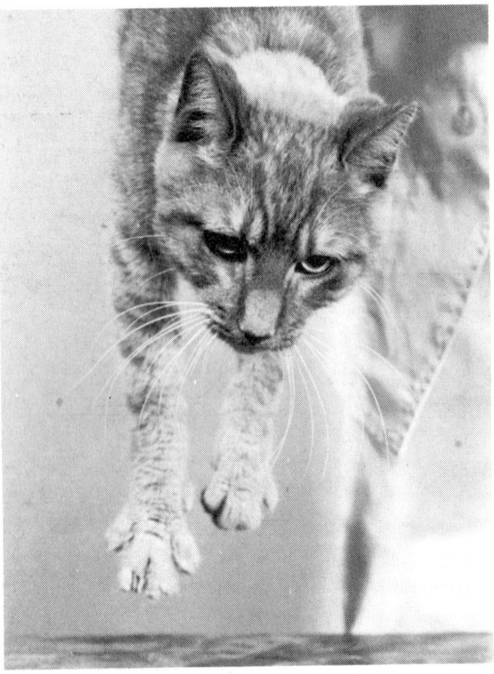

Fig 27. Alternative method of testing the righting reflex.

in Figure 26. Although normal cats can land on their feet, an abnormal one may not. This does not impress the client.

Another useful reflex, especially in depressed animals, is to suspend the animal with its head down and see if it reaches out with its paws and tries to look forward (Fig 27). This is another way of testing a combination of righting and visual placing responses. If the cat is forced to walk in this way, just on its forelimbs, it is called wheelbarrowing.

Seizures

A seizure or convulsion (ictus or fit) is best defined as the intermittent presence of all, any number or any combination of the following signs: loss or derangement of consciousness (unconscious, dull, glassy-eyed, excited); loss of or excess muscle tone or movement (constant rigidity or tonus, intermittent rigidity or clonus, paddling, flaccidity); alteration of sensation (pain, pruritus, self-mutilation), including hallucinations of special senses (sounds, vision, taste); changes in the autonomic nervous system (urination, salivation, defecation, vagal bradycardia, rapid peristalsis with diarrhea, vomiting); and behavioral signs (nonrecognition of owner, crying, disorientation, viciousness, pacing, running in circles, chasing imaginary objects).

These 5 general types of signs are caused by intermittent (paroxysmal) intracranial dysrhythmias (abnormal electrical activity) that do not produce the signs every time the dysrhythmias occur. The primary molecular disturbance that triggers the dysrhythmias is as poorly understood as the mechanism that permits the dysrhythmia to cause signs at some times but not at others. However, a number of factors are known to influence this process, including anticonvulsants, estrogens, pruritus, otitis externa and emotions.

There are many causes of seizures but one cause that requires careful definition is epilepsy (Table 5). Epilepsy is simply defined as a state of repetitive seizures. Hence, epilepsy is not a true disease; it is a state or syndrome. It is customary not to refer to animals with seizures from brain tumors or acute encephalitis as epileptics. There is also no sharp demarcation, in regard to time, between acutely traumatized animals with seizures and those with post-traumatic epilepsy; when the acute problem persists longer than a few weeks, it is called epilepsy.

The major mistakes made by clinicians managing seizure cases are failing to recognize a seizure, failing to use adequate diagnostic tests, failing to discuss the case with the client, and failing to use drugs correctly.

Recognizing a Seizure: The clinician must pay careful attention to all possibilities that the definition of seizures presents. The most frequent signs seen in convulsion are, in order of their occurrence: loss of consciousness, complete rigidity (tonus), intermittent rigidity/relaxation (clonus), salivation, urination, paddling and a few minutes of disorientation after recovery. The whole episode takes 1-5 minutes. Prior to the full generalized seizure, one leg may go stiff and be raised or the head may turn. These localizing signs tend to indicate which area of the brain is affected first and are not "Jacksonian seizures." Abnormal behavior (quietness, hyperactivity, anxiety) for minutes or hours before a seizure is called an aura. After the seizure the cat may not recognize the owner, may be blind, may be ataxic or may wander and pace aimlessly for hours or several days; these are called postictal signs. Some cats maay eat and drink excessively after a seizure; these are interpreted as hypothalamic effects of the seizure.

Most recognition problems arise when only a few signs are seen or with psychomotor seizures. Some animals may have diarrhea and/or vomiting as the only evidence of a seizure. Others may wake up from a normal sleep disorientated and glassy-eyed or may attack something for no apparent reason. Some may only collapse and get up, although this is more typical of narcolepsy or cardiac syncope. One of the rarest types of seizure in people involves unusual hypothalamic signs, such as fever; however, this is not to be attributed to every cat with paroxysmal fever of unknown origin.

Minor episodes of jaw-champing, facial twitches or twitches of one limb or the limbs on one side are called "focal seizures" and are not referred to as petit mal. Likely causes are encephalitis, meningioma or stroke.

When considering that an episode may be a seizure, one must look for evidence of intermittent occurrence and some of the signs listed in the definition of convulsions. Some syndromes in cats seem not to fall into any one category, such as behavior, epilepsy or sleep disorders. One such entity is the feline hyperesthesia syndrome.

Differential Diagnosis of Seizures: Table 5 lists the causes of seizures in cats, as well as the methods of diagnosing the cause. The most common causes are FIP and toxicity. The history may be helpful (Table 6).

The average diagnostic workup includes a CBC, blood chemistry profile, including glucose, Ca, BUN, creatinine, SGPT, alkaline phosphatase, and blood protein, a blood Pb determination run on heparinized blood, and perhaps CSF analysis and an electroencephalogram. Other tests may be indicated, such as serologic tests for FIP or toxoplasmosis, FeLV tests, electrolyte determinations, a glucagon- or ammonia-tolerance test, radiography, electrocardiography, microbiologic tests and biopsy. We recommend routine use of the first 3 and a serologic test for FIP, with a CSF pressure and analysis only if a brain tumor or recent encephalitis is suspected. An EEG is a helpful tool if available but is not essential. Institutional clinics may be able to run isotope and computerized axial tomography (CAT) scans.

The clinician must be satisfied with a diagnosis by elimination in many seizure cases because the cause of seizures is often labeled as "idiopathic." There is no positive blood test for epilepsy. Only the EEG shows abnormal brain electrical activity, and not in every case.

It is not wise to regard any pattern or age of onset of seizures as diagnostic; one can only suspect a diagnosis with such information. For example, sudden onset of many seizures suggests stroke, toxicity or infection (especially FIP).

The types of epilepsy are discussed in more detail later in the chapter.

Organic Behavioral Problems

Behavioral changes caused by brain lesions may be constant or paroxysmal (intermittent). Self-mutilation and changes in habits of urination and defecation may accompany organic or neurotic variations in brain function but may also be produced by diseases of the peripheral nervous system or the viscera. All options must be considered before assuming the lesion is organic, behavioral or in one particular organ.

Changes in behavior may be caused by nonneurologic causes (Table 7). Estrous behavior is commonly misinterpreted. Urine spraying by a cat previously well trained and neutered or loss of housetraining may be due to cystitis and urethral irritation. Chronic renal disease or diabetes mellitus may result in polyuria that may be interpreted as loss of habitual behavior. Many young cats and some older ones frequently run as if chasing or stalking prey; this may be confused with hallucinations or the feline hyperesthesia syndrome. Old cats may become intolerant of an owner's attentions, which may be misinterpreted as a pathologic change.

Some intracranial organic diseases cause behavioral changes, such as nonrecognition of the owner, viciousness, sudden friendliness or dullness. These are often progressive and usually accompanied by other neurologic deficits or convulsions, which are better indications of the cause. Cerebrovascular lesions often produce severe behavioral changes (viciousness) and may even produce only behavioral changes. Brain tumors may initially cause no other clinical signs than changes in behavior. With vague or problem cases, it often is more rewarding to wait for any progression of clinical signs if a cause is not apparent after the initial examinations.

Encephalitis, as in FIP, can produce marked behavioral changes. Although rabies is a well-known cause of behavioral changes early in its course and is usually a rapidly progressive disease, it is often misdiagnosed. Either acute or chronic hepatic disease can cause behavioral changes, ranging from depression to convulsions with distinct psychomotor signs.

Hallucinogenic drug toxicosis is perhaps more frequent than is generally suspected. Affected

Table 5. Differential Diagnosis of Seizures

Causes	Means of Diagnosis
Acquired Epilepsy (also called secondary or partial epilepsy)	Elimination of other causes: C,H,CR,E,CSF,OP
Postencephalitis (rare in the cat, most common cause is active FIP and this is progressive)	
Birth injury or anoxia	
Head trauma	
Postanoxia (*eg,* anesthesia or cardiac arrest)	
Postcerebrovascular accident	
Idiopathic Epilepsy (*eg,* causes hard to document via history or EEG such as migrating larvae, microemboli or genetic?)	Elimination of other causes: C,H,CP,E,CSF,OP
Acute Encephalitis	C,H,CSF,E,CP,S,B,OP
Feline infectious peritonitis	
Toxoplasmosis	
Feline leukemia viremia ?	
Rabies	
Other viruses or bacteria	
Feline Hyperesthesia Syndrome	C,H,CP,OP,E,S
Toxicity (exogenous)	C,H,CP,E,T
Chlorinated hydrocarbon or organophosphate derivatives	
Lead	
Strychnine	
Ethylene glycol	
Others	
Toxicity (endogenous)	
Hepatic encephalopathy; (portacaval shunt, chronic liver insufficiency, (*eg,* cirrhosis, urea cycle enzyme deficiency, hepatic lipidosis)	C,H,PR,CR,B
Azotemia (usually terminal)	C,H,CP
Hydrocephalus	C,H,E,PR,CR
Brain Tumor	C,H,CSF,E,CP of skull (rare), chest (primary focus)
Primary (often meningioma)	
Metastatic	
Multifocal (lymphoma)	
Hypoglycemia (insulinoma, chronic hepatic insufficiency, liver tumor, juvenile enzyme immaturity, endotoxic or septic shock)	C,H,CP
Hypocalcemia (eclampsia)	C,H,CP

CODE: **B**—biopsy, aspiration or necropsy; **C**—clinical signs and examination (includes neurologic examination); **CP**—clinical pathologic examination; **CR**—contrast radiography; **CSF**—cerebrospinal fluid analysis; **E**—electrophysiologic examination (EEG, EMG, ECG, ERG, isotope brain scan, CAT scan); **H**—history; **M**—microbiologic examination; **OP**—ophthalmologic examination; **PR**—plain radiography; **S**—serologic examination, skin tests, FeLV slide test (paired serum samples often needed); **T**—treatment.

Table 5 (continued)

Causes	Means of Diagnosis
Acute Meningitis Bacterial Fungal Viral (FIP)	C,H,CP,CSF,E,M,S,OP
Acute Cranial Trauma (including projectile)	C,H,CSF,E,PR
Acute Cerebrovascular Accident (or feline ischemic encephalopathy)	C,H,CSF,E
Acute Anoxias Cardiac Pulmonic Vascular	C,H,PR,E
Thiamin Deficiency (thiaminase toxicity)	C,H,T
Hyperthermia (106 F+)	Usually caused by the seizure and not the reverse
Flashing Lights	H
Other Inherited Lysosomal Enzyme Deficiency or CNS Degenerative Diseases	C,H,CSF,E,S,B
Narcolepsy (not a true seizure but a collapse)	C,H,E,T
Electrical Injury (*eg*, bit electric cord)	C,H,PR (chest)

Table 6. Association of History and Possible Causes of Seizures

Circumstances of Seizure	Possible Cause
cat less than 1 year old	FIP, endogenous or exogenous toxin
cat 1-5 years old	FIP, injury at birth
cat 5 or more years old	FIP, brain tumor, hypoglycemia
with stress or activity	hypoglycemia
during sleep	epilepsy
focal-motor type	epilepsy, FIP, tumor
cat chews or licks objects	lead poisoning
multi-cat household	FIP
severe head trauma	post-traumatic epilepsy
status epilepticus at onset	toxicity, stroke
steady increase in seizure activity	FIP any age, epilepsy if young, brain tumor if older
associated with food intake	hypoglycemia, hepatic encephalopathy
previously ill	FIP

cats respond well to temporary sedation but diagnosis is difficult.

Postanesthetic behavioral changes may result from anoxia, but confirmation is rarely possible without an early EEG.

With lysosomal enzyme deficiency or other inherited CNS diseases, ataxia and paresis occur in cats under a year of age. There may be behavioral changes. The progession of clinical signs should help in making this diagnosis.

Table 7. Some Organic Causes of Changes in Behavior

(This table ignores all neurotic or psychotic causes of behavioral problems seen either in the cat or its owner. Always consider the relationship between the cat and other animals, the owner and other people when diagnosing a behavioral problem.)

Cause of Behavior Change	Methods of Diagnosis
CNS	
Brain tumor (including FeLV-positive cats)	C,H,PR,CSF,CR,E,S
Feline hyperesthesia syndrome	C,H,CP,OP,E,S
Acute brain trauma (including projectile)	C,H,PR,CSF,E
Cerebrovascular accident	C,H,CSF,E
Rabies	C,H,B
Minor convulsive episodes (especially psychomotor)	C,H,CP,E,T
Postictal (postseizure) (see Table 5)	C,H,EM,CP,E
FIP, FeLV and toxoplasmosis	C,H,E,CSF,M,S,CP,OP
Intracranial meningitis (bacterial, fungal or algal)	C,H,E,CSF,OP,M,S
Acute cerebral anoxia of respiratory, cardiac, or vascular origin	C,H,CP
Postanoxia, post-trauma, or postcerebrovascular accident	C,H,E
Lysosomal enzyme deficiency diseases or other inherited CNS degenerations	C,H,E,B
Lead poisoning or other toxicities	C,H,CP,E,PR

Table 7 (continued)

Cause of Behavior Change	Methods of Diagnosis
Hepatic encephalopathy	C,H,CP,E,PR,CR
Sedatives, tranquilizers or anticonvulsants	C,H,CP,E,T
Hallucinogenic drugs	C,H,E,T
Idiopathic senile brain degenerations	C,H,E,OP,CP,CSF,S
Idiopathic focal or generalized encephalopathies	C,H,E,OP,CP,CSF,S
Fractures of L_7-S_1, sacrum or S_3-C_1 (bowel habits)	C,H,PR
Non-CNS	
Estrus behavior	C,H
Hyperthyroidism	C,H,CP,B
Owner's misinterpretation of normal activities	C,H
Any organic cause of change in bowel or urinary habits (*eg*, cystitis)	C,H,CP,PR,CR,E
Postpuberty	C,H
Old age	C,H,CP
Pain (see Table 2)	
Any cause of depression (see Table 8) (non-CNS)	

CODE: **B**—biopsy, aspiration or necropsy; **C**—clinical signs and examination (includes neurologic examination); **CP**—clinical pathologic examination; **CR**—contrast radiography; **CSF**—cerebrospinal fluid analysis; **E**—electrophysiologic examination (EEG, EMG, ECG, ERG, isotope brain scan, CAT scan); **H**—history; **M**—microbiologic examination; **OP**—ophthalmologic examination; **PR**—plain radiography; **S**—serologic examination, skin tests, FeLV slide test (paired serum samples often needed); **T**—Treatment.

Fractures or lesions of L_7 to S_1, the sacrum or S_3 to Co_1 may not affect normal walking but may cause incontinence. Without radiographs, the diagnosis may be missed because some clinicians expect more severe signs with spinal lesions.

A cat's personality may be pleasant or nasty. There is not necessarily an organic or inorganic behavioral explanation for the nasty personality. Such natural personalities may not become apparent until 1-2 years of age, after reproductive puberty. Some of these cats, especially if the "nasty streak" is episodic, may be exhibiting the feline hyperesthesia syndrome (see below).

Pacing aimlessly and performing a fixed behavior pattern are indications of personality blunting or mental or extreme environmental pressures. This is a characteristic of many focal or generalized brain diseases. It may occur temporarily after anesthesia, tranquilization or a seizure, and may be associated with a brain tumor, encephalitis or senile degeneration. Corticosteroids are more helpful than sedatives, which can worsen fixed motor activity.

Hyperesthesia caused by morphine and amphetamine derivatives is a well-known problem in cats but similar activity may be caused by tranquilizers, encephalitis, meningitis, stroke or toxicity.

Depression and Coma

Depression or coma is an indication for urgent treatment. The initial breakdown of the differential diagnosis of the causes of depression or coma is into intracranial or extracranial, but the state of the animal may necessitate immediate life-saving treatments before an extensive history or an accurate diagnosis is obtained (Table 6). This extreme usually only applies when the animal is in a true coma (no or minimal response to noxious stimuli, but with swallowing, blinking and segmental spinal reflexes intact). In this state the clinician must ensure adequate respiratory minute volume, heart rate, tissue perfusion, blood volume and body temperature as soon as possible. Blood samples for diagnosis are obtained when an IV catheter is inserted.

Blood electrolyte changes (Na, K, Ca), uremia (azotemia), hypoadrenocorticism, toxicity, hypoglycemia, ketoacidosis and blood hyperosmolality (hyperglycemia) are all potential critical states in coma subjects; treatments for these conditions are often incompatible. The clinician must also be aware that the patient may be anesthetized or under the influence of sedatives or hallucinogens. An ECG is a useful guide to plasma K status and can detect arrhythmias. The ECG, combined with urine ketone and glucose estimations, should quickly eliminate the incompatible therapy situations mentioned above.

Once the cardiovascular, electrolyte, renal, respiratory and blood glucose status of the patient is reasonable, the detailed differential diagnosis can be considered and other diagnostic tests performed, such as an EEG or CSF tap. Coma is similar to cardiac arrest—an already prepared chart of how to handle the case needs to be readily available.

An unconscious animal that can only be aroused by extreme stimuli (yelling in its ear or hitting it hard) is described as stuporous. If the animal is just about awake but extremely dull, it is showing obtundation. Lethargic describes all other less depressed animals. These last 3 states are expressions of potential coma and their differential diagnosis is handled similarly. Many of the conditions in Table 8 can induce any state from lethargy to coma.

The signs of brain pressure cones or herniations, decerebration and intracranial pressure rises are discussed in the section on brain trauma. Interpretation of these signs is vital to the management of depressed animals.

Neuritis

Neuritis is a change in the physiologic status of a spinal (or cranial) nerve such that abnormal sensations (paresthesia, dysesthesia, flashing pains) occur, abnormal motor discharges (fasciculations, fibrillations, spasms) are seen or function is lost (anesthesia, analgesia, muscle atrophy, paralysis). Any or all signs may be paroxysmal (intermittent), constant or seen in any combinations. A total loss of nerve function is usually called paralysis or a deficit rather than neuritis.

The use of electromyography and electroneurography is critical in the accurate diagnosis of many causes of neuritis or nerve damage. These electrical means of studying the peripheral nervous system and its musculature have helped identify new types of peripheral nervous system and muscle diseases. Table 9 lists most of the causes of neuritis and nerve damage or deficits. Table 10 lists the sensory area, muscles innervated, and signs of damage to each major spinal nerve. Table 4 similarly lists the cranial nerves. Note that combinations of nerves or their nerve roots may be damaged entirely or partially, which may complicate the clinical diagnosis.

Table 8. Some Causes of Depression or Coma

Causes	Methods of Diagnosis
Intracranial	
Brain trauma (including projectile)	C,H,PR,CSF,E
Toxicity (hallucinogens, sedatives, anticonvulsants, ethylene glycol)	C,H,CP,E
Hepatic encephalopathy	C,H,CP,E,PR,CR
Cerebrovascular accident	C,H,E,CSF,CP
Encephalitis (FIP, toxoplasmosis, rabies, vaccinal, pseudorabies)	C,H,E,OP,CSF,S
Brain tumor	C,H,E,CSF
Bacterial, cryptococcal, other fungal or algal meningitis	C,H,E,OP,CSF,M,S
Hydrocephalus	C,H,E,PR,CR
Lysosomal enzyme deficiency diseases or other inherited CNS degenerations	C,H,E,B
Seizures or postictal (see Table 5)	
Idiopathic senile brain degenerations	C,H,E,OP,CP,CSF
Idiopathic encephalopathies	C,H,CP,E,CSF
Narcolepsy (collapses might be misinterpreted)	C,H,E,T
Non-CNS	
Shock	C,H,CP
Anemia	C,H,CP
Addison's disease	C,H,E,CP
Diabetic ketoacidosis	C,H,CP
Azotemia	C,H,CP
Hypoglycemia, hyperglycemia (hyperosmolar)	C,H,CP
Hypocalcemia	C,H,CP
Cardiac arrhythmia or insufficiency	C,H,E
Pyrexia, septicemia, viremia	C,H,CP
Pulmonary, pleural and percardial disease	C,H,PR,E,B
Anoxia (respiratory)	C,H,CP,PR
Other systemic diseases or injury	C,H,CP,PR,CR
Cachexia	C,H,CP
Pain (see Table 2)	

CODE: **B**—biopsy, aspiration or necropsy; **C**—clinical signs and examination (includes neurologic examination); **CP**—clinical pathologic examination; **CR**—contrast radiography; **CSF**—cerebrospinal fluid analysis; **E**—electrophysiologic examination (EEG, EMG, ECG, ERG, isotope brain scan, CAT scan); **H**—history; **M**—microbiologic examination; **OP**—ophthalmologic examination; **PR**—plain radiography; **S**—serologic examination, skin tests, FeLV slide test (paired serum samples often needed); **T**—treatment.

Confusing cases usually involve multiple peripheral nervous system lesions that lead to the mistaken diagnosis of a spinal lesion (*eg,* polyradiculoneuritis), muscle atrophy, which can result from disuse (orthopedic problem) or upper motor neuron (spinal or brain) lesions, or vague pain in a limb. Upper motor neuron atrophy is much slower in developing (1-2 months) as compared to lower motor neuron atrophy (2-3 weeks), never progresses as far as lower motor neuron atrophy (fibrosis and total loss), and is characterized by the presence of segmental spinal reflexes. Nerve root and spinal pain from a tumor or trauma may cause the cat to carry the leg. This is an exception to the general rule that neurologic lesions cause limbs to be dragged rather than carried. A carried leg usually but not always indicates a nonneurologic lesion.

Muscle Spasms, Twitches, Tremors and Fasciculations

These muscle activities may be constant or intermittent. Their causes are listed in Table 11. Intermittent spasms or limb twitches are called myoclonus but are rare in cats, and are usually not regular as in canine distemper myoclonus ("chorea"). They are usually seen as a feature of focal motor seizures.

A clinician must always be wary of interpreting tremors and must first ask if the cat trembles at home as much as it does on the examination table. Nervousness, discomfort, cold and fever are all more likely causes of trembling. Virtually any cause of paresis can induce trembling. Senile tremors rarely occur in cats as compared to dogs. Intention tremors indicate a cerebellar lesion and are a feature of cerebellar hypoplasia (neonatal onset, static) or FIP cerebellitis (mature onset, progressive). Intention tremors are absent at rest or when the cat is restrained and are worse when voluntary movements are attempted (placing reflexes).

The clinician's attention should be drawn to spasms or fasciculations of lower motor neuron origin caused by spinal cord inflammation, such as trauma, hypoxia and myelitis.

Lower motor neuron rigidity usually masks the knee jerk and withdrawal reflexes and blocks all limb movements. Fasciculations are a common feature of myelitis and encephalitis in cats but are not a pathognomonic observation because they may be seen with toxicity, electrolyte changes, hypoglycemia and seizures.

Episodic Weakness

Episodic weakness in cats is more commonly due to an intrathoracic disease (heart, lungs) than a neuromuscular one. One must look closely for evidence of dyspnea and handle the cat carefully until the cardiopulmonary functions have been shown to be normal. Neurologic causes of episodic weakness are difficult to diagnose without electromyography and none is acutely life-threatening. Therefore, cage rest and elimination of the non-neurologic diseases as causes are the first priorities (Table 9). Early use of neostigmine or edrophonium to diagnose myasthenia gravis is contraindicated since it may kill the cat. Improved motor ability with use of these drugs is not absolute proof of myasthenia because polymyositis can produce the same result.

Central Blindness

Central blindness is a term usually applied to a loss of visual perception, appreciation and understanding that leaves the pupillary light reflexes intact (Fig 18). It can be produced by a variety of lesions in the midbrain and occipital hemispheres (Table 13). Most such causes are diffuse diseases (hypoxia, trauma, inflammation) but occasionally a suitably situated tumor (lymphoma, ependymoma, meningioma, pinealoma) can produce apparent central blindness. Some centrally blind cats have a crude appreciation of light and dark. This is interpreted as cortical damage, with the midbrain (colliculus) circuits intact.

Optic nerve, optic chiasma and optic tract lesions (tumor, trauma, meningitis, reticulosis, lead) cause loss of the corresponding pupillary light reflex. The causes listed in Table 13 are not often detected by examination of the eye. Lesions in these sites may also be referred to as "central blindness" in some texts, although the pupillary light reflexes are abnormal.

Amaurosis is a term applied to blindness from any cause. However, in neurology texts it is often reserved to describe any blindness not involving the eyeball or a central blindness with intact pupillary light reflexes. Hence, the term "amaurotic idiocy" to describe a CNS degeneration characterized by central blindness and mental deterioration.

Deafness

The cause of deafness is very difficult to diagnose in cats (Table 14). Repeated auditory-evoked brain potentials, which are computer

Table 9. Some Causes of "Neuritis"
(Nerve irritation, inflammation or damage seen as muscle spasms, muscle fasciculations, dysesthesia, pain or paralysis)*

Causes	Methods of Diagnosis†
Cranial and spinal nerves (including their CNS cell bodies, nuclei or nerve roots)	
Trauma (including projectile)	C,H,PR,E
Injection injury	C,H,E
Tumor (nerve, brain, cord, adjacent structures, meninges, metastasis)	C,H,E,PR,CR
Nerve regenerations and neuroma	C,H,E,T
Immune (brachial neuritis, polyradiculoneuritis, sensory polyneuropathies)	C,H,E,T
Metabolic (diabetes, hypothyroid, uremia)	C,H,CP,E,B
Toxic (lead, organophosphates, ticks, acrylamide)	C,H,CP,E,B
Inherited lysosomal enzyme deficiencies (various types usually causing paresis or paralysis)	C,H,CP,E,B
Exostosis pinching nerve (hypervitaminosis A)	C,H,PR
Bacterial inflammation (abscess, cellulitis, osteomyelitis, otitis media)	C,H,CP,E,PR
Encephalitis or myelitis (FIP, toxoplasmosis, rabies, pseudorabies, vaccinal)	C,H,CP,E,OP,CSF,S,B
Implanted materials	C,H,PR
Postsurgical reaction around nerve	C,H,T
7th Nerve neuropathy (compression in stylomastoid canal)	C,H,PR,E
Botulism	C,H,CP,E,S
Non-PNS (that are commonly misdiagnosed as neuritis)	
Pain—see Table 3	
Mild psychomotor type seizure—see Table 4	
Lick granulomas	C,H
Feline hyperesthesia syndrome	C,H,CP,OP,E,S
Anal gland inflammation	C,H
Any pruritic dermatitis (*eg*, miliary, flea bite and hyperthermic dermititis)	C,H,S,B,T
Steatitis	C,H,B
Hallucinogenic drugs	C,H,T
Arthritis	C,H,PR,CP
Partial aortic saddle embolus or unilateral femoral artery embolus	C,H,CR

* *Warning:* Rabies may cause self-mutilation, twitching, paresis or paralysis, any of which may initially be interpreted as signs of neuritis.

† For Key, see Table 11.

Table 10. Signs of Some Spinal Peripheral Nerve Lesions

Nerves*	Loss of Sensation Best Detected in:	Muscles Affected	Gait	Reflexes Lost
Suprascapular (C_6-C_7)	This nerve is not sensory	Supra- and infraspinatus	No variation	None
Musculocutaneous (C_7)	Dorsomedial side of foreleg	Biceps and brachialis (flex elbow)	No variation	Foreleg flexor withdrawal
Radial (C_7-C_8-T_1)	Dorsolateral side of foreleg	Extensors of elbow and carpus	Limb in flexion held off ground, unable to bear weight	Triceps reflex
Median and Ulnar (C_8-T_1)	Ventral aspects of paw and foreleg and the whole 5th digit	Flexor muscles of carpus and digits	Slight carpal drop may be seen	Flexor withdrawal variable
Entire brachial plexus (C_6-T_1)	Entire foreleg from mid-humerus distad	All limb muscles	Leg dragged on ground	All
Femoral (L_4-L_6)	Medial side of thigh and distal leg to medial digit (varies in distal extent)	Quadriceps group of muscles (extensors of stifle)	Unable to fix stifle	Knee jerk
Sciatic (both peroneal and tibial branches) (L_6-S_2)	Whole leg distal to mid-thigh except medial side	Hock flexors and extensors, digit flexors and extensors	Flexion of hock and knuckling of digits	Flexor withdrawal lost
Peroneal branch alone	Dorsal (cranial) distal leg and paw	Hock flexors and digit extensors	Straightening of hock, knuckling of digits	Variable flexor withdrawal response
Tibial branch alone	Ventral (caudal) distal leg and paw	Flexors of paw and extensors of hock	Flexion of hock	Variable flexor withdrawal response
Pudendal (S_1-S_3)	Perineum	Anal sphincter, urethra	No variation	Anal reflex (urinary and fecal incontinence)
C_8T_1 (Dorsal branch of nerves)	Undetectible	Panniculus	—	Panniculus totally lost on affected side
T_1-T_2-T_3**	None	Sympathetic to ipsilateral neck and face	—	Horner's syndrome on affected side

* Their respective spinal cord segments and spinal cord nerve root number are in parentheses.
** Initial segment of spinal nerve, rami communicans, vagosympathetic trunk, cranial cervical ganglion or sympathetic nerves via ear to eye

Table 11. Some Causes of Constant or Intermittent Muscle Spasms, Tremors, Twitches or Fasciculations

Causes or Signs	Methods of Diagnosis
Inflammation from trauma or hemorrhage in cord	C,H,PR,CSF,CR
Feline hyperesthesia syndrome (skin twitches on back)	C,H,CP,OP,E,S
Lower motor neuron irritation of myelitis or meningitis (FIP, toxoplasmosis, rabies, pseudorabies, vaccinal)	C,H,CP,E,S
Tetanus	C,H,CP
Toxicity (*eg*, strychnine, organophosphates, chlorinated hydrocarbons, thiaminase)	C,H,CP
Hypocalcemia/hypercalcemia	C,H,CP
Myositis (immune, toxoplasmosis, nutritional, traumatic, projectile)	C,H,E,OP,CP,S,B
Muscle or spinal cord anoxia (vascular occlusion or cardiac arrhythmia cramps)	C,H,E,CP
Spinal lesions causing involuntary rigidity or spastic paralysis (see Table 1)	
Brain tumor (especially meningiomas)	C,H,E,CSF
Encephalitis or meningitis (FIP, toxoplasma, rabies, pseudorabies, vaccinal)	C,H,CSF,E,S,B
Stroke (cerebrovascular accident, feline ischemic encephalopathy)	C,H,E,CSF
Focal motor seizures (see Table 5)	
Any cause of neuritis (see Table 9)	
Any cause of paresis (trembling) (see Table 1)	
Schiff-Sherrington sign	C,H,PR,CR
Cerebellar hypoplasia and FIP cerebellitis (tremors)	C,H,S,CSF
Spinal walking	C,H,PR,E,CSF
Decerebrate rigidity	C,H,PR,E,CSF
Hypoglycemia (muscle fasciculations)	C,H,CP
Stilted gait seen with pain of many causes (see Table 2)	
Myasthenia gravis (fasciculations)	C,H,E,CP,T
Senile tremors of limbs	C,H,E,CP
Torticollis (upper motor neuron/lower motor neuron/idiopathic)	C,H,PR,CR,CSF,E,S
Polymyositis, corticosteroid myopathy or muscular dystrophy, with advanced fibrotic replacement, stiff limbs	C,H,E,OP,CP,B

CODE: **B**—biopsy, aspiration or necropsy; **C**—clinical signs and examination (includes neurologic examination); **CP**—clinical pathologic examination; **CR**—contrast radiography; **CSF**—cerebrospinal fluid analysis; **E**—electrophysiologic examination (EEG, EMG, ECG, ERG, isotope brain scan, CAT scan); **H**—history; **M**—microbiologic examination; **OP**—ophthalmologic examination; **PR**—plain radiography; **S**—serologic examination, skin tests, FeLV slide test (paired serum samples often needed); **T**—treatment.

Table 12. Causes of Episodic Weakness

Causes	Methods of Diagnosis
Myasthenia gravis	C,H,E,T
Polymyositis (immune; toxoplasmosis)	C,H,E,CP,B
Hypoglycemia	C,H,CP
Hypokalemia (chronic vomiting, insulin)	C,H,CP
Hyperkalemia (uremia, Addison's disease)	C,H,CP
Cardiac (failure, cardiomyopathy, 3rd-degree block, severe arrhythmias, sinus syncope, severe congenital shunts or stenoses, heartworms, hypercalcemic or vagal bradycardia)	C,H,E,PR,CR
Respiratory (pleural, pericardial effusion, diaphragmatic hernia, lymphoma, thymoma, cardiac tumor, pulmonary edema, asthma)	C,H,PR,CP,CR,B
Vascular (anemia, erythrocyte anomaly, blood parasites, hemoconcentration, coarctation of aorta)	C,H,CP,B,CR
Energy pathway enzyme deficiencies (pyruvate dehydrogenase)	C,H,CP,B
Brain (epilepsy, narcolepsy)	C,H,E
Hypothyroidism	C,H,CP
Arthropathies (secondary arthritis, immune and infectious polyarthritis)	C,H,PR,B,CP
Myotonias (metabolic, *eg,* Cushing's disease)	C,H,CP,E
Any chronic debilitating disease	C,H,CP
Recovery phase from any severe disease	C,H
Pyrexia (abscess, heat stroke)	C,H

CODE: **B**—biopsy, aspiration or necropsy; **C**—clinical signs and examination (includes neurologic examination); **CP**—clinical pathologic examination; **CR**—contrast radiography; **CSF**—cerebrospinal fluid analysis; **E**—electrophysiologic examination (EEG, EMG, ECG, ERG, isotope brain scan, CAT scan); **H**—history; **M**—microbiologic examination; **OP**—ophthalmologic examination; **PR**—plain radiography; **S**—serologic examination, skin tests, FeLV slide test (paired serum samples often needed); **T**—treatment.

averaged, can be used to localize the lesion to the cochlea, eighth nerve, brainstem, midbrain or cerebral cortex and help select the most likely cause (see Chapter 18). Diagnosis is difficult unless the cat is white, or other signs are present, or the history (trauma, hypoxia, toxicity) is helpful. Most deafness in nonwhite cats is labeled idiopathic. White cats are usually thought to have a cochlear hair cell problem.

Principles of Prognosis and Treatment of Neurologic Diseases

Prognosis

Multiple factors are always involved in the subjective estimation of a prognosis. It is rarely possible to give exact percentages in a prognosis, even if the results of controlled studies of the disease in question are available. The clinician must use the words "excellent," "good," "guarded" or "poor" and should avoid extremes in prognosis. A guaranteed recovery is never applicable to any situation and many cats with a prognosis described as hopeless have lived on, to the embarrassment of the veterinarian involved. One should consider the following factors in giving a prognosis: the condition diagnosed and its variable effects; the functional degree and anatomic extent of the nervous system lesion; the duration of signs and the rate of progression of signs; the cat's age, breed, size and personality; other diseases of a clinical or subclinical nature; the na-

Table 13. Some Causes of Blindness of CNS Origin
(optic nerves and brain but not the eye)

Causes	Methods of Diagnosis*
Optic neuritis	C,H,OP,E,CP,CSF
Lead toxicity	C,H,OP,CP
Hepatic encephalopathy	C,H,OP,CP,PR,CR
Trauma to optic nerve	C,H,OP,E
Brain trauma/brain edema	C,H,OP,E,CSF,CP
Cerebrovascular accident (stroke), ischemic encephalopathy	C,H,OP,E,CP,CSF
Encephalitis (FIP, toxoplasmosis, vaccinal)	C,H,OP,E,CSF,CP,S,M
Meningitis (bacterial, fungal or algal)	C,H,OP,E,CSF,CP,S,M
Cerebral anoxia (acute or post)	C,H,OP,E,CSF
Postictal (see Table 5)	
Brain tumor (meningioma, reticulosis, lymphoma)	C,H,OP,E,CSF
Hydrocephalus	C,H,OP,E,PR,CR
Idiopathic, senile brain degenerations	C,H,OP,E,CSF
Lysosomal enzyme deficiency and other inherited CNS degenerative diseases	C,H,OP,E,CSF,B
Migrating parasites	C,H,CP,CSF,B

*For Key, see Table 12.

ture of any infection and the animal's immune status; the state of any malignancy and possibility of metastasis or multifocal origin; the accurate selection of treatments and compatibility of such treatments with concurrent diseases or medication; factors limiting treatment, such as the cost and need for special equipment; and the effective enforcement of treatment by your staff or the owner.

Treatment

Principles of treatment apply equally to medical or surgical methods, whether used alone or in combination. Extradural pressure on the brain, spinal cord or peripheral nerves should be reduced by laminectomy or slotting and intradural pressure by use of mannitol or corticosteroids. Inflammation and pain should be combatted with corticosteroids, aspirin or cage confinement. Infection should be prevented or treated. Vertebral movement or bone fragments should be stabilized to prevent further injury.

Formation of decubiti should be prevented with the use of slings, pads, sawdust, straw, a dry cage and frequent changing of the recumbent animal's position. Use of urinary catheters should be avoided; the bladder should be completely expressed often. Physical therapy, in the form of massage, swimming or faradization, and rehabilitation, as with the use of carts, aid recovery or adapt the animal to its deficits. Further injury can be prevented by limiting exercise, preventing the animal from roaming, castration, and advising the owner on proper care.

Special Diagnostic Tests

It is not the objective of this chapter to discuss all of the special neurodiagnostic technics. Myelography and CSF taps are described because they are reasonably simple to perform, require minimal equipment, and provide large amounts of otherwise unobtainable practical information. The other technics require expensive equipment, are time-consuming, are only in the clinical development stage or are of minimal practical significance in selection of therapy. They all require careful interpretation by an experienced operator. Any practitioner wishing to perform these

Table 14. Some Causes of Deafness

Causes	Methods of Diagnosis
Congenital or juvenile (white cat)	C,H,E
Postictal (see Table 5)	
Acute or post-CNS anoxia	C,H,E
Cerebrovascular accident (stroke)	C,H,E
Toxicity (antibiotics) and hepatic encephalopathy	C,H,E,CP
Hydrocephalus	C,H,E,PR,CR
Encephalitis or meningitis (FIP)	C,H,E,OP,CP,CSF
Lysosomal enzyme deficiency diseases and other inherited CNS degenerations	C,H,E,B
Senile brain degenerations	C,H,E,CP,CSF
Trauma to ears or brain	C,H,PR,E
Idiopathic	C,H,E,CP,CSF

CODE: **B**—biopsy, aspiration or necropsy; **C**—clinical signs and examination (includes neurologic examination); **CP**—clinical pathologic examination; **CR**—contrast radiography; **CSF**—cerebrospinal fluid analysis; **E**—electrophysiologic examination (EEG, EMG, ECG, ERG, isotope brain scan, CAT scan); **H**—history; **M**—microbiologic examination; **OP**—ophthalmologic examination; **PR**—plain radiography; **S**—serologic examination, skin tests, FeLV slide test (paired serum samples often needed); **T**—treatment.

tests should first observe clinicians actually using suitable equipment before purchasing it.

Cerebrospinal Fluid Analysis

Performing contrast myelography and collecting CSF involves entering the subarachnoid space. The usual routes of entry are the cisterna magna (cisterna cerebellomedullaris) between the base of the skull and the first cervical vertebra, the dorsal lumbar intervertebral spaces, or the dorsal lumbosacral space. Another route used less frequently is through the skull into a lateral ventricle.

The CSF pulsates and flows, and can have variable pressure or composition in the presence of CNS disease or damage. As blood samples are taken for diagnosis of systemic diseases, so is CSF sampled for evidence of CNS disease.

The CSF serves as a cushion to the brain and is also a transport medium, at least to the epen-

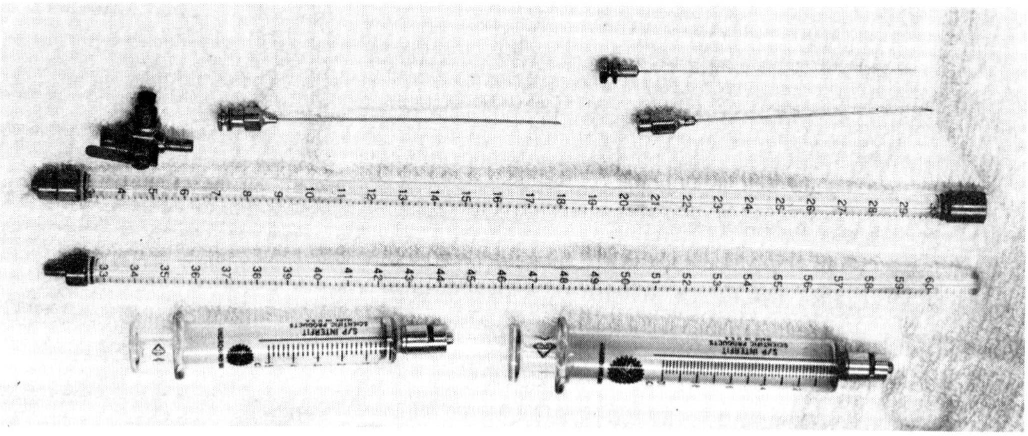

Fig 28. Instruments for CSF sampling and pressure measurements: screw-ended glass syringes, manometer and 3-way stopcock, spinal needles and stylets.

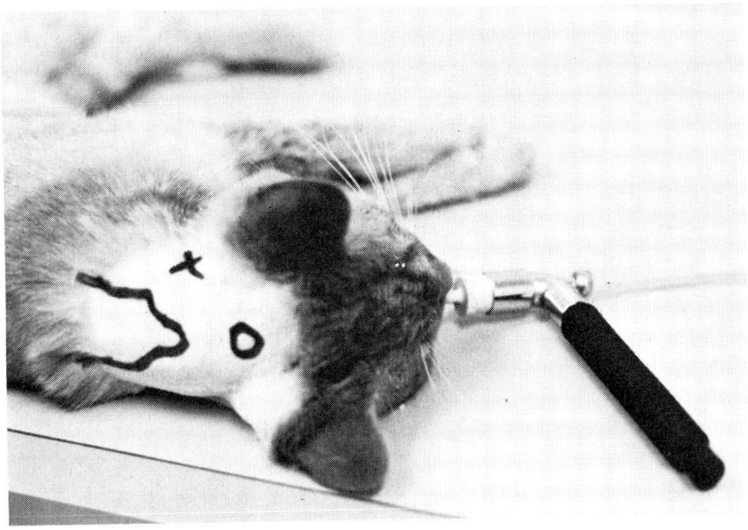

Fig 29. Cat prepared for a cisterna magna tap. An Ayers T-piece anesthetic circuit is being used. The positions of the axis, wing of the atlas (x), and occipital crest (o) are marked on the skin.

dymal cells lining the ventricles. It is formed in 4 choroid plexi located in the left and right lateral ventricles, the roof of the third ventricle, and the roof of the fourth ventricle. It is also formed to a lesser extent in the Virchow-Robin spaces around blood vessels as they enter the brain. The CSF is absorbed directly from the ventricles, as well as from the meninges of the spinal cord and brain.

The CSF flows from the lateral ventricles via the 2 foramina of Monro into the third ventricle, then via the cerebral aqueduct (aqueduct of Sylvius or mesencephalic aqueduct) into the fourth ventricle, and then to the cisterna magna via the 2 lateral foramina of Luschka (lateral apertures), which are small openings in the lateral portions of the brainstem. The cisterna magna is an enlarged portion of the subarachnoid space in the triangle between the caudal part of the brainstem and cerebellum. It can be entered dorsad between the occiput and the first cervical vertebra.

From the cisterna magna, CSF flows over the surface of the brain in the subarachnoid space or down the spinal cord in the spinal subarachnoid space. The flow of CSF is not smooth; intracranial pressure rises and falls with each arterial pulse and respiration. With each cardiac systole, a small volume of CSF rushes from the fourth ventricle into the cisterna magna and sometimes returns during each diastole.

The dura mater of the brain lies directly against the bones of the skull. In the spinal cord, the dura is separated from bones of the vertebral canal by epidural fat. The arachnoid mater is not attached at all points to the dura but is in such close apposition to it that the space between the 2 is only theoretical in normal animals. The

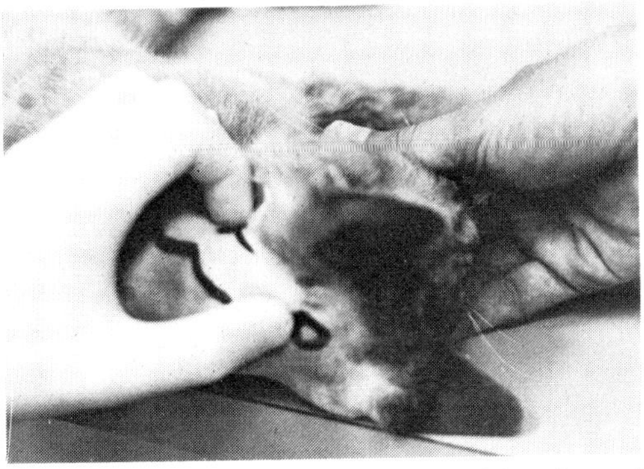

Fig 30. The index finger is on one wing of the atlas and the thumb is on the occipital crest.

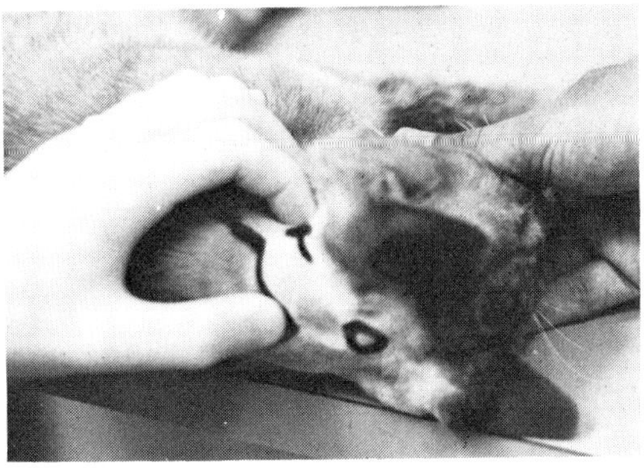

Fig 31. The thumb is palpating the rostral extent of the dorsal arch of the axis.

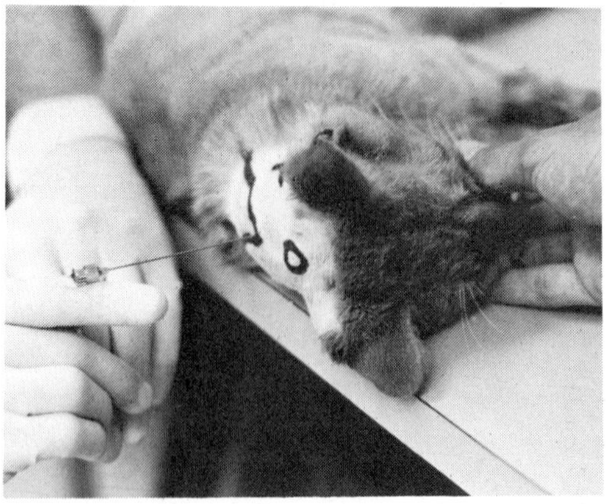

Fig 32. The needle is in the cisterna magna and CSF has begun to flow.

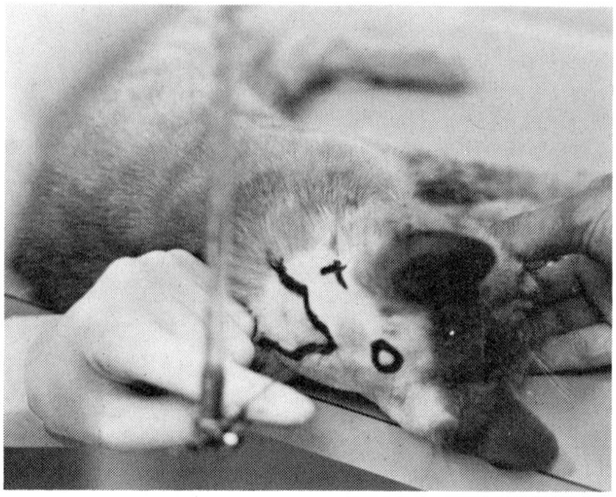

Fig 34. A manometer is connected to the needle in the cisterna magna.

pia mater is attached to the surface of the brain and spinal cord, and is joined to the arachnoid by many small trabeculae that cross the subarachnoid space, which is filled with CSF and many small veins and arteries.

When the cisterna magna is punctured, small 1- to 2-mm fluctuations should be seen in the column of fluid in the manometer. Slightly larger fluctuations, synchronous with respiration are also seen. The yield of CSF from a lumbar tap in cats is so low that pressure recordings are of little value.

Because of the direction of CSF flow, fluid from the cisterna magna is not useful in diagnosing disease in the thoracolumbar area. A lumbar tap is necessary if CSF is to assist diagnosis of thoracolumbar disease.

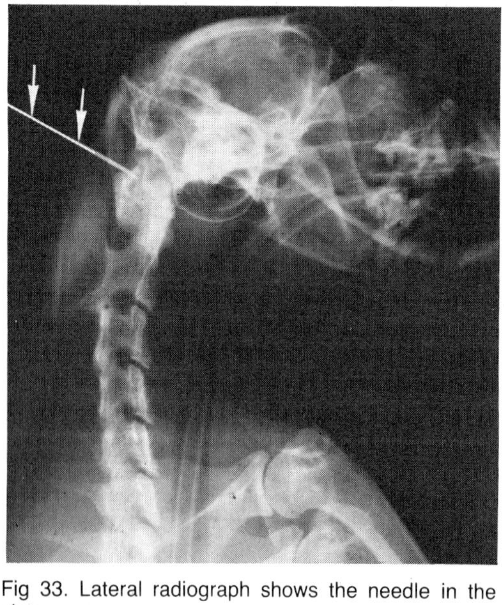

Fig 33. Lateral radiograph shows the needle in the cisterna magna.

Cisternal Tap: The equipment required for puncture of the cisterna magna is shown in Figure 28. Anesthesia is preferably induced with a short-acting barbiturate. The animal is then placed in lateral recumbency and intubated, and the area is prepared for aseptic penetration. The palpable landmarks used when performing the tap are shown in Figure 29.

The cat's neck is fully flexed and its nose is held parallel to the table by an assistant. The fingers of the clinician's left hand are placed on the wing of the atlas and the thumb on the occipital crest (Fig 30). A spinal needle (1- to 2-inch, 20- or 22-ga) is inserted on the midline between the occipital crest and wings of the atlas, just cranial to the dorsal spine of the second cervical vertebra, which can easily be palpated (Fig 31). The tip is directed toward the cat's nose. As the needle penetrates each fascial plane, a sudden release in resistance is felt; the stylet should be withdrawn from the needle each time to determine if the subarachnoid space was penetrated. Individuals used to performing this tap on dogs should be warned that the distance the needle must penetrate in a cat is surprisingly short. When the needle tip encounters bone, it is withdrawn slightly and redirected craniad or caudad. A jerk of the neck muscles is usually noticed when the needle penetrates the subarachnoid space. The CSF flows from the needle when the stylet is withdrawn (Figs 32, 33). A 3-way stopcock and manometer are attached to the needle and CSF pressure is measured immediately (Fig 34). Normal pressure in cats prepared as described ranges from 60 to 120 mm. A sample of fluid can then be withdrawn for analysis or culture. The point of the needle's entry is shown on a skeleton in Figure 35.

CSF Analysis: Only 2-3 ml CSF are required for most laboratory procedures. The fluid is examined visually. Normal CSF looks like water. A red discoloration indicates the presence of fresh blood from a vessel injured during the tap or recent CNS hemorrhage. If the fluid is bloody, the RBC and WBC in the CSF should be present in the same ratio as in circulating blood. The latter ratio can be used to estimate the number of WBC in the CSF from the bloody tap, and thus the number of WBC present in the first place. A brown-yellow discoloration (xanthochromia) reflects the presence of hemoglobin pigments, usually from CNS hemorrhage that occurred 12 hours or more previously. If fresh blood discolors the fluid because the needle hit a blood vessel or if an earlier CNS hemorrhage is continuing, immediate centrifugation removes the red color from the fresh blood, leaving any xanthochromia from the earlier hemorrhage apparent. A cloudy white turbidity reflects an increase in cells or debris in the CSF, which normally is clear and does not clot.

The CSF is analyzed for protein content and examined microscopically for cellular composition. It can also be cultured. A smear of centrifuged or filtered CSF sediment is made to determine the types of cells present, as well as any bacteria or fungi.

If the cisternal tap has been made to obtain a myelogram or pneumoventriculogram, air or contrast material is injected into the cisterna magna (see Myelography). Occasionally antibiotics are injected into the subarachnoid space.

Counting the WBC in CSF must be done within a half hour after the sample is obtained or the cells lyse. The WBC pipette is used to draw diluent to the "1" mark. The pipette is then filled to the "11" mark with CSF. The diluent is prepared with 10 ml glacial acetic acid, 0.1 g crystal violet and 90 ml water. The hemacytometer is filled with dilute CSF and all WBC within the 9 outer 1-mm squares of the grid are counted. The total is multiplied by 1.2 to obtain the number of cells per mm^3 (normal is 0-10).

The differential counting of WBC involves centrifuging the CSF and staining 0.25 ml of sediment with 1 drop of methylene blue. A drop of the mixture is put on a slide and covered with a coverslip. In addition to serving for a differential WBC count, the slide preparation can be examined for bacteria, fungi and abnormal cells.

An estimation of total protein content in a CSF sample is best obtained with a photometer

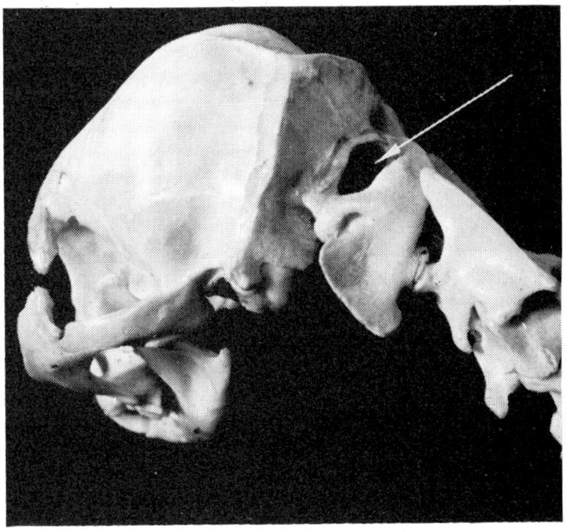

Fig 35. Major landmarks for a cisternal tap.

(normal 0-20 mg/dl). If one is not available, the Pandy test for increased globulin is a fairly reliable substitute to detect moderate or large elevations in protein content. This test is performed by adding 3-4 drops of CSF to 1 ml Pandy reagent (10 g crystalline carbolic acid in 100 ml water) and shaking. An increased globulin content produces a white turbidity. Normal fluid may have a faint white tinge.

Changes in CSF: In cases of bacterial meningitis the CSF is usually turbid, but it is clear or only moderately turbid in viral encephalitis. There is marked rise (250 mm H_2O) in CSF pressure in meningitis but only a moderate rise with encephalitis (150-200 mm). In both encephalitis and meningitis, the WBC count is increased. With viral infections, the increase is in lymphocyte numbers (20-100/mm^3). Neutrophilia reflects bacterial infection (50-500/mm^3). In mycoses, lymphocyte and/or neutrophil numbers are increased. With CNS inflammations, the protein content (especially globulin) of CSF is increased (30-200 mg/dl).

In cats with brain tumors, the CSF pressure is increased (150-200 mm). The fluid remains clear and the WBC count is rarely increased. Tumor cells may be found in CSF sediment. The protein content is rarely increased.

Following trauma to the CNS, xanthochromia or fresh blood may be observed, but the CSF remains clear if there is only brain edema. The pressure is nearly always elevated and sometimes extremely so. The RBC count in CSF is elevated only if RBC are entering the ventricular system. With CNS trauma, the protein content of CSF is usually increased but this is variable, depending on the presence of blood in

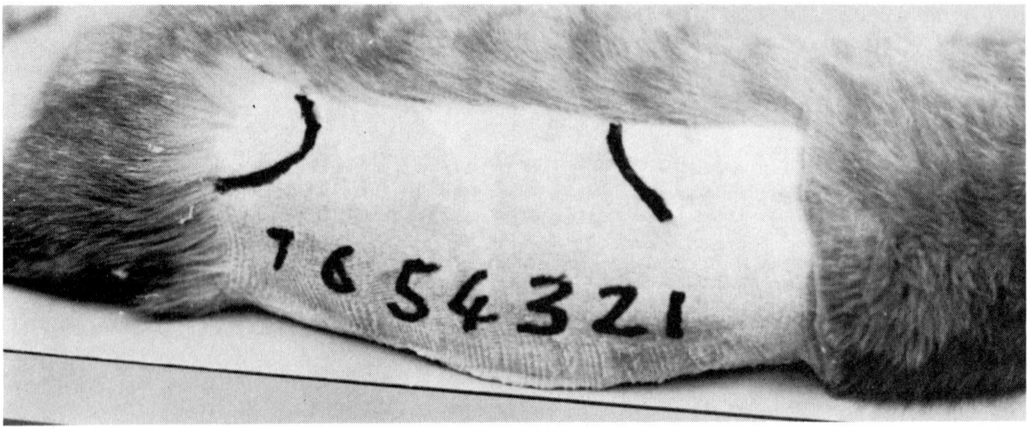

Fig 36. Landmarks for a lumbar tap: the wing of the ilium, the last rib, and the dorsal spines of the lumbar vertebrae.

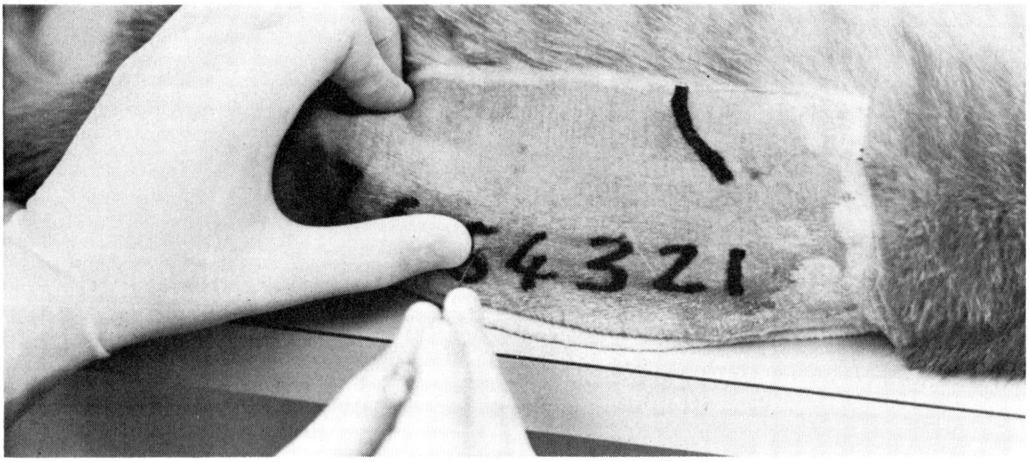

Fig 37. The fingers are placed on the wing of the ilium and the thumb is used to palpate the dorsal spine of the vertebra selected (L_5 in this case). The needle is directed horizontally on the midline and angled about 10° caudad from a right angle to the spine.

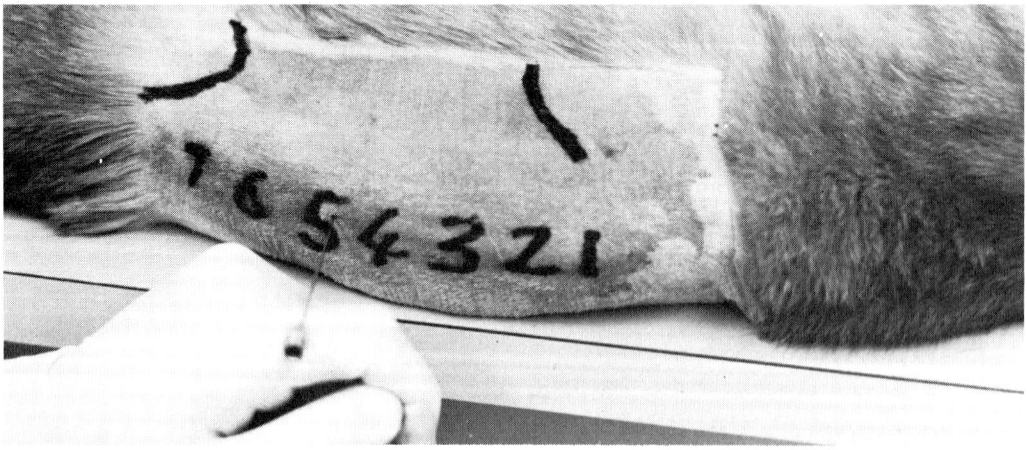

Fig 38. The needle in position.

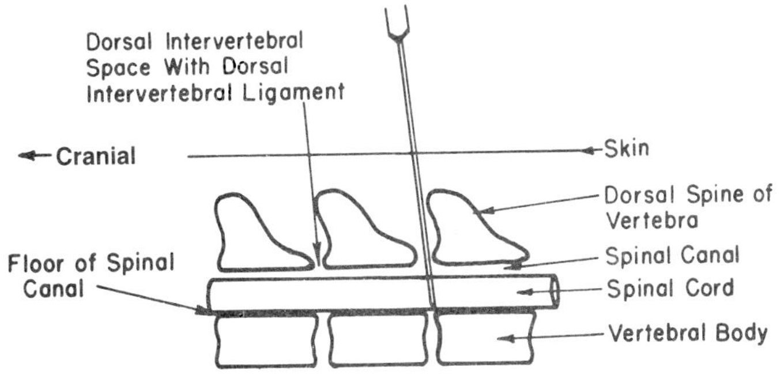

the ventricles and the severity of the edema.

In hydrocephalic animals, the CSF is normal but the pressure is variable.

With convulsive disorders, including lead poisoning, uremia and hypoglycemia, a moderate rise in CSF content (20-30 mg/dl) and pressure (150 mm) may occur.

When CNS trauma has occurred and a high CSF pressure (250 mm) is detected, one should never remove more CSF fluid than is absolutely necessary; the amount needed for analysis should be removed slowly. This prevents a sharp fall in subtentorial pressure within the skull. If the subtentorial pressure falls when the supratentorial pressure is elevated, a tentorial pressure cone develops, leading to severe damage of the midbrain.

Myelography

Myelography involves the use of contrast material to outline the spinal cord. The contrast material can produce a positive image (Pantopaque:La Fayette, Skiodan:Winthrop, Amipaque:Winthrop) or a negative image (air) on the radiograph. Air is rarely employed. The contrast medium is injected into the subarachnoid space at the cisterna magna, at the lumbosacral space or between 2 lumbar vertebrae (usually L_3-L_4 or L_4-L_5).

Pantopaque is an oily, nonabsorbable contrast medium that gives results inferior to those provided by absorbable, aqueous contrast materials, such as Skiodan or Amipaque.

When a contrast medium is injected, the animal should be under general anesthesia and should remain anesthetized for one hour thereafter to avoid convulsions after contrast medium injection. If convulsions do occur, diazepam (Valium) should be given IV to effect (5-30 mg) and/or phenobarbital (30-100 mg). Fewer convulsions occur with use of Amipaque than with Skiodan.

The cat should be intubated and on a nonrebreathing anesthetic circuit. Care must be taken to ventilate the animal because respiratory depression may occur after the contrast medium is injected.

Technic: We prefer to have the cat in lateral recumbency on the radiography table. To flex the back, the hindlegs are pulled rostrad between the forelegs. For thoracolumbar myelograms, the dorsal lumbar region is prepared for aseptic penetration. We inject the cisterna magna for cervical myelography.

The subarachnoid space of the feline spinal cord usually ends at the L_7-S_1 junction (Fig 36). In 50% of cats, a lumbosacral puncture yields CSF. A 22-ga, 3-inch needle, with a stylet and a short tip, is used. For interlumbar injections the needle is inserted percutaneously, in the midline just cranial to the dorsal spine of a lumbar vertebra and pushed down to the dorsal arch

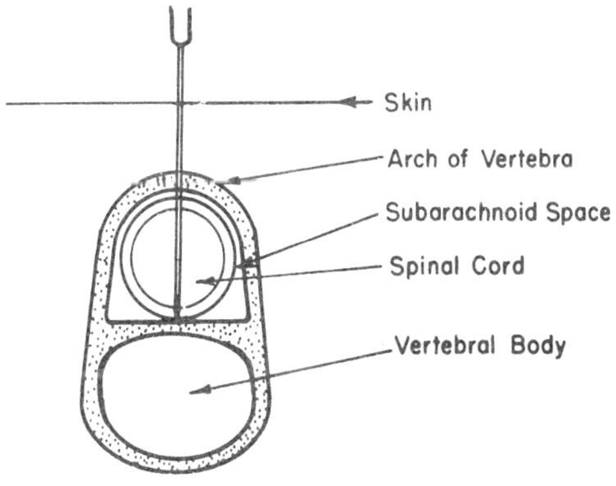

Fig 40. Diagram of a lumbar tap, frontal view.

(Fig 37). After the intervertebral space is entered, the needle is pushed to the ventral floor of the spinal canal. A sudden release in resistance is felt as the needle goes through the dorsal intervertebral ligament. The hindlegs twitch as the needle passes through the spinal cord and then the needle meets the bone of the canal's floor. These 3 signs are good indications of successful entry. The bevel of the needle is turned craniad and the stylet is removed (Figs 38-40).

In at least 50% of the cases, CSF drips slowly from the needle. If this does not happen, a radiograph can be obtained to determine the needle's position or a small amount of contrast medium can be injected. There is mild resistance to injection of contrast medium; the lumbar muscles should twitch and respirations become irregular if the needle's placement is correct.

The most suitable contrast medium currently available seems to be Amipaque (metrizamide). The medical-grade medium is expensive but the analytic (chemical) grade is much cheaper and can be used in cats as follows: 3.75 g metrizamide is mixed with 8.9 ml distilled sterile water to make 10 ml isotonic solution with 170 mg iodine/ml. An alternative diluting solution is 0.005% $NaHCO_3$. The shelf life of the powder is long but once in solution reportedly degenerates. The solution contains no preservative and hence can be contaminated. The solution should be injected from one syringe through a Milex filter into another syringe to remove particles before use. The dosage is 0.3 ml/kg body weight.

Some people cannot procure metrizamide or prefer methiodal sodium (Skiodan). We suggest using a 20% solution of Skiodan (Skiodan 40% diluted with saline) with 0.1% lidocaine. The dosage is 0.3 ml/kg body weight if only thoracolumbar films are required, and 0.5 ml/kg if good cervical films are needed from a lumbar injection.

Skiodan is more irritative than metrizamide and more likely to cause seizures. It is also absorbed more rapidly from the subarachnoid space than metrizamide. Metrizamide can be induced to flow by gravity up or down the spine by raising one end of the cat. One has about 15-20 minutes to perform these manipulations. Neither agent causes significant meningeal irritation and both are completely absorbed. Pantopaque is not absorbed and must be removed.

After the operator is sure that the needle is in the correct position, the contrast medium can be injected, taking about 4 seconds to inject 2 ml. One film (lateral lumbar) should be exposed as the contrast is injected (a cassette and grid should be used). The other films are exposed after completing the injection and removing the needle (one more lateral lumbar, a ventrodorsal lumbar, lateral thoracic, ventrodorsal thoracic, lateral cervical and ventrodorsal cervical, as needed). Normal myelograms of the lumbar, thoracic and cervical regions are illustrated in Figures 41-43.

Interpretation of Myelograms: The main purpose of a myelogram is to outline compression of the cord by intra- and extradural masses (Fig 44). A myelogram is of particular value in the following circumstances: with paralysis, when localization by clinical tests is inconclusive or differs from the evidence in plain radiographs; when plain radiographs reveal no evidence of the cause of compressive cord disease; when paralysis is only partial (clinical localization is poor), when the plain films provide inconclusive evidence, and yet surgery is necessary; and to demonstrate the presence or absence of pressure on the cord when the cause of spinal paralysis is unknown.

Myelography may result in extension of localized infection in the subarachnoid space further up the cord, even into the ventricles. When spinal meningitis is suspected, CSF examination should precede myelography to assist detection of segmental meningitis before it is converted into extensive infection.

The trans-spinal approach for myelography, as described here, has been criticized because of the dangers of cord damage. In our clinical and experimental experience with this technic, we have not observed permanent cord damage unless the contrast medium was injected into the spinal cord instead of the subarachnoid space. In such cases, a contrast haze is seen in the cord tissue on radiography.

Electroencephalography

The electroencephalogram (EEG) is valuable to the neurologist as it permits a noninvasive study of cerebrocortical function. Cerebral function is modified by systemic problems (hypoglycemia, anoxia), generalized CNS disease (FIP), focal cerebral disease (spike focus, tumor, cerebrovascular accident, hematoma), epilepsy and hydrocephalus. The EEG must be interpreted with the help of a good history and physical examination because cerebral changes are rarely specific for one disease entity. Animals less than

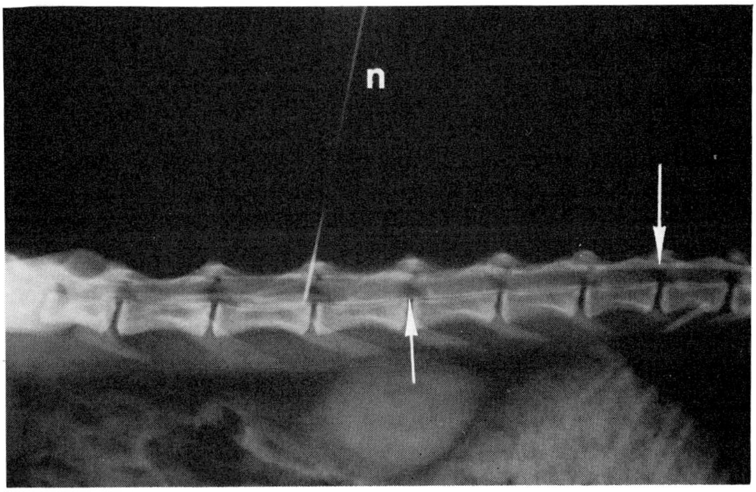

Fig 41. Normal lumbar myelogram. The contrast medium appears as 2 lines (dorsal and ventral) in the subarachnoid space (arrows). The needle (n) is in position at the injection site.

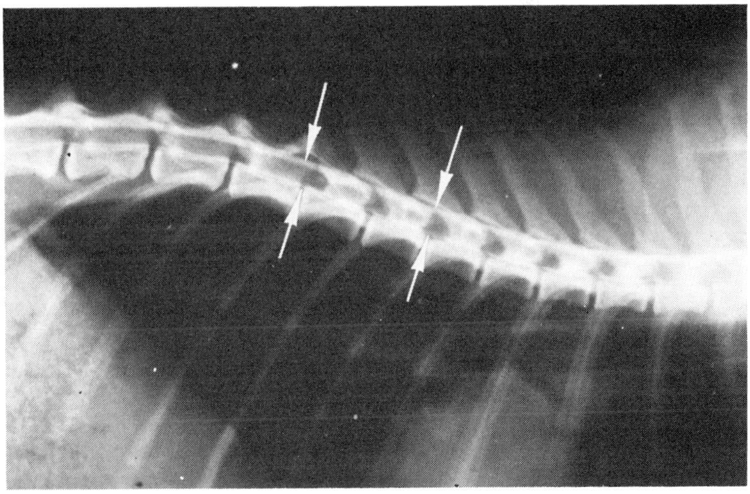

Fig 42. Normal thoracic myelogram. The dorsal and ventral contrast columns are indicated by arrows.

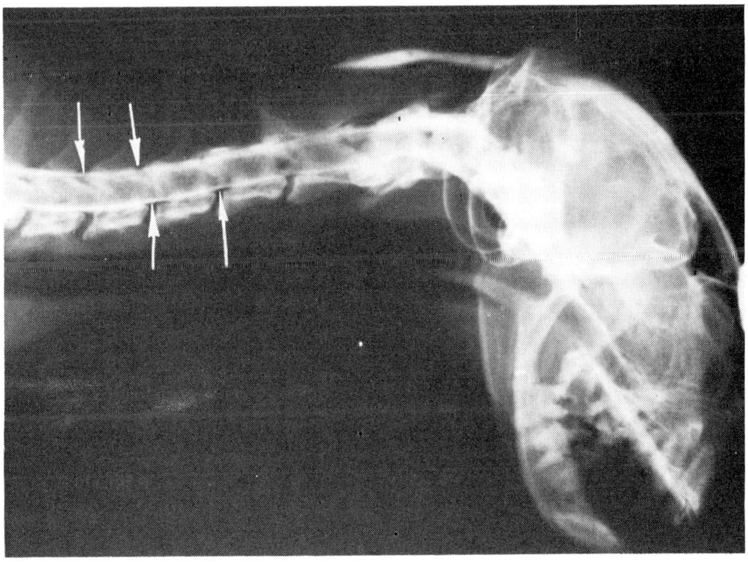

Fig 43. Normal cervical myelogram. The dorsal and ventral contrast columns are indicated by arrows.

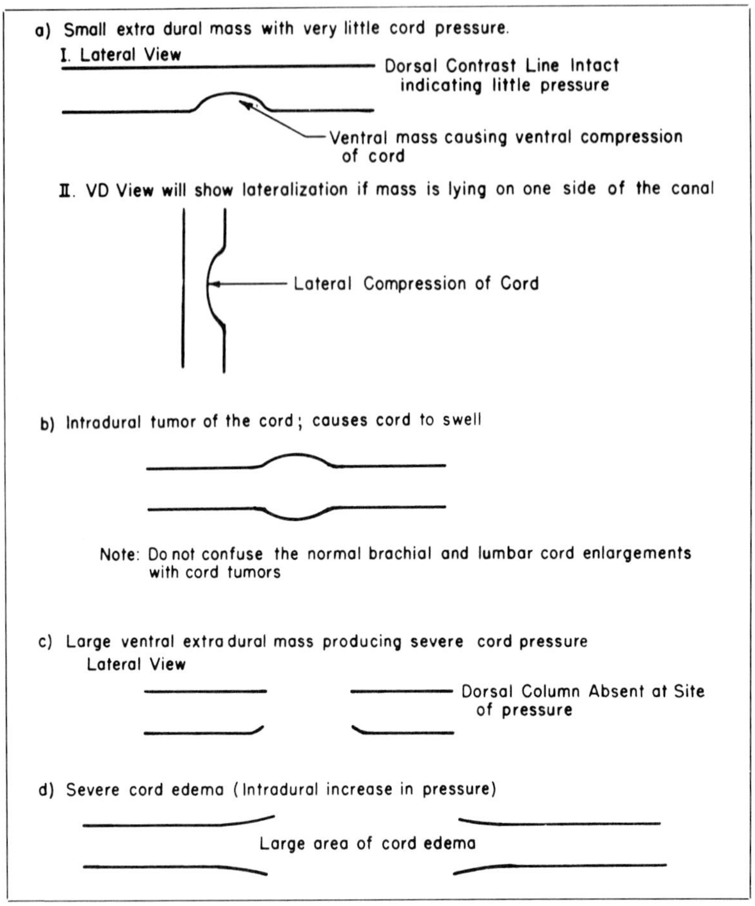

Fig 44. Myelographic abnormalities.

6 months of age have an immature EEG, which renders interpretation difficult. In encephalitis, the character of the recording changes with the stage and cause of the disease.

Despite these limitations, we have found the EEG invaluable in handling neurologic cases. It is of particular use in identifying sites of cerebral dysfunction, differentiating cats with coma associated with cerebral edema from cats anesthetized by ingestion of unknown drugs, estimating cerebral status after anesthetic emergencies or diagnosing meningitis and acute encephalitis without a history.

The EEG is a specialist's tool. The equipment is expensive, delicate to operate, and it requires considerable skill to interpret the recordings. Generalists should be aware of what the test can do and when to refer a case for electroencephalography.

Electromyography and Electroneurography

These technics permit identification of diseases affecting the spinal or cranial lower motor neuron cell body (myelitis, trauma), its nerve root in the peripheral nerve (trauma, injection), or its axon (polyradiculoneuritis), as well as the neuromuscular junction (botulism, myasthenia gravis) and the voluntary muscle fibers themselves (myositis, myotonia). It is also possible to study the function of a variety of smooth muscles and to study more complex reflex circuits, as is done in evoked anal electromyography. Electroneurography is particularly useful in measuring the conduction velocity of motor or sensory peripheral nerves, which permits diagnosis of the various neuritides. Electromyography is gaining acceptance as a method, both for identifying affected peripheral nerves (neuropathies) and muscles (myopathies) and for localizing segments of spinal cord in which the lower motor neuron function is affected. It may augment or replace myelography in some cases. Electromyography and electroneurography are also preferred initial technics to muscle or nerve biopsy.

Performance and interpretation of the electromyogram and the electroneurogram require considerable skill. The reader is referred to other texts for detailed discussions.[1] Basically the electromyographer listens to the sounds on a speaker and looks at the oscilloscope picture of the muscle's electrical activity as a needle is inserted or nerves are stimulated. Various electrical activities found at insertion of the needle when the muscle is at rest or upon stimulation suggest the absence or type of disease in either the muscle, its motor nerve supply or a sensory nerve.

Electromyography and electroneurography are more suited to a group practice than is electroencephalography, but the skill necessary for their use is still considerable. The equipment involved in electromyography and electroneurography costs about 30% of that required for electroencephalography and probably yields about the same amount of useful data.

Lumbosacral Venography

This procedure is used to delineate any obstruction to venous flow in the L_7-S_1 spinal cord segments. Myelography cannot do this because the spinal cord ends cranial to this level.

An 18-ga needle is inserted percutaneously into the body of the vertebra L_7 from a lateral approach just ventral to the wing of the ilium and 3-5 ml of an angiographic contrast agent are injected. The contrast medium normally fills the lumbar and sacral veins within the spinal canal. Lesions in the canal in the L_7-S_1 area deviate or obstruct caudal flow of the material.

Cerebral Arteriography

This procedure is mainly used prior to intracranial surgery. In our experience, it is difficult to perform in cats because the internal carotid arteries do not supply the brain. Common carotid artery injections yield poor results because the arteriogram is of the whole head, not just of the brain. An alternative technic is to catheterize a vertebral artery via the femoral artery. The vertebral route has problems because the basilar artery's blood flow is caudal in the cat. Hence, even pressure injections do not fill the circle of Willis or hemispheres very well. In theory, the site and extent of an intracranial tumor or other space-occupying lesion may be delineated, enabling performance of a craniotomy in the right place. Theoretically, cerebral angiography also distinguishes cerebral artery occlusion from embolism or thrombosis. In reality, cerebral arteriography is unrewarding in cats.

Cerebral Venography

Cerebral venography is more easily performed but rarely provides useful information. It delineates only the lesions that are inaccessible surgically. Such lesions usually produce deficiencies in one or more cranial nerve functions and can actually be localized just as well with this evidence. Cerebral venography is performed by injecting contrast into the facial vein (or more rarely into the dorsal midline sinus inside the cranial vault) and obtaining several radiographs during injection. The intracranial veins and their major anastomoses are delineated. This is the easiest of the catheterization technics to perform but the least helpful clinically.

Ventriculography

Filling of the ventricles of the brain with air (pneumoventriculography) or a water-soluble contrast agent is an aid to diagnosis of hydrocephalus (enlarged ventricles) or a space-occupying lesion deforming the normal-sized ventricles. Use of aseptic technic is vital in performing ventriculography.

Most injections are made into the lateral ventricles. With the animal in sternal recumbency, the skull is penetrated 1 cm lateral to the midline in the mid-parietal region and the needle (with stylet) is inserted vertically into one lateral ventricle. Some CSF is withdrawn before and during injection of air or positive-contrast agent. Radiographs can be taken in lateral, ventrodorsal, anteroposterior or oblique positions to delineate any lesion. The animal should be under anesthesia and intubated during the procedure. If a positive-contrast agent is used, the anesthesia may have to be prolonged for 1-2 hours and diazepam or phenobarbital given to control seizures. Air should be used as the contrast agent if possible.

The clinical value of ventriculograms in cats is minimal. Their risk (with air) is not great but they are time-consuming. The only use we find is to prove the size of the ventricles in cases of suspected hydrocephalus.

Radioisotope Scintigraphy

This is not even a specialist's tool; it belongs in research. The cost of the equipment is high and the skill in running it is considerable. Scintigraphy involves injecting radioactive isotopes systemically, waiting a few hours for tissue distribution, then scanning the brain with a gamma (Anger) camera. A computer is used to average a large number of scans in the anteroposterior or lateral dimension as an oscilloscope image. In this way, "hot" or "cold" areas of the brain can be detected. Artifacts may be a problem and the images are not crisp in the small brain of a cat. Cerebral vascular lesions and tumors can be detected with reasonable accuracy.

A few colleges of veterinary medicine have the facilities to perform scintigraphy but they find more use for their equipment scanning other parts of the body.

Computerized Axial Tomography

The CAT scan is popular in human medicine but the equipment is very expensive. A few practices, institutions and veterinary schools have access to CAT scanners. The small size of a cat brain limits the usefulness of the scanners because of resolution problems. The scan demonstrates changes in density in the soft tissue of the brain, such as edema, enlarged ventricles, tissue displacement, calcification, vascular anomalies and tumors. It is perhaps the most useful special procedure before surgical attempts to remove a brain tumor are made.

The CAT scanner uses a computer to build up an oscilloscope image of a cross-section of the body. Although x-rays are used, the image shows brain tissue very well. The anode and x-ray detector rotate about the plane of the body selected for study. Many exposures are made and analyzed to produce the image. Several successive cross-sectional images of the brain and skull, from rostral to caudal, can be made. Images can be enhanced by use of contrast media.

Averaged Evoked Sensory Potentials

With the advent of small, cheap signal-averaging computers, a new clinical field has opened up. Sensory stimuli (noise, light, nerve stimuli) evoke small electrical changes in the brain and/or spinal cord that can be detected with skin electrodes. Such changes are normally lost among the normal electrical noise of the brain. However, if they are time-locked to the event that caused them and if enough of them are averaged together, using the stimulus to start the recording sweep each time, the time-locked events are additive and the random noise is averaged out.

By producing clicks in the ear canal with a small earphone, the auditory-evoked potentials can be measured using subdermal electrodes. Similarly, not only can a single-sweep electroretinogram be performed, but averaged visual-evoked potentials in the brain can be studied. Other potentials can be recorded from the spinal cord (dorsal root- or dorsal horn-evoked potentials) in response to peripheral nerve stimuli. These stimuli also evoke spinal, brainstem and cerebral activity (evoked cortical potentials).

No similar motor circuit tests exist for structures in the CNS.

These tests are used to evaluate the function of points along the CNS sensory pathways. Their use is mainly academic but a few practical uses are being found for them. The most useful one seems to be the auditory-evoked potential.

These tests require moderately expensive equipment, the operation of which is fairly simple but time-consuming. They are available in

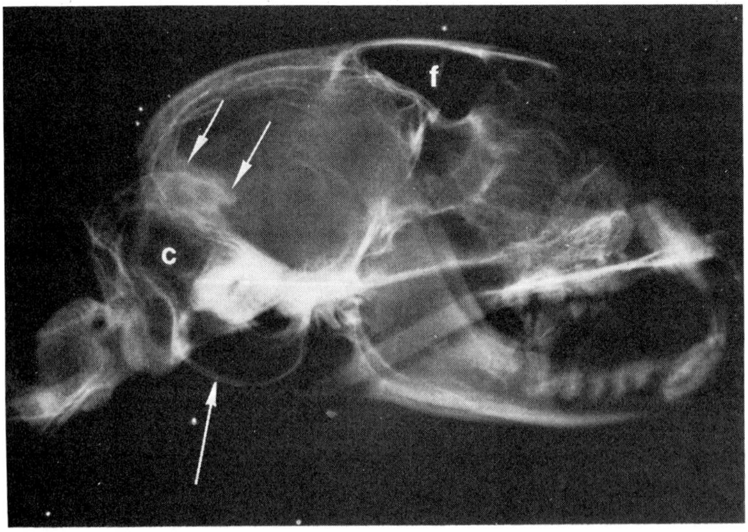

Fig 45. Lateral radiograph of a normal cat's skull. Notice the shape of the tentorium (double arrows) and the delicate tympanic bullae (single arrow), the frontal sinuses (f), and position of the cerebellum (c).

many colleges of veterinary medicine. Their use in practice is of questionable value.

THE BRAIN AND GENERALIZED DISEASES

Trauma

Cause: Trauma to the head may be caused by projectiles or blunt-object impart (car, fall, club). Projectiles (bullets, pellets, rocks, etc) may not penetrate the skull, in which case the injury is similar to that from a blow. If they penetrate the skull, infection is a likely complication, with almost certain laceration and hemorrhage.

Pathophysiology: Blows to the head can result in concussion, contusion, laceration, hemorrhage, increases in intracranial pressure, and edema. All can occur with or without skull fractures. Concussion has been referred to as a molecular shakeup of brain cells. Contusion is a bruising of brain tissue. Hemorrhage with the cranial vault can be diffuse or localized, but its localization as a clot is not common in cats. Edema and increased intracranial pressure are the most serious changes. Edema can be caused by trauma, anoxia, toxins, thrombosis and infection. This swelling of brain cells with fluid interferes with cellular respiration and causes a rise in intracranial pressure. An increase in pressure also occurs with intracranial space-occupying lesions, hydrocephalus and meningitis. The systemic blood pressure rises as intracranial pressure rises (Cushing's reflex or response), causing bradycardia.

Clinically one judges a cat's prognosis and treatment by its neurologic state. Treatment should not be based entirely on the form of brain injury. Brain injury may immediately damage cranial nerves, cause unconsciousness, affect vital centers (respiration, vasomotor) or cause mild concussion. If the cat survives the initial injury and the clinician controls vascular, respiratory and renal functions, the cat's survival depends on the medical management of subsequent brain swelling. Brain swelling is caused by hemorrhage, vascular bed swelling and CSF accumulation, but most importantly by edema. Brain edema is the major killer in brain trauma. Most types of therapy are designed to prevent or limit brain edema.

Brain edema may be an intracellular or cytotoxic process (Na rushes into cells, followed by water, caused by loss of the ATP-dependent Na pump) or an extracellular-intercellular vasogenic process (increased permeability of brain capillary endothelium). Both processes may occur simultaneously. Brain swelling is a vicious spiral; as it develops, it worsens local hypoxia, which leads to more edema.[2]

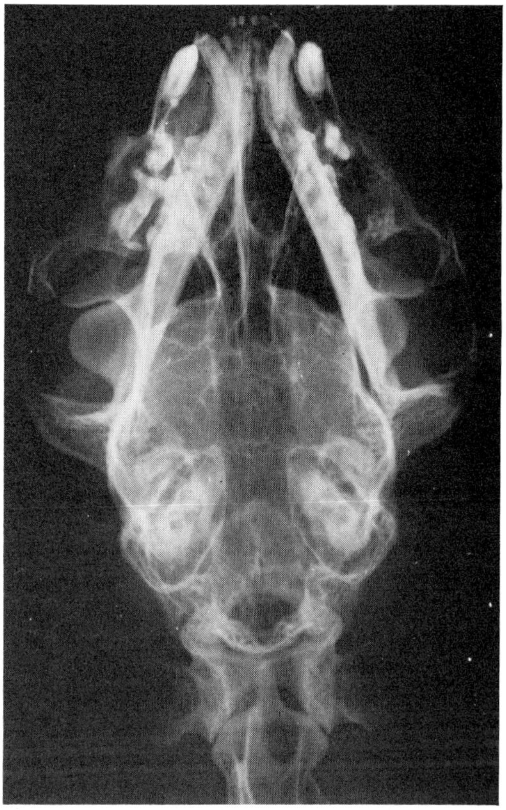

Fig 46. Ventrodorsal radiograph of a normal cat's skull.

The part of the skull encasing the brain (the calvarium) protects the brain from the environment but is its worst enemy once brain swelling starts (Figs 45, 46). The brain has a certain amount of compliance and, as edema develops, the ventricles and vascular bed may decrease in size; however, eventually the only thing that can happen is gross movement of brain tissue. The brain has no supporting connective tissue so it cannot resist deformation. Parts of it are squeezed out of their normal position, which leads to tearing of blood vessels and hemorrhage, as well as tissue deformation.

The 2 places where this process causes major problems are the tentorium and foramen magnum (Fig 47). The tissue distortion is referred to as a pressure cone. A tentorial pressure cone develops because the tentorium creates a narrow

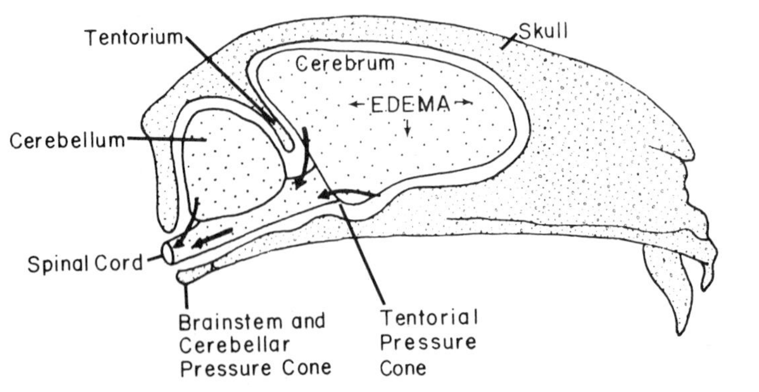

Fig 47. Diagram of the major sites of pressure cones in the skull.

ring of bone at the level of the midbrain. There is a large amount of brain mass (hemispheres) that is supratentorial. This tissue swells and moves the midbrain caudad. The brainstem and cerebellum may be partially squeezed out of the foramen magnum as well. Deformation of the midbrain leads to decerebrate rigidity, pupil constriction and depression, all of which can be easily monitored as they progress.

Large subdural hematomas are common in people but seem to be rare in cats. We have seen subdural clots after subdural hemorrhage in cats, but usually such hemorrhage is diffuse. Therefore, we believe medical reduction of brain edema should be the primary objective of treatment in most cases; surgery is not indicated. When a detectible skull fracture is in a surgically accessible site and the injured animal is not responding to medical therapy, surgical decompression should be considered.

However, the site of the brain laceration and perhaps hemorrhage may not be at the fracture site. It may be at the diagonally opposite point in the brain (contrecoup injury). The objective of any surgery is to clean up a penetrating wound, remove blood clots, reduce hemorrhage and decompress a compression fracture. It may not be wise in all cases to operate. Figure 48 shows a cat with a midline compression fracture (hammer blow) of the parietal bone. The dorsal sagittal sinus is in the midline and bleeds easily; damage to it worsens edema. The cat was successfully managed medically.

Electrical injuries usually occur because the cat, usually a kitten, bites into an electrical cord. Unconsciousness and tonic or clonic seizures may occur. Mouth burns and pulmonary edema are likely. Whether the edema is neurogenic or not is unknown, but it seems likely.

Treatment: Brain trauma is managed medically by maintaining a low-normal body temperature, maintaining good tissue oxygenation, and using corticosteroids, osmotic diuretics, metabolic diuretics and pentobarbital anesthesia. Each facet of treatment must be initiated at the earliest opportunity and each may result in complications. Monitoring the patient depends on visual observations; a generalist cannot monitor intracranial pressure, blood flow, oxygenation and brain compliance.

Maintaining a low-normal body temperature seems contraindicated in shock, but a rise in body temperature of 2-3 degrees F may increase the degree of brain edema by half.[3]

Initial management of brain trauma involves ensuring a patent airway, and thus adequate oxygenation by endotracheal intubation. In rare instances, a tracheotomy may be necessary. In addition, an O_2 cage may be needed.

Corticosteroids and diuretics are used to reduce brain inflammation and edema.[4] Massive doses can be given initially, but the dosage should be rapidly reduced within 1-2 days. Dexamethasone dosages of 0.05-0.1 mg/kg, repeated BID, can be continued for 2 weeks. Dexamethasone (up to 3 mg/kg repeated TID) during the first day of treatment is perhaps one of the most effective drugs for reducing some types of intracranial edema.[2]

If given alone, nonosmotic diuretics seem to have little effect on brain edema; however sodium ethacrynate (Sodium Edecrin:Merck), at 1 mg/kg, has a synergistic effect if given 10-60 minutes before mannitol.[5] Sodium ethacrynate blocks Na ion resorption in the renal tubules and promotes its excretion. It may affect cerebral membranes similarly and thus reduces Na and water entry into the brain cells after injury. Furosemide may be equally effective.

Mannitol is the osmotic diuretic of choice because it has minimal "rebound" effect when reducing raised intracranial pressure. It is given IV as a fast drip at 250 mg/kg in a 10-20% solution. The dose can be repeated every 6-8 hours. Its maximum effect occurs 1/2-2 hours after administration. Mannitol also appears to act synergistically with dexamethasone to reduce brain edema.[6] Should shock develop, giving mannitol can be dangerous.[7] In such cases, whole blood or plasma should be given initially to return the central venous pressure to normal. In any case, the central venous pressure should be monitored during infusion of mannitol and the infusion terminated if the central venous pressure rises by more than 10 cm H_2O. Cats are more susceptible than dogs to developing pulmonary edema during rapid IV infusions.

Deep barbiturate anesthesia reduces irreversible brain cell damage and perhaps edema. The mechanism of action is not completely understood but may involve depressed cell metabolism and constriction of cerebral blood vessels. Anesthesia is maintained for 12-24 hours, with careful pulmonary ventilation.[8]

The treatment for a specific cat that has suffered brain trauma should be based on clinical signs. A cat that is slightly dazed or disoriented but has no deficits in any higher reflex and is only slightly ataxic should only be given dexamethasone at a low dosage (0.05-0.1 mg/kg BID) for 1-3 days. Even in mild cases, the owners should be told about the signs of possible deterioration due to intracranial hemorrhage or edema and secondary infection. Although hospitalization is not essential, it is preferable for at least a day. Radiographs are not necessary, but the skull should be palpated for evidence of fractures. Some cats may have temporary irregularity in pupil size. Anisocoria or temporary constriction of the pupils is often considered an indication of concussion.

Marked ataxia, loss of a higher reflex, or loss of voluntary motor function and/or conscious proprioception suggests more serious brain injury. Provided consciousness is not lost for longer than a few minutes, these signs reflect moderate and localized brain damage and do not indicate life-endangering edema or increased intracranial pressure. For such cats, dexamethasone is all that is required; it should be given at 1 mg/kg TID for the first day. The dosage can be reduced to 0.1 mg/kg TID for the next 3 days, then reduced gradually until suspension of treatment by the end of a week.

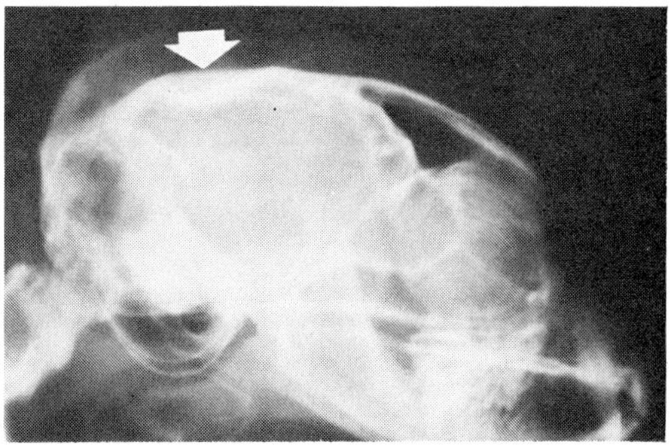

Fig 48. Lateral radiograph of the skull reveals a dorsal parietal mid-line compression fracture (arrow).

Prognosis for full recovery is good, but the owner should be warned of possible hemorrhage and edema that can develop within 24 hours and possibly be fatal or produce permanent damage. The pupils of affected cats vary in size but, provided that at least one pupil has a good response to light, this is not a cause for alarm. Full recovery may be delayed, even in mild cases, for as long as 2 months. There are 2 major exceptions to this generalization. Cats with a head tilt attributable to a vestibular lesion may be left with a permanent head tilt, for which they usually learn to compensate. Cats with optic nerve or optic chiasma lesions may be permanently blind in one or both eyes.

Injured animals with quadriplegia, decerebrate rigidity or loss of consciousness for an hour or more should be assumed to have suffered severe brain injury. Decerebrate rigidity refers to extensor rigidity of all 4 limbs and the spine. It is produced by severe, but not necessarily irreversible, midbrain damage. Although some cats that remain comatose for as long as 24 hours may make a sudden, complete recovery, they are exceptions. Prognosis for these cases should be very guarded until the animals regain consciousness and can stand and move to a limited degree. If improvement is not noticeable within a week, the prognosis is poor. Once improvement is noticed, most cats make a reasonable recovery or learn to adapt to minor deficiencies. Recovery may continue as long as 3 months and the required nursing may become tedious to the owner.

Animals in this group and those that deteriorate rapidly require dexamethasone at 3 mg/kg TID for the first 24 hours. The dosage is reduced to 0.5 mg/kg TID on the second day, and then 0.05-0.1 mg/kg TID can be given for as long as 2 weeks. These cats should be kept in an O_2 cage; tracheal intubation may be needed if they become comatose. Their body temperature must be kept to low-normal. Pentobarbital anesthesia is probably indicated for 12 hours. Mannitol should also be given, along with sodium ethacrynate (or a diuretic with similar mechanisms of action), as soon as possible and repeated TID during the first treatment day at 250 mg/kg.

Major signs of increasing intracranial pressure are increasing degrees of decerebrate rigidity, decreasing consciousness and increasingly pinpoint pupils. In some cases, only one pupil is miotic, which perhaps indicates unilateral inflammation in the midbrain on that side. Unilateral miosis usually indicates less extensive and less life-endangering changes than bilaterally constricted pupils. As the increase in pressure becomes severe, the pupils constrict to pinpoints and consciousness becomes severely impaired (it may have been lost initially at the time of trauma).

If the pressure rises further, the pupils dilate completely just before death. Cisternal removal of CSF may be dangerous in such cases because it can result in a sudden drop of subtentorial pressure.

If there is definite history of trauma, there is little practical advantage to further diagnostic procedures. If a definite history is not available, additional tests may be rewarding. Toxemia, cerebral infarction, tumor or infections may produce acute signs similar to those caused by trauma. Skull radiographs reveal some fractures with minimal displacement and most compression fractures. Good technic is required to detect skull fractures with minimal displacement. Figures 45 and 46 show a normal cat's skull.

When injured animals are deteriorating rapidly and the site of the lesion has not been determined by manual or radiographic examination, an electroencephalogram may enable localization of the lesion. Speculative attempts to find the site of suspected hemorrhage are unjustified because the bleeding is often diffuse or only severe edema has occurred. The chances of exposing a site of localized bleeding are thus low, and it is almost certain that brain tissue will ooze from the trephine hole after the dura is cut (this is another form of pressure cone called a transcalvarial cone).

Projectiles produce effects similar to other forms of brain trauma, but are unsterile and may carry debris into the brain. Therefore, high dosages of ampicillin or chloramphenicol (100-300 mg/kg TID for 4 days) should be used. An attempt to remove the projectile surgically may be indicated if it is accessible.

Sequelae: The long-term complications of head trauma are surprisingly few. If they live, a few animals may be left with a weakness of one or more limbs. If they recover consciousness and show improvement within a week, most recover well. The permanent sequelae associated with vestibular and optic nerve lesions have been mentioned. Behavioral changes also occur and can be permanent. Seizures that may start months later can occasionally be attributed to the trauma.

Neurogenic pulmonary edema sometimes develops after moderate to severe head injury. It generally develops a few hours after the acute injury and often develops as the systemic arterial pressure rises (Cushing's response), paralleling rises in intracranial pressure. Although the 2 processes were thought to be connected, they usually are not. The pulmonary edema can be independent of systemic arterial pressure and is more dependent on increased sympathetic tone to the lungs, caused directly by the brain injury (edema, hypoxia). This produces profound pulmonary artery hypertension and a serum-like edema fluid.[9] Treatment of severe cases is difficult, but diuretics, bronchodilators, corticosteroids and an O_2 cage are helpful.

The treatment for electrical injuries, once the electricity is turned off, is the same as for neurogenic pulmonary edema.[10,11] The seizures are self-limiting.

Infections

Inflammation of brain tissue (parenchyma) is referred to as an encephalitis. Inflammation of the meninges covering the brain is a meningitis. When both occur together, it is called meningoencephalitis. Similar inflammations of the spinal cord are myelitis or meningomyelitis.

The clinical signs of encephalitis depend on the site of inflammation. There usually is evidence of more than one focus (multifocal) of CNS damage: facial muscle or mandibular paralysis, facial twitching, dysphagia, head tilt, circling, blindness, variable nystagmus, pupil reflex changes, ataxia, hypermetria, loss of conscious proprioception in one or more limbs, limb paralysis, convulsions, depression and changes in behavior. Neurologic examination should reveal damage to upper motor neurons, lower motor neurons and/or higher reflexes. Signs develop over a few days in acute infections, but in FIP the onset may be insidious. There is often a slight elevation of temperature. Electroencephalography and CSF analysis are performed to confirm the diagnosis.

Viral infections: Feline infectious peritonitis is a curious viral disease. Many cats exposed to the virus do not become ill but develop an immunity to it. Others seem to develop an exuberant inflammatory response to viral infection. The latter response is mainly a vasculitis and is the apparently infectious disease called FIP. The effusive response leads to the classic peritoneal "wet" form, with fluid accumulation in the abdomen. This has been attributed to B-lymphocyte disease. The "dry" or noneffusive form is attributed to T-lymphocyte disease. In the dry form, the vasculitis often affects the nervous system, although CNS signs may occur with the wet form. The onset may be acute, over a few days, but more commonly is insidious, with the multifocal CNS signs developing over a period of months.

Any neurologic sign may be seen, including seizures, nystagmus, cranial nerve paralysis, facial spasm, head tilt, cerebellar signs (hypermetria, tremors), ataxia, neuritis, limb paralysis and behavioral changes. Obstruction to CSF drainage may lead to hydrocephalus.[12]

Uveitis (hypopyon, flare) is often present. In fact, in any cat with CNS and ocular signs, the major differential diagnosis is FIP, followed by leukemia, fungal agents and toxoplasmosis. Many cats have FIP and are carriers of FeLV.

Determination of serum titers against FIP virus is a reasonable diagnostic guide if interpreted carefully and if clinical signs are progressive. Electroencephalographic evidence and CSF analysis are also helpful to confirm the type of inflammation (polymorphonuclear lymphocytes, with much globulin) and its multifocal nature. The vasculitis lesions are histologically pyogranulomatous and usually involve the meninges and brain tissue. Occasionally a lesion may resemble a tumor.

Treatment with prednisolone (0.5-2 mg/kg daily or every other day) slows the development of clinical signs, often for 1-2 years. Seizures can be controlled with phenobarbital but they tend to become more frequent. More vigorous therapy can be modelled on anticancer regimens (cyclophosphamide, phenylalanine mustard, interferon). One must remember, however, that FIP usually is a multisystemic disease with a poor prognosis (see Chapter 4).

Feline leukemia is a generally well-understood disease that seems to be involved in CNS disease directly and indirectly. Detection of the replicating virus in cats (FeLV positive) usually represents an acute or carrier state, especially if the state persists several months and if protective antibodies do not appear in the blood. Among many possible systemic problems, these carrier cats may also have pupil changes (anisocoria), with ciliary ganglion lesions attributed to infiltration by lymphocytes.[13] Their status renders them susceptible to other infections, such as FIP. In addition, other entities may be associated with FeLV-positive cats. Demyelination of the spinal cord has been observed in FeLV-positive cats with no other apparent disease.[14] Immune complexes with FeLV antigen have been found in the nervous system of FeLV-positive cats with neurologic signs attributable to such lesions. Carriers of FeLV may have behavioral changes, seizures, limb ataxia or lower motor neuron paralysis that may be reversed temporarily or permanently with corticosteroids and phenobarbital. At necropsy, no lesions to account for the signs are evident on light microscopy. Polioencephalomyelitis has also been observed in FeLV-positive cats.

Feline leukemia virus can affect the nervous system directly or indirectly; the explanation of the mechanisms is not yet available. Clinically one should not be surprised to find neurologic signs in cats that are only FeLV-positive. Many of these animals respond well but usually only temporarily to corticosteroids. Chapter 4 contains more information on FeLV infection.

Polioencephalomyelitis may be associated with FeLV infection. Affected animals are often ataxic initially. Cranial nerve deficits are rare except for slow pupillary light reflexes. Hallucinatory sleep seizures (cats wake up hissing and biting) may occur. The signs usually progress slowly to paralysis of all limbs. Only a limited response to corticosteroids is seen. Hyperesthesia may be observed. At necropsy, changes in the brain and spinal cord involve neuronal degeneration, gliosis and perivascular cuffing with mononuclear cells.[15]

Rabies is a well-known disease of cats and unfortunately fairly common because of the frequent failure of owners to vaccinate cats against it. The neurologic signs vary from sudden friendliness, biting objects or self-mutilation and rage, to dysphagia and limb paralysis.

The Negri body is not specific for rabies; brains of suspect cats should be tested by fluorescent antibody technics or mouse inoculation. The onset of CNS signs after exposure is not automatic; some cats have naturally acquired protective titers against rabies virus. Some cats may incubate the disease many months. Others may have CNS signs for 20 days before dying. It is not known if cats can survive once CNS signs have appeared, as a few dogs can.

The important things for clinicians to note are that rabies in cats can begin with paralysis of just one limb (apparent injury) or as dysphagia (apparent needle in throat) and CNS signs can be present for over 10-days before death occurs.

Vaccine-induced rabies is a problem in cats. Both the modified-live Flury and Street Alabama Dufferin virus strain vaccines have been incriminated.[16] The low-egg passage vaccines have long been known to cause problems in cats but clinicians are now faced with the fact that any modified-live rabies vaccine is a risk in cats. It may not always be the vaccine but may be the cat's depressed immune response (FeLV, FIP). Annual use of inactivated rabies vaccines is advised for cats.

Most cats show the first CNS sign 2-4 weeks after vaccination. Some cats seem to recover from apparent postvaccinal problems. A frequent feature of these cases is rear-limb (often unilateral at first) weakness. It is not known if the cats excrete the virus or if the virus is dangerous to people.

Pseudorabies (Aujeszky's disease) is a peracute encephalitis that causes death within 2-3 days of the onset of signs. Signs include pruritus, dysphagia and convulsions. Contact with pigs or uncooked pork or pig offal is the usual source. Infected cats usually live on farms housing infected pigs.

Other viral diseases that experimentally cause encephalitis in cats include Newcastle disease and eastern equine encephalomyelitis.

Bacterial Infections: Bacteria rarely infect the cranial vaults of cats. When they do, it usually is an extension of chronic sinusitis, otitis interna and osteomyelitis or by hematogenous infection. Bacterial infections almost invariably cause meningitis. Progression of clinical signs occurs over 2-10 days. There is no constant pattern of clinical signs seen in intracranial meningitis in cats. With spinal meningitis, however, there usually is evidence of pain. Signs associated with intracranial meningitis in cats observed by the authors have been either depression or hyperesthesia and convulsions. Blindness, ataxia, paralysis and behavioral changes may also occur. The febrile and bone marrow responses may not be marked. Analysis of CSF is important in diagnosis because the common signs occur in other conditions as well. The CSF usually shows a marked increase in pressure, polymorphonuclear leukocyte numbers and protein content. It is wise to make gram-stained smears and to culture the CSF of cats with suspected meningitis.

As chloramphenicol and ampicillin pass the intact blood-brain barrier and reach therapeutic levels in the CSF, they are the most commonly used antibiotics for treatment of meningitis in cats. There is evidence that other antibiotics, including penicillin at 20,000-50,000 IU/kg daily, reach therapeutic levels if the blood-brain barrier is rendered more permeable by inflammation.[17] Both chloramphenicol and ampicillin are given in dosages as high as 100-300 mg/kg TID for 4-5 days. Such large doses of chloramphenicol should be given cautiously because dosages of 50 mg/kg daily have been toxic to cats after one week and fatal after 3 weeks.[18]

Inappropriate use of corticosteroids often causes improvement for 1-2 days in cats with bacterial or fungal meningitis before sudden CNS collapse occurs. Meningitis from FIP responds well to corticosteroids. Hence, it is necessary to perform a CSF tap before corticosteroids are used if a bacterial or fungal etiology is suspected.

Fungal or Algal Infection: Once CNS signs develop, the prognosis with any fungal or algal disease is poor. Surgical removal may be possible if the lesion is focal.

Cryptococcus neoformans is a small (20μ diameter), saprophytic, budding yeast-like fungus with a thick capsule. It has a reputation for being spread by pigeons and has a predilection for the nose, lung, CNS and skin of cats. Cryptococcosis may be the most common fungal disease of cats.

Immunodeficiency (specific or general) of the host probably plays a large part in successful infection with all the fungae and algae. Affected cats are likely to be FeLV or FIP positive.

Chronic nasal discharge, sneezing, lymphadenopathy, retinal detachment, uveitis, optic neuritis and skin nodules are systemic signs of cryptococcosis. When the CNS becomes infected there may be depression, blindness, circling, head tilt, nystagmus, ataxia, seizures, coma, hypermetria, pain or limb paralysis, depending on the route of infection. Penetration from the nose is a common route, directly via the ethmoid plate or via veins, into the cranium. Cats so infected develop CNS signs over a few days; such signs often involve cranial nerves 2 through 6. A few cats with CNS signs develop signs much more slowly over 2-4 weeks.

Treatment seems pointless once CNS signs appear, although some success with amphotericin B and newer antifungal agents has been reported in limited (skin, nose) infections.[19,20] Intrathecal (cisternal or ventricular) injections of these agents have not proved successful in treating CNS infections.

Diagnosis of cryptococcosis is easy. *Cryptococcus neoformans* can be detected by most staining methods in tissues, smears, aspirates and CSF using India ink preparation. Caution should be used in culturing any fungal agent since most produce large numbers of spores, which are released when the culture is opened for inspection. Susceptible humans could become infected. The CSF pressure in cats with CNS infection may be extremely high (400 mm H_2O). Serologic and skin tests are unreliable.

The eye lesions may contain organisms or the retinal detachments may just be the result of serous fluid accumulations behind the retina. Cats with only eye lesions may be treated with corticosteroids if cryptococcosis is not suspected. Temporary improvement may be noticed before dissemination develops.

Histoplasma capsulatum is an intracellular (often in macrophages of all types), yeast-like agent 2-4 μ in diameter that rarely affects cats. Infection by inhalation leads to pulmonary disease that may spread to the CNS and eyes. Occasionally gut involvement may occur. The CNS signs are similar to those of cryptococcosis.[21] Diagnosis is a little more difficult because the agent is small and intracellular. Serologic tests are reasonably sensitive and reliable. Circulating monocytes and polymorphonuclear leukocytes may be found containing the agent. Bone marrow aspirates may also be diagnostic. When cultured it is pathogenic to people. Treatment is slightly more rewarding than with cryptococcosis but not if CNS signs are present. Infection is occasionally associated with exposure to neighboring flocks of birds.

Blastomyces dermatitidis rarely causes disease in cats and is usually found in skin lesions.[22] Rarely it may involve the eye, bone and CNS. Inhalation and pulmonary infection does not seem common in cats. Stained smears of skin discharges, aspirates and CSF are usually diagnostic. The agent of blastomycosis is 7-15 μ in diameter and a budding, yeast-like organism in tissues. It is sensitive to amphotericin B. Serologic tests are reliable.

Coccidioides immitis infection is endemic in the desert areas of the southwestern US but cases may occur in any geographic area if the owners have traveled with their cats through endemic areas. However, cats are rarely affected. Inhalation seems to be the route of infection, with pulmonary and bone lesions the most common. Infection of the CNS has apparently not been observed in cats but is known in dogs. The agent should never be cultured as it is highly pathogenic for people in this form. In aspirates or biopsies of lesions, cyst-like sporangia may be seen, with some containing many endospores. Skin testing animals in endemic areas is useless, since about 50% of normal animals react.[23]

Prototheca spp are achlorophyllic, saprophytic algae with a thick cell wall. They are occasionally responsible for disseminated or focal granulomatous CNS disease in many species but have not yet been reported to affect the CNS of cats. Infection by *Prototheca* is an example of an opportunistic infection. Other fungal and algal agents are probably capable of similar actions, such as penicilliosis, paecilomycosis and cladosporiosis. The clinician should always make smears of any available fluid or cells, take biopsies and beware of culturing unknown agents of this type unless strict precautions are taken. Most cats with CNS signs from fungal or algal disease are unlikely to respond to treatment.

Chapter 5 contains more information on these diseases.

Protozoal Infection: Toxoplasma gondii is a coccidial parasite for which the cat is the definitive host. It multiplies in the gut mucosa and its oocysts are shed in the feces. Clinical signs of this are usually not observed. Direct ingestion of oocysts or infected rodents completes the life cycle. The role of the cat in human toxoplasmosis seems much overrated.[24] Most cats shed oocysts as kittens and intermittently as adults.

A few cats, either as kittens or adults, develop a disseminated form of toxoplasmosis. The agent multiplies in many tissues (liver, lung, spleen), as well as in the CNS and eye. Tachyzoites, small free forms that may be seen in groups, and bradyzoites (cysts) are found surrounded by inflammatory reactions. Lymphadenopathy is common. The disseminated infection can be inapparent and may leave only a few retinal scars. It may cause mild signs, such as depression, or may be overwhelming.[25,26] The CNS disease may be similar. Fresh ocular signs (small retinal hemorrhages) are common in CNS cases. The CNS signs vary from posterior paresis to ataxia, head tilt and behavioral changes, but do not often include seizures. Diagnosis is difficult in the form limited to the CNS but CSF analysis, electroencephalography and serologic examination of paired serum samples can help.

Treatment of the CNS form of toxoplasmosis is controversial. Some cases are self-limiting. Use of antiprotozoal agents may be helpful in the disseminated form but does not seem so in the CNS form. Most of the drugs used are especially toxic to cats. We use corticosteroids (prednisolone at 0.5-1 mg/kg daily or every second day) to reduce the inflammation as is done for the ocular form. This usually controls CNS signs but the cats may require treatment for 6 months. Relapses may occur. The signs of the CNS form may be due as much to an exuberant immune response as to the actual organism.

Other protozoa, such as *Babesia, Trypanosoma* and encephalitozoan species, cause encephalitis and/or meningitis but not usually in the US.

Parasitism

Dirofilaria immitis (canine heartworm) can mature in the cat's heart and may migrate at any stage to the spinal canal or cranial vault, where it may cause acute or progressive CNS signs (circling, head tilt, ataxia, depression). The adult worms, 8-10 cm long, are usually found in the lateral ventricles and may cause some degree of hydrocephalus.[27,28] No successful treatment has been reported. Diagnosis has been by necropsy, but high eosinophil counts in blood and CSF suggest metazoan parasite migration.

Toxocara spp larvae (visceral larval migrans) can migrate through the CNS of cats, causing low-grade encephalitis (depression, ataxia). It is usually a self-limiting problem and the signs are often responsive to corticosteroids. Thiabendazole has been given orally at up to 200 mg/kg but may be hepatotoxic. Corticosteroids may do more good by reducing inflammation. Definitive diagnosis is not possible except at necropsy unless a migrating larva is found in the CSF. High eosinophil counts in CSF and blood are strongly suggestive.

Angiostrongylus cantonensis, the rat lungworm of Southeast Asia, North Australia and Hawaii, is a well-known cause of eosinophilic meningitis in animals other than rats (inappropriate hosts). The intermediate hosts are slugs, snails, prawns and crabs. Fever and generalized CNS signs are seen. Eosinophilia and a high CSF eosinophil count are highly suggestive in endemic areas. Thiabendazole and mebendazole are of limited value and toxic but corticosteroids (*eg,* prednisolone at 1-2 mg/kg daily) are valuable in reducing inflammation.

Cuterebra spp flies have parasitic larvae that can penetrate the skin of the host and migrate in the body. *Cuterebra americana* affects cats, rodents, rabbits and people. If a larva migrates into the CNS, it may have devastating effects (hyperesthesia, circling, seizures) and kill the host. Such cases are reported but the diagnosis is by necropsy unless a focal spinal lesion is detected and explored surgically. Treatment is otherwise ineffective.[29]

Metabolic disorders

Hypoglycemia: Hypoglycemia is not common in cats and may be associated with a pancreatic tumor. Weakness, trembling, excessive salivation and convulsions accompany hypoglycemia. The blood glucose level usually falls below 40 mg/dl if an insulinoma is responsible for the signs. Simultaneous blood glucose and insulin assays can be used to calculate the amended insulin:glucose ratio:

$$\text{AIGR} = \frac{\text{insulin (units/ml) x 100}}{\text{glucose (mg/dl) - 30}}$$

Any ratio over 30 indicates inappropriate secretion of insulin. Treatment is by surgery and/or use of diazoxide (*eg,* Hyperstat:Schering), at 10-50 mg/kg/day in divided doses, if metastatic disease is present.

Other causes of hypoglycemia are endotoxic shock, hepatic tumors, portocaval shunts, hepatic cirrhosis, pregnancy toxemia and glycogen storage diseases, few of which have been observed in cats.

Hypocalcemia: Hypocalcemia can cause generalized muscle spasms and even convulsions, with variable ataxia and loss of consciousness.[30] Such signs are only seen in late pregnancy or up to 8 weeks portpartum (eclampsia) and are controlled rapidly by giving calcium borogluconate solution IV or IM. During IV infusion of 5% calcium borogluconate, the heart rate must be monitored and the infusion stopped if the rate changes sharply. Approximately 5-10 ml are needed to abolish acute clinical signs. An equal volume should be given SC and oral supplementation should be supplied. The kittens should be removed from the queen and hand-reared if clinical signs recur.

Thiamin Deficiency: A deficiency of thiamin causes small hemorrhages, malacia and edema of the brainstem in cats. Clinical signs include head-weaving, flexed neck posture (often as spasms), ataxia, muscle tremors, mydriasis, hypersensitivity, behavioral changes, head tilt, loss of righting reflexes, circling, convulsions and death. Many of these signs suggest vestibular damage.[31] The diets of affected cats usually have adequate thiamin but also contain thiaminase. Several varieties of raw fish have a high thiaminase content. Affected animals on such a diet are said to have Chastek paralysis. Outbreaks of Chastek paralysis may occur if commercial cat food contains sufficient thiaminase.[32] As treatment, thiamin is supplied and the high-thiaminase foods are avoided. The prognosis for recovery generally is good, except for severely affected animals. Occasionally cats with signs of Chastek paralysis have been fed a diet in which no source of thiaminase can be found.[33]

Porphyria: Porphyria can produce behavioral signs in people and is reportedly inherited in cats as an autosomal recessive trait.[34,35] Affected animals have a brown discoloration of their teeth and urine that fluoresces. No CNS signs were reported in affected cats.

Hepatic Encephalopathy: This disease can result from severe hepatic cirrhosis, hepatic lipidosis, toxic destruction of the liver, genetic enzyme deficiencies in the Krebs-Henseleit (ammonia to urea) cycle in the liver, and from congenital or acquired portocaval shunts. A few cases of portocaval shunts have been observed in cats.[36] These shunts bypass the portal blood around the liver into the systemic circulation. Any combination of small stature, recurrent systemic infections, small liver size, hypoalbuminemia, mild hypoglycemia, low BUN level, prolonged recovery from anesthesia, intolerance of organophosphate products and sedatives, cyclic behavioral changes, depression, ataxia, blindness and seizures are seen in young cats.

Diagnosis is by detection of the chemical ans anatomic changes listed above, ammonia-tolerance test and portal angiography (Fig 49). The treatment can be daily oral antibiotics neomycin), small doses of lactulose (Cephulac: Merrell-National) (up to 1 tsp TID until stool is slightly soft) and a low-protein diet in mild cases. Severe cases require a single or graduated attempt(s) to totally or partially ligate the shunt in the hope that the portal blood flow to the liver will increase.

The actual chemicals responsible for the CNS signs are not completely understood. Hyperammonemia causes encephalomalacia but other chemicals are also involved in the process, such as mercaptens and abnormal neurotransmitters.

Glycogen-Storage Diseases: These have rarely been observed in cats. Hepatomegaly and hypoglycemia are the clinical features of such diseases. In severe variants, muscle weakness and neurologic signs appear early. They are usually the result of inherited enzyme deficiencies or temporary juvenile immaturity in the lysosomal enzyme pathways that release glucose from glycogen, as in deficiency of alpha glucosidase.[37]

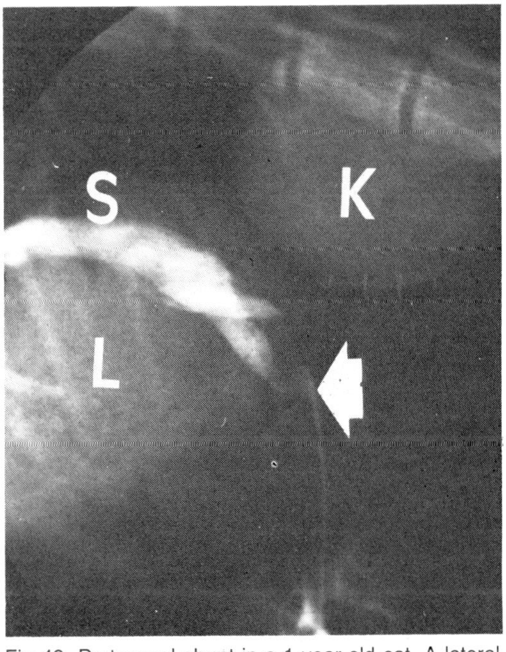

Fig 49. Portacaval shunt in a 1-year-old cat. A lateral view of a mesenteric vein injection angiogram (arrow) reveals an anomalous vessel (S) shunting portal blood around the liver (L) into the vena cava. K = kidney.

Table 15. Some Lysosomal Enzyme Deficiency Diseases of Cats

Name and Enzyme Deficient	Substrate that Accumulates	Reference
Glycogen Catabolism		
Pompe's disease (alpha glucosidase)	Glycogen	37
Glycoprotein Catabolism		
Mannosidosis	Not known in cats	
Glycolipid Catabolism		
Type-1 ganglosidosis (beta galactosidase)	Gangliosides	38,41,42
Type-2 gangliosidosis (partial beta galactosidase)	Gangliosides	37,41,51
Tay Sachs disease (hexosaminidase A)	Gangliosides	37
Nieman-Pick disease (sphinomyelinase)	Sphingomyelin	39,40,50
Metachromatic leukodystrophy (arylsulfatase A)	Sulfatide	37
Krabbe's globoid-cell leukodystrophy (beta galactocerebrosidase)	Galactocerebroside	49
Lipofuscin Accumulations (lysosomal enzyme deficiency ?)		
Neuronal ceroid lipofuscinosis	Ceroid and lipofuscin	37,38
Mucopolysaccharidosis		
Mucopolysaccharidosis 1—Hurler's syndrome (alpha L-iduronidase)	Glycosaminoglycan	43
Mucopolysaccharidosis V1—Maroteaux-Lamy syndrome (arylsulfatase B)	Glycosaminoglycan	44,45

Inherited Disorders

This classification is really an extension of the previous section on metabolic disorders because most inherited disorders are actually metabolic in nature and vice versa.

Many enzymes in cells are contained within small organelles called lysosomes. They are involved in a variety of catabolic processes and in tissue or substrate turnover (mainly degradation) pathways. Lysosomal enzyme deficiencies fall into several groups (Table 15): glycogen-storage diseases discussed above; glycoprotein-catabolism diseases of membranes (*eg*, mannosidosis), which have not been observed in cats; glycolipid-catabolism diseases of neurons and myelin, of which several occur in cats; lipofuscin-storage diseases, which may not involve lysosomes and are observed rarely in cats; and mucopolysaccharidoses, some of which are well documented in cats. The list of these identified hydrolase enzyme deficiencies is continually growing for all species.[38-45] The names given to each disease may reflect its discoverer, the enzyme deficiency or the substrate that accumulates. Entities are reclassified or subdivided frequently. The major research significance of these diseases is that they offer a model for the disease in people.

The clinically significant facts can be summarized as follows: Most are autosomal recessives (both parents are carriers). They tend to occur in lines or pure breeds but occasional exceptions can occur. Diagnosis is by tissue, serum and/or urine chemistry. Signs develop early in life, often at 2-6 months of age, and are progressive and painless but incapacitating. Central nervous system signs (ataxia, proprioception loss, loss of reflexes, hypermetria, tremors, stupidity, blindness, circling, loss of balance, seizures) are common but hepatic and splenic enlargement can occur, as well as distortion of the facial features (in the mucopolysaccharidoses). There may be small retinal lesions (grey spots) and/or a cloudy cornea. There is no treatment. Tissues at necropsy should be fresh for histochemistry as well as for formalin fixation. In some instances, carrier states can be identified. All of these diseases are rare. Most have their clinical effects by leading to intralysosomal or intracellular accumulations of large amounts of the substrate of the missing enzyme.[46-49]

Other unknown degenerations of CNS cells are known to be inherited but their mechanisms are not known. Early death of viable cells for unknown reasons is called abiotrophy but this name is rarely applied to any CNS diseases of cats. Two other poorly understood inherited diseases of cats are inherited tremor and neuroaxonal dystrophy, both of which are autosomal recessives, with onset of progressive CNS signs at an early age. The inherited tremor condition causes problems in eating and affected cats die young.[50] This could represent hypomyelinogenesis or dysmyelinogenesis, which are often temporary phenomena. The neuroaxonal dystrophy causes progressive ataxia, tremors, incoordination, poor vision and a curious lilac coat color.[51]

Developmental Defects

Cerebellar hypoplasia and hydrocephalus are the only major developmental abnormalities of the cat's brain.

Cerebellar Hypoplasia: Cerebellar hypoplasia is caused by prenatal or early neonatal infection by feline panleukopenia virus. The clinical signs in kittens are ataxia, tremors, wide-based stance and hypermetria. Signs are apparent as soon as the kitten walks and are not progressive. Affected kittens need not be euthanized. Necropsy is the only diagnostic test. No proof for genetic transmission has ever been offered despite statements in the literature to the contrary.

Hydrocephalus: Hydrocephalus in cats is not as common as in dogs.[52] We have seen 2 forms. The first is the juvenile variety, characterized by a domed skull, open dorsal fontanelle and variable combinations of blindness, ataxia, depression, coma and convulsions. Most cats affected die at an early age but a few survive. Although such kittens are usually the result of nongenetic birth defects, this form apparently has a genetic factor in its etiology in some instances.[52] The other form is acquired at any age as a consequence of brain trauma, inflammation, hemorrhage or tumor, in which CSF flow is obstructed. Cats in the latter group have the usual signs associated with a rapid rise in intracranial pressure: pinpoint pupils, ataxia, depression, blindness, coma and convulsions terminating in death.

The only drugs that relieve the signs of hydrocephalus are diuretics and corticosteroids. They are only temporarily effective unless the CSF obstruction is alleviated. In acute cases, direct taps of the lateral ventricles may relieve the pressure until the inflammatory obstruction is reduced medically.

Generally it is pointless to put a ventriculoperitoneal shunt in a young animal with hydrocephalus. If not due to a tumor, the adult form could be treated with a shunt; however, we know of no cases in which a cat was treated successfully by this method.

Toxicities

Central nervous system signs can result from endogenous or exogenous toxins. The major examples of diseases caused by endogenous toxins are hepatic encephalopathy, uremia and bacterial endotoxemia. Uremia rarely causes more than depression in cats, although severe hypokalemia may produce muscle weakness. Seizures, precipitated by hypocalcemia, may occur before or during treatment of uremia. Bacterial endotoxins have direct CNS-depressive effects and indirect effects via hypoglycemia (muscle tremors, seizures).

There are many exogenous toxins that affect the CNS but only a few are mentioned here. Lead poisoning is not as common in cats as in dogs. Clinical signs include anorexia, emesis, gingivitis, hemorrhagic enteritis, nasal discharge, anemia, depression, frenzy and convulsions or coma.[53] Measuring the lead level in blood is a good method of diagnosis in the live animal; more than 0.5 ppm is proof of toxicity, from 0.35 to 0.5 ppm is the questionable range, and less than 0.35 ppm is considered nontoxic. Radiographs of the gut may show evidence of lead particles. Urinary levels of delta aminolevulinic acid are also diagnostic (normal up to 40 μmol/L). Calcium EDTA is used for treatment (50 mg/kg TID given IV). Symptomatic therapy, such as use of anticonvulsants, is often needed. High urine levels of lead after therapy can be used to confirm the diagnosis. Relapses can be expected if the exposure to lead has been chronic (lead in the bones) or if the source of the lead is not found.

Diphenylhydantoin (Dilantin:Parke-Davis) is not metabolized well by cats. At human or canine dosages, it accumulates and causes ataxia and sedation (see Seizures).

Popular hallucinogenic drugs have occasionally produced clinical signs in cats.[54] Cats are exposed accidentally as well as deliberately to such drugs. The clinical signs vary and include vomiting, ataxia, sudden onset of abnormal behavior (catching imaginary flies), sedation, hyperesthesia and even convulsions. Few owners admit that such drugs are in the cat's environment and it is difficult to prove the drug is in the cat's body. Therefore, suspected cases may be unconfirmed. Tranquilizers or sedatives, such as chlorpromazine or phenobarbital, are used as needed to suppress signs.

Chlorinated hydrocarbon and organophosphate toxicities are common. The large number of such compounds and their varied uses, overuses and inappropriate uses result in difficult diagnostic and therapeutic problems. The clinical signs of organophosphate toxicity include muscular tremors, ataxia, vomiting, salivation, diarrhea, miosis and rapid, shallow respiration. Chlorinated hydrocarbon toxicity is frequently accompanied by convulsions and hypersensitivity to touch as well as many of the signs associated with organophosphate toxicity.[55] Treatment of chlorinated hydrocarbon toxicity involves IV administration of phenobarbital to effect and 10-20 ml of 5% calcium borogluconate. For organophosphate toxicity, atropine (1 mg repeated as needed) is given along with specific antidotes, such as pralidoxime chloride (Protopam:Ayerst) at 10-20 mg/kg. As in any poisoning by ingestion, use of an emetic or gastric lavage may be indicated. If the exposure has been external, the hair and skin should be rinsed well.

Flea collars containing organophosphates have been blamed for many clinical signs in cats. Excluding the contact dermatitis that may accompany their use, there is little evidence to support the contention that they frequently intoxicate cats. This may happen when a cat with a new collar has been confined in a box and has absorbed an excess of the chemical or if the cat has been exposed to other related chemicals. The clinical signs are usually ataxia and salivation.

The anticancer drug 5-fluorouracil reportedly causes CNS signs (hyperexcitability, tremors, coma, seizures) at doses not far above recommended doses. Cats may be excessively sensitive to this drug.[56]

Barbiturate overdose is not common in cats. Ataxia, coma and even respiratory arrest may occur. Use of a respirator may be necessary. Central nervous system stimulants, such as bemegride (Mikedimide:Parlam) or amphetamine, are the only specific therapeutic agents.

Benzoic acid is a commonly used meat preservative in some countries and is toxic to cats. It causes ataxia, hyperesthesia, marked behavioral abnormalities (hallucinations or even aggression), and convulsions.[57] No specific antidote is available.

Ingestion of soft plastic toys made in Hong Kong has reportedly intoxicated cats.[58,59] Incoordination, muscle fasciculations, vomiting, lacrimation, photophobia and even convulsions or coma are the clinical signs. Treatment is symptomatic and recovery occurs in a few days. A noxious agent could not be isolated from the toys, but the cut surface of the plastic was damp and smelled strongly until it had dried.[58]

Strychnine toxicity is usually manifested by tonic convulsions, especially upon sensory stimulation (sound, touch). The site of action of this toxin is the inhibitory Renshaw cell, where the toxin blocks the cell's inhibitory neurotransmitter (glycine) by competitive blockade at the lower motor neuron. Treatment is with pentobarbital or phenobarbital given IV to effect. Administration of 25 ml of 5% calcium borogluconate is also beneficial.

Mercury poisoning has become a topic of international interest after outbreaks in Japan and Iraq. Mercury salts are used to treat seed grain, which may be eaten by people or by birds and rodents that are eaten by cats. Inorganic mercury salts can also be converted to organic salts and enter food chains via fish. Cats were the first species affected in the Japanese outbreaks of "Minamata disease." Signs included paresthesia, loss of sensation in the extremities, ataxia, blindness, behavioral changes, coma, convulsions and death. The best treatment is dimercaprol (BAL:Hynson), given IM at 3-5 mg/kg every 4-8 hours, to effect, along with supportive therapy for up to 10 days. This treatment is not very effective in cases of chronic mercury toxicity.

Ethylene glycol poisoning is not common in cats. Coma and convulsions occur in poisoning with this chemical. These signs may be related to primary renal damage, direct CNS effects of metabolites or osmotic effects of this agent.

Vascular Disease

Apart from rare cases of arteriovenous malformations or shunts, most intracranial vascular problems are referred to as "strokes," "cerebrovascular accidents" or "ischemic encephalopathies." The term "stroke" includes spontaneous intracranial hemorrhage as well as thrombotic or embolic occlusion of intracranial blood vessels. Apoplexy is another term of mixed usage, although originally it only meant intracranial hemorrhage. The most popular term in people is cerebrovascular accident, although use of the word stroke to the lay public is perhaps better.

Embolic occlusion of an intracranial artery occurs rarely in cases of right-to-left cardiac shunt when clots from the venous circulation enter the arterial side. It may also occur in cases of cardiomyopathy, left-sided endocarditis or during carotid artery catheterization.

Traumatic intracranial hemorrhage is not uncommon but spontaneous intracranial hemorrhage is very rare. It may be produced by a brain tumor, particularly hemangiosarcoma, or embolic bacterial masses in septicemias.

Cerebral vasospasm (transient cerebral ischemia) has been a misused term in the human literature and there is no evidence that it occurs in cats. However, since proof of its spontaneous occurrence is almost impossible to obtain, there is no reason to deny its existence. Transient ischemia has been ascribed to small emboli or thrombi that rapidly disperse transient generalized hypotension, or focal cerebral vasospasm. Signs of CNS involvement develop rapidly in people but also resolve completely in a few days. Such clinical episodes occur in older cats but what they represent is unknown. They may be mild cerebrovascular accidents or mild versions of the massive cerebral hemisphere stroke lesions as in the feline ischemic encephalopathy syndrome.

Occlusion of an intracranial artery appears to be the most common cause of spontaneous cerebrovascular accident.[60] Atherosclerosis is rare in cats and does not appear to be the underlying cause. Atherosclerosis occurs more often in hypothyroid individuals and should perhaps be considered in cases of stroke.

Feline ischemic encephalopathy is a well-defined apparently thrombotic stroke condition of cats and mainly affects the middle cerebral artery.[61,62] Its cause is unknown but FIP and migrating nematode parasites have been suggested.[61,63] It affects cats of any age over 2 years, of either sex and more commonly in the winter. There may be a regional incidence, with more cases occurring in the northeastern US. It is not identical to the idiopathic feline vestibular syndrome, which is a peripheral vestibular (labyrinthitis) disease.

The onset of signs is acute, only progressive for a few hours, and of variable severity. Even severely affected cats often recover most functions in a few days. The signs may start with or progress to seizures, circling, head tilt, twitching (sometimes unilateral face and limbs), behavioral changes (often aggression), dilated pupils, optic nerve (pupillary light reflexes lost) or cortical blindness (loss of the menace response in one eye, with normal pupillary light reflex) and loss of higher (placing) reflexes. The lesion is usually unilateral, involving one cerebral hemisphere, especially the temporal (behavior) lobe, and often extending to the optic chiasma. Localizing the lesion is an exercise in simple anatomy; the affected cortex supplies the contralateral limbs and face with upper motor neurons (reflexes, twitches) and the contralateral visual field (menace reflex lost). The head tilt and circling are to the side of the lesion.

Diagnosis is based on acute onset of signs and a CSF tap showing a rise in the number of cells (10-200 mm^3), which are mainly mononuclear with perhaps some RBC, a rise in protein content (20-100 mg/dl) and a slight rise in pressure. In some cases, especially after a few days, no changes are seen. Electroencephalography can pinpoint the lesion but not its cause. Isotope scintigraphy can also localize fresh lesions.[62]

Treatment with dexamethasone, at 2 mg/kg TID for 1 day, then 0.1 mg/kg daily for a week, may help reduce peripheral edema but does not help ischemic brain cells. The affected cortex atrophies. If seizures occur (status epilepticus is often seen), phenobarbital and/or diazepam, given to effect (see Seizures), is required. Megestrol acetate (Ovaban:Schering) and time may help cats with persistent behavioral problems.

The term "cerebral" is used almost synonymously with "brain" at times, despite its anatomic identification with the cerebral hemispheres. Most cerebrovascular accidents in people occur in arteries in the connections of the midbrain to the cerebral hemispheres (the internal capsule) and thus the adjective "cerebral" is overused. Cerebrovascular accident does not mean that all such accidents occur only in the cerebral hemispheres.

Stroke lesions may occasionally directly or indirectly affect other areas of the brain. Midbrain involvement is indicated by paralyzing rigidity of muscles on one side of the body (hemiplegia), with the other side partially affected (in severe cases, this progresses to decerebrate rigidity), coma and small pupils (miosis). Such signs may be mainly secondary to cerebral lesions. The cerebral lesions cause edema which, if extensive, may produce a tentorial pressure cone and midbrain distortion.

Brainstem lesions cause a variety of cranial nerve signs, such as seventh nerve paralysis, dysphagia, head tilt, circling and coma. While primary brainstem cerebrovascular accident lesions can occur, brainstem signs also occur with cerebral lesions. In such cases, they are apparently caused by a tentorial or foramen magnum pressure cone.

Neoplasia

The most common intracranial neoplasm in cats is the meningioma.[64,65] Lymphoreticular (lymphoma, reticulosis) tumors are about half as common.[66,67] Other types of tumors (pituitary adenomas, ependymomas, gliomas) are much less common in cats than in dogs.[68-70] Choroid plexus papillomas can affect CSF drainage and induce hydrocephalus, with associated depression, seizures and ataxia.

Lymphomas affect the CNS in only 5% of lymphoma cases.[67] Affected cats are usually FeLV-positive. Signs are progressive over at least a few weeks. Pupil changes and midbrain/brainstem signs are common.

Meningiomas are usually slow-growing, with a 1-year progression not unusual. They mainly occur in cats over 10 years of age and usually are supratentorial and sometimes asymptomatic, even when large. Signs include circling, head tilt, depression, behavioral changes, ataxia, coma, loss of proprioception and higher reflexes unilaterally, hemiparesis or eventual tetraparesis, nystagmus (often only seen if the position of the cat's head is changed) and seizures. Seizures from tumors are, however, not common in cats.

Diagnosis is by history, CSF analysis (pressure elevated, cell counts and protein normal). A CAT scan is the best localizing tool, although isotope scintigraphy is useful and electroencephalography is reasonable. Ipsilateral sclerosis of overlying parietal bone may occur with hemispheric meningiomas. Rostrocaudal radiographs of the skull may reveal this diagnostic sign and its location. The cause of the sclerosis is unknown. Surgical removal of feline meningiomas should be considered because some are superficial, over the hemispheres and accessible. Prolonged response (1 year) to anticonvulsants and corticosteroids can be obtained in some cases.

Seizures

The definition of a seizure, its signs and differential diagnosis, and the tests for seizure cases have been discussed in the section on seizures (Table 5).

Epilepsy is defined as "repeated seizures." It is thus a state or syndrome rather than a disease. It is uncommon in cats because they have not been shown to have genetic epilepsy and do not suffer from epileptogenic diseases, such as canine distemper. Tumors and FIP are progressive diseases. Even so, most of the causes of acquired epilepsy have been observed in cats (Table 5). Occasionally a family incidence suggests a genetic etiology, but in most cases the term idiopathic is applied because the cause of the epilepsy cannot be found. Epilepsy is thus not just a state of repeated seizures but is also a state in which seizures are the only problem; there is no progressive organic disease, except perhaps for an increase in frequency of seizures.

In people the types of epilepsy are classified largely on the basis of results of electroencephalography. Terms such as "petit mal" and "grand mal" have very specific meanings. Common mistakes made by veterinarians are to refer to minor focal seizures (*eg*, champing) as "petit mal," localizing signs as "Jacksonian seizures," and any generalized seizure as "grand mal." It is best not to apply the human terms in veterinary medicine. Petit mal seizures in people are short muscle jerks or mental lapses characterized by specific electroencephalographic changes rarely found in animals. Jacksonian seizures are caused by specific motor cortex lesions and the human motor cortex is much larger and physiologically very different from the cat's. Grand mal seizures are "primary" generalized seizures, of a frequently inherited type in people, caused by deep lesions in the brain, *ie*, there is not a cerebral focus that starts them.

Classifications of epilepsy are cumbersome and of little clinical significance in veterinary medicine. Rather, it is best to recognize the following signs: focal seizures (limited to one area of the body) or generalized seizures (affecting the whole body); localizing signs, aura and postictal signs; and psychomotor seizures, which are characterized by considerable personality or behavioral changes (hallucinations, abnormal but coordinated movements, viciousness, etc) during or just after the seizure.

Age of Onset of Seizures: Insulinomas and other tumors tend to occur in middle-aged to older animals and hence a late onset of seizures suggests such a cause. However, several causes of acquired epilepsy or seizures (trauma, cerebrovascular accident, postencephalitis, postmeningitis) can affect older animals as well. The animal under a year of age is a prime candidate for toxicity or encephalitis. Cases with congenital, neonatal or genetic causes of epilepsy usu ally have their first seizure between 1 and 4 years of age. Cerebrovascular accidents can cause seizures in cats of any age.

Seizure Patterns: Seizure patterns often surprise owners and veterinarians. An accurate summary is to state that seizure patterns can vary markedly. Some epileptics start with irregular short seizures that become more frequent and longer over the first year. Others start with status epilepticus. However, status epilepticus suggests some cause other than epilepsy, such as feline ischemic encephalopathy or toxicity. Some animals have fewer seizures as they get older and others have more. Some have seizures irregularly and others at exactly the same time of day or at exact intervals of a few days or weeks. Gastrointestinal irritation, pruritic conditions, estrus, pseudocyesis, pregnancy, use of stilbestrol, excitement and boredom can all be associated in some cases with an increased number of seizures.

Client Education: The education of the client about epilepsy is critical in patient management. It is necessary to explain to the client what a seizure is, what epilepsy is, how epilepsy is diagnosed by elimination, what is meant by "idiopathic," that epilepsy is controlled not cured, that not all cats are controlled and that there are various causes of apparent epilepsy, including progressive diseases. Neutering makes seizure control easier. Explanations of the varied seizure patterns, the aura, postictal signs, and the absence of pain during a seizure are also necessary. The clients must be particularly advised to keep their hands out of the animal's mouth during a seizure; animals do not swallow their tongues or dentures. Carefully advise the client when to call you after a seizure and specify at once if the seizure lasts longer than 10 minutes. Explain all side effects of anticonvulsants, the need to give doses several times a day and the need not to miss doses.

Treatment: For a convulsion in progress less than 5 minutes, wait for recovery but ensure the cat is breathing effectively. If respiration is inadequate, treat the cat as for status epilepticus. Obtain necessary blood samples at once and perhaps give phenobarbital (5-10 mg/kg); do not use phenothiazine tranquilizers since they can cause seizures in epileptics. Do not treat these cats chronically unless diagnostic efforts have been made or the animal's seizure pattern is known and control is needed. Do not treat chronically after the first seizure unless the client demands it. If results of physical, neurologic and blood examinations are normal, wait to see the seizure pattern develop.

Status epilepticus is a seizure lasting longer than 10-15 minutes. This is inappropriate ter minology because few cats in status epilepticus are epileptics; more likely they are suffering from toxicities, cerebrovascular accidents or encephalitis. Use IV diazepam (5-30 mg total dose) to abolish the seizure. If this is not effective, use IV phenobarbital, 30-180 mg given slowly to effect. The diazepam dose may need to be repeated hourly if the abnormal electrical activity persists. The phenobarbital dose may be repeated every 4-6 hours in the same situation. Pentobarbital, thiopental or thiamylal are only used if phenobarbital is not available since they have no anticonvulsant effects except via anesthesia. Seizures may begin again when the plane of anesthesia lightens. Phenobarbital permits a lighter plane of sedation/anesthesia to control seizures; therefore, it is much easier to wean affected cats from IV to oral medication. Any animal in status epilepticus should be weaned to oral phenobarbital, at 4-10 mg/kg in divided doses BID or TID as soon as possible. Supplementation with IV phenobarbital may be necessary until the correct dosage is achieved. Err on the side of oversedation initially. Status epilepticus is a life-threatening situation and an indication for immediate chronic therapy even after the first seizure, at least until a diagnosis is made.

Once the status epilepticus is controlled and the animal is breathing well, blood samples should be taken. Glucose (20-30 ml of 10% solution) and calcium gluconate (1-3 ml of 5% solution) should be given slowly IV once samples have been taken. Animals with suspected hypoglycemia can be given IV glucose before the anticonvulsant but preferably not before a blood sample is obtained to confirm the diagnosis. Use of IV dexamethasone (2-4 mg/kg) after long seizures may reduce hypoxic brain swelling. Use of hyperosmotic agents is not indicated. Lower dosages of dexamethasone (0.1-0.5 mg/kg) can be repeated SID or BID for several days as needed. The possibility of exposure to toxic materials must be considered and appropriate treatments provided in cases of status epilepticus.

Cats with repeated seizures of a known frequency should be treated if the client requests it. Most clients cannot tolerate more than 6 seizures a year but some do not want the bother of treatment until the seizures are more frequent. It is a personal decision because occasional short seizures are not life-threatening. We advise treatment if the seizures occur 6 or more times a year, are lasting longer, occur more often or if status epilepticus has occurred. If laboratory tests show no evidence of abnormality and the history and results of physical and neurologic examinations are normal, such animals can be treated as "epileptics."

The aim of treatment is control of the seizures. Control is defined as an absence of seizures or a greatly reduced incidence, limited only to short single seizures, with minimal postictal signs and no tendency to develop status epilepticus. Not all seizures are controlled by treatment. Some owners may be satisfied with less than total control but others demand perfection; the owner's criteria are thus the significant factors. Once the seizures are controlled, the cat may appear to improve in general attitude and often becomes more playful.

Phenothiazine derivatives (antihistamines, antiemetics or tranquilizers) should not be given to epileptics because they may cause seizures. Doses of anticonvulsants must always be split BID, TID or QID, and higher fractions of the dose can be given at night when most seizures occur. This trick is best reserved for cats that require large doses.

Cats require smaller doses of some anticonvulsants than do people or dogs and are almost intolerant of some drugs. Phenobarbital is the drug of choice, given at 4-10 mg/kg divided BID or TID initially and increased as indicated (up to 20 mg/kg may rarely be needed). Diazepam is the second-choice drug given at 2-5 mg/kg divided TID or QID. Diphenylhydantoin (phenytoin) is poorly metabolized by the cat's liver and should not be used unless blood levels are assayed. Cats can sometimes tolerate 1-5 mg/kg/day.[71,72] Primidone can be given to cats (5-30 mg/kg/day) but may cause liver problems. Labels of the veterinary products carry warnings against use in cats. If phenobarbital or diazepam do not control the neurologic signs, the diagnosis may be FIP or another disease, not epilepsy. Thiamin should be given to any cat with acute onset of seizures or any acute severe CNS signs.

Narcolepsy and Sleep Disorders

Narcolepsy is a primary sleep disorder. In people it is characterized by suddenly falling asleep and showing rapid eye movement at inopportune moments, cataplexy or sudden flaccid loss of all voluntary control of limb muscles, without loss of consciousness, for a few seconds to a few minutes, intense, vivid hallucinations while going to sleep (hypnagogic hallucinations), and sleep paralysis (inability to move while falling asleep).

In dogs, in which genetic narcolepsy is well documented, cataplexy is the only clinical sign noted by owners. Sudden lapses into sleep may occur but special sleep tests must be used to diagnose it. Hallucinations and sleep paralysis could hardly be diagnosed in an animal.

Narcolepsy is uncommon in cats and has rarely been documented.[73]

The cataplectic attacks are the most diagnostic features of narcolepsy. Electroencephalographic confirmation is difficult. Diagnosis depends on ruling out other causes of episodic weakness and epilepsy, careful study of the collapse episodes, and challenge tests. There should be no defecation, urination or excessive salivation during the episodes. They tend to occur at times of excitement and when eating. The eyes are usually open and can often track objects, and the menace reflex is intact. Petting the animal should help it recover partially. There are no tonic/clonic/paddling episodes, although a few twitches or cries might occur. Consciousness is not usually lost. Signs begin suddenly at 2-24 months of age. Attacks last a few seconds or minutes and several attacks may occur each day. Sleep centers in the brainstem normally suppress spinal neurons and reflexes in sleep. Cataplexy is an abnormal switching on of this suppression. Careful electroencephalographic study may reveal that these animals go from an alert state to rapid-eye-movement sleep, with minimal or no nonrapid-eye-movement sleep preceding the rapid-eye-movement sleep. This is not a clinical diagnostic tool. Challenge tests involve exposing the fasted cat to a line of food morsels (not many cats cooperate as do dogs) spaced a foot apart across a room (try pieces of shrimp). A cataplectic cat usually collapses several times as it tries to eat its way across the room and takes longer to eat than a normal cat. Another challenge test is to give imipramine (Tofranil:Geigy) IV at 0.5 mg/kg and count the collapse episodes for half an hour before and after exciting activity (play). Imipramine greatly reduces the number of collapses.

Cataplexy is treated with stimulants, such as oral methylphenidate (Ritalin:Ciba) at 0.1-0.5 mg/kg TID and/or antidepressives, such as oral imipramine at 0.1-2 mg/kg TID. Both of these drugs have serious side effects, including hyperkinesis and cardiac arrhythmias. Doses must be small initially. If only a few attacks occur each day, it is better not to treat. Rarely can all signs be abolished.

Other sleep disorders have been observed in cats.[74] Excessively violent spasms or apparent seizures occurring only during sleep are occasionally seen in cats. If the cat can be easily aroused from these episodes, incontinence is not seen and response to anticonvulsants is minimal, one should consider it a sleep disorder. Lesions in the brainstem sleep centers can experimentally produce such signs.

Nocturnal enuresis (urination during sleep) is occasionally another result of sleep disorders.

Anoxia

Central nervous system anoxia can result from obstruction of respiration, paralysis of the respiratory muscles, damaged hemoglobin, massive fall in arterial pressure, cardiac fibrillation or arrest, obstruction of arteries of the CNS, edema of the CNS, or interference with cellular uptake of O_2. The most common cause of severe CNS anoxia survived by cats is cardiac arrest from anesthetic overdosage.

We have seen few cases in which CNS anoxia from respiratory obstruction, without cardiac arrest, has produced significant signs. Cats that suffer cardiac arrest frequently show signs of CNS damage if they survive.[75,76] It rarely is possible to know for how long cardiac arrest existed; prognosis and treatment are based on clinical signs. There is considerable individual variation among cats as to their ability to withstand cardiac arrest.[76]

When cardiac arrest has occurred and has been reversed, administration of a corticosteroid should be started immediately. For example, dexamethasone can be given at 2 mg/kg TID for a day, then gradually reduced to zero in the following week.

The cat should be examined when the effects of any anesthetic have disappeared. Signs of severe brain damage are fixed dilated pupils (atropine causes this sign but the effects of atropine are gone in most cats within 24 hours), coma and extensor rigidity (delayed recovery from anesthesia is accompanied by the last 2 signs). Appearance of these signs should prompt a guarded prognosis, but their absence does not mean that there has been no CNS damage because the cat may show only behavioral signs. The behavioral signs are usually mild and temporary (disorientation), but in some cases they can be permanent and serious (viciousness, loss of elimination habits). If the behavioral changes continue, phenobarbital (2-10 mg/kg TID) can be given in a therapeutic trial or megestrol acetate (1 mg/kg/day). Electroencephalography is not initially helpful in giving an accurate prognosis because cats that recover fully may have flat (isoelectric) recordings for a few days. Normal EEG activity on day 1 is a good sign.

Cats with fixed dilated pupils and extensor rigidity, and in a coma need supportive therapy. Some begin to improve within a few days and make a full recovery. Others remain in essentially this condition, although the rigidity may decrease, and either die or are euthanized. The rest make various degrees of recovery and may remain blind, epileptic, ataxic or antisocial.

The brains of cats that have suffered CNS anoxia contain areas of malacia, necrosis and minor hemorrhage. The location of the lesion(s) can usually be correlated with the signs.

Organic Behavioral Diseases

Most of the organic diseases discussed so far can induce changes in behavior. Non-neurologic diseases can also induce marked behavioral changes. For example, hyperthyroid cats are often nervous and hyperactive, and hepatic disease may cause hepatic encephalopathy (see Metabolic Diseases).[77]

Clinicians should remember that owners often misinterpret normal cat behavior (especially during estrus) and the decreased activity of old age as signs of disease.

Feline Hyperesthesia Syndrome: The feline hyperesthesia syndrome is a specific entity in cats that seems to be increasing in incidence. It has been referred to as neurodermatitis, rippling, rolling or twitchy-skin syndrome, neuritis and even hyperkinesis. It is a complex problem and probably an external manifestation of a number of problems. It is doubtful there is just one cause.

The signs can develop at any age but usually begin between 1-4 years of age. Most of the signs are exhibited in moderation by many normal cats; however, in cats with the hyperesthesia syndrome the signs are carried to extremes so that normal activities are curtailed. Signs observed include rippling of the skin of the dorsum, biting or licking at the tail, flank or pelvis, apparent hallucinations, glassy eyes with widely dilated pupils, frantic meowing, swishing of the tail, sudden violent licking when running, walking or eating, running crazily around the house, and attacking objects, including the owner, without provocation. The cats may even have generalized seizures and associated social problems, such as urinating outside the litterbox. Signs may last a few seconds to a few minutes, occur at a specific time of day, vary in incidence from month to month, and occur once every few days or almost constantly all day. Between episodes the cats may be normal or slightly agitated. Once asleep, these cats seem peaceful but may wake up suddenly at night and attack their owners. Both sexes, neutered or intact, are affected.

Because many normal cats, especially kittens, do some of these things, the diagnosis of feline hyperesthesia syndrome is probably overused. Diagnosis is difficult and is based largely on the history and ruling out other differential diagnoses (Tables 7, 9). Many affected cats exhibit an excessive response (glassy eyes, dilated pupils, biting themselves or the clinician, licking the flanks, twitching the back muscles) when scratched by a finger over the L_7-S_3 area on the midline. Normal cats react similarly but to a lesser extent to this stimulation.

Affected cats may have a fever (less than 106 F) but exhibit no WBC number changes. In a few severe cases, marked electroencephalographic changes disappear if treatment is successful. No significant lesions have been found at necropsy.

There are a few things that this disease is not; it is not from lesions of the tail, anal glands, flank, back, skin, gut, ovarian or uterine stumps, ligatures or hemostatic clips. Topical local therapy is pointless. The most likely causes seem to involve an interaction of the cat's basic personality (affected cats are often nervous, loners, hyperexcitable), frustrations (not being allowed outside, boredom, being ignored) and environmental pressures (overcrowding, sexual competition, another cat has cystitis or is spraying). The signs seem to be manifestations of mental problems. Rarely is any systemic disease the cause. However, some cats have obvious electroencephalographic abnormalities (slow waves, dysrhythmias, spike discharges) that disappear when treated. Some cats seem to respond to a simpler diet with fewer preservatives. Hence, it is likely that the feline hyperesthesia syndrome is caused by a combination or variety of single factors. The syndrome may also have or be exacerbated by organic causes (toxins, dietary preservatives, minimal brain damage). It is in an area with sleep, dreaming, behavior, hallucinations and epilepsy.

Treatment involves test therapy with all, a combination or one of the following: megestrol acetate at 1 mg/kg/day, prednisolone at 1-2 mg/kg/day, phenobarbital at 4-10 mg/kg/day in divided doses and diazepam 2-5 mg/kg/day in divided doses. Behavioral or environmental pressures should be reduced and food with fewer preservatives fed. In some cats, we have found that more attention when the cat behaves normally, combined with a whack on the rump or spray of water when signs appear, helps reduce the problem. Once a successful treatment is found, the dosage of the drug(s) should be reduced as much as possible. The dosage of megestrol acetate can usually be cut to 1 mg/kg given every 3-4 days and prednisolone to 1-2 mg/kg given every 2-3 days. Drug administration can often be stopped for prolonged periods but signs usually recur at irregular intervals. The client should be advised of the side effects of these drugs, which include polyphagia, polydipsia, polyuria, obesity and diabetes mellitus.

NEUROLOGIC DISEASE OF THE SPECIAL SENSES

Diseases of Vision

Nystagmus was discussed earlier in this chapter and in Chapter 17. Some Siamese and other purebred cats have a cerebellar type of nystagmus in which there is horizontal trembling of the eyes in both directions, without a slow phase. The nystagmus worsens when affected cats are excited. Some are only affected when they are frightened. The condition does not seem to bother the cats and is untreatable.

Horner's syndrome (sympathetic ophthalmoplegia) is characterized by unilateral miosis, ptosis of the upper eyelid, eyeball retraction and protrusion of the third eyelid (see Chapter 17). It is not surprising that sympathetic innervation to an eye can be lost because the nerve tracts originate in the hypothalamus and travel via the brainstem, cervical spinal cord, cervical sympathetic ganglia and vagosympathetic trunk to the orbits via the ear. Spinal cord lesions, T_1-T_3 nerve root lesions, cranial mediastinal tumors, trauma of the tympanic bulla or neck, otitis media and surgery along the neural route can all cause Horner's syndrome.[78]

There is no specific treatment for Horner's syndrome, although the causative lesion can sometimes be treated effectively. Few affected cats, except those injured during carotid artery catheterization, regain full sympathetic function. Affected cats can live normally with the condition. If the site of the lesion is unknown (which is rare), it is possible, by measuring the pupil diameter in the affected and normal eyes after instillation of epinephrine and then cocaine into both eyes, to identify which part of the sympathetic tract the lesion is affecting.[79]

The mechanism of Siamese cat strabismus (convergent squint) has been studied in detail and is reported to be an attempt of the oculomotor positioning reflexes to compensate for abnormalities in the position of neurons in the "retinal map" of the tectum (a region of the midbrain).[80,81] The squint is not present when kittens first open their eyes but develops by the time of weaning. There is no treatment but the condition does not appear to affect the cat's activities.

Strabismus, conjugate eye movements and central blindness are discussed in the section on Differential Diagnosis (Tables 3, 13, Fig 18).

Auditory and Vestibular Diseases

The eighth cranial nerve has auditory and vestibular branches. The branches and their respective sensory devices may be damaged independently or at the same time. The left and right auditory structures consist of the external ear canal, tympanum, small middle ear bones and cochlea. The auditory branch of the eighth nerve enters the brainstem and information is then sent to the posterior colliculi, thalamus and cerebral cortex. The left and right vestibular structures consist of the semicircular canals, utricle and saccule. The vestibular branch of the eighth nerve also enters the brainstem to reach the ipsilateral vestibular nuclei. Information is then sent to the limbs (vestibulospinal tract), eye muscles, thalamus, cerebral cortex and cerebellum.

Damage to the auditory branch, its sensory apparatus or brain structures may result in deafness. Damage to the nerve or the cochlea results in nerve deafness, in which no sounds can be perceived, even those produced by a vibrating tuning fork applied to the skull near the ear. Damage to the rest of the sensory apparatus may result in conduction deafness, in which sounds arriving by air are not heard but the cochlea can still detect sounds vibrating against the skull.

Cats can be rendered deaf by several processes (Table 14). Toxicity is uncommon but dihydrostreptomycin, streptomycin and the other aminoglycosides, neomycin, neomycin B, kanamycin, viomycin and vancomycin can damage the auditory apparatus when given by injection. There may be a latent period of several months before evidence of the damage appears.

Trauma is a rare cause of deafness in any species and has not yet been observed in cats.

Senile degenerations of the brain or cochlea may be responsible for deafness for no apparent reason in old cats. Brain tumors have not yet been reported to cause deafness but encephalitis (FIP) is a recognized cause. Severe strokes and hydrocephalus may also be causes.

Congenital or neonatal deafness of cats has been studied extensively because of its similarity to some human forms of deafness. The lesion producing the deafness is a progressive degeneration of the cochlea's organ of Corti and the stria vascularis. The degeneration starts in the first week of life and is thought to be caused or aggravated by rapid cyclic osmotic changes within the body. Deaf or normal white cats can have either 2 blue eyes, 2 yellow eyes or 1 of each color. Therefore, eye color is not an absolute indication of deafness.[83-85] Both sexes are affected. The gene for white hair color in cats is dominant and has 100% penetrance. The same gene is apparently responsible for the deafness but for deafness it has a much lower penetrance. In the general population of white cats, 20% are deaf but the incidence rises to 80% if one of the parents is deaf. Longhaired white cats are more likely to be deaf than shorthaired white cats. The gene can be expressed as a bilateral or unilateral deafness or there may be no abnormality.[86] The term "Waardenburg syndrome" may be applied to deaf cats with white fur and blue eyes. It is sometimes claimed that only blue-eyed cats can be deaf, or only cats with one blue eye; but there are exceptions to all these rules. Although there is no treatment for this condition, affected cats can live normally.

Damage to the vestibular branch of the eighth cranial nerve, its organs of sensation or its vestibular nuclei in the brainstem can produce essentially similar clinical signs, including head tilt (which, when severe, may be a continuous rolling movement of the whole body), falling to one side, nystagmus, ataxia, circling and strabismus (Fig 50). These signs are collectively called the vestibular syndrome (see Differential Diagnosis section on head tilt, circling and nystagmus).

If the lesion is outside the cranial vault, it is called a peripheral vestibular lesion. Peripheral lesions usually cause a constant horizontal or rotatory nystagmus, with the fast phase away from the affected side. Horner's syndrome and seventh nerve facial paralysis, spasm, fasciculations or contracture may be seen with peripheral lesions. The ipsilateral limbs may be slightly

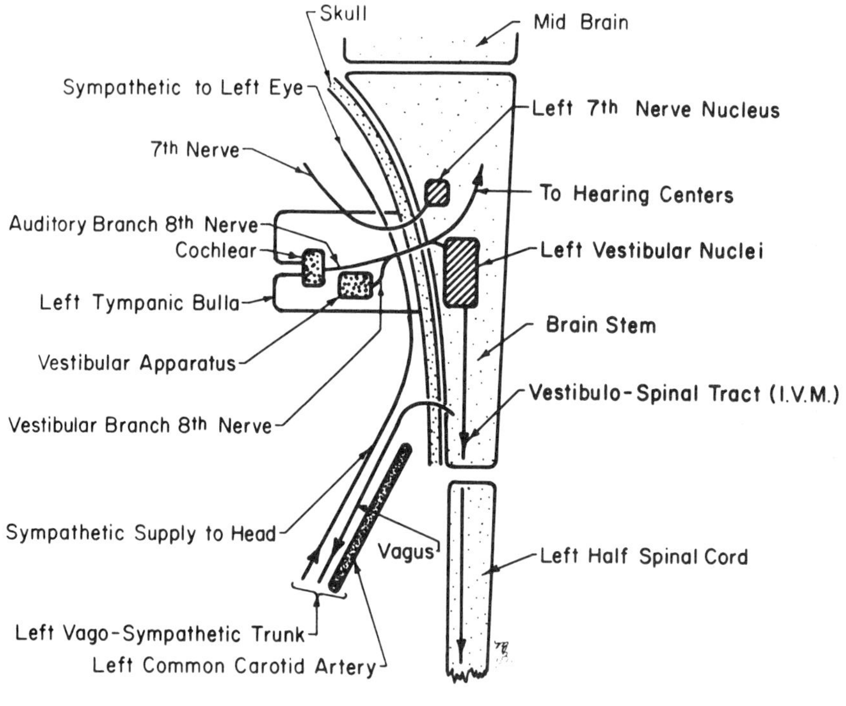

Fig 50. Clinically significant structures associated with the vestibular system.

stiff. Lesions inside the cranial vault are called central vestibular lesions and produce a variable diagonal, vertical or rotatory nystagmus. Central vestibular lesions usually cause circling and head tilt toward the affected side. Conscious proprioception or motor function may be lost on the affected side and seventh nerve paralysis or fasciculations may be seen with the central form.

With either peripheral or central vestibular lesions, the nystagmus is often compensated for rapidly and may not be present after 1-2 weeks. The ataxia may be partially compensated for, but the head tilt may be permanent or remain until the lesion is healed. Vomiting may occur during the acute stages. Severe bilateral lesions abolish all vestibular reflexes and the animal is unable to stand. Unless rolling or circling develops, most of the vestibular reflexes are maintained with unilateral lesions, although careful examination or observation reveals a deficiency.

Causes of central vestibular disease are head trauma, stroke, brainstem tumor and intracranial infection (Table 3). Causes of peripheral vestibular disease are otitis media/interna, tumors, inner ear trauma and the idiopathic feline vestibular syndrome. Toxic damage to the peripheral vestibular system from injection of streptomycin or other aminoglycosides is rare and usually bilateral.[87,88]

The treatment and prognosis of these causes are discussed elsewhere in this chapter. Trauma affecting the inner ear is treated with large doses of corticosteroids as for brain trauma. Animals with prolonged head tilt caused by demonstrable middle ear infection that is unresponsive to antibiotics and corticosteroids alone or combined with ear resection and myingotomy may benefit from curettage of the middle ear and a month's treatment with antibiotics and corticosteroids. We have had some success with this procedure, but hearing in the treated ear is sacrificed.

Idiopathic Feline Vestibular Syndrome: This syndrome is an acute peripheral vestibular disease (labyrinthitis) that affects cats of all ages. The cats are often affected when out at night. There is a spring and fall seasonal incidence. Affected cats have nystagmus, ataxia and head tilt, and may vomit (nausea?). Circling is rare. Occasionally the signs are apparently bilateral and cats so affected lie flat on the ground. Not much has been added to our knowledge of this condition since it was first reported.[61] There is no specific diagnostic test but any test of vestibular function reveals the problem and the side affected. The major differential diagnoses are trauma and toxicity, but physical examination usually reveals no depression, pain or other signs of injury. No treatment seems to help but many cats are given corticosteroids and diuretics for a few days. Most cats improve in a few hours and recover completely in 1-2 weeks. Some cats may have permanent mild deficits or suffer a repeated episode.

Motion Sickness

Cats are usually good travelers, even in cars, but a few individuals become highly agitated or vomit. The cause of motion sickness is not completely understood, but vertical movements of a rhythmic nature are primarily responsible. The detection of such movement is mainly via vestibular impulses but ocular impulses (peripheral visual field movements) are also important. Odors (auto emissions) may also play a part in induction of the syndrome. Ultimately, the chemoreceptor trigger zone on the floor of the fourth ventricle and the vomition center in the brainstem are affected.

Treatment of motion sickness should include medication, training and feeding. The owner should be advised to fast the cat prior to short trips or feed a light, fat-free meal 2 hours before long trips. Short trips to acclimate the cat to automobile travel may be beneficial, especially if the cat has had motion sickness previously. The car should be stopped as soon as signs of sickness develop and the cat walked on a leash or taken out of the car in a carrier. When the signs disappear, the journey can be resumed. As with seasickness in people, the cat usually becomes tolerant of the motion. Bumpy roads and a constant speed should be avoided initially. The cat should be spoken to, petted and kept calm on the front seat (less bumpy) during training sessions. Most cats do not need training and adapt quickly.

Drugs are much more effective if used before the signs develop. The most commonly used drugs are the tranquilizers/antihistamines, such as chlorpromazine or promethazine (phenothiazine derivatives) or diazepam. The effective oral dosage of each drug is 1-2 mg/kg, but there is considerable variation in the effect among individuals. The drug should be given about an hour before travel and its effects last 6-8 hours. The dosage for SC or IM injection of these drugs is about half the oral dosage; the effect occurs within 5-15 minutes after injection.

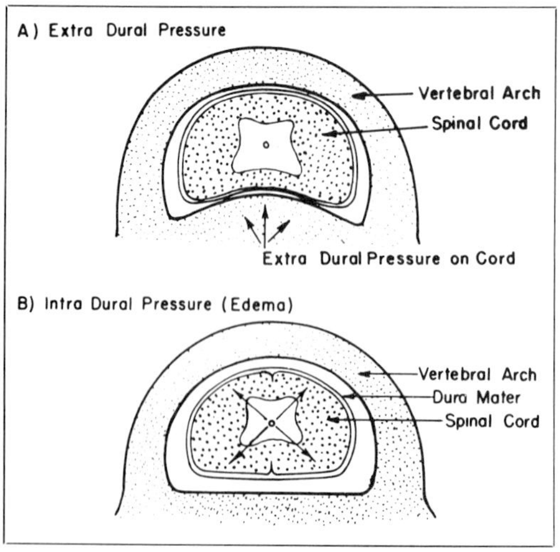

Fig 51. Extradural (A) and intradural (B) spinal cord compression.

A few cats may become excited and/or disoriented when given phenothiazine derivatives, and these drugs may cause convulsions in epileptics. For these reasons it is important to give diazepam or phenobarbital to epileptics and to give test doses several days before a trip to determine the dosage needed to slightly tranquilize the cat. The owner should be told about such side effects as ataxia, weakness, protrusion of the third eyelid and conjunctival erythema. Good ventilation is also important. The owner should also be told that tranquilized or sedated cats have a reduced ability to control their body temperature. The occurrence of heat stroke is therefore more likely and its prevention and treatment should be discussed.

SPINAL CORD LESIONS

Trauma

Trauma to the spine can cause cord contusion, laceration or severance, hemorrhage and edema. The vertebrae may be dislocated or fractured. Trauma may also result in rupture of an intervertebral disc.

The outer meningeal layer (dura mater) is semielastic and serves as a barrier to infection. As in the cranial cavity, the inner layer (pia mater) is thin and vascular. Between the 2 layers is the reticular-like arachnoid mater, which forms the subarachnoid space in which CSF flows. The cord and its meninges lie in the spinal canal. The inner lining of the vertebrae is periosteum, from which the dura is separated by a space that contains fat. This differs from the arrangement in the cranial cavity, where the dura is in direct contact with the bone.

Masses or swellings that compress the spinal cord are referred to as extradural or intradural (Fig 51). Intradural swelling (cord edema is the most common cause) raises the intradural pressure of the spinal cord mainly because of the dura mater's resistance to expansion. Extradural masses also compress the cord against the walls of the spinal canal. Increases in either extradural or intradural pressure restricts the blood supply to the spinal cord. The main objective in diagnosis and treatment of cord trauma is to identify the degree and site of any compression or inflammation and to relieve it.

When trauma is known to have occurred, it is not necessary initially to determine whether cord contusion, laceration, disc rupture or edema is present. The initial treatment and prognosis are based on the clinical signs and radiographic findings. The necessary parts of the neurologic examination must be performed before the cat is anesthetized. Care must be taken to minimize movement of the cat and avoid a struggle. Lateral and ventrodorsal radiographs of the affected spinal region must be obtained. The results of testing cord tract function and segmental reflexes, together with the radiographic evidence, are then considered in deciding about future management of the animal. If there is a question about whether trauma actually occurred, other possible differential diagnoses must be considered first.

Cats with total functional cord damage and in which radiographs show a fracture or fracture-luxation and overriding of the vertebrae or fragments to the extent that the cord is obviously severed, should be destroyed (Figs 52, 53).

Cats with partial functional cord damage, such as loss of conscious proprioception or the presence of involuntary rigidity, and in which radiographs reveal only subluxation, fracture-luxation, compression fracture or no fracture-luxation have a good prognosis (Figs 52, 54). Affected cats should be confined to a cage for a month and given short-term corticosteroid therapy. Because the cat may make violent movements before a callus forms, the best treatment for animals in this group with a fracture is decompressive laminectomy and internal stabilization of the fracture as soon as possible. Although a body cast can be used if surgery is not performed, cats do not tolerate such casts very well.

The greater the loss of spinal tract functions, the more imperative is surgery; the prognosis worsens the longer surgery is delayed.

Cats with total functional cord damage and in which radiographs reveal a subluxation or compression fracture must be given a guarded prognosis until an exploratory laminectomy has been performed to determine the severity of cord damage. Surgery should be immediate.

Dexamethasone should be given at 1 mg/kg TID while preparations for surgery are made. There is little evidence that diuretics help these cats. If the cord is only contused, stretched or edematous, the decompression provided by laminectomy, together with internal fixation of the fracture, may help recovery. With severe cord edema, the dura mater can be incised longitudinally to see if the cord is necrotic. If it is, the prognosis is hopeless. Durotomy is not a form of treatment.[90] It may even cause mild damage itself. The prognosis when the cord is intact and not necrotic is uncertain, but many animals recover if treated promptly. Delaying treatment more than 24 hours greatly reduces the chances for recovery. Use of dexamethasone should be continued at 0.1 mg/kg/day for one week only. If there is no improvement by 3 months, recovery is unlikely

Cats with total functional cord damage but no radiographic evidence of damage have suffered a spinal cord contusion, intervertebral disc prolapse or a fracture, with a luxation that corrected itself before radiographs were obtained. Localization of the spinal lesion in cats with total functional cord damage is not difficult with the help of the panniculus and other spinal reflexes. Close examination of radiographs of the area in question may reveal evidence of the prolapsed disc (lateral view) or small fracture lines in dorsal vertebral articulations (ventrodorsal view). In either case, prompt decompressive treatment and an exploratory laminectomy are necessary. If present, prolapsed disc material can be removed. If the cord is torn or bruised, the cat can be treated as those with total functional cord damage and partial fracture-dislocations. Myelography is often necessary for cats in this group.

If no radiographic signs of damage can be found, especially if the cord appears swollen on the myelogram, the spinal cord may have only been bruised by shear waves. With corticosteroid therapy (dexamethasone at 1 mg/kg TID), and cage rest, affected animals often recover in 1-2 weeks. Most animals with only spinal cord contusion have at least deep pain function intact in the affected limbs.

Pellet, Shot and Bullet Wounds: These wounds of the spinal cord are diagnosed similarly. If the cord is obviously severed by a bullet and there is total functional cord damage, euthanasia is

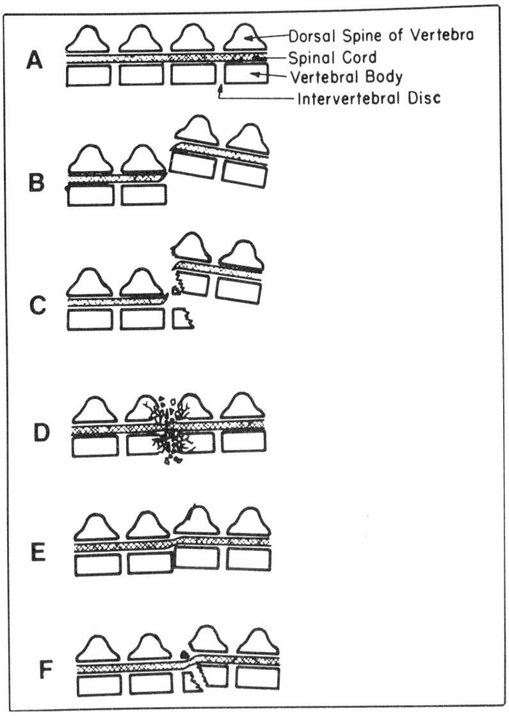

Fig 52. Diagram of various spinal fractures or fracture-dislocations: (A) normal, (B) total luxation, (C) fracture-luxation, (D) compression fracture, (E) subluxation, (F) fracture-subluxation.

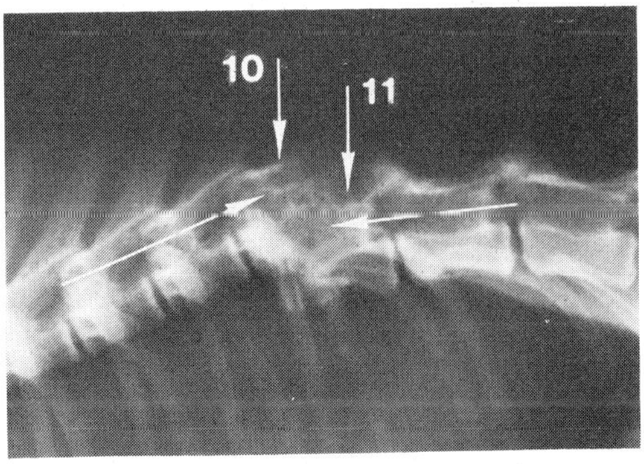

Fig 53. Spinal fracture-luxation, with compression of vertebrae T_{10} and T_{11}. The cat had total functional cord damage and at surgery the cord was found to be severed.

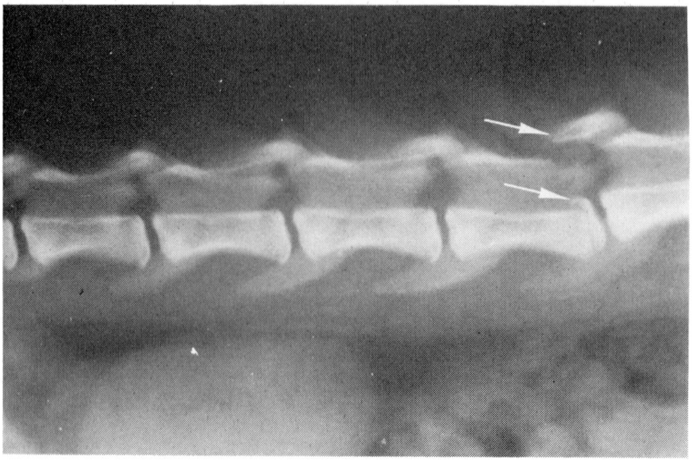

Fig 54. Fracture of vertebra L_5 (arrows). The hindlimbs were paretic.

indicated. In all other cases, especially those with only partial functional cord damage, an exploratory laminectomy should be performed (Fig 55). Pellets, shot and bullets may carry debris into the spinal canal. This should be removed if possible and large doses of ampicillin or chloramphenicol given postoperatively.

On rare occasions a pellet or bullet may enter the pulmonary veins or the left ventricle of the heart without killing the animal and be carried distad in an artery as an embolus.[89] If the aorta is affected, obstruction at the pelvic bifurcation may result in bilateral hindlimb paralysis from apparent thoracic or unknown trauma. All trauma victims must be radiographed, with views obtained of all areas that might contain a lesion responsible for the clinical signs.

Traumatic Disc Rupture: These cases are handled as if they were partial fracture cases. Mildly affected cats need cage rest and corticosteroids; severely affected cats need surgery.

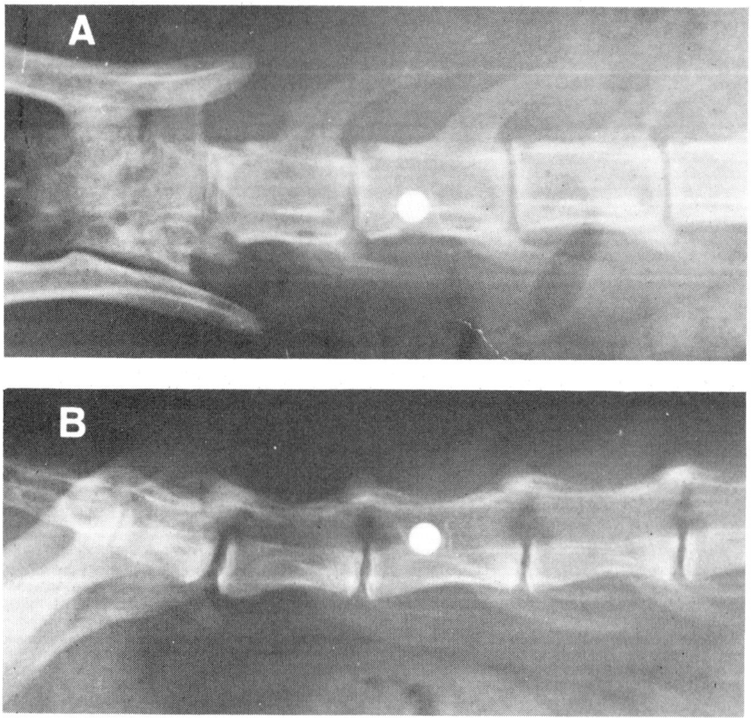

Fig 55. Ventrodorsal (A) and lateral (B) radiographs of the lumbosacral spine of a cat with partial functional cord damage reveal a pellet within the spinal canal.

Paralyzed cats need special nursing care. The bladder must be expressed manually twice or three times a day while there is no voluntary control; catheterization is unnecessary and may result in urethrocystitis. Soft bedding (fine wood shavings are excellent) is essential to reduce the chance of decubital ulcers. Slings that support the animal vertically and allow the legs to dangle are especially useful when the animal is temporarily quadriplegic. Massage, faradization and manipulation of the limbs are beneficial during long-term paralysis, especially if there is lower motor neuron damage.

Unlike in the dog, there is no indication for fenestration of neighboring discs when a laminectomy is performed on a cat.

A fracture of L_7-S_1, the sacrum or S_3-coccyx can damage the sacral nerve roots to the pudendal nerves, which innervate the perineal skin, anal ring and bladder. Because nerve roots are more elastic than the spinal cord, they can remain intact with considerable vertebral displacement. Affected cats may only have a temporary hindlimb weakness, but have no voluntary control of urine or fecal eliminations. It is very difficult to predict the outcome of these cases, but most do not do well. If the tail is paralyzed and cannot be kept clean in the long term, it should be removed. In most cases, a laminectomy should be performed and the fracture stabilized. If recovery is to occur, most affected cats have begun to improve in the first month but some may be delayed up to 3 months. During the recovery period, it may be necessary to use either propantheline bromide (7.5-15 mg BID) for cats with urethral and bladder sphincter spasms or urecholine (5-10 mg BID for cats with atonic bladders.

Of current interest is the use of normothermic or hypothermic saline solution to irrigate a surgically exposed spinal cord in animals with severe cord injury. Midline myelotomy and use of reserpine, dimethylsulfoxide or epsilon amino caproic acid have also been suggested as means of therapy. Most of them have been shown in clinical situations to be of no more benefit for severe spinal cord damage than dexamethasone and prompt decompressive surgery.[91-95] Only normothermic irrigation provides any real benefit and then only if initiated within about 4 hours of injury.

The reason for the interest in these other drugs and treatment is the elucidation over the last 15 years of some of the events that occur in a severely injured spinal cord. Within minutes, the process of cell destruction begins in the spinal cord grey matter and capillaries begin to break down. Most of the irreversible damage is complete in 12-24 hours. The chemical or reflex instigators of this process are not yet known. Various theories have been proposed in the last decade about which chemicals or neurotransmitters (*eg*, norepinephrine, dopamine, prostaglandins) are responsible. Unlucky and sometimes poorly designed research led to some of the early misunderstandings about which treatments would work clinically.[96,97] The idea of hypothermic irrigation was to cool the traumatized spinal cord segments. The cold was ineffective but the dialysis helped; hence, normothermic irrigation came into vogue. However, it can rarely be initiated early enough to be of much value. Some drugs are useful if given before experimental trauma but not if given afterwards. These studies are merely steps along the way to understanding the chemical causes of spinal cord necrosis (or hemorrhagic necrosis) following trauma; they are of no current clinical use.

Spontaneous Intervertebral Disc Disease

Spontaneous disc bulges and ruptures are common in cats but rarely cause clinical signs.[98,99] One paper that claimed to report clinical signs of a disc lesion is open to challenge.[99] Another paper substantiated its claim with surgery and radiographs.[98] We have seen a few older cats with acute onset of cervical or thoracolumbar pain and paresis and radiographic evidence of disc disease; however, we have not operated on them nor have we necropsied them to confirm the diagnosis. The presence of disc lesions radiographically is not proof, even if clinical signs are present.[100,101] Most cases improve rapidly with corticosteroids and cage rest.

Postmortem studies of the incidence of disc disease in cats have disclosed that, in asymptomatic cats 1-20 years of age, both disc prolapse (rupture) and disc protrusion (bulging) occur. Protrusions have been found in cats as young as 6 years of age. Prolapsed discs occur mainly in cats over 15 years old. Cats 6-15 years of age usually have protruded discs, mainly in the cervical region, whereas older cats suffer rupture of the lumbar discs.[100] Approximately 30-50% of middle-aged cats have disc protrusions, whereas almost 100% of old cats have either disc protrusion or prolapse.[101] These postmortem findings suggest that clinical signs of cervical disc prolapse (cervical pain, quadriataxia, forelimb paresis) could be commonly expected in middle-aged cats and signs of lumbar disc protrusions or rupture (lumbar pain, posterior paresis or paralysis) in older cats. Such cases are rarely documented.

To satisfactorily diagnose spontaneous disc rupture in a cat, one must have the appropriate clinical signs (pain, paresis, paralysis), radiographic evidence (calcified material in the canal, narrowed disc) that agrees with the neurologic localization (or a myelogram), and surgical or postmortem demonstration of the prolapsed disc material. Slow onset of signs makes the diagnosis less likely. In our experience and in one published case, most apparent disc ruptures causing clinical signs in cats involve already calcified discs, *ie,* the involved disc calcified before it ruptured.[98]

Infectious and Parasitic Diseases

Viral Infection: Viral diseases that cause spinal ataxia (spinal and/or brain lesions) are FIP (most common), FeLV infection, an unknown entity called feline polioencephalomyelitis, rabies, rabies vaccination and pseudorabies. When the spinal cord is affected, it is called myelitis. When the meninges are involved, it is meningitis. Feline infectious peritonitis often leads to meningomyelitis but rarely causes pain or discomfort. Feline polioencephalomyelitis, FeLV infection and FIP usually cause slowly progressive (months) signs of ataxia or even lower motor neuron deficits. Rabies and cats vaccinated for rabies usually have a more rapid course (days to weeks). Pseudorabies is peracute in onset (2-3-days).

Bacterial Infections: Bacterial infections of the spinal canal are rare because the dura is an efficient barrier to infection. Occasional cases of epidural abscess have been reported.[102] These have usually been associated with previous or current abscesses near the spine. They cause pain, hyperesthesia and even paresis. Diagnosis is difficult and a myelogram may be necessary.

Bacteria rarely penetrate the meninges to cause meningitis. Hematogenous spread during septicemia is more likely. Bacterial meningitis usually spreads rapidly (3-10 days) and causes pain, paresis, paralysis, fever and eventually death when the brainstem becomes involved. Diagnosis is by analysis of CSF obtained from a lumbar or cisternal tap and by counts of circulating WBC. In such cases, the immune status of the cat must also be questioned (FeLV infection, FIP). Treatment is with the appropriate antibiotic, although most antibiotics cross the weakened blood-brain barrier when infection is present.

Discospondylitis (intervertebral disc infection) or spondylitis (vertebral infection) is usually caused by bacteria. A foreign body may be involved (missile, grass seed, needle, splinter) but local spread from an abscess and hematogenous invasion during septicemia may also initiate it.[103] Diagnosis is by radiography. Treatment involves vigorous use of antibiotics for 4-8 weeks, preferably after a direct needle aspirate (culture) or surgical exploration and drainage.

Fungal and Algal Infections: Fungae and algae are extremely rare causes of epidural abscesses, meningitis or spondylitis in cats. The immunocompetency of any affected cat must be questioned. Each of these sites of infection is diagnosed exactly as for bacterial infection. The clinical signs are similar but usually slower in developing. Treatment is difficult. Antifungals may help if the vertebrae are involved; however treatment is virtually pointless once such infections penetrate the meninges. Infected granulomas or masses occasionally can be identified in the epidural space by myelography. Surgical removal may then be possible.

Parasitism: The protozoon *Toxoplasma gondii* is a well-known cause of spinal ataxia in cats. Affected cats can develop myelitis from this agent at any age. Signs are usually slowly progressive, involve the rear legs first, are often asymmetric, and are distinctly corticosteroid-responsive. Prednisolone treatment may be required for 6 months at 1 mg/kg every second or third day. Diagnosis is by lumbar CSF analysis, serologic examination and occasionally by necropsy. The lesions may be diffuse or segmental, involving the brain and spinal cord. The diagnosis may be confused with FIP, FeLV infection or feline polioencephalomyelitis initially. The diagnostic tests are not completely accurate and the clinician may have to resort to test therapy with corticosteroids. Cats with FIP usually respond to corticosteroids for up to a year. The response to corticosteroids of cats with any of the group of diseases caused by FeLV varies from minimal to excellent, with even an apparent complete remission on occasion. Cats with feline polioencephalomyelitis do not show more than a minimal response.

Metazoan parasites may be encountered in many abnormal locations in the body. When large parasites (*Dirofilaria immitis, Cuterebra*) invade the spinal canal, the signs are usually dramatic, such as transverse myelopathy of a fairly acute nature. Diagnosis is by myelography but the total circulating eosinophil count may offer a clue as to the etiology. When migrating larvae invade the cord (*Toxocara* spp, *Angiostrongylus cantonensis*), the process resembles meningomyelitis and is diagnosed by CSF analysis and circulating eosinophil counts.

Metabolic and Inherited Diseases

Few of these generalized diseases are limited to the spinal cord but their initial signs often suggest spinal cord disease (hindleg paresis or ataxia). They have been fully discussed in the Brain and Generalized Disease section of this chapter. One 4-week-old kitten had lower motor neuron weakness of all 4 limbs.[104] The signs progressed rapidly (tremors, paralysis) in about a week. Muscle atrophy, hyporeflexia and flaccid paralysis were present. The large lower motor neurons of the limbs were found to be degenerative at necropsy. Thus, the condition could be termed a "spinal lower motor neuron" disease of cats.

Vascular Diseases

The most common vascular lesion of a cat's limbs is aortic embolus. Trauma or hemorrhagic disease may lead to focal (hematoma) or diffuse spinal vascular accidents. Cats with cardiomyopathy may shed small emboli into the spinal cord arteries, leading to obstructive spinal vascular accidents. We have had cats with acute bilateral or unilateral spinal cord signs (paresis, paralysis) that exhibited no focal pain. When such signs cannot be attributed to trauma or any other disease, a spinal vascular accident should be suspected. However, proof is only to be found at necropsy. Mildly affected cats may slowly recover in a few weeks, but some permanent deficit may remain. We have not yet encountered a cat with a fibrocartilagenous embolus in the spinal arteries as seen in dogs. The cats we have seen have only had unexplained focal malacia of the spinal cord.

Developmental Abnormalities

The major developmental abnormality of the feline spinal cord is spina bifida, which is a general term for several conditions involving various degrees of nonfusion of the neural tube and vertebral arches (spinal dysraphism). The term "spina bifida occulta" refers to simple nonfusion of the vertebral laminae; "meningocele" refers to protrusion of the meninges through the defect; "meningomyelocele" indicates protrusion of meninges and spinal cord. Either of the last 2 protrusions may or may not be covered by intact skin. The open form of this defect has been observed in a Siamese cat.[105]

Tailless cats (Manx) can be affected by a variety of spinal defects, including true spina bifida occulta, absence of all vertebrae caudal to S_1, cervical or lumbar vertebral fusion and shortening, and pelvic abnormalities.[106-110] There has been discussion about whether the Manx is a breed of cat. It theoretically cannot be considered a breed because it does not breed true, *ie*, it does not reproduce offspring of similar phenotypic appearance. There is good evidence that taillessness in cats can be inherited as an autosomal dominant gene (M), called the Manx factor.[109-111] Manx cats do not breed true and have small litters when inbred. The homozygous genotype (MM) is apparently a lethal genotype.[110] All cats with the Manx factor are Mm; normal cats are mm. The Manx factor is expressed in at least 4 ways: absence of the tail, one inch or less of immovable coccygeal vertebrae, 2-3 inches of movable tail, or a longer tail that is still not of normal length. Breeders use such terms as "rumpy," "rumpy riser" and "stumpy" to describe these variations. Because of the urinary and fecal incontinence, constipation and secondary infections in some of these cats, the Manx factor can also be considered semilethal, *ie*, it causes a reduced life span, even in heterozygotes. Because of the tail variations, there must be phenotypic (nongenetic) factors involved in expression of the Manx factor in affected (Mm) cats. Cats with tail variations do not breed true and seem to be variations of one genotype.[112]

The signs seen in some cats with the Manx factor are urogenital malformations, absence of bowel and bladder control, megacolon (cord segments S_1-S_3 involved), hindlimb weakness, and loss of hindlimb coordination (cord segments L_6-S_3). Some affected cats may hop instead of run. Most are untreatable and should be neutered or euthanized. Occasionally reports of surgical corrections appear but the success rate is not good.[113] Similar clinical signs can be expected with spina bifida of the lumbrosacral junction

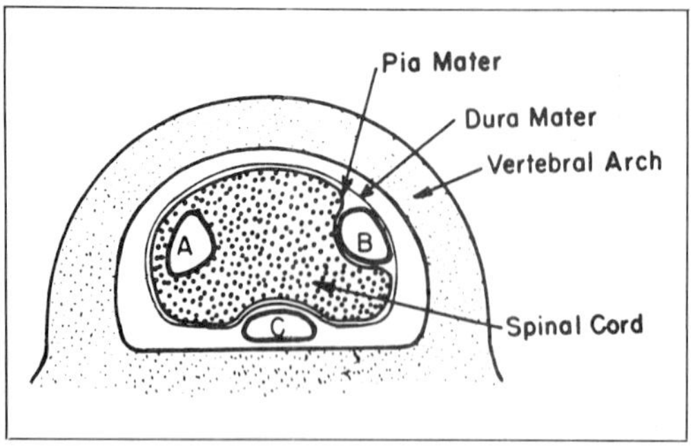

Fig 56. Diagram of the 3 sites for a spinal tumor: intradural and intramedullary (A), intradural but extramedullary (B), extradural (C).

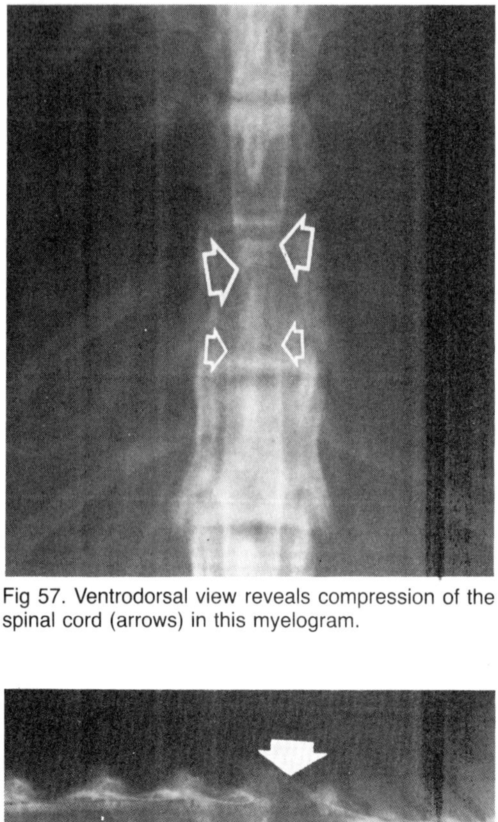

Fig 57. Ventrodorsal view reveals compression of the spinal cord (arrows) in this myelogram.

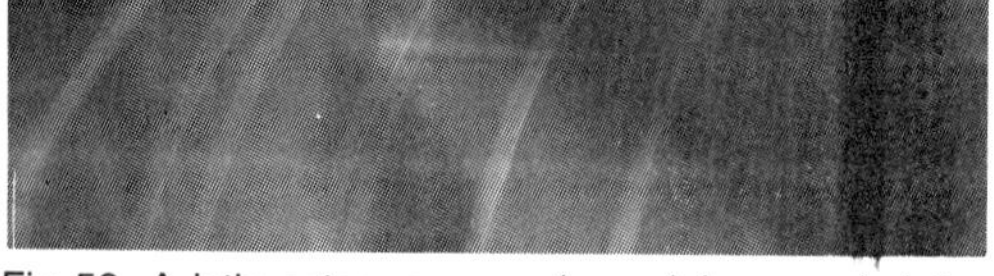

Fig 58. A lytic osteosarcoma (arrow) has eroded the lamina of vertebra T_{11}. A myelogram reveals spinal cord compression.

or other spinal dysraphisms (sacral cord agenesis) in cats that are not Manx.[114,115] When spina bifida occurs in other areas of the spine, the signs resemble those of a focal transverse cord lesion at that point. Other cord defects, such as cavitation (syringomyelia), occur with the Manx factor or spina bifida. Brain deformity has been reported in Manx cats.[116]

Hemivertebrae are occasionally encountered in otherwise normal cats or Manx cats. They are the result of abnormal development of the growth centers of vertebral bodies. The vertebral body may be wedge-shaped or residual. The point of the wedge is usually ventral. The abnormality rarely causes gross spinal curvature, is not palpable or painful, has no callus around it, and rarely causes clinical signs. It is usually an incidental finding on a radiograph. The nature of the deformity usually is recognized if lateral and ventrodorsal views are obtained.

Butterfly vertebrae are even rarer and similarly cause no problems. They are the result of incomplete midline fusion of the vertebral laminae and body. The cranial and caudal ends of the vertebrae are unfused. This produces the "butterfly" shape on ventrodorsal radiographs.

Block vertebrae are also asymptomatic and merely represent the failure of an embryonic body somite to split in the production of the vertebrae. Usually only 2 vertebrae are joined together.

Acquired Spinal Deformities

Hypervitaminosis A: Cats fed an excess of vitamin A (*eg*, raw liver) may develop extensive hyperostosis and ankylosis of vertebrae and joints, particularly of the cervical vertebrae and elbows.[117,118] Clinical signs include pain or manipulation, abnormal gait, hyperesthesia, lick granulomas, general depression and muscle wasting. The muscle loss is attributed to injury of spinal nerve roots by the vertebral lesions.

Diagnosis of hypervitaminosis A is based on the history and radiographic evidence of extensive hyperostosis. Serum or liver biopsy levels of vitamin A can be assayed. The normal plasma level of vitamin A is about 200 IU or µg/dl and in liver is up to 10,000 IU or µg/g (wet weight). The serum Ca level also is elevated to 130-150% of normal. The only treatment is to change the diet; the ankylosis is usually irreversible. Mildly affected cats lose their hyperesthesia and improve within several months after being fed a low-vitamin A diet. Lost muscle may not be replaced in severely affected animals. Because vitamin A is stored in the liver, some cats may continue to have an elevated serum vitamin A level for as long as 2 years after being put on a low-vitamin A diet.[117]

Spondylosis: Spondylosis is a noninflammatory exostosis of the vertebral bodies. Spondylosis of vertebral bodies is the general term for the condition, but individual exostoses may be called vertebral osteophytes.[119,120] They develop laterad and ventrad from vertebral bodies, eventually interlock and may bridge the intervertebral spaces, but do not obliterate the intervertebral disc. The exostoses may fuse to form ankylosed vertebrae. We have not observed clinical signs demonstrated to have been directly caused by vertebral body spondylosis.

Clinicians should not confuse spondylosis with spondylitis. Spondylitis is an inflammatory process due to bacteria or fungi.

Neoplasia

Extradural lymphosarcoma is the most common spinal canal tumor in cats.[69,70,121] Other types of spinal tumors are rare (reticulosis, glioma, neurilemmoma, sarcoma, metastases).[122] Tumors (chondroma, chondrosarcoma, osteoma, osteosarcoma) of the vertebrae are also uncommon.[123] Unlike the high incidence of intracranial meningiomas in cats, the incidence of meningiomas in the spinal canal is very low.[70] Therefore, if a spinal tumor is suspected, an FeLV test, thoracic radiography and lymph node aspiration should be performed before myelography to more easily obtain the likely diagnosis.

The 3 major sites for spinal tumors are shown in Figure 56. In the extradural location, lymphomas, vertebral tumors, metastases, neurilemmomas, and perhaps lipomas and meningiomas are found (Figs 57, 58). In the intradural but extramedullary site, lymphomas, meningiomas and metastases are found (Fig 59). In the intradural and intramedullary sites, the tumors are gliomas and ependymomas.

The clinical signs caused by spinal cord tumors are typically those of slowly progressive (weeks or months) transverse cord syndrome, with ataxia, paresis and paralysis in limbs caudal to the lesion. Focal pain is rare. Occasionally a rapid course may be seen with lymphomas; paralysis may appear in 1-2 days and be associated with focal pain. Diagnosis is by myelography; plain radiographs do not show the lesion.

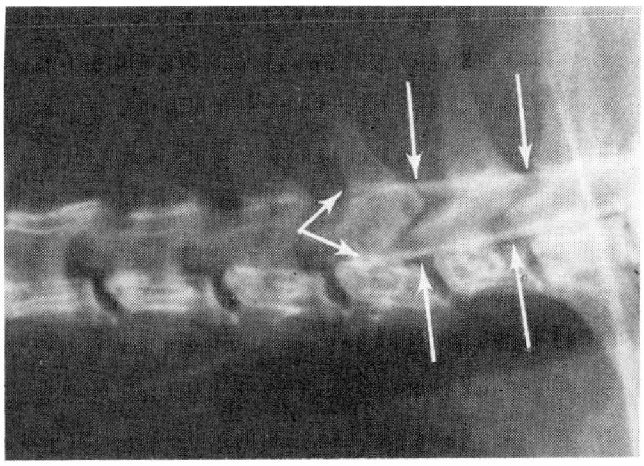

Fig 59. Cervical myelogram reveals an intradural enlargement of the spinal cord within vertebrae C_5-C_6. This was a lymphoid tumor. The parallel arrows indicate the dorsal and ventral contrast columns. The divergent arrows indicate the cranial end of the cord enlargement.

Vertebral tumors can more easily be diagnosed with plain radiographs. They cause clinical signs similar to those of spinal cord tumors but discomfort or pain is usually present.

Treatment of any tumor is by surgical excision. Lymphomas warrant a grave prognosis. Most affected cats have evidence of lymphoma elsewhere. Other tumors are more amenable to removal, even vertebral tumors.[123] Thoracic radiographs should be obtained before any surgery to make sure the spinal lesion is not a metastatic lesion.

PERIPHERAL NERVOUS SYSTEM DISEASES

The peripheral nervous system is composed of the cranial and spinal nerves.

Trauma

Trauma is the most common cause of peripheral nervous system dysfunction. Injury to the cranial nerves alone is rare; they are usually injured in association with brain trauma. One seventh nerve may be injured with a blow to the side of the head or during facial surgery (facial paralysis). One fifth nerve may be injured by fractures of the vertical ramus of the mandible (atrophy of the ipsilateral temporal and masseter muscles follows). Vestibular and optic nerve lesions were previously discussed.

The only therapy for trauma of any cranial nerve is administration of a corticosteroid in small doses, such as dexamethasone at 0.05-0.1 mg/kg daily, for 1-2 weeks. It is doubtful if this

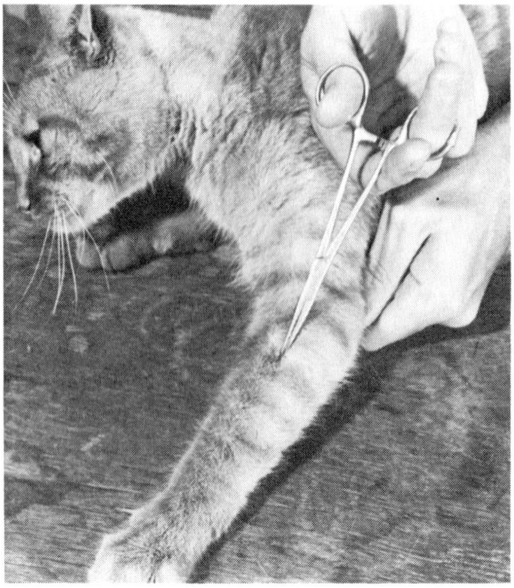

Fig 60. Testing the area of radial nerve innervation to the dorsolateral foreleg.

treatment really helps. The prognosis should be guarded, although some cats with facial nerve paralysis caused by trauma recover within a few hours. There is no easy way to find out if a damaged nerve is severed or bruised. Thus, less seriously affected animals cannot be identified except by their eventual recovery. As an arbitrary period, we allow 3 months before a final judgment is made. Cats are very adaptable and those with seventh or fifth unilateral nerve damage can live with the disability. Those with vestibular problems may have slightly more difficulty for a longer period. Unilaterally or bilaterally blind cats do well.

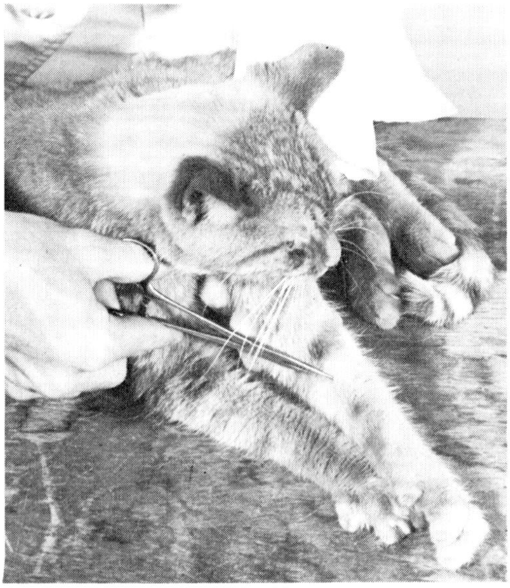

Fig 61. Testing the area of musculocutaneous innervation to the mediodorsal foreleg.

Spinal nerves are injured by being stretched or torn as the limb is jerked, severed by bone fragments, cut by scalpels and damaged by injections. The injury is usually unilateral except in sacral or multiple pelvic fractures.

Foreleg: The nerves to each forelimb are derived from the spinal nerves C_6-C_8 and T_1 (Table 10). These nerves form the brachial plexus between the scapula and ribs on each side of the body. When a cat is hit by a vehicle, any of the nerves comprising the plexus may be bruised, stretched or severed at their nerve roots as they leave the spinal cord (most common), around the first rib, in the plexus, or damaged around the humerus by a fracture or a tourniquet applied proximal to the elbow. The clinically significant and easily tested nerves of the plexus are the suprascapular, musculocutaneous, radial, median and ulnar, arranged in that order cranial to caudal (Table 10).

Several syndromes may occur after trauma to nerves or nerve roots of the forelimb. Brachial paralysis refers to loss of all motor and sensory function by nerves of a forelimb. There is total loss of sensation distal to the elbow. The limb is flaccid and drags on the ground because the cat cannot raise it. The 3 sensory testing sites distal to the elbow are shown in Figures 60-62.

The foreleg sensory area supplied solely by the radial nerve is a dorsolateral strip (Fig 60). The musculocutaneous nerve solely supplies a dorsomedial strip (Fig 61). The median/ulnar nerve (clinically one might as well regard them as 2 branches of the same nerve) is tested ventrad (Fig 62). Each of these testing areas does not represent the whole area supplied by each of the nerves; there is considerable overlapping by each of the sensory nerves. To confirm total sensory loss, one should pinch the medial and then lateral digits in a pair of hemostats. This tests crude (deep) pain in the median, radial and ulnar nerves. Motor function is tested by observing the cat move, palpating muscles for tone or atrophy, and percussing muscles or their tendons for a normal muscle reflex (myotactic) contraction (Table 10).

In many road accidents, the cat suffers tearing of the nerve roots (C_6-T_1) before they have combined their motor and sensory components to form the peripheral nerves (radial, musculocutaneous, etc), resulting in a nerve root syndrome. This may lead to confusion if only a few nerve roots are injured or if the sensory and motor losses do not correspond to each other or to any one of the forelimb nerves.

Injury of the T_1-T_3 nerve roots close to the cord before the sympathetic rami communicans branch off results in an ipsilateral Horner's syndrome. If the C_8-T_1 nerve roots are similarly injured before their dorsal branches separate from the ventral branches which form the brachial plexus, an ipsilateral loss of the panniculus reflex occurs, although skin sensation to the back remains intact. These are 2 useful observations to help decide if a nerve root or proximal lesion exists in nerves C_8-T_3.

In the musculocutaneous syndrome, there is total brachial paralysis except that the musculocutaneous nerve is not affected. This is attributed to its length and partial isolation from others in the plexus or to survival of the C_6 nerve roots. The limb is desensitized distal to the elbow except for a strip of the mediodorsal foreleg and occasionally the medial digit. The cat can flex its elbow and hold its paw off the ground.

Radial paralysis refers to damage to only the radial nerve. In high radial paralysis, the whole nerve is damaged. Because the triceps and extensors of the carpus are denervated, the limb cannot be voluntarily extended. The elbow is usually flexed and held off the ground as the cat moves; the paw is rested (usually knuckled over) on the ground when the cat is stationary. If the limb is not carried flexed, the paw knuckles over and the elbow collapses at every step. There is loss of sensation to a narrow strip of the dorsolateral forearm and to the dorsal carpus and paw.

In low radial paralysis, only the leg distal to the elbow is affected. The same area as with high paralysis is desensitized but the triceps is unaffected; only the carpal and digit extensors are denervated. Initially the cat often knuckles over on the affected paw but can walk. Within a few days, most cats learn to flick the affected paw forward as they walk, and the muscle atrophy is easily overlooked. With fractures of the humerus, the radial nerve may be severed or bruised as it runs caudad and laterad to the humerus (Fig 63).[124] The nerve may also be bruised by blows to the foreleg or by a tourniquet placed proximal to the elbow. The superficial branch of the radial nerve is sensory to the dorsolateral foreleg and the deep branch is motor to extensors of the carpus and digits. Care must be taken during repair of humeral fractures to avoid stretching or severing the radial nerve or incorporating it in the fracture repair. Unfortunately, iatrogenic injury of this nerve is common. The deep branch is the critical one because

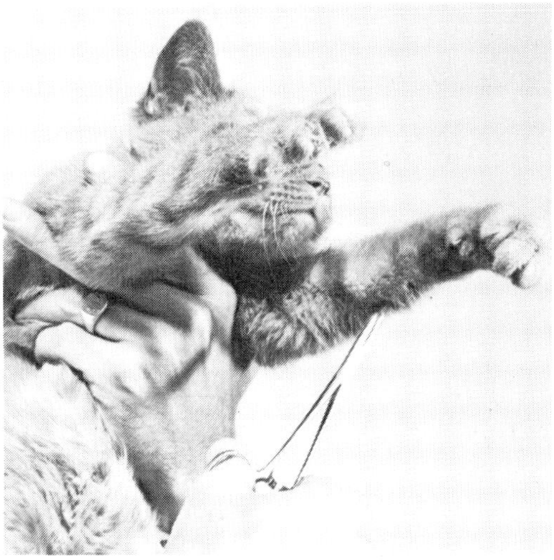

Fig 62. Testing the area of ulnar nerve innervation to the ventral foreleg.

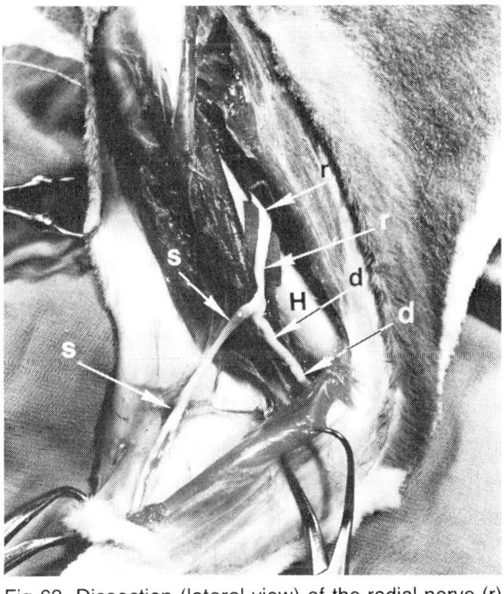

Fig 63. Dissection (lateral view) of the radial nerve (r) shows its proximity to the humerus (H), as well as its terminal deep (d) and superficial (s) branches.

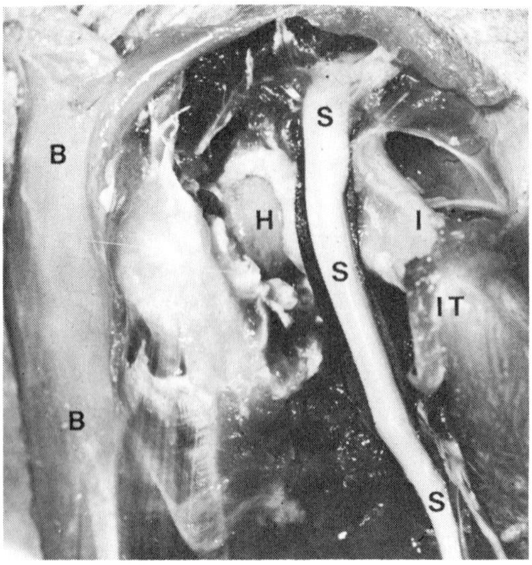

Fig 64. Dissection of the proximal part of the sciatic nerve (S) shows its proximity to the head of the femur (H), ischium (I) and ischial tuberosity (IT). The biceps femoris (B) muscle is reflected craniad.

the superficial branch can be severed with impunity and is often used for nerve biopsies.

Further diagnosis of nerve injuries depends on electromyography and electroneurography (motor and sensory), but radiographs of the scapula, first rib and humerus should be obtained.

The prognosis for nerve lesions of the forelimb is problematic. With severance of a nerve, the prospect of regaining function is zero unless it is promptly repaired. Even if the damaged nerve is accessible and repaired by competent surgeons, the chance of recovery is poor. Although the function of bruised or stretched nerves may be regained in 1-3 months, it is not possible to initially identify those that will recover. We wait for 6 months before a final judgment is made. However, if recovery is not apparent in the first month, less than 10% of affected cats recover from brachial injuries thereafter. Amputation may be necessary when neural function is not regained and the cat drags a limb, thus damaging the paw. If the limb contracts to a flexed position, the owner must decide about amputation. Because 3-legged cats manage quite well, euthanasia is unnecessary.

For the first week after injury, small doses of a corticosteroid may help reduce inflammation. Fractures must be repaired and stabilized, with nerves protected from the callus. During the waiting period, the limb should be flexed, extended and massaged for a half hour daily to retard atrophy and fibrosis of the denervated muscles. A muscle faradizer (electric stimulator) can also be used for 10-minute periods BID if there is brachial paralysis. The disc electrodes are dipped in saline solution and taped to either side of the forearm; 60-100 volts are intermittently applied to stimulate twitching of the foreleg muscles. If there is any sensation below the elbow, electrical stimulation obviously will not be tolerated. As neural function returns, the cat may lick at the paw; sensory function often returns before motor. If fibrotic contracture of muscles has occurred, the limb will be useless unless some muscles remain functional and the fibrotic ones are severed. In some cases, tendons can be transposed to regain function of some joints.

Some cats with brachial paralysis recover within a few days; others require several months. Those that recover in a few days have presumably suffered a nerve bruise. Patients that require months to recover have presumably suffered axon degeneration, followed by regrowth of axons within the intact nerve sheaths. Recoveries that require a month are attributed to remyelination of damaged segments of nerve. Generally, the more nerves that survive the injury, the better is the prognosis. Thus, there is a better chance for recovery from high radial paralysis than from the musculocutaneous syndrome. Cats can compensate rapidly for low radial paralysis, even if no recovery occurs.

Hindleg: Nerves of the hindlimb and perineum are derived from L_4-L_7 and S_1-S_3. Femoral nerve damage in cats has not been reported except from severe pelvic (ilium) fractures. The sciatic nerves are commonly traumatized. With ischial fractures, the sciatic nerve may be damaged where it lies between the head of the femur and point of the ischium (Fig 64). The nerve may also be damaged during a careless surgical approach to the femoral head, during internal fixation of ischial fractures and by injection. The pudendal nerves, which rarely are damaged unilaterally, often are injured in conjunction with sacral or sacrococcygeal fractures. The 2 branches of the sciatic nerve (tibial and peroneal) are rarely injured separately. A lateral blow to the stifle or a carelessly lateral approach to the stifle or the cranial third of the tibia may injure the peroneal (fibular) branch (Fig 65).

The femoral nerve is solely sensory to a thin medial strip of the distal leg and usually to the medial side of the first digit and is motor to the extensors of the stifle (Table 10). The sciatic nerve supplies the rest of the distal limb and is motor to all muscles distal to the stifle. The pudendal nerve is sensory to the perineum and motor to the anus and bladder.

The remarkable fact about sciatic paralysis is the degree of use remaining in an affected leg. The muscles innervated by the femoral nerve fix the stifle, and thus the leg can bear weight. However, the paw knuckles over, the hock sinks and the leg is rarely carried. As a consequence, severe ulcers develop on the dorsum of the paw unless the cat is confined until recovery, or either amputation or arthrodesis is performed. Peroneal paralysis produces only knuckling of the paw, to which the cat can adapt reasonably well. It usually does not require amputation but may require tendon transposition.

Sensation is lost only distal to the hock when the sciatic branches are injured at the stifle and only distal to the stifle when injured at the head of the femur. For these reasons, most clinicians commonly underestimate the severity of sciatic injuries.

Cats with evidence of sciatic nerve injury should be examined radiographically to determine if an ischial fracture has occurred. If there is no fracture and no skin wound, it is reasonable to assume that the nerve is intact and that surgical exploration is not necessary. The only treatment for cats with sciatic paralysis after hip surgery, trauma with ischial fractures, or peroneal nerve paralysis after stifle surgery is surgical exploration of the likely site to examine the nerve, relieve pressure of fracture fragments and attempt repair if the nerve has been severed. The prognosis is guarded and if recovery occurs, it may take 6 months.

With only bruising or stretching of the sciatic or peroneal nerves, recovery may occur in a few days, 1-3 months or not at all. While waiting for recovery, small doses of a corticosteroid and physiotherapy can be given as outlined for foreleg nerve injuries. Electrical stimulation for sciatic paralysis is not easy because the femoral nerve is sensory to the medial surface of the leg.

Injury to the sciatic nerve by needle penetration and irritant injections is common. The position of this nerve is shown in Figure 65. It is preferable to make injections cranial to the femur and thus avoid injuring the sciatic nerve. The signs of neural damage may be immediate (sharp pain, then paralysis) or delayed a few hours (secondary inflammation and spread of the solution). The resultant paralysis may be complete or partial. There may only be evidence of sensory neuritis and no paralysis.

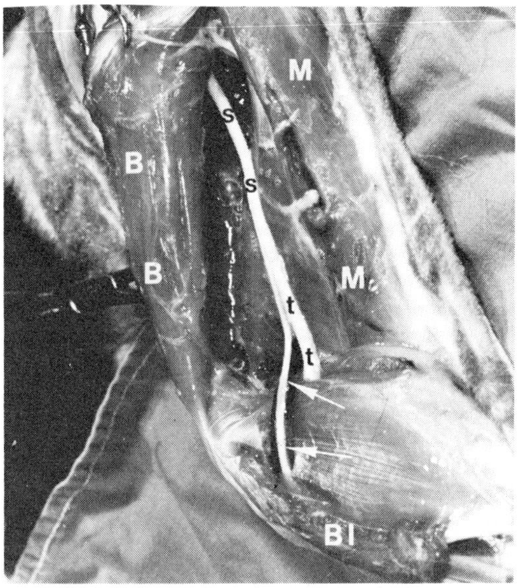

Fig 65. Dissection (lateral view) of the distal part of the sciatic nerve (S) shows its relationship to the biceps femoris (B) and semitendinosus (M) muscles, as well as its terminal peroneal (arrows) and tibial (t) branches. The insertion of the biceps femoris muscle (BI) is also indicated. The biceps femoris muscle has been reflected craniad.

If the injected material contains a local anesthetic, function may return within 1-2 days. Function may also return rapidly if the effects of the injection were mild or due to secondary inflammation. We have observed some cats that recovered after 1-3 months (remyelination?) and have also seen animals that did not recover. Therefore, we advise surgical exposure of the injection site to remove (saline flush, no corticosteroids) the injected material. The sooner this can be done, the better are the results.

Neoplasia

Tumors of the feline peripheral nervous system are rare. Even infiltration or local compression of a nerve or nerve root by lymphoma is uncommon. Tumors of the nerve sheath (schwannoma, neurofibroma, neurilemmoma) have occasionally been reported.[70,121,122,125] Tumors of bone (osteosarcoma) and surrounding tissue may involve peripheral nerves (spinal and cranial) or their roots.[126] Radiography usually reveals these tumors but is rarely helpful with tumors of nerves. Myelography rarely demonstrates nerve root tumors. Slowly progressive clinical signs, palpable masses if present, and electroneurography and electromyography are necessary for diagnosis of nerve or nerve root tumors. The only treatment is surgery but it is rarely successful; the affected nerves or roots must usually be sacrificed.

Toxic, Immune, Hormonal and Idiopathic Diseases

Traumatic and neoplastic diseases of the peripheral nervous system are usually mononeuropathies involving one nerve or perhaps a plexus (regional polyneuropathy). Generalized diseases of the peripheral nervous system usually produce polyneuropathy (sensory, motor or mixed neuropathies). If nerve roots are the primary site of the lesions, it is polyradiculoneuropathy. Nerves may be stripped of their myelin (demyelination), leaving the axons intact and allowing remyelination to occur. Demyelination effectively blocks nerve conduction; remyelination returns it to normal. The distal portion of a severed nerve undergoes Wallerian degeneration, in which the severed axon dies distad, the distal myelin is phagocytosed, but the Schwann cells survive to remyelinate regrowing axons if the nerve ends are successfully joined and axon sheaths survive. If an axon is cut too close (in a nerve root) to its lower motor neuron cell body, the entire neuron dies. Axons may degenerate starting distad and progressing proximad toward their cell body. The myelin may also be involved. This is called a dying-back neuropathy, distal denervating disease, or a distal axonopathy. Axons tend to swell along part of their length when their metabolism (inherited or toxic) is affected, which is referred to as a giant axonal neuropathy. Polyneuropathies may be acute, chronic or relapsing.

Polyneuropathies have rarely been observed in cats. Lead toxicity can cause segmental demyelination. Several chemicals can cause a dying-back neuropathy. Diabetes mellitus, hypothyroidism, and intoxication with organophosphates or chlorinated hydrocarbons can cause a variety of polyneuropathies. When no etiology can be found, the cases are termed idiopathic. Some inherited diseases also cause polyneuropathies (Krabbe's globoid-cell leukodystrophy).

The immune system seems to be able to recognize different types of myeline (sensory vs motor nerve root, cranial vs spinal nerve) and may attack any part of the peripheral nervous system accordingly. Some initiating factors (antigens) are known to be responsible for starting this process in a variety of species. Brachial plexus neuropathy has been recognized and attributed to recent (1-4 weeks) rabies vaccination.[127] The affected cat made a rapid recovery. Dietary antigens (meats), injected antigens (serum, vaccines) or previous infections (virus) may also be initiating factors. Note how the rabies vaccine virus may trigger the immune attack as an alternative mechanism to actually causing a vaccinal encephalomyelitis itself.

The clinical signs of polyneuropathies are varied. Those of immune origin tend to be rapid in onset (1-3 days). Those of toxic origin are slower (1-4 weeks and progressive until the toxin is removed), and those of hormonal origin tend to progress slowly over months. Polyneuropathy of immune origin tends to affect motor roots and produce mainly motor signs (polyradiculoneuropathies), such as paresis, hyporeflexia and lower motor neuron paralysis. The rear limbs tend to be affected first but not in brachial plexus neuropathy. Toxic and hormonal neuropathies are often mixed, with sensory dysesthesia or paresthesia (abnormal sensations) a common feature.

Pure sensory neuropathies are extremely difficult to recognize or diagnose except by electroneurography and nerve biopsies. Motor polyneuropathies or polyradiculoneuropathies are easier to recognize because of their motor signs but electromyography is necessary for diagnosis. They may be confused clinically with myasthenia gravis, botulism, tick paralysis, polymyositis (generalized muscle inflammation) or muscular dystrophies.

Treatment of polyneuropathies is aimed at correcting the underlying cause. Inherited diseases are slowly progressive and nonresponsive. Slowly progressive chronic or relapsing idiopathic ones are unresponsive. Immune cases usually recover in a few weeks, sometimes more rapidly. It is doubtful if corticosteroids have any effect but it is customary to use them (*eg*, prednisolone at 2 mg/kg/day for 1-2 weeks).

Hemifacial spasm is a condition in which the seventh cranial nerve or its nucleus is irritated. Spasm and fasciculation of the facial muscles may produce a "grin." If the irritative process worsens, facial paralysis (droop) results. Hemifacial spasm can be caused by encephalitis or otitis media/interna. Treatment is with corticosteroids and/or alleviation of the otitis.

Contracture of the face results if the seventh nerve is destroyed and the facial muscles fibrose. This results in a permanent grin unlike the variable one of hemifacial spasm, which also usually leaves the orbital and eyelid blink reflex intact.

Tetanus: Cats are highly resistant to the exotoxin of the *Clostridium tetani* bacillus but occasional cases are seen.[128] The usual clinical signs are a grin, stiff limbs, elevated tail (even vertically), third eyelid protrusion, intermittent muscle spasms, and opisthotonus. Severely affected animals are rigidly paralyzed. Mildly affected cats can usually walk stiffly.

Tetanus is diagnosed by recognition of the clinical signs. Recovery of the toxin from serum or the bacterium from a necrotic wound is not easy. There may be no visible wound nor even a history of one. Any wound should be flushed with hydrogen peroxide (*Cl tetani* is an anaerobe) and left open. The cat should be given penicillin at 50,000 IU/kg twice a day for a week. Equine-origin tetanus antitoxin (10,000 units/kg) should be given IV on day one an hour after a small SC test dose (horse serum anaphylaxis may occur) and should be repeated for 5 days at 1000 units/kg/day given SC. Diazepam or chlorpromazine (1-5 mg/kg), repeated 4 times a day or as a continuous infusion, or methocarbamol (20-50 mg/kg BID) can be given for muscle relaxation. Pentobarbital sedation may help the phenothiazines or diazepam function by reducing upper motor neuron activity. Affected cats require turning if they are unable to rise and may require bladder catheterization, parenteral fluids and nasogastric stomach tubing for feeding soup. Our feline tetanus cases have all been mild and responded in a few days. Severely affected cats, if treated effectively, may require 1-2 months to recover. The success rate is good even in these cats.

The tetanus toxin is adsorbed onto axons and transported up and down them to its sites of action, the interneurons, in the spinal cord, where it interferes with the release of these cells' lower motor neuron inhibitory neurotransmitter glycine, and at the neuromuscular junction. Once the toxin is adsorbed onto the membranes, the antitoxin has little effect. One must wait for the natural turnover of membranes to occur.

NEUROMUSCULAR DISEASES

Aortic Embolism

The effects of an aortic embolus have been described as an ischemic neuromyopathy.[129] Both the peripheral nerves and the muscles in the hindlimbs are affected.

Cause: The etiology is an embolus that originates in the left side of the heart and lodges in or at the origin of the external iliac arteries, forming a "saddle" embolus. Most affected cats have cardiomyopathy. If the terminal aorta is experimentally ligated, cats do not have hindleg paralysis and in minutes have an adequate collateral circulation. In aortic embolism, the clot itself is responsible for the failure of collateral circulation. Studies with antiserotonergic drugs have shown that serotonin released from platelets in the clot seems to be the chemical instigator of the vasoconstrictive failure of collateral circulation.[130]

Clinical Signs: The ischemic muscles of the hindlimbs have a stiff, dough-like feel on palpation. The paws are cold, the limbs have no sensation from mid-thigh distad, and limb reflexes are absent. The tail may have normal motor and sensory function, and functions of the anus and perineum are almost always normal.

Diagnosis: Diagnosis is by clinical signs. If more information is needed, a nonselective bolus angiogram (cephalic vein injection) of the distal aorta is adequate. The heart should be closely examined.

Treatment: Many affected cats recover in 3-6 weeks without suffering skin necrosis. Treatment seems of little additional value. Surgical removal of the clot is unnecessary. The big clinical problem is recurrence because of the underlying cardiomyopathy. Some cats have such large emboli that the renal or mesenteric arteries also are affected. Death is rapid in such cats if the embolism is not immediately recognized (anuria).

Affected muscles have patchy necrosis and affected nerves (distal sciatic and femoral) have patchy demyelination (remyelination usually occurs in 3-4 weeks), as well as axonal degeneration (2-3 months to recover) and spared axons, which can function in a few days once the collateral circulation develops. These muscle and nerve changes account for the permanent partial muscle atrophy in affected cats, the early improvement (days) in some cats, the improvement in 3-4 weeks in most, and the delayed or lack of recovery in others.

Myasthenia Gravis

Myasthenia gravis in cats has rarely been reported.[131,132] Affected cats have episodic weakness and can walk well after a rest, but tire, take unstable stilted steps, and sit or lie down frequently. The hindlimbs may be the more severely affected. The mucous membranes remain pink and affected cats rarely are dyspneic. Their voice is weak and they have no pain or cramping. After a few minutes of rest, they can get up. Megaesophagus and inhalation of vomitus are associated problems. In rare cases a thymoma may be present.

The heart, lungs and blood gases (including pH) should be evaluated. Blood electrolytes and glucose should be tested. Once metabolic, respiratory, electrolyte, and cardiovascular causes have been ruled out, the cat should be examined electromyographically to detect a decremental evoked muscle response to repeated nerve stimulation and its reversal after IV injection of edrophonium (Tensilon:Roche).

If electromyography is not available, the following drugs can be used as test therapy. In 5-10 minutes after IM injection of 0.25-0.5 mg neostigmine, cats with myasthenia gravis have a normal gait for 1-2 hours, in addition to salivation, peristalsis and small pupils. In 1-2 minutes after IV injection of 0.25-0.5 mg edrophonium, cats with myasthenia gravis have a normal gait for 10-20 minutes, in addition to salivation, peristalsis and small pupils. If no responses are seen in the appropriate times, equal amounts can be given again until the visceral effects are noticed. Failure of the animal to walk well after the second injection suggests the diagnosis is wrong. Atropine should be used to effect to block the parasympathetic effects if dyspnea (bronchiolar constriction) develops.

Drugs for long-term treatment include oral pyridostigmine (Mestinon:Roche) at 5-10 mg SID or BID, or 1-5 mg neostigmine BID. In either instance, atropine (0.1-0.2 mg) may have to be given simultaneously or shortly before the other drugs to block their muscarinic effects (salivation, bronchial, diarrhea); pyridostigmine has fewer muscarinic effects.

In dogs and people, acquired myasthenia is associated occasionally with thymomas and often with circulating acetylcholine-receptor antibodies. Serum can be tested for these antibodies. This has not been observed in cats.

Botulism

Botulism occurs occasionally in cats and is the result of ingesting contaminated food or waste products. The clinical signs are those of acute (within 1-2 days) lower motor neuron paresis or paralysis, with no focal pain or loss of pain sensation. Differential diagnoses include polyneuritis and tick paralysis. Diagnosis is by electromyography (depressed or no evoked muscle potentials, with normal nerve conduction velocity) because the exotoxin of *Clostridium botulinum* blocks release of acetylcholine from the motor endplate. Occasionally one of the botulinum toxins can be recovered from vomitus, feces or serum of the affected animal. Treatment is with polyvalent antitoxin and supportive care. The prognosis is guarded and any recovery occurs in 1-2 weeks.

Tick Paralysis

Tick paralysis affects cats but not as commonly as dogs. The cause in the US is the salivary neurotoxin of the female common wood tick, *Dermacentor variabilis*. Other species of ticks may also be responsible. The clinical signs are those of a rapidly progressive (within 1-2 days), painless lower motor neuron paresis or paralysis affecting the hindlegs first. Ticks in other parts of the world may produce a much more severe disease (*eg, Ixodes holocyclus* in Australia) involving autonomic (cardiac, vascular) signs as well as somatic motor signs. Diagnosis is by finding a feeding female tick on the cat or suspicion of tick infestation, followed by rapid recovery in 1-3 days upon removal of the ticks. Affected cats should be sprayed thoroughly against ticks. Electromyography reveals depressed evoked muscle potentials and slowed transmission near or across the neuromuscular junction, with secondary reduction of acetylcholine release.

Polymyopathies

Polymyopathies are very rare in cats. A generalized, patchy, ossifying myositis in a cat has been described.[133] Generalized inflammatory disease of muscle (immune or idiopathic) is referred to as polymyositis. Slowly progressive muscle weakness (often episodic) and atrophy are the common signs. Muscle enzyme activity (CPK, SGOT, LDH) is often elevated, the electromyelogram is highly abnormal, and immune tests (antinuclear antibody, Coombs, lupus erythematosus preparation) may be abnormal. Muscle biopsy is diagnostic. Noninflammatory, nonneurogenic muscle degenerations may cause similar signs and may be called muscular dystrophies or idiopathic myopathies. Excessive use of corticosteroids can lead to a similar corticosteroid myopathy. They are diagnosed by electromyography and muscle biopsy.

References

1. Hoerlein, BF: Canine Neurology. WB Saunders, Philadelphia, 1978.
2. Fishman, RA. N Engl J Med **293** (1975) 706.
3. Clasen, RA *et al.* J Neurosurg **41**(1974) 576.
4. Tornheim, PA and McLaurin, RL. J Neurosurg **48** (1978) 220.
5. Wilkinson, H *et al.* J Neurosurg **34** (1971) 203.
6. Rosomoff, HL. Acta Anaesth Scand **Suppl 29** (1968) 75.
7. Parker, AJ. Am J Vet Res **34** (1973) 1523.
8. Kassell, NV *et al.* J Neurosurg **54** (1981) 615.
9. Garcia-Uria, J *et al.* J Neurosurg **54** (1981) 632.
10. Bradley, RL and Keating, ML. Fed Proc **9(3)** (1979) 26.
11. Kolata, RJ and Burrows, CF. JAAHA **17** (1981) 219.
12. Kornegay, JN. JAAHA **14** (1978) 580.
13. Brightman, AH *et al.* Fed Proc **7(6)** (1977) 23.
14. Mesfin, GM *et al.* JAVMA **176** (1980) 62.
15. Vandevelde, M and Braund, KG. Vet Path **16** (1979) 420.
16. Erlewein, DL. Fed Proc **11(2)** (1981) 16.
17. Lithander, A and Lithander, B. Acta Path Microbiol Scand **60** (1964) 117.
18. Penny, R *et al.* Br Vet J **123** (1967) 145.
19. Wilkinson, GT. J Sm Anim Pract **20** (1979) 749.
20. Rosenthal, JJ *et al.* JAAHA **17** (1981) 307.
21. Peiffer, RL. Feline Pract **9(4)** (1979) 24.
22. Campbell, KL *et al.* Feline Pract **10(3)** (1980) 28.
23. Kaplan, W. JAVMA **163** (1973) 1043.
24. Reif, JS. Comp Cont Educ Pract Vet **2** (1980) 810.
25. Feeney, DA *et al.* JAAHA **17** (1981) 311.
26. Petrak, M and Carpenter, J. JAVMA **146** (1965) 728.
27. Cusick, PK *et al.* JAAHA **12** (1976) 490.
28. Linquist, WD and Winters, KD. Feline Pract **11(2)** (1981) 37.
29. McKenzie, BE *et al.* JAVMA **172** (1978) 173.
30. Edney, AT. J Sm Anim Pract **10** (1969) 231.
31. Jubb, KV *et al.* J Comp Path **66** (1956) 217.
32. Loew, F *et al.* Can Vet J **11** (1970) 109.
33. Munday, BL and King, SJ. N Zeal Vet J **20** (1972) 80.
34. Glenn, B *et al.* Am J Vet Res **29** (1968) 1953.
35. Tobias, G. JAVMA **145** (1964) 462.
36. Vulgamott, JC *et al.* JAAHA **16** (1980) 915.
37. de Lahunta, A. Vet Clin No Am **10** (1980) 91.
38. Jolly, RD and Blakemore, WF. Vet Rec **92** (1973) 391.
39. Blakemore, WF. Vet Clin No Am **10** (1980) 81.
40. Wenger, DA *et al.* Science **208** (1980) 1471.
41. Blakemore, WF. J Comp Path **82** (1972) 179.
42. Murray, JA *et al.* J Sm Anim Pract **18** (1977) 1.
43. Haskins, ME *et al.* JAVMA **175** (1979) 384.
44. Langweiler, M *et al.* JAAHA **14** (1978) 748.
45. Cowell, KR *et al.* JAVMA **169** (1976) 334.
46. Percy, DH and Jortner, BS. Arch Path **92** (1971) 136.
47. Johnson, KH. JAVMA **157** (1970) 2057.
48. Chrisp, CE *et al.* JAVMA **156** (1970) 616.
49. Baker, HJ and Lensey, JR. Am J Path **74** (1974) 649.
50. Norby, DE and Thuline, HC. Nature **227** (1970) 1261.
51. Woodward, JC *et al.* Am J Path **74** (1974) 560.
52. Silson, M and Robinson, R. Vet Rec **84** (1969) 477.
53. Watson, ADJ. J Sm Anim Pract **22** (1981) 85.
54. Holliday, TA. Vet Clin No Am **1** (1971) 367.
55. Wilkinson, GT. Vet Rec **92** (1973) 510.
56. Henness, AM *et al.* JAVMA **171** (1977) 692.
57. Bedford, PG and Clarke, EG. Vet Rec **90** (1972) 53.
58. Brockis, DC. Vet Rec **83** (1968) 206.
59. Unwin, DD. Vet Rec **83** (1968) 552.
60. Fankhauser, R *et al.* Ann NY Acad Sci **127** (1965) 817.
61. de Lahunta, A: Veterinary Neuroanatomy and Clinical Neurology, WB Saunders, Philadelphia, 1977.
62. Kallfelz, FA *et al.* JAVMA **172** (1978) 589.
63. Zaki, FA and Nafe, LA. J Sm Anim Pract **21** (1980) 429.
64. Nafe, LA. JAVMA **174** (1979) 1224.
65. Luginbuhl, H. Am J Vet Res **22** (1961) 1030.
66. Barker, J and Greenwood, AG. J Sm Anim Pract **14** (1973) 15.
67. Meincke, J *et al.* JAVMA **160** (1972) 1093.
68. Fox, J *et al.* J Sm Anim Pract **14** (1973) 23.
69. Zaki, FA and Liu, SK. Vet Path **10** (1973) 232.
70. Zaki, FA and Hurvitz, AI. J Sm Anim Pract **17** (1976) 773.
71. Roye, OB *et al.* AJVR **34** (1973) 947.
72. Tobin, T *et al.* AJVR **34** (1973) 951.
73. Knecht, CD *et al.* JAVMA **162** (1973) 1052.
74. Hendricks, JC. JAVMA **178** (1981) 55.
75. Palmer, AC and Walker, RG. J Sm Anim Pract **11** (1970) 779.
76. Hossmann, KA and Sato, K. Science **168** (1970) 375.
77. O'Brien, SE *et al.* Vet Rec **107** (1980) 199.
78. Kneller, SK *et al.* J Sm Anim Pract **13** (1972) 595.
79. Bistner, S *et al.* JAVMA **157** (1970) 1220.
80. Berman, N and Cynader, M. J Physiol **224** (1972) 363.
81. Kalil, RE *et al.* Science **174** (1971) 302.
82. Leach, W. J Laryn Otol **76** (1962) 744.
83. Bamber, RC. J Genetics **27** (1933) 407.
84. Little, CC. Nature **133** (1934) 215.
85. Whiting, PW. J Exp Zool **25** (1918) 539.
86. Bosher, SK and Hallpike, CS. Proc Royal Soc **162B** (1965) 147.

87. Winston, J *et al.* Ann Otol Rhin Laryng **57** (1948) 738.
88. Winston, J *et al.* Ann Otol Rhin Laryng **62** (1953) 121.
89. Wehrung, GD, JAVMA **178** (1981) 153.
90. Parker, AJ and Smith, CW. Res Vet Sci **18** (1975) 110.
91. Smith, CW and Parker, AJ. Res Vet Sci **19** (1975) 224.
92. Parker, AJ and Smith, CW. Res Vet Sci **21** (1976) 246.
93. Parker, AJ and Smith, CW. Res Vet Sci **27** (1979) 253.
94. Swain, SF *et al.* Vet Surg **8** (1979) 119.
95. Teague, HD and Brasmer, TH. Am J Vet Res **39** (1978) 1584.
96. Albin, MS *et al.* J Neurosurg **29** (1968) 113.
97. Osterholm, JL. J Neurosurg **40** (1974) 5.
98. Seim, HB and Nafe, LA. JAAHA **17** (1981) 201.
99. Heavner, JE. JAVMA **159** (1971) 425.
100. King, AS and Smith, RN. Vet Rec **72** (1960) 381.
101. King, AS and Smith, RN. Acta Orthoped Scand **34** (1964) 139.
102. Stowater, JL *et al.* Feline Pract **8(1)** (1978) 26.
103. Norsworthy, GD. Feline Pract **9(1)** (1979) 39.
104. Vandevelde, M *et al.* Vet Path **13** (1976) 428.
105. Frye, FL and McFarland, LZ. JAVMA **146** (1965) 481.
106. Kerruish, DW. J Cat Genetics **1** (1964) 16.
107. Martin, HA. Vet Path **8** (1971) 232.
108. Frye, FL. JAAHA **3** (1967) 238.
109. Robinson, R: Genetics for Cat Breeders. Pergamon Press, Oxford, 1971.
110. Todd, NB. J Hered **55** (1964) 225.
111. Howell, J and Siegel, P. J Hered **57** (1966) 100.
112. Deforest, ME and Basrur, PK. Can Vet J **20** (1979) 304.
113. Dorn, AS and Joiner, RW. Feline Pract **6(6)** (1976) 40.
114. Segedy, AK *et al.* JAVMA **174** (1979) 510.
115. Leipold, HW. JAVMA **164** (1974) 520.
116. Field, B and Wanner, RA. Vet Rec **96** (1975) 42.
117. English, PB. J Sm Anim Pract **10** (1969) 207.
118. Seawright, A *et al.* J Comp Path **77** (1967) 29.
119. Beadman, RM *et al.* Vet Rec **76** (1964) 1005.
120. Read, RM and Smith, RN. J Sm Anim Pract **9** (1968) 159.
121. Northington, JW and Juliana, MM. J Sm Anim Pract **19** (1978) 409.
122. Luttgen, PJ *et al.* J Sm Anim Pract **21** (1980) 213.
123. O'Brien, DP *et al.* JAAHA **16** (1980) 497.
124. Evers, WH. JAVMA **152** (1968) 1671.
125. Schaer, M *et al.* JAVMA **174** (1979) 513.
126. Rendano, VT *et al.* JAAHA **16** (1980) 921.
127. Bright, RM *et al.* JAAHA **14** (1978) 612.
128. Killingsworth, C *et al.* JAAHA **13** (1977) 209.
129. Griffiths, IR and Duncan, ID. Vet Rec **104** (1979) 518.
130. Olmstead, ML and Butler, HC. J Sm Anim Pract **18** (1977) 247.
131. Dawson, JR. Vet Rec **86** (1970) 562.
132. Mason, KV. J Sm Anim Pract **17** (1976) 467.
133. Norris, AM *et al.* JAAHA **16** (1980) 659.

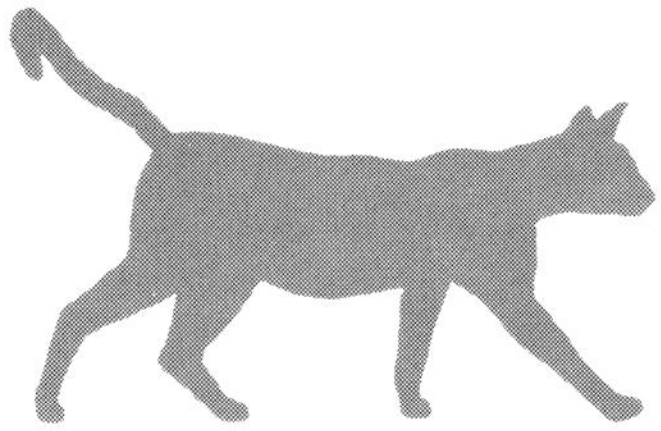

15 the reproductive system

E.D. COLBY AND B.S. STEIN

THE FEMALE REPRODUCTIVE TRACT

Hormonal Influences

Follicle-stimulating hormone (FSH) is released from the anterior hypothalamus after mating. The target organ of FSH is the ovary, where its action results in follicle growth and maturation. Rising serum levels of estrogen inhibit further release of FSH. In males, FSH induces cellular growth in the seminiferous tubules.

Luteinizing hormone (LH) is also produced by the anterior hypophysis and its release is probably regulated by LH-releasing hormone.[1] That it may be influenced by the estrogen feedback mechanism is not proven. The LH-releasing hormone causes release of high levels of LH in both estrous and anestrous cats and induces ovulation in estrous animals. It also maintains a significantly higher-than-normal level of LH in estrous cats, which has practical value for those practicing artificial induction of estrus and ovulation, as well as for purposes of ovulation during artificial insemination.

The primary source of progesterone is the corpus luteum of the ovary, with an additional source located in the placenta. The action of progesterone is primarily upon the uterine endothelium in preparation for implantation of the blastocyst and for maintenance of pregnancy. It is essentially antagonistic to estrogen in its action. Because of placental production of progesterone, queens may be ovariectomized after about 50 days of pregnancy without causing abortion due to a lack of progesterone.

The active estrogen compound in cats, 17-beta estradiol, originates within the ovary and is secreted into the ovarian follicle. It produces the physical, behavioral and cytologic characteristics of estrus in the queen. It sensitizes the smooth muscle of the reproductive tract, is essential for sperm transport and may be given in excess (exogenous estradiol cypionate) to prevent pregnancy immediately (see Mismating).

The Estrous Cycle

Domestic cats are seasonally polyestrous, with 2, or less commonly, 3 cycles per year.[2-5] Usually there are several estrous periods within each cycle, although there may be some variation among individuals, especially purebreds. Some differences also may be observed between the northern and southern latitudes of the US.

Anestrus

Anestrus is the quiescent phase of the estrous cycle. It usually occurs from mid- or late September to late December or early January. During this time females exhibit no reproductive activity or no associated reproductive behavior patterns. Anestrus may be identified by vaginal cytology. The anestrous state may be altered if animals have access to increasingly longer periods of artificial light of natural intensity over a period of weeks.[6,7]

Proestrus

This state represents a period of follicular growth and maturation as well as an increase in size and volume of the other reproductive organs. The ovary is under the influence of FSH from the anterior pituitary gland, and estrogen produced by the ovarian follicle is responsible for other reproductive organ changes.[8] Only rarely are behavioral changes associated with this phase of the cycle indicative of approaching estrus. Vaginal cytologic changes are significant as proestrus progresses. The true period of proestrus is thought to last only 3-5 days.

Estrus

The onset of estrus, signifying puberty, occurs at 5-9 months of age. Cats as young as 4 months, however, have shown signs of estrus and conceived. Some purebred cats, such as Persians, may be slow maturing and often do not have estrous cycles until they are 1-1½ years old. The time of year that sexual maturity is reached can influence the onset of estrus. Cats that mature in late fall may not show overt signs of estrus until spring, whereas cats maturing in the spring are often younger when they first show signs of estrus.

A study of ovarian and behavioral cyclicity in laboratory queens revealed that the mean length of estrus in nonovulating, mated ovulating and induced ovulating (HCG) cats was 5.8, 6.5 and 10 days, respectively.[9] Ovaries of cats showing no estrous behavior were also visually (laparoscopy) noted to have patterns of development and regression at 14- to 19-day intervals. It is significant that behavioral patterns alone are not always an indicator of ovarian cyclicity.

Laparoscopy is a technic by which the ovary and other abdominal organs may be visualized and photographed. It is relatively easy to perform, effective and done under light general anesthesia with ketamine.[10]

The common signs of estrus may be minimal during the first heat, and estrus may be brief. It is not unusual for a small amount of mucoid vulvar discharge to be present just before the first estrus. It should not prompt any therapy. Cats expecting their first estrus may be anorectic, withdrawn and easily excited due to normal hormonal effects.

The usual signs of estrus are behavioral and exhibited by posturing, frequent urination, vocalizing and other changes. There are very few, if any, external anatomic signs of estrus. There is rarely a vaginal discharge, although mucus is present in the vagina at this time. Cytologic examination of the vaginal epithelium reveals significant change (see Vaginal Cytology).

When handled, estrous queens often posture, roll over and not infrequently strike out at the handler. If the animal is patted or stroked in the region of the tailhead or the perineum, it arches its back and treads. Rough handling of the genital area can induce ovulation in the well-stimulated and fully estrous animal. Following handling of this type, estrous animals often roll over and exhibit postmating behavior. Some queens spray urine during this period; frequent urination or use of the litter box may resemble the behavior of cats with cystitis or the feline urologic syndrome.

In fully estrous queens, the rostral portion of the animal, in contrast to the rear quarters, is close to the floor, with the elbows and forelimbs down. When grasped by the scruff of the neck, estrous cats often posture in the mating position. Treading is common when estrous cats are handled in this manner.

When handled, cats in full estrus flag, *ie,* the tail is placed to one side to facilitate mounting and intromission by the male.

Coital Behavior: The female's acceptance of the male may be first expressed by rubbing her face and body against inanimate objects and then the male. The queen may twist and roll her body and turn her rear quarters toward the male, allowing him to approach and smell her. The tomcat may emit a characteristic mating call; it is unlike the harsh, unpleasant call of the female in estrus. After limited foreplay, the male attempts to mount the female and grasp her dorsal neck surface with his teeth. The female may tread with her rear legs as the male mounts. Intromission is accomplished after a few pelvic thrusts and ejaculation is almost immediate. Some males, if trained to mate when an estrous female is placed in their cage, may not release the neck after intromission and may mate again.

It is important to ensure that the animals are physically compatible and that the male can mate successfully when the neck is grasped. Pairing short-bodied males with long-bodied females, or vice versa, may cause the mating act to be prolonged or may interfere with it entirely. If the male trusts the handler, he may mount under adverse physical conditions without using the neck grasp.

Coitus is very brief, lasting 10 seconds, and may be repeated within 5-15 minutes. As the tomcat withdraws his penis from the female, she emits a characteristic cry, possibly induced by the pressure applied against the vaginal wall by the sharp, reversed spinal processes of the penis. Immediately after coitus, the female's pupils dilate widely and she springs away from the male and may attack him. She then rolls around on the ground several times, splays her forefeet, with the nails exposed, and kneads. Meanwhile, the male usually watches from a short distance. Postcoital behavior of the female also includes persistent licking and cleansing of the anogenital area.

The duration of estrus is variable. In the absence of a tomcat, estrus continues for 10-14 days and occasionally up to 3 weeks, and may recur again every 2-3 weeks. If a male cat is present and coitus occurs, estrus usually lasts 4-6 days, with the female being most likely to accept the male on the third and fourth days. Estrus may continue for 24 hours after coitus (related to the delay associated with ovulation), and then end fairly abruptly. The female usually accepts the male(s) for several breedings each day.

About 10% of pregnant queens display typical estrous behavior during the third and sixth weeks of gestation.[11] These pregnant queens copulate, which may result in superfetation.

Estrus during advancing age tends to be exhibited by irregularity of estrous cycles, with lengthened interestrus intervals. The numbers of maturing follicles diminish but old cats have produced live, vigorous young. By the same token, the incidence of fetal death, mummification and shortened pregnancies is more frequent in older cats. Based on the results of hormone studies, the optimum age for breeding is 1-7 years. Beyond 7 years of age, queens become more erratic in their response to administration of sex hormones.[12]

Queens should be taken to the cage or the environment of the male for mating. Queens in full estrus may terminate estrus if transported any distance, although the animal may cycle again in less than the normal 2-3 weeks.

Reproduction in female cats should be considered on an individual case basis. Case records of previous breeding history may be important in the determination of a breeding problem. Occasional females exhibit no external signs of heat, even when handled, and yet accept the male, conceive and carry a litter to term. Cycling may be influenced by environmental changes, such as introduction of another cat, territorial conflicts or a new owner. Certain males may not be acceptable to individual queens. In the latter case, if the queen can be handled easily, she may be grasped by the scruff of the neck and presented to the male in this manner. Experienced males successfully mount females so restrained. Females occasionally fight the male when placed together. This action may temporarily inhibit the male from mating; therefore, the cats should be observed closely during the first mating act if they are unfamiliar with each other.

Lack of the queen's receptivity of the male usually signals the end of estrus.

Induction of Estrus: Estrus must be induced with care. A complete history is necessary to include previous breeding experience and behavior, and environmental changes. A physical examination should be done to rule out the presence of infectious diseases, such as FeLV infection, FIP and hemobartonellosis. The animal should have current vaccinations and the nutritional status should be known.

Estrus may be induced by placing the queen with normal cycling females for 4-5 weeks. Occasionally, association with an experienced tom is enough to initiate cycling, although time must be allowed for estrus to occur. Illumination may be prolonged for up to 18 hours per day, although illumination for 14-16 hours per day is more commonly used. Use of prolonged illumination should be gradual and at least 50 days should be allowed for the effect to be successful. When using supplemental illumination, one must take into account the natural light available. Rheostatically controlled lights have been used to lengthen illumination as natural daylight fades.

Exogenous hormones may be given if psychologic and environmental stimuli do not induce estrus. It should be remembered that not all hormone preparations are approved for use in cats. Hormones should not be given to female cats under a year of age. It is preferable to ensure that thyroid activity is normal before instituting such therapy.

Administration of estrogens, such as 50 μg estradiol benzoate or 0.25 mg estradiol cypionate given IM and repeated in 48 hours, induces estrus in most cats.[13,14] Because excessive use of estrogens may induce a toxic state, no more than 8 mg of estradiol cypionate equivalent should be used within a 4-month period.

Cats are also one of the few animals in which a single injection of testosterone (20 mg testosterone propionate given IM) initiates estrus.[13] Estrus usually occurs within 2-5 days after administration of either estrogen or testosterone and persists 2-4 weeks, unless mating occurs.

Estrus initiated with estradiol benzoate, estradiol cypionate, testosterone or stilbestrol does not induce ovarian follicle production as they do not act directly on the ovary. Pregnant mare serum gonadotropin (PMSG) (Gestyl:Organon Labs) and FSH (FSH-P:Burns-Biotec) act directly on the ovary to cause follicle production.

Estrus may be induced by the use of PMSG, which is primarily follicle-stimulating in character but may have some luteinizing activity, and by use of FSH, which is derived from pituitary gland material and is reportedly free of LH contamination.[12] Follicle-stimulating hormone has been approved for cats but PMSG has not.

Pregnant mare serum gonadotropin acts directly on the ovary to induce follicle growth. The amount needed varies with the season and whether or not the cat is or has been cycling. A dose of 100 IU is given IM on the first day, followed by 50 IU on each succeeding day. The animal should be handled daily to facilitate identification of early estrous behavior, at which time the dosage is reduced or administration is stopped. As estrous behavior begins to manifest itself, the queen is placed with the male; if she is not receptive, additional PMSG is given. It usually takes 7 days for mating behavior to appear and for the queen to be receptive to the male. The drug should not be given for more than 8 days since excessive PMSG may cause superovulation and subsequent problems during gestation.

This method has been used successfully in several laboratory breeding situations over a period of years and in cats that have failed to cycle. There is a tendency for PMSG to produce excessive numbers of follicles in animals during their first estrus or in animals less than a year of age. This therapy appears to work best in queens that previously have cycled and been bred.

Follicle-stimulating hormone has been used to induce estrus, with a dose of 2 mg/day until estrus is observed.[15,16] It usually takes 5 days to induce estrus but may take longer if the FSH is given during the animal's anestrous season. A single IM dose of 50-100 IU of LH should be given at mating. Use of FSH induces maturation of 3-5 ova.

Control of Estrus: There is no licensed chemical method of estrus control for cats.[17] Megestrol acetate (Ovaban:Schering) has been used experimentally at a dose of 5 mg daily PO until estrus ceases, followed by 5 mg weekly for 10 weeks.[18] There have been no significant problems associated with return to estrus after megestrol use. The mechanism is thought to be negative-feedback suppression of pituitary gonadotropins. Megestrol acetate has a half-life of 8 days in dogs and may have a similar half-life in cats.

Mibolerone, an anabolic androgen, has been used to control feline estrus by administration of 50 μg daily for 180 days.[19,20] Although treated queens returned to estrus, there were some undesirable side effects.

Many other hormones have been studied for their effects of estrus suppression.[21-27]

The advent of the radioimmunoassay for the study of reproductive hormones has led to an increasing number of articles on circulating levels of estrogen, progesterone, LH and testosterone in domestic cats.[28-31] These hormones have been studied in relation to estrus and the associated behavioral and vaginal cytologic changes during polyestrus, pregnancy and pseudopregnancy and in relation to specific changes associated with the reproductive organs.

Suppression of Estrus: Estrus has been supressed in cats by a variety of means.[32-35] However, many of the drugs used are not approved for use in cats. Before any such activity is initiated, the owner must be advised of possible side effects. Subsequent estrual periods may be delayed for extended periods. The animal must be closely followed clinically while under such treatment; owner cooperation is essential. Side effects include prolonged anestrus, hydrometra, chronic endometritis, cystic endometrial hyperplasia, pyometra, mammary neoplasia and stillbirths. Such an impressive list of undesirable complications does not indicate that in every case such treatment fails but should be a reminder that this type of therapy has not been thoroughly investigated.

Testosterone has been used experimentally to suppress estrus when given before the onset of true estrus.[36] However, use of this hormone is contraindicated because of its secondary masculinizing effects and the unpredictability of subsequent estrous cycles.

Pilocarpine has been used orally in a 1% solution to suppress estrus. However, use of pilocarpine in this manner induces considerable salivation. Its mechanism of action is not understood. Many treated cats have delayed cycles and some have failed to cycle after treatment.

Postpartum Estrus: Postpartum estrus is rare in domestic queens. However, enough queens have been found pregnant at ovariohysterectomy 3-4 weeks postpartum to make the condition a reality.[5] Queens have exhibited signs of estrus from 18-36 hours after parturition to 7-10 days later.[26,37] This variance in the observation of estrous behavior may be due to more than one estrual cycle during the lactation period. Early removal of nursing kittens usually results in estrus recurring in 3-4 weeks.[38,39]

Metestrus

The metestrous period varies among queens during the regular estrous season. This period is one of aloofness from the male and not characterized by estrous behavior. Cytologic examination of vaginal smears reflects changes associated with metestrus (see Vaginal Cytology). This period is followed by proestrus and recycling or by anestrus.

Vaginal Cytology

Two technics are routinely used to obtain cells from the epithelium of the vaginal wall: the swab technic and use of a short-tipped medicine dropper.[5,40,41] Regardless of the technic used, procedures to obtain material for vaginal cytologic examination induce ovulation after 24 hours in most queens.

The materials used must be sterile. The cotton swab is moistened with a few drops of normal saline and inserted through the vaginal opening. Contact with clitoral fossa during insertion is preferred but not easily accomplished in most estrous cats. The swab is gently rotated and then removed. It is then rolled gently on a clean microscope slide, which is then air dried and stained. The amount of saline on the swab influences the number of cells retained; excessive saline produces fewer cells.

The medicine dropper technic is essentially the same. A few drops of sterile saline are taken into the tip of the dropper, which is inserted into the vagina. The rubber bulb is then squeezed several times to expel and agitate the saline solution. The solution is then taken back into the dropper and the dropper tip removed from the vagina. The material is then placed on a glass slide, which is air dried before staining. This method of obtaining vaginal epithelial cells almost always induces ovulation. When the dropper is withdrawn from a cat in full estrus, the cloudiness (cellular debris) of the saline often indicates estrus to the trained observer.

Only the surface epithelial cells are required when making a vaginal smear. Violent agitation with the swab or medicine dropper causes sloughing of the underlying epithelium, which could result in error in proper diagnosis of the exact stage of the estrous cycle.

The most commonly used stain is Wright's stain. The smear may be treated the same as a blood smear with regard to the staining process. The smears should be dried in a dust-free area and preferably in a covered environment. The smear may be microscopically examined while wet or dry after staining. Other stains occasionally are used but cellular detail is best with Wright's stain.

Proestrus is recognized by a mixture of basal and epithelial cells. The nucleus is prominent and the nucleus:cytoplasm (N:C) ratio is 1:1 or greater. As the full estrous state is approached, the epithelial cells tend to enlarge, the nucleus becomes smaller and more pyknotic, and the proportion of nucleus to cytoplasm is less. Cellular debris often is noted during proestrus and is recognized as debris with no particular staining characteristics or cellular morphology. Sheets of cells occasionally are observed when the method of obtaining the smear has been excessively rough.

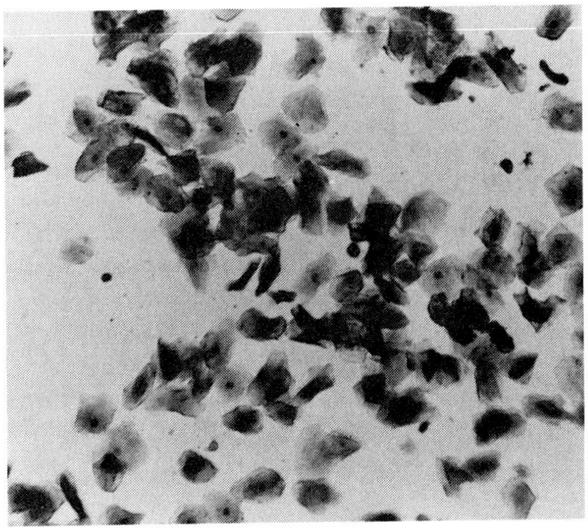

Fig. 1. Estrous vaginal smear stained with Wright's stain. Note the pyknotic nuclei, irregular cell shapes and the low nucleus:cytoplasm ratio.

An estrous smear contains predominantly cells with pyknotic nuclei, with a N:C ratio such as 1:6 or 1:10 (Fig 1). The edges of the cells often are curled and irregular.[42] The staining characteristics of the cytoplasm of these cells are almost negligible. Occasional blood cells are observed, but an abundance of them indicates rough handling during the swabbing technic.

Cornified cells, with a ragged, indistinct cytoplasmic outline, are still present during the first few days of metestrus; this is followed by the appearance of WBC, bacteria and nucleated epithelial cells.[43] The presence of large vacuoles within nucleated epithelial cells 3-4 days after copulation may be diagnostic of pregnancy but cannot be identifed accurately.[44]

Anestrus is characterized by the presence of mainly small, dark-staining nucleated epithelial cells with smooth, usually oval borders. Amorphous material, noncellular debris and polymorphonuclear WBC, the number of which is probably related to the vaginal bacterial flora, may also be found.

The relatively short duration of proestrus, estrus and metestrus in cats necessitates serial examinations of vaginal smears. The numbers of cell types are only relative.

In a study of the vaginal epithelial cycle in estrous laboratory cats, the length of the estrous cycle was greatest in the spring, with the shortest period occurring in the fall or late estrous cycle.[41] The number of estrous cycles per year ranges from 4 to 25, with an average of 13. The estrous vaginal smear exhibited the same seasonal variation. Considering the known variations in estrogen surges during a given cycle, the variation in estrous smears and the number of periods per year, and the varying length of the cycle with a given season, it is important to use more than one criterion to determine the true estrous period of female cats.

Ovulation

Ovulation in cats is a reflex act, mainly neuronal in nature. Release of LH from the anterior pituitary gland lasts only a matter of hours. Release of LH causes production of estrogen within the ovarian follicle, which results in rupture and release of the ovum about 24 hours after mating.[4,5,43,45,46] The cat is thus termed a reflex or postcoital ovulator. Denervation of the vagina and uterus, followed by coital stimulation, has provided further proof that ovulation occurs only after mating.

Ova are fertilized in the proximal third (nearest the ovary) of the oviduct. The fertilized ova reach the uterus on the fifth or sixth day after ovulation.[43] Implantation occurs 11-14 days after ova release. Secretions of the uterus apparently nourish the blastocyst before implantation.

An average of 4 eggs is discharged at each ovulation; they lose their ability to be fertilized within 24 hours after ovulation.[47]

There is no regular alternation in functioning of the ovaries.

After ovulation, there is no hemorrhage in the follicular cavity but the follicular wall becomes deeply invaginated.[48] Activity of the corpora lutea due to the effect of LH is immediate. The corpora lutea that form after ovulation reach their maximum size (0.3 cm) at about 17-21 days, after which there is a natural regression until about days 40-44 of pregnancy, at which time they cease to function. Removal of the ovaries before this time results in abortion; removal after 50 days' gestation often results in no interruption of pregnancy.

Ovulation may be induced by vaginal stimulation with a glass rod, coitus with a vasectomised male and rarely by the stimulation of handling, *ie,* grasping behind the neck and manipulation of the genital area. Older nulliparous cats may rarely ovulate spontaneously.

Implantation of the trophoblast into the endometrial lining begins about day 13 after coitus and is fully underway by day 14.[49]

Mismating

Abortifacients have been used in female cats but few are approved for clinical use.[50] If such drugs are used, they should be handled with extreme care and the owner advised of the side effects. A single IM dose of only 250 μg (0.25 mg) estradiol cypionate (ECP:Upjohn) given 40 hours postcoitus prevents pregnancy by blocking the entry of the fertilized ovum into the uterus in what is known as tubal blocking.[43] It has also been used, in a limited study, up to 14 days after initial coitus, after entry of the ovum into the uterus. A serious side effect of estradiol cypionate is continued estrous behavior. Another complication can be pyometra as a result of continuous cervical distension and ascending bacterial infection during estrus.

Repository stilbestrol (2 mg) has also been used IM on the second or third day after coitus, with the same dose repeated on the seventh to tenth day. Signs of estrus are prolonged as with the use of estradiol cypionate.

Use of hormones as abortifacients in cats is not recommended if the time of uterine implantation has passed. There have been no studies to support this type of endeavor. Two 10-mg doses of repository stilbestrol, given IM 10 days apart, may prevent implantation, as does estradiol cypionate, with all of the undesirable side effects of continuous estrus. Normal recycling may be delayed as a result of the continued high level of circulating estrogen.

False Pregnancy

In the absence of coitus, there is no luteal phase in the feline estrous cycle. If a sterile mating occurs, ovulation is induced, corpora lutea form and endometrial changes similar to those in pregnancy develop.[51] Unlike in a normal pregnancy, the corpora lutea persist for only 20 days and then regress. The signs of most false pregnancies (pseudocyesis) subside after 37 days and are rarely seen 45 days after copulation.[38] Depending on the season of the year, cats may show signs of estrus within a week after regression of the corpora lutea.

Mammary changes associated with pseudocyesis, more prominent in other species, are rarely noted in cats. Parturient behavior also is not observed.

Hormonal therapy seldom is necessary due to the early decrease in corpus luteum activity. If indicated, respository testosterone (1 mg/lb) or repository stilbestrol (0.25 mg/lb) can be administered and repeated if necessary after a week. If the psychologic manifestations are severe, mild tranquilization may help.

Some animals in pseudopregnancy may gain weight. On palpation the uterus feels enlarged and doughy until about day 35. The enlargement is consistent with that of pregnancy but without the resiliency of the pregnant uterus.

PREGNANCY

The normal gestation period of cats is 58-70 days, with 63-65 days the standard.[37] Larger breeds often have a gestation period closer to 70 days.[52] Kittens born before 58 days' gestation have little chance of survival. Siamese, Abyssinians and certain females of any breed may have extended gestation periods.

The first day of mating usually is considered the first day of pregnancy. This date often is not known in free-ranging cats and can only be determined with some accuracy among cat breeders. Cats with exceptionally large litters, of perhaps 8 or more kittens, may have slightly shortened gestation periods, but this has not been well documented. This usually occurs among free-ranging cats in which the date of the first mating is not known. Nutrition and stress during first-time pregnancy also may have considerable bearing on the length of gestation.

Pregnancy Diagnosis

Early signs (1-3 weeks) of pregnancy include partial anorexia, decreased activity, occasional mild vomiting, and withdrawal from people and other cats. Many cats do not display any such signs and remain normal in all respects.

There may be changes in the nipples about 16 days after mating, especially in primiparous cats. The nipples become more prominent, darker pink and more erect than in unbred females.

The most significant and reliable means of pregnancy diagnosis is by palpation and radiographic examination. Palpation may be done as early as 14 days by experienced clinicians. By 17 days even inexperienced examiners may palpate the fetuses as firm uterine enlargements about 1.5-2 cm in diameter.

At 21 days the uterus has begun to elongate but is still fairly firm and readily palpable. By 25 days the fetuses are fully formed; caution must be used during palpation at this time. Rough handling may damage the fetus severely enough to result in death and resorption. Abortion rarely occurs unless most of the fetuses have been damaged.

Between 25 and 45 days, the fetuses may not be palpable and the enlarged uterus is doughy in consistency. At about 45 days, when the uterus has become the sole support of progesterone to sustain pregnancy, the fetal heads may be felt.

The usual procedure for palpation is to place the thumb and middle finger together over the spinous processes and slowly withdraw them to the floor of the abdomen while holding the animal by the scruff of the neck with the other hand. After the rectum slips through the fingers, the body of the uterus may be identified and the horns may be followed from this point. The uterus is turgid during estrus and does not become firm until about day 14 of gestation. The ovaries are rarely palpable and there is no reason to attempt to do so as they are small and easily damaged.

Radiographic determination of pregnancy may be made after 35-38 days of gestation.[53] As in other species, exposure to x-rays during the first third of pregnancy should be avoided due to possible teratologic effects. The crown-rump fetal dimensions on radiographs can be used to determine fetal age. Finally, the appearance of various areas of ossification on radiographs can also be used to estimate fetal age (Table 1).[53]

Another method of pregnancy diagnosis is by ultrasonography.[15] This technic identified the fetal pulse and placental blood flow after the fourth week of gestation but the number of fetuses could not be determined.

Due to the extremely low levels of chorionic gonadotropins in blood and urine, early verification of feline pregnancy by laboratory analysis has not been accomplished.

Table 1. Time of Ossification of Various Fetal Tissues [46]

Day 38:	Mandible, frontal, maxillary and parietal bones, scapula, femur vertebrae, ribs
Day 41:	Radius, ulna
Day 43:	Tibia, fibula, ilium, ischium, occipital bone
Day 47:	Interparietal bones
Day 49:	Metacarpals, metatarsals
Day 52:	Sternebrae, phalanges
Day 53:	Entire digits, fibular tarsal bone, tympanic bullae
Day 56:	Molars in alveoli, tibial tarsal bone

It is possible to estimate the age of kittens from the neonatal period through a year of age by observing the appearance and fusion of ossification centers.[54,55]

Hemogram During Pregnancy

A mild degree of normocytic normochromic anemia occurs during the last third of pregnancy in cats. The decreased RBC count, hemoglobin concentration and PCV return to normal within a week after parturition. There is little variation during lactation. Reticulocytosis, in response to anemia, is normal in late pregnancy; reticulocyte numbers begin to decrease and return to normal within 24 hours after parturition. Leukocyte counts, both total and differential, as well as total plasma protein level, remain constant during pregnancy and lactation.[56]

Superfecundation

Superfecundation refers to fertilization of separate ova by sperm cells of different males during the same estrous period. After initial coitus induces ovulation, liberated ova not immediately fertilized remain viable for several hours and may be fertilized in subsequent matings.

Superfecundation is not unusual in cats, especially if the female is allowed to roam. The queen may allow multiple matings by several tomcats during the peak of estrus. The resulting pregnancy can include fetuses of different male parentage.

Superfetation

Superfetation refers to development of 2 or more fetuses of different ages due to separate matings during different estrous periods (Fig 2).[47,57] Although the incidence of superfetation is low, it is most common in cats. Histologic verification is the most reliable means of differentiating between early maceration and superfetation, especially since a dead fetus can remain in the uterus for several days with only minimal deterioration. When 2 full-term kittens were born to a queen 13 days after parturition of other full-term kittens, laparotomy helped verify the case as one of superfetation. One uterine horn had undergone involution and the other horn was larger and contained 2 implantation sites. Likewise, the ovary on the side of the larger uterine horn had corpora lutea, while the other ovary did not.

The exact mechanism by which superfetation occurs is not known, but the following conjecture is offered. Insufficient progesterone production by the corpora lutea may allow some activity of FSH and subsequent formation of mature follicles. As cats can have coitus up to 6 weeks after conception, ovulation may thus be induced. Sensitization of the uterus, either due to the existing pregnancy or the hormonal influence of ovulation and fertilization, then enables implantation and embryonic development.

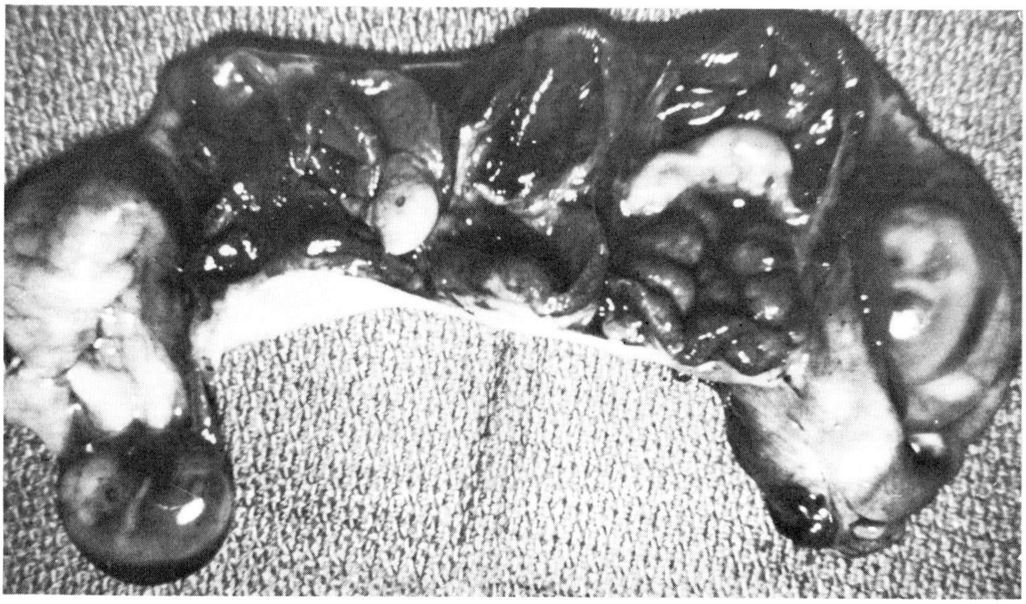

Fig 2. Uterus with hyperplastic endometritis. The 2 fetuses at the ends of the horns were viable and had intact fetal membranes. The 2 fetuses located centrally were necrotic and had no fetal membranes.

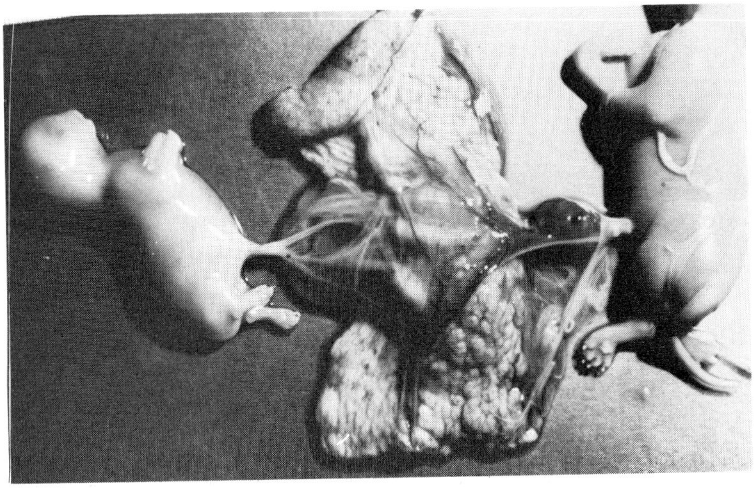

Fig 3. Synchorial littermates. The kitten on the left died at about 35 days. The kitten on the right, with an inguinal hernia, was alive when taken at 42 days.

Superovulation

Superovulation refers to ovulation of a greater-than-normal number of ova after copulation. The average number of ova shed during a normal estrous cycle is thought to be 4-7. Superovulation can be a natural as well as an induced phenomenon and is most commonly recognized at parturition by superfetation.

Superovulation usually results in fetal deaths at various times during gestation. As maceration is slow to occur *in utero,* the age of the fetuses may be fairly accurately determined. What initiates the death at various ages is not known. It may be related to overcrowding, unavailability of nutrition, uterine distension or other factors. Disease usually is not a consideration when fetuses of this type are born.

Use of exogenous hormones to induce estrus may result in superovulation if they are given in excessive amounts without regard to the activity of the recipient female or if they are not given according to a predetermined dosage schedule.

Twinning

Twinning probably occurs in domestic cats but evidence for positive identification of this phenomenon is lacking. Cats are polyovulatory and thus the chance for twinning is increased. To prove this in neonatal kittens requires genetic studies of the chromosomes of animals in any given litter. Coat color is not a sufficient criterion for distinguishing twinning.[58] Cases of possible twinning usually are observed at necropsy or cesarean section.

Twinning commonly is characterized by one zonary placenta containing 2 fetuses. The fetuses may be contained in the same amniotic sac or 2 sacs may have fused together early in embryonic life. The chorions usually are separate, as is the blood supply. Fetuses that share the same blood supply are called synchorial littermates.[59] If observed in late gestation, one or both will be dead and their different size indicates different survival times (Fig 3). Both may be the same size if observed at 25-30 days. The fact that 2 fetuses are in the same placental sac does not indicate they are monozygotic twins.

Polyovular follicles, *ie,* those containing more than one ovum, are not uncommon in cats.[60] Perhaps if more ovaries were observed histologically after ovariohysterectomy, more polyovular follicles would be noted. Such follicles have 1-3 ova in the antrum. There is no known relationship between polyovular follicles and twinning. Prepubertal histologic examination of the ovary reveals up to 6 layers of closely packed primordial cells that later develop into mature ova. This primordial crowding may result in polyovular follicles as the individual follicles mature and expand.

Ectopic Pregnancy

Ectopic or extrauterine pregnancy is being observed more commonly in cats.[61-63] It may occur as a primary circumstance, in which the fertilized ovum is released into the abdominal cavity, or as a secondary condition, in which the uterus has ruptured and the fetus continues its growth outside the confines of the uterus.[64]

Extrauterine implantation occurs most commonly on the peritoneum but may also occur on the mesentery. The usual limiting factor to continued growth is the blood supply as the fetus may be walled off and have the radiographic appearance of an abnormal growth. Bony material may be observed within these structures or free within the queen's abdominal cavity. The queen's abdominal cavity may contain a brownish fluid as a result of the maceration process.

Abdominal enlargement may not be significant if intrauterine or other ectopic fetuses are not present. The first sign of ectopic pregnancy may be onset of estrus during what would appear to be mid-gestation or at the time of expected parturition. Occasionally such masses are palpated incidentally during routine physical examination of free-ranging cats.

Secondary ectopic pregnancy has been diagnosed up to 18 months after ovariohysterectomy. During surgical manipulation of a recently bred cat, the ova could conceivably be released into the abdominal cavity and continue to grow for a limited time within the omental tissue. For this reason, ovariohysterectomy should be delayed until after implantation (at least 14 days postcoitus) to prevent possible release of ova into the abdominal cavity.[43,65]

Prebreeding and Early Pregnancy Examination

One of the important aspects of feline reproduction is a thorough prebreeding examination. This procedure should be a part of the routine preventive medicine program. The history is perhaps the most important item and should include genetic background as well as parental and individual breeding performance.

Cats of indeterminate age occasionally are presented for examination. In such cases the age can be estimated by assessing the numbers and positions of the teeth.[66]

A history of reproductive performance should include frequency of estrus, behavior before, during and after the estrous cycle, mating characteristics, number of previous litters, number of kittens produced, number of stillbirths or other abnormal fetuses, parturition sequence and postpartum complications. Attention should also be given to the start of the next estrous cycle after weaning of the kittens.

The physical examination should include palpation of the uterine horns and body, and palpation and inspection of the mammary tissue, nipples and external genitalia. Laboratory tests should include a CBC, and FeLV and FIP testing. An attempt should be made to examine the vagina. A smear indicates the cellular detail of the epithelial lining (see Vaginal Cytology).

Dietary habits should be noted and vaccinations updated. The presence of other household animals should be raised with respect to their health status and contact with the queen. When problems arise with other cats in the household, it may be advisable to segregate the queen during pregnancy and lactation. Male cats other than the selected sire should be removed or the queen isolated. It should be remembered that the estrous cycle lasts several days and that post-implantation estrus can occur in some animals. Keeping the owner informed about the process of feline reproduction saves considerable time should a problem arise. The date of the first mating should be recorded. Parasitic examination should be done and treatment given, if necessary, before breeding and parturition.

Pregnancy examination should be performed 17-21 days after the first mating. The fetuses are palpable at this time, although this method of diagnosis is not infallible. Radiographic diagnosis of pregnancy also may not be 100% accurate at this early stage.

Late Pregnancy Examination

A second or late pregnancy examination is not always necessary unless requested by the owner or the animal has a history of dystocia or abortion. Such an examination should be performed about the eighth week of pregnancy. The queen's abdomen can be radiographically examined at this time. A lateral or ventrodorsal view alone should not be used to count the number of fetuses, especially if many are present. Both views should be obtained to be reasonably sure of the number involved.

It may be advisable to have the owner clip the perineal hair before parturition, especially in long-haired breeds.

Complications of Pregnancy

Abortion

Expulsion of a fetus before the completion of normal gestation and before viability can be maintained is a common complication of feline pregnancy. Abortion may terminate the pregnancy before it is even suspected or confirmed. Kittens born before 8 weeks of gestation rarely survive; births between 55 and 60 days are considered premature but survival is possible. Causes of abortion in cats may be classified as noninfectious or infectious.

Noninfectious Causes: These causes of abortion include trauma, nutritional imbalances before or during pregnancy, physical abnormalities of the genital tract, acute or chronic illness not specifically related to pregnancy, psychologic disturbances, especially in response to stress or changes in environment, exposure to toxins, abnormalities of the fetuses or placenta, and endocrine deficiencies.[67]

Repeated abortions, especially if they occur at nearly the same stage of gestation, may be caused by improper development or premature regression of the corpora lutea of pregnancy. Treatment consists of IM administration of repository progesterone (*eg*, Depo-Provera:Upjohn), at 0.5-1.0 mg/lb, beginning 7-10 days before the time of previous abortions and repeated at weekly intervals until 5-7 days before the anticipated date of parturition. Overdosage of progesterone may result in masculinization of female kittens and prolonged gestation, thus requiring cesarean section.[68]

Elimination of other common causes of abortion, both infectious and noninfectious, should precede hormonal therapy. If a queen has a history of 2 abortions, one at 28 days of gestation and the other at 45 days, the cause probably is not hormonal since endocrine-related abortions recur at almost the same time in each pregnancy.

Infectious Causes: There are a variety of infectious causes of abortion, premature birth and stillbirth. The history may incriminate something other than an infectious cause for the problem. Superfetation and superfecundation, in which young may be delivered undeveloped and in a macerated state, have made owners fear something is wrong with the queen.

Bacterial infections of the uterus are mostly due to coliforms, especially *E coli* and to a lesser extent staphylococci and streptococci.[69] These organisms may not interfere with estrus, conception or early pregnancy unless they are present as the result of a previous pyometra and thus could interfere with conception and early pregnancy if the uterine endothelium has been damaged by the bacterial invasion and subsequent treatment. *Salmonella choleraesuis* has caused abortion in cats.[70] Some investigators believe cats are refractory to natural infections of *Brucella* spp.[71]

Toxoplasmosis rarely causes abortion in cats. Because controlled experiments involving pregnant cats and natural or artificial infection with *Toxoplasma gondii* have not been performed, abortion due to toxoplasmosis can only be assumed to happen on the basis of clinical observation. It is not known if the disease must be in the acute stage in the pregnant queen or if the queen may be chronically infected after implantation and asymptomatic, or merely shedding occysts for the organism to cause abortion.[72-75]

Toxoplasmosis should be considered when enzootic abortion cannot be attributed to other causes. Paired serum samples obtained 14-21 days apart, together with a history of the abortion sequence, should be submitted for determination of *Toxoplasma* titers by the Sabin-Feldman dye test or the indirect fluorescent antibody technic. The titers of both samples should be compared on the basis of the same serologic examination. A 3- or 4-fold rise in titer is considered presumptive evidence of active infection. A single titer should not be correlated with a clinical illness.

Antibodies to toxoplasmosis develop slowly in cats in comparison with other species. Clinical toxoplasmosis may be present in young cats with no identifiable titers. Affected kittens may die with only very low titers. The presence of antibody suggests the cat may be immune, whereas a lack of antibody usually indicates the cat is susceptible to toxoplasmosis and is likely to shed oocysts if infected. During the period when affected cats shed infectious feces, serologic tests usually are negative.

Fecal specimens should be submitted for examination and identification of *Toxoplasma* oocysts. Oocysts may be identified in the feces but must be differentiated from those of coccidians, namely *Isospora felis* and *I rivolta*.[76,77] *Toxoplasma* oocysts are 10-12 μ in diameter, whereas oocysts of the coccidian *I rivolta* are 20-25 μ in diameter.

Transplacental transmission of toxoplasmosis has not been documented in cats. As carnivorism is the most common means of infection in domestic cats, in the absence of proven transplacental transmission, kittens probably are only infected when they are fed rodents by the queen as the kittens reach weaning age.

Queens that are positive or have questionable titers should not be bred and should be eliminated from the colony. It is not known if immunity subsequent to infection is sufficient to protect the fetuses of future pregnancies.

More details on toxoplasmosis are found in Chapter 4 and in 2 review articles.[78,79]

Many viruses cause abortion or fetal death with or without expulsion. Inoculation of panleukopenia virus into susceptible pregnant cats produced abortion, mummification and stillbirths.

Feline rhinotracheitis virus (FVR), a herpesvirus, causes abortion. Intranasal or IV inocu-

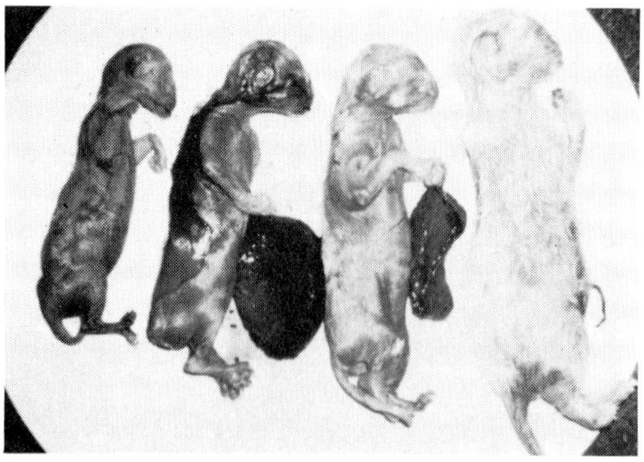

Fig 4. Litter of mummified fetuses delivered by a queen inoculated with panleukopenia virus during pregnancy. (Courtesy of Dr F.W. Scott)

lation of pregnant queens with FVR virus during the sixth week of gestation resulted in abortion, dead fetuses and placental lesions.[80-82] Intranasal inoculation produced abortion within 2-3 weeks, although FVR virus could not be isolated from the fetuses or placental lesions. Intravenous inoculation of FVR virus produced detectible virus particles in the uterus, placenta, amniotic fluid and vagina. This suggests that viral-induced placental lesions may lead to abortion or fetal death. Unvaccinated cats naturally infected with FVR usually abort the fetus and placenta intact. The fetuses appear about 40 days of age, according to crown-rump distances, and the placentas are mottled. There is almost always vulvar bleeding but never to the point where corrective measures are required.

There is no indication that feline picornavirus infection produces abortion. This is also true for other members of the feline respiratory disease complex. Debilitation of pregnant females may cause abortion regardless of the viral agent present. Some agents, viral, bacterial or other, may thus indirectly contribute to fetal death.

Feline leukemia virus has been responsible for fetal death, perhaps because it prevents implantation. The virus has been isolated from the endometrium of queens infected with FeLV.[83]

Feline T-strain mycoplasmas have been incriminated as a cause of abortion.[84] When *Mycoplasma gatae* was inoculated into pregnant cats during various stages of pregnancy, some cats aborted and some carried to term. All kittens died and the organism could be isolated from the kittens. The queens were febrile, anorectic, listless and dehydrated, and one died after abortion. The fact that mycoplasmas have been incriminated as a cause of abortion should indicate the need for bacteriologic testing for *Mycoplasma*. Abortion should not be attributed to other more common causes.

Attempts to culture an infectious agent may be unrewarding in queens that habitually abort during the third or fourth week of pregnancy. Some of these animals have multifocal placental necrosis, beginning with the syncytial trophoblastic cells and extending throughout the labyrinth. This type of abortion resembles that caused by certain viruses (herpesvirus), but no viruses were isolated from many affected cats.

Kitten Mortality Complex/ Fading Kitten Syndrome

This problem continues to be an enigma. The role of FIP virus in the kitten mortality complex has been studied. However, FIP virus has not been substantiated as the cause of all facets of the kitten mortality complex. In studies of breeder colonies and of feline research colonies in which cats have died from FIP or had antibody titers to the virus, the problem was first observed as reproductive failures or kitten mortality. Interestingly, virus isolations from affected kittens and adults revealed no cytopathic viruses.

The reproductive failures associated with the kitten mortality complex range from repeat breedings, fetal resorption at 4-6 weeks, abortions during the last half of gestation, stillbirths and congenital malformation.[85]

Fading kittens often are born underweight (normal birthweight is about 90 g for females and 100 g for males). They may appear emaciated and fail to nurse or have any significant vitality. Conversely, they may be born normal in appearance and live normally for a few days or even weeks before dying without apparent cause. Kittens that live for more than a few days have a rather rapid downhill course and become anorectic, depressed and dehydrated.

Acute congestive cardiomyopathy, with severe dyspnea, cyanosis and subsequent death, may affect kittens that have lived for days or weeks. The percentage of kittens that may die with this condition is not known nor are there data for a conclusion to be drawn relative to percentage of deaths from acute congestive cardiomyopathy.

In a kitten mortality survey of 3468 kittens in 790 litters, 10.2% were stillborn, of which two-thirds were males.[86] Of the remaining 3116 kittens born alive, 6.7% died within 24 hours, 3.6% died within 48 hours, 4.9% died by the end of 7 days and 34% died before a year of age. Malformations occurred in 6.8% of the kittens and abortions in 17 of the queens. Fetal resorption was reported in 6 instances. The greatest num-

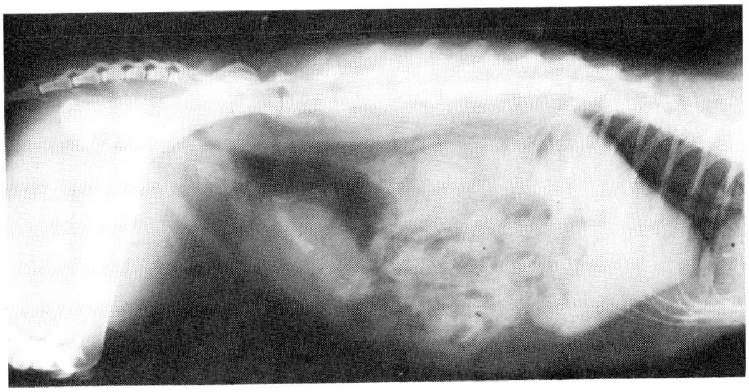

Fig 5. Lateral radiograph of a pregnant queen reveals advanced fetal maceration.

ber of abortions occurred during the seventh and eighth weeks of pregnancy. Attempts were not made to account for the cause of the kitten deaths.

Fetal Mummification

The occurrence of fetal mummification in cats is second only to that in cattle. Papyraceous mummification of a fetus can occur at any time during gestation and may involve only one fetus while the others develop normally. The dead fetus slowly dehydrates and the fetal membranes become closely wrapped around the fetus so they are almost indistinguishable from the fetus.[87] There is no placental hemorrhage or active infection and no signs are exhibited by the queen.

The mummified fetus may be expelled along with viable kittens at term, go unnoticed and may be consumed by the female, or be readily identified among placental tissue and other debris (Fig 4). More than one mummified fetus may be delivered at term or a single mummified fetus may be the only result of the pregnancy. Depending upon the stage of fetal development at which death occurs, the fetus may be expelled or resorbed.

Mummification may be induced by uterine torsion or some other means that limits the blood supply to a portion of the uterus.[87] Mummified fetuses may also be found in the abdominal cavity, either intact or attached to various abdominal organs, after uterine rupture.[88,89] A brownish fluid often is observed in the abdominal cavity in such cases. Mummification may occur late enough in gestation so that the scattered skeletal remains may be identified in radiographs in various areas of the abdominal cavity.

Fetal Maceration

Fetal maceration is a process of decomposition often associated with various pathogenic bacteria. Infection within the fetus may be established via the hematogenous route as a result of systemic infection originating elsewhere in the queen's body, as a result of low-grade endometritis at the time of mating and subsequent implantation, and via ascending infection through a dilated cervix as might occur during prolonged estrus, with excessive use of exogenous hormones to induce estrus or prevent mismating, or as the result of an abortion with only one fetus expelled and the rest carried to term.

The signs exhibited by the queen under these circumstances may go unnoticed, depending upon the rapidity of maceration. When maceration has been preceded by an abortion in which one or more fetuses have been expelled, the discharge from the vagina varies from serosanguineous to purulent to dark red. The queen may be afebrile if the infection is mild and the maceration process slow because only a few bacteria are present.

Continuous deterioration of the fetus may make the remains almost indistinguishable if delivered along with normal kittens at parturition. Depending upon at what stage of development the fetus died, only hair, bones and skin may be delivered.[90] Occasionally the fetal remnants must be removed surgically to have successful subsequent pregnancies.

The fetus may undergo emphysematous changes during the first 48-72 hours after fetal death if the cervix remains open. This process may involve the entire uterus. Affected queens usually are depressed and febrile during this type of fetal deterioration. Crepitation of the fetus may be detected by palpation, and the gas-filled fetus(es) and uterus may be readily observed radiographically (Fig 5). Fetal maceration in the absence of emphysema may not be apparent radiographically if the bones have not developed to the point of radiopacity.

To what extent spontaneous chromosomal abnormalities are responsible for feline abortion, maceration and mummification is not known.

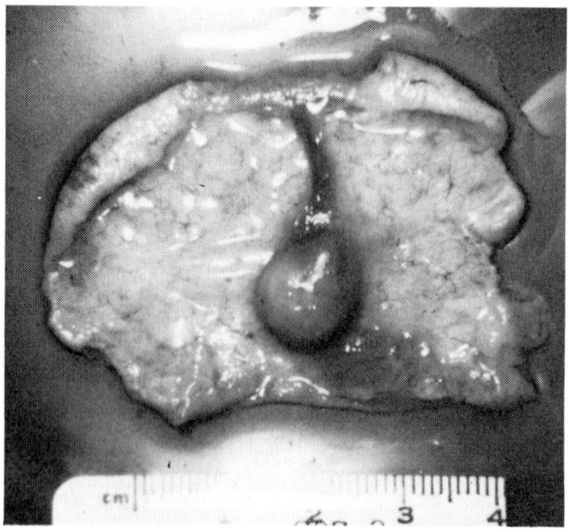

Fig 6. Placenta with resorbed fetus from a queen inoculated with feline panleukopenia virus on the seventeenth day of gestation. (Courtesy of Dr F.W. Scott)

Uniparous pregnancies of aneuploid zygotes are readily aborted. The presence of other fetuses (littermates) with normal chromosomal numbers and composition may prevent expulsion of the abnormal fetus.[91]

Neonatal Infection Secondary to Maternal Infection

Panleukopenia: Cerebellar hypoplasia is caused by late prenatal or early postnatal infection with panleukopenia virus and is not a heritable defect. Pregnancy may be terminated spontaneously if infection occurs early in gestation (Fig 6). If infection occurs during mid-gestation, the kittens may be born depressed and die rapidly with few, if any, clinical signs. Hemorrhagic areas in the cerebellum of such kittens may be evident at necropsy.

Some kittens exposed to panleukopenia virus as fetuses are normal at birth, but littermates may have signs of cerebellar ataxia.[92] Some infected queens remain asymptomatic, although localization of the virus in the placenta results in some or all of the kittens being affected. Queens with subclinical infections may bear kittens with cerebellar hypoplasia and immediately ingest them, thus obscuring the diagnosis of panleukopenia.[93]

The cerebellum of ataxic cats is not always grossly hypoplastic but may be reduced to a fifth of its normal mass. There is no correlation between the size of the cerebellum and severity of ataxia. Therefore, "cerebellar degeneration" may be a more appropriate term.

The external granular layers of the cerebellum are particularly susceptible because of the affinity of the panleukopenia virus for tissue undergoing rapid mitosis. In addition, the Purkinje cells of the cerebellum often are decreased in number or lacking in kittens with viral ataxia. Multiple CNS lesions, including hydrocephalus, scattered spinal cord demyelination, focal neuronal degeneration of cerebral white matter and focal meningitis, have been found along with renal and testicular hypoplasia in affected kittens.

The normal incoordination of kittens may mask the condition in affected individuals until they are 3-4 weeks of age. Some kittens are wobbly and weak, and others have a staggering gait that becomes more pronounced with age. Hypermetria may be pronounced in the forelegs and can involve the hindlimbs also. Affected kittens usually are able to eat and masticate. The condition is painless and there is no effective treatment. Some affected kittens may continue to shed the active virus and thus should be isolated from susceptible animals. In view of this, kittens less than 4 weeks of age and pregnant cats should not be vaccinated with modified-live panleukopenia virus under any circumstances. Because the cells of the CNS multiply rapidly in neonatal kittens, panleukopenia virus infection is particularly detrimental at that time.[94,95]

Herpesvirus Infection: Experimental infection of queens with herpesvirus (FVR) during the last trimester of pregnancy results in congenital herpesvirus infection. The severity of the disease is greatest in kittens born within a few days of the queen's exposure to the virus.

Affected kittens show signs of respiratory disease and may cry continuously. Histopathologically, the disease is manifested as fibrinosuppurative rhinitis, tracheitis, bronchopneumonia and focal hepatic necrosis. To what degree genital infection occurs naturally in conjunction with respiratory infections by FVR virus is unknown.[96]

Differentiation of the causative viruses of the upper respiratory complex is important in cattery and laboratory populations. Viral isolation, serologic and immunofluorescent testing may confirm the diagnosis.

Eradication of FVR from a cattery is difficult. If the carriers can be identified and moved out of the colony, the rest of the colony can be temporarily moved and the animal quarters disinfected with Clorox (4 oz/gal water). The quarters should then be left vacant for 2-4 weeks before restocking the colony with cats negative for herpesvirus. Use of FVR vaccines helps control the disease. Vaccinations must be kept current and contact with animal handlers must be controlled when they handle cats outside the colony.

In a study of feline reproductive failures, 39% of the animals had problems associated with the reproductive tract and the remaining 61% had no obvious reproductive tract anomalies.[97] Cystic endometrial hyperplasia, ovarian cysts, infantile reproductive tracts and villus hyperplasia of the oviducts were the most frequent causes of reproductive failure. That the remaining animals had no obvious lesions indicates there may be a significant number of causes of reproductive failure other than those directly associated with physical changes in the reproductive tract.

Congenital Defects

Although the placenta was once thought to be an impervious barrier against the influence of foreign substances on the embryo, overwhelming evidence indicates otherwise. There is transplacental conveyance of not only several diseases but of vaccines, antibiotics, sedatives and corticosteroids. Although some drugs can have a beneficial effect on the fetus, they are more likely to result in abortion, stillbirth or fetal malformations.

Severe congenital defects, including hydrocephalus, atresia ani, antresia coli, anophthalmia, spina bifida, cleft palate, cyclopia and fusion of hindlimb phalanges, have been associated with griseofulvin administration during pregnancy (Fig 7).[98] Because of this drug's widespread and often indiscriminate use in catteries containing cats with chronic dermatophytoses, owners should be advised to avoid griseofulvin therapy in pregnant queens.

An infinite variety of possible congenital defects may occur in kittens (Fig 8, Table 2).[99] Pseudohermaphroditism may or may not occur in cats. Some anomalies may resemble pseudohermaphroditism but in one the gonads are missing.[100] In true pseudohermaphroditism, all organs are present.

PARTURITION

As parturition nears, physical and behavioral changes become more evident. The queen may be noticeably restless because of her cumbersome abdominal distension and may frequently alternate sides while reclining or prefer a sitting position. Fetal movements may distress or confuse her, and she may quickly turn her head toward her flank in response. The muscles in the perineal area become flaccid as parturition nears. The nipples of the swollen mammary glands become deep pink and prominent.

During the last week of pregnancy, the queen's activity lessens and she may begin to investigate dark, quiet areas. At this time, a suitable location should be chosen for the queening box and the queen placed in it often. The queen should be placed in the selected queening location at least 2 weeks before the expected time of parturition, preferably with some familiar items, such as a litter box, blanket or pad. Hospitalization for routine queening is unnecessary. The queen may be acclimated to a selected area by essentially locking the animal in the space for increasingly longer periods, with considerable

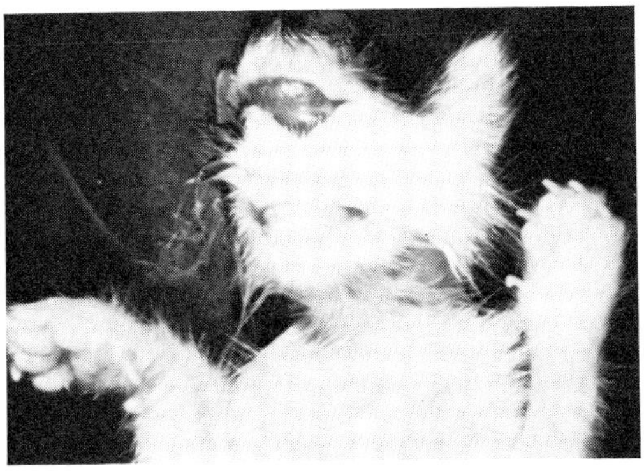

Fig 7. Cyclops fetus from queen treated with griseofulvin during pregnancy. (Courtesy of Dr F.W. Scott)

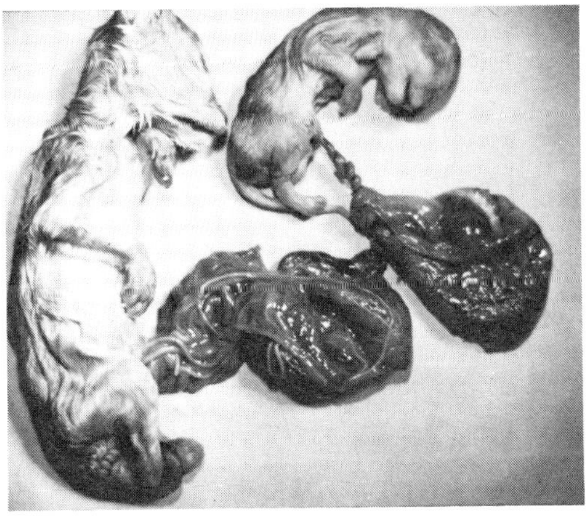

Fig 8. Dead, abnormal fetuses carried to term by an Abyssinian queen. The fetus on the left has an umbilical hernia containing abdominal viscera. Umbilical cord torsion in the fetus on the right resulted in arrested development.

Table 2. Congenital Defects in Kittens[99]

Monstrosities: dipygus (double pelvis), diprosopus (double head), schistocormia (cleft trunk)

Skeletal Defects: radial hemimelia (absent radius), cleft palate, anodontia (absent teeth), polydactyly*, hip dysplasia, spina bifida, anury (absent tail)*, pectus excavatum, kink tail*, peromelus ascelus (absent rear limbs), ectrodactyly (absent digit or part of digit)

Gastrointestinal Defects: achalasia*, hepatic cysts, atresia ani, pyloric stenosis

Cardiovascular Defects: endocardial fibroelastosis, tetralogy of Fallot, patent ductus arteriosus, interatrial septal defect, interventricular septal defect, agenesis of aortic and pulmonary valves, supravalvular aortic and pulmonary valves, persistent right aortic arch, persistent truncus arteriosus, persistent common atrioventricular canal, pulmonary stenosis

Urogenital Defects: unilateral renal hypoplasia, unilateral renal agenesis, persistent urachus, fusion of kidneys, polycystic kidneys, uterus unicornis (one horn absent), cryptorchidism*, sterility of male tortoiseshells, intersexuality

Respiratory Defects: peritoneopericardial diaphragmatic hernia, internal branchial fistula

CNS Defects: deafness in blue-eyed, white cats*, globoid leukodystrophy*, sphingomyelin lipidosis*, metachromatic leukodystrophy*, gangliosidosis*, glycogenosis*, hydrocephalus, cerebellar hypoplasia, double ears*

Ocular Defects: anophthalmos*, microphthalmos, hydrophthalmos, cyclopia, infantile glaucoma, heterochromia, retinal detachment, infantile cataract*, persistent pupillary membrane, eyelid agenesis, entropion, conjunctival adhesions, lacrimal system defects, nictitating membrane defects, strabismus

Miscellaneous Defects: congenital alopecia, porphyria

* May be hereditary

affection given between the episodes of isolation. Despite these efforts, cats frequently choose their own queening site.

The desire for human contact may diminish during the period before parturition. Cats that seek human companionship before parturition make it very obvious by vocalizing and seeking constant attention. These animals often are primigravid cats having some difficulty adjusting to the changes associated with gestation and parturition. Human contact should be quiet, gentle and without fanfare.

When psychologic attempts fail to calm an overwrought pregnant queen, the animal may be mildly tranquilized with acepromazine at 0.125-0.250 mg/lb body weight, given IM, SC or PO. Use of higher dosages is not recommended because of approaching labor and because acepromazine may severely depress blood pressure. The cat must retain the ability to respond to muscular contraction should labor start during this excitement phase.

Changes in the pregnant queen's environment immediately prepartum should be avoided. Such changes may hasten or delay delivery, with either result having a detrimental effect upon the offspring. Introduction of new animals into a queen's environment immediately preceding or after parturition is contraindicated. Some queens resent the proximity of another cat and may be psychologically stressed by its presence.

The client should be instructed not to bring the queen to the hospital for examination near the time of parturition. This may increase the anxiety of the animal and initiate the first stage of labor due to stress. Information on abnormal behavior, delayed parturition or problems with delivery may be relayed by telephone.

Any required examination of the queen at term should be done in a quiet environment. She should not be kept waiting in a reception room full of other animals. The little finger of a sterile gloved hand may be inserted into the vagina of most adult queens to note dilation of the cervix. Lubrication of the vagina by glandular secretions may also be assessed. Abdominal palpation provides some indication of uterine tone. A full colon or bladder should be emptied if possible before attempting extraction of a kitten or guidance of one through the birth canal. Queens rarely require help unless they are purebreds with a high calvaria, such as Persians.

LABOR

Stage 1 (Onset of Labor)

From a few hours to 24 hours before queening, the female may be increasingly restless, and may pace and vocalize. In response to early contractions, she may squat in the litter box, strain and leave without voiding. In her queening box she may do some scratching, and shredding and rearranging of nesting material. Some queens lose their appetite a day before parturition and others continue to eat until the kittens are born and eat during intervals between delivery of kittens. A decrease in body temperature to 99-100 F (37.2-37.8 C) occurs in some queens 12-24 hours prepartum.

Stage 2 (Fetal Delivery)

This is the period during which the kittens are actually born. The queen may begin panting and abdominal contractions can be seen as well as felt. The queen may lie on her side or sternum, with the hindlimbs extended at the side, and begin to strain as uterine contractions intensify. She may occasionally get up and assume a squatting position. When the fetus enters the pelvic canal, intense muscular contractions may cause the queen to groan or cry. Vocalization seldom occurs after the first kitten is born.

The perineal area may be moistened by rupture of the amniotic sac ("water bag") of the first kitten. The queen may respond by putting her head under a rear leg and licking vigorously at the perineum.[101]

If the amniotic sac is intact, the fluid-filled, balloon-like structure may be noticed at the vulva before the kitten is expelled. More often the sac is torn as the kitten enters the pelvic canal and the kitten's head, limbs or tail may first be seen at the vulva. At this point, the queen may aid delivery by biting and tugging at the membranes or kitten.

The queen's vigorous licking of the newborn not only tears the amniotic sac, if it is still intact, and liberates the kitten, but also aids in stimulating its respiration. This innate licking behavior is not in response to the kitten per se but rather to the amniotic fluids that soiled the queen's body and environment. Some queens lick and cleanse themselves before giving any attention to the newborn kittens. Others sever the umbilical cord as soon as the kitten is born but do not continue any further. In these instances, human intervention is needed to prevent death of the neonate.

Cannibalism of normal kittens is rare despite the intensity with which the queen may lick and clean the newborn. Cannibalism appears to be instinctive when macerated fetuses or severe congenital anomalies exist.

After vigorous contractions have begun, the first kitten may be presented within 3-4 minutes or 30-60 minutes may pass before the first birth. Often 2 kittens are born, one immediately after the other, and then 10-90 minutes elapse before another birth. The fetuses are expelled from the uterus in an irregular order; the first kitten may be from one horn, the next 3 from the other horn, and the last from the first horn.

After the birth of the first kitten(s), some queens have a physiologic interruption of parturition that lasts 12-48 hours. Contractions cease, no kittens are present at the pelvic outlet, and the queen is content to quietly nurse her first kittens. Although other fetuses are palpable in the uterus, the queen acts as though parturition has been completed and assumes normal postparturient eating, resting and lactation. When labor begins again, the remaining kittens are delivered normally. The cause of interrupted parturition is unknown, but it must be differentiated from dystocia.

The second stage of labor varies in duration but usually is complete within 2-6 hours. Indications of dystocia are imprecise but the following should prompt examination by a veterinarian: strong contractions that are unproductive after 4 hours' duration; continuation of intense contractions 2-4 hours after delivery of the first kitten(s); weak, diminished contractions in place of true second-stage labor; partial delivery of a kitten, followed by cessation of labor; and passage of bright- to dark-red vaginal discharge, without the onset of labor.

Stage 3 (Placental Delivery)

Passage of the placental membranes constitutes the third stage of delivery. This brownish-pink tissue usually is expelled by mild, infrequent contractions shortly after each kitten is born, if not at the same time. When 2 kittens are born within a few minutes of each other, both placental membranes may be extruded shortly afterward. If the queen is actively licking at the amniotic sac, kitten and umbilical cord as parturition occurs, the placental membranes are more likely to be separated immediately.

Many, but far from all, queens ingest the placental membranes soon after they are delivered. Although this is not harmful to the queen, it is not necessary. If the membranes are gently removed from the queening box without upsetting or distracting the queen, postpartum diarrhea may be prevented in that the membranes are thought to have a laxative effect.

The feline placenta is zonary, with the chorionic villi distributed in a band-like pattern around the center of the chorionic sac. This area of fetal-maternal junction is classified as endotheliochorial, *ie,* the endothelium of maternal blood vessels is in direct contact with the fetal chorion.[102,103]

Queening usually is completed within 4-6 hours. Newborn kittens attempt to nurse within 1-2 hours, if not immediately.[104] Depending on the number of kittens in the litter, the ease of delivery, and previous experience, the queen may allow the kittens to nurse for brief periods between births. Others do not allow suckling until the last fetus is delivered.

Complications of Parturition

Maternal Dystocia

Osseous Deformity: Physical deformities of the queen, specifically those involving the pelvis, may significantly contribute to dystocia. Healed pelvic fractures can markedly narrow the pelvic outlet. This should be considered when valuable queens are first presented for treatment of pelvic trauma. Similarly, pathologic fractures of the pelvis from secondary nutritional hyperparathyroidism may affect the future breeding capabilities of a young queen.

For most cats with a history of severe pelvic injury and radiographic verification of consequent pelvic distortion, ovariohysterectomy is the obvious means of preventing complications of parturition. However, if the animal is already pregnant or its breeding is strongly desired by the owner, radiographs obtained 1-3 days prepartum may help determine if a cesarean section will be required. If the pelvic deformity clearly prohibits fetal expulsion, cesarean section should be performed before labor begins.

To what extent deformities created by hypervitaminosis A, as seen in cats fed excessive amounts of liver, may complicate parturition is unknown.[105] Although vitamin A intoxication does not appear to affect the fertility of female cats, it may result in sacroiliac ankylosis and pelvic exostoses that could interfere with normal queening (see Chapter 13).

Soft-Tissue Deformity: In addition to osseous deformities that may cause maternal dystocia, soft-tissue abnormalities of the queen may likewise result in parturient complications. A congenital abnormality of the queen's reproductive tract, such as uterus unicornus, can result in dystocia. Congenital or acquired inguinal hernias may include the gravid uterus and prevent normal expulsion of the fetuses. If the queen has a history of dystocia, layers of fibrous scar tissue may result in stenosis of the birth canal.

Illness: Serious illness during pregnancy may result in dystocia. Debilitating diseases can result in anemia and poor body condition. Cats so affected may have poor uterine tone and decreased stamina, leading to dystocia.

Age and Size: The age and size of the queen are other factors in maternal dystocia. The correct age at which to breed a female cat should be determined on the basis of body size as well as chronologic age and can vary considerably among breeds. Although many 4- and 5-month-old females show signs of estrus, they have not attained full body size or development. As a consequence, dystocia is not unusual in 6- or 7-month-old queens.

Uterine Inertia: Queening complications arising from uterine inertia or atony are not rare and can be anticipated in primigravid cats over 5 years old and multiparous queens over 8 years old. Uterine atony is more likely to occur if prolonged gestation results in a small litter of excessively large kittens.

Primary uterine inertia in obese queens is probably the most common form of maternal dystocia. Passage of the fetus may be impeded by intrapelvic or perivulvar fat deposits and diminished uterine muscular tone, resulting in poor contractions. Many obese cats, especially longhaired breeds, suffer chronic constipation; the impacted colon may interfere with normal uterine and fetal motility during parturition. Treatment of dystocia in these cats should begin with evacuation of the bladder and colon.

Although less common, secondary uterine inertia may develop in multiparous queens if parturition is unusually difficult or prolonged. Both the animal and uterine musculature become exhausted. Before uterine inertia is complete, the intensity of contractions may be increased by "feathering" or digital stroking of the dorsal vaginal wall. This technic may also hasten passage of the next kitten.

When uterine inertia is suspected, oxytocic drugs should be used judiciously. Injection of 3-5 units of oxytocin SC may initiate normal uterine contractions. The injection can be repeated in 30-45 minutes if necessary. Sensitization of the uterus can be increased by slow IV administration of 5 ml of 10% Ca gluconate solution. Larger doses of oxytocic drugs are contraindicated as intense uterine contractions, coupled with insufficient cervical dilation, can result in uterine rupture.

If contractions are not induced within 30 minutes of the second oxytocin injection, prompt cesarotomy is indicated. After the kittens are surgically removed from the uterus, the uterus should involute normally. If atony persists, gentle kneading of the uterus and IV administration of oxytocin may stimulate contractions. Failure of the uterus to regain tone and undergo involution after these measures necessitates immediate ovariohysterectomy to prevent metritis.

Uterine Rupture: As mentioned previously, the uterus may rupture immediately before or during parturition. Primary rupture is most likely if normal contractions begin but the kittens cannot be expelled due to fetal or maternal factors. Secondary rupture may occur as a result of trauma to the distended uterus (blow to the abdomen), injudicious use of oxytocic drugs without ensuring patency of the birth canal, and forceful manipulative efforts applied abdominally to maneuver fetuses through the cervix.

Fetal Dystocia

Fetal Malformation: When severe enough to result in a monstrosity, abnormal fetal development may interfere with normal parturition. Examples of such deformities include gross enlargement of the head, as in congenital hydrocephalus or cyclopia, and partial duplication of the body, as in dipygus (double pelvis) or diprosopus (double head).

Kitten Size: Rarely is kitten size a complicating factor in parturition unless gestation is prolonged. This is more apt to occur if the litter is composed of only 1 or 2 kittens. Difference in size between the queen and stud seldom, if ever, results in kittens that are too large to be born naturally.

Abnormal Presentation: Abnormal presentation is seldom a complicating factor in feline parturition. Because 45-50% of kittens are born in breech presentation, this should be considered normal. Vertex presentation (top of head) does not necessarily result in difficult delivery.

Because of the restrictions imposed by the small size of the feline birth canal, it is often impossible to determine the exact presentation of a kitten. If the fetal head and mouth can be palpated, it usually can be determined if the fetus is in a dorsosacral or dorsopubic position.

One of the simplest means of managing dystocia caused by abnormal presentation and aggravated by inadequate lubrication due to the loss of fetal fluids is to instill 5-10 ml of sterile lubricant (light mineral oil or nitrofurazone solution) via soft plastic tubing advanced into the cranial portion of the vagina toward the dilated cervix. This is contraindicated, however, if uterine rupture is suspected.

If additional lubrication does not ease passage of the fetus, delivery must be facilitated by manipulation and instrumentation. A technic involving use of an ovariectomy hook and digital traction to extract the fetus without endometrial trauma has been described.[106] The ovariectomy hook is positioned immediately parallel and adjacent to the operator's middle finger. The hook portion is directed dorsad and the middle finger is pressed into its curvature so the open tip rests against the operator's middle fingernail. Assuming the fetus to be in a dorsosacral position, the hook and finger are inserted through the queen's vagina and into the uterus until both have entered the mouth of the fetus. The middle finger is left in the mouth as the hook is gently withdrawn and redirected into the soft area between the horizontal rami of the mandible. The finger is again pressed into the open portion of the hook, achieving a pincerlike grip on the mandibular symphysis. Gentle traction is applied in a dorsocaudal direction until the fetal head clears the pelvis. Traction is then directed caudad and slightly ventrad to clear the fetal pelvis from the maternal pelvis.

If the fetus is in posterior presentation, the same technic can be used by holding the tail and the hook with a finger. Traction is again applied caudodorsad until the fetal pelvis clears the maternal pelvis; it is then directed caudad and slightly ventrad to clear the fetal head. The risk of trauma in this method of delivery is greater to the fetus than to the endometrium, as would be the case if forceps were used.

If a third of the fetus has cleared the bony pelvis before difficulty occurs, it may be helpful to grasp the exposed portion of the fetus with a dry gauze sponge. The sponge can be introduced into the vagina while held with 2 fingers, and then applied around the fetus to exert traction.

Another method for delivering a fetus after it has reached the pelvis is by careful digital manipulation through the queen's rectum. Because of limitations imposed by the size of the queen and the clinician's hands, other manipulations often are impossible.

Umbilical Cord Torsion

Umbilical cord torsion probably is related to rapid delivery of 2 or more kittens in a manner that allows the umbilical cords to be wrapped around various parts of the individual kitten (Fig 8). Sometimes the female does not attempt to clean the kittens but leaves them alone and they are found dead. Usually the queen cleans the kittens but does not attempt to sever the umbilical cords. If the cords are not removed immediately, strangulation may result in death or loss of a leg. Placentas, whole or partially removed, may be found among the kittens. Separation of the kittens immediately, before damage due to strangulation, and presentation to the queen usually results in resumption of maternal attention.

Postpartum Examination

If the need exists for postpartum examination, it should be done 12-48 hours after delivery. When taken to the hospital, the kittens should arrive in the same box with the queen to minimize the queen's anxiety and give the practitioner a chance to examine the kittens as well. The postpartum examination should be similar to the prepartum examination, and the mammary tissue should receive extra attention at this time. Owners of animals with a history of postpartum complications should be advised to report anorexia that persists for over 24 hours, any malodorous vulvar discharge, and a body temperature above 103 F (39.4 C).

The kittens should be nursing freely; subnormal temperature in a kitten older than one day should be cause for concern. Use of oxytocin for removal of placental tissue may be necessary. Animals that are anxious 24-48 hours postpartum should be examined for evidence of retained kittens (dead or alive) or fetal membranes and treated accordingly, keeping in mind that reproductive organs are more friable immediately postpartum.

Postpartum Complications

Postpartum Rejection

This type of behavior may be noted as total rejection at birth, in which case the kittens are not cleaned or otherwise cared for, or the kittens may be cleaned but not allowed to nurse. This type of behavior is most common in primiparous or timid queens. The queen may reject kittens with birth defects even though the defect may not be obvious. Environmental disturbances and the presence of other animals also inhibit maternal care, although this is more common with first litters and reticent queens. A lack of progesterone in the queen has been suggested as a possible cause for this type of behavior as well as for molestation of the kittens by the queen. Neither a lack of progesterone nor failure to deliver the placental membranes has been proven as a cause of such behavior.

Litter Relocation

Queens may frequently move the kittens from one secluded place to another. This is not unusual when the kittens are 3-4 weeks old and may be common among free-ranging queens.[101]

Postpartum Hemorrhage

The normal postpartum vulvar discharge is slight and lasts 3-5 days. The fastidious nature of queens makes this discharge difficult to observe, even when the labia are parted. Any hemorrhage usually is the result of some degree of dystocia or improper uterine involution. Bright-red secretions indicate inspection of the vaginal mucosa for lacerations.

If the discharge is copious, considerable attention should be given to proper care of the queen. The body temperature should be monitored and the reproductive organs thoroughly examined. An IM injection of 0.1 mg ergonovine maleate produces tetanic contractions of the uterus. This may be sufficient to constrict the bleeding capillaries of the uterine endometrium. Use of ergonovine maleate is not recommended for queens with a vulvar discharge of material other than blood or in which there is a significantly elevated body temperature. If the latter is not the case, injection of ergonovine maleate may be repeated within 20-30 minutes. Simultaneous administration of 5 ml of 10% Ca gluconate solution, given slowly IV, may also enhance the uterine muscular tone. The uterine contractions produced by oxytocin are rhythmic and therefore may not be as effective as ergonovine in treatment of uterine hemorrhage.

Uterine hemorrhage uncontrolled by drugs should be surgically investigated without delay. Ovariohysterectomy is the treatment of choice. Supportive therapy to control shock should be instituted subsequent to surgery.

Retained Fetal Membranes

The placentas usually are delivered in a random sequence, some with the fetus, some following delivery of one or more fetuses, and a few several hours after delivery of kittens has been completed. Unless one actually observes the delivery, it may be impossible to tell if the tissues have been expelled in that some are consumed by the queen. The first clue that some have been retained may be an excessive, dark-red to brownish vulvar discharge. The queen may or may not exhibit abnormal behavior during this time. Constant licking of the perineal area also may indicate a greater-than-normal postparturient discharge.

Abdominal palpation may disclose the membranes in the enlarged uterus, which is rather firm at the point of retention. Radiography may aid in their identification. Intrauterine infusion of a positive-contrast agent (25% Hypaque: Winthrop) has been used to identify retained placental membranes, although such infusions should be considered a last resort.[107] Rarely the retained membranes go unnoticed for several weeks, which may result in low-grade endometritis or pyometra that may only become evident as sterility at subsequent mating.

Treatment of retained placental membranes depends upon the condition of the queen, the desire for subsequent litters and the number of placentas retained. Ergonovine maleate may be used PO at 0.05 mg BID for 3 days to increase uterine involution and facilitate expulsion of the membranes. Antibiotic and other supportive therapy should be instituted. When the placental tissues have been retained for days or weeks, the usual solution is removal of the placentas by hysterotomy and continued supportive therapy postoperatively. Ovariohysterectomy may be performed if visual inspection of the endometrium reveals complications necessitating treatment beyond removal of the placental tissues.

Other Complications

Other postpartum complications include uterine prolapse, metritis, mastitis and lactational tetany, all of which are discussed elsewhere in this chapter.

THE MAMMARY GLANDS

Cats normally have 4 pairs of mammary glands. Additional glands and supernumerary teats (polythelia) are observed occasionally. Some of the former are functional as a fifth or sixth mammary gland. Each normal teat contains 4-8 galactophores. Rarely a single mammary gland may have several functional teats.

Lactation

During lactation it is not unusual for a queen to require 150-300% more food than usual, depending on the age, size and number of kittens she is nursing, and her prelactational body condition. In addition to the regular diet, the queen should receive increased amounts of high-quality protein, such as organ meats and cooked eggs. Cow's milk should not be fed because many cats cannot tolerate its high lactate content. Diarrhea is a common result. Rather than milk, a milk replacer (*eg,* KMR:Borden) should be diluted 1:1 with warm water. Multiple-vitamin supplements may be fed if the nutritional status is unknown or obviously deficient. Despite such dietary additions, most heavily lactating queens lose significant amounts of body weight and have poor haircoats by the time the kittens are weaned.

Most kittens establish a priority for a particular nipple from which to suckle within the first few days of life. Attempts to nurse other nipples usually are limited, especially if a dominant kitten uses that nipple. The smallest, most timid kittens in large litters should be allowed to nurse independently or their diet should be supplemented with an artificial milk formula (*eg,* KMR:Borden) (see Chapter 1). Neonates suckle 2-3 ml milk several times each hour.

In addition to providing nutrients and antibodies, maternal milk may be the source of pathogens. For example, FeLV is transmitted in queens' milk, although endometrial infection of the fetus is likely to precede lactational infection. Various parasites, such as ascarids and *Toxoplasma,* also may be transferred during nursing.[108]

Most queens make themselves less accessible to the kittens by the third week of lactation. They no longer readily roll on their side when a kitten approaches. However, most queens allow occasional nursing for 6-8 weeks. In this natural process of weaning, no drugs are indicated to help suppress milk formation. The queen's food and water intake should be gradually reduced during this period.

When a litter of kittens dies shortly after parturition, the mammary glands may become engorged with milk and cause much discomfort. Owners should be cautioned not to "milk out" the glands because this stimulates production of more milk. When necessary, repository testosterone (*eg,* Depo-Testosterone:Upjohn) can be given IM at 1 mg/lb to hasten galactostasis.

Diseases of the Mammary Glands

Mammary Hyperplasia

Mammary hyperplasia occurs in a significant number of young cats after the first estrous period.[109] The mammary glands may become very enlarged, turgid, warm and painful. The hyperplasia may affect one or more glands in a paired or random fashion. Expressed fluid from affected glands usually is dark brown. Severe cases may result in rupture through the skin over the mammary tissue, but this is not common. Purulent drainage, under these conditions, is uncommon, at least initially.

Cause: Cats with mammary hyperplasia have vaginal smears exhibiting most cornified epithelial cells, indicative of high estrogen levels and a state of estrus. The presence of cystic endometrial hyperplasia along with mammary hyperplasia also suggests high estrogen levels and thus a hormonal cause.[110]

Treatment: Treatment of mammary hyperplasia usually involves ovariohysterectomy because the condition often recurs after each estrous period. Mammary engorgement should be reduced by use of diuretics and corticosteroids before ovariohysterectomy is attempted unless the surgical approach is via a flank rather than a midline incision.[111] Results obtained with use of repository testosterone are variable.

Primary Acute Mastitis

Cause: Acute mastitis usually is associated with parturition and lactation. The most commonly affected glands are the caudal (inguinal) pair. There appears to be no relationship among the glands affected as they may appear only on one side. The most common causes of infection are staphylococci and streptococci.[112] The most common route of infection is via the teat orifices rather than via the blood or lymphatics. Any relationship between acute mastitis and metritis or retained placental tissues is speculative.

Clinical Signs: Primary acute mastitis may be masked and not recognized except when kittens die or if weak, cold and crying kittens are noted. Examination reveals the warm, swollen, reddened and sensitive glands. Affected queens are anorectic, febrile and depressed; vomiting may be noted. The infection may become more localized with time and may form abscesses.

Secretions from affected glands may be flocculent and grey to brown. Smears of this material reveal a preponderance of bacteria and toxic neutrophils. The pH is alkaline instead of the normal slightly acidic pH. A hemogram reveals an absolute leukocytosis.[113]

Treatment: Treatment of acute mastitis usually involves the use of broad-spectrum antibiotics for at least 7-10 days, with additional supportive therapy as needed. Surgical drainage of any abscesses may be necessary. Bandages should be applied to the infected glands to prevent nursing. Kittens are allowed access to the queen to continue the maternal relationship.

The kittens of affected queens should also receive antibiotic therapy. If they cannot be fed by another nursing queen, they must be fed a formula because the lactose concentration in cow's milk usually causes scours (see Chapter 1). Attention should be paid to the kittens' warmth and body temperature. Excessive and direct heat usually results in kitten mortality.

Secondary Acute Mastitis

Cause: Secondary acute mastitis usually is observed after the kittens are about 2 weeks old and is caused by the trauma of nursing. Clipping the nails of the kittens may assist in recovery. More severe cases may be handled as with primary acute mastitis. Evaluation of the milk from affected glands may assist in differentiating secondary from primary acute mastitis.

Treatment: The kittens may be removed from the queen and their diet supplemented or they may be allowed to continue nursing, with the affected glands wrapped for protection.

Clipping the hair around the mammary tissue of longhaired cats is of questionable necessity. The hair affords some protection against secondary acute mastitis problems; however, unless the queen is unkempt, problems rarely develop. Because some longhaired queens do not clean themselves sufficiently after parturition, especially if it has been difficult, cleansing of the lower abdomen may be necessary.

Chronic Mastitis

Clinical Signs: Chronic mastitis rarely follows acute mastitis in household cats but occasionally may be noted in free-ranging cats. Chronic mastitis usually is an incidental finding associated with older queens. Mammary tissue in this condition usually is not active and the inflammatory reaction is minimal or not obvious. There may be an abnormal bacterial population in the inspissated milk in the gland. Small but firm nodules may be palpated or the entire gland may feel firm and nodular.[114] The tissues are not sensitive to palpation and a small amount of watery fluid may be expressed. This material should be cultured.

Mammary cysts may also be found and usually are the result of duct closure preventing the escape of milk. The volume of milk in the gland increases until back-pressure prevents formation of more milk within the gland.

Treatment: Treatment depends upon the state of the mammary tissue. Mastectomy is the treatment of choice but may not be necessary in all cases due to consolidation of the mammary tissue. If neoplasia is suspected, biopsy is recommended and histopathologic diagnosis is necessary. Complete or partial mastectomy should be based upon the condition of the queen, anticipated subsequent pregnancies and the condition of the mammary tissue.

Neoplasia

Mammary gland neoplasia is not common in cats. Mammary tissue should always be palpated in any physical examination, with special attention to the mammary gland in the pre-estrus, postestrus and postpartum examinations.

Mammary gland neoplasia has been noted with increasing frequency as the life span of cats has lengthened and the percentage of cats examined by veterinarians has increased. Neoplastic mammary tissue in cats has a high incidence of malignancy and thus warrants a guarded prognosis. The most common mammary neoplasm in cats is the adenocarcinoma (Fig 9).[115,116] Such tumors grow rapidly and are very invasive. They are epithelial in origin, often regrow after excision and are very prone to metastasis. Histologically, these tumors are classified as scirrhous, ductal or papillary. More than one morphologic type may develop in one gland although usually not simultaneously.

There appears to be no relationship between sexual maturity or the presence of the female reproductive organs and mammary neoplasia. There is some indication that sexually intact cats have a greater incidence (7-fold increase) of mammary neoplasia than do neutered animals.[117] Earlier studies have contradicted this finding as it appeared that mammary malignancy was independent of hormonal stimulation.[118] Neutering, simultaneous with partial mastectomy, did not lessen the recurrence of neoplasia or retard the progress of malignancy. It may only be theorized, in the absence of sufficient study, that ovariohysterectomy has no positive effect after a malignancy has developed but it may be a factor in preventing or retarding development of neoplasia.

The cause of feline mammary neoplasia remains unknown. Virus-like particles have been noted in the cell membranes and intercellular spaces of some mammary carcinomas but their presence or identification has yet to be associated with the tumor itself.

Mammary tumors are most often noted in cats 7 years of age and older, although they also occur in young cats. The tumors tend to ulcerate early

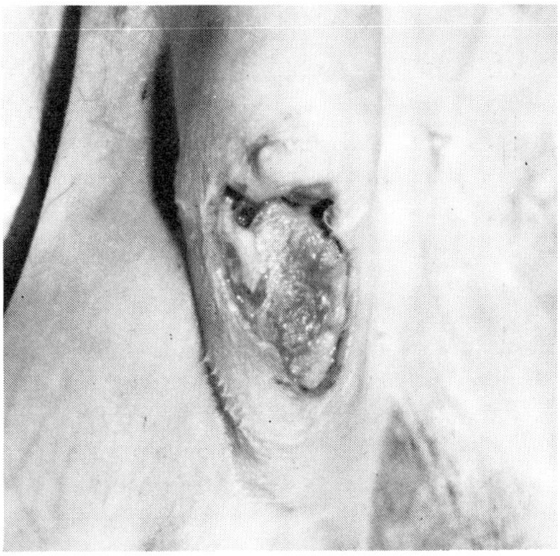

Fig 9. Mammary adenocarcinoma, with ulceration.

in their growth, usually are noted in only one gland and often are mistaken for abscesses. Seeding to another gland may be natural or encouraged by frequent palpation. Cytologic examination of secretions expressed from the teat or of the ulcerous area reveals malignant cells.[119]

Neoplasms have been found in all areas of the mammary tissue. Some surveys have indicated a predilection for the pectoral glands and others have indicated an equal distribution between the cranial and caudal glands. The observations of these and other authors indicate a higher incidence in the caudal or inguinal glands.

Mastectomy is the preferred treatment. Before this is attempted, the cat should be thoroughly examined, including thoracic radiographs and palpation of area lymph nodes. The lymph nodes and lungs are the most common sites for metastasis; the kidney, spleen, pleura, brain and liver may be involved (Fig 10).[120]

Adenocarcinomas are the most common type of mammary tumor, but other types, including mixed tumors containing osteoid material, spindle-cell sarcomas and fibrosarcomas, have also been observed. Benign mammary tumors are not common and include lipomas, adenomas, duct papillomas and fibroadenomas.

Galactostasis

Inspissation of milk within a mammary gland, with subsequent lack of secretion (galactostasis), usually affects the cranial glands and usually is due to insufficient nursing. The condition may be precipitated by inverted nipples that prevent the kittens from nursing those glands.

Warm, moist, topical applications and gentle massage of the gland help soften the inspissated

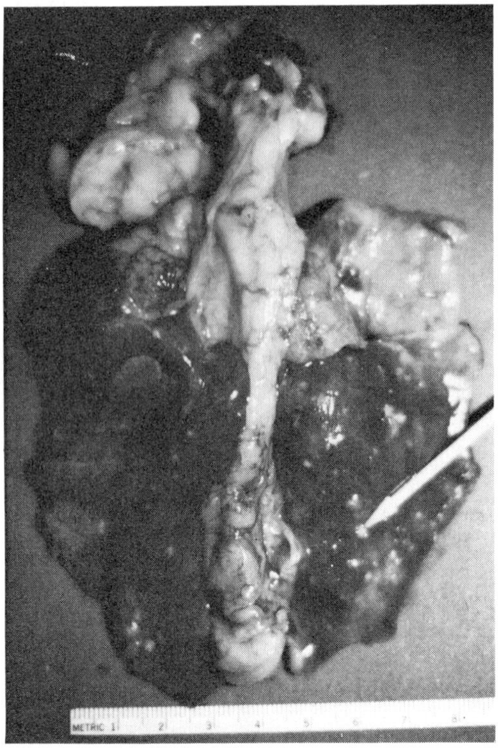

Fig 10. Pulmonary metastases from the mammary adenocarcinoma in Figure 9.

milk and stimulate milk secretion. Mild diuretics may also reduce edema. After milk flow is reestablished, kittens should be encouraged to suckle that gland when possible.

If teat inversion is noticed during pregnancy, the owner should be instructed to gently evert and massage the nipple daily in an attempt to permanently evert it before lactation.

Agalactia

True agalactia is uncommon in cats. More often, a primiparous queen is restless, confused and reluctant to stay with her litter for more than a few minutes, and appears to be either unwilling or unable to nurse her kittens.

Providing a quiet environment and reassurance usually results in release of milk. Administration of acepromazine at 0.125-0.25 mg/lb PO occasionally helps calm nervous queens and encourages their willingness to nurse the kittens. Only 1 or 2 doses usually are necessary. If the queen is willing to nurse but milk secretion is slow, owners can be instructed to administer minute doses of oxytocin in the form of a nasal spray (Syntocinon:Sandoz). Small amounts of this drug can be instilled in the queen's nostrils several times daily. Milk is released within a few minutes.

Puerperal Tetany

Although not a disease of the mammary glands, puerperal tetany (lactational tetany, eclampsia) is related to depletion of body Ca during heavy lactation. The resulting hypocalcemia, if untreated, may result in clonic convulsions and death. Considering the common occurrence of parturition and lactation, the incidence of lactational tetany in cats is very low.[121]

Cause: The condition is seen more often in multiparous queens nursing a litter of 5 or more kittens. However, puerperal tetany has occurred in cats 14 months to 6 years of age, nursing only 1 or 2 kittens. The onset usually corresponds with the peak of the kittens' requirements for milk, *ie,* 2-4 weeks after parturition. Cases of preparturient lactational tetany have been seen.

Careful distinction should be made between use of the term "eclampsia," as applied to the hypocalcemic condition of dogs and cats, and its use in human medicine to describe a toxemia of pregnancy, characterized by hypertension, edema and proteinuria. Although the cause of lactational hypocalcemia in cats is unknown, hypoparathyroidism has been incriminated.[122]

Clinical Signs: In the early stages of puerperal tetany, the queen usually is restless, unwilling to stay with her litter and anorectic, and may stumble or appear unusually awkward when moving. As the condition worsens, vomiting, polydipsia, hyperpnea and progressive ataxia may be noted. As the hypocalcemia becomes more severe during the next 2-8 hours, intense muscular spasms, in the form of tremors and twitching, develop and eventually lead to clonic convulsions. During this period there may be profuse salivation, panting and fever of up to 108 F (42.4 C). Collapse and coma soon follow if treatment is not begun. Queens presented for treatment in the advanced stages of hypocalcemia show signs of shock, including dilated pupils, subnormal body temperature, and dry, pale mucosae.

Diagnosis: A serum Ca level below 7 mg/dl is evidence of puerperal tetany. Because the urgency of treatment may not allow time to determine the serum Ca level, the diagnosis is almost always made on the basis of a history of recent parturition and lactation, along with the typical tetanic signs. The diagnosis is confirmed by the rapid response to administration of Ca.

Treatment: Because most cats with lactational tetany are in the advanced stages when presented, treatment consists of slowly giving 10% Ca gluconate solution IV to effect over a 5-minute period. If the Ca is administered slowly, cardiac disturbances are unlikely. The average dose of a 10% Ca gluconate solution is 2-5 ml; however, some cats require double that amount before responding.

In the few cats that do not immediately respond to IV Ca therapy, 10% dextrose solution also may be given IV. The rationale for such therapy is that the intense hypocalcemia and resultant muscular tremors may have caused hypoglycemia, particularly in very thin, nutritionally deficient cats.

If the cat is in the early stages of hypocalcemia when presented and is only slightly incoordinated, 5-10 ml of an isotonic Ca solution (Calphosan:Carlton) can be given SC.[123] Most queens can be treated as outpatients and sent home after the signs have subsided. Home therapy should consist of 300-325 mg Ca (as lactate or gluconate), given as tablets daily for a week. The queen's diet should also be evaluated and improved if necessary, including vitamin supplementation.

Another rare complication of lactational tetany that may partially account for a poor response to Ca therapy is distortion of the acid-base balance. If the cat is febrile and has been hyperventilating during development of hypocalcemia, respiratory alkalosis may develop due to carbonic acid deficit. Alkaline blood (pH over 7.45) and urine confirm the diagnosis. Therapy consists of replacing the bicarbonate ion with chloride in the form of an IV normal saline solution (see Chapter 2). Although correction of acid-base imbalance is seldom necessary in treating lactational tetany, its existence should be considered whenever the response to routine therapy is incomplete. Serum electrolyte levels should also be measured in unresponsive cases.

Control of convulsions with IV barbiturates is rarely necessary after Ca therapy is initiated. Tranquilization with phenothiazine tranquilizers is contraindicated during the acute stages of hypocalcemia.

Prevention: To prevent recurrence, kittens over 3 weeks of age should be weaned promptly and not allowed to nurse the queen. The queen should not be totally isolated from her kittens, however, as this results in behavioral and psychologic abnormalities in the kittens. To prevent nursing, a body bandage may be applied to the queen until lactation has ceased. Alternatively, periods of maternal contact might be allowed under close supervision.

If the kittens are less than a week old and no "wet-nurse" queen is available, limited nursing may be allowed provided the queen's condition quickly stabilizes. At least half of the kittens' daily caloric requirements should be provided as a substitute milk formula (see Chapter 1). The owner should be advised of the possible recurrence of the condition. Should lactational hypocalcemia develop a second time in the same lactation, the kittens must be removed.

Some clinicians believe that refractory or recurrent hypocalcemic states may respond to corticosteroid administration. The exact mechanism of the corticosteroid action is unclear. In fact, corticosteroids would seem to be contraindicated because they inhibit intestinal absorption of Ca and enhance renal excretion of Ca. Perhaps the usefulness of corticosteroids in treating and preventing recurrence of lactational tetany may be related to the stress of parturition and nursing, and to the subsequent increased requirements for corticosteroids that are not met by the adrenal output. Corticosteroids may be especially indicated if the queen continues to nurse her kittens. An oral dose of 5 mg prednisolone given BID during the remainder of lactation may help prevent recurrence of hypocalcemia.

THE UTERUS

Diseases of the Uterus

Earlier literature cited hyperestrogenism as the cause of a variety of uterine problems.[48] Recent research has proven this is not necessarily the case. Cystic endometrial hyperplasia, hydrometra and pyometra are considerably influenced by high progesterone levels.[124,125]

Progesterone is produced by the corpus luteum soon after involution of the ruptured ovarian follicle. Maximum production is probably at the time of maximum growth of the corpus luteum about 3 weeks after ovulation. Slow regression of the corpus luteum begins at about 21 days after ovulation and is complete at 45-50 days, when pseudopregnancy ends. Ovariectomy in pregnant queens at about this time usually does not result in abortion.

Progesterone has multiple effects on the uterus, including increasing secretory activity of the endometrial glands, inhibition of myometrial activity and closure of the cervix. Estrogen, on the other hand, has effects opposite to those of progesterone: the myometrium is sensitized, the cervix is dilated, the uterine blood supply is increased and neutrophils migrate toward the

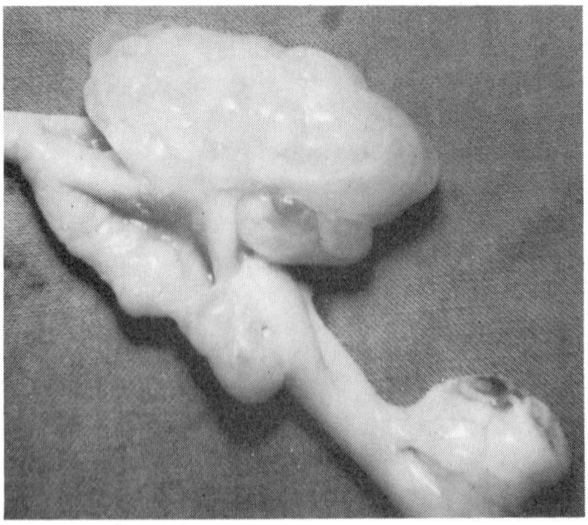

Fig 11. Cystic hyperplasia of a uterine horn. The cauliflower-like mass was greyish-white and glistening.

uterine lumen. This last activity helps create a bactericidal environment and supports the concept that high estrogen levels are an advantage in the treatment of bacterial invasion of the uterus. The progestational phase appears to encourage bacterial activity, making the uterus more susceptible to infection.[126]

Cystic Endometrial Hyperplasia

Clinical Signs: Mild cystic endometrial hyperplasia may not be recognized except at necropsy or ovariohysterectomy.[71] The cysts may be small and only observed microscopically. Successful mating and ovulation may not result in implantation under these conditions. Palpation of the uterus may not reveal anything abnormal. Histopathologically, this form of cystic endometrial hyperplasia may appear as only a pathologic extension of a normal process of uterine proliferation in preparation for blastocyst implantation.

The more common form of cystic endometrial hyperplasia is characterized by a large number of cysts ranging in size from several millimeters to several centimeters and containing clear fluid (Figs 11, 12). They resemble water-filled sacs. The cysts may course along the endometrial lining or be attached by a single pedicle. These cysts may be palpated as an enlarged uterus; however, care should be exercised during palpation since rough treatment may result in hemorrhage if the cysts are torn away from the endometrial lining. The cervix usually is closed under these conditions and hemorrhage may not be readily identified unless sufficient pressure is exerted to allow release of the fluid. The fluid is almost always sterile.

Treatment: Ovariohysterectomy is the treatment of choice. The ovaries usually have large cysts filled with fluid of high estrogen content. Treatment by aspiration of these cysts with subsequent pregnancy has not been successful in the author's hands.

Hydrometra

Cause: Hydrometra is an accumulation of watery or mucous fluid in the uterus. It is uncommon and most often observed at necropsy or ovariohysterectomy. It is related to the increased secretory activity of the endometrial glands as stimulated by progesterone. The accumulated fluid typically is sterile.

Clinical Signs: The condition may be recognized radiographically as uterine enlargements indicative of pregnancy except that the enlargements remain the same size and shape as time passes or may become elongated.

On palpation, the mucus-filled uterine enlargements are less firm than early fetuses and are more doughy in consistency. When the accumulated material is watery, the uterus may become distended. The uterus is thin-walled and palpation should be done with great care. Compression of the uterus rarely dilates the cervix but may express fluid in the direction of the ovary and into the abdominal cavity through the ovarian bursa.

Treatment: Medical treatment of hydrometra is unrewarding. Ovariohysterectomy is the treatment of choice.

Pyometra

Pyometra refers to accumulation of purulent material in the uterus, with the cervix closed. When the cervix is open, the condition should be referred to as purulent metritis; however, this condition usually is discussed synonomously with pyometra, closed or open. Pyometra is enhanced by the effects of progesterone upon the uterus. It is most common in nulliparous queens and has occurred in cats in which a significant portion of the uterus was not removed at ovariohysterectomy.

Cause: The exact pathogenesis of pyometra is poorly understood but it is probably related to the effects of both estrogen and progesterone, with the latter being the dominant factor. High circulating levels of progesterone normally are present during metestrus. Prolonged release of this hormone may be related to retained and cystic corpora lutea. The normal function of progesterone is development and proliferation of the endometrial glands. In the face of sustained progesterone production, cystic endometrial hyperplasia may develop. Progesterone is also responsible for the secretory activity of the endometrial glands, which, under excessive progestational influence, continue to produce large quantities of fluid. The distended uterine glands often are noted as large sacs associated with cystic endometrial hyperplasia. Progesterone also inhibits activity by the myometrium and effectively maintains a closed cervix, which prevents drainage of fluid from the uterus. In other species, progesterone has been associated with the development of an inflammatory component within the endometrium, thus providing the necessary medium for bacterial growth. Withdrawal of the progesterone influence causes regression of the inflammation.

In attempting to understand the pyometra complex, one must remember that estrogen plays an important role. Estrogen increases the vascularity of the uterus and promotes growth of the endometrium, uterus and cervix. It is also responsible for relaxation and dilation of the cervix, as well as for sensitization of the myometrium for contractility. In addition to the above mentioned antagonistic actions to progesterone, estrogen also causes migration of neutrophils toward the uterine lumen, increasing the bactericidal potential. Thus it is obvious that under normal conditions, estrogenic activity must precede the progesterone influence for pyometra to develop.

Escherichia coli is the most commonly isolated agent from the uterus of affected queens.[127] The purulent accumulation is sterile in about 15% of the cases. In attempts to produce pyometra by intrauterine inoculation with *E coli* and daily injections of progesterone, only 25% of the cats developed pyometra.[124] In the same study, the bactericidal effect of estrogen was reflected by failure of the inoculated organisms to survive in the uterus of cats receiving estrogen injections simultaneously.

Clinical Signs: The signs of pyometra may or may not be conspicuous, depending upon the severity of uterine involvement. Mild anorexia and depression may be the only sign recognized by the owner until the condition is well advanced. Infertility after repeated matings is a common complaint.

The estrous cycles may occur in a normal sequence; however, mating and ovulation may not result in pregnancy, depending upon the extent of the uterine involvement. There may be no obvious vulvar discharge and cervical dilation during a subsequent estrous period. The discharge may be consumed by the fastidious queen or may be limited and not evident. The only clue to a problem may be the lack of pregnancy. As a result of the next estrous cycle and mating, the uterine involvement may increase as progesterone levels again influence the intrauterine environment. The term chronic pyometra may be applied to cats so affected.

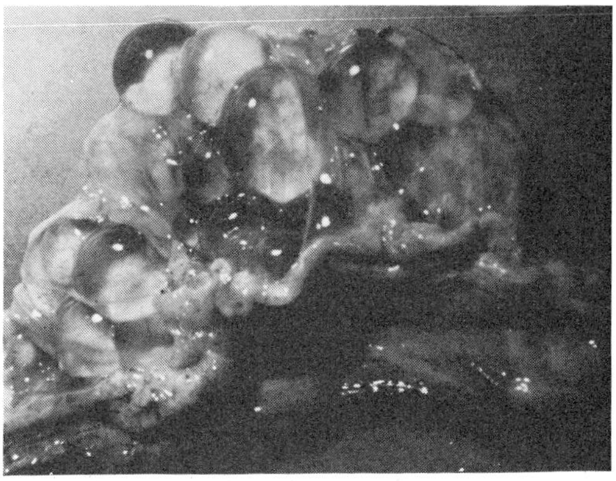

Fig 12. Cystic endometrial hyperplasia.

Severe cases are characterized by vulvar discharge, listlessness, anorexia, depression and fever. Toxemia may become a problem in cases in which the infection is active and the cervix is closed. The few cats with sterile pyometra may be asymptomatic. The vulvar discharge varies in color from off-white to dark red and brown. It is usually of relatively thick consistency and may be malodorous. The perineum may be soiled by the discharge, the vulva slightly edematous and the vaginal mucosa slightly erythemic.

Cats that have recurrence of pyometra often have cyclic signs. During the active inflammatory stages of uterine engorgement with purulent exudate, the cat is noticeably ill. Following evacuation of the uterus the condition of the queen improves but the uterus remains incapable of maintaining pregnancy.

Abdominal distension often is not recognized by the owner. When accompanied by weight loss secondary to anorexia and anemia, however, the distension becomes more obvious. Polyuria and polydipsia often are unnoticed by the owner. Vomiting may occur, especially as toxemia increases and renal function is disturbed. Dehydration may be evident and accentuated by preexisting renal disease. Weakness of the rear

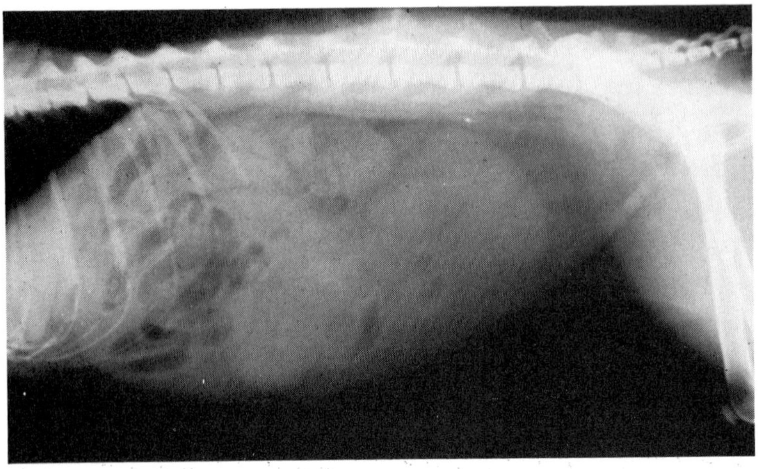

Fig 13. Cranial displacement of other abdominal viscera and distension of the uterus in a lateral radiograph of a queen with pyometra.

limbs is seen occasionally. Fever is an inconsistent sign of pyometra, and a subnormal body temperature may indicate profound debilitation and toxemia. Pain is not a common sign.

Diagnosis: Radiographic examination may reveal an elongated uterus or segmentation suggestive of 4-week-old fetuses (Fig 13). The density of the enlargements is homogeneous. Uterine rupture results in a ground-glass appearance of the abdomen on radiographs.

Hematologic examination reveals an overwhelming absolute neutrophilia, with as much as 30% immature forms.[128] The total WBC count may range from 20,000/mm^3 to over 100,000/mm^3 and depends upon cervical patency and the degree of bacterial activity, endometrial necrosis and duration of inflammation. The leukocytosis is accompanied by increased medullary activity and extramedullary myelopoiesis. In untreated or chronic pyometra the WBC count may fall to normal or subnormal levels. At this stage mature neutrophils predominate and may contain toxic granules. Marked leukopenia indicates severe toxemia and should prompt a guarded prognosis. Sterile pyometra may cause no elevation in WBC numbers.

About 50% of affected queens have a normocytic, normochromic anemia, the cause of which is unknown. Dehydration may mask the severity of the anemia initially. An increase in the myeloid:erythroid (M:E) ratio is due to hyperplasia of the myeloid elements and depression of the erythroid series.

One of the most common diseases to be differentiated from pyometra is FIP, which may be manifested chiefly by ascites. Analysis of abdominal fluid obtained by paracentesis, abdominal radiographs, blood chemistry (serum gamma globulin) assay and an indirect fluorescent antibody test can be used for differentiation.

Vaginitis can be easily differentiated from pyometra by examination of vaginal smears. Although WBC are present in both conditions, the number seen with pyometra far exceeds that associated with bacterial vaginitis. In pyometra, large aggregates of WBC and bacteria completely obliterate the presence of other cell types, such as noncornified vaginal epithelial cells.

Any disease accompanied by hypoproteinemia and subsequent ascites, such as hepatic and renal dysfunction or severe malnutrition, must be differentiated by pyometra. Likewise, the polyuria and polydipsia associated with cystitis or diabetes mellitus may mimic that of pyometra. Rupture of an abdominal organ, such as the bladder or intestine, and the resultant peritonitis must also be considered. If the breeding history is unknown, normal pregnancy could constitute a differential diagnosis (Fig 14). Concurrent pyometra of one cornu and viable pregnancy in another has also been reported.[129]

Treatment: The treatment of choice for cats with pyometra is ovariohysterectomy. Surgery must be performed promptly and in conjunction with supportive treatment before, during and after surgery.

Depending on the cat's condition and the results of the laboratory evaluations, presurgical treatment may include IV replacement fluids, electrolyte solutions, blood and broad-spectrum antibiotics. Very depressed and toxic cats benefit from IV corticosteroids immediately before and during surgery. Delaying surgery for several days while attempting to improve the cat's condition is futile.

During surgery, the patient should be given an electrolyte solution IV. It may be helpful to induce diuresis during surgery by giving 10% dextrose, 20% mannitol or ethacrynic acid.[126]

Administration of fluids usually is warranted for at least 24 hours after surgery. After the cat's condition is stable, often within a day after surgery, the patient should be sent home for the needed nursing care and oral medication. Prolonged hospitalization is contraindicated unless complications arise.

One of the most serious complications during surgery is rupture or tearing of the friable uterus. To minimize the chances of peritonitis and adhesions as a consequence of contamination by uterine contents, the peritoneal cavity should be thoroughly flushed with warm lactated Ringer's solution and water-soluble antibiotics instilled into the peritoneal cavity. Adhesions of the uterine stump, bladder, intestines, ureters or kidneys may also develop if there is leakage from any portion of the uterus when it is excised.

Gross examination of the excised uterus reveals areas of petechial hemorrhage interspersed among patches of cystic hyperplasia, resulting in variable thickness of the mucosa (Fig 15). The serosal surface usually is a darker red-blue than normal, and the superficial vessels are prominent and distended.[71]

If the patient is a valuable breeding queen, ovariohysterectomy may not be desired. Alternate treatments can be tried, but if they are unsuccessful or if the cat is severely debilitated and toxic, removal of the uterus and ovaries may be the only way of saving the animal's life.

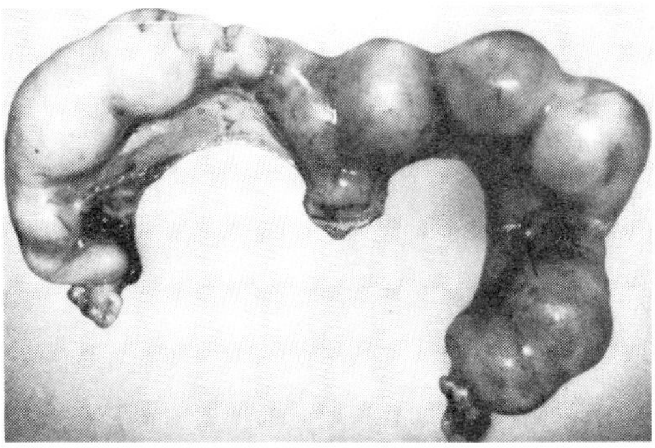

Fig 14. Uterine dilations in pyometra may be mistaken for fetuses on abdominal palpation.

Mildly affected cats have been successfully treated by uterine lavage and parenteral antibiotic therapy, with successful delivery of a subsequent litter. Recurrence of pyometra is common and necessitates either ovariohysterectomy or repeated lavage. Rarely has more than one litter been successfuly obtained after uterine lavage.

Medical treatment of pyometra requires that the cervix be dilated and drainage established. Dilation of the cervix is necessary for the insertion of a catheter for lavage. Cervical dilation is initiated by IM administration of 5 mg repository estradiol (*eg,* ECP:Upjohn), repeated in 5 days. Also, the resultant increased myometrial activity increases flow of fluids from the uterus. Systemic antibiotics also should be given.

When the cervix has dilated, a flexible plastic catheter may be carefully inserted into each horn of the uterus and the uterus flushed daily with nitrofurazone solution or a combination antibiotic-estrogen (Utonex:Schering).

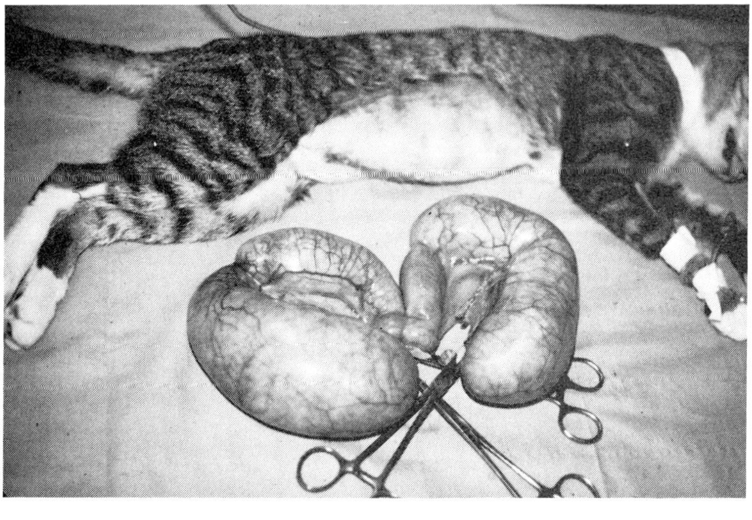

Fig 15. Grossly distended uterus removed from a queen with pyometra.

If the cervix remains closed, the uterus may be flushed via hysterotomy.[130] However, this is not recommended as the chance of leaving small pockets of pus still remains and the potential for abdominal contamination and consequent peritonitis is increased. Through a midline laparotomy incision, the uterus is incised and its contents removed. The cervix is dilated by retrograde insertion of forceps and a catheter inserted. The material removed from the uterus should be cultured. This is a high-risk method of treatment and the chances of successful reproduction thereafter are small.

The uterus must be flushed very gently, with the animal heavily sedated or lightly anesthetized and the cat's condition considered. Excessive pressure from forced fluids may rupture the uterus, resulting in peritonitis. Small perforations may go unnoticed until signs of peritonitis develop. Fluids may also be forced into the abdominal cavity through the ovarian bursa, producing similarly disastrous results.

Chronic Endometritis

Chronic endometritis is a common low-grade bacterial infection of the gravid or nongravid uterus. It may develop after recovery from acute metritis associated with parturition or may be the final stage of progesterone dysfunction that began as cystic endometrial hypererplasia.

Cats with chronic endometritis usually are asymptomatic except for their inability to have healthy litters. The estrous cycles of nulliparous affected cats may be infrequent and irregular. Once bred, the queen may conceive but aborts within a few weeks. If abortion does not occur, stillbirths and neonatal deaths are common, with 1-2 kittens occasionally surviving. In mature cats with a history of normal parturition, chronic endometritis results in smaller litters. After repeated breedings, the queen may fail to conceive or not even show signs of estrus.[37]

Diagnosis: In diagnosis of chronic endometritis, much emphasis is placed on the history and past breeding performance. If cystic endometrial hyperplasia is suspected, the cervix should be examined for patency. If the cervix is not patent, a uterine culture should be obtained with the cat heavily sedated or under light general anesthesia during a subsequent estrous period or during early metestrus.

Uterine cultures should be negative before infusion of a radiopaque material (*eg,* 25% Hypaque:Winthrop) to assist in the radiographic visualization of the uterus. Repository stilbestrol (2-3 mg IM) or estradiol cypionate (ECP:Upjohn) (0.25 mg IM) may be used to induce cervical dilation to facilitate infusion of the radiopaque material. Cervical dilation by the use of hormones may take 1-3 days. More than one view of the uterus should be obtained, preferably a ventrodorsal and a lateral. Irregularity of the uterine lumen, as outlined by the contrast material, may indicate cystic endometrial hyperplasia or hydrometra.

The most frequently cultured organism in cases of chronic endometritis is *E coli.* After the bacterial isolate has been identified and sensitivity tests performed, the appropriate antibiotics should be given systemically for at least 2 weeks. The cervix is rarely dilated sufficiently to permit intrauterine instillation of antibiotics. Concurrent hormonal therapy is contraindicated. If the cat is in estrus at the time antibiotic therapy is initiated, breeding should be delayed until the following estrus.

Systemic antibiotics should be administered again during the last 10 days of pregnancy and the first week after parturition. After weaning, another cervical specimen should be cultured to determine if additional antibiotic therapy is needed. Should abortion occur, long-term antibiotic therapy should be given again.

No antibiotics should be given to a queen immediately after breeding or during early to mid-pregnancy because of possible teratogenic effects. If specifically indicated by sensitivity test results, tetracyclines should be given only in the initial treatment of nonpregnant cats.

Cats with chronic endometritis unresponsive to antibiotic therapy should be treated by ovariohysterectomy.

Acute Metritis

Cause: Acute metritis may be life-threatening if left untreated. It may occur naturally after an estrous cycle or as a result of artificial insemination and excessive matings allowed by the queen during an extended estrous cycle. Regardless of the method by which the condition is induced, it is generally the direct result of an ascending infection via the cervix.

Acute metritis may also be noted after prolonged labor or dystocia, manipulation to remove a fetus, digital examination of the vagina without proper cleansing of the external genitalia and use of nonsterile materials during the exploratory process (Fig 16). Retention of placental membranes may also be a prime source of infection. Failure of longhaired cats to clean themselves after parturition may also contribute to the problem.

Clinical Signs: Acute metritis should be suspected when a queen fails to take care of the kittens and they are found weak, cold and improperly cleaned after parturition. The queen is ill and listless, and attempts to remove herself from the presence of the offspring. Because acute mastitis frequently accompanies acute metritis, the mammary glands should be examined before allowing the kittens to nurse cats with metritis. Bacterial contamination of the colostrum and milk may cause death of the kittens.

Because acute metritis usually involves the entire endometrial lining, the extent of involvement is reflected in the physical condition of the queen. Affected queens usually have a body temperature well above the normal postpartum temperature of 103 F (39.4 C). Vomiting, diarrhea, dehydration and inactivity are usual signs. There may be a dark-red to light-brown, thick, malodorous vulvar discharge that the queen does not attempt to clean. The discharge must be distinguished from that associated with retained placental membranes.

Abdominal palpation is painful and must be done with care to prevent greater damage to the very friable uterus. The danger of uterine rupture is not great except in protracted and untreated cases. The uterus has a doughy consistency and is significantly larger than in early metestrus. A CBC reveals a slight to moderate absolute leukocytosis, depending upon the severity of the infection. Serum creatinine and BUN values should be determined to assist in definition of a successful treatment regimen. Radiographic examination usually is not necessary unless fetal retention is suspected. Infusion of radiopaque material to assist in visualization of the uterus is contraindicated.

Treatment: Because streptococci, staphylococci and *E coli* are the most frequently isolated organisms, a broad-spectrum antibiotic should be given until the results of culture and sensitivity tests on the vulvar discharge are obtained. The uterus and vagina may be cleansed by gentle flushing with nitrofurazone (Furacin Solution:Eaton) or an estrogen-antibiotic combination (Utonex:Schering). Flushing by hysterotomy is not indicated unless the queen's condition is very stable and the results of all blood tests are normal. Care must be taken with this technic because of the possibility of bacterial contamination of the abdominal cavity. Evacuation of the uterus may be aided by the use of 0.1 mg ergonovine maleate (Ergonil:Pitman-Moore) given IM, followed by 0.05 mg given PO BID for 3 days.

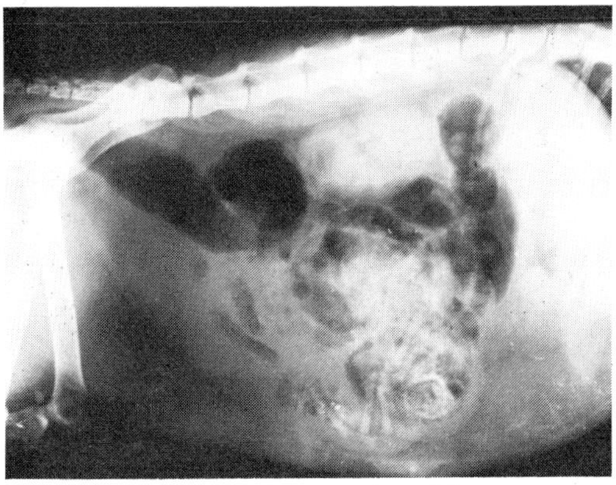

Fig 16. Retention of emphysematous fetuses.

Supportive therapy must be given to the debilitated queens, including force-feeding if necessary. In severely debilitated animals, an esophagostomy tube may be placed for feeding and removed after the health of the animal improves. Placement of the tube requires general anesthesia and care must be used in the choice and administration of the anesthetic used (see Chapter 2).

Queens that do not respond to therapy after 24 hours should be spayed, which may be risky but the only chance for the queen's survival. Any live kittens should be foster-nursed or hand-fed. Queens with a history of reproductive problems should be watched closely for 2-3 days after parturition to ensure a normal postpartum recovery and that kittens are progressing well and their food supply is plentiful and not contaminated.

Pyometra, peritonitis secondary to uterine rupture, chronic endometritis and sterility are possible sequelae of acute metritis not treated vigorously. Queens that recover should not be bred for at least 6 months and then only after cervical cultures obtained before breeding are negative. Educating the client on the nature of the problem is essential.

Uterine Prolapse

Only one horn of the uterus or the entire organ may prolapse anytime during parturition and up to 48 hours later. The cat may expel the fetuses from one horn, which subsequently prolapses, while the other horn is still gravid.[131] Usually, however, all of the kittens have been born before the prolapse occurs.

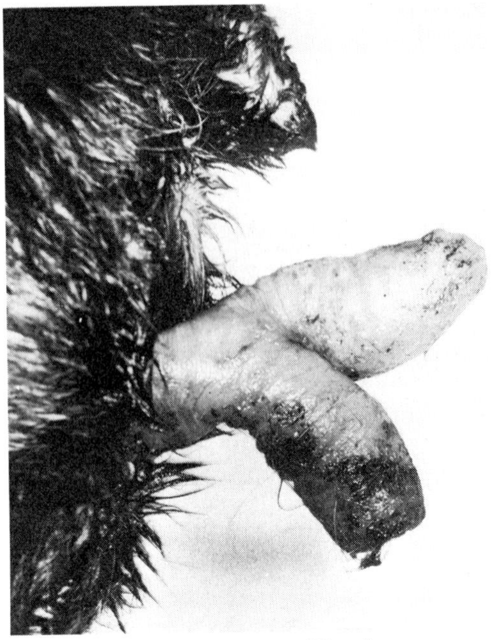
Fig 17. Postparturient prolapse of the uterus.

Primiparous or previously unaffected multiparous queens may have a uterine prolapse. The age range of affected cats has been 10 months to 8 years. Several kittens or one large kitten are born alive and active but may not survive because affected queens are reluctant to nurse.

Cause: The cause of uterine prolapse is unknown. Several possibilities have been proposed, including over-relaxation and stretching of the pelvic musculature, uterine atony due to metritis, incomplete separation of placental attachments, trauma resulting in bruising and small lacerations of the uterus, extreme and prolonged tenesmus accompanying dystocia, and postpartum contractions intensified by oxytocin release during lactation.[114,132,133]

Clinical Signs: The presence of 1 or 2 turgid, erythematous, tubular structures at the vulva is obvious (Fig 17). Litter, feces or placental membranes may be encrusted upon the surface. Ulcerations and hemorrhage of the endometrium develop from licking if the prolapse is not replaced promptly. The degree of tenesmus is variable. Pain during abdominal palpation, anxiety and polypnea may precede shock.

Treatment: If the prolapse has just occurred, manual reduction should be attempted provided that injury to the exposed organ is not extensive. After administration of general or epidural anesthesia, the cat is placed in lateral recumbency and the exposed uterus is cleansed with warm saline solution and rinsed with a mild antibacterial wash. A small amount of water-soluble lubricant is then applied to the exposed uterus and the uterus is replaced to its normal position by gentle manipulation with a gloved finger, sterile smooth syringe plunger or similar atraumatic instrument. If the tissues are too edematous to be replaced into the abdominal cavity, applying cold 50% dextrose solution topically for a short period may decrease the swelling sufficiently to allow replacement. The position of the uterus after replacement in the abdominal cavity can be determined by abdominal palpation. The hindlimbs are then elevated and each uterine horn is infused with an antibiotic-estrogen solution (Utonex:Schering). Vulvar sutures are not necessary because uterine prolapse does not tend to recur in cats.

Complications due to sepsis are avoided by administering an antibiotic after manual reduction. Use of oxytocin may be indicated if the replaced uterus remains atonic and flaccid. After successful reduction of a prolapsed uterus, the cat may be bred 6 months later and usually bears kittens without complications.

When manipulative reduction of a prolapsed uterus is not possible or if the prolapse has occurred many hours before presentation, one of several surgical procedures may be employed. If a laparotomy is performed, combining external with internal manual manipulation may be successful in replacing the uterus. The necessity of an ovariohysterectomy depends on the condition of the uterus. If ovariohysterectomy is not performed, fixation of the uterine horns to the abdominal wall (hysteropexy) is of questionable necessity in preventing recurrence.

If reduction cannot be accomplished with the uterus intact, after laparotomy the ventral aspect of the prolapsed uterine surface can be incised past the cervix and the one freed portion manipulated into the abdomen for ligation. After ligating the uterine vessels, the remaining portion of uterus is excised through the vaginal exposure after first applying a pursestring suture to the uterine stump. The ovaries should also be removed before the abdominal incision is closed.

Most queens recover with antibiotic therapy and routine postoperative care. Unless severely weakened, they usually resume nursing.

Uterine Torsion

Uterine torsion is a complication of mid- to late gestation. Usually only one uterine horn is rotated 90° along its long axis, in a clockwise or counterclockwise direction (Fig 18).[134-137]

Although rare, uterine torsion may occur in cats with pyometra, in which the uterine horns are greatly enlarged and distended. Uterine torsion also may result in uterine rupture.

Cause: The cause of uterine torsion is unknown. Careful questioning of the owner may reveal a history of a period of excitement, rough handling or similar activity during pregnancy. Fetal movement, uterine contraction and abortion may be contributing factors. The numbers and size of the fetuses may also be of some importance.

Clinical Signs: The signs of uterine torsion are not specific except that they reflect abdominal pain and are acute in onset. Depression, restlessness, anorexia and vomiting may be noticed early. Some affected cats may crouch and strain as though in labor; others frequently go to the litter box as if to urinate or defecate. There may be prior delivery of a healthy or dead kitten from one horn.

As the condition worsens, the cat may run excitedly for no reason or lie on her side and vigorously kick her legs; these are probably indications of pain. After a few hours, the onset of shock may be indicated by a subnormal temperature, pale mucous membranes and polypnea. A vaginal discharge may be serosanguineous or mucoid, or there may be none. The abdomen is tense and sensitive on palpation, and palpation of the uterus is difficult. There may be free fluid within the abdomen as a result of venous stasis and occlusion of major vessels. The abdomen is soon distended beyond that associated with normal pregnancy.

Vaginal examination may aid diagnosis if the cervix is sufficiently dilated to allow digital palpation of the caudal aspect of the rotated organ. Radiographs reveal the enlarged and possibly air- and fluid-filled uterus.

Although uterine torsion usually represents an acute, life-threatening crisis, the condition may exist for several days. In 2 such cases, the cats were only moderately depressed, had aborted kittens within the past 2-3 days and were afebrile. Following abdominal palpation and consideration of the radiographic findings, a laparotomy was performed. One cat had a 180° torsion of a gravid cornu. The other cornu had been the source of the previously expelled fetus and appeared to be involuting normally. Approximately 200 ml of serous fluid were present in the abdominal cavity. As the 7-week-old fetus

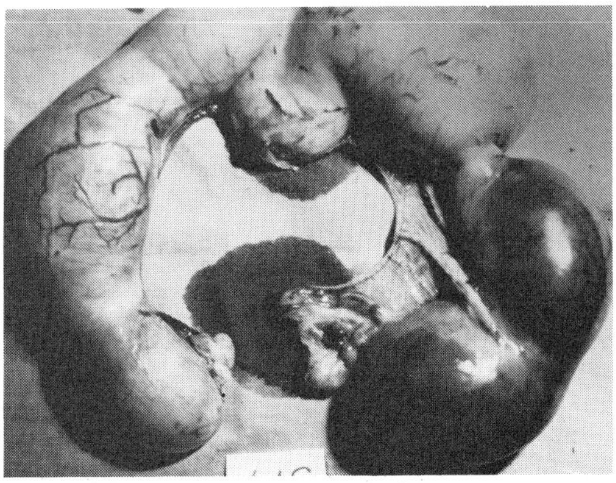

Fig 18. Torsion of one uterine horn involved 2 of 6 fetuses.

within the twisted horn was assumed to be dead, an ovariohysterectomy was performed. In the second cat the cornu from which the fetus had already been expelled was twisted 180°; the other horn had not been gravid.

Clinical signs vary with the extent of uterine involvement, the duration of the torsion and the stage of gestation at which it occurs. Depression, anorexia and vomiting may be noted early. Abdominal pain is evident and some affected queens frequent the litter box as if to urinate or defecate. The lack of fetal expulsion at parturition, coupled with obvious attempts by the queen to pass the remaining fetuses, may corroborate the diagnosis. Shock may follow. Pale mucous membranes, with or without a mucous vulvar discharge, are observed.

Treatment: The diagnosis of uterine torsion is confirmed at laparotomy and an ovariohysterectomy is performed. Supportive care must be provided during surgery, including IV administration of fluids, electrolytes, corticosteroids and antibiotics. If the cat is not in severe shock before surgery, the chances for complete recovery are fair. Death usually is attributed to severe shock but may also be due to massive hemorrhage from the engorged placenta.

Uterine Rupture

Cause: Rupture of the gravid uterus usually is related to trauma during mid- or late gestation. The uterus may rupture during parturition, especially if there is some degree of dystocia. Indiscriminate use of oxytocin under certain conditions, such as uterine atony or abnormal fetal size, anatomy or placement, at the time of parturition could be a predisposing factor.

Diagnosis: Diagnosis of uterine rupture may be based on the immediate history and the clinical signs. Radiographic examination of the abdominal cavity may be used to confirm the diagnosis. When trauma is suspected as the cause of uterine rupture, other abdominal organs must be evaluated for damage before treatment is instituted.

Clinical Signs: Evidence of uterine rupture may be found during routine ovariohysterectomy. Displacement of fetuses into the abdominal cavity results in their death. They may be found with or without intact fetal membranes and placental tissue. The fetuses are in various stages of decomposition and there may be fluid in the abdominal cavity. Healing of the uterine perforation with heavy scar tissue could prevent subsequent pregnancies, especially with rupture of both horns.

Treatment: Laparotomy may reveal a uterine torsion, with expulsion of the fetus and fluid accumulation in the uterus. Leakage of this fluid into the abdominal cavity is easily recognized. The horn from which the fluid has leaked is rarely torn but the fluid may enter the abdominal cavity through the ovarian bursa. One cat had a torsion of about 180° of one horn containing a fetus, while the other horn was the source of an expelled fetus. There were about 200 ml of fluid in the abdominal cavity. In another queen, a single fetus had been expelled and a uterine horn was twisted about 180°

The treatment of choice is ovariohysterectomy, with rigorous supportive care. Intravenous administration of fluids, electrolytes, corticosteroids and antibiotics is recommended. The uterus should be inspected for evidence of hemorrhage due to an engorged placenta. There is no evidence that uterine torsions may be corrected. The vascular involvement and stasis over an extended period prohibits successful correction.

A history of uterine rupture warrants a guarded prognosis during subsequent pregnancies since the uterus may rupture again at the same site. It is best not to immediately breed valuable queens during the next heat cycle. Depending upon the season of the year, the next estrous period could occur within 2-3 weeks, which would leave only a 2- to 3-week healing period for the uterine tissues.

Neoplasia

The incidence of feline uterine neoplasia is obscured by the fact that so many queens are altered at a relatively young age. Uterine neoplasia should be considered as a differential diagnosis in animals that do not become pregnant after successful mating. Uterine neoplasia has been most often reported in cats over 10 years of age. It may occur in nulliparous and multiparous cats.

Cats in which a partial ovariohysterectomy has been performed may develop uterine neoplasia. In one cat, the uterine horns had been severed 2 cm cranial to the uterine bifurcation. The cat died 4 years later when an endometrial adenocarcinoma developed.[138] The animal had also suffered chronic arsenic poisoning, a carcinogen with an affinity for the endometrium, 2 years previously.

Benign neoplasms of the uterus include fibroma, lipoma and leiomyoma, the last being the most common. Endometrial adenocarcinoma is the most common malignant tumor. Squamous-cell carcinomas are of vaginal or vulvar origin.

Uterine tumors may be singular or multiple. Metastasis of uterine tumors is not common but may involve a wide variety of organs, including the CNS and eyes.

Clinical Signs: Clinical signs indicative of uterine neoplasia are nonspecific but may include alteration of the estrous cycle, polydipsia, polyuria and abdominal distension.[138,139] Ascending pyometra may occur when a neoplasm causes the cervix to remain open.

Diagosis: The diagnosis of uterine neoplasia is aided by obtaining a complete reproductive history, abdominal palpation and radiography. Contrast radiography (pneumoperitoneogram) may be of some assistance.

Treatment: Ovariohysterectomy is the best treatment for uterine neoplasia. Multiple ovarian cysts are commonly noted in such cases. The relationship between ovarian cysts and uterine neoplasia is unknown.

Congenital Anomalies

Congenital anomalies of the uterus are uncommon in cats. Uterus unicornis and abnormal junction of the uterine body and horns have been reported.[140] Partial fusion of the horns has been observed, with their junction resembling an elongated uterine body extending craniad from the cervix. Unilateral uterine horn agenesis, with corresponding renal agenesis, has been observed in cats with a normal opposite ovary and uterine horn.

It is more important to realize that these abnormalities occur than to remember exactly what they were with regard to problems associated with estrus and subsequent pregnancy. Examination of the reproductive organs in problem queens should be complete, including exploratory laparotomy in some cases.

THE OVARIES

Diseases of the Ovaries

Ovarian Cysts

Cysts arising from the mature or atretic follicle and from the corpus luteum are the most common abnormalities of the feline ovary. Cysts arising from distension of mature follicles usually are singular and unilateral (Fig 19). They usually do not produce clinical signs and are most often incidental findings at ovariohysterectomy. Cysts arising from atretic follicles are multiple and often bilateral, and vary widely in size and shape. These cysts often are functional and may result in prolonged estrus, with signs of nymphomania. These queens are hard to handle, refuse to breed and may even become aggressive. Breeding rarely results in pregnancy.

Ovarian cysts are thin-walled and contain varying amounts of clear, watery fluid. The cysts apparently arise from excessive FSH production. Cats may be predisposed to development of ovarian cysts because ovulation and subsequent LH release are not spontaneous.

Treatment: Use of exogenous LH for resolution of ovarian cysts is not successful, but may depend somewhat on the size of the follicles and the numbers involved. Before such treatment is instituted, the ovaries should be examined at laparotomy. If the follicles are numerous and large, ovariohysterectomy should be performed. Cysts related to the corpora lutea should not be treated medically because their progestational activity may be the cause of metestral diseases. In general, ovariohysterectomy is the treatment of choice for any ovarian cyst.

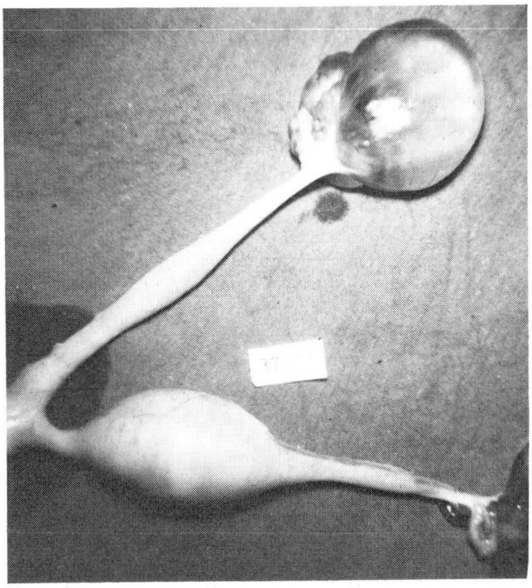

Fig 19. Ovarian cysts (top) and focal cystic endometrial hyperplasia (bottom). The queen was asymptomatic.

Ovarian Remnant Syndrome

The ovarian remnant syndrome refers to estrus in a cat that supposedly was spayed. The most frequent cause is failure to remove a small portion of the ovarian cortex at ovariohysterectomy. Whether this portion is left attached to the ovarian pedicle or falls free into the abdominal cavity makes no difference. Estrus after ovariohysterectomy is not always the result of faulty surgical technic. Functional ovarian tissue adjacent to the ovarian pedicle or at the broad ligament may also cause estrus in animals that have been properly neutered.

Depending upon the size of the amount of tissue remaining, follicles may mature and cysts may develop (Fig 20). The tissue develops a blood supply within the abdominal cavity relatively easily and continues its endocrine functions. The availability of the blood supply dictates whether ovarian endocrine function ceases altogether, is delayed or is resumed soon after ovariohysterectomy, with the associated behavioral signs of estrus. These signs are accompanied by the usual changes in the vaginal epithelium indicative of estrus (see Vaginal Cytology). The queen may mate but cannot conceive.

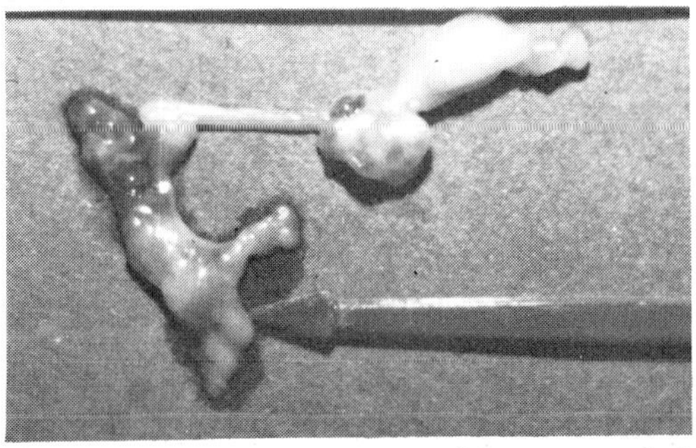

Fig 20. Ovarian remnants removed from queen that showed signs of estrus after incomplete ovariohysterectomy.

Hormonal alopecia may develop, beginning along the dorsum in the region of the tail head. The signs of estrus and alopecia usually develop simultaneously.

Treatment: Treatment involves a search of the abdominal cavity for the ovarian remnant. However, it usually is impossible to find. The ovarian stump should first be examined and then the abdominal cavity completely examined. Rarely is the offending tissue found unless it happens to be large enough to be spotted easily or unless cysts have developed that make the tissue recognizable. Because a disproportionate number of cats with this problem have been spayed through a flank incision, a midline incision should be used for ovariohysterectomy.

Neoplasia: The granulosa-cell tumor is the most common ovarian neoplasm in cats.[141] The abdominal mass usually is palpable and some degree of hyperestrogenism is evident, such as prolonged estrus and alopecia. The tumors typically are unilateral, yellow and cystic. Granulosa-cell tumors are malignant and commonly metastasize to the peritoneum and lungs.

Germ-cell tumors of the ovary include malignant dysgerminomas and malignant and benign teratomas. Other malignant ovarian tumors include the papillary adenocarcinoma, adenocarcinoma with spindle-cell formation and multiple metastases, and metastatic bilateral carcinoma of endometrial origin.[141] The last 2 neoplasms were accompanied by ascites. A lipid-cell tumor of the ovary caused masculinization, evidenced by a deepened vocal tone and enlargement of the head and neck musculature.[141]

THE VAGINA

Diseases of the Vagina

Vaginitis

Cause: Primary vaginitis is not common in cats and usually occurs in prepubertal females. Secondary vaginitis occurs in sexually mature cats of all ages. A wide variety of causes includes excessive mating during an abnormally long estrous period, coital injury, injury to vaginal tissue due to manipulative delivery of a lodged fetus, pyometra, cystitis and possibly viral rhinotracheitis.

Clinical Signs: A slight discharge may be evident, although it may not be evident because of the fastidious nature of cats.[142] Reddening of the vulva from constant licking may be a clue to the problem, which may become obvious upon close inspection of the tissues around the vagina and vulva. Frequent micturition is not uncommon with vaginitis but is more often associated with other problems, such as cystitis.

The amount of vaginal discharge usually is related to the extent of the vaginitis and its duration. Acute cases involve more inflammation and are readily recognizable. Chronic cases are more serious and more difficult to diagnose, with the vaginal mucosa appearing grey.

Diagnosis: A hemogram and abdominal radiograph should be done to assess the extent of the infection and to ensure that extension of the inflammation to the uterus has not occurred. Urinalysis should be performed in all cases of vaginitis to rule out concomitant cystitis. The urine sample should be obtained only after flushing and cleansing of the vagina, and then by catheterization if possible or by obtaining a midstream sample. Finding large numbers of WBC and only a few cornified epithelial cells on a vaginal smear stained with Wright's stain may assist in differentiating vaginitis from estrus. Culture and antibiotic sensitivity tests should dictate the appropriate medical management of the condition.

Treatment: Treatment consists of thorough flushing of the vagina with warm sterile saline, preferably with the queen sedated or lightly anesthetized so that struggling does not impede adequate treatment. A dilute (1:10,000) potassium permanganate solution may be used with a curved tip flushing syringe to lavage the vagina after most of the mucoid material has been removed. After use of the permanganate solution, the vagina should be rinsed with warm saline so as not to leave the permanganate in prolonged contact with the vaginal epithelium. The vagina may also be flushed with nitrofurazone, chlorhexidine (Nolvasan:Fort Dodge) or a variety of other compounds with similar results. Regardless of the solution used, the flushing must be gentle, the solution warm and flushing repeated until the vaginal wash is clean. Occasional application of an oil-based antibiotic (*eg*, Furacin Solution:Eaton) on a swab to coat the vaginal mucosa may be beneficial.

Broad-spectrum antibiotics may be used parenterally until specific treatment is indicated by identification of the proper antibiotic. If the cat is in estrus, further mating is not recommended until the next cycle or the condition has cleared sufficiently. A painful mating may make the

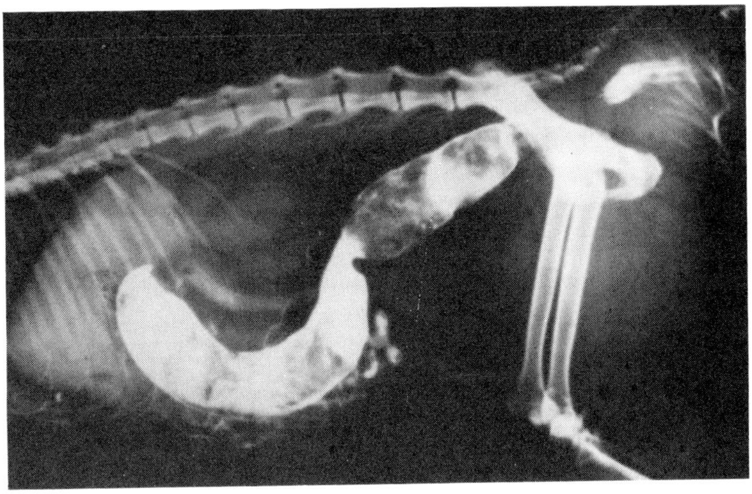

Fig 21. Compression of the barium-filled colon by a vaginal leiomyoma.

queen less than receptive during subsequent estrous cycles.

Neoplasia

The most common vaginal neoplasm is the leiomyoma. The vagina of any queen with a history of breeding problems or failure of intromission by the male should be examined to determine if a vaginal tumor is the cause of such problems. Vaginal tumors also may cause chronic constipation and perineal swelling. Extension of cervical cancer should also be considered when vaginal tumors are noted.

Contrast radiography may aid diagnosis, depending upon the location of the obstructing tumor and its type (Figs 21, 22). Rather than total excision, if possible, biopsy of vaginal tumors is recommended. Subsequent histopathologic examination may be used to determine the tumor's potency for metastasis. Ovariohysterectomy may be necessary if the cervix is involved, if the vagina is nearly obliterated by the tumor or if the tumor has a high metastatic potential.

THE MALE REPRODUCTIVE TRACT

Anatomy and Physiology

The testes are fully descended in male kittens at birth. Leydig cells are active within the testes at birth but become quiescent until the kitten is about 3 months of age. These cells normally mature at about 5 months and by the sixth month, early spermatogenesis may be observed histologically. Sperm cells usually are present within the testes by 7 months.

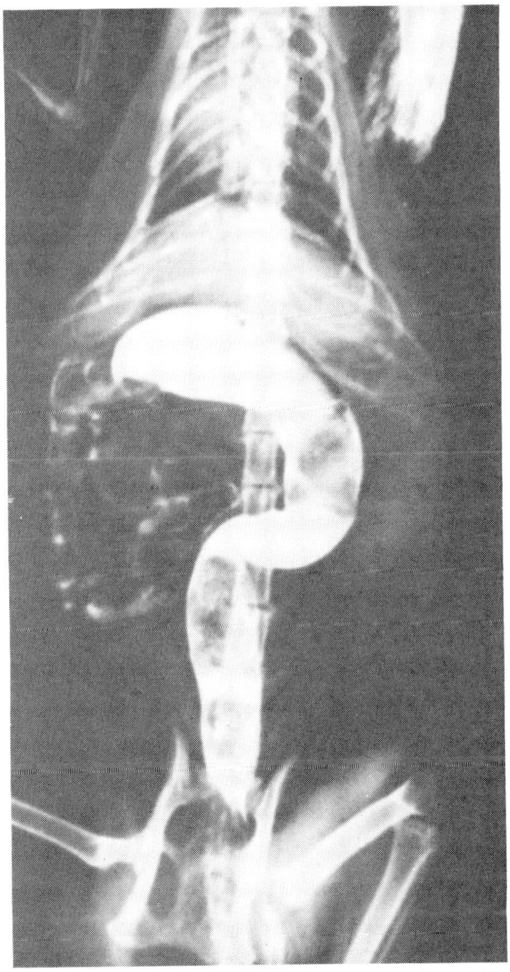

Fig 22. In this ventrodorsal view of the cat in Figure 21, the colon is displaced laterad and contains no barium at the tumor site.

Male cats are sexually mature at 9-12 months of age and remain fertile throughout the year, although some physiologists believe there is a seasonal variability in the fertility of male cats. Most breeding activity is nocturnal. A few male cats have a rudimentary os penis, 3-5 mm long and located dorsal to the urethra.

The distal shaft of the penis is covered with about 120 spines facing the base of the penis (craniad). The spines may stimulate release of LH by the queen during the mating process when they are in contact with the vaginal epithelium. The presence of the spines depends upon the presence of androgen, as they disappear 2-4 months after castration. They are not essential for mating but do add to stimulation of the female. Ablation of the cutaneous mechanoreceptors of the glans penis anesthetizes the penis and results in aberrant mounting and disoriented thrusting.[143,144]

Semen Characteristics

The ejaculate volume varies from 0.03 ml to 0.3 ml, with an average of 0.05 ml. The total numbers of sperm in an ejaculate ranges from 60×10^6 to 15×10^8, varying with the frequency of ejaculation.[46,145,146]

The normal proportion of motile sperm is 80-90%. The proportion of sperm with club tails is 3-5% and with cytoplasmic droplets is 1-4%. The pH of semen is 7.4. These values are based on collection by electroejaculation or with an artificial vagina.

Semen may readily be examined by removal from the vagina after mating. A saline-moistened, cotton-tipped applicator stick or a medicine dropper with 1-2 drops of warm (body temperature) saline may be used. The sample is transferred to a glass slide for microscopic examination of sperm numbers, shape and motility. When obtaining the sample, it is important to remember that the semen will be diluted and that sperm cells are easily damaged. Care must be used in obtaining the sample. The smears may be examined with or without the use of a coverslip and staining. Use of stains diminishes the motility and soon kills the cells. Regardless of the technic used, it is important to examine the slide immediately since exposure to room temperature significantly decreases the motility.

Semen is deposited in the vagina near the cervix. The method by which sperm cells reach the oviduct is a complicated process involving muscular and ciliary activity, neurohumoral influences and sperm motility.[147] High circulating levels of estrogen in the queen enhance the efficiency of sperm transport. Only 40-120 sperm reach the oviduct when deposited in numbers of about 56×10^6.

The life span of the feline sperm cell in the reproductive tract of the female is not greater than 50 hours. The shorter the estrous period, the shorter the survival time of the sperm cells in the female reproductive tract. The life span of an ovulated ovum is only 24 hours. Because the female normally ovulates 24 hours postcoitus, more than one mating is advocated to ensure sufficient numbers of sperm to fertilize all ovulated ova.

Feline sperm cells require capacitation before they can penetrate the egg, as in other species. Eggs cultured with fresh semen are not fertilized. The sperm cells appear to require 1-2 hours *in utero* for capacitation and 1-2 hours to migrate from the site of deposition to the oviduct.

Castration

Castration is the most common surgical procedure performed on male cats. It is used as a method of population control, and it makes the male cat a better pet by reducing urine odor, straying tendencies, and territorial fighting and marking (spraying). The veterinarian should be aware, however, that castration does not always completely eliminate such undesirable behavior.

Castration of the adult cat is 80-90% effective in causing either a rapid or gradual decline in fighting, roaming and urine spraying.[148] A rapid decline in one objectionable behavioral pattern is not always followed by the same rate of decline of another. Thus, fighting and roaming may be reduced at similar rates, while fighting and spraying are not. Differences in decline of various behavior are not due to residual testosterone since testosterone levels become undetectible within 6 hours after castration; nor is there compensatory adrenal production of androgen.[148]

Male cats that have displayed the most intense sexual behavior for the longest periods are the ones in which such activities persist for the longest periods after castration.[148] This is not meant to imply, however, that these cats indefinitely continue to exhibit objectionable sexual behavior after castration. Most veterinarians have seen sexually active cats that, after being castrated at 9-10 years of age, lost typical male behavioral patterns and became good pets.

The effects of castration are not based on elimination of the masculine neural substrate, but on elimination of testosterone that activates the substrate. Retention of the masculine neural substrate explains occasional urine spraying for territorial marking by a castrated cat.[148]

The veterinarian should advise the owner that certain nonsexual aggressive behavior, such as predatory or fear-induced aggression, is unaffected by castration.[148]

There is no evidence that castration causes obesity. Decreased roaming should prompt substantial reduction of food offered, however.

Cats that continue to spray urine after castration may respond to IM injection of 10 mg medroxyprogesterone acetate (Depo-Provera: Upjohn). Repeated doses occasionally are required before the habit is abolished.

The preferred age at which to castrate a male cat has been a controversial subject among veterinarians. At one time it was felt that early castration (5 months) was preferred to reduce the likelihood of undesirable behavioral patterns, such as urine spraying, fighting, and roaming. The opponents of early castration held that the subsequent failure of normal urethral development increased the possibility of urethral obstruction. It has since been shown that prepubertal castration does not alter urethral circumference.[149] However, preputial adhesions to the penis are more likely in prepubertally castrated cats.[150] Such adhesions prevent full extrusion of the penis for urination and routine grooming. Accumulation of debris and urine in the resultant fold increases the possibility of ascending urinary infections.

There appears to be an increase in body fat laid down subcutaneously, with the characteristic location being the inguinal skin folds. Diet, in relation to activity, can be used to control this effect in most animals if the owner can be convinced of the necessity. Failure of development of the secondary sex characteristic of the "thick skin" at various sites, particularly around the neck as noted in old intact toms, may occur in cats prepubertally castrated. Certain changes in hair growth, with eventual hair loss on the ventral body, have been attributed to early castration. Treatment by SC implantation of 25 mg testosterone cypionate (Depo-Testosterone: Upjohn) has been a successful method of treatment. The cat must be watched for undesirable side effects, such as restlessness, or excessive vocalization, while under treatment with testosterone. Use of estrogens for this type of condition is contraindicated.

Castration before 6 months of age is not recommended. Veterinarians associated with the field of feline reproduction usually recommend castration at 7 months or even 10 months of age unless there are extenuating circumstances. Each cat to be castrated should be considered individually with regard to full development of secondary characteristics. Some males, especially purebred animals such as Persians, mature very slowly and should not be castrated before 1½ years of age. Altered male cats may be shown or exhibited and thus must be fully mature before castration so as not to remove male characteristics upon which they may be judged.

Other Methods of Sterilization

Although not frequently performed in cats, vasectomy is a simple and reliable procedure. Vasectomy may not decrease libido, especially in experienced breeding toms. Mating of estrous females by vasectomized males induces ovulation and may prolong the period between estrous cycles because of development of pseudocyesis.

Chemical sterilization is strictly experimental and must be used with that in mind. Use of alphachlorohydrin decreases the motility of the sperm cells, thereby accomplishing sterility.[151]

Diseases of the Male Genitalia

Aside from the feline urologic syndrome (see Chapter 12), diseases and physical anomalies of the male genital tract are not common. The most common problems are related to trauma.

Penile Hematoma

Penile hematoma is a common consequence of urethral obstruction. Gentle manipulation or careful catheterization and flushing may be used to remove an obstruction from the urethra, often related to the feline urologic syndrome (see Chapter 12).

Penile Hair Ring

During mating, friction of the penile spines against perineal and back hair of the female may result in accumulation of hair around the base of the glans penis. As the hair ring enlarges after repeated mountings, intromission and successful mating may be impossible.[152] Cats with penile hair rings display persistent mounting activity, with prolonged pelvic thrusting (Fig 23).

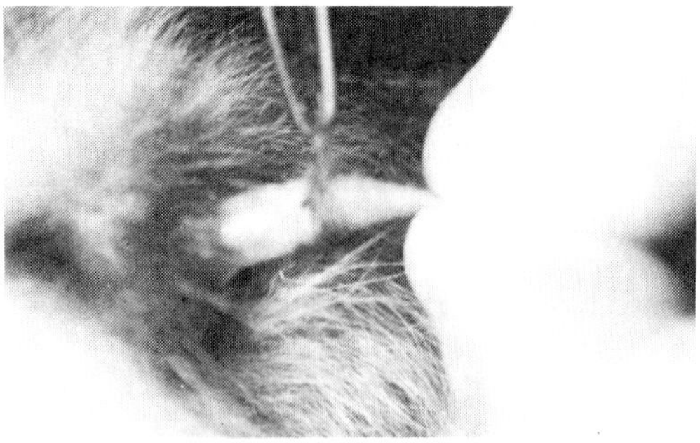

Fig 23. Hair ring encircling the glans penis. (Courtesy of Dr B.L. Hart and Lab Anim Sci)

Often the male cat removes the hair ring during routine grooming. Otherwise, it is easily removed with forceps by retracting the preputial sheath and sliding the hair ring over the glans. Successful mating is then immediately possible.

Cryptorchidism

The testes of kittens are descended at birth. They are palpated only with great difficulty at that time but are readily palpated at 4-6 weeks of age. When a testis has not descended at birth and remains undescended for 4-6 months, it rarely descends on its own and should be removed by laparotomy. Administration of exogenous hormones of any type has been unsuccessful in initiating testicular descent in such cases.

The incidence of this condition is higher in purebred cats than in mixed-breeds. This may be due, in part, to the care given to these animals versus those cats that are free-roaming and in which breeding is not a predeterminant. Cryptorchids may have more feminine characteristics than the average male. Monorchism is more common than cryptorchidism. Monorchids can mate and produce normal offspring. There is no evidence that either of these conditions is an inherited trait in cats.

In cases of so-called "yo-yo" testis, one testis is retracted into the inguinal canal except during periods of hormonal stimulation related to the mating season. When the male is placed with an estrous female, the retracted testis descends. It retracts when the male is isolated or removed from the presence of a female in estrus. Movement of the testis is relatively rapid, *ie,* retraction takes only hours. These animals can mate and produce offspring, and appear to have no significant decrease in libido.

Treatment: Because of the increased risk of neoplasia in retained testes, cryptorchids or monorchids should be castrated as young adults. Occasionally the retained testes cannot be found at laparotomy. Usually they are located in or near the inguinal canal. If the cat has reached puberty, the retained testes are soft and atrophic, with a tortuous vas deferens. The relatively high temperature in the abdominal cavity causes degeneration of the seminiferous tubules and subsequent aspermatogenesis.

The animal's history of past reproduction should be considered. If other males in the lineage have had similar problems, the male in question should be castrated.

Scrotal Inflammation

The position and anatomy of the scrotum of cats afford great protection to the male reproductive organs. Bite wounds or inflammation of the scrotum due to chemical or physical injury are rare. Injuries that prevent the male cat from lifting its tail may result in inflammation from accumulation of feces and urine on the scrotum.

Cats with scrotal inflammation are febrile and often reluctant to move. The perineal area is painful to the touch. Licking, in an effort to alleviate the problem, may add to the problem due to the spinous processes of the tongue. Scrotal edema is occasionally noted.

Treatment: The scrotum should be gently cleaned and the cause of the inflammation determined, if possible. Cool, moist packs should be applied and broad-spectrum antibiotics given parenterally for at least 24 hours before castration. Application of an Elizabethan collar may be required to prevent the animal from licking the affected area and interfering with treatment.

Scrotal Hematoma

Scrotal hematomas occasionally occur due to inadequate hemostasis during castration. The scrotum should be reopened and adequate hemostasis achieved after cleaning the scrotum thoroughly. Antibiotic powder may be administered through the incision site to control infection at the discretion of the surgeon.

Scrotal Distension

Scrotal distension that is cool, painless and fluctuating may be observed in cases of FIP. The fluctuation may be due to fluid draining from the peritoneal cavity since it is continuous with the scrotum through the inguinal canal.

Orchitis

Orchitis due to *Brucella* infection has only been observed once in a cat.[71] Some investigators believe cats have a natural resistance to *Brucella* infection.

Neoplasia

Testicular neoplasms in cats are rare. There are reports of Sertoli-cell tumors, with and without metastasis, in the literature.[153] The low incidence of testicular tumors may in part be due to the infrequent observation of old, intact males or the fact that a high proportion of male cats are castrated.

An adenocarcinoma in the prostate gland of an old cat caused urinary obstruction.[133]

Infertility in Male Cats

Infertility in males may be related to psychologic problems, physical injury or hormonal insufficiency. The psychologic problems usually are related to the environment or a previous mating experience (see Chapter 19). Physical problems may be related to retained testes, penile hair rings and possibly hormonal disorders, such as hypothyroidism, although the last is not well documented. Improper administration of estrogens may cause testicular atrophy and subsequent infertility. A complete history must be obtained and physical examination performed to help determine the cause of infertility.

Artificial Insemination

Artificial insemination is currently practiced in laboratory colonies, with excellent results.[46] Semen is collected from trained males in an artificial vagina, diluted and used immediately. Semen has also been frozen, thawed and successfully used for insemination.[161] Use of frozen semen may be advantageous to some owners of purebred cats. These technics have been used in naturally estrous cats and those in which estrus has been induced through use of exogenous hormones. Artificial insemination requires time and patience, and should only be performed by those trained in the technic.

The simplest method of semen collection is with an artificial vagina. A teaser queen usually is used to help train the male. The queen may be one in natural estrus or one in which estrus has been induced by administration of FSH or PMSG (see Induction of Estrus). Properly trained males may not need the teaser queen and can be induced to mount the artificial vagina in the queen's absence.

The artificial vagina is constructed by placing a 2-ml rubber pipette bulb, with the bulb tip removed, over a 2 x 44-mm test tube. The tube assembly is placed inside a water jacket made from a 35 x 75-mm (60-ml) polyethylene bottle, and the rolled end of the pipette bulb is stretched over the rim of the water bottle jacket. The semen is kept viable by maintaining a temperature of 125.6 F (52 C) inside the water jacket that in turn provides a semen temperature of 111.2-114.8 F (44-46 C).

A small amount of water-soluble lubricant is applied to the artificial vagina, which is then easily slipped onto the erect penis of the tomcat as he mounts the female. After collection and careful removal of the test tube from the rest of the system to avoid contamination of the water jacket, the semen is diluted. The usual ejaculate (0.05 ml containing 50-60 x 10^6 spermatozoa) is diluted with sufficient warm (52 C, 126 F) normal saline to produce 0.1-ml aliquots, each containing about 10 x 10^6 spermatozoa.[42]

Semen has also been collected by electroejaculation, with the animal anesthetized with ketamine.[155] The volumes collected are about the same as those collected with an artificial vagina. A special rectal probe, which delivers a specific voltage in a sequence of stimuli, is used for electroejaculation.

Kittens have been successfully born from pregnancies initiated by insemination with sperm collected in this manner, either directly after collection or after freezing and thawing. The latter has important ramifications for purebred breeders in that the semen of prominent or rare males may be preserved for considerable periods. This also increases the possibility of shipping the semen for insemination rather than transporting the estrous queen for mating. Although use of artificial insemination has just begun in cats, the portent is great if one considers what has happened in other domestic species.

Male cats have been ejaculated at various intervals to observe the animal's libido, numbers of normal and abnormal sperm, and ejaculate volume.[46] Weekly collection resulted in a variation in volume and total sperm count, while collection 3 times a week resulted in a relatively constant ejaculate volume, with the sperm count nearly equaling the normal weekly total. Daily ejaculation sharply reduced the sperm count by the fourth day, at which time it leveled off. This appeared to indicate that the numbers of sperm cells recovered after the fourth day of the daily routine would be the normal sperm production for the animal. There were no significant changes in the numbers of abnormal sperm cells, even when semen was collected daily.

When the queen is showing signs of estrus, as confirmed by a vaginal smear, the diluted semen is instilled just caudal to the cervix with a bulb-tipped, 9-cm, 20-ga spinal needle on a 0.25-ml syringe.[46] Ovulation is induced by administering 50 IU of human chorionic gonadotrophin (HCG) IM at the time of the first insemination. A second insemination 24 hours later results in a conception rate of 75%. If the queen is inseminated again, an additional 10 IU of HCG are given.

Tomcats used for artificial insemination can be ejaculated 2-3 times weekly without lowering the sperm count. Thus, with the double insemination method, one tomcat can service 12-15 queens weekly through semen dilution. Under normal breeding circumstances, which would include 2-3 breedings per queen on successive days, only 2 queens could be bred weekly by tomcats without lowering the sperm count per ejaculate.

Litter size is slightly lower (2-4 kittens) with artificial insemination than with normal breeding, although this may be due to use of only virgin queens. Gestation may be slightly prolonged (65-72 days).[46]

Homosexuality

Homosexual behavior in male or female cats is not uncommon. It is not true homosexuality in that sexual activity with the same sex is not preferred to the exclusion of that with the opposite sex.[156] Homosexual behavior, such as mounting, grasping the neck with the teeth and pelvic thrusting, usually occurs in the absence of an intact cat of the opposite sex. When an estrous queen is present, homosexual activity between males is quickly diverted and interest is given to her. Mounting may also occur among queens in estrus in the absence of tomcats.

Prepubertal kittens of both sexes often engage in homosexual play. Mounting may be an expression of territorial dominance and usually is accepted passively by the less dominant male.[157]

References

1. Chakraborty, PK *et al.* Lab Anim Sci **29** (1979) 338.
2. Pond, G: The Cat Encyclopedia. Crown Publishers, New York, 1972.
3. Jemmett, JE and Evans, JM. J Sm Anim Pract **18** (1977) 31.
4. McDonald, LE: Veterinary Endocrinology and Reproduction. 1st ed. Lea & Febiger, Philadelphia, 1969.
5. Herron, MA. Vet Clin No Am **7** (1977) 715.
6. Dawson, AB. Endocrin **28** (1941) 907.
7. Scott, PP and Lloyd-Jacob, MA. Nature **184** (1959) 2022.
8. Crandall, EE *et al.* J Neurosurg **25** (1966) 140.
9. Wildt, DE *et al.* Horm Behav **10** (1978) 251.
10. Wildt, DE *et al.* Am J Vet Res **38** (1977) 1429.
11. Scott, in Hafez: Reproduction and Breeding Techniques for Laboratory Animals. Lea & Febiger, Philadelphia, 1970.
12. Colby, ED. Lab Anim Care **30** (1970) 1075.
13. Whalen, RE and Hardy, DF. Physiol Behav **5** (1970) 529.
14. Hart, BL. Physiol Behav **7** (1971) 675.
15. Herron, MA. Feline Pract **3(4)** (1973) 4.
16. Wildt, DE *et al.* Lab Anim Sci **28** (1978) 301.
17. Burke, TJ. Feline Pract **5(6)** (1975) 16.
18. Oen, EO. Nord Vet-Med **29** (1977) 287.
19. Burke, TJ *et al.* Am J Vet Res **38** (1977) 469.
20. Sokolowski, JH. Mod Vet Pract **55** (1974) 505.
21. Burke, TJ. Vet Clin No Am **7** (1977) 669.
22. Gerber, HA and Sulman, FG. Vet Rec **76** (1964) 1089.
23. Colton, MW. Mod Vet Pract **46(6)** (1965) 53.
24. Newman, MS. Feline Pract **10(4)** (1980) 6.
25. Jochle, W. Canine Pract **1(5)** (1974) 8.
26. Djerassi, C *et al.* Bull Atom Sci, Jan (1973) 10.
27. Schille, VM and Stabenfeldt, GH. Biol Reprod **21** (1979) 1217.
28. Verhage, HG *et al.* Biol Reprod **14** (1976) 579.
29. West, NB *et al.* Biol Reprod **17** (1977) 138.
30. Schille, VM *et al.* Biol Reprod **21** (1979) 953.
31. West, NB *et al.* Endocrin **99** (1976) 1010.
32. Gerber, HA *et al.* J Sm Anim Pract **14** (1973) 151.
33. Harris, W and Wolchuk, N. Am J Vet Res **24** (1963) 1003.
34. Moltzen, H. Nord Vet-Med **14** (1962) 69.
35. Sulman, FG. Vet Med **56** (1961) 513.
36. Russe, M and Jochle, W. Kleintier-Praxis **8** (1963) 87.
37. Joshua, JO: The Clinical Aspects of Some Diseases of Cats. JB Lippincott, Philadelphia, 1965.
38. Arthur, GH: Wright's Veterinary Obstetrics. 3rd ed. Williams & Wilkins, Baltimore, 1964.
39. Roberts, SJ: Veterinary Obstetrics and Genital Diseases. 3rd ed. Edwards Bros., Ann Arbor, MI, 1961.
40. Mills, JN. Can Vet J **20** (1979) 95.
41. Cline, EM *et al.* Feline Pract **10(2)** (1980) 47.
42. Sojka, NJ. Norden News, Fall (1970) 1.
43. Herron, MA and Sis, RF. Am J Vet Res **35** (1974) 1277.
44. Foster, MA and Hisaw, FL. Anat Rec **62** (1935) 75.
45. Greulick, WW. Anat Rec **58** (1934) 217.
46. Sojka, NJ. Lab Anim Care **20** (1970) 199.
47. Hoogeweg, JH and Folkers, ER. JAVMA **156** (1970) 73.
48. Bloom, F: Pathology of the Dog and Cat. American Veterinary Publications, Santa Barbara, 1954.

49. Denker, HW *et al.* Anat Embryol **154** (1978) 39.
50. Catcott, EJ. Mod Vet Pract **53(7)** (1972) 7.
51. Paape, SR *et al.* Biol Reprod **13** (1975) 470.
52. Prescott, CW. Aust Vet J **49** (1973) 126.
53. Boyd, JS. J Sm Anim Pract **12** (1971) 501.
54. Smith, RN. J Sm Anim Pract **9** (1968) 497.
55. Smith, RN. J Sm Anim Pract **10** (1969) 523.
56. Berman, E. Am J Vet Res **35** (1974) 457.
57. Beaver, BG. Feline Pract **3(5)**(1973) 24.
58. Smithcors, JF. Mod Vet Pract **47(4)** (1966) 25.
59. Wislocki, GB and Hamlett, GWD. Anat Rec **61** (1934-1935) 97.
60. Dederer, PH. Anat Rec **60** (1934) 391.
61. De Nooy, PP. VM/SAC **74** (1979) 349.
62. Hansen, JS. VM/SAC **69** (1974) 1135.
63. Tomlinson, J *et al.* Feline Pract **10(5)** (1980) 18.
64. Carrig, CB *et al.* JAVMA **160** (1972) 308.
65. Gilbride, AP. Feline Pract **2(5)** (1972) 5.
66. Berman, E *et al.* Lab Anim Care **17** (1967) 511.
67. Dawson, AB and Kosters, BA. Am J Anat **75(1)** (1944) 1.
68. Stein, BS. Mod Vet Pract **55** (1974) 597.
69. Walton, TE and Gillespie, JH. Cornell Vet **60** (1970) 215.
70. Hemsley, LA. Vet Rec **68** (1956) 152.
71. Jubb, KV and Kennedy, PC: Pathology of Domestic Animals. 2nd ed. Academic Press, New York, 1970.
72. Petrak, M and Carpenter, J. JAVMA **146** (1965) 728.
73. Frenkel, JK. Paper presented at Am Assoc Feline Pract seminar, 1974.
74. Gilbride, AP. Feline Pract **2(1)** (1972) 10.
75. McKinney, HR. VM/SAC **68** (1973) 493.
76. Dubey, JP. Feline Pract **3(5)** (1973) 14.
77. Frenkel, JK *et al.* Science **167** (1970) 893.
78. Frenkel, JK. Comp Immun Microbiol Infect Dis **1** (1978) 15.
79. Willard, MD and Crow, SE. Comp Cont Ed AHT **2** (1981) 158.
80. Scott, FW and Gillespie, JH. Vet Scope **17(1)** (1973) 1.
81. Scott, FW and Gillespie, JH. Proc 36th Ann Mtg AAHA, 1969.
82. Hoover, EA and Griesemer, RA. JAVMA **158** (1971) 929.
83. Hardy, WD. Vet Clin No Am **4** (1974) 133.
84. Tan, RJS and Miles, JAR. Aust Vet J **50** (1974) 142.
85. Scott, FW *et al.* Feline Pract **9(2)** (1979) 44.
86. Scott, FW and Geissinger, C. Feline Pract **8(6)** (1976) 31.
87. Brooks, C and Murray, JG. JAVMA **170** (1977) 1413.
88. Sekeles, HBE and Marcus, R. Feline Pract **10(3)** (1980) 44.
89. Hannon, CA. Mod Vet Pract **62** (1981) 133.
90. Hansen, J. VM/SAC **65** (1970) 1077.
91. Benirschke, K *et al.* Am J Vet Res **35** (1974) 257.
92. Kilham, L *et al.* JAVMA **158** (1971) 889.
93. Csiza, CK *et al.* Cornell Vet **61** (1971) 423.
94. Csiza, CK *et al.* Am J Vet Res **32** (1971) 419.
95. Scott, FW. JAVMA **158** (1971) 910.
96. Bittle, JL and Peckham, JC. JAVMA **158** (1971) 927.
97. Cline, EM *et al.* Feline Pract **11(3)**) (1981) 10.
98. Scott, FW *et al.* Terat **11** (1975) 79.
99. Stein, in Catcott: Feline Medicine and Surgery. 2nd ed. American Veterinary Publications, Santa Barbara, 1975.
100. Diegmann, FG *et al.* Feline Pract **8(5)** (1978) 45.
101. Hart, BL. Feline Pract **2(5)** (1972) 6.
102. Harbutt, PR. Aust Vet J **39** (1963) 401.
103. McDonald, LE: Veterinary Endocrinology and Reproduction. 2nd ed. Lea & Febiger, Philadelphia, 1975.
104. Hart, BL. Feline Pract **2(6)** (1972) 6.
105. Scott, PA and Scott, MG. J Reprod Fert **7** (1964) 270.
106. Collins, DR. VM/SAC **61** (1966) 455.
107. Reid, JS and Frank, RJ. JAAHA **9** (1973) 367.
108. Swerczek, TW *et al.* Am J Vet Res **32** (1971) 189.
109. Mandel, M. VM/SAC **70** (1975) 846.
110. Hardy, WD. Paper presented at Ohio VMA mtg, 1971.
111. Krzaczynski, J. VM/SAC **69** (1974) 572.
112. Heidrich, HJ and Renk, W. Diseases of the Mammary Glands of Domestic Animals. WB Saunders, Philadelphia, 1967.
113. Burke, TJ, Univ I11; Personal communication, 1974.
114. Wilkinson, GT: Diseases of the Cat. Pergamon Press, New York, 1966.
115. Brodey, RS. Adv Vet Sci Comp Med **14** (1970) 309.
116. Hayden, DW and Nielsen, SW. J Sm Anim Pract **12** (1971) 687.
117. Dorn, CR *et al.* J Nat Cancer Inst **40** (1968) 295.
118. Nielsen, SW. No Am Vet **33** (1962) 245.
119. Engle, CG. Feline Pract **3(5)** (1973) 9.
120. Paster, MB. JAVMA **153** (1968) 700.
121. Lawler, DC. Vet Rec **75** (1963) 811.
122. Lorenz, MD. Vet Clin No Am **2** (1972) 331.
123. Cartwright, C. Mod Vet Pract **54** (1973) 95.
124. Dow, C. J Comp Path **72** (1962) 303.
125. Thornton, DAK. Vet Rec **80** (1967) 380.
126. Hardy, RM and Osborne, CA. JAAHA **10** (1974) 245.
127. Dow, C. Vet Rec **74** (1962) 141.
128. Bradley, RL and Olson, P. Feline Pract **9(5)** (1979) 17.
129. Wilson, HC. Vet Rec **76** (1964) 438.
130. Catcott, EJ. Mod Vet Pract **54(5)** (1973) 21.
131. Bruinsma, DL. VM/SAC **76** (1981) 60.
132. Wallace, LJ *et al.* VM/SAC **65** (1970) 595.
133. Whitehead, in Catcott: Feline Medicine and Surgery. 1st ed. American Veterinary Publications, Santa Barbara, 1964.
134. Young, RC and Hiscock, R. Vet Rec **75** (1963) 872.
135. Kudale, ML. Indian Vet J **49** (1972) 1148.
136. Newman, MA. Vet Rec **73** (1961) 1269.
137. Singer, A. JAVMA **137** (1960) 290.
138. Meier, H. Cornell Vet **46** (1956) 188.
139. O'Rourke, MD and Geib, LW. Cornell Vet **60** (1970) 598.
140. Hansen, JS. VM/SAC **69** (1974) 1135.

141. Norris, HJ *et al.* J Path **97** (1969) 138.
142. Shehata, R. Acta Anat **84** (1973) 52.
143. Cooper, KK. Physiol Behav **8** (1972) 793.
144. Semans, JH and Langworthy, OR. J Urol **40** (1938) 836.
145. Coles, HH and Cupps, PT: Reproduction in Domestic Animals. 2nd ed. Academic Press, New York, 1969.
146. Berman, in Morrow: Current Therapy in Theriogenology. WB Saunders, Philadelphia, 1980.
147. Hamner, CE: The Regulation of Mammalian Reproduction. Charles C Thomas, Springfield, IL, 1973.
148. Hart, BL. Feline Pract **3(2)** (1973) 10.
149. Herron, MA. JAVMA **160** (1972) 208.
150. Herron, MA. Feline Pract **1(1)** (1971) 17.
151. Schille, VM. Proc 41st Ann Mtg AAHA, 1974.
152. Hart, BL and Peterson, DM. Lab Anim Sci **21** (1971) 422.
153. Meier, H. No Am Vet **37** (1956) 979.
154. Platz, CC *et al.* J Reprod Fert **52** (1978) 279.
155. Platz, CC and Seager, SWJ. JAVMA **173** (1978) 1353.
156. Barton, A. Vet Med **54** (1959) 155.
157. Michael, RP. Behav **18** (1961) 1.

16

the skin

ANATOMY AND PHYSIOLOGY OF THE SKIN AND HAIR
By S.I. Reinke and P.J. Ihrke

The skin is composed of the epidermis, dermis and subcutis. It prevents loss of fluid and electrolytes from the deeper tissues and protects against physical, chemical and microbiologic assaults. It is also involved in sensory perception, secretion via its glands, temperature regulation, production of keratinized structures, such as the hair and nails, insulation, and Vitamin D synthesis.[1] The skin of the cat is thickest dorsad and thinnest ventrad.

The epidermis is composed of 5 layers and is thickest in the footpads and planum nasale. The most superficial layer is the stratum corneum, which is thicker in sparsely haired or hairless areas. The next layer is the stratum lucidum (in footpads and planum nasale only), followed by the stratum granulosum, stratum spinosum and stratum basale. The basement membrane zone, which is thin and indistinct in cats, separates the epidermis from the dermis.

The dermis contains collagen, elastin, ground substance, sebaceous and apocrine glands, blood and lymph vessels, nervous tissue, and arrector pili muscles. (Eccrine sweat glands are restricted to the footpads.) The dermal elements provide nourishment and support for the epidermis. The subcutis contains primarily fat tissue, with interwoven collagen and elastin fibers.

Cats have both primary (guard) and secondary (undercoat) hairs. The secondary hairs considerably outnumber the primary hairs and emerge from the same follicular orifice as the primary hair they surround.

The hair is composed of the inner medulla, the cortex and the outer cuticle. Pigment contained in the cortex gives the hair its color. Except in a few specialized areas, there is very little pigment in the haired skin.

There are 2 specialized types of tactile hairs in cats. Sinus hairs on the face and upper eyelids, and in tufts on the ventral carpi are thought to function as slow-adapting mechanoreceptors. Tylotrich hairs, found individually in small knob-like enlargements (tylotrich pads), may function as rapid-adapting mechanoreceptors.[2]

Hair does not grow continuously but has a period of active growth (anagen) and a resting stage (telogen). Maximal hair growth occurs in late spring, whereas minimal hair growth occurs in midwinter. Outdoor cats, particularly those in cold climates, shed twice a year, primarily in spring and fall. Indoor cats may shed continuously. Shedding may also occur during disease since more hairs enter the resting stage during internal pathologic processes.

CLINICAL EVALUATION OF SKIN DISEASE
by P.J. Ihrke

As in any other area of medicine, an accurate, complete history and a thorough physical examination are necessary in establishing the etiology of a skin disease. In addition, various laboratory tests and, occasionally, trial therapy may be used in establishing a diagnosis.

Data Base and Past History

The age, breed and sex of a cat should be noted as this data may be useful in directing an index of suspicion toward certain likely diseases. As an example, seborrhea sicca associated with endoparasites is a more likely diagnosis in a young cat, while seborrhea in older cats is more commonly associated with internal metabolic problems or a poor diet. Ringworm is diagnosed more frequently in kittens than in adult cats.

In an evaluation of hospital population-corrected breed predilections for feline skin diseases, longhaired cats, such as the Angora, Persian, Himalayan and Maine coon cat, and Burmese, a shorthaired cat, were found to be at higher risk.[2] Of more important clinical significance, definite breed predilections are also seen for certain diseases. For example, Siamese, Burmese and Abyssinians account for over 90% of the cases of feline psychogenic alopecia and dermatitis. Feline endocrine alopecia is seen almost exclusively in domestic shorthaired cats, while "stud tail" is at least presented to veterinarians much more commonly in purebred cats.

Most feline skin diseases do not show any sexual bias in incidence. As an exception, abscessation and cellulitis are seen most commonly in intact fighting males that are allowed to roam. In feline endocrine alopecia, neutering is a significant factor as all reported cases have been in neutered animals. In addition, 90% of the cases of this disease are seen in males.

The term "past history" may be used to encompass all prior medical problems, the general health of the animal, dietary history, environment and a history of skin problems in people or other animals in the household.

Diet may be important in several feline dermatoses. A fat-deficient diet can be an underlying cause of seborrhea. Food allergy should be considered in the differential diagnosis of any case of pruritus. It is important to record brand names and approximate percentages of various foods involved.

Environment may be extremely important in establishing the likelihood of various diseases. Ectoparasitic and fungal diseases are more common in "in and out" cats that roam or in outdoor cats. Obviously, flea-allergy dermatitis would be a much less likely underlying cause of miliary eczema in a strictly indoor animal without other animal contacts. Conversely, flea infestation, cheyletiellosis and notoedric mange (in enzootic areas) are all more common in cats with many animal contacts. The geographic prevalence of disease should also be considered since notoedric mange and intermediate and deep mycoses occur most frequently in certain areas.

The involvement or lack of involvement of other household pets may offer a clue as to the potential contagious nature of a disease. Where it exists in isolated, enzootic concentrations, notoedric mange is reportedly highly contagious among cats. The author has seen cheyletiellosis rapidly spread to involve 20 cats in a cattery after several cats returned from a cat show. Asymptomatic carriers as well as clinically affected animals were seen. Dermatophytosis may also spread in a cattery in a similar manner.

Feline ringworm is one of the most common zoonoses seen in small animal practice. In up to one-third of the cases of this disease, a family member exhibited signs of the disease.

Current History

Information as to the onset, progression and duration of the skin disease is often valuable. A rapid onset is more common with ectoparasitism and other diseases of external causation. Conversely, the onset of clinical signs may be considerably slower in diseases of internal causation. The initial site of the lesion and the progression may afford valuable clues long after a disease has become more generalized. Generalized alopecia or miliary eczema may have begun as localized ringworm on a predisposed site, such as the pinna or face. The duration of the lesions is also important as secondary, chronic changes may have obscured the original character of the disease. Any pattern to the disease noted by the owner may be helpful since some pruritic disease, such as flea allergy, atopy or trombiculiasis, may be seasonal.

Physical Examination

An orderly, systematic approach is mandatory in the physical examination of animals with dermatologic disease. The animal's general demeanor and signs of pruritus should be evaluated while the clinician is taking the history. Proper lighting in the examination room is especially important in dermatology. The entire surface of the cat should be palpated through the pelage. The coat quality, length of hair and coat thickness should be noted. Patterns of symmetry to alopecia may sometimes be noted more readily if the animal is examined at arm's length. The ventrum may be examined by lifting the cat by its axillae and the caudal aspect should be examined by displacing the tail dorsad and lifting the animal by its thighs. The clinician should part the hair, and view the underlying skin. Examination of the mucocutaneous junctions, oral cavity, ears, genitals and lymph nodes should be emphasized during the examination.

If skin lesions are present, an attempt should be made to characterize them morphologically.

Are macules, papules, pustules, nodules, erosions, ulcers, plaques or miliary crusts present? Is self-trauma evident and if alopecia is present, is it naturally occurring or traumatic in origin? Unfortunately, one difficulty in feline dermatology is that cat skin reacts to a wide variety of insults, both external and internal, in a very similar morphologic pattern known as the "miliary eczema complex." Consequently, evaluation of rather subtle morphologic differences and correlation of physical examination findings with history and laboratory evaluation are extremely important.

Lesion Distribution

The localization of lesions has valuable diagnostic significance in dermatology. Familiarity with the most common sites of various diseases is necessary in determining the most likely diagnosis among a list of differentials. As examples, the head and neck region of cats is often a pruritic focus in food allergy; immune-mediated diseases often involve the face and mucocutaneous junctions. Distribution patterns commonly seen with various pruritic or alopecia-inducing diseases are presented in Tables 1-3 and elsewhere.[3]

Diagnostic Technics by P.J. Ihrke

Certain laboratory procedures are used routinely by clinicians in evaluation of skin diseases. These methods include skin scrapings, Wood's lamp analysis, fungal and bacterial cultures, and skin biopsy. Other potentially valuable procedures, such as elimination diets, cellophane tape stripping, impression smears, aspiration of vesicles or bullae, and environmental restrictions, should be performed more often than currently practiced. More involved procedures, such as intradermal skin testing, are usually performed by referral dermatologists or clinicians with a special interest in dermatology.

Skin Scrapings

Skin scrapings should be part of the minimum data base collected in most feline skin diseases. The skin of every pruritic cat should be scraped. Notoedric mange, cheyletiellosis, demodicosis and trombiculiasis are all diagnosed by skin scrapings. The clinician should clip the affected area to obtain a good representative scraping. A #10 scalpel blade is dipped in medium-grade mineral oil and the scraping is accomplished best by moving in the direction of hair growth, with the blade held perpendicular to the skin. Several scrapings should always be obtained. In general, all feline skin mites are more readily demonstrated on scrapings than scabies mites are in dogs. Because of this, these feline skin diseases are not usually treated based upon clinical impressions alone. An exception would be the treatment of other cats in a household if either cheyletiellosis or notoedric mange had been identified in one cat. Scrapings in suspected cases of ringworm are considerably more difficult to interpret. Microscopic evaluation of hair stubble in affected areas, using either 10% KOH or chlorphenolac (50 g chloral hydrate, 25 ml liquid phenol, 25 ml 85-90% USP feed-grade lactic acid), may be a valuable tool for a clinician adept at this procedure. Without special training, clinicans will not find skin scrapings a valuable tool for diagnosis of ringworm.

Wood's Lamp Analysis

The Wood's lamp is probably the most frequently abused tool in veterinary medicine. Its use in cats is more valuable than in other species since 98% of feline ringworm is caused by *Microsporum canis*, and about two-thirds of *M canis* infections fluoresce. The major source of inaccuracy with respect to this test is that many scales, crusts and topical medications fluoresce, giving false-positive results. True-positive fluorescence due to a tryptophan metabolite of *M canis* is blue-green and restricted in distribution to the surface of affected hairs. The most common falsely interpreted fluorescence is a yellowish glow associated with crusty lesions.

Fungal Cultures

Fungal cultures are the most consistently accurate method of diagnosing ringworm. Because of the extreme variability of presentation of both localized and generalized ringworm in cats, a fungal culture should be performed on all feline dermatologic cases in which another etiology has not been definitely proven. Since ringworm may coexist with other diseases, culture should also be obtained in cats not responding to specific medication for another diagnosed skin disease. The most common error associated with interpretation of culture growth and color change is too infrequent checking of the culture. All fungal cultures should be observed daily (see Superficial Mycoses).

Bacterial Cultures

In general, bacterial culture of skin lesions is less useful in feline than in canine dermatology, primarily because feline bacterial skin diseases, with fight wound abscessation and cellulitis as an exception, are rather rare. In addition, the pathogenic bacteria most commonly isolated from feline skin diseases are quite sensitive to many antibiotics. *Pasteurella multocida* and beta-hemolytic streptococci usually are quite susceptible to penicillin, amoxicillin, ampicillin and hetacillin.

Since intact pustules are extremely rare in cats, the most common clinical situation requiring a culture would be a draining abscess that had not responded to one of the above antibiotics (see Bacterial Skin Diseases).

Biopsy

A skin biopsy may be quite useful if a representative area is selected and the biopsy is interpreted properly. Biopsy of primary lesions, early lesions and lesions without superimposed self-trauma are most likely to be beneficial. Biopsy of chronic, traumatized lesions may lead to the unsatisfactory diagnosis, "chronic nonspecific dermatitis."

Use of a disposable 4- or 6-mm Keyes cutaneous biopsy punch (Baker Laboratories) is an easy method of obtaining a specimen. After the sample has been obtained, it is of equal importance to submit the specimen to a veterinary histopathologist with an interest in dermatology because of the morphologic similarities among many feline skin diseases.

Elimination Diets

Elimination diets are useful in ascertaining if an allergy to food is an underlying cause of pruritus. Since most pet foods share common protein antigens, dyes, preservatives and stabilizers, a restrictive "home-cooked" elimination diet is necessary. Mutton or chicken alone or mixed with rice is the most frequently employed test diet for cats. Chicken or mutton commercial baby food may also be used. Feeding the totally restrictive test diet for at least 3 weeks is recommended.

Cellophane Tape Stripping

As an alternative to skin scrapings for *Cheyletiella*, the clinician may use clear cellophane tape to collect scales and debris from the skin surface of cats with seborrhea or miliary eczema.

Table 1. Localized Alopecia*

Disease	Prevalence	Site	Lesion	Predilection
Physiologic preauricular partial alopecia	Very common	Preauricular temporal region, bilaterally symmetric	Thinning of hair	None, but more apparent in black cats
Stud tail	Common	Dorsal tail, symmetric midline band	Alopecia, comedones, scaling, waxiness	Primarily purebreds?
Ringworm	Very common	Face, ears, extremities, anywhere	Alopecia, stubble, circular, expanding border	None
Flea-collar dermatitis	Rare	Neck, symmetric, occasionally generalized?	Alopecia, erythema, edema, scaling, crusting	None
Demodicosis	Very rare	Face (periorbital), forelegs	Alopecia, scaling, follicular obstruction	None
Psychogenic alopecia and dermatitis	Uncommon	Extremity, abdomen, flank	Solitary, alopectic, excoriated lesion; skin changes variable	Siamese, Burmese, Abyssinian

* This table is limited to diseases in which focal alopecia is associated with minimal visible skin changes. Many other diseases may cause focal alopecia if the normal follicular architecture is severely disturbed or ablated.

Table 2. Generalized Alopecia

Disease	Prevalence	Site	Lesions	Predilection
Psychogenic alopecia	Somewhat common	1 or 2 dorsal stripes, perineal, genital, caudomedial thighs, rarely forelegs, somewhat bilaterally symmetric	Stubbled hairs not easily epilated, looks clipped, broken, dry, disheveled hairs	Siamese, Burmese, Abyssinian
Feline endocrine alopecia	Uncommon	Genital, perineal, caudomedial thighs, ventral abdomen, chronic cases—severe ventral involvement but spare dorsum, bilaterally symmetric	Diffuse thinning of hair, hairs epilate easily	Primarily domestic shorthaired cats, 90% males
Generalized ringworm	Uncommon	Thorax, head, limbs, ears, can be remarkably symmetric	Diffuse alopecia, scaling, hyper-pigmentation, stubble	None
Generalized demodicosis	Rare	Focal, multi-focal or generalized	Alopecia, scaling, follicular plugging, papules, crusts, pigmentary changes	None
Hyperadreno-corticism	Very rare	Thorax, bilaterally symmetric	Thin hypotonic easily torn skin, scaling, diffuse thinning of hair	None
Notoedric mange	Generally rare, but enzootic areas	Head, neck, ears occasionally paws, generalized	Severe alopecia, thick yellowish crusts, erythema, scaling	None
Contact dermatitis	Rare	Contact site, may be generalized with liquids (especially petroleum products)	Alopecia scaling, pigmentary changes	Siamese??
Telogen effluvium	Uncommon	Generalized	Diffuse thinning of hair	After gestation, fever, severe illness
Excessive physiologic shedding	Common	Generalized	Loss of undercoat, primary hairs do not epilate easily	Spring and fall in outdoor cats
Hereditary hypotrichosis	Very rare	Almost total alopecia	Alopecia	Siamese (autosomal recessive)
Alopecia universalis	Rare	Almost total alopecia, stubble on face	Alopecia, seborrhea oleosa, comedones	Bred as sphinx or Canadian hairless cats

The tape is then placed on a drop of mineral oil on a slide and used as a cover slip. Both mites and eggs may be gathered by this procedure.[4]

Impression Smears

Glass slides may be applied to exudative lesions, draining tracts or excised nodules and stained with either gram or acid-fast stain. In many cases, initially almost as much information may be gained from an impression smear as from a bacterial culture and antibiotic sensitivity. For example, common bacterial pathogens, acid-fast bacteria or organisms causing deep mycoses may be identified this way.

Vesicle Aspiration (Tzank Test)

A fine needle aspirate may be taken of bullae or vesicles, stained with Giemsa stain, and evaluated microscopically. The presence of acantholytic cells (rounded, detached keratinocytes) may indicate an immune-mediated disease. Unfortunately, most bullae or vesicles in feline skin disease are quite transient and rupture readily due to the thinness of feline skin. Consequently, this test has limited application in cats unless a clinician is fortunate enough to see the cat at the exactly ideal time.

Environmental Restriction

Considering that allergic contact dermatitis is probably quite rare in cats and that irritant contact dermatitis from unidentified sources is also rather uncommon, environmental restriction as a diagnostic tool is used infrequently in feline dermatology. If contact dermatitis is suspected, the cat may be housed for 7-10 days in a water-rinsed cage for controlled contactant exposure.

Intradermal Skin Testing

Intradermal skin testing has been a neglected diagnostic tool in cats. The difficulties inherent in feline restraint, coupled with problems in interpretation due to the resultant flat wheals, have led to this neglect. Atopy occurs in cats and may be manifested as pruritus without primary lesions or as a miliary eczematous condition. More work is needed to document the incidence and scope of feline atopy.

Differential Diagnosis of Alopecia by P.J. Ihrke

Alopecia is a partial or complete loss of hair. It may be focal or diffuse, localized or generalized, partial or complete, and transient or permanent. Although alopecia is a common clinical sign associated with many diverse diseases, it is much less likely than pruritus to be the primary reason for presentation to a veterinarian. Consequently, although alopecia may be a major clinical feature of a disease, other clinical signs may be more important to the clinician in arriving at a diagnosis. While focal alopecia may be associated with discrete lesions, such as various neoplasms or diseases in the eosinophilic granuloma complex, it is seen less commonly as a solitary clinical sign (Table 1). Furthermore, generalized alopecia is not an especially common reason for presentation of a cat for examination (Table 2).

After evaluating the extent of the alopecia, the clinician should determine if the hair is being chewed or pulled out or if it is falling out. As discussed in the sections on feline endocrine alopecia and psychogenic dermatosis, it is important to pluck hairs from the cat and examine them microscopically since disheveled, jagged ends usually indicate self-trauma. If hairs are easily epilated and have normal ends when viewed microscopically, a disease that causes excessive shedding, such as feline endocrine alopecia, should be suspected.

A biopsy is frequently beneficial if other diagnostic technics have not been successful in determining the cause of alopecia.

Differential Diagnosis of Pruritus by P.J. Ihrke

Pruritus is defined as an uneasy sensation of irritation within the skin or any sensation that elicits the desire to scratch. It is one of the most common clinical signs associated with skin disease in any species. It may occur in conjunction with significant skin lesions or as a solitary clinical sign with or without self-trauma. Unfortunately, pruritus is one of the most frustrating manifestations of skin diseases.

Clinical signs associated with feline pruritus include alopecia, broken brittle hairs, general dullness of the pelage, postinflammatory pigmentary changes, excoriation, ulcers, and also discrete traumatic lesions from chewing or scratching. The manifestations of pruritus reported by owners vary. Licking, chewing and scratching may occur constantly or intermittently. Pruritic cats frequently withdraw from social contact with owners or other pets. A general irritability or personality change may be

Table 3. Pruritic Feline Dermatoses[3]

Disease	Site	Lesions
Flea-allergy dermatitis	Neck, especially dorsal, lumbosacral, caudal and medial thighs, ventral abdomen, head, ears	Papules, crusts, alopecia, miliary eczema, erosions, ulcers
Food allergy	Head, neck, ears, generalized	Miliary eczema, alopecia, seborrhea, erythema, papules
Psychogenic alopecia	Symmetric stripe(s) on back, caudal thighs, ventral abdomen, perineum	Alopecia, stubbles of hair, usually symmetric, normal skin
Psychogenic dermatitis	Extremities, abdomen, flank	Erosion or ulcer
Cheyletiellosis	Dorsal thorax	Seborrhea, miliary eczema
Dermatophytosis	Thorax, neck, head, ears	Erythema, alopecia, stubbles of hair, miliary eczema, scaling, hyperpigmentation
Intestinal parasitism	Thorax, neck, head, generalized	Miliary eczema
Eosinophilic plaque	Ventral abdomen, medial thighs, anywhere	Raised, ulcerated, erythematous plaques
Otodectic mange	Ears, head, neck, rarely generalized	Erythema, scales, crusts, miliary eczema
Notoedric mange	Head, neck, rarely generalized	Erythema, scales, crusts, alopecia

noticed. Another manifestation of pruritus, peculiar to cats, is a rather curious twitching of the back muscles, termed "hyperesthesia." Owners may report that affected cats began twitching and then sporadically began racing around the house, seemingly without cause.

The concept of threshold for pruritus is very important in diagnosis of the underlying cause. Since all contributing causes of pruritus are additive in effect, a number of unrelated diseases, each causing mild pruritus, may push an animal above its own individual pruritic threshold. Consequently, it is not always sufficient to document only one cause of itching since the problem may be multifactorial. All potential causes of pruritus should be explored.

An accurate, complete history and a thorough physical examination are essential in determining the cause of pruritus. This process is made somewhat more difficult in cats since many pruritic skin diseases of diverse etiologies have remarkably similar morphologic characteristics. Miliary eczematous lesions and coat changes caused by excessive grooming appear virtually identical, regardless of the underlying cause.

Certain generalizations may be useful in evaluating pruritic cats. In many cases, the rapidity of onset, in conjunction with the appearance of primary lesions, should focus the clinician's attention on the possibility of ectoparasitism or other diseases of external causation. For example, trombiculiasis, pediculosis, cheyletiellosis, notoedric mange, ear mite infestation and contact dermatitis usually are diseases of rapid onset. Diseases of internal causation, such as allergies, are more likely to be insidious in onset. In cases of flea-allergy dermatitis, food allergy or feline atopy, it is unlikely that the owner will be able to recall when the problem began.

Seasonality, periodicity or any predictability may be a valuable clue in determining a cause of pruritus. For example, flea-allergy dermatitis and atopy may be seasonal, and psychogenic dermatosis may be correlated with stress. The ability to predict episodes of pruritus may lead the owner and the clinician to a diagnosis of food allergy or contact dermatitis.

If the clinician is familiar with the most common sites and lesions associated with the more common pruritic skin diseases, tests applicable to each disease may be used to arrive at a diagnosis from multiple differential diagnoses (Table 3).

INFECTIOUS SKIN DISEASES
Bacterial Diseases
By E.J. Rosser, Jr. and P.J. Ihrke

The incidence of bacterial infections in the skin of cats is relatively rare when compared with that in dogs. This may be due to a lower bacterial population on the skin and haircoat of cats because of their regular grooming habits. In support of this, qualitative studies suggest a low or absent bacterial population from various regions of the cat's body. However, quantitative studies to determine the resident bacterial flora of feline skin and haircoat from different regions of the body have not been performed and must be before any generalizations can be made. When the skin from the interscapular region of 6 normal adult cats was cultured, 5 cats had no growth of bacteria and only one had a light growth of a nonhemolytic staphylococci.[5] Other qualitative work done on 10 cats with swabs taken from 7 different sites showed no bacterial growth in half of the sites cultured.[6] Of the organisms isolated, alpha-hemolytic streptococci, *Micrococcus* spp and *Acinetobacter* spp were the most common. The chin region had the most frequent positive bacterial cultures.

The hair on the top of the head produced positive cultures of *Staphylococcus aureus* in 98 out of 100 cats.[7] This finding is of interest since cats cannot groom this area as effectively as other parts of their body. These results may have been due to use of cats residing in pet shops and the data may have been biased due to a contaminated environment. However, in a study of randomly selected, healthy outpatient dogs at the University of California, samples from the same area of the head also produced predominantly pure cultures of *Staphylococcus aureus*.

Interestingly, these studies suggest a difference in the potential resident bacterial flora of the skin vs hair. Quantitative studies should be performed and would be most beneficial if the skin and hair were examined separately.

Abscessation and Cellulitis

Cause: Abscesses and cellulitis are among the most common dermatologic problems in cats. Most frequently they develop secondary to a cat bite that inoculates bacteria under the skin. Therefore, the organisms isolated from cat bite wound abscesses are those most commonly isolated from the mouths of cats and include *Pasteurella multocida,* beta-hemolytic streptococci and anaerobic *Fusiformis* spp.[8] In addition, *Escherichia coli* and the anaerobe *Bacteroides melaninogenicus* can be isolated.[8,9] Of these organisms, *Pasteurella multocida* is the major pyogenic organism and is almost invariably present in cat bite wounds.

After the bacteria are inoculated into the wound, either an abscess or cellulitis may develop. Abscessation is most likely where the subcutaneous connective tissues are loose, such as the trunk (Fig 1). In contrast, where the subcutaneous connective tissues have more tension on them, such as the limbs, cellulitis is more likely to develop.[2]

Clinical Signs: Abscesses and cellulitis are most often seen in intact males that spend at least some time outdoors. The lesions may be located anywhere on the body but frequently involve the face, limbs, base of the tail and back. When an abscess forms, there is usually a soft, fluctuant swelling, with evidence of puncture wounds. This area is frequently painful and may spontaneously rupture and appear as a draining wound rather than as a swelling. In cellulitis, the area of inflammation is poorly defined compared with an abscess. The cat may be presented for pain and disuse of the affected area. Upon closer inspection, multiple small puncture wounds may be discovered after the area is clipped.

The systemic effects of these infections often include anorexia, depression and pyrexia. Occasionally a cat appears normal in all respects except for the abscess or cellulitis.

Treatment: In cats with well-defined abscesses, the area should be clipped, cleansed and lanced both dorsal and ventral to the lesion. Debridement may be necessary. Surgical drains can be used to facilitate drainage. Initially the abscess cavity should be flushed with an antiseptic solution, such as hydrogen peroxide. Thereafter the wound may be flushed with a povidone iodine solution (Betadine:Purdue Frederick) or chlorhexidine solution (Nolvasan:Fort Dodge) 2-3 times daily until the wound has begun to granulate. Any surgical drains used should be removed 2-3 days after placement.

If cellulitis is present and an abscess has not developed, hot packs should be applied to the area for 10-15 minutes 2-3 times daily. The cellulitis may resolve with this therapy or the heat may induce formation of an abscess.

Use of systemic antibiotics is recommended for these subcutaneous infections. Unlike for dogs, penicillin and its derivatives, (hetacillin, ampicillin and amoxicillin), are the antibiotics of choice since *Pasteurella multocida* is the most common isolate from these wounds and is usually sensitive to these antibiotics.

When a cat fights often and has a history of abscess formation, preventive measures may be considered. Cats presented within 24 hours of a known cat fight can be given a single injection of procaine penicillin G, which may prevent development of an abscess or cellulitis.[10] In addition, if the cat is an intact male, castration may decrease roaming and fighting and therefore reduce the incidence of fight wounds.

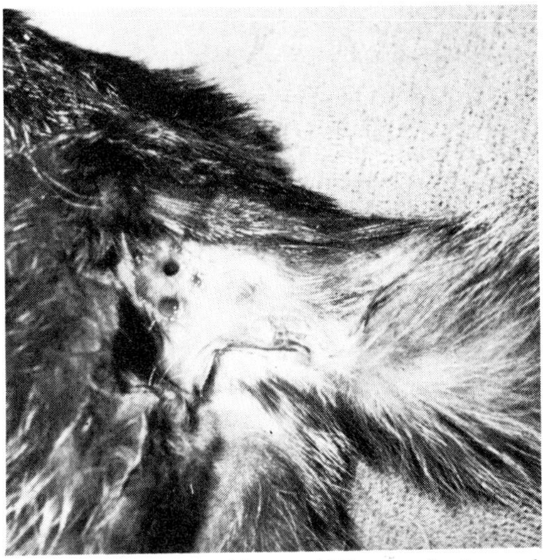

Fig 1. Abscess caused by a cat bite near the base of the tail. (Courtesy of Dr D.W. Scott and AAHA)

Folliculitis

Cause: Folliculitis is a very rare type of bacterial skin infection in cats. The bacteria initially invade hair follicles, causing an inflammatory response. If the infected follicles rupture and involve the dermis, the disease may be termed furunculosis. The bacterial organisms isolated from feline folliculitis have included beta-hemolytic streptococci, *Staphylococcus aureus* and *Pasteurella multocida*.[2]

Clinical Signs: The primary lesions reported have been papules and pustules. In severe cases, focal erosions, crusts, alopecia and occasional draining tracts also may be seen. The chin region is most commonly affected as this condition may be seen as a sequela to feline acne. Occasionally a more generalized folliculitis may be manifested as miliary eczema (see Miliary Eczema).[2]

Diagnosis: A biopsy is necessary to confirm folliculitis of the chin or to differentiate among the various causes of miliary eczema. Skin scrapings and fungal cultures should be performed to rule out feline demodicosis and dermatophytosis as possible underlying problems.

Treatment: Topical therapy should be initiated by gently cleansing the affected area with 2.5% benzoyl peroxide shampoo (OxyDex Shampoo:DVM) or chlorhexidine shampoo (Nolvasan Shampoo:Fort Dodge) once or twice daily for 5 minutes. Systemic antibiotics, such as penicillin, amoxicillin, ampicillin and hetacillin, may be used empirically. In cases that are recurrent or refractory to initial therapy, use of culture and sensitivity tests of an intact pustule is recommended. The appropriate antibiotics should be given for at least 14 days or until the lesions have been completely resolved for 1-2 weeks.

Feline Acne

Cause: The cause of feline acne is unknown. However, the term "feline acne" is useful clinically since the term "acne" connotes the disease in people, in which control rather than cure is the realistic goal. This syndrome is discussed under bacterial diseases because of the folliculitis and furunculosis often associated with it. However, feline acne is not considered a primary pyoderma. Feline acne has some similarities to human acne but is not an identical syndrome. Feline acne may develop in cats that do not clean their chin sufficiently. A genetic predilection may also be important.[1,2,11] Affected cats develop hair follicles obstructed with lipids and keratinous debris, forming the classic comedones (blackheads) of acne.

Clinical Signs: Feline acne is characterized by comedones localized to the chin and lower lips. It can affects cats of any age and has no sex or breed predisposition. The early stage of the disease does not seem to bother the cats but may be noticed by the owner. When secondary bacterial infections occur, *Pasteurella multocida* or beta-hemolytic streptococci are most commonly isolated.[2] In such cases, papules, pustules and occasional draining tracts may be seen along with the comedones.

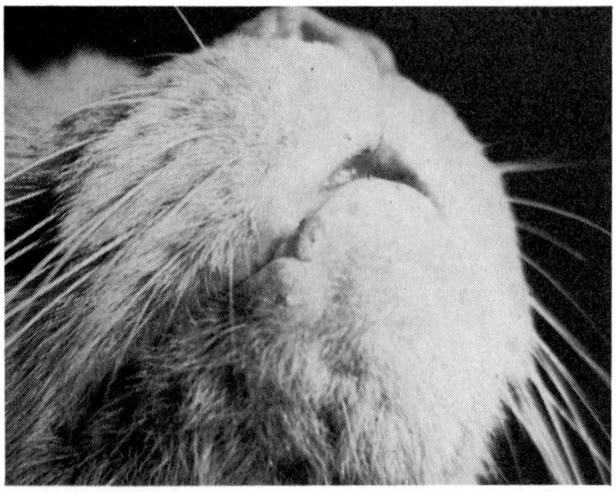

Fig 2. Moderately severe feline acne. (Courtesy of Compend Cont Ed)

Diagnosis: The physical appearance of feline acne is usually sufficient for diagnosis (Fig 2). However, if excessive swelling or severe lesions are present, a skin biopsy can aid in determining the primary problem. Histopathologic examination should demonstrate follicular obstruction due to keratinous debris associated with a dilated hair follicle. Additionally, perifolliculitis, folliculitis and furunculosis may be present histologically. As mentioned previously, skin scrapings and fungal cultures are indicated to rule out underlying demodicosis or dermatophytosis in refractory cases.

Treatment: For cats with comedones, the chin region can be washed gently with 2.5% benzoyl peroxide shampoo (OxyDex Shampoo:D.V.M.) once daily. Benzoyl peroxide shampoos possess a "follicle-flushing" action and have been most useful for this condition. Occasionally a cat may respond more favorably to use of benzoyl peroxide gel (OxyDex Gel:DVM). Megestrol acetate (Ovaban:Schering, Megace:Mead-Johnson) may be useful as an anti-inflammatory drug in difficult cases. Since this condition may affect some cats on a lifelong basis, the owner should be advised that intermittent maintenance therapy may be required to control the disease.

Any secondary bacterial infection should be treated as for folliculitis.

Paronychia

Paronychia is an inflammation of the nail fold; however, the term is often used specifically to designate bacterial infections. This condition is very rare in cats and is thought to be secondary to other diseases. Underlying diseases reported to cause paronychia include foreign bodies, trauma, osteomyelitis, declawing regrowths, dermatophytosis, chemical irritants, demodicosis, neoplasms and various diseases associated with immunodeficiency, such as FeLV infection and systemic lupus erythematosus. Bacteria isolated on culture include *Escherichia coli* alone or with beta-hemolytic streptococci, *Enterococcus* spp or *Staphylococcus aureus.*[2]

Clinical Signs: Affected cats often are presented for pain and inflammation of the nail bed region, associated with licking of the affected digit, and mild to severe lameness. Crusting and exudation of the nail bed are evident on physical examination (Fig 3). One or multiple digits may be involved. The claws may become brittle, cracked and malformed. Occasionally the entire claw may slough.

Diagnosis: Vigorous efforts should be made to rule out the various underlying conditions commonly seen in association with paronychia. An evaluation should include skin scrapings, fungal cultures, bacterial cultures, radiography, direct smears of exudate, FeLV testing and an antinuclear antibody test.

Treatment: The underlying cause of paronychia must be identified and, if possible, corrected. Any loose nails should be avulsed from the nail bed before initiating therapy. The affected feet are then soaked in warm water and povidone iodine solution or chlorhexidine solution for 10-15 minutes 2-3 times daily. If chronic licking is a problem, an Elizabethan collar may be used. If necessary, systemic antibiotics are best chosen based on culture and sensitivity tests, and administered for 4-6 weeks.

Actinomycosis

Cause: Actinomycosis is a rare disease of cats caused by various species of *Actinomyces.* The most common isolate has been *Actinomyces bovis.*[12] These bacteria are gram-positive, non-acid-fast, filamentous organisms capable of branching and breaking up into coccobacillary forms. They are anaerobic and microaerophilic in their O_2 requirements. *Actinomyces* spp are normal inhabitants of the oral cavity and bowel of animals and have a worldwide distribution. Infections usually occur subsequent to a penetrating wound, particularly the inhalation or cutaneous penetration of various plant awns (especially foxtails). This results in a pyogranulomatous and suppurative process commonly affecting the skin and subcutaneous tissues, lungs, pleura and vertebrae. *Actinomyces* spp may require the presence of other bacteria to produce infection, and cultures performed almost always reveal other organisms, especially *Bacteroides* spp.[12,13]

Clinical Signs: Cutaneous actinomycosis is characterized by abscesses, cellulitis and nodular lesions that usually develop draining tracts. Lesions can occur anywhere on the body, with the limbs most commonly affected. The exudate from draining tracts varies in appearance and is often thick and red-brown, with yellow granules ("sulfur granules," "mycelial clumps").

Diagnosis: Actinomycosis can be diagnosed by direct smears, culture and biopsy of lesions. Nocardiosis may be clinically similar to actinomycosis but these 2 diseases must be differentiated because their treatments differ. Direct smears of the exudate and granules should be examined with gram and acid-fast stains. *Actinomyces* spp are gram-positive, branching filaments that are not acid-fast. When submitting the exudate for culture, the granules, which are clumps of organisms, must be submitted since the organism often cannot be found in the fluid alone.[13] The cultures should be grown under aerobic, anaerobic and microaerophilic conditions. Biopsy of lesions reveals a pyogranulomatous reaction, usually with "sulfur granules" within the tissues.

Treatment: Therapy should be initiated by surgically probing the abscess and draining tracts for evidence of any plant awns, especially foxtails, or other foreign bodies. If the lesion is localized, total surgical excision may be attempted. Antibiotics should be administered after these procedures, with penicillin the drug of choice. High dosages of penicillin must be given (100,000 IU/kg/day IM) for 4 weeks beyond clinical remission.[2] Although this usually means 2-4 months of continuous therapy, this long regimen is necessary to avoid relapses. In cats allergic to penicillin, use of tetracyclines, chloramphenicol, lincomycin, erythromycin and triple sulfas has been effective.

Nocardiosis

Cause: Nocardiosis is a rare disease caused by various *Nocardia* spp. The most common species isolated are *Nocardia asteroides* and *N brasiliensis*.[12,13] These bacteria are aerobic, gram-positive, branching, beaded filaments. Most species are acid-fast or partially acid-fast. *Nocardia* spp are common soil inhabitants and have a worldwide distribution, except for *Nocardia brasiliensis*, which is localized to Mexico and Central and South America. Infection usually develops after inhalation, ingestion or subcutaneous inoculation via a penetrating wound. Pyogranulomatous and suppurative disease subsequently develops, usually in the skin, subcutaneous tissue and lungs. Infection with *N asteroides* has occurred in patients with depressed immune function, which may be a predisposing factor for infection with this organism. Therefore, tests to evaluate immunocompetency may be required when *N asteroides* is isolated.

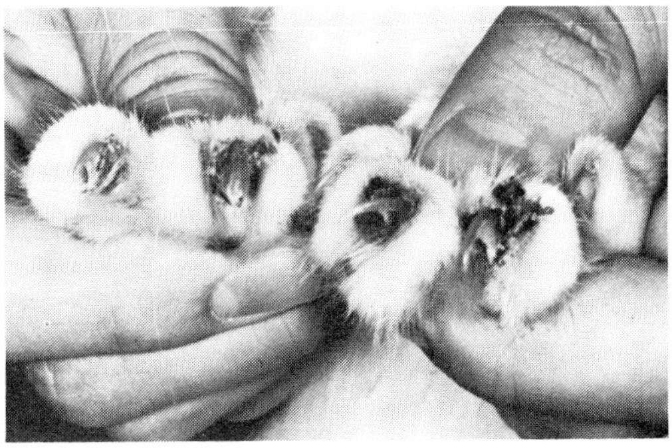

Fig 3. Paronychia caused by *E coli* in an FeLV-positive cat. (Courtesy of Dr D.W. Scott and AAHA)

Clinical Signs: Cutaneous nocardiosis can be manifested as abscesses, cellulitis and granulomatous lesions that ulcerate and develop draining tracts. Lesions most commonly occur on the limbs. The exudate from the draining tracts is often described as resembling tomato soup in appearance. "Sulfur granules" can be seen in the exudate, as in actinomycosis, but are less common in cases involving *N asteroides*.

Diagnosis: The diagnostic tests performed are the same as for actinomycosis. Direct smears of the exudate and granules reveal gram-positive, branching, beaded filaments that are usually acid-fast or partially acid-fast. However, some *Nocardia* spp are not acid-fast.[13] This stresses the importance of culturing for this organism to differentiate it from *Actinomyces* spp. Biopsy of lesions reveals the same type of pyogranulomatous reaction, with or without granules, as seen in actinomycosis.

Treatment: Therapy often requires surgical establishment of good drainage, followed by chemotherapeutics. High dosages of penicillin (100,000 IU/kg/day IM) are given initially until substantial clinical improvement is seen, usually in 9-11 days. At the end of penicillin therapy, sulfadiazine (40 mg/kg TID) or sulfadimethoxine (24 mg/kg SID) should be given orally for 4 weeks beyond clinical remission, which usually requires 2-4 months of continuous therapy.[2]

Mycobacterial Diseases
By S.D. White, P.J. Ihrke and A.A. Stannard

Mycobacterial skin diseases are rare in cats, although asymptomatic cats undoubtedly exist. The pathogens may be divided into the tuberculous and the nontuberculous mycobacteria.

Tuberculosis

Cause: Tuberculosis in cats usually is caused by *Mycobacterium bovis,* although other mycobacteria have been implicated. Transmission is thought to be primarily from contaminated cow's milk. Other sources of infection may be sputum from infected people and bite or scratch wounds from infected cats. Skin lesions are usually nodules and/or ulcers, and may be solitary or multiple. Concomitant illness may be present. An asymptomatic carrier state is thought to exist.[14] Differential diagnoses include other mycobacterial infections, deep mycoses and neoplasia.

Diagnosis: Direct smears and biopsies of skin lesions may reveal acid-fast mycobacterial bacilli.[2] Cultures and laboratory animal inoculation are required to differentiate tuberculosis from other mycobacterial infections. Mycobacteria that cause tuberculosis grow on special media, usually within 6 weeks but not before 3 weeks. Guinea pig inoculation leads to the animal's death in 6-8 weeks.[15] Cats with tuberculosis should be euthanized and public health authorities notified.

Feline Leprosy

Cause: A mycobacterium closely resembling *M lepramurium,* the causative agent of murine leprosy, has been isolated from skin lesions in cats. This rare condition has been termed "feline leprosy" and may have been recognized in Australia, Canada, Great Britain, New Zealand, the Netherlands and the US.[16,17] The exact mode of transmission is unknown, although the bite of infected rats has been postulated as a cause. Differential diagnoses include sporotrichosis, deep mycoses, neoplasia and other mycobacterial infections.

Clinical Signs: Clinical signs include nodular or occasionally ulcerative skin lesions, with no site predilection. No evidence of systemic illness has been reported.

Diagnosis: Diagnosis of feline leprosy may be difficult. Acid-fast bacilli usually can be demonstrated on biopsy. *Mycobacterium lepramurium* has only recently been grown on artificial culture media.[78] Inoculation of guinea pigs does not cause death but produces characteristic localized lesions.[17] Inoculation of rats and mice causes characteristic but more generalized lesions and may cause their death.[18] Unfortunately, these transmission studies have not always been reproducible or attempted in all cases of suspected feline leprosy.[19]

Treatment: Treatment has usually been limited to surgical excision. The lesions occasionally recur after surgery. Since most antileprosy drugs used in people are potentially toxic for cats, a veterinary dermatologist should be consulted before medical therapy is attempted. Many of the cats described in the literature were eventually euthanized for aesthetic reasons.

Atypical Mycobacterial Infections

Cause: Other mycobacteria implicated in feline skin disease are categorized as atypical (Runyan groups I-IV) mycobacteria. Pathogens most commonly isolated are in Runyan group IV, the fast-growing mycobacteria. Most of these organisms are found in the environment and infections may be the result of opportunistic invasion of wounds.

Clinical Signs: Skin lesions may include cutaneous or subcutaneous nodules, ulcerations and draining tracts. These lesions seem to occur more commonly on the ventral abdomen or thorax (Fig 4).

Diagnosis: Acid-fast mycobacteria may be seen on impression smears of nodules, in exudates or on histopathologic examination. Final identification is on the basis of culture and biochemical tests. Group-IV mycobacteria usually grow on blood agar culture medium within 2-4 days.[15] The authors are aware of at least 4 cases of infection with a group-IV mycobacterium in which the organisms were demonstrable on impression smears of subcutaneous nodules, were grown on culture medium and in experimental animals, and yet were not demonstrable on histopathologic examination of the same nodule. Inoculation is not fatal in guinea pigs.[15] Other mycobacterial diseases, deep mycoses and nodular panniculitis should be considered as differential diagnoses.

Treatment: If bacterial cultures are successful, antibiotic sensitivity testing should be performed. Atypical mycobacteria occasionally are sensitive to chloramphenicol or tetracycline. Dosages vary tremendously. The recommended dosage for chloramphenicol is 333 mg given orally TID and for tetracycline is 12.5 mg/kg BID to 50 mg/kg TID given orally. Surgical excision of isolated lesions may be attempted but these may recur. Since in people these conditions may spontaneously regress, various "cures" reported for cats may be suspect.[20,21]

The public health significance of feline leprosy and atypical mycobacterial infections is unknown. One report of suspected feline leprosy cases noted histopathologic lesions similar to those caused by *M leprae*, the agent causing human leprosy.[19] Studies of the atypical mycobacteria have not shown conclusive evidence of transmission from animals to people.

The classification of atypical mycobacteria in human medicine does not include *M lepramurium*.[15] The terms "feline leprosy" and "atypical mycobacterial infections" describe 2 different types of infections and should not be used interchangeably.

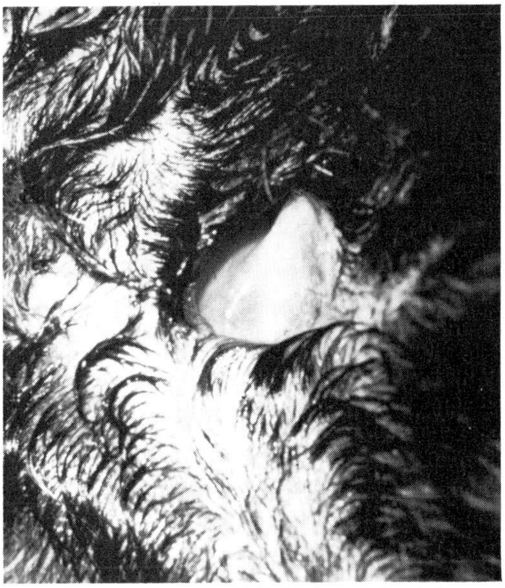

Fig 4. Atypical mycobacterial infection on the abdomen.

Superficial Fungal Infections by C.A. Sousa and P.J. Ihrke

Ringworm

Dermatophyte infections are some of the most commonly overdiagnosed and misdiagnosed diseases in feline dermatology. They are probably also the most common small animal dermatologic zoonoses. Cats of any age can be affected, although kittens are more susceptible. The disease shows no sex or breed predilection.

Dermatophytes are fungi that invade the keratinized layers of skin, hair and occasionally nails. Fungal hyphae cannot survive in living tissue. Infection is established by contact with infected hairs and keratin scales. Microtrauma to the hair or skin may be needed for infection to become established. The incubation period of ringworm is variable but is usually between 4 days and 4 weeks.

Dermatophyte growth begins in the hair or in the stratum corneum around the hair follicle. It proceeds down the hair shaft and stops at the junction between dead and living tissue. Since the germinal hair cells are not affected, the hair follicle is not destroyed and hair can regrow unless a deep fungal folliculitis develops.

The fungi release toxins and potential allergens that penetrate the dermis and cause an inflammatory reaction. The toxins can cause mild erythema and scaling. A biologic contact hypersensitivity is thought to develop in the more inflammatory cases. Desquamation also occurs within the hair follicle, obstructing it and giving the area a papular appearance. Since the dermatophyte cannot survive in an area of inflammation, new growth spreads peripherally to adjacent follicles, giving the lesion its expanding, circular appearance. With a severe inflammatory reaction, as caused by a zoophilic dermatophyte, there may be edema, suppuration and necrosis. This type of lesion is known as kerion ringworm.

Fungal growth weakens the hair and often causes breakage, leaving short stubble. Ringworm is primarily disseminated by contaminated broken hairs. Inflammation may lead to

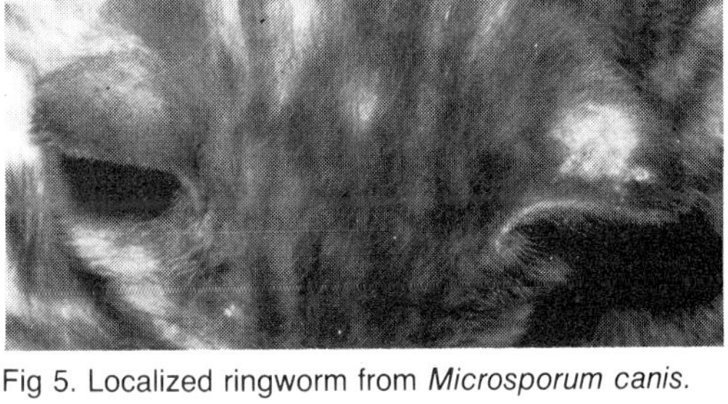

Fig 5. Localized ringworm from *Microsporum canis*.

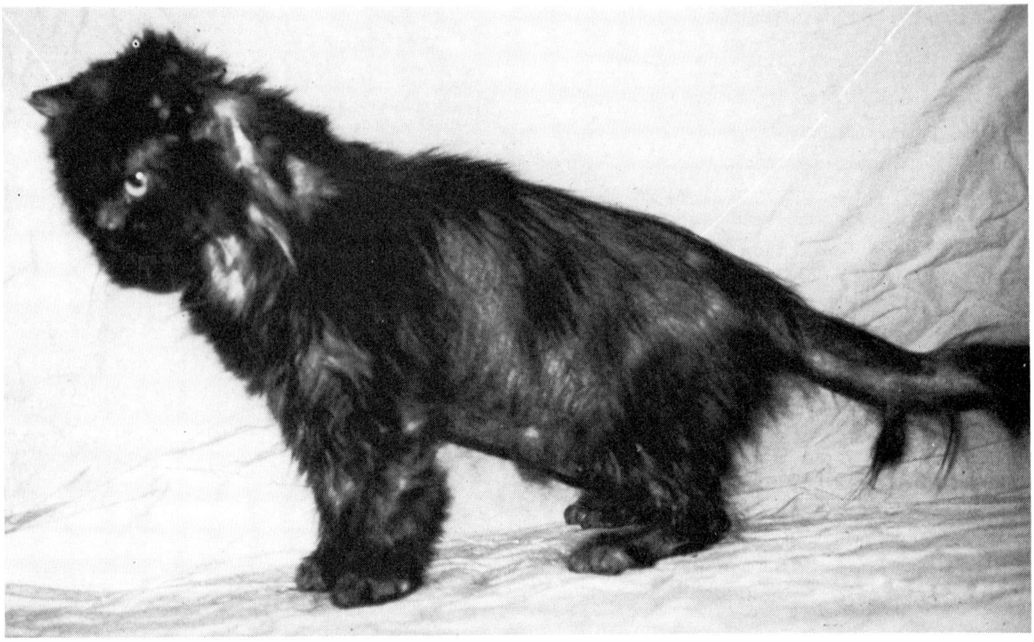

Fig 6. Extensive, somewhat symmetric alopecia in generalized ringworm caused by *Microsporum canis*.

increased scaling, which also aids in spread of the dermatophyte.

Cause: Microsporum canis causes 98% of the dermatophytoses seen in cats. *Microsporum gypseum* and *Trichophyton mentagrophytes* account for most of the remaining cases.[2,22,23]

Microsporum canis is a zoophilic fungus for which the cat is the natural host. It also may infect dogs, people and other animals. Because this dermatophyte is so well adapted to cats, there are many asymptomatic carriers. Direct microscopic examination, using the high-dry objective, of infected hairs cleared with 10% KOH reveals the fungus in grape-like clusters on the outside of the hair shaft. Examination of a culture under the microscope reveals many thick-walled, long, spindle-shaped macroaleuriospores. These have a rough surface, usually an asymmetric knob at each end and more than 6 compartments.[24,25]

Microsporum gypseum is a geophilic fungus for which the main habitat is soil. It too grows on the outside of the hair shaft. Macroaleuriospores are thin-walled ellipsoids with a rough surface and up to 6 compartments.

Trichophyton mentagrophytes is a zoophilic dermatophyte that rarely infects cats. Asymptomatic carriers have been reported. Chains of large arthrospores can be seen on cleared hairs under the low-power objective of the microscope. In culture, many spherical microaleuriospores are produced in grape-like clusters, along with a few club-shaped macroaleuriospores. Spiral hyphae are also found in abundance.[24,25]

Clinical Signs: The classic lesion of ringworm consists of a circular, expanding area of alopecia, with broken hairs, crusting, scaling and an erythematous border. The most commonly affected sites are the face, ears and extremities (Fig 5). Some affected cats may have extensive alopecia, seborrhea sicca, a papulovesicular rash, paronychia (onchomycosis), pigmentary changes of the hair or skin, folliculitis, furunculosis or simply pruritus (Fig 6).

Diagnosis: A diagnosis of dermatophytosis is based on the history, physical examination, microscopic examination of hair, Wood's light examination, fungal culture, or a biopsy.

Hair and debris plucked from the edge of a lesion can be cleared with KOH or other cleaning solutions and examined for arthrospores. Scrapings of hair and scales can be mixed with 10% KOH and briefly heated. The slide is then microscopically examined under the high-dry objective after 5-20 minutes. Every common pathogenic fungus of veterinary importance is an ectothrix, *ie*, produces arthrospores on the outside of hair shafts. The KOH preparation has the disadvantage of difficulty in interpretation. Even to the trained mycologist it is only 60-70% accurate as compared with fungal cultures.[2]

The Wood's light emits ultraviolet light filtered through a nickel oxide filter. In veterinary dermatology its primary use is in diagnosis of *M canis* infections. The organisms break down keratin, producing a tryptophan metabolite that fluoresces apple-green. Up to 60% of feline *M canis* infections fluoresce when examined carefully. The Wood's light examination should be done in a darkened room and the entire body should be checked. Broken hairs should be plucked and the intrafollicular portion examined. False-positive fluorescence can be caused by sebum crusts, scales, medication and lint.

Dermatophyte culture is the most accurate test for the diagnosis of ringworm. A few broken hairs or, if Wood's lamp positive, fluorescent hairs are selected. The area is gently blotted with alcohol and allowed to air dry. Lesions that have been recently medicated should not be cultured as dermatophyte growth may be delayed for up to 130 days.[26]

Dermatophytes can be grown on Sabouraud's dextrose agar. Unfortunately many of these cultures are difficult to interpret due to overgrowth of nonpathogenic fungi. Sabouraud's medium has been combined with chlortetracycline and gentamicin to inhibit bacterial growth, cyclohexamide to inhibit saprophytic fungi, and phenol red as a pH indicator. This useful medium is called Dermatophyte Test Medium (Pitman-Moore). Pathogenic fungi digest the protein in the medium, producing alkaline metabolites that turn the medium red, usually within 72 hours. Saprophytes initially cause no color change as they digest the carbohydrates and produce acid or neutral metabolites. The culture medium is observed for a color change from amber to red that coincides with the first signs of fungal growth (Fig C1). Any growth eventually changes the color indicator. Growth of any pathogenic fungus usually is seen within 7-10 days.

After the fungus has grown, an attempt should be made to identify it by examining the thallus stained with lactophenol cotton blue. Because fungi do not sporulate well on a Dermatophyte Test Medium culture, a second culture on an appropriate medium may be necessary.

A skin biopsy may occasionally be useful in the diagnosis of dermatophytosis. It is reportedly about 80% accurate.[2] Special stains (gram or periodic acid-Schiff) may be useful in identification of fungal elements.

Asymptomatic carriers may be identified by brushing the cat with a sterile toothbrush, then pressing the bristles gently onto agar medium (MacKenzie brush technic). About 25-30% of families with a pet with ringworm have at least one member of the family affected with the disease. Generally children and the elderly are at higher risk.

Treatment: There are many methods of treating feline dermatophytosis. However, it should be remembered that ringworm frequently is a self-limiting disease that undergoes spontaneous remission within 1-6 months. It is impossible to estimate how many cases of "successfully treated" ringworm actually underwent spontaneous remission.

Systemic griseofulvin (Fulvicin:Schering) has been used extensively in cats. It acts by inhibition of nucleic acid synthesis and is therefore fungistatic. The manufacturer's recommended oral dosages are 20-132 mg/kg SID. Unfortunately, the manufacturer's recommended dosages are based on data extrapolated from other species. Until further research is done in cats, our current recommendation is 88-132 mg/kg/day. Griseofulvin should be given with a high-fat meal (oil) to increase intestinal absorption and minimize vomiting.[2]

Therapy should be continued until fungal cultures are negative or for 2 weeks beyond clinical recovery. The average cat is treated for 6 weeks. Nailbed ringworm (onchomycosis) may require treatment for 6 months or longer. Griseofulvin is highly teratogenic and should never be used in pregnant queens. Other potential side effects include anemia, leukopenia and depression.

There are many products available for topical use. The most success had been obtained with a 2% lime sulfur solution (Lym Dyp:DVM, Lime Sulfur:Woolfolk Chemical, Orthothrix:Chevron) or a 2.25% captan suspension (Orthocide:Chevron) at a 1:200 dilution or 2 tbsp/gal. Either treatment is fairly inexpensive, antifungal and quite safe. The liquids should be applied as a total body rinse weekly until 2 weeks beyond clinical remission. This treatment regimen can also be followed for animals with localized lesions. Due to the odor of lime sulfur products, captan is more aesthetically acceptable to most owners. Since captan is known to be a potent contact sensitizer in people, rubber gloves should be worn during treatment.[27] If desired, topical miconazole (Conofite:Pitman-Moore) may be applied twice daily for spot treatment of isolated focal lesions. The medication should be rubbed well into the areas of normal hair and skin around the lesion. However, whole body rinses generally are more effective and less expensive.

Clothing, bedding, cages, utensils and other environmental objects must also be treated. Disinfectants, such as chlorhexidine (Nolvasan: Fort Dodge), sodium hypochlorite (Clorox, 1:10 dilution) and steam can be used.

Intermediate Fungal Infections by S.I. Reinke, P.J. Ihrke and A.A. Stannard

Sporotrichosis

Cause: Sporotrichosis is a chronic, granulomatous fungal disease caused by the dimorphic soil saprophyte, *Sporothrix schenckii.* This rare disease in cats usually is the result of wound contamination as the fungus is common in nature. It is not generally regarded as contagious; yet transmission from animals to people has occurred from handling of infected cats. The disease is most common in the coastal areas and river valleys of the southeastern US.

Clinical Signs: The cutaneolymphatic form of the disease is most common. Affected cats have firm, tender nodules, often on the extremities or face, that may ulcerate and discharge a brownish-red pus (Fig C2). The nodules may extend along the draining lymphatic chain. A second primary cutaneous form reportedly begins dorsad and spreads randomly, with no lymphatic involvement. Sporotrichosis may also be seen as a disseminated systemic disease.

Diagnosis: Due to the small number of organisms in the exudate, it is difficult to demonstrate the organism by impression smear. The most effective means of diagnosis is culture on Sabouraud's dextrose agar (Dermatophyte Test Medium contains selective inhibitors of saprophytic fungi). However, the tissue form of the fungus must be identified to demonstrate pathogenicity.[2]

Treatment: Recommended treatment of the cutaneolymphatic and cutaneous forms of the disease is with 20% aqueous solution of sodium iodide given PO at 0.5-1.0 ml/5 kg every 12-24 hours.[13] Treatment should be continued for one month beyond clinical remission. Caution should be exercised since cats are very sensitive to iodine toxicity.

Phaeohyphomycosis

Cause: Phaeohyphomycosis (chromomycosis) is a rare, chronic pyogranulomatous infection caused by the saprophytic dematiaceous fungi that form pigmented, septate hyphae in host tissues.[13] *Dreschlera* and *Phialophora* are most frequently isolated. Infection is by wound contamination. Lesions usually begin as solitary nodules that may later ulcerate and form fistulas.

Diagnosis: Direct examination of exudate or tissue in 10-20% KOH reveals black, septate hyphae. Modified Sabouraud's dextrose agar must be used for culture as Dermatophyte Test Medium contains selective inhibitors of saprophytic fungi.

Treatment: Surgical excision is the treatment of choice. Advanced cases may require more extensive surgery, such as limb amputation. No information regarding successful medical treatment in cats is available; however, amphotericin B or miconazole might prove useful.[28]

Mycetoma

Cause: Mycetomas (maduromycosis) are chronic, pyogranulomatous infections, with granules appearing in the exudate. The granules (or grains) are actually colonies of the organisms. Two types of mycetoma have been identified in cats. Actinomycotic mycetomas are caused by *Actinomyces, Nocardia* and *Streptomyces.* Eumycotic mycetomas are caused by various species of fungi in animals, but *Brachicladium* has been the only species isolated from cats.[2] These saprophytes are all ubiquitous in nature. Infection usually occurs via wound contamination.

Clinical Signs: Clinically the "triad of tumefaction, draining tracts and granules" is present.[13] Lesions usually are singular and found on the extremities.

Diagnosis: The granules should be crushed and examined in 10-20% KOH to demonstrate the hyphae and chlamydospores of eumycotic mycetomas. A gram stain reveals the gram-positive filaments of an actinomycotic mycetoma. Culture of the granules on modified Sabouraud's dextrose agar and on blood agar should be made since correct identification of the type of mycetoma determines the therapy.

Treatment: Surgical excision or amputation of the entire affected area is the only current therapy for eumycotic mycetoma. The treatment of choice for the actinomycotic mycetomas is oral sulfa drugs, such as trimethoprim-sulfadiazine (Tribrissen:Wellcome).

Parasitic Diseases
by S.D. White and P.J. Ihrke

Flea Infestation

Cause: Fleas are the most important feline ectoparasite. *Ctenocephalides felis* is the most common flea affecting cats and dogs in most parts of the US.

Fleas spend most of their time in the environment and only jump on the cat to feed (suck blood) and breed; eggs are laid on the skin or in the environment. The larvae hatch and feed on adult flea fecal casts, dried blood, feces and tapeworm (*Dipylidium caninum*) eggs. Depending on the environment, the life cycle may be 3 weeks to over a year.

Either an irritant or an allergic reaction to the flea may occur in cats. In simple flea infestation, flea saliva may have an irritant action. In flea-allergy dermatitis, it is postulated that both immediate and delayed hypersensitivities occur in cats as in other species.

Clinical Signs: Clinical signs vary considerably. A mild to severe papular-crusting miliary eruption may be seen around the neck, periaurally or along the dorsal lumbosacral region. Occasionally the entire body may be involved. Some pruritus usually is present. In severe cases, pruritus may lead to excoriation and pyotraumatic dermatitis (Fig 7). Fleas or flea dirt (excreta) often may be found.

Diagnosis: Diagnosis is based on history and physical examination. The absence of fleas or flea dirt does not preclude a diagnosis of flea infestation or flea-allergy dermatitis since fleas spend most of their time in the environment and cats are fastidious groomers. Cats that become hypersensitive to flea saliva may manifest clinical signs after only a small number of flea bites. (see Flea-Allergy Dermatitis). Flea dirt may be demonstrated to the owner by placing the dark brown casts on a white background and adding a drop of water. Red streaks and stains of blood readily appear as the cast dissolves. Tapeworm segments are also of diagnostic significance since the flea serves as the intermediate host for *D caninum*.

Treatment: Any treatment regimen should include vigorous flea control for the animal and environment. Our current recommendation in northern California is use of a 5% carbamate powder applied every other day. All cats and dogs in the household should be treated regardless of the presence or absence of clinical signs. As an alternative to powdering, powder may be taken in the gloved hands and "petted" into the animal's coat. Sprays and shampoos have little residual effect. Dips are messy and potentially toxic to cats. Collars alone are ineffective in all but the mildest infestations in a closed environment. No scientific evidence is available to support the use of thiamin (vitamin B_1) as a flea infestation preventive.

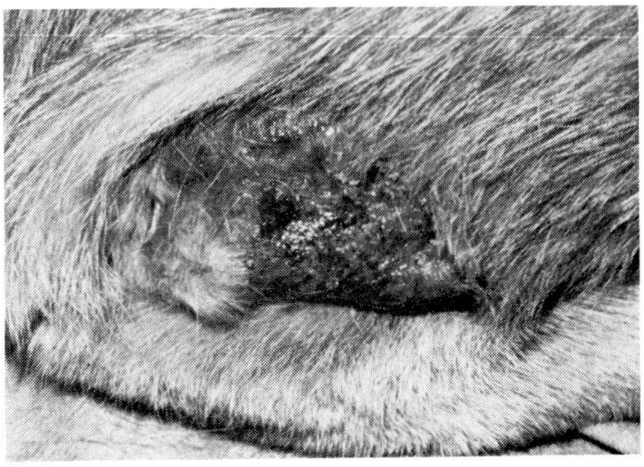

Fig 7. Excoriation from flea-allergy dermatitis.

Oral prednisone or prednisolone may be necessary in severe cases to control pruritus for several weeks until flea control becomes effective. Corticosteroid therapy is covered in more detail in the section on Flea-Allergy Dermatitis.

Control: Flea control in the house should consist of insecticide spraying and frequent vacuuming. Foggers ("bug bombs") or professional exterminators are effective in killing a large percentage of the flea population in a house. Residual action is usually limited to less than a week and flea eggs are unaffected. Use of foggers, therefore, must be repeated at least once several weeks after the initial use. Using a pyrethrin spray weekly under sinks and around floorboards and as a light area spray is helpful. Vacuuming at least once weekly is very important. A 5% carbamate powder should be vacuumed into the bag or the bag thrown out after each vacuuming. This is to prevent proliferation and hatching of fleas and flea eggs vacuumed into the bag.

Fleas in the outside environment are more difficult to control since cats frequently roam. Yards may be sprayed with malathion or carbamate spray twice monthly.

Notoedric Mange

Cause: Notoedric mange or feline scabies is caused by the sarcoptid mite, *Notoedres cati*. The disease is rare in most parts of the US but often is found in localized enzootic areas.

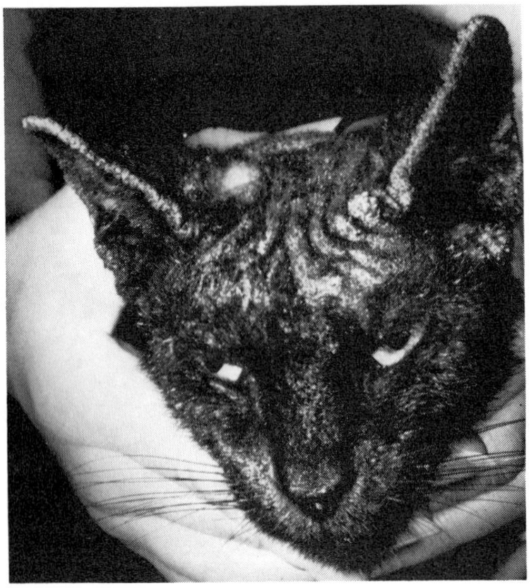

Fig 8. Notoedric mange. (Courtesy of Dr I. Ameti)

The life cycle of the mite is completed in 2-3 weeks and is spent entirely on the host. Transmission is by direct contact. The disease is highly contagious and other species, including dogs and people, can be affected.

Clinical Signs: Clinical signs generally include intense pruritus, especially around the head, ears and neck (Fig 8).[1] Erythema and a papular eruption, progressing to crusts, scales, excoriations and lichenification, are the usual lesions. Lesions may also occur on the paws and genitalia, and rarely may be more generalized.

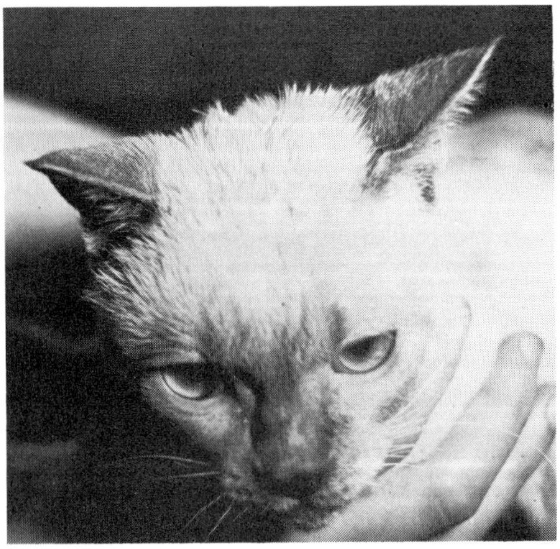

Fig 9. Cheyletiellosis. Note the disheveled appearance of the hair on the head.

Diagnosis: Diagnosis is based on history, physical examination and skin scrapings. The mite usually is easy to find and is somewhat smaller than the canine scabies mite. A dorsal anus rather than a terminal anus differentiates this mite from the canine scabies mite.[29] Differential diagnoses include any pruritic condition, especially food allergy, which also has a predilection for the head region.

Treatment: Parasiticidal dips may be used weekly on all animals in the household until 2 weeks past clinical remissions (usually 3-4 weeks total). A lime sulfur preparation (Orthothrix:Chevron, Sulpho-Dip:California Veterinary Supply), diluted to a 2% solution with water, is safe and economical. Alternatively, a carbaryl shampoo (Mycodex with Carbaryl: Beecham) may be used weekly. The affected animals should be clipped gently and any crusts cleansed off before application of the insecticide. Systemic corticosteroids may be used to control pruritus. Since *Notoedres* cannot live long in the environment, one thorough cleaning of the habitat is sufficient.

The disease in dogs reportedly resembles canine scabies. Affected people may have a pruritic papular eruption on the arms and trunk similar to that in infestations with canine scabies. Since the mites probably cannot reproduce on people, the condition regresses within 3 weeks after elimination of the source of infection.[2]

Cheyletiellosis

Cause: The 3 species of *Cheyletiella* mites that affect cats are *Cheyletiella blakei, C yasguri* (more common on dogs), and *C parasitovorax* (more common on rabbits).[1] These mites do not burrow but are surface dwellers thought to live on tissue debris. The eggs are laid attached at one end to a hair shaft and may be visible. Authorities disagree as to how long the mite may live in the environment.[1,2] Indirect transmission from fomites may be as important as direct transmission.

Clinical Signs: Clinical signs are variable. Focal dorsal seborrhea or miliary eczema is most common (Figs 9, 10). Pruritus may be present. Some cats may be asymptomatic carriers.

Diagnosis: Diagnosis is based on history, physical examination and demonstration of the mites. The last is done by microscopically examining superficial skin scrapings taken from large areas. Alternatively, clear cellophane adhesive

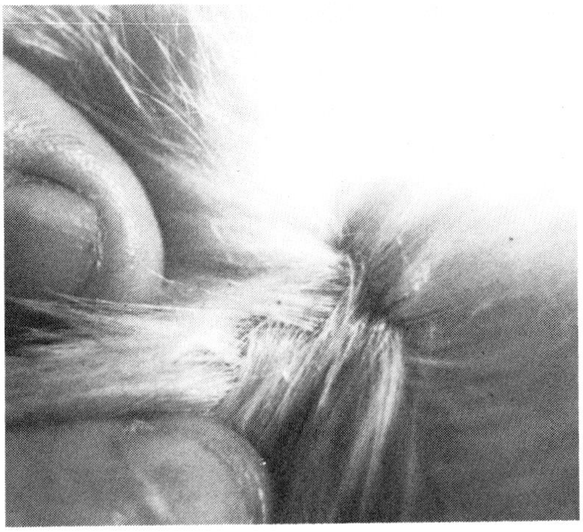

Fig 10. Localized areas of scaling in cheyletiellosis.

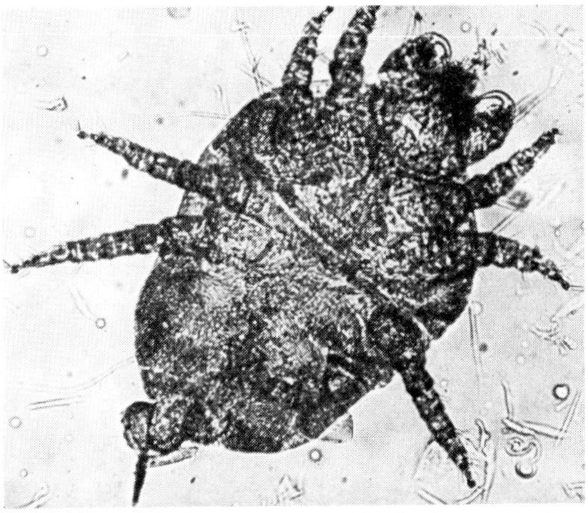

Fig 11. Adult *Cheyletiella* mite. (Original magnification 100X) (Courtesy of Compend Cont Ed)

tape may be applied to the skin in crusty areas and then placed on a drop of mineral oil on a slide for microscopic visualization (see Diagnostic Technics). A hand lens also may be used to view the mites. Occasionally mites or their eggs may be identified on fecal flotation. *Cheyletiella* mites usually are found without difficulty but multiple scrapings should be performed in all suspected cases.[29] Microscopically the mites are characterized by large palpal hooks on the accessory mouthparts and an elongated body relative to that of sarcoptic mites (Fig 11).[29]

Treatment: Cheyletiella mites are susceptible to a wide spectrum of parasiticides, including powders, shampoos and dips. A carbaryl shampoo (Mycodex with Carbaryl:Beecham) used weekly for a month usually is curative. Alternatively, lime sulfur may be used as noted above. All animals in the household should be shampooed because of the potential for development of asymptomatic carriers. The environment should be thoroughly cleaned at least once weekly for 3 weeks. Bedding should be disposed of or cleansed.

Cheyletiella mites are not very species specific and may infest people. The condition in people is intensely pruritic, usually affecting the trunk and arms, and may progress from a macular-papular stage to pustules and crusting. The mites are not thought to reproduce on people and once the animal is treated, the lesions regress within 3 weeks.[2,29]

Demodicosis

Cause: Feline demodicosis is rare. *Demodex cati* is thought to be a resident, in small numbers, on the skin of normal cats. Occasionally these mites may proliferate and cause localized or generalized disease. It is tempting to extrapolate from data on canine demodicosis and hypothesize that cats with clinical demodicosis also have concurrent endogenous and/or exogenous immunosuppression of some sort.[2]

Clinical Signs: The most common clinical signs are single or multiple areas of alopecia and erythema around the head, ears and neck (Fig 12). Pruritus, papules and scaling may or may not be present. A generalized dermatosis and ceruminous otitis externa has been reported (Fig 13).[2] Generalized demodicosis has been observed in cats positive for FeLV and in cats with generalized debilitating diseases, such as diabetes

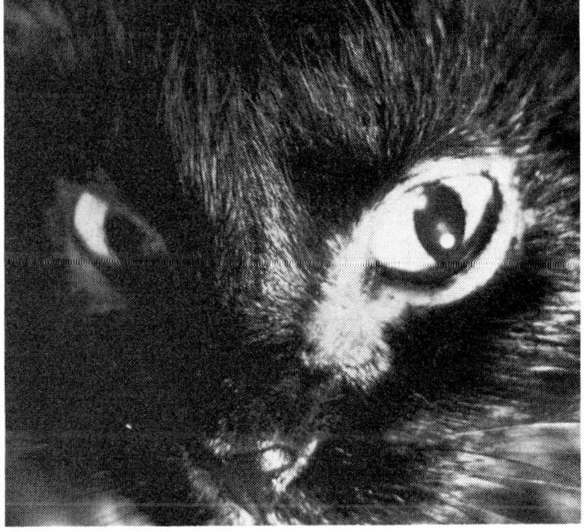

Fig 12. Well-circumscribed periorbital alopecia in localized demodicosis.

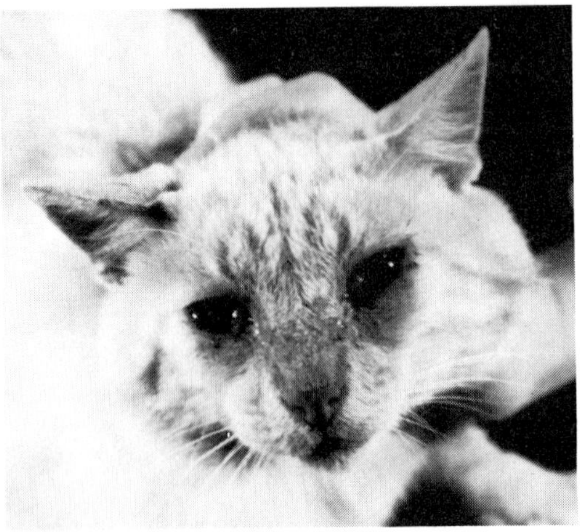

Fig 13. Patchy alopecia and mild generalized scaling in generalized demodicosis.

mellitus. Consequently, cats with generalized demodicosis should be tested for FeLV and other possible underlying causes of immunosuppression. One of the authors has seen 2 generalized cases of feline demodicosis in which no underlying immunosuppressive cause was demonstrated. The disease regressed without treatment over the course of several months.

Diagnosis: Diagnosis is based on history, physical examination, skin scrapings and ear swabs, if otitis is present. As in canine demodicosis, scrapings should be deep enough to cause capillary oozing (Fig 14).

Treatment: Therapy of localized demodicosis is probably unnecessary since most of these cases regress without treatment. Unlike its canine counterpart, *D cati* may be susceptible to 2% lime sulfur dips. Because the disease may occur only in immunosuppressed cats, corticosteroids are contraindicated. Use of a parasiticidal corticosteroid-antibiotic solution (Tresaderm:Merck) for otitis externa would be an exception.

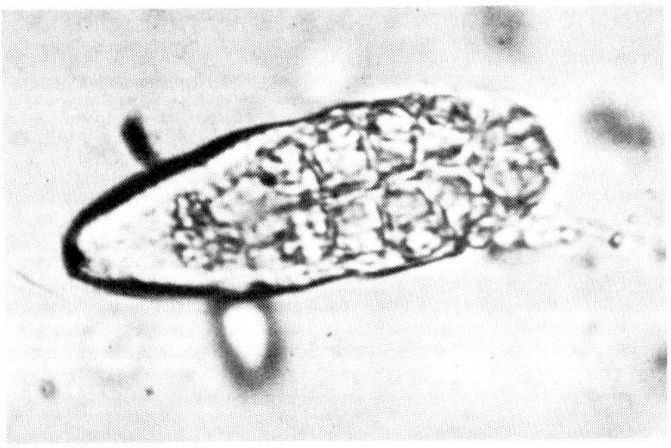

Fig 14. *Demodex* in a skin scraping. (Original magnification 100X)

Trombiculiasis

Cause: The parasitic larvae of the trombiculid mites (chigger or harvest mite) rarely affect cats. In North America the involved mite usually is *Eutrombicula alfreddugesi*. The adult mites are free-living or parasitize plants or arthropods. Eggs are laid on soil. The larvae hatch, parasitize a vertebrate host, then drop off to become nymphs and subsequently adults. The 6-legged larvae may stay on the cat from several hours to 7 days.[1,2] Transmission is through contact with an environment inhabited by the mite.

Clinical Signs: Chiggers produce a papular eruption, with scaling and alopecia, most noticeably around the head, ears and interdigital regions. The lesions may become generalized. Classically described as an intensely pruritic disease, trombiculiasis may be present without pruritus.[2,29] Since the pruritus may outlast the presence of the mites, a hypersensitivity reaction to the mites' saliva has been postulated.[2,29]

Diagnosis: On physical examination, the small orange-red mites may be seen as dots within papules. In parts of the country where chiggers are present, cats that roam in rural areas in late summer and fall are most commonly affected. Chiggers may be seen on skin scrapings.

Treatment: Treatment should include a single parasiticidal dip (2% lime sulfur) or an insecticidal shampoo (pyrethrin or carbaryl) and corticosteroids for pruritus. Avoidance of re-exposure is an important aspect of client education.

Otodectic Mange

Cause: Otodectes cynotis, the ear mite, is the primary cause of otitis externa in cats. The 3-week life cycle is spent entirely on the host, on which the mites live on superficial epidermal debris and fluids. Ear mites are highly contagious among cats, rabbits and dogs. People may be transiently affected with a papular eruption of the arms and trunk.[2] This disappears upon treatment of the affected animal.

Clinical Signs: The mite causes variable degrees of pruritus and irritation due both to mechanical injury of the ear canal and to mite saliva, which can cause an inflammatory and probably a hypersensitivity reaction. Some cats seem to tolerate great numbers of mites in the ear canal with minimal clinical signs, while others develop pruritus from relatively small numbers. Young animals seem to be more commonly affected.

A thick, crusty, crumbly, brown-black exudate occurs in classic otitis externa due to *O cynotis*. The pruritus associated with these mites may result in severe self-excoriation, head-shaking and aural hematomas. Secondary bacterial otitis may be present. Otitis media and otitis interna may rarely result.

Diagnosis: Diagnosis is based on physical examination, history and the presence of mites in the ear canal. The mites may be seen with an otoscope or a mineral oil preparation of the exudate observed microscopically. The mites are large, white and mobile. Their absence does not preclude the diagnosis since they may be killed by inflammatory debris. Otitis externa in cats should be considered as due to *O cynotis* until proven otherwise.

Treatment: Treatment consists of gentle cleaning of the ears with a ceruminolytic agent, such as dioctyl sodium sulfosuccinate, if necessary, and instillation of an acaricide, such as Tresaderm (Merck), with 3 drops applied BID for 10 days. Tresaderm is the only otic product in the management of otoacariasis that one of the authors has not seen cause contact dermatitis in susceptible cats. In addition to the miticidal effects of the thiabendazole, the dexamethasone in Tresaderm helps control inflammation. The cat also should be treated with either an insecticidal shampoo (Mycodex with Carbaryl: Beecham) or powder (5% carbamate) to kill mites living outside the ears. All other animals on the premises should be treated, even in the absence of clinical signs.

Tick Infestation

Cause: Ticks are arachnids that occasionally parasitize cats. They can be divided into the soft-shelled ticks (Argasidae) and the hard-shelled ticks (Ixodidae). They usually are not species specific.[1]

The most important argasid tick is *Otobius megnini*, the spinous ear tick. Found primarily in the southwest US, the larval and nymphal stages are parasitic and inhabit the external ear canal, in which they feed on blood and other fluids. The parasitic stage may last 2-6 months before the second stage nymphs drop off and molt into nonparasitic adults.[2,30] The eggs are laid in the environment and hatching larvae must find a host within 3 months.

Several ixodid ticks have been reported to infest cats. The important distinction among the various species reported is that *Rhipicephalus sanguineus* (brown dog tick) inhabits buildings and urban areas, while the other species are found in wooded environments.[2,30] Ixodid tick infestation in cats is uncommon. Infestation generally is associated with debilitation and inability of the cat to remove the tick.

Clinical Signs: Clinical signs of argasid tick infestation are relative to otitis externa and include head-shaking, ear-scratching and aural hematomas. In severe cases, otitis media, otitis interna and even meningitis may result.

Ixodid tick bites are irritating and may induce areas of local inflammation. Heavy infestations may cause anemia. In one cat seen by the authors, the left side of the face and left leg became acutely edematous and subsequently partially necrotic. Two ixodid ticks were removed from this cat's neck and left front paw.

Diagnosis: Diagnosis of argasid tick infestation is based on the history and finding the ticks on otoscopic examination. Ixodid tick infestation is diagnosed by identification of the tick after removal with alligator forceps.

Treatment: Treatment of argasid tick infestation consists of manually removing the ticks with alligator forceps and application of a corticosteroid-antibiotic-parasiticide medication (Tresaderm:Merck) in the ear. Since these ticks may be difficult to eradicate from the environment, the area should be sprayed with a pesticide at least once a month.[30] All animals (cats, dogs, cattle) in contact with affected cats should be treated.

Solitary ixodid ticks may be removed by grasping the head of the tick, as close to the skin as possible, with forceps and pulling with firm, gentle traction. In cats with many ticks, a parasiticidal dip, such as 2% lime sulfur, may be necessary. Care should be taken with the use of any insecticide in a debilitated, anemic animal. Blood transfusions and other supportive therapy may be necessary in some cases. Since flea and tick collars have been disappointing in their ability to prevent reinfestation, avoidance of ticks and tick habitats is probably the best prophylaxis. If the tick is identified as *R sanguineus*, household foggers or professional exterminators are necessary to eliminate it.

Pediculosis

Cause: Pediculosis (lice infestation) is uncommon in cats. *Felicola subrostratus*, a biting louse, is the only cat louse seen with any frequency and usually is associated with debilitation and unsanitary conditions. Pediculosis is contagious, with transmission by direct contact or possibly fomites, such as grooming materials. Lice infestation seems to occur more commonly in the winter, when animals have closer contact with one another and may have longer haircoats. Lice tend to be species specific; *F subrostratus* has little public health significance.

The life cycle is spent entirely on the cat and is complete in 3-4 weeks. Unlike *Cheyletiella* eggs, lice eggs (nits) are attached to the hair shafts along their entire length.

Clinical Signs: Clinical signs include seborrhea sicca, miliary dermatitis, mild to severe pruritus, and a disheveled haircoat. Asymptomatic carriers may also be seen.

Diagnosis: Diagnosis is based on history, physical examination and careful visual evaluation with a hand lens. Skin scrapings, plucked hairs and clear cellophane tape application (see Diagnostic Technics) may also be used.

Treatment: Since lice are susceptible to most parasiticides, almost any total-body parasiticide is effective. Carbaryl shampoos or 2% lime sulfur dips should be applied weekly for a month to the affected animal and all animals in contact with affected cats. Corticosteroids may be used to relieve pruritus. Underlying causes for debilitation or poor environmental conditions should be corrected. As lice do not live long in the environment, one thorough cleaning of the area is sufficient.

Cuterebriasis

Cause: Although rabbits and rodents are considered the primary hosts for *Cuterebra*, cats occasionally are affected. The adult female *Cuterebra* (one of the blowflies) lays its eggs in soil, usually near rodent or rabbit burrows. The larvae hatch, penetrate the skin of the host, develop in subcutaneous nodules for a month, and drop to the ground to pupate. The disease is seen most often in the summer.[2,29]

Clinical Signs: Skin lesions of cuterebriasis are subcutaneous nodules, usually in the cervical region. Occasionally they may involve other skin regions, the nostrils or the CNS.[30] Early lesions are firm upon palpation. As the brown, spiny larvae mature, a small breathing pore is cut by the larvae through which they may be seen. The nodules may cause no problems or may abscess.

Diagnosis: Diagnosis is based on the history and finding the nodular lesions with or without the larvae.

Treatment: The treatment of choice is gentle removal of the larva with forceps after enlargment of the breathing pore, if necessary. The procedure should be performed gently to avoid rupturing of the larva since anaphylactoid reactions have been reported.[2,30] The wound should be cared for as an open wound but healing often is slow.

Myiasis

Cause: Myiasis (flystrike, maggot infestation) is rare in domestic cats and usually seen in debilitated or neglected animals. Various fleshflies and blowflies are attracted to moisture, feces, urine and wound exudates, and deposit their eggs in devitalized areas.[30] The perineum and truncal wounds are the most common sites of feline myiasis. Larvae hatch within 12 hours and create ulcerated, exudative, punched-out, macerated skin lesions. The larvae feed for a week, causing extensive damage, and then pupate. Subcutaneous necrosis and a foul odor are often associated with myiasis.

Diagnosis: Diagnosis is by observation of maggots in the wound.

Treatment: Treatment should include resolving the primary underlying conditions. The affected area should be gently clipped and cleaned with a dilute povidone iodine or chlorhexidine solution. As many larvae as possible should be removed from the skin, subcutaneous tissue and draining tracts by flushing with saline, manual removal with forceps, or with careful topical application of ether. Application of strong disinfectants or insecticides onto the wound should be avoided. Necrotic tissue must be debrided. General supportive therapy is extremely important as these animals may be extremely debilitated. Too-vigorous initial manipulation may lead to demise of the animal during maggot removal.

Viral Diseases
by C.A. Sousa and P.J. Ihrke

Feline Leukemia Virus Infection

A number of cutaneous disorders in cats are thought to be associated with FeLV infection. Many are believed to occur secondary to the immunosuppressive effects of the virus, but there is little published data available to substantiate these presumptions.[1,2,31]

Nonhealing wounds or abscesses, recurrent bacterial or fungal infections and paronychia have occurred in cats infected with FeLV. The virus has also been associated with eosinophilic ulcers, seborrhea sicca and idiopathic pruritus, as well as cutaneous lymphosarcoma, fibrosarcoma and liposarcoma.

Treatment of some of these conditions may be aided by use of corticosteroids, such as prednisolone at 0.5 mg/kg divided BID initially, with a gradually decreasing dosage until the cat is receiving 0.25-0.5 mg/kg every other day. The mechanism of action as to why corticosteroids are beneficial in viral immunosuppressive skin diseases is not understood. They may have an immunomodulatory effect that could decrease the effect of a serum immunosuppressive factor. Potentially immunosuppressive drugs, such as corticosteroids, should be used cautiously in treating cats with an infectious disease.

Other Viral Infections

Herpesvirus, calicivirus and cowpox virus have all been implicated in ulcerative dermatoses in a small number of cats. The clinical importance of these conditions has yet to be determined.

IMMUNE-MEDIATED SKIN DISEASES by S.D. White and P.J. Ihrke

The immune system normally functions to protect the body from infectious disease. Immunologic responsiveness ultimately depends upon the activity of small lymphocytes derived from stem-cell precursors. In postnatal life these lymphocytes differentiate in the bone marrow into 2 main populations, one thymus-dependent (T-cells) and the other thymus-independent (B-cells). The T-cells require either temporary residence in the thymus or exposure to a humoral factor produced by the thymus to become fully functional. The immune system functions via cell-mediated mechanisms involving T-cells and humoral antibodies derived from B-cells.

Immunodeficiencies result from absence or depression of the humoral or cellular functions of the immune system. Immunodeficiency is discussed throughout this chapter as it relates to individual diseases.

Inappropriate or excessive reaction by the immune system to exogenous substances or autogenous substances (self) produces allergic or autoimmune diseases, respectively. There are 4 types of hypersensitivity reactions. A type-I reaction, also known as immediate hypersensitivity or anaphylaxis, is mediated by IgE antibody. The IgE reacts with mast cells and basophils when an allergen combines with it on the surface of these cells. Subsequent degranulation of the mast cells and basophils releases various vasoactive amines. Feline atopy and some parasite hypersensitivities, food allergies and drug reactions are examples of type-I reactions.

Type II or cytotoxic reactions are mediated by IgG and IgM, and lead to direct destruction of cutaneous proteins, such as intracellular cement. Bullous immune-mediated diseases and cold agglutinin disease are examples of type-II reactions. A type-III reaction or immune-complex hypersensitivity is mediated by antibody-antigen complex activation of complement, with subsequent cell lysis, neutrophil chemotaxis and release of lysosomal enzymes from neutrophils. Systemic lupus erythematosus is a type-III hypersensitivity.

A type-IV reaction or cell-mediated hypersensitivity is mediated by sensitized T-lymphocytes that, when stimulated by certain antigens, release lymphokines and other effectors of tissue and vascular necrosis.[32] Allergic contact dermatitis and some parasite hypersensitivities are examples of type-IV reactions.

Investigation of immunologic disorders in cats is still in its early stages. As more species-specific diagnostic tests are developed, more immune-mediated skin diseases will be documented.

Allergic Diseases by S.D. White and P.J. Ihrke

Flea-Allergy Dermatitis

Cause: Flea-allergy dermatitis is the most common allergic skin disorder in cats. Flea saliva contains antigens thought to cause type-I or type-IV hypersensitivity reactions with dermatologic manifestations.

Clinical Signs: Pruritus, often with a miliary papular eruption, usually is present. Secondary alopecia and pyotraumatic dermatitis also may be present. Clinical signs may be limited to the head and neck, dorsal lumbosacral area or ventral abdomen (Fig 15). Involvement of the entire body occasionally is seen. When head and neck lesions predominate, food allergy and *Notoedres* infestation are important differential diagnoses. *Cheyletiella* infestation and other causes of the miliary eczema complex should be considered as

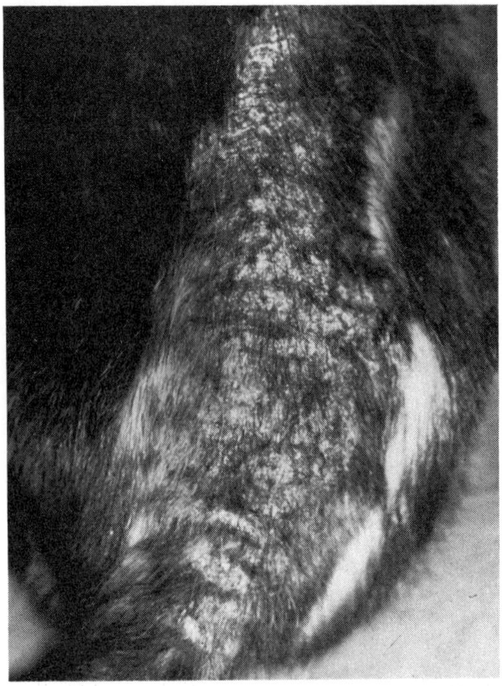

Fig 15. Severe flea-allergy dermatitis. The dorsal lumbosacral area has been shaved.

differential diagnoses in cats with primarily dorsal involvement. Generalized cases of flea-allergy dermatitis must be differentiated from most other causes of pruritus.

Diagnosis: Diagnosis is based upon history, physical examination and response to therapy. Failure to demonstrate fleas or flea dirt (excreta) on the cat does not preclude the diagnosis of flea-allergy dermatitis. Fleas spend most of their time off the cat in the environment, jumping on the animal only to feed. The cat's fastidious grooming habits may make finding flea dirt less likely than in dogs. Intradermal skin testing with commercial flea allergens, while quite impressive if positive, often gives false-negative results, possibly due to the lack of specificity of the allergens in the preparations.

Treatment: Therapy of flea allergy should include corticosteroids to control pruritus, and flea control. Severity of the allergy or lack of client compliance with flea control occasionally necessitates long-term corticosteroid use. The authors prefer prednisone or prednisolone at an initial dosage of 2 mg/kg daily, with the dosage tapered to the lowest alternate-day dosage sufficient to control clinical signs. A dose of 20 mg methylprednisolone acetate (Depo-Medrol:Upjohn) may be used if an initial repository injection is desired while the owners are beginning flea control. Hyposensitization for flea-allergy dermatitis in cats is still very much in the investigative state; too little information is available for the authors to make any recommendations.

Food-Allergy Dermatitis

Cause: Food-allergy dermatitis is uncommon in cats. Theories of immunologic mechanisms are controversial, but probably a type-I or type-III (and possibly a type-IV) hypersensitivity reaction is involved. The offending allergen is often one to which the cat has been exposed for a long period.

Clinical Signs: Pruritus is the most consistent clinical sign. Papules, urticaria, edema and secondary ulcerations may also be present. A predilection for the head and neck is often seen, although the signs may become generalized (Fig C3). Associated GI signs are uncommon and respiratory signs are rare. The history often reveals a gradual onset of signs limited to one cat in the household. Differential diagnoses of head and neck lesions should include flea-allergy dermatitis and *Notoedres* infestation.

Diagnosis: Diagnosis can only be made by feeding the cat an elimination diet. Most commercial cat foods contain many of the same preservatives, additives and protein constituents. Therefore, switching from one commercial cat food to another is unlikely to halt clinical signs. With the advent of "fast food" chicken franchises, many chicken by-products are used in commercial pet foods, especially as bone meal. This makes chicken a less satisfactory component of an elimination diet than in the past. An elimination diet ideally should consist of foods to which the cat has not been exposed previously. The authors prefer lamb (stewing lamb or mutton), with white, long-grain rice (not "Minute" quick-cooking rice) or boiled potatoes. In cases of adverse reactions (vomiting, diarrhea) to the lamb, chicken may be used. The cat should be fed this diet for 3 weeks. Absolutely no other foods should be given to the cat during that time. Since client education and compliance is vital for the success of an elimination diet as a diagnostic tool, we often recommend a family conference to encourage all people in the household to cooperate. While cats may manifest improvement within 3 days, sometimes the entire 21 days are necessary before a response is seen.

Ingestion of the offending allergen causes recurrence of clinical signs within 3 days.

Control: Occasionally a cat manifests such severe clinical signs that symptomatic therapy is necessary while an elimination diet is initiated. Prednisone or prednisolone, at 2 mg/kg SID for 1-2 weeks, or 20 mg methylprednisolone acetate (Depo-Medrol:Upjohn), given once IM, is the authors' choice. Corticosteroids make the initial evaluation of an elimination diet difficult but are sometimes necessary to ensure comfort of the patient and the cooperation of the client.

Once an elimination diet is found that does not cause pruritus, the next step is to add various foods to the diet at weekly intervals. Foods that do not lead to recurrence of clinical signs may be used as permanent dietary components. Unfortunately, many pet owners are unable or unwilling to go through this laborious process. As an alternative, switching to a predominantly chicken commercial cat food occasionally is successful. A commercial lamb-based dog food (d/d: Hill's) may be used for cats, with the addition of 2 boiled eggs per can. Usually the original elimination diet is used with vitamin, mineral and fatty acid supplements. Taurine, an amino acid essential for retinal function in cats, should be supplied by the daily addition of ½ tsp of the juice from canned clams.

For the cat owner unwilling or unable to experiment with various diets, corticosteroids, such as prednisone or prednisolone, may be used palliatively. Unfortunately, food-allergy dermatitis may respond poorly to corticosteroids, and establishing a safe, low, alternate-day dosage may be difficult.

Drug Eruption

Cause: Any drug, whether ingested, injected, inhaled or applied topically, may elicit an adverse dermatologic reaction. Immunologic mechanisms have not been elucidated in cats. The current inclusion of all 4 types of hypersensitivity reactions in the pathogenesis of drug eruption in cats probably reflects uncertainty as well as multiple possible causes.

Clinical Signs: Clinical manifestations of such reactions are quite variable but may include erythema, pruritus, urticaria, edema, papules, alopecia and the miliary eczema complex.

Diagnosis: Diagnosis is based upon ruling out other possible causes, a history of drug administration, and response to withdrawal of the medication. The offending drug may be a substance not usually thought by the owners to be a drug, such as vitamins, aspirin, antihistamines and other pharmaceuticals.

Treatment: While withdrawal of a suspected drug often causes abatement of clinical signs within 2 weeks, signs may persist for months. Challenge testing is undesirable and dangerous. The hematopoietic, renal and other systems should be evaluated, and chemically similar drugs should be avoided. Corticosteroids in immunosuppressive dosages, such as prednisone at 2-4 mg/kg daily, are indicated for symptomatic relief. In cases of anaphylaxis, therapy for shock, with epinephrine, antihistamines and supportive care, should be given.

Contact Allergy

Cause: Contact allergies are rare in cats. No cases have ever been confirmed using patch testing, the most frequent diagnostic test used in human medicine. Contact allergies in people are type-IV (delayed) hypersensitivity reactions.

Clinical Signs: Clinical signs should be limited to the glabrous (unhaired) portions of the skin unless the allergen was in liquid or aerosolized form. Pruritus, erythema and papules have been reported.[33]

Diagnosis: Diagnosis is often difficult. A thorough history of the cat's environment, particularly those substances most likely to be contacted, is essential. Differential diagnosis must include contact irritant dermatitis. In general, contact allergens cause a dermatologic reaction only in selected individuals of a species, whereas a contact irritant affects most members of the species. Patch testing in cats is technically difficult, usually impractical and not at all standardized.

Treatment: Therapy is removal of the offending substance and use of corticosteroids for relief of clinical signs. In the authors' experience, only certain flea collar-induced skin eruptions have been likely candidates for true contact allergies.

Miscellaneous Allergic Dermatoses

Allergy to intestinal parasites has been reported as a possible cause of various skin problems in young cats. Roundworms, tapeworms and hookworms have been implicated. Clinical signs include seborrhea, pruritus and a miliary eczematous eruption. Diagnosis is on the basis of fecal examination, plus a response to elimination of the parasite.

Inhalant allergy (atopy) is probably underdiagnosed in cats since skin testing is not routinely done. Clinical signs may include pruritus, alopecia and a miliary eczematous eruption. Diagnosis is based on positive intradermal skin testing with inhaled allergens. Corticosteroids may be used palliatively and hyposensitization has been successful in a few cases. More investigative work is needed in this field.

Toxic epidermal necrolysis has been observed in 4 cats.[2] All cases were subsequent to drug or vaccine administration. Clinical signs included ulceration, blister formation, variable cutaneous pain, febrile episodes, anorexia and a positive Nikolsky sign (ability to manually rub off apparently normal epidermis). The pathogenesis is unknown. Of the reported cases in people, 50% are due to drug eruptions, 25% are due to underlying systemic disease and 25% are idiopathic. Diagnosis is based on history, physical examination and biopsy. The last reveals full-thickness coagulation necrosis of the epidermis. Therapy involves correction of the underlying cause, large doses of corticosteroids, and supportive care. All reported cases plus the one case seen by one of the authors were severe, rapidly fulminating and life-threatening.

An allergic mechanism has been postulated but not proven in certain cases of highly inflammatory feline ringworm. The kerion form of a dermatophyte infection may be an allergic response to fungal elements or by-products. Further studies are needed in both of these areas.

Autoimmune Diseases by E.J. Rosser, Jr, P.J. Ihrke and A.A. Stannard

Systemic Lupus Erythematosus

Systemic lupus erythematosus is an autoimmune disease that can affect numerous organ systems. In people, several manifestations include polyarthritis, glomerulonephritis, anemia, thrombocytopenia, cutaneous lesions, myopathies, neuropathies, convulsions, pleuritis, pericarditis, retinopathies and persistent fevers. Systemic lupus erythematosus also has been observed in dogs and most commonly causes any combination of 4 clinical syndromes: autoimmune hemolytic anemia, immune-mediated thrombocytopenia, nonerosive polyarthritis, and immune-complex glomerulonephritis. Skin lesions, pericarditis, myocarditis, neuropathies and myopathies also can be associated with systemic lupus erythematosus in dogs. The disease was recently observed in cats.[34-36] The clinical signs included cutaneous lesions, autoimmune hemolytic anemia and immune-complex glomerulonephritis.

Cause: The cause of systemic lupus erythematosus is unknown. Most evidence in people suggests that heritability, viral infections, photostimulation and immunologic disorders are contributing factors. The basic defect is the formation of autoantibodies against various substances in the body. In the cutaneous manifestations of the disease, the basement membrane zone (dermoepidermal junction) is the primary area affected by this altered state of immunity. Antibodies to basement membrane substance and/or circulating antigen-antibody complexes are deposited at the dermoepidermal junction.[37,38] The circulating antigen-antibody complexes are predominantly antinuclear antibodies to double-stranded DNA. A viral source of DNA nuclear material may be responsible for this altered antigenicity. In addition, ultraviolet light exposure can alter DNA so that specific antibodies are directed against it.[38]

In people with systemic lupus erythematosus, there is also impaired cell-mediated immunity. Specifically there is an inhibitory serum factor (an IgG antibody) and a deficiency in the number of suppressor T-cells.[38,39] These suppressor T-cells are responsible for modifying and reducing antibody production by B-lymphocyte-induced plasma cells. With a decreased number of suppressor T-cells, the result is a population of overactive B-cells and possible excessive autoantibody production. This is rare in cats.

Diagnosis and Clinical Signs: Numerous criteria have been described for diagnosis of systemic lupus erythematosus in people, but many of these criteria are not applicable to domestic animals.[40] A modified scheme suggested for diagnosis of the disease in dogs could serve as a guideline in cats.[41] To diagnose cutaneous lesions related to systemic lupus erythematosus in cats, the skin disease should resemble systemic lupus erythematosus clinically, histologically and immunologically as seen in people and dogs. In any species, the lesions usually affect the face (predominantly nasal and periorbital region) and ears, and are of gradual onset. The specific type of lesion produced is quite variable. Alopecia, erythema, depigmentation, scales, crusts, ulcers and rarely vesicles or bullae may be seen. The skin lesions tend to be symmetric and may or may not be pruritic. In addition, the feet and mucocutaneous junctions may be involved. Oral lesions are much less common.

To document a diagnosis of feline systemic lupus erythematosus, the most commonly affected systems should be screened for evidence of disease. These include: autoimmune hemolytic anemia, which is Coombs positive; immune-mediated thrombocytopenia, which is platelet factor III positive; nonerosive polyarthritis; and immune-complex glomerulonephritis, with proteinuria and positive direct immunofluorescence of the basement membrane of the renal glomeruli, using IgG and complement.

Many cutaneous histopathologic changes have been observed in affected people and dogs and some have been suggested for cats.[34,42-44] The most consistent lesion observed in all species is hydropic degeneration of the basal cell layer of the epidermis (liquefactive degeneration). There also may be evidence of thickening of the basement membrane zone, a mononuclear cell infiltrate around the cutaneous appendages (hair follicles, apocrine glands, sebaceous glands), and pigmentary incontinence (loss of melanin from the basal cell layer and phagocytosis by dermal macrophages). Intraepidermal or subepidermal bullae are observed less commonly.

When submitting a skin biopsy for diagnosis of systemic lupus erythematosus, select a recent and inflamed lesion for fixation in formalin. If a vesicle or bulla is present, submit this lesion as well, being careful not to rupture the bulla when removing it.

Specific tests should be done to support the immunologic aspects of this disease. A positive antinuclear antibody test should be demonstrated in all cases of systemic lupus erythematosus. However, this test can also be positive in other diseases as well as in certain drug interactions. More than one antinuclear antibody test may be required since some cats may initially be negative but turn positive as the disease progresses. Direct immunofluorescence tests should be performed on samples of affected skin as well as normal skin adjacent to the lesion. This should demonstrate deposition of IgG at the basement membrane zone (dermoepidermal junction), known as a positive lupus band test. The lesion selected should be more chronic in nature than the one selected for routine histopathologic examination. Preferably a lesion at least 3 weeks old from an area most exposed to sunlight can be submitted in Michel's transport media to an immunology laboratory equipped to do this testing.

Treatment: Immunosuppressive dosages of corticosteroids are currently the treatment of choice for feline systemic lupus erythematosus. Since cats require higher dosages of corticosteroids than dogs to produce immunosuppression, use of oral prednisolone at 2-6 mg/kg, divided BID, is recommended. Once improvement is noticed, the dosage should be gradually decreased approximately every 2 weeks. Eventually an attempt should be made to establish an alternate-day regimen of prednisolone using the lowest dosage possible to prevent recurrence of skin lesions. In cats that are nonresponsive or that become refractory to corticosteroids, use of cyclophosphamide (Cytoxan:Mead Johnson) plus prednisolone could be considered.

Feline Pemphigus Complex

The pemphigus complex is a group of skin diseases associated with autoantibody production directed against the intercellular cement of the epidermis. This results in a chronic blistering disease that may involve the mucocutaneous junctions, mucosal surfaces and skin. In both people and dogs, 4 variants have been described: pemphigus vulgaris, pemphigus vegetans, pemphigus foliaceus and pemphigus erythematosus. The only variant not yet recognized in cats is pemphigus vegetans.

Cause: The cause of pemphigus diseases is unknown. In the development of these skin diseases, circulating autoantibodies are directed against the intercellular cement of keratinocytes in the epidermis. The circulating autoantibodies then become bound within the epidermis, resulting in loss of cohesion between epidermal cells due to destruction of the intercellular cement. Subsequently, intraepidermal bullae form and rupture, leaving erosions in the epidermis or mucosal surface.

There may be genetically predisposed people who develop antibodies against their own intercellular cement.[38] Various triggering factors are thought to be involved, such as certain drugs or exposure to ultraviolet light. This causes release of an antigenic material into the intercellular space, with resultant autoantibody formation against that substance.

Pemphigus Vulgaris: Pemphigus vulgaris in people and dogs has been well described and is characterized by bullae formation on the oral mucosa and mucocutaneous junctions.[45-47] The

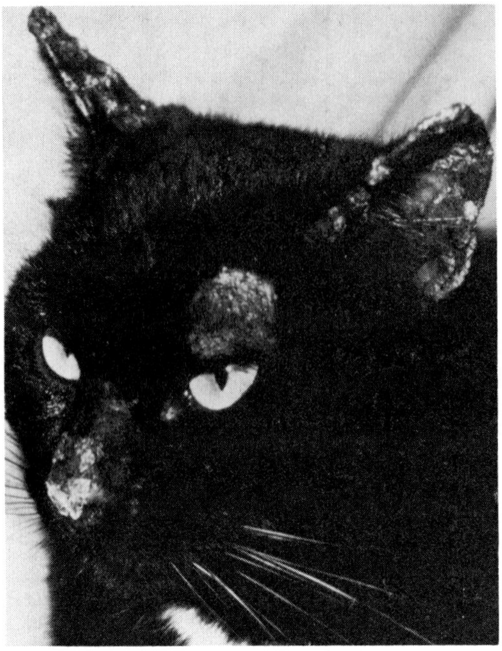

Fig 16. Somewhat symmetric scaling and crusting on the ears and face in pemphigus foliaceus.

skin is less commonly involved. Inflammation of the nail bed may lead to shedding of the nails. Due to the thin epidermis and mucosa in dogs, these bullae are very transient and rapidly form deep erosions and ulcers. The ulcers develop overlying crusts and secondary infection of the lesions is common. Pemphigus vulgaris may be associated with a febrile response and may cause systemic illness.

In the single case of pemphigus vulgaris observed in a cat, there were chronic ulcerations of the oral mucosa and mucocutaneous junctions of the lips and nares.[2]

The characteristic histologic feature of pemphigus vulgaris is acantholysis (loss of cohesiveness between epidermal cells). This results in formation of an intraepidermal bulla in the suprabasal region (prickle cell layer/basal cell layer interface). Therefore, the floor of the bulla should have intact basal cells, forming a "tombstone" appearance.[46] Within the bulla there are individual acantholytic cells (free-floating, rounded keratinocytes) or "rafts" of keratinocytes as a result of acantholysis. Acantholysis may also be seen within the epithelium of the external root sheath of the hair follicles. The underlying dermis usually contains an inflammatory cell infiltrate of plasma cells and lymphocytes. Best results are obtained histologically by selecting a recent lesion for biopsy and, if possible, an intact bulla.

Direct immunofluorescence performed on affected skin or mucous membranes should reveal deposition of IgG and complement within the intercellular spaces. This pattern usually is throughout all layers of the epidermis or mucosa but may involve the deeper epidermal or mucosal cells only. Due to species specificity, only antifeline antibodies may be used.

Serum autoantibodies against intercellular cement may be demonstrable by indirect immunofluorescence. This finding has not been as constant in dogs as in people and was not performed on the single affected cat.

Pemphigus Foliaceus: Pemphigus foliaceus, as described in dogs, is a crusting, scaling skin disease that often begins on the face (nasal planum and periorbital and ears) and often becomes generalized.[47-49] Mucocutaneous junctions can be involved but oral mucosal lesions are very rare. Vesicles and pustules may be observed as the disease develops but these rapidly rupture, resulting in superficial erosions with overlying crusts. Alopecia subsequently develops and epidermal collarettes often are formed. Affected animals commonly are presented for a chronic skin problem without any evidence of systemic illness.

Two cases of pemphigus foliaceus have been observed in cats. Lesions included crusts, scales, superficial erosions, erythema and epidermal collarettes involving the trunk, abdomen and paws (Fig 16).

Upon histopathologic examination, acantholysis occurs more superficially within the epidermis, in contrast to that seen in pemphigus vulgaris, and results in subcorneal pustules. Numerous acantholytic cells and a large number of neutrophils may be found within the pustule.[48,49] This process frequently involves hair follicles.

The pattern of direct immunofluorescence in affected skin usually is identical to the pattern seen in pemphigus vulgaris. However, in people and dogs the intercellular deposition of IgG occasionally is more specifically deposited only in the upper half of the epidermis. Indirect immunofluorescence can be performed but may be negative as frequently occurs in canine pemphigus foliaceus.

Pemphigus Erythematosus: Pemphigus erythematosus, as described in people and dogs, is considered an abortive localized variant of pemphigus foliaceus.[45] The types of lesions observed are identical to those seen in pemphigus foliaceus, but only the face and ears are involved.

A cat with documented pemphigus erythematosus had erythema, alopecia, erosions, epidermal collarettes, vesicopustules, crusting and scaling localized to the face and ears (Fig C4). In addition to the skin lesions, the cat was febrile and depressed, neither of which is a characteristic finding of this disease in dogs and people.

The histopathologic changes in pemphigus erythematosus are identical to those in pemphigus foliaceus. Results of direct immunofluorescence performed on skin lesions are the same as for pemphigus foliaceus but also may reveal deposition of IgG along the basement membrane zone. Indirect immunofluorescence, as performed in the few canine and feline cases reported, has produced negative results for detection of circulating autoantibodies.

As an aid in diagnosing this variant of pemphigus, an antinuclear antibody test should be submitted since it is often positive at a low titer. This finding, along with deposition of IgG at the basement zone, suggests the possibility of a relationship between this disease and lupus erythematosus.

Treatment: The feline pemphigus complex is treated with immunosuppressive dosages of corticosteroids as discussed under systemic lupus erythematosus. More recently, chrysotherapy (use of gold salts) has been used to treat pemphigus diseases in dogs and cats.[49,50] Aurothioglucose (Solganal:Schering) is administered IM at weekly intervals, beginning with test doses of 1-2 mg. The cat is re-examined weekly and samples for urinalysis and a CBC submitted to monitor for any evidence of glomerulonephritis or blood dyscrasias (reported in people treated with gold salts). The cat also should be inspected for stomatitis or any new pruritic, erythematous areas of exfoliative dermatitis since these reactions have also occurred in people when initiating chrysotherapy. The cats and dogs treated thus far with gold salts have not shown these side effects and have tolerated the drug well. After the first 2 weekly test doses of aurothioglucose are given, a dosage of 1 mg/kg is administered IM once weekly until the skin lesion resolves. At this time the frequency of injection is decreased to bimonthly, then monthly intervals while the skin lesions are in remission.

HORMONAL AND METABOLIC SKIN DISEASES

by C.A. Sousa and P.J. Ihrke

Feline Endocrine Alopecia

Cause: The term feline endocrine alopecia has been used to denote an uncommon skin disease thought to be caused by hormonal aberration. The etiology of this disease is unknown but an absolute deficiency or imbalance of sex hormones in neutered cats has been postulated, based upon an apparent response to various mixtures of sex hormones given parenterally. No clinicopathologic data are available to support this contention. Other authors have implicated hypothyroidism as the underlying cause of this condition. The diagnosis of feline endocrine alopecia as a specific disease entity is suspect; all conjectured cases seen in the past 5 years by the authors have either been cases of psychogenic alopecia or symmetric alopecia associated with an underlying pruritic disease.

Feline endocrine alopecia has been reportedly seen most commonly in male cats neutered at an early age. It has also been reported less commonly in spayed females.

Clinical Signs: The most common clinical signs include bilaterally symmetric alopecia of the genital area that may extend to the ventral abdomen, medial thighs, flank and lateral thorax (Fig 17). The dorsum is usually unaffected. The hair in affected areas is epilated easily. Microscopic examination of easily epilated hairs reveals them to be in the telogen phase. Pruritus,

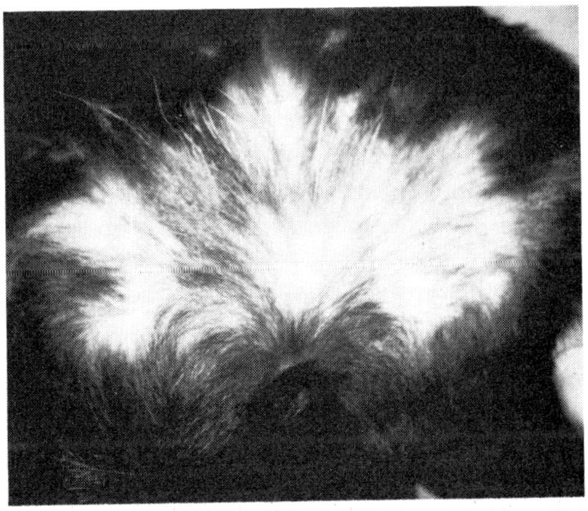

Fig 17. Possible feline endocrine alopecia. Note the symmetry of the alopecia and the lack of underlying skin changes.

as evidenced by excessive licking, grooming or hair-pulling, is reportedly absent.

Diagnosis: Diagnosis is based upon history, physical examination, examination of the hair from the affected areas and a response to therapy. Histopathologic examination suggested an endocrine alopecia. Care must be taken to rule out potential cases of psychogenic alopecia or alopecia secondary to excessive grooming associated with an underlying pruritic disease before feline endocrine alopecia is considered.

Treatment: Various endocrinologic treatments have been deemed effective. A daily oral dose of 2.5 mg megestrol acetate (Ovaban:Schering, Megace:Mead Johnson) has been given until hair regrowth has occurred. Maintenance therapy of 2.5 mg given every 3-7 days has been suggested to maintain a normal coat.

Before a response to female sex hormone is used as the prime indicator of an underlying endocrine disease, it should be stressed that progestational compounds have potent anti-inflammatory and mood-changing effects in cats. An oral dose of 0.05-0.1 mg sodium levothyroxine (Synthroid:Flint) has been given twice daily, by some veterinary dermatologists despite normal thyroid function tests. Obviously, considering the divergence of opinions with respect to this disease, more research is needed to definitively document or disprove its existence.

Hyperadrenocorticism

Cushing's disease is very rare in cats. Only 3 naturally occurring cases have been reported.[2,51,52] Cats appear to be much more resistant to the side effects of corticosteroids than people or dogs. In addition, it is very difficult to create iatrogenic Cushing's disease in cats, even intentionally.[53]

Clinical Signs: Clinical signs include polydipsia, polyuria, polyphagia, lethargy, a pendulous abdomen and bilaterally symmetric alopecia. The skin is thin and easily torn, and may be hyperpigmented or scaly.

Diagnosis: The diagnosis is based on the history, physical examination and laboratory data. As in dogs, laboratory data in cats may reveal lymphopenia, elevated SGPT activity, hyperglycemia and glucosuria. Baseline cortisol levels are not of diagnostic significance. Consequently, use of an ACTH-response test is recommended. Histopathologic examination of the skin in the reported cases was compatible with endocrine dermatosis.

Treatment: The most logical treatment of hyperadrenocorticism in cats would be surgical removal of the adrenal glands. Mitotane (Lysodren:Burns) should not be used because of the recognized toxicity of chlorinated hydrocarbons in this species.

Hypothyroidism

A well-documented case of feline hypothyroidism has not been reported.

Clinical Signs: Cats suspected of having hypothyroidism are obese and lethargic, and have a poor haircoat and bilaterally symmetric alopecia over the lateral thorax and abdomen.

Diagnosis: A diagnosis of hypothyroidism should be based on history, physical examination, a TSH-reponse test, preferably measuring both serum T_4 and T_3 levels by radioimmunoassay, and a thyroid biopsy. Histopathologic examination of the skin should reveal changes consistent with those of an endocrinopathy.

Treatment: If a definitive diagnosis of feline hypothyroidism is made, therapy should parallel that for canine hypothyroidism.

PHYSICOCHEMICAL SKIN DISEASES by S.I. Reinke and P.J. Ihrke

Irritant Contact Dermatitis

Cause: Irritant contact dermatitis, an uncommon condition in cats, is an inflammatory reaction of the skin after direct contact with an irritating agent. The agent damages the skin by direct toxic action rather than any immunologic mechanism. Allergic contact dermatitis has not been documented in cats. Until further evidence is presented, it is presumed that most if not all cases of contact dermatitis in cats are irritant rather than allergic in nature.

Factors affecting the severity of damage include moisture, which decreases the normal skin barrier and increases the contact surface, concentration of the agent, the period of contact, and previously irritated or traumatized skin.

Common precipitating agents include topical medications (coal tar shampoos or creams, selenium shampoos, neomycin, sulfur compounds, otic miticides, benzoyl peroxide), flea collars, road tar, asphalt, kerosene and other petroleum distillates, turpentine, paint, acids, alkalies, household chemicals (detergents, soaps, floor cleaners, polishes, waxes), fertilizers and insecticides (Figs 18, 19).[2] Many of these agents are less of a problem in cats than in dogs, perhaps due to the more fastidious nature of cats.

Clinical Signs: Lesions usually are localized to the hairless or sparsely haired areas that commonly contact surfaces, such as the footpads, interdigital areas, axillae and ventral abdomen. More densely haired areas are spared unless the offending agent is a liquid or aerosol.

In the acute stage, signs vary from mild erythema, alopecia, pruritus and occasional papules and vesicles, to serous exudation, ulceration and sloughing. Chronically affected cats have alopecia, lichenification, hyperpigmentation and mottled erythema with or without pruritus.

Diagnosis: Diagnosis is based on history, clinical signs, and isolation and provocative testing. The cat can be hospitalized for 7 days in a highly controlled environment and, if improvement is noted, gradually reintroduced into different areas of its normal environment. Patch testing, the method of choice in people, is impractical in cats.

Treatment: Therapy ideally should consist of avoidance of the offending agent if it can be identified. Otherwise, topical and systemic corticosteroids may be palliative. Flea-collar dermatitis rarely may require many months of therapy with corticosteroids. If the offending agent is still present on the cat, warm-water soaks and a gentle shampoo may be used to remove the offending substance. This is necessary not only to prevent continued damage to the skin but also to protect the cat from possible systemic intoxication by ingestion. Petroleum distillates and insecticides are major offenders.

Road tar, asphalt and dried paint can be removed by trimming the hair with scissors. If this is impossible, dioctyl sulfosuccinate or vegetable oil may help soften the tar or asphalt so it can be removed by wiping or shampooing.

Solar Dermatitis

Cause: Feline solar dermatitis is a chronic cutaneous response to repeated exposure to the sun. It is seen primarily in white cats in sunny areas of the country.

Clinical Signs: The most common site of involvement is the ear margins and tips. Occasionally the nose and eyelids may also be involved. Frequently a seasonality is noted as the lesions worsen in the summer and become more quiescent in the winter. Erythema and scaling are the most common early signs. As exposure continues, the lesions may progress to a pruritic, alopecic, crusting, ulcerative condition and may subsequently progress to squamous-cell carcinoma. Neoplastic transformation is more common in cats over 7 years of age but may occur as early as 3 years of age.[2]

Treatment: Treatment consists of keeping the cat out of the sun, especially between 10 am and 4 pm in the summer. If the cat must be outside, topical sunscreens, such as Sundown (Johnson & Johnson) or Presun (Westwood) may be applied. Topical and systemic corticosteroids often are palliative. If ulceration occurs, bilateral amputation of the pinnae should be considered. After hair regrowth, the cosmetic result is surprisingly acceptable.

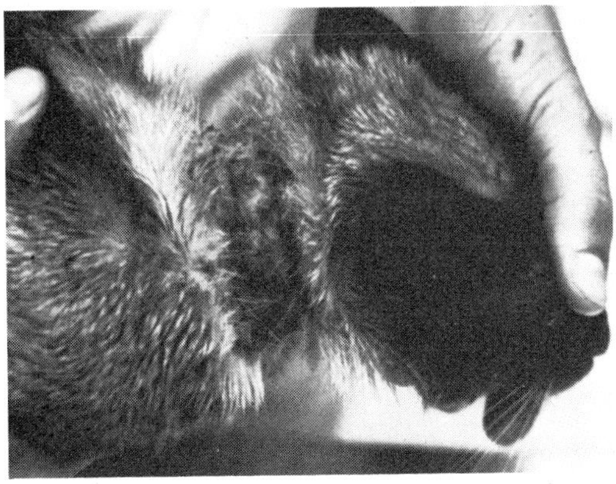

Fig 18. Flea-collar dermatitis. Note the severe ulceration and crusting associated with the band of alopecia around the neck. (Courtesy of Dr C. Griffin)

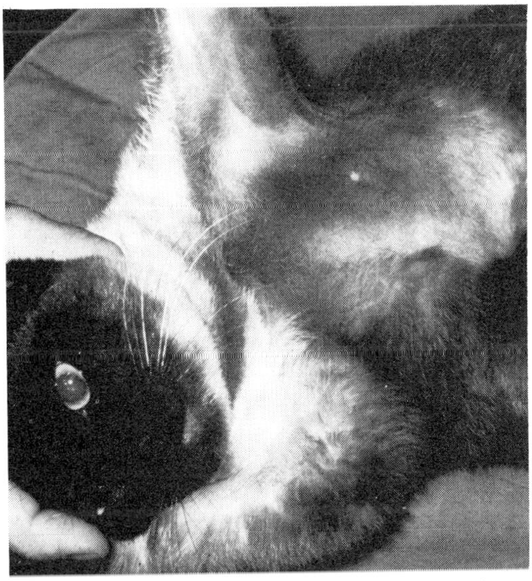

Fig 19. Severe reaction to contact with a petroleum distillate. Hyperpigmentation and alopecia persisted several months after the incident.

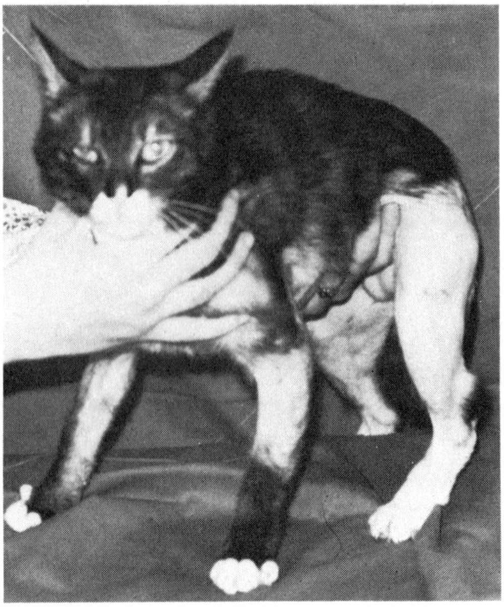

Fig 20. Psychogenic alopecia. Note the symmetric alopecia and the lack of underlying skin changes.

Temperature-Dependent Hair Color Changes

Siamese and Himalayan cats have a temperature-dependent enzyme system that converts melanin precursors into melanin by oxidation.[54] External factors, such as climate, may cause Siamese cats living in colder areas to have darker points and coat, whereas Siamese cats living in warmer areas may have lighter points and coat color.

Physiologic factors also may influence coat color. Hair regrowth may be lighter in areas after abscessation or inflammation and darker in areas that have been clipped. Fortunately, the hair frequently returns to its normal color during the next hair growth cycle.[2]

PSYCHOGENIC DERMATOSIS by C.A. Sousa and P.J. Ihrke

Cause: Psychogenic alopecia and dermatitis, or idiopathic neurodermatitis, is caused by excessive licking or grooming.

Any breed of cat may be affected but the disease is most common in high-strung or nervous cats, especially Siamese, Burmese and Abyssinians. House cats are affected more often than outdoor cats.

In some cases a "psychologic insult" initiates the licking. Such insults may be difficult to identify or may be obvious, such as moving to a new home, addition of a new pet or a baby to the household, or discord in the household.

Clinical Signs: The dermatitic form of the disease usually is characterized by a well-demarcated, erythematous, alopecic, ulcerated plaque generally located on the abdomen or flank. Occasionally a lesion may be present on an extremity. Localized psychogenic dermatitis is much less common than psychogenic alopecia and must be differentiated from an eosinophilic ulcer or plaque.

Occasionally such diseases as generalized dermatophytosis or flea-allergy dermatitis may mimic psychogenic alopecia. Other underlying causes of pruritus also should be explored in any case of apparent psychogenic alopecia since chronic pruritus of any origin may contribute to the psychologic insult.

Diagnosis: A history of excessive grooming is a valuable aid in establishing the diagnosis. Unfortunately, most owners are either unaware of the excessive grooming or the licking and chewing is performed out of sight. Usually affected cats are presented with a somewhat bilaterally symmetric alopecia. The hair loss may extend down the middle of the back or involve the perineal, genital, caudomedial thigh or abdominal area (Fig 20). Inflammation usually is not present. A uniform stubble may give the impression the affected area has been shaved. Upon microscopic examination, the ends of the hairs are ragged and appear to have been bitten off. Telogen hairs usually are not in excess.

Psychogenic alopecia must be differentiated from feline endocrine alopecia. A history of excessive grooming, the lack of the ability to easily epilate hair and the presence of a short stubble of hair in the affected areas are the most valuable aids in differentiating this condition from feline endocrine alopecia. Cases of psychogenic alopecia are frequently misdiagnosed as presumptive feline endocrine alopecia that has not responded to therapy.

Treatment: The determination and correction, if possible, of the psychologic insult is the most important aspect of therapy. When this is not possible, long-term maintenance with antianxiety drugs may be palliative. If the psychologic insult can be determined and corrected, antianxiety drugs, such as phenobarbital ¼ gr BID or TID orally), diazepam (Valium:Roche at 1.25-2.5 mg orally BID) or megestrol acetate (Ovaban:Schering, Megace:Mead-Johnson at 2.5 mg daily orally) should be given for 4-6 weeks to break the habit of licking. The duration of therapy required varies from cat to cat. Combination therapy with phenobarbital and megestrol acetate occasionally may be beneficial when neither drug alone has been beneficial.

DISEASES OF KERATINIZATION by P.J. Ihrke

Diseases involving a defect in the keratinization process generally are much less common in cats than in dogs. With the exception of "stud tail," most keratinization problems in cats tend to be generalized.

Seborrhea

Seborrheic skin diseases of any type are uncommon in cats. Most evidence indicates that an alteration in the keratinization process is probably more important than disturbances in sebaceous function despite the implications of the term "seborrhea."

Clinical Signs: Seborrhea sicca, the dry form of the disease complex, is the most common form in cats. Clinical signs usually include generalized, excessive scaling or dandruff and a dry coat, with dry underlying skin. Pruritus and inflammation often are absent. The most common underlying causes of seborrhea sicca include ectoparasitism (especially cheyletiellosis and pediculosis), endoparasitism (especially in young cats), dermatophytosis, malnutrition and fat deficiency (implied by response to fat supplementation). Many systemic illnesses, such as diabetes mellitus, may also cause dry seborrhea, often noted as an incidental finding upon physical examination for more severe systemic clinical signs. Diminished grooming associated with chronic debilitating disease may be causative. Less severe seasonal dandruff may occur during the winter in colder climates and is thought to be associated with low humidity in the household. In contrast to the prevalence in dogs, idiopathic seborrhea is quite rare in cats.

Diagnosis: The minimum data base for diagnosis of seborrhea sicca should include fecal flotation, skin scrapings, a dermatophyte culture and tests indicated by other clinical signs.

Treatment: Therapy usually is limited to correction of the underlying disease. If no underlying disease is found, fat supplementation with both animal fat (pork fat) and vegetable fat (corn oil) as trial therapy is recommended. Use of most antiseborrheic shampoos should be avoided since coal tars may cause toxicity. Chlorhexidine (Nolvasan Pet Shampoo:Fort Dodge) or other shampoos (Allergroom:Allerderm, HyLyt EFA:D.V.M., Veterinary Shampoo:Neutrogena) may be used as a palliative measure.

Seborrhea oleosa and seborrheic dermatitis are quite rare in cats. Greasiness, crusting, alopecia, erythema and pruritus are seen in both of these forms of the seborrheic disease complex. Erythema and pruritus often are more profound and more localized with seborrheic dermatitis. Infection with FeLV is by far the most common underlying cause of both seborrhea oleosa and seborrheic dermatitis. Greasy seborrhea lesions have also been associated with pemphigus foliaceus, systemic lupus erythematosus and chronic liver disease.

A test for FeLV infection, a hemogram, a serum chemistry panel and an antinuclear antibody test should be performed in all such cases. Palliative therapy has not been beneficial.

Stud Tail

Stud tail is a seborrheic disorder manifested by greasy, waxy accumulations of debris on the skin and hair, and comedones on the dorsal surface of the tail in the area of the preen gland (Fig 21). Stud tail is otherwise asymptomatic

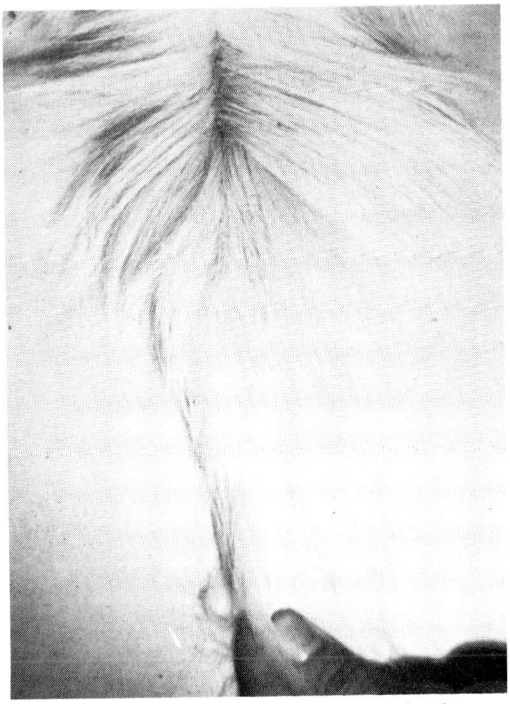

Fig 21. Symmetric seborrheic deposits on the dorsum of the tail in stud tail.

and most frequently presented as a "cosmetic problem." It is most common in sexually active males but may also occur in castrated males, intact females and spayed females. Purebred cats, such as Persians and Siamese, seem to be more commonly affected but the condition may also occur in domestic shorthaired cats. The higher incidence in purebred cats may reflect a statistical bias due to breeder concern for this condition in their show studs.

No therapy is required unless the owner wishes treatment for cosmetic reasons. Shampoos containing benzoyl peroxide (OxyDex: D.V.M.) or sulfur (Sultex:Derma) may be used cautiously to provide symptomatic relief. Progestational compounds (Ovaban:Schering, Megace:Mead Johnson), are quite effective but caution should be exercised in treating males intended for breeding (see Dermatologic Therapeutics). Castration usually is not effective.

THE EOSINOPHILIC GRANULOMA COMPLEX by E.J. Rosser, Jr., P.J. Ihrke and A.A. Stannard

It is useful to group a number of skin and oral cavity lesions in cats under the category of the eosinophilic granuloma complex.[1,2,55] The most commonly used terms include eosinophilic granuloma, eosinophilic ulcer, rodent ulcer, lip ulcer, labial granuloma, intradermal granuloma and feline lick granuloma. On a clinical and histologic basis, the conditions should be referred to as eosinophilic ulcer, eosinophilic plaque and linear granuloma.[55] The justification for grouping these conditions is their similarity as to methods of treatment and response to therapy. In addition, some cats have various combinations of these lesions simultaneously.

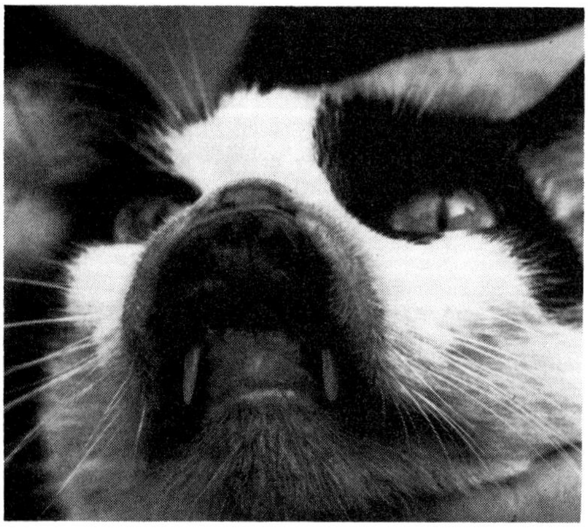

Fig 22. Severe eosinophilic ulcer involving much of the upper lip. This condition must be differentiated from squamous-cell carcinoma.

Eosinophilic Ulcer

An eosinophilic ulcer (eosinophilic granuloma, rodent ulcer, lip ulcer) is most commonly found on the upper lip margin as a unilateral lesion (Fig C5). It also can occur as bilaterally symmetric lesions on the lips or appear on the lower lip or nose, in the oral cavity or virtually anywhere on the skin (Fig 22). This form appears as a reddish-brown erosion or ulcer and has a slightly raised, well-demarcated border. The ulcer usually is not associated with any pain or pruritus. Hemograms usually do not reveal circulating eosinophilia.

Histologically there is ulceration, loss of the epidermis and generally a superficial layer of serum and necrotic debris. The dermis contains a mixed infiltrate of neutrophils, lymphocytes, plasma cells and fibroblasts. Despite its common name, this condition is characterized neither by tissue eosinophilia nor a granulomatous reaction. These ulcers have progressed to squamous-cell carcinomas or fibrosarcomas. Consequently, biopsy of these lesions is recommended, especially if there is no response to conventional therapy. Pseudoepitheliomatous hyperplasia occasionally is seen, which might suggest a squamous-cell carcinoma but actually is a sign of severe inflammatory response.[57]

Eosinophilic Plaque

An eosinophilic plaque (eosinophilic granuloma, lick granuloma) most commonly occurs in the inguinal and abdominal regions and on the medial aspect of the rear limbs (Figs 23, 24). It also occurs in various other locations on the skin and in the oral cavity. An eosinophilic plaque is a raised, well-circumscribed, plaque-like lesion that is moist and erythematous. Affected cats appear intensely pruritic and continuously lick the affected area. Hemograms generally reveal mild to marked circulating eosinophilia.

The most common histologic findings are widespread spongiosis of both the epidermis and the upper portion of the hair follicles and heavy infiltration of the dermis with eosinophils.[53] Acanthosis and intraepidermal microvesicles containing eosinophils also are seen.[2,56] This form is most consistently characterized by tissue

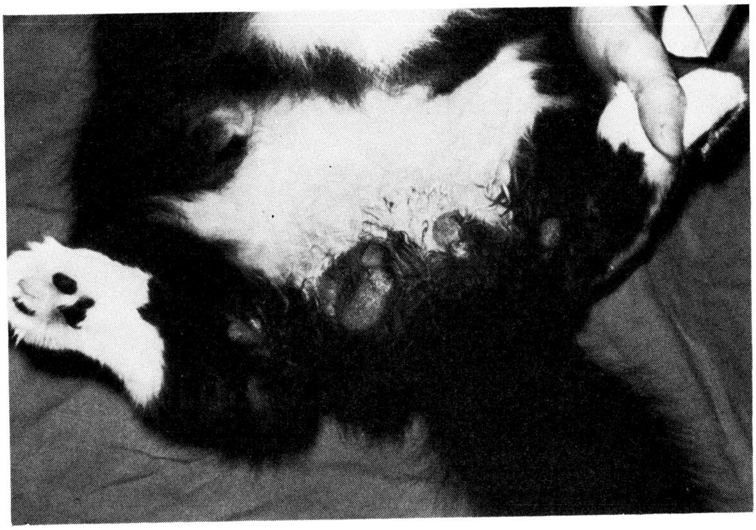

Fig 23. Early, well-demarcated eosinophilic plaques in the groin area.

eosinophilia but does not cause a granulomatous reaction.

Linear Granuloma

Two somewhat distinct forms of linear granuloma (eosinophilic granuloma, intradermal granuloma) exist: one with cutaneous lesions and the other with oral lesions. The cutaneous form most commonly occurs on the caudal or medial aspect of the rear limbs (Figs C6, C7). Linear granulomas have been observed less frequently on the medial aspect of the front limbs and lateral aspects of the thorax. This type of granuloma is linear in configuration and appears as sharply demarcated, raised, firm, yellowish-pink lesions. Usually it is asymptomatic and often discovered accidentally. Occasionally a cat licks excessively at these areas, resulting in irritation and additional alopecia. Hemograms usually do not indicate circulating eosinophilia. This condition is more common in young cats (less than 1 year of age) and many cases undergo spontaneous remission.[55]

The oral form most commonly occurs on the lower lip, tongue, gingivae and palate.[1] The characteristic lesions are raised, firm, yellowish-pink nodules that may ulcerate (Fig C8). In contrast to hemograms in cats with the cutaneous form of linear granuloma, hemograms in cats with the oral form often reveal circulating eosinophilia.

The oral and cutaneous forms are basically identical on histologic examination. The most significant finding is multiple areas of necrobiotic (degenerating) collagen. This change elicits a foreign-body reaction and the dermis becomes infiltrated with histiocytes and giant cells. Therefore, this form actually demonstrates a granulomatous reaction. The presence of tissue eosinophilia is quite variable but is more common with the oral form.

Cause: The cause of these diseases is unknown. Numerous attempts at isolating pathogenic bacteria, fungi, viruses and parasites have been unsuccessful. Other proposed mechanisms, such as chronic self-induced trauma, allergy and chronic pyoderma, have not been substantiated. Recently it was shown that lesions can be transmitted from one area to another on the same cat with autologous transplants.[2] Lesions also have been induced in experimental animals by intradermal injections of antigen-antibody com-

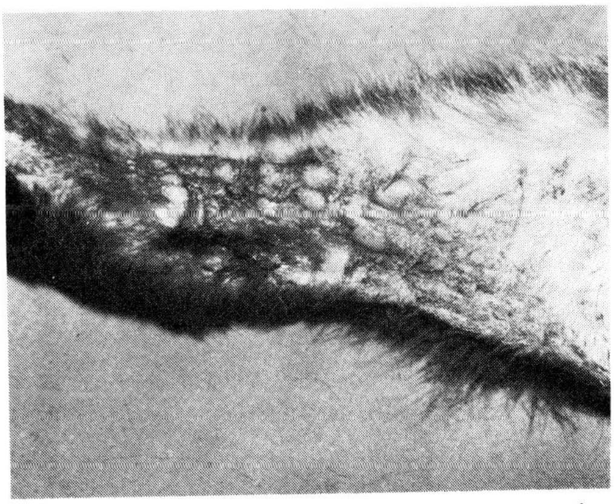

Fig 24. Diffuse, multifocal eosinophilic plaques on the medial thigh.

plexes.[56] These findings suggest a hypersensitivity reaction involving any of several immunologically mediated pathways. In one instance, 3 related cats developed linear granulomas, which suggests some possible hereditary factors.[55] Varying percentages of cats with each of the conditions in the complex have been positive for FeLV. The eosinophilic granuloma complex usually is the only clinical problem present, with no other apparent syndromes associated with FeLV. The significance of this finding is not understood.

Treatment: In general, all forms of the eosinophilic granuloma complex respond to the same mode of therapy. Corticosteroids are the drugs of choice upon initial presentation. The most effective and easiest method is to give 20 mg methylprednisolone acetate (Depo-Medrol: Upjohn) IM or SC.[2] This dose has been well tolerated by cats and is relatively free of side effects.[53] One of the authors has occasionally observed a granulomatous reaction to SC injection of Depo-Medrol. This results in a local irritation manifested by continuous licking at the injection site. Local alopecia, cutaneous atrophy and hair color change also have been observed when the drug is administered SC. The cat should be reexamined in 2 weeks. Even if complete remission is observed, a second injection of 20 mg methylprednisolone acetate should be given. This seems to have decreased the frequency with which these lesions recur.

In cases refractory to corticosteroids, use of progestational compounds is recommended. Corticosteroid tachyphylaxis occurs most commonly when the drugs have been used previously and the lesion has recurred. Megestrol acetate can be given PO at 2.5 mg daily or 5 mg every other day for 4-6 weeks. The rationale for the duration of therapy is an attempt to decrease the percentage of recurrence. If oral medication cannot be used, use of long-acting progesterone (*eg*, Depo-Provera:Upjohn), could be considered.[2] When using progestational compounds, the potential side effects must be considered and explained to the client. They include polyuria, polydipsia, polyphagia, weight gain, pyometra, diabetes mellitus, possible increased incidence of mammary neoplasia and hyperplasia, and infertility. In addition, focal hair color change, alopecia and cutaneous atrophy have resulted from use of injectable forms.

When recurrence is a problem and the lesion can be treated effectively with corticosteroids or progestational compounds, maintenance therapy may be considered. After remission, oral administration of prednisolone at 1-2 mg/kg on an alternate-day basis or 2.5-5 mg megestrol acetate every 3-7 days may be beneficial.

In cats that do not respond to these regimens, corticosteroids and progestational compounds may be used concurrently. For refractory or chronic eosinophilic ulcers of the lip, 0.5 ml of 6 mg/ml triamcinolone (Vetalog:Squibb) may be injected intralesionally once a week for 3-4 weeks. This procedure is painful and may require sedation or anesthesia.

Some success also has been achieved with use of imidazoles as immunostimulants.[56] Use of levamisole (Pitman-Moore, 100-mg tablets) has been recommended and can be given PO at 5 mg/kg on alternate days until 75-100% regression occurs (4-6 weeks) and weekly thereafter for at least 2 weeks.

Radiation therapy may be another alternative. Eosinophilic granulomas that did not respond to conventional medical therapy have shown improvement in 30-50% of the cases treated in one study.[58] Use of 300-500 rads once weekly over 4-8 weeks was most effective on solitary lesions. Multifocal lesions have been successfully treated using strontium-90 beta-ray therapy. Radiation therapy requires general anesthesia and generally is not available to practitioners.

A system of patient classification has been developed to provide the cat owner with a more accurate prognosis.[56] Stage-I patients have received no previous therapy. Stage-II patients have responded to previous theapy but have developed a recurrent lesion. Stage-III patients are refractory to conventional therapy (corticosteroids). Based on this system, stage-I patients that have received proper therapy should show complete remission of the lesion, with only a 10-25% rate of recurrence in 6 months. Stage-II and stage-III patients have a 50% rate of recurrence in 6 months regardless of the method of therapy. Therefore, it should be emphasized that proper therapy of adequate duration, while monitoring the progress of the patient, is most important. Inadequate initial therapy may lead to subsequent failure.

Specific prognostic comments also can be offered in regard to various lesions of the eosinophilic granuloma complex. The cutaneous form of linear granuloma can undergo spontaneous remission and rarely becomes a recurrent problem when treated. The long-term prognosis of the eosinophilic ulcer is good when treated early while the lesion is small. As the lesion becomes larger, more erosive and chronic, the chance for total remission is reduced. The oral form of linear granuloma has the most guarded prognosis of all the subgroups in this disease complex.

CONGENITAL AND HEREDITARY SKIN DISEASES by C.A. Sousa and P.J. Ihrke

Cutaneous Asthenia

Clinical Signs: Cutaneous asthenia (Ehler-Danlos syndrome) is a rare hereditary disease characterized by skin that is hyperextensible and easily torn (Fig 25).[59,60] Affected cats usually have a history of frequent lacerations, often from unknown or minor trauma. However, considerable variations in skin fragility occur in various cats with this condition. Simple procedures, such as clipping or venipuncture, may result in large wounds with minimal bleeding.

The skin of affected cats may feel soft and "spongy." Healing is often accompanied by hypopigmented scars. Several biochemical collagen defects have been documented.

Treatment: Avoidance of trauma and careful surgical closure of wounds is the only recommended therapy. These cats should not be bred.

Chediak-Higashi Syndrome

Chediak-Higashi Syndrome is an autosomal recessive genetic disease of Persian cats with yellow eyes and "blue smoke" hair. The syndrome is characterized by partial oculocutaneous albinism, photophobia, increased susceptibility to infection and a hemorrhagic tendency. The basis for the partial albinism is formation of large, irregular clumps of melanin in the hair shafts.[61,62]

No treatment is effective. Breeding of affected and suspected carriers should be discouraged.

Epitheliogenesis Imperfecta

Clinical Signs: Epitheliogenesis imperfecta occurs only rarely in kittens. Affected animals are presented with gross defects in epithelial integrity, mimicking extensive ulcerations of the skin or mucous membranes. The lesions tend to be secondarily infected, which may predispose to septicemia. Death is the frequent result.

The hereditary aspects of the disease have not been studied in cats but are well known in calves, piglets and foals.

Treatment: There is no effective therapy. Suspected carriers should not be bred.[63]

Alopecia Universalis

Clinical Signs: Alopecia universalis is a rare hereditary disorder for which cats have been selectively bred to produce a virtually hairless cat popularized as the "sphinx" or "Canadian hairless cat."[1] Some facial hair and whiskers may be present but most affected cats have no body hair. The cats feel oily and have an unpleasant seborrheic odor. Comedones and patchy, greasy lipid deposits may be present.

Treatment: Some symptomatic treatment for the greasiness, odor and comedones may be

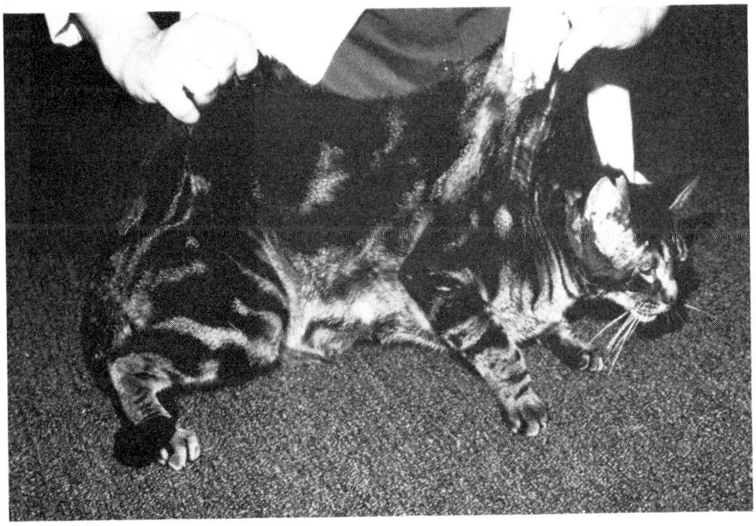

Fig 25. Hyperextensibility of the skin in cutaneous asthenia.

achieved with periodic antiseborrheic shampoos that do not contain coal tars.

Hypotrichosis

Clinical Signs: Hereditary hypotrichosis is a very rare autosomal recessive condition observed in Siamese cats. Affected kittens have soft, downy hair that is lost within 2 weeks after birth. Although transient, hair regrowth may occur. Almost total alopecia results at about 6 months of age.

Treatment: Affected cats and their relatives should not be bred. No treatment is effective.[2]

NUTRITIONAL SKIN DISEASES by C.A. Sousa and P.J. Ihrke

The average house cat is fed a balanced diet of commercial cat food. Consequently, true nutritional deficiencies are uncommon and most nutritional problems are the result of a dietary imbalance. Dermatologic signs of any dietary deficiency or imbalance are rare in cats.

Vitamin E Deficiency

Cause: Vitamin E is required in the diet for its antioxidant properties in association with highly unsaturated fatty acids. A deficiency usually is caused by diets primarily of red tuna or other types of fish, or high dietary levels of cod liver oil.[64,65]

Clinical Signs: Affected cats have a history of anorexia and lameness. Palpation of the skin on the back and abdomen may cause pain. Many affected cats are febrile.

Diagnosis: Diagnosis is based on the history and physical examination. The hemogram usually reveals leukocytosis, with neutrophilia and occasionally eosinopenia. Histopathologic examination of affected fat reveals fat necrosis, edema and a neutrophilic infiltrate within connective tissue between fat cells.

Treatment: Affected cats should be given 18.5-55.5 mg (25-75 IU) vitamin E (alpha tocopherol) PO twice daily.[2] In suspected cases, therapy should be initiated before laboratory confirmation of the deficiency. Prednisone, at 1 mg/kg BID, may be helpful initially in stimulating the appetite and decreasing inflammation. Obviously, correction of the offending diet is mandatory. In some cats a gradual dietary transition may be necessary.

Fatty Acid-Responsive Dermatosis

A condition characterized by a dull, dry, seborrheic haircoat has been seen occasionally in cats fed an apparently good commercial cat food. A fatty-acid deficiency has not been documented in these cats but the response to oral fat supplementation (1/4 tsp pork fat daily) has been dramatic within 8 weeks. Diagnosis is based upon physical examination and response to fat supplementation.

Vitamin A Deficiency

A few cases of vitamin A deficiency in cats have been reported. Affected cats had anorexia, weight loss, muscle wasting, patchy alopecia and scaly skin. Many also had ocular and reproductive abnormalities.

Treatment consisted of adjustment of the diet and IM injection of 12,500-25,000 IU vitamin A. Oral carotenes cannot be metabolized by cats.[2]

Biotin Deficiency

Development of a naturally occurring biotin deficiency is unlikely. This had been suggested as a cause of miliary eczema in cats. Experimental biotin deficiency causes a thin haircoat and dry, scaly skin. The lesions progress to ulcerations on the lips, neck, thorax and legs.

Injections of 0.25 mg biotin every other day caused remission of clinical signs in experimental animals.

SKIN TUMORS by S.D. White and P.J. Ihrke

Cutaneous neoplasms are an important part of feline dermatology. Early diagnosis is essential in the effective management of feline skin tumors. A biopsy or a fine-needle aspirate of a suspected neoplasm is a valuable early diagnostic procedure. Unfortunately, practitioners often fall into the familiar trap of "This feels (or looks) like a . . ." as an alternative to pursuing a definitive diagnosis. There is no substitute for cytologic or histopathologic evaluation.

A thorough physical examination, plus a minimal diagnostic workup, should not be forgotten when evaluating a patient with a skin tumor. Particular attention should be given to examination of the lymph nodes, lungs and the hematopoietic system for potential metastases. Once a diagnosis has been reached, alternatives of therapy can be discussed with the client.

Common tumors are discussed in this section. The reader is referred to a text on veterinary cancer medicine for more information.[66]

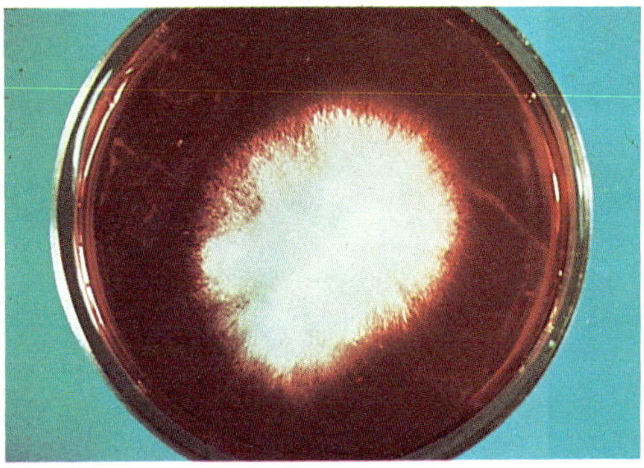

Fig C1. White *Microsporum canis* growing on Dermatophyte Test Medium. (Courtesy of Pitman-Moore)

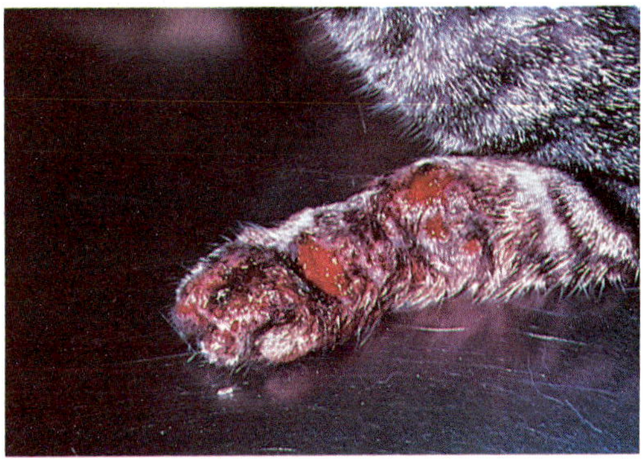

Fig C2. Severe ulceration and exudation in sporotrichosis. (Courtesy of Dr N. Gulbas)

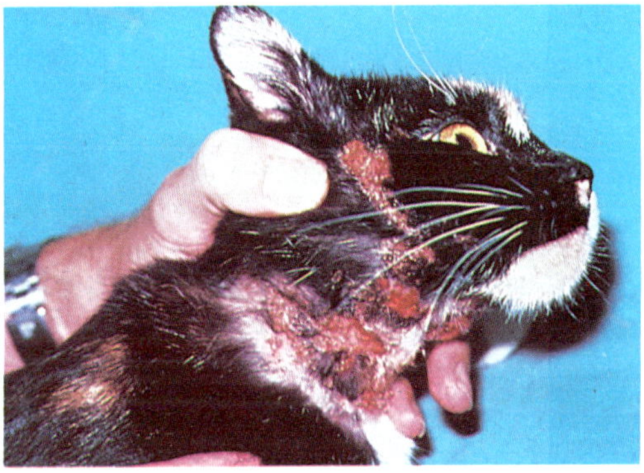

Fig C3. Extensive traumatic lesions from self-trauma in food allergy.

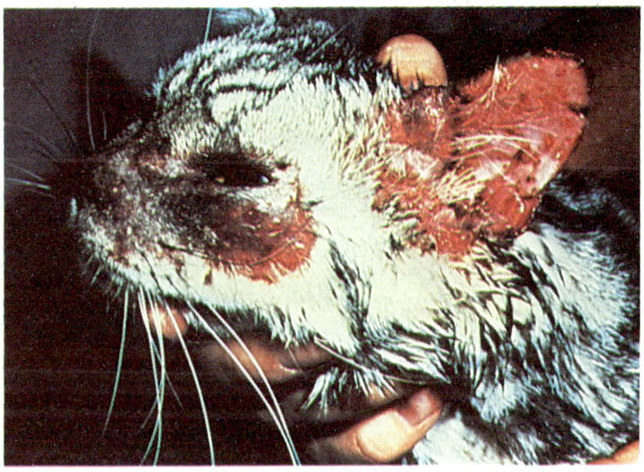

Fig C4. Severe scaling, crusting and ulceration in pemphigus erythematosus. (Courtesy of AAHA and Drs D.W. Scott and T. Manning)

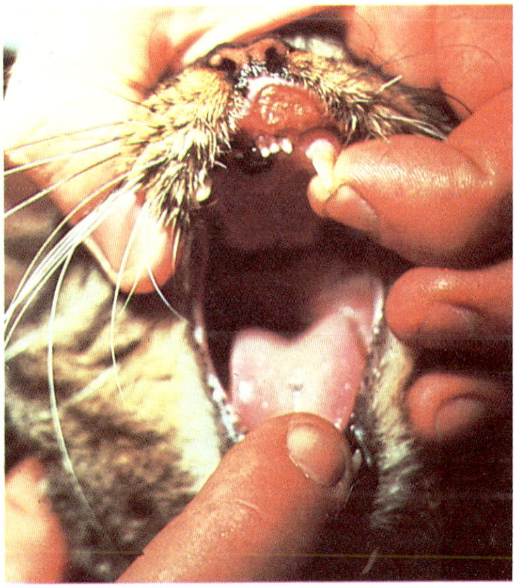

Fig C5. Unilateral eosinophilic ulcer. Note the slightly raised, well-demarcated border.

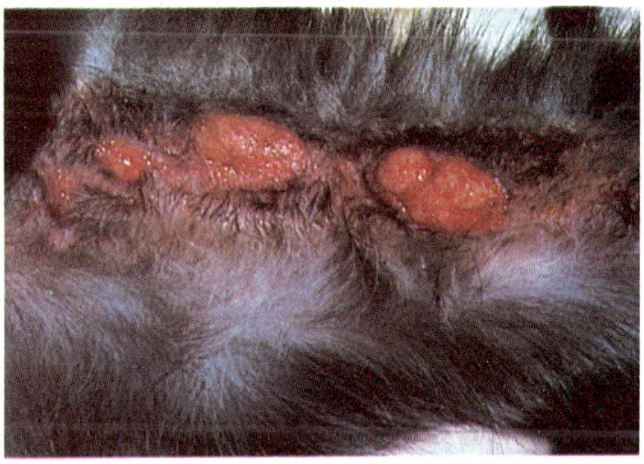

Fig C6. Linear arrangement of eosinophilic plaques on the medial aspect of the rear limb. This lesion may have developed from an earlier linear granuloma.

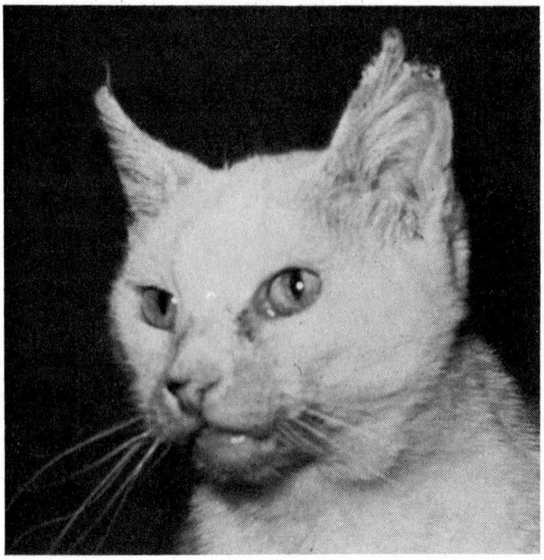

Fig 26. Eroded, irregular margins of the ear in squamous-cell carcinoma in a white cat.

Epithelial Tumors

Squamous-Cell Carcinoma

Squamous-cell carcinoma is one of the most common feline skin tumors. (Squamous-cell carcinoma, basal-cell tumor and fibrosarcoma together account for 67-85% of all feline skin tumors). Squamous-cell carcinoma has a strong predilection for the nose, pinnae, eyelids and lips (Figs 26, C9). White cats or those lacking pigment in the predisposed sites are at greater risk. Most affected cats are 5 years of age or older. Many investigators believe that exposure to sunlight is a predisposing factor and that feline solar dermatitis can progress to squamous-cell carcinoma.[1,2]

Clinical Signs: The affected area may first develop erythema, crusting and scaling, progressing to an ulcerative, firm, poorly circumscribed lesion. The tumor may be proliferative in appearance and the firm, fibrous base may be closely adherent to the underlying tissues. Although this tumor usually is solitary, multiple tumors (especially on both pinnae) have been seen. In their early stages, these tumors may mimic an inflammatory lesion, such as solar dermatitis. Later, the eosinophilic granuloma complex can be an important differential diagnosis. (Some authors have reported transformation of eosinophilic ulcers to squamous-cell carcinomas.[2]) Most squamous-cell carcinomas tend to be highly invasive locally but late to metastasize. When metastasis does occur, usually it is to the regional lymph nodes and lungs. Therefore, early biopsy of suspected lesions is essential. Histologic interpretation is of clinical importance since the more differentiated the tumor is, the less likely it is to metastasize and the more likely it is to respond to therapy.

Treatment: Treatment of squamous-cell carcinoma generally involves radical surgical excision and/or radiotherapy. The surgeon should attempt to excise at least a 1-cm margin of healthy tissue beyond the perimeter of the tumor. Surgical removal is often curative and is the therapy most often employed by practitioners. Good results have been obtained with cryosurgery and hyperthermia.[67,68] Use of radiotherapy is limited to medical institutions with appropriate facilities. Excellent results can be obtained with radiotherapy, either used alone or in conjunction with surgical excision, especially after recurrence. If regional lymph node involvement is suspected, thoracic radiographs are indicated to check for metastasis before therapy is initiated.

An important adjunct to all therapy is severely limiting the patient's exposure to sunlight. Use of sunscreens, such as Sundown (Johnson & Johnson), may be effective but tattooing has not been beneficial. If lesions are classified histopathologically as "premalignant," avoidance of sunlight may prevent further progression to neoplasia.

Basal-Cell Tumors

Basal-cell tumors are relatively common in cats. They can occur anywhere on the body but show a predilection for the head and neck, and usually are found in cats older than 6 years. They are circumscribed, solitary firm masses attached to the skin and usually are less than 2.5 cm in diameter (Fig C10). Occasionally those tumors are large, ulcerated or cystic structures containing enough melanin to be grossly indistinguishable from melanomas. Basal-cell tumors usually are benign despite the fact that their high mitotic index may give the false impression of a highly malignant neoplasm. Consequently, interpretation of the biopsy by a veterinary pathologist is important. The various histologic patterns of these tumor cells hold no prognostic significance.

Because basal-cell tumors rarely metastasize, surgical excision usually is curative. Since basal-cell tumors are sensitive to radiation therapy,

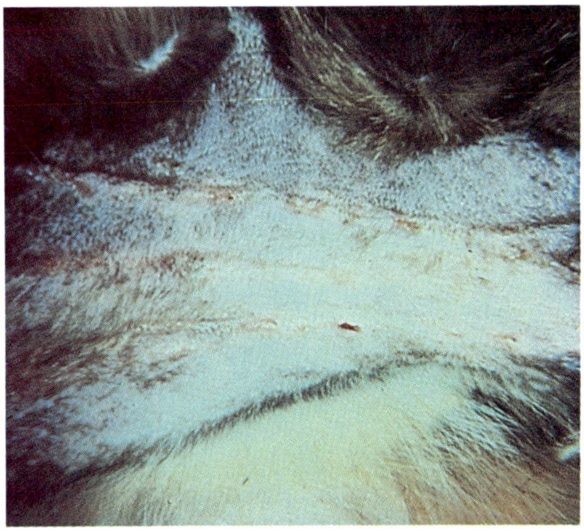

Fig C7. Typical linear granuloma on the caudal aspect of the thigh. Note the raised, yellow-pink lesions.

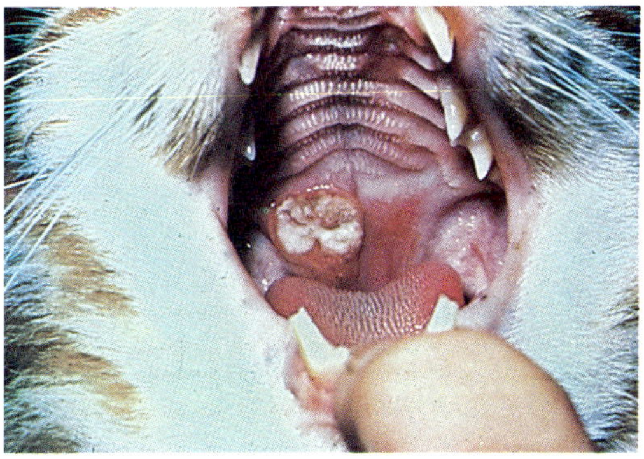

Fig C8. Well-demarcated, raised oral linear granuloma.

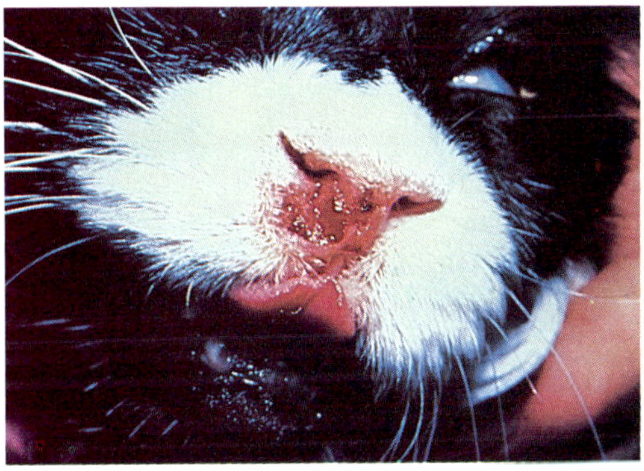

Fig C9. A severe, erosive squamous-cell carcinoma.

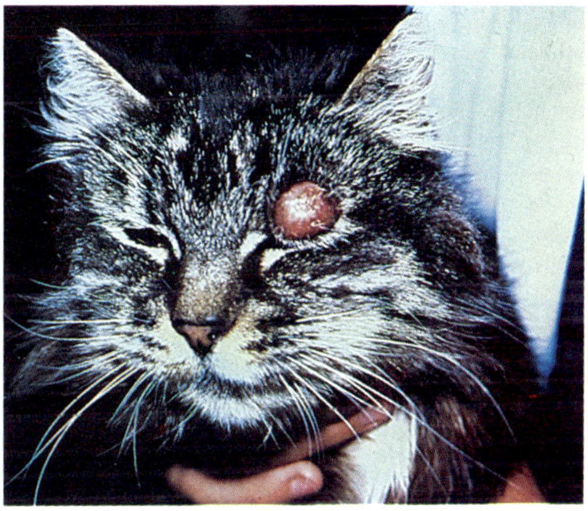

Fig C10. Basal-cell tumor. Note typical circular shape. (Courtesy of Dr B. Brewer)

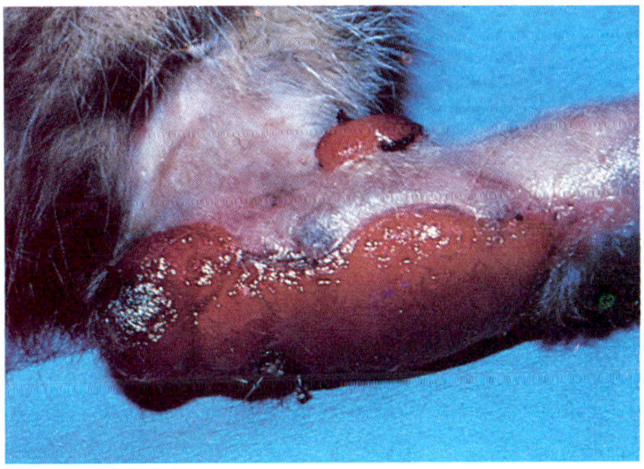

Fig C11. Fibrosarcoma on the rear foot.

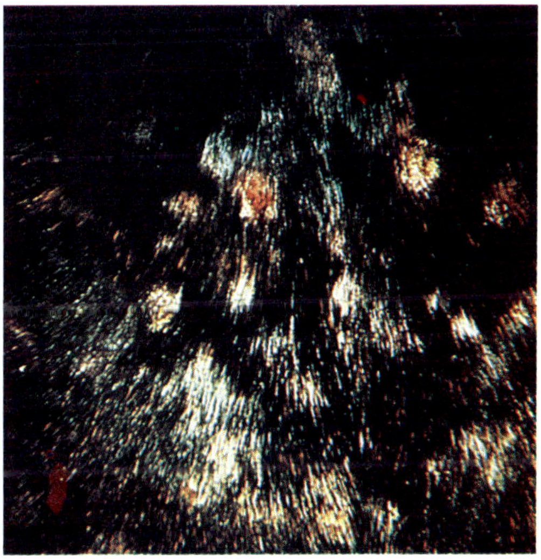

Fig C12. Papules, scales and crusts in a cat with miliary eczema. (Courtesy of Dr R. Halliwell)

this type of treatment may be used in the rare cases of recurrent malignant basal-cell tumors or if surgery would be disfiguring.

Cerumen-Gland Tumors

The cerumen glands in the external ear canal usually are modified apocrine sweat glands. Tumors arising from these glands are not common but occur more often in cats than in other domestic species. They should be considered in the differential diagnosis of chronic otitis externa. Cerumen-gland tumors tend to be unilateral and usually occur in cats older than 8 years of age. Males appear to be at higher risk.[2] The rate of malignancy seems to be high (50-65%) but this may reflect a sampling bias. Cerumen-gland adenocarcinomas can metastasize to regional lymph nodes and the lungs.

Clinical Signs: Cerumen-gland tumors usually appear as chronic otitis externa, characterized by seropurulent discharge, head-shaking and ear-scratching. Drainage occasionally may occur in the parotid region, mimicking a parotid gland tumor or an abscess.[2] On otoscopic examination, they are small, pink, well-circumscribed and often ulcerated masses near the tympanic membrane. Since they often cannot be distinguished grossly from glandular hyperplasia or inflammatory granulation tissue, a biopsy is important diagnostically. Any mass in an older cat's ear should be biopsied if no response is seen to standard treatment for otitis externa within 3 weeks.

Treatment: Surgical excision is the treatment of choice. Because of the anatomic location, lateral ear resection or total ablation of the ear canal often is necessary. Radiotherapy has been used successfully on localized adenocarcinomas. Cytotoxic drugs have been used in conjunction with surgery in metastatic adenocarcinomas. Regional lymph node and thoracic radiographic evaluation for metastases should be done before initiating therapy. Because of the surgical difficulty associated with the anatomic location of these tumors, the prognosis is fair to good with benign tumors and very guarded with the malignant form.

Other Epithelial Tumors

Other feline epithelial neoplasms include epidermoid and dermoid cysts, sebaceous-gland adenomas and adenocarcinomas, apocrine sweat-gland adenomas and adenocarcinomas, trichoepitheliomas, keratoacanthomas and papillomas. Epidermoid cysts (commonly called "sebaceous-gland" cysts or adenomas) and dermoid cysts (developmental defects usually found along the dorsal midline) generally cause no clinical problems. They may provoke an inflammatory response if they rupture into surrounding tissues.

The other tumors mentioned usually are found in older cats. No viral etiology has been shown for feline papillomas. The apocrine-gland adenocarcinoma is more common than the sebaceous-gland adenocarcinoma, but both are aggressive tumors that may metastasize to regional lymph nodes and the lungs. In any solitary skin tumor, excisional biopsy is recommended. Prognosis usually is good except for the aggressive adenocarcinoma, which is guarded.[2,66]

Mesenchymal Tumors

Fibrosarcomas

Fibrosarcomas in cats may be either multiple or solitary. The multiple form tends to occur in young cats and kittens. About half of the cats affected with the multiple form are infected with the feline sarcoma virus, a type-C oncornavirus.[66] These cats are also FeLV positive.[2] Unlike FeLV, of which it is a mutant, the feline sarcoma virus has not been shown to be horizontally transmissible by contact.[66] Unfortunately, there is no simple test for feline sarcoma virus.

The solitary form of fibrosarcoma affects older cats. It apparently is not associated with the feline sarcoma virus of FeLV.

Clinical Signs: Fibrosarcomas are variably sized, poorly circumscribed, frequently ulcerated masses attached to the overlying skin. They may have a slight predilection for the face and extremities (Fig C11). The multiple form often occurs on the trunk. Fibrosarcomas are locally invasive and highly variable as to when during the clinical course they will metastasize. Metastasis usually occurs by hematogenous spread to the lungs and liver. Lymphatic metastasis to regional and distal lymph nodes may occur.

Diagnosis: Biopsy is mandatory for diagnosis because these tumors must be differentiated from fibromas and other mesenchymal tumors. Due to the difficulty in dislodging tumor cells from the collagenous stroma, fine-needle aspirates are unrewarding.[66]

Treatment: Surgical excision is the treatment of choice. However, these tumors frequently recur. Radiation therapy may be effective when used in conjunction with surgery. Following partial excision, the mitotic index of these tumors increases, thus making them more susceptible to radiation. A new promising treatment is hyperthermia. Before instituting therapy, thoracic radiographs to check for metastasis are indicated. The prognosis is guarded, especially in cases of metastasis or recurrence. On rare occasions the multiple form may spontaneously regress.[2]

Solitary fibrosarcomas on the extremities of older cats (not associated with feline sarcoma virus) can be treated by amputation. These tumors metastasize late in their clinical course, giving a good prognosis with amputation.

Other Mesenchymal Tumors

Other neoplasms of mesenchymal origin have occasionally been observed in cats. These include lipomas, liposarcomas, myxomas, myxosarcomas, neurofibromas and cutaneous lymphosarcomas. These tumors generally occur in older cats and tend to be solitary lesions. Cutaneous lymphosarcoma may also occur in a multiple form, with either nodules or pruritic, ulcerative plaques.[2] The only accurate diagnostic technic is biopsy. Needle aspiration may not distinguish between the benign and malignant forms of these tumors.

Surgical excision of benign mesenchymal tumors is optional. Radical surgical excision is indicated in malignant mesenchymal tumors but local recurrence and metastasis are common. Feline cutaneous lymphoma often has concomitant internal involvement and often is refractory to treatment.

Tumors of Miscellaneous Origin

Mast-Cell Tumors

Clinical Signs: Mast-cell tumors (mastocytomas) have no size or age predilection. They can occur as solitary or multiple raised, firm, variably sized masses, often fixed to the underlying tissue (Fig 27). Occasionally they may be ulcerative and pruritic.

Mast-cell tumors may arise in conjunction with visceral mast-cell tumors or may be independent of any internal involvement. However, the latter usually metastasize via the lymphatics to the viscera within 3-6 months. Since mastocythemia may be seen, buffy coat smears may be evaluated for circulating mast cells. When vomiting is present, it is presumably in response to the histamine release from the mast cells. Bleeding diatheses (due to the heparin the mast cells contain) appear to be rare.

Diagnosis: Since the variability of clinical presentation is extreme, the clinician should not rely on appearance alone for a diagnosis. A fine-needle aspirate of the neoplasm, stained with new methylene blue or Romanowsky stain, can be diagnostic. Mast cells appear as mononuclear cells with dark granules. Poorly differentiated tumor cells have large, irregular nuclei with hyperchromatophilic staining cytoplasm. The more malignant the tumor, the larger and more poorly staining are the cytoplasmic granules. If there are only a few mast cells as the only cellular component in an aspirate of a neoplasm, a diagnosis of mast-cell tumor is justified. If these few mast cells are only part of a large

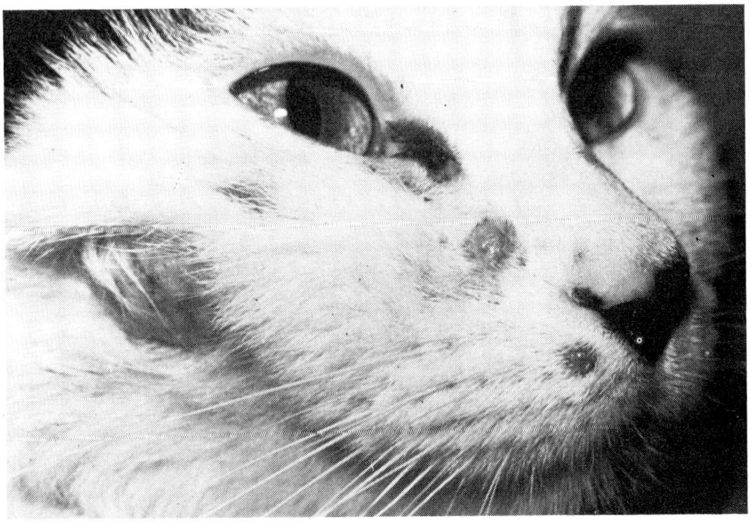

Fig 27. Multiple mast-cell tumors.

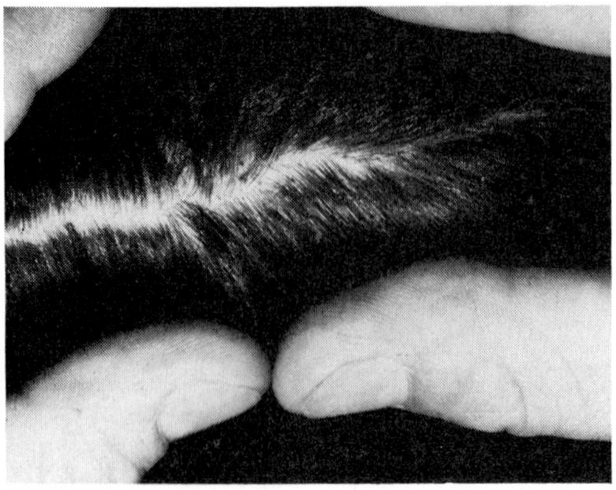

Fig 28. Miliary eczema. Note the small crusts where the hair is parted.

inflammatory response or if any uncertainty exists, the clinician should biopsy the tumor. The pathologist should be made aware of the suspicion of mast-cell tumor since special stains often are necessary for the histopathologic diagnosis of a mast-cell tumor. Differential diagnoses of mast-cell tumors are other neoplasms, inflammatory lesions and the eosinophilic granuloma complex.

Treatment: Therapy of solitary mast-cell tumors consists of surgical excision, cryosurgery or radiation therapy.[67] The multiple form may be treated palliatively with corticosteroids, such as prednisone at 1 mg/lb BID. Unfortunately, mast-cell tumors in cats usually are advanced at presentation and often involve internal organs. Despite the fact that the lesions may not be painful, the ulceration and exudation are often distressing to the client, especially if the tumors are multiple. Although a recent article reports success in treating mast-cell tumors with splenectomy, none of the reported cats had cutaneous involvement.[69] It is uncertain what effect splenectomy would have on a cat with both cutaneous and visceral mast-cell tumors. Cimetidine (Tagamet:Smith Kline), given PO at 25 mg/kg divided QID, may alleviate vomiting. Mast-cell tumors, especially the multiple form, must be given a guarded prognosis.

Melanomas and Melanocytomas

Melanomas (malignant melanomas) are quite rare in cats and usually occur in older animals. They usually appear as solitary, brown or black nodules of variable size and shape. Metastasis via the lymphatics to the lungs is common. Radical excisional biopsy is recommended for suspected lesions as both a diagnostic technic and the therapy of choice. The differential diagnosis includes other neoplasms, particularly basal-cell tumors. The prognosis is poor due to frequent metastasis.

Melanocytomas (nevi, moles) are benign, congenital growths consisting of "altered" melanocytes. They occur in the dermis or at the dermoepidermal junction. They are rare in cats. Their principal importance is as a differential diagnosis for melanomas. Previously reported benign melanomas may in fact have been nevi. Surgical excision is optional.[2,66,70]

Mammary Tumors

Mammary glands are modified apocrine sweat glands. Tumors of these glands usually affect the cranial pair of the 4 pairs of glands in cats.[66] Mammary tumors occur most often in older females and rarely in castrated males. Early ovariectomy is of great value in reducing the incidence of mammary tumors in later life. In one study, spayed queens had 7 times less likelihood of developing mammary cancer than their unspayed counterparts.[71]

Most mammary tumors in cats are carcinomas, mainly of the glandular type, and metastases are very common. The histologic appearance of the tumor has prognostic significance. Cats with more differentiated, less malignant-appearing, smaller tumors survive longer than those with poorly differentiated, large and more malignant-appearing tumors.[72]

Treatment: The treatment of choice is radical surgical excision of the affected glands. A delay in surgery decreases postsurgical survival time. Chemotherapy in conjunction with surgery has been attempted but its value has yet to be determined. Ovariectomy at the time of mastectomy has had no effect on recurrence.[66] In general, feline mammary tumors tend to be more malignant and aggressive than their canine counterparts, and this is reflected in a poorer prognosis.

Benign neoplasms of the feline mammary gland are rare (15-20%). Another condition, benign fibroglandular proliferation of one or more of the mammary glands, has been seen in young, intact and often-pregnant queens. Since regression occurs after ovariectomy, resection is not required.[73] Non-neoplastic hypertrophy of the mammary gland has been associated with medroxyprogesterone acetate (Depo-Provera:Upjohn) therapy.[74] Both of these conditions are quite dramatic and should be considered important differential diagnoses of mammary neoplasia.

THE MILIARY ECZEMA COMPLEX by P.J. Ihrke

Miliary eczema is a common clinical sign associated with a number of diverse diseases and should not be considered a single disease entity. It is often impossible to determine the underlying cause of miliary eczema based upon physical examination alone since the lesions may be morphologically identical despite different underlying causes.

Cause: The most commonly recognized causes of miliary eczema are generally thought to be flea-allergy dermatitis, food allergy, dermatophytosis and cheyletiellosis. Most authors consider flea allergy the most common cause of feline miliary eczema.[1,2,75,76] In parts of the country where fleas cause significant problems, they may be responsible for greater than 90% of all cases of miliary eczema. Pediculosis, intestinal parasitism, drug eruption, fatty acid deficiency, folliculitis and irritant contact dermatitis have all been reported to cause miliary eczema in a few cases. One investigator recently reported that 15% of cases of miliary eczema are idiopathic.[2] The perentage of idiopathic cases is probably lower in areas of the country with a more significant flea population than where fleas are not such a problem.

Clinical Signs: No age, breed or sex predilections are seen with miliary eczema.[2] Miliary eczema or miliary dermatitis is characterized by a crusting, papular rash often localized to the neck, head and area at the base of the tail (Figs 28, C12). Chronic cases may be generalized. The degree of pruritus depends upon the underlying cause. Personality changes and sudden twitching of the skin of the dorsum, followed by rapid motion, have been observed in chronic cases.

Diagnosis: Diagnosis of the miliary eczema complex should be based initially on elimination of the most common causes for this condition. For example, a thorough history should be obtained, with emphasis on other animal contacts, possible seasonality of occurrence and any associated problems, such as GI disease. A careful physical examination, with emphasis on detection of ectoparasites, should be followed by a dermatophyte culture, skin scrapings and fecal flotation. If these procedures do not establish a likely diagnosis, an elimination diet, withdrawal of any medication, and a biopsy should be considered. Miliary eczema should be deemed idiopathic only after all known causes of the syndrome have been ruled out.

Treatment: Since miliary eczema is of multifactorial etiology, therapy depends upon the underlying cause. Therapy for the specific diseases that can cause miliary eczema is discussed in the sections dealing with that disease.

Progestational compounds (Ovaban, Megace) are the drugs of choice for idiopathic miliary eczema. Recommended dosages parallel those for other disease, *ie,* 2.5-5 mg/day PO initially, then 2.5-5 mg PO every 4-10 days for maintenance. Maintenance therapy generally is required for life since recurrence is common within a month after cessation of therapy. Corticosteroids usually are not effective in controlling idiopathic miliary eczema.

DERMATOLOGIC THERAPEUTICS by P.J. Ihrke

As a generalization, fewer drugs both topical and systemic, are used in feline dermatology than in canine dermatology. The most obvious factors governing this generalization are that cat skin is more sensitive than dog skin to many topical products and far more diseases requiring systemic therapy have been identified in canine dermatology.

Topical Therapy

The basic principles of topical therapy have been reviewed elsewhere.[2,27,77] Before any topical product is recommended for a feline patient, the clinician should determine if the product is recommended for feline use or if the product contains any of the most common agents contraindicated for use in cats. Products containing chlorinated hydrocarbons (*eg,* lindane), coal tars, selenium disulfide or phenol derivatives, such as resorcinol, should not be used.

Localized topical therapy is rarely indicated in cats. Notable exceptions are in the treatment of otitis externa and feline acne. If localized treatment is used for other purposes, an increased interest in the grooming of the lesion may cause significant self-trauma. Generalized topical application of shampoos, rinses and powders are the most effective methods of topical therapy in cats.

Tresaderm (Merck) should be considered the drug of choice in treating ear mite infestation. Whereas other otic preparations are often implicated as exacerbating feline otitis, the author has not had any adverse reactions to Tresaderm. The thiabendazole is probably responsible for the preparation's miticidal activity and the dexamethasone seems to significantly decrease inflammation.

Topical corticosteroids are not commonly used in cats. Flea-collar dermatitis is the only localized feline dermatosis for which topical corticosteroids are recommended as routine therapy. If localized therapy for treatment of contact dermatitis, an eosinophilic plaque or pyotraumatic dermatitis is desired, a potent topical corticosteroid, such as desoximetasone (Topicort:Hoechst-Roussel) or betamethasone valerate (Valisone: Schering) may be used.

Benzoyl peroxide gel (OxyDex Gel:D.V.M.) may be used gently once daily for feline acne but use of benzoyl peroxide shampoo is recommended initially due to ease of application and a lesser likelihood of irritation.

For gentle whole-body cleansing, Allergroom (Allerderm), Veterinary Shampoo (Neutrogena) and HyLyt EFA (D.V.M.) may be used. Either of these products or Nolvasan Pet Shampoo (Fort Dodge) may be helpful in palliative treatment of some seborrheic cats. Unfortunately, most antiseborrheic shampoos contain either coal tar or salicylic acid, both of which can cause significant problems in cats. Benzoyl peroxide shampoos (OxyDex Shampoo:D.V.M.) are effective in seborrhea oleosa but frequently are irritating. Consequently, benzoyl peroxide shampoos are only recommended for application to limited areas in cases of feline acne or stud tail.

Rinses are an effective method of applying antiparasitic and antifungal preparations. Lime sulfur (1-2%) is an excellent, safe parasiticide in cats (Orthorix:Chevron; LymDyp:D.V.M.; Vlem-Dome:Dome) and captan wettable powder (Orthocide:Chevron, 2 tbsp/gal water) is an excellent product for feline ringworm.

Powders containing 5% carbaryl are still effective for flea control in many parts of the US. Insecticidal resistance is emerging as a major problem in certain areas. Pyrethrins and pyrethroids may be used in young kittens due to their very low toxicity. Other insecticides should be used with extreme caution in cats.

Systemic Therapy

Corticosteroids and progestational compounds deserve special mention due to their frequent use in feline dermatology. Systemic corticosteroids often are used in cats for their antipruritic and anti-inflammatory effects. Rarely they may also be used for their immunosuppressive and immunomodulatory effect. Older reports on a poor response to oral corticosteroids in cats were probably due to the use of excessively low dosages similar to those used in canine regimens. In general, cats require considerably higher dosages per unit weight than do dogs. If oral medication is desirable, a typical initial antipruritic or anti-inflammatory dosage would be 2-4 mg/kg daily, divided BID. Cats appear more resistant to the side effects of corticosteroids than are dogs or people.[2] Because of its safety for short-term use, ease of administration and consistency of effect, methylprednisolone acetate (Depo-Medrol:Upjohn) is the corticosteroid of choice in cats. The average dose used is 20 mg, which is considerably higher than the manufacturer's recommendation.

Progestational compounds (Ovaban:Schering; Megace:Mead Johnson) are effective in management of a wide variety of unrelated feline dermatoses. Definite antigonadotrophic and antiandrogenic effects, as well as anti-inflammatory actions, are documented. In addition, progestational compounds seem to have a "mood-elevating" effect, which may be due to actions on the hypothalamus and limbic system. Consequently, the dramatic response to this drug in cases of feline endocrine alopecia, eosinophilic granuloma complex, psychogenic alopecia, idiopathic miliary eczema, and even flea-allergy dermatitis is probably due to multiple actions.

Dosage recommendations vary considerably among clinicians. A typical regimen for many of the diseases listed above would be 2.5 mg megestrol acetate given daily for 2-3 weeks or until substantial improvement is noted, followed by a gradual decrease to a maintenance dosage. Typical maintenance therapy usually varies from 2.5 mg given every 3 days to every 7 days. In general, diseases in the eosinophilic granuloma complex require higher dosages than do other feline dermatoses listed.

The veterinary product, Ovaban, is considerably more palatable than Megace and its use is preferred in cats that are difficult to medicate.

Otherwise, differences between the products have not been noted.

Unfortunately, the side effects of progestational drugs may be significant. Polyphagia, weight gain, polydipsia and personality changes are common. Mammary hyperplasia, mammary neoplasia and diabetes mellitus are less common but have more severe side effects.[2] Consequently, caution should be exercised when recommending use of these drugs for long-term maintenance therapy. However, most reported cases of severe side effects seem to be associated with use of higher dosages.

References

1. Muller, GH and Kirk, RW: Small Animal Dermatology. 2nd ed. WB Saunders, Philadelphia, 1976.
2. Scott, DW. JAAHA **16** (1980) 331 *et seqq.*
3. Ihrke, in Ettinger: Textbook of Veterinary Internal Medicine. WB Saunders, Philadelphia, *In press*, 1982.
4. Ihrke, PJ. Compend Cont Ed AHT **2** (1981) 5.
5. Baker, KP. Vet Rec **86** (1970) 62.
6. Krough, HV and Kristensen, S. Nord Vet Med **28** (1976) 459.
7. Hearst, BR. VM/SAC **62** (1967) 475.
8. Smith, JE. J Sm Anim Pract **5** (1964) 517.
9. Biberstein, EL and England, K. JAVMA **53** (1968) 1045.
10. Joshua, JO. Feline Pract **1(2)** (1971) 9.
11. Dorring, GG. Vet Clin No Am **6** (1976) 468.
12. Scott, in Kirk: Current Veterinary Therapy VI. WB Saunders, Philadelphia, 1977.
13. Attleberger, in Kirk: Current Veterinary Therapy VII. WB Saunders, Philadelphia, 1980.
14. Snider, WR *et al.* Am Rev Resp Dis **104** (1971) 866.
15. Carter, GR: Essentials of Veterinary Bacteriology and Mycology. Michigan State Univ Press, Ann Arbor, 1976.
16. Lawrence, WE and Wickham, N. Aust Vet J **39** (1963) 390.
17. Wilkinson, in Kirk: Current Veterinary Therapy VI. WB Saunders, Philadelphia, 1977.
18. Peolma, FG and Leiker, DL. Int J Leprosy **42** (1974) 307.
19. Shiefer, B *et al.* JAVMA **165** (1974) 1085.
20. Dewevre, P *et al.* JAAHA **13** (1977) 68.
21. Wilkinson, GT *et al.* J Sm Anim Pract **9** (1978) 357.
22. Blakemore, in Kirk: Current Veterinary Therapy V. WB Saunders, Philadelphia, 1974.
23. Chester, DK. Compend Cont Ed Pract Vet **12** (1979) 910.
24. Rebell, G and Taplin, D: Dermatophytes: Their Recognition and Identification. Univ Miami Press, Coral Gables, FL, 1970.
25. Blakemore, JC. Pract Vet **46(6)** (1974) 15.
26. Blakemore, JC. Pract Vet **47(1)** (1975) 8.
27. Ihrke, PJ. Compend Cont Ed Prac Vet **2** (1980) 156.
28. Attleberger, MH, Auburn Univ: Personal communication, 1981.
29. Fadok, VA. Compend Cont Ed Pract Vet **2** (1980) 782.
30. Fadok, VA. Compend Cont Ed Pract Vet **2** (1980) 707.
31. Cotter, in Kirk: Current Veterinary Therapy VI. WB Saunders, Philadelphia, 1977.
32. Robbins, SL and Angell, M: Basic Pathology. 2nd ed. WB Saunders, Philadelphia, 1976.
33. Walton, in Kirk: Current Veterinary Therapy VI. WB Saunders, Philadelphia, 1977.
34. Scott, DW *et al.* JAAHA **15** (1979) 157.
35. Slauson, DO *et al.* J Path **103** (1971) 131.
36. Heise, SC *et al.* Feline Pract **3(3)** (1973) 14.
37. Wierzchowiechi, MO *et al.* Arth Rheum **18** (1975) 77.
38. Fellner, MJ: Immunology of Skin Diseases. Elsevier, New York, 1980.
39. Abdou, NJ *et al.* Clin Immun Immunopath **6** (1976) 192.
40. Cohen, AS and Canoso, JJ. Arth Rheum **15** (1972) 540.
41. Halliwell, REW. Adv Vet Sci Comp Med **22** (1978) 237.
42. Scott, DW *et al.* Vet Path **17** (1980) 264.
43. Lever, WF and Shaumburg-Lever, G: Histopathology of the Skin. JB Lippincott, Philadelphia, 1975.
44. Ohun, MR and Edelstein, LM: Gross and Microscopic Pathology of the Skin. Dermatopathology Foundation Press, Boston, 1976.
45. Moschella, in Moschella, SL *et al:* Dermatology. WB Saunders, Philadelphia, 1975.
46. Stannard, AA *et al.* JAVMA **166** (1975) 575.
47. Halliwell, REW. Adv Vet Sci Comp Med **22** (1978) 249.
48. Halliwell, REW and Goldschmidt, MH. JAAHA **13** (1977) 43.
49. Manning, TO *et al.* JAAHA **16** (1980) 189.
50. Scott, DW *et al.* JAAHA **16** (1980) 815.
51. Fox, JG and Beatty, JO. JAAHA **11** (1975) 129.
52. Swift, GA and Brown, RH. Vet Rec (1976) 374.
53. Scott, DW *et al.* Cornell Vet **69** (1969) 104.
54. Kirk, in Kirk: Current Veterinary Therapy VII. WB Saunders, Philadelphia, 1980.
55. Scott, DW. JAAHA **11** (1975) 261.
56. Hess and MacEwen, in Kirk: Current Veterinary Therapy VI. WB Saunders, Philadelphia, 1977.
57. Conroy, in Catcott: Feline Medicine and Surgery. 1st ed. American Veterinary Publications, Santa Barbara, 1964.
58. Biery, in Kirk: Current Veterinary Therapy VI. WB Saunders, Philadelphia, 1977.
59. Butler, WF. Res Vet Sci **19** (1975) 213.
60. Patterson, DF and Minor, RR. Lab Invest **37** (1977) 170.
61. Kramer, JW *et al.* Lab Invest **36** (1977) 554.
62. Sorry, WB and Collier, LL. Am J Path **90** (1978) 533.
63. Munday, BL. Br Vet J **126** (1970) 47.
64. Holzworth, in Kirk: Current Veterinary Therapy IV. WB Saunders, Philadelphia, 1971.

65. Scott, in Catcott: Feline Medicine and Surgery. 2nd ed. American Veterinary Publications, Santa Barbara, 1975.
66. Theilen, GH and Madewell, BR: Veterinary Cancer Medicine. Lea & Febiger, Philadelphia, 1979.
67. Winthrow, SJ. Vet Clin No Am **10** (1980) 755.
68. Grier, RL *et al.* JAVMA **177** (1980) 55.
69. Liska, WP *et al.* JAAHA **15** (1979) 589.
70. Stannard and Pulley, in Moulton: Tumors in Domestic Animals. 2nd ed. Univ Calif Press, Berkeley, 1978.
71. Dorn, CR *et al.* J Nat Cancer Inst **48** (1968) 307.
72. Bostock, in Kirk: Current Veterinary Therapy VI. WB Saunders, Philadelphia, 1977.
73. Allen, HL. Vet Path **10** (1973) 501.
74. Hinton, M and Gaskell, CJ. Vet Rec **100** (1977) 277.
75. Willemse, in Kirk: Current Veterinary Therapy VII. WB Saunders, Philadelphia, 1980.
76. Reedy, LM. Compend Cont Ed Pract Vet **2** (1980) 833.
77. Ihrke, PJ. Compend Cont Ed Pract Vet **2** (1980) 28.
78. Pattyn, SR and Portaels, F. Int J Leprosy **48** (1980) 7.

BURNS AND FROSTBITE
by P.J. McKeever

Thermal Burns

Causes

Thermal burns to the skin of cats generally are due to friction, direct heat or flames. Friction burns usually result from the animal being hurled or dragged over the pavement after being struck by a car. Direct thermal burns develop from such situations as cats walking over hot stove burners, prolonged contact with heating pads, hot liquids spilled on the animal, and malfunction of hair-drying equipment. Flame burns may result from fires in homes or automobile accidents.

Extent of Tissue Damage

The extent of a burn is related to the area exposed to the heat source. The severity of a burn depends on the duration of the thermal insult and maximum temperature the tissue attains. These are influenced by such variables as the temperature and mass of the burning agent, the mass, specific heat and thermal conductivity of the burned body, the temperature of the environment in which postburn cooling takes place, and the amount of heat convection in the surrounding medium.[1]

Water and tissues of which water is the main component are characterized by a high specific heat (large amount of heat required to raise the temperature) and low thermal conductivity (heat slow to dissipate). Therefore, tissues become overheated slowly but are also slow in cooling. The duration of tissue overheating extends beyond the contact time with the burning agent.[1] Immediate cooling of the burned area can decrease tissue damage by shortening the duration of tissue overheating.[2]

Tissue damage from overheating proceeds in a graduated manner. Threshold overheating of tissue causes inapparent, reversible cell damage. Further overheating produces foci of irreversibly damaged cells scattered among reversibly damaged and uninjured cells. Finally, when a critical threshold is exceeded, necrosis of the entire tissue occurs.[2]

Because the transition from necrotic skin to healthy skin is gradual, regeneration of skin defects proceeds not from healthy tissue but from partly damaged tissue. This is one of the major reasons why burn wounds take longer than mechanical injuries to heal.

Burn Classification

Burns in people have been classified as follows: first degree, with erythema and some damage to the epidermis but no blistering; second degree, with blistering and complete necrosis of the epidermis and varying degrees of damage to the dermis; and third degree, with total loss of all elements of the skin.[2]

Application of this classification to cats in a clinical situation is difficult because feline skin does not blister as easily as does human skin. However, because of the need to excise necrotic tissue, early assessment of burn severity often is required. For this determination, it is more practical to use a simplified classification that differentiates burns into 2 types. Partial-thickness burns are characterized by incomplete destruction of the skin and epithelialization from local epidermal elements. Full-thickness burns are characterized by complete destruction of all elements of the skin and epithelialization through migration of epidermal cells from the edges of the defect.

Clinically, partial-thickness burns are distinguished by erythema, local edema, evidence of persistent capillary circulation, and partial sensation to touch. Full-thickness burns are distinguished by lack of superficial blood flow, insensitivity of the skin to touch, and easy epilation of hair.

Sequelae

Infection: Infections of burn wounds generally are caused by microorganisms found in the normal microflora of the skin. They are opportunists in the burn wound because damaged tissue is a good medium for bacterial growth. In severe burns, the immunologic competency of the animal is impaired.[2]

The bacteria most frequently isolated from burn wounds in people include *Staphylococcus, Streptococcus, Proteus, Pseudomonas, E coli* and *Klebsiella.*[3] Too few samples from burn wounds in cats have been cultured and reported to confirm the presence of similar bacteria.

Systemic infection is rare in small and medium-sized burns. However, in extensive burns involving 15-30% of the body, septicemia and invasive spread of local infection are frequent complications. Extensive local infection may also convert superficial skin necrosis into a full-thickness defect.[2]

Shock: Burn shock is defined as a set of signs occurring when the autoregulative mechanisms of the body are unable to allow normal blood flow to vital tissue and organs.[2] It is characteristically associated with hypovolemia that begins very soon after the animal is burned and is typically most severe after several hours.[2] The hypovolemia is due to an immediate, transient vascular leakage from venules and a delayed, prolonged leakage from capillaries or from medium and small venules. The immediate leakage is mediated by histamine liberated in response to the complement cascade, which is activated by heat-modified protein.[1] Delayed permeability is mediated by prostaglandins and accounts for the most leakage.[1]

Hypovolemic shock associated with burns is not as severe in cats as in people because less fluid and plasma protein are lost due to infrequent development of vesicles and bullae. However, it may be important clinically if over 20% of the body surface is burned. Chapter 2 discusses treatment for hypovolemia.

Respiratory Disorders: Ventilation may be affected by inspiration of hot air and gases, which burn the upper respiratory tract and cause laryngeal and pharyngeal edema and bronchospasm. This may be followed by hypersecretion by the bronchial mucosa and subsequent plasma exudation, which impairs respiration and reduces the vital capacity of the lungs. Focal atelectasis and infectious pulmonary complications may appear in 5-6 days.[2]

Treatment

Standard principles for the treatment of small traumatic lesions of the skin may be applied to minor burns. Experimental studies in animals and clinical studies in people have not demonstrated a particular treatment that has distinct advantages.[2]

Depending on the extent of the wounds, the treatment of severe burns involves reversal of shock, cooling the tissue, cleansing and debriding the wound, topical and systemic antibacterial therapy, and skin grafting, if necessary.

Shock: Initial evaluation and treatment of the burned patient should be similar to that used in animals treated for other severe trauma. Airways should be examined for patency, any serious hemorrhage controlled, and the animal evaluated for hypovolemic shock. If necessary, the hypovolemia should be treated as outlined in Chapter 2. If hypovolemia is not present or if the animal's condition is stabilized, evaluation and treatment of devitalized skin may be started.

Cooling: If the burn occurred within the last 2 hours, cooling may have a beneficial effect. It reduces the pain, edema and depth of the burn wound. Cold compresses can be applied or affected areas may be immersed in cold water. The optimal temperature for the cooling water or compresses is 3-17 C (37-63 F).[2]

Cleansing and Debridement: Hair should be clipped from all affected areas. Contamination and loose devitalized tissue may be removed by flushing with saline or washing with povidone iodine soap.

As indicated previously, determining the extent of burn wounds in cats is difficult and generally the extent of the damage is underestimated. Final confirmation of the extent of a burn may not be possible until about 10 days later, when the normal and necrotic skin begin to separate.

All devitalized tissue should be excised as it provides a good growth medium for bacteria. Baths are also helpful to soak off exudates, crusts and necrotic tissue. If possible, immersion of the affected areas in a tepid whirlpool bath for 15-20 minutes twice daily is effective.

Topical Antibacterial Treatment: Silver sulfadiazine cream (Silvadene Cream:Marion Labs) is one of the most effective antibacterial drugs for topical therapy of burns.[4] It has antibacterial properties, is nonirritating to exposed tissues, has no systemic side effects, and is easily applied to the wound. A method for its use is as follows. After initial cleansing and debridement of the burned skin, silver sulfadiazine cream is applied liberally to the affected areas with a gloved hand or tongue depressor and the area is bandaged with loose mesh gauze. Dressings are changed twice daily. During dressing changes, any necessary debridement is performed, and the lesion is cleansed by irrigation with saline or immersion in a whirlpool bath.

Systemic Antibacterial Treatment: The efficacy of systemic antibiotics in the treatment of severe burns is questionable. Studies on animals and human burn patients show that systemic antibiotic therapy does not favorably influence mortality, resolution of fever or the rate of healing.[2] Systemic use of antibiotics probably should be limited to confirmed cases of bacterial septicemia. In such cases, antibiotic selection should be determined by sensitivity tests.

Skin Grafts: Before surgical intervention, severe burn wounds should be treated as previously described until all necrotic tissue has been separated from viable tissue, infection is controlled, and granulation tissue has developed. Feline skin is very elastic and loose subcutaneous tissue allows a great degree of stretching. Therefore, most skin defects can be closed by direct apposition or by one of several reconstructive technics using skin flaps.[5] If the defect is too large for primary closure, a free, autogenous graft, either full thickness or partial thickness may be used.

Chemical Burns

Chemical burns are rare in cats and most frequently due to acid or alkali spills. However, the author has seen skin severely damaged by improperly diluted pesticides.

Acids

When strong acids react with skin they coagulate protein and cause tissue to dehydrate, contract and darken. Contact with acids usually results in severe pain; however, phenol or chromic or hydrofluoric acid, if contact is limited, may produce transient local anesthesia.[6]

All acid burns necessitate immediate dilution and flushing with water. The general therapeutic management parallels that required for thermal burns.

Alkalis

Strong ammonia solutions and lye are common household products that can cause burns in cats. Alkalis liquefy skin proteins and change the skin color to white or brown. Affected skin develops a characteristic soft, gelatinous, slippery feel.[6]

Alkali burns should be thoroughly flushed with water. The general therapeutic management parallels that required for thermal burns.

Frostbite

Frostbite of the ear tips is common in cats allowed outside in cold regions. In mild cases, depigmentation of the hair may be the only noticeable finding. In severe cases, the ends of the pinnae may slough. Affected ears seldom need treatment.

Gross freezing, with resultant massive necrosis of skin, is rare in cats. Initial treatment would consist of rapid thawing in water at 40 C (104 F).[6] During warming, the frozen part should not be massaged or handled excessively. After warming, the patient should be carefully monitored to assure that self-mutilation does not occur. Further therapeutic management of necrotic skin and resulting defect parallels that of thermal injury.

References

1. Arthurson, G. Ann Chir Gynaecol **69** (1980) 178.
2. Rudowski, W *et al:* Burn Therapy and Research. Johns Hopkins Univ Press, Baltimore, 1976.
3. Sevitt, S. J Trauma **19** (1979) 358.
4. Monafo, WW. J Trauma **19** (1979) 879.
5. Swaim, SF: Surgery of Traumatized Skin. WB Saunders, Philadelphia, 1980.
6. Daniels, in Fitzpatrick: Dermatology in General Medicine, McGraw-Hill, New York, 1979.

17

the eye

A.H. BRIGHTMAN

The cat, although domesticated over the centuries, still retains the highly specialized vision of a predator. The visual system of domestic cats is similar to that of most other mammals yet has many unique characteristics. The frontal placement of the eyeballs, combined with large corneas and lenses, give cats a large area of stereoscopic vision. Extraocular muscles do not provide great motility to the globes; however, this is compensated for by rapid head movements when tracking an object. The nictitating membrane, controlled by the sixth cranial nerve, is mobile and helps protect the globe.

The visual system of cats helps the animal in nocturnal activities. In darkened conditions, the pupil fully dilates and the "light-gathering" effect of the tapetum lucidum combines to provide maximum illumination to the retina. Conversely, in bright light the pupil forms a narrow vertical slit, which may aid both depth perception and depth of field.

Diseases of the feline eye can be divided into those that are common to any mammal, such as trauma and ulceration, and those unique to domestic cats. In this chapter, I have limited the in-depth coverage of ocular diseases to those commonly found only in cats.

EXAMINATION OF THE EYE

The ophthalmic examination should be conducted in a quiet room with a lighting system that can be dimmed by a rheostat. The examiner should seat himself at the head of the table while the assistant restrains the cat. Usually, holding the cat near the edge of the table by the back of the neck is all that is necessary.

With the room fully illuminated, the cat should be observed for any orbital swelling, drooping of the lids and epiphora. The presence or absence of coordinated eye movements and the ability to track objects should be noted.

With the lights dimmed, the examiner should use a loupe (Donagan Optivisor with 2.5X magnification) and a focal light source (Finoff Transilluminator:Welch-Allyn) to examine the lids and anterior segment of the eye. The anterior segment consists of the conjunctiva, cornea, anterior chamber, iris and lens.

Before proceeding with the examination or placing any drops in the eyes, tear production should be measured with the Schirmer tear test (see Epiphora). After completing the Schirmer tear test, one must decide if dilation of the pupil is necessary to facilitate further examination of the lens, vitreous or retina. If pupillary dilation is deemed important, one drop of tropicamide solution (1% Mydriacyl:Alcon) is applied to dilate the cat's pupil in 5-10 minutes.

If the area of concern seems to be the cornea, fluorescein dye may be applied to facilitate detection of ulcerations. Examination with the slit-lamp biomicroscope (Kowa) also helps localize lesions within the cornea.

After pupillary dilation, the lens may be examined with the slit lamp or with a direct ophthalmoscope set on the +10 diopter setting.

The direct or indirect ophthalmoscope are both useful in examination of the retina and optic nerve. The direct ophthalmoscope has the advantage of being inexpensive and easy to use. However, its disadvantage is that it provides only monocular images and therefore provides the examiner with little depth perception.

Usually the cat retina can be visualized at a setting on the direct ophthalmoscope ranging from 0 to −3 diopters. The indirect ophthalmoscope has the advantage of giving the observer binocular stereoscopic vision. The disad-

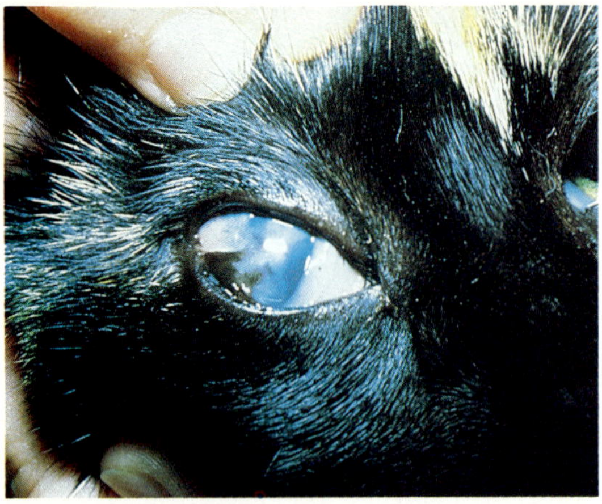

Fig C1. Symblepharon in a 6-month-old cat that had herpesvirus keratitis at 2 months of age.

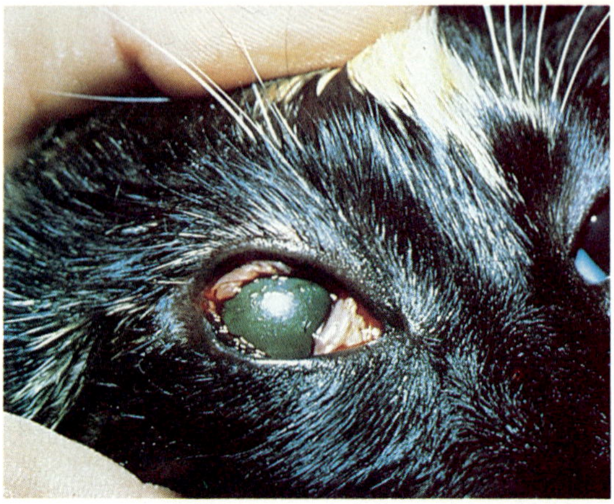

Fig C2. Postoperative appearance of the eye of the cat in Figure C1 after keratectomy and conjunctival resection.

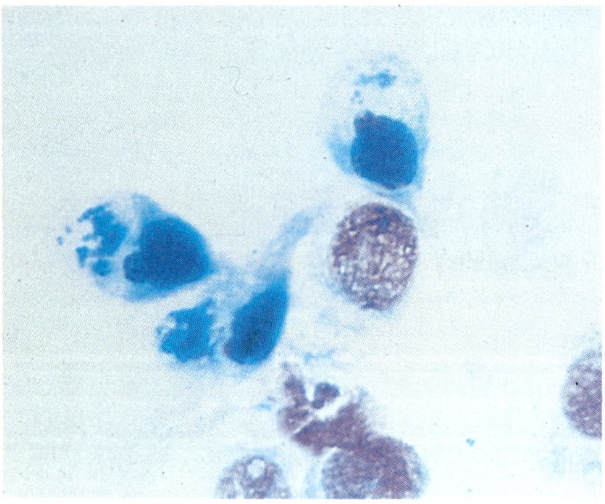

Fig C3. Intraepithelial cell inclusions characteristic of chlamydial conjunctivitis. Initial and elementary bodies are near the nucleus. Giemsa stain, original magnification 1000X. (Courtesy of Dr L. Campbell and Lea & Febiger)

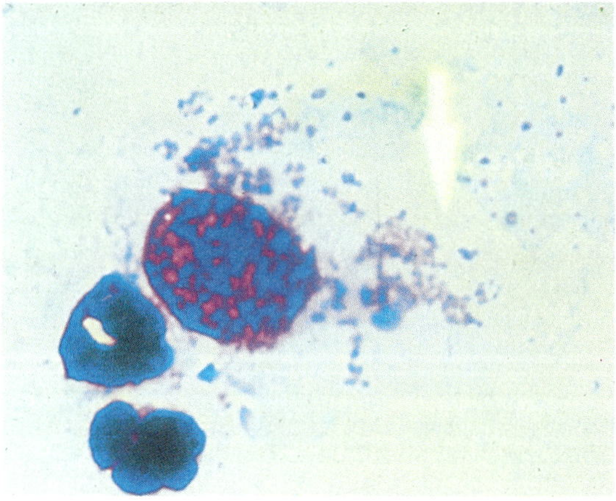

Fig C4. Small inclusion bodies on the epithelial cell surface are characteristic of mycoplasmal infection. Original magnification 1000X. (Courtesy of Dr L. Campbell and Lea & Febiger)

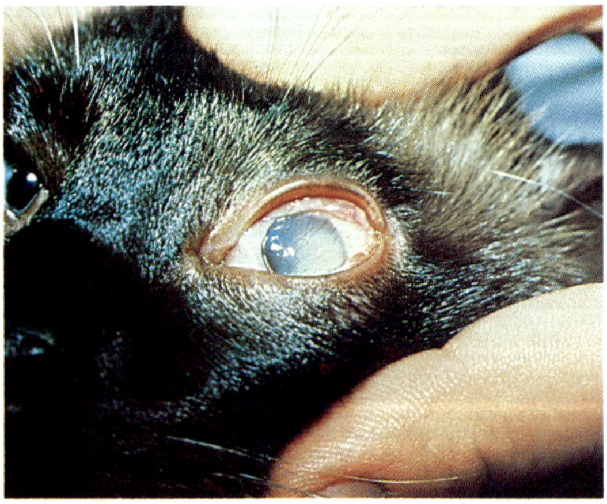

Fig C5. Neovascularity and a dendritic ulcer in a 4-month-old Siamese with unilateral herpesvirus keratitis.

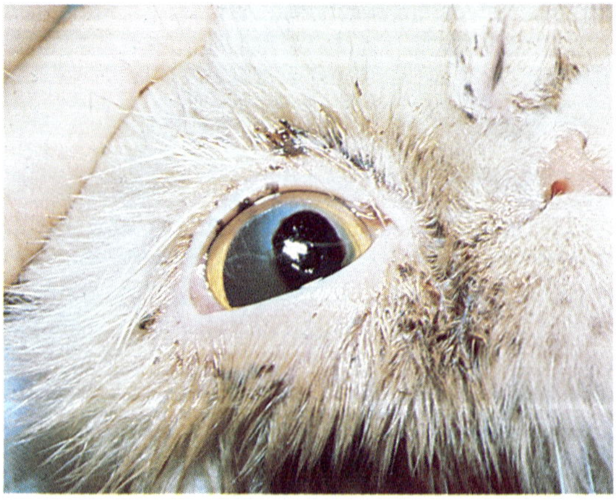

Fig C6. Corneal sequestration in a 5-year-old female. Corneal edema and neovascularity are present.

vantages of indirect ophthalmoscopes are expense and the fact that a period of training is required to acquire the skill necessary to use them.

After completion of the ophthalmoscopic examination, intraocular pressures may be recorded by using the Schiotz tonometer. Topical anesthesia is necessary for this test.

The visual ability of the cat may be assessed by several methods, in combination with the case history. Menacing gestures with the hand may elicit a response but generally the cat is too frightened to react or merely reacts to the air currents generated. A far simpler method is to place the cat on the floor in a maze of obstacles and observe the animal as it navigates the course.

This simple examination procedure generally provides a base line of information from which an accurate diagnosis can be made.

THE GLOBE AND ORBIT

Anatomy

The eye of the cat rests in the rostral portion of the orbit. The orbit is not a complete bony orbit, as in people and other primates, but rather is formed from the sphenoid, maxillary, lacrimal, zygomatic and frontal bones.[1] There is no bone covering the dorsolateral or ventral orbit. The soft tissue structures filling the orbit include the globe, extraocular muscles, lacrimal gland, optic nerve, nictitating membrane, and the vessels and nerves that supply these structures. Trauma, infection, inflammation or neoplasia of the orbit can cause rostral displacement of the globe (exophthalmos). Exophthalmos is often accompanied by chemosis of the conjunctiva, and edema and elevation of the nictitating membrane.[2]

Diseases of the Globe and Orbit

Microphthalmia

Microphthalmia, or a smaller than normal globe, is generally considered a developmental abnormality and congenital disease. Congenital narrowing of the palpebral tissue may coexist with this condition. Many microphthalmic eyes also have other congenital defects, such as persistent pupillary membrane and persistent hypoplastic primary vitreous, with cataracts. There is no medical or surgical treatment for this condition and a guarded prognosis for vision should be considered until proven otherwise.

Congenital microphthalmia must always be differentiated from phthisis bulbi, a shrunken, fibrotic globe. Phthisis bulbi may occur at any age, whereas microphthalmia is present at birth. A phthisical globe generally is the result of overwhelming trauma or infection, from which the eye loses its ability to produce enough aqueous humor to maintain its normal shape and size. Entropion and conjunctivitis usually are found secondary to phthisis bulbi. Enucleation is generally the recommended treatment for phthisis bulbi.[3]

Retrobulbar Abscess

Cause: Bacterial infections of the orbit are common in cats. Bite wounds, penetrating foreign bodies and diseased upper molars are among the most probable causes.[4]

Clinical Signs: The typical clinical signs of a retrobulbar abscess include pain on opening the mouth, exophthalmos, and swelling in both the orbital area and the area caudal to the last molar. Anorexia and fever often accompany the disease. Occasionally a small draining tract develops near the nasal canthus.

Treatment: The recommended treatment is to establish ventral drainage by bluntly dissecting into the orbit through an incision behind the last molar. To avoid inhalation pneumonia, general anesthesia with endotracheal intubation should be accomplished before opening the abscess. Establishing drainage and initiating appropriate systemic antibiotic therapy generally resolve clinical signs. Persistent orbital cellulitis may warrant radiographic examination of the orbit, in which case surgical exploration of the orbit should not be attempted unless a foreign body is evident.

Orbital Neoplasia

The orbit may be a primary or metastatic site for tumors (Fig 1), such as lymphosarcoma, carcinoma, fibroma, adenoma or melanoma.[5]

It is important to differentiate orbital neoplasia from orbital abscesses. Neoplasia generally causes no pain on opening the mouth or on palpation of the globe, and the cat is afebrile. The prognosis must always be considered guarded, and a physical examination and thoracic radiography should be completed before any attempts at excisional biopsy.

Orbital Parasites

Subcutaneous infection with the larvae of the fly *Cuterebra* usually is seen in rabbits, mice and chipmunks, but cats also appear to be a rela-

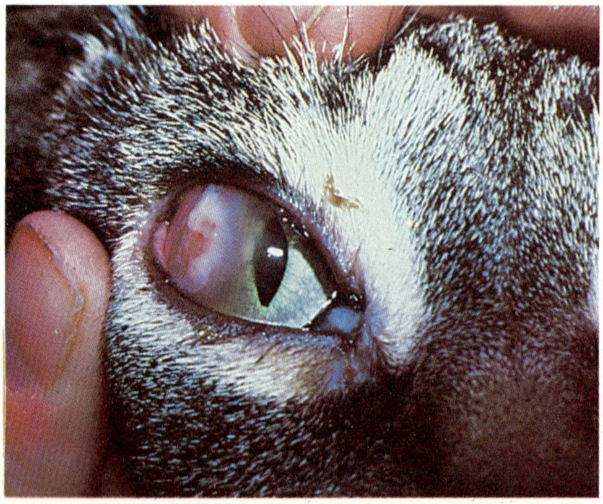

Fig C7. Eosinophilic keratitis of the lateral portion of the cornea in a 3-year-old cat. The lesion cleared completely after megestrol therapy.

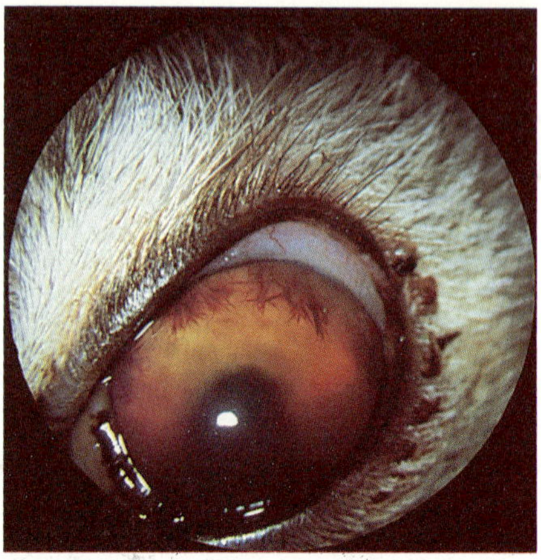

Fig C8. Interstitial keratitis, vessel infiltration of the stroma, in a cat with generalized FIP.

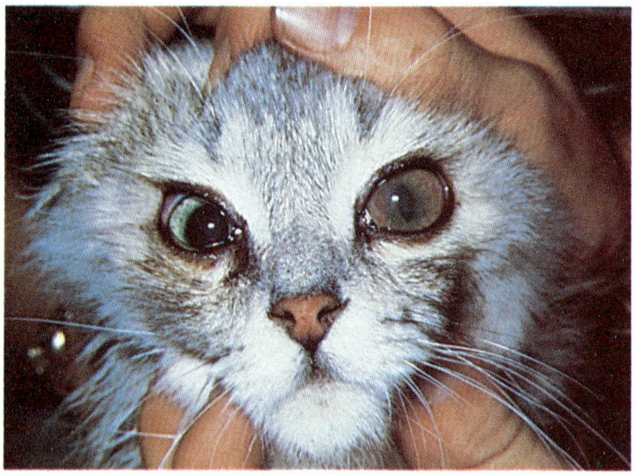

Fig C9. Unilateral anterior uveitis. Miosis, hyperemia of the iris and subnormal intraocular pressure were present.

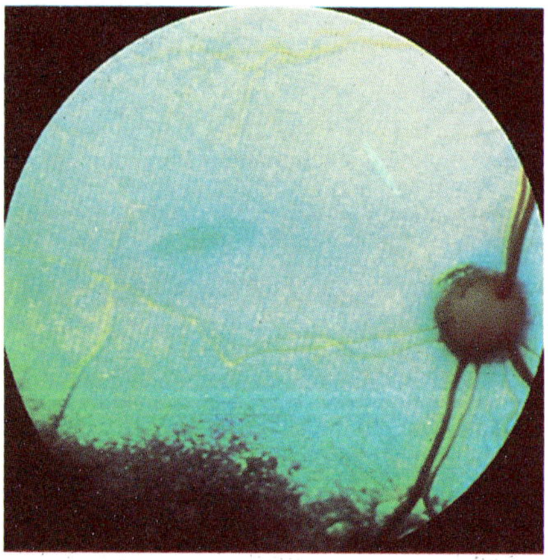

Fig C10. Area of retinal degeneration in the area centralis of a kitten on a taurine-free diet.

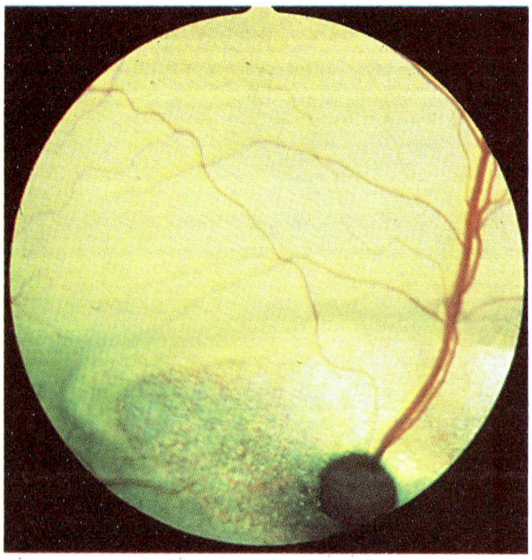

Fig C11. Retinal degeneration in a taurine-deficient cat. The large atrophic area surrounds the optic nerve.

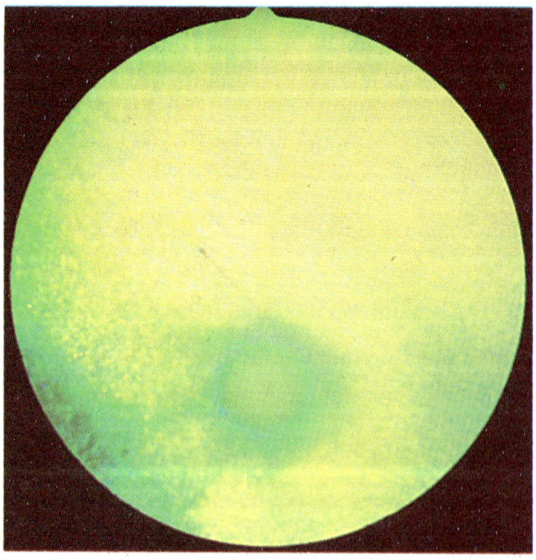

Fig C12. Total retinal degeneration, with loss of vessels, atrophy of the neurosensory retina, and a pale optic disk.

tively common host.[6] The larvae penetrate the skin to mature in the tissues and cause a draining tract in the conjunctiva or eyelids. The larvae, which may be several centimeters long are easily removed surgically.

Proptosis

Cause: When the globe is pushed from the orbit and trapped rostral to the eyelids, it can be considered proptosed. Proptosis usually follows high-velocity trauma to the orbit, as in road accidents and dog bites. Subsequent orbital hemorrhage and edema are common sequelae and serve to further displace the globe.

Treatment: Immediate medical and/or surgical therapy should be instituted. After careful evaluation of the pupillary light responses and examination of the eye, the cornea should be covered with a heavy layer of antibiotic ointment to prevent exposure keratitis. Proptosed eyes that have ruptured generally are very soft on palpation, while intact globes have normal to higher than normal intraocular pressure.[7] Eyes with dilated, unresponsive pupils may have suffered irreversible damage to the optic nerves and thus have a poor prognosis for vision. A miotic pupil generally indicates uveitis and warrants a more favorable prognosis.

Treatment is based on the cat's general physical condition. Surgical replacement of the globe should be accomplished as soon as possible. Tarsorrhaphy sutures should be left in place for 3-4 weeks to allow for resolution of orbital edema. Chloramphenicol ointment applied 2-3 times a day helps prevent corneal infection, and atropine ointment applied twice daily relieves pain and prevents synechia formation associated with uveitis. Topical corticosteroids should be used only when the cornea does not retain fluorescein dye. Systemic antibiotics and corticosteroids are generally not indicated.

Sequelae that may appear from days to weeks after proptosis include keratoconjunctivitis, lagophthalmos, cataract formation and retinal degeneration. Therefore, re-evaluation of the eye several months after the incident should include tear testing, fluorescein staining of the cornea, and funduscopic examination.

THE EYELIDS

Anatomy

The eyelids protect the eye and spread the tear film to prevent drying. The eyelids are composed of 4 layers. The external layer is normal skin. The next layer consists of the orbicularis oculi muscle, innervated by the seventh cranial nerve. A thin stromal layer is covered by the last layer, the conjunctiva.

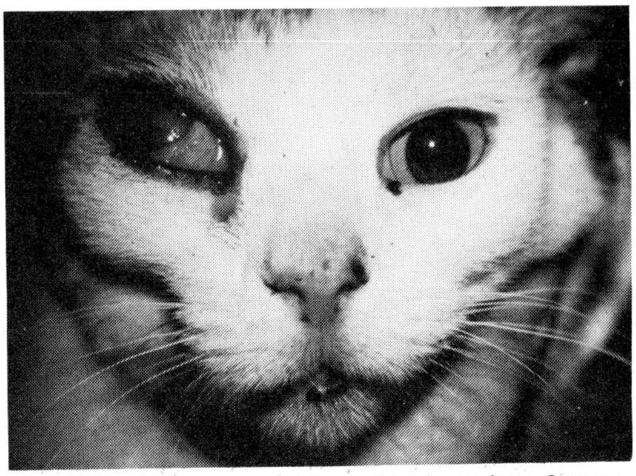

Fig 1. Exophthalmos and lagophthalmos in a 9-year-old male cat, caused by orbital and intraocular lymphosarcoma.

The lid margins contain numerous tactile hairs or cilia. Associated with the roots of these cilia are accessory sweat glands (glands of Moll) and small sebaceous glands (glands of Zeis). Caudal to the cilia is a row of openings of the Meibomian glands. The sebaceous glands contribute to the "oily" component to the tear film.

The third eyelid (nictitating membrane) of cats is similar to that of other species in that it contains serous glands, with a supporting cartilage that provides a small percentage of the aqueous portion of the tear film. The third eyelid can be voluntarily elevated by muscles innervated by the sixth cranial nerve.

Diseases of the Eyelids

Agenesis of the Upper Eyelid

A congenital absence or coloboma of all layers of the upper eyelid is uncommon in cats. When seen, the defect may be unilateral or bilateral and most often affects the lateral portion of the upper eyelid (Fig 2). The diagnosis usually is obvious. Secondary keratitis associated with exposure or trichiasis may also be observed. Surgical reconstruction of the defect is the only acceptable treatment.[8]

Ankloblepharon

Ankloblepharon is the union of the upper and lower eyelids and is normal in kittens for the first 10-12 days of life.[5] Several conditions warrant manual separation of the eyelids. First, if

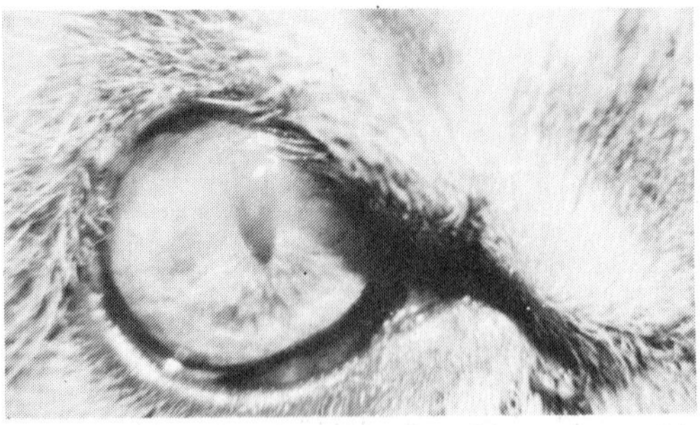

Fig 2. Agenesis of the lateral portion of the upper eyelid. The condition was bilateral in this cat.

a viral or bacterial infection of the conjunctiva or cornea (neonatal keratoconjunctivitis) should occur before normal separation at 10-12 days of age, a mucopurulent discharge appears at the nasal canthus of one or both eyes. Separation of the eyelids with a blunt instrument, careful inspection for corneal ulceration, and administration of a broad-spectrum ophthalmic antibiotic preparation constitute the treatment of choice. Second, should the lids not separate naturally by 14 days of age, they should be gently opened. The most likely cause for this delayed opening is subclinical neonatal keratoconjunctivitis. After separation of the lids, careful inspection of the cornea for ulceration is indicated.

Entropion

Congenital entropion is rare in cats. Persians, however, seem to be more often affected than other breeds. Congenital entropion usually occurs laterad on the lower eyelid. Clinical signs of blepharospasm, lacrimation and ulcerative keratitis are consistent with a diagnosis of entropion. Spastic entropion, a result of primary corneal disease, can be differentiated from congenital entropion by applying 1-2 drops of topical anesthesia, which alleviates the blepharospasm. Elimination of spastic entropion is accomplished by use of a third-eyelid flap to protect the cornea. Congenital entropion is corrected surgically by removing a crescent-shaped wedge 2-3 mm ventral to the involved lid margin.[8]

Ectropion

The eversion of the lower lid margin in cats is almost always associated with cicatricial healing of a wound or chronic inflammatory conjunctivitis, as in herpesvirus infection. Often no medical or surgical treatment is required for ectropion. Should chronic exposure conjunctivitis be associated with the lid deformity, application of an antibiotic-corticosteroid ointment usually alleviates the problem. Surgical correction of ectropion is accomplished using the V to Y technic described for dogs.[8]

Blepharitis

Inflammation of the skin of the eyelid, blepharitis, may be a result of trauma or infection. On examination, the skin on the eyelids may be red, moist or scaly. Alopecia also is a common finding.

Acute bacterial blepharitis often is associated with staphylococcal infection secondary to puncture wounds from cat fights. The affected eyelid is moist and hyperemic. Underlying edema may also be seen. Application of moist hot packs 4-6 times a day and a broad-spectrum ophthalmic antibiotic ointment usually effect a rapid cure. Systemic antibiotics may be indicated in treatment of eyelid abscesses.

Chronic blepharitis associated with encrusted, scaly skin and alopecia may indicate a parasitic or mycotic etiology. Skin scrapings, mycotic cultures and KOH preparations help differentiate mycotic from parasitic blepharitis (see Chapters 5, 16). Cats are very susceptible to infection with the rabbit mite, *Notoedres cati*. Cases of *Demodex* infestation are rare in cats. Parasitic blepharitis generally is associated with other areas of cutaneous involvement on the head and neck. Treatment with a 2.5% solution of lime sulfur, rotenone ointment or 0.25% physostigmine sulfate ophthalmic ointment usually is curative.

Mycotic blepharitis associated with *Microsporum canis* infection causes a circular lesion, with little or no pruritus. After confirming the diagnosis with a fungal culture, treatment should start with oral griseofulvin at 50 mg/kg daily for 2-4 weeks and topical tolnaftate twice daily until the lesion resolves.[4]

Granulomatous lesions unresponsive to conservative therapy should be biopsied. Infections with both *Mycobacterium* spp and lepromatous-like acid-fast bacteria have been reported. Cats with confirmed tuberculosis represent a public health hazard since the disease may be transmissible to people.

Neoplasia

Squamous-cell carcinoma is the most common tumor involving the eyelids of cats. Its occurrence seems to be related to actinic radiation exposure in lightly pigmented cats. Excisional or partial biopsy should be used to confirm the diagnosis. Cryotherapy with liquid nitrogen is currently the treatment of choice for this type of squamous-cell carcinoma.

THE LACRIMAL SYSTEM

Anatomy

The lacrimal system consists of the lacrimal gland, tear film, lacrimal puncta, canaliculi and nasolacrimal ducts. The aqueous portion of the tear film is produced in the lacrimal gland, which is located dorsolateral in the orbit. The gland of the third eyelid also contributes a small percentage to the tear volume. The aqueous tears pass through small microductules in the upper conjunctival fornix and are distributed over the cornea by blinking. Once tears have pooled in the lower conjunctival sac, blinking forces the excess into 2 small openings or puncta located just inside the lid margins both ventrad and dorsad. The tears then move down the ductuli canaliculi, which join just as they enter the lacrimal bone to form the nasolacrimal duct. The nasolacrimal ducts run bilaterally from the lacrimal bone to open in the nasopharynx. As they exit the nasolacrimal duct, tears are either swallowed or run from the nose.

Diseases of the Lacrimal System

Epiphora

Epiphora is a condition in which tears overflow the eyelid margin onto the face. It is usually a chronic condition and, although not a serious problem, often causes owners some concern. If the lacrimal puncta or canaliculi are congenitally absent or sealed by symblepharon, epiphora may result. This problem usually involves the ventral punctum or canaliculus. Atresia of the punctum may be diagnosed by flushing the dorsal canaliculus with a 25-ga blunt needle and locating the bulging conjunctiva over the ventral punctum. Incision of the conjunctiva re-establishes ventral drainage. The scarring associated with symblepharon subsequent to severe conjunctival infections generally is irreparable. A procedure involving the creation of a new nasolacrimal duct from the eye to the nasal passages, dacryocystorhinostomy, can be considered in extreme cases but has not proven a reliable procedure in cats.

In white cats, especially Persians, epiphora may result in brown discoloration of the facial hair. The epiphora may either be a result of irreversible damage to the nasolacrimal system or something as subtle as a slightly misplaced punctum. Although the practitioner may not wish to surgically correct the problem of inadequate drainage, staining of the facial hair can be eliminated through the use of tetracyclines. For reasons not yet understood, the staining property of tears is eliminated by giving the cat 5-10 mg of oral tetracycline once daily.

Keratoconjunctivitis Sicca

Cause: The absence of tears results in a condition known as "dry eye" or keratoconjunctivitis sicca. Decreased lacrimation has many causes, the most common of which is direct trauma to the lacrimal gland located dorsolateral to the globe. Severe conjunctivitis may result in edema or scarring, which in turn stops the flow of tears through the microtubules from the lacrimal gland to the upper fornix. Neurologic dysfunction of the parasympathetic (seventh cranial) nerves supplying the lacrimal gland can also cause decreased lacrimation.

Clinical Signs: The presenting signs include a thick, ropy mucous discharge, conjunctivitis and keratitis. Ulceration may also occur later in the course of the disease. The confirmatory test is the Schirmer tear test.

The Schirmer tear test is conducted by placing a strip of sterile filter paper (Cooper Labs) over the lower lid. Each strip has a notch at which the strip is folded at a right angle to facilitate placement in the eye. The strip is left in the unanesthetized eye for one minute and is then removed, and the amount of wetting is recorded in millimeters per minute.

The normal Schirmer tear test value for cats is 16.9 mm $\pm$ 5.7 mm of wetting in one minute. Values of 5 mm/min or less are diagnostic for keratoconjunctivitis sicca.

Treatment: Treatment is aimed at supplementing lacrimation by application of artificial tears 6-10 times a day and reducing the conjunctivitis with antibiotic-corticosteroid drops 3 times a day. Corticosteroids are used only if the cornea does not retain fluorescein dye. The lacrimal gland can be stimulated with parasympathomimetics. A 1% solution of pilocarpine is placed on the food at a dosage of 2 drops/4.5 kg (10 lb) twice daily. Cats with no tear production have a poor prognosis for restoration of function, whereas those with tear test readings of 2-5 mm/min usually respond to medical therapy. Should the condition of the cornea deteriorate during treatment or the owner's compliance with therapy wane, parotid duct transposition is a surgical alternative to life-long medication.[8] Affected cats should be re-evaluated at least 4 times a year after a satisfactory medical or surgical correction has been achieved.

THE CONJUNCTIVA

Anatomy

The conjunctiva can be divided into the portion that lines the eyelids (palpebral conjunctiva) and that which covers the globe (bulbar conjunctiva). These 2 areas of conjunctiva are continuous and meet ventrad and dorsad to form the fornix.

The conjunctiva itself is composed of layered, nonkeratinizing, squamous epithelial cells. Goblet cells, which produce the mucous portion of the tear film, are found throughout the conjunctiva. With inflammation of the conjunctiva, these cells hypertrophy and produce the excess mucus associated with external ocular disease.

The deeper layers of the conjunctiva contain lymph channels, arteries and veins. The sensory innervation of the conjunctiva is provided by the ophthalmic branch of the fifth cranial nerve.

Diseases of the Conjunctiva

Conjunctivitis

Inflammation and infection of the conjunctiva of cats is common. Conjunctivitis can be acute or chronic and may become a major problem in breeding colonies. Clinical signs of acute conjunctivitis include marked chemosis, mucopurulent ocular discharge and blepharospasm. These signs often are associated with rhinitis and glossitis caused by a herpesvirus or calicivirus infection. Secondary bacterial infections often coexist with viral, chlamydial and mycoplasmal conjunctivitis.

Irritation from foreign bodies and chemicals is rare. However, the eye worm, *Thelazia californiensis,* reportedly causes catarrhal conjunctivitis in cats in the western US.[9]

Viral Conjunctivitis: Viral conjunctivitis is usually associated with upper respiratory disease. Herpesvirus is the most common viral agent encountered and is widespread in the feline population. The virus seems to most severely affect young cats, causing mucopurulent rhinitis, conjunctivitis and corneal ulceration.[10] Severe symblepharon can result from acute herpetic conjunctivitis in young cats. (Figs C1, C2).

The clinical signs of viral conjunctivitis vary from a serous to purulent discharge, chemosis, hyperemia and/or blepharospasm. Chronic cases may involve symblepharon, which can result in chronic epiphora. In the early stages of the disease, only one eye may be infected, but the other usually becomes involved in 7-10 days.[11]

Conjunctivitis from herpesvirus infection is often associated with severe respiratory disease, while mild respiratory signs and ulceration of the oral mucosa indicate a probable calicivirus infection. Conjunctival cytologic examination and viral cultures help confirm the diagnosis. Viral cultures can be submitted in either Eagle's medium or sterile skim milk. Microscopic examination of Giemsa-stained conjunctival scrapings may reveal giant epithelial cells, RBC and neutrophils. The absence of mycoplasmal or chlamydial inclusions in these is additional evidence of a viral etiology, but this is not pathognomonic.

Treatment consists of application of idoxuridine ointment (*eg,* Stoxil:Smith Kline) 5 times a day or drops every 2 hours for 20-30 days. Adenine arabinoside (*eg,* Vira-A 3%:Parke-Davis) may be substituted for idoxuridine. Broad-spectrum antibiotic drops or ointments should be used along with the antiviral drugs to prevent secondary bacterial infection. Corticosteroids are not used if corneal ulceration is present. Their use in viral conjunctivitis is controversial, but may help some individuals. Isolation of infected cats during treatment is indicated.

Viral conjunctivitis runs a course that may last 2-8 weeks. Although some cats have recurrence of the disease, most recover completely with treatment.

Chlamydial Conjunctivitis: Chlamydial conjunctivitis is caused by *Chlamydia psittaci,* probably the most common cause of conjunctivitis in cats.[7] Although *Chlamydia* can cause rhinitis, this rarely is a concurrent finding in chlamydial conjunctivitis.

The disease occurs in cats of all ages and usually starts with unilateral involvement, the other eye becoming infected in 7-10 days. Chemosis and blepharospasm usually are less severe than with herpetic conjunctivitis, but chronic chlamydial conjunctivitis may lead to development of follicles on both the palpebral and bulbar sides of the nictitating membrane. The cause can be determined during the first several weeks by detection of intracytoplasmic inclusion bodies in Giemsa-stained conjunctival epithelial cells on cytologic examination (Fig C3). Culture of the organism requires inoculation of chick embryos and often is not performed by local laboratories.

Treatment consists of topically applied oxytetracycline ointment 4 times a day for 1-2 weeks. Other antibiotics, such as chloramphenicol and gentamicin, can also be prescribed, but tetracyclines are probably most effective. If treated early, the disease has a course of 4-6 days. If left untreated, however, it may last several months and the cat may remain a carrier.

Mycoplasmal Conjunctivitis: Mycoplasma gatae and *M felis* can cause conjunctivitis in cats. They may be either primary agents or secondary invaders. The conjunctivitis produced by *Mycoplasma* is less severe than that caused by herpesvirus and *Chlamydia,* the extent of invasion seeming directly related to the amount of stress on the cat. As with the previously discussed organisms, it may involve one or both eyes but ultimately becomes bilateral. The discharge associated with mycoplasmal conjunctivitis is mucopurulent and a pseudomembrane may form on the conjunctiva.

Diagnosis can be confirmed by culture or cytologic examination. Numerous small, basophilic inclusions on the surface of Giemsa-stained epithelial cells are highly suggestive of mycoplasmal infection (Fig C4).[12]

Treatment with topical tetracycline or chloramphenicol ointment 4 times a day for 7-10 days usually resolves the disease. If untreated, the disease is generally self-limiting and resolves in about a month.

THE CORNEA

Anatomy

The feline cornea is similar to that of most other domestic animals. It is transparent and oval. The 4 layers that compose the cornea are the epithelium, stroma, Descemet's membrane and endothelium. The 6- to 8-cell-thick epithelium composes the most external layer. The cells in the epithelium consist of basal cells, wing cells and superficial squamous cells. The superficial squamous cells have numerous microvilli that help bind the 8-micron-thick tear layer to the epithelium.

The thickest layer of the cornea is the stroma (substantia propria), which is composed of laminated layers of spacially arranged collagen fibers and fibroblasts (keratocytes).

Descemet's membrane is actually the thick basement membrane of the endothelial layer. The single layer of cells that line the inside of the cornea are derived from mesodermal tissue but are conventionally referred to as endothelial cells. They have poor regenerative ability in cats and healing of a wound in this layer is accomplished by the spreading of existing cells into any defects rather than by new cell growth.

Both the epithelium and endothelium are selective to fat-soluble materials and both layers actively pump fluid from the hydroscopic stroma. Thus, any loss of epithelium or endothelium results in overhydration of the cornea and a clinically "hazy" appearance.

Diseases of the Cornea

The feline cornea is rarely affected by congenital abnormalities, such as microcornea, keratoconus or dermoid cysts. Superficial keratitis and ulceration are common and similar to that in other species in clinical findings and treatment. However, cats are affected by several corneal diseases essentially unique to that species.

Herpetic Keratitis

Cause: The herpesvirus that causes rhinotracheitis and conjunctivitis is also associated with ulcerative keratitis, the corneal form being less prevalent than the conjunctival form. Herpetic keratitis can infect cats of any age but, unlike the conjunctival form, is more common in adults. Ulceration of one cornea is not necessarily followed by involvement of the other as is the case with herpetic conjunctivitis.

Clinical Signs: As the virus replicates in the corneal epithelial cells, it has a cytopathic effect that eventually destroys the cells. An early clinical sign is small, punctate ulcers that may or may not retain fluorescein dye. As the virus infects more cells, the small lesions coalesce to form a linear or branching pattern. This branching pattern is the "dendritic ulcer" so typical of this disease.[11] The deeper stroma may also become involved if secondary bacterial infection occurs. Superficial neovascularity of the cornea is common in chronic cases and superficial corneal scarring may occur after the lesion has healed (Fig C5).

The herpesvirus seems to survive indefinitely in the small nerve fibers or ganglion of the fifth cranial nerve (trigeminal). In animal models of herpetic keratitis, the virus seems to become reactivated during times of stress or corticosteroid therapy. This also appears to be the case in cats, as the disease may recur in times of stress.

Treatment: Treatment with antiviral agents is indicated. Idoxuridine ointment should be applied 5 times a day for 30 days. Idoxuridine drops must be used every 1-2 hours. As an alternative treatment, topical application of a solution made of 1 part povidone iodine solution and 4 parts sterile saline, 1 drop applied every 2-3 hours, has proven an inexpensive and effective substitute for idoxuridine.

A broad-spectrum topical antibiotic should also be used to help prevent secondary bacterial infection. If the cat is exhibiting discomfort, atropine ointment can be applied twice daily for its cycloplegic effect. After the cornea no longer retains fluorescein dye, topical corticosteroids may be administered to eliminate the vascular infiltration and minimize scarring.

Corneal Sequestration

A corneal disease, unique to cats, that is usually manifested as a hard, raised brown-black plaque on the central cornea has been referred to as corneal sequestration, corneal mummification, or simply a "black spot."[13] Persians and Siamese seem to have a higher than average predisposition, suggesting a genetic propensity for this disease.

Cause: The cause of corneal sequestration is unknown. It is thought by some that a previous injury may initiate deposition of pigmented material within the anterior corneal stroma. Others think an abnormal metabolic pathway involving endogenous epinephrine may underlie the cause.

Clinical Signs: The early phase of the disease is characterized by a small, brown deposit of material in the center of the cornea. The material is subepithelial and spreads within the anterior stroma. As the sequestration grows in size, the overlying epithelium is lost and the cat has the typical signs of ulcerative keratitis. The lesion itself does not retain fluorescein. After a period of weeks to months, the lesion becomes elevated and black (Fig C6). The stroma surrounding the lesion usually undergoes necrosis and the cornea becomes neovascularized. Occasionally a secondary bacterial or fungal infection develops and must be treated accordingly.

Treatment: In some cases the sequestrum sloughs spontaneously, but few owners are willing to wait for this to occur. Therefore, keratectomy is the treatment of choice. In most cases, however, the pigment has invaded so deeply into the stroma that complete removal is impossible. Postsurgical treatment should consist of topical antibiotics until healing has occurred. The cornea should then be treated with a topical antibiotic-corticosteroid preparation until the neovascularity has resolved. Unfortunately, even after surgery the sequestration may recur in the same eye or may develop in the other eye.

Eosinophilic Keratitis

A keratitis clinically resembling pannus in German Shepherd dogs has been observed in cats.[14] The disease is characterized by a chronic, invasive infiltration of the superficial cornea by a granulomatous mass (Fig C7). A corneal scraping or excisional biopsy can differentiate the disease from tumors, such as fibrous histiocytomas, and other diseases. Large numbers of eosinophils in a corneal scraping or biopsy are pathognomonic for eosinophilic keratitis.

Treatment with topical corticosteroids has been effective in some cases; however, dramatic regression of the disease can be achieved with oral megestrol acetate (Ovaban:Schering). Daily treatment at 0.5 mg/kg for 10 days usually causes complete remission of the lesions. In some cases, megestrol acetate must be given once or twice weekly indefinitely to prevent recurrence. It has been suggested that eosinophilic keratitis is part of the eosinophilic granuloma complex; however, no cats with ocular involvement seem to manifest other signs of the complex.

Corneal Dystrophy

The deposition of lipids, cholesterol, Ca or combinations of these materials results in opacification and degeneration of the cornea, referred to as corneal dystrophy. Cats can have many types of corneal dystrophy, 2 of which are unique to the species.

A hereditary corneal dystrophy has been observed in stump-tailed Manx cats. The dystrophy is first evident at about 4 months of age.[15] Initially there is slight edema of the anterior corneal stroma. Over a period of a year, the epithelium becomes more edematous and bullous keratopathy develops (Fig 3). By 2 years of age the bullae begin to degenerate, leading to rupture and loss of the globe. The degenerative process appears to be irreversible and treatment is unrewarding. As the disease apparently is an autosomal recessive trait, genetic counseling and test breeding to eliminate the trait are indicated in a breeding colony. Affected cats have a poor prognosis for recovery and eventually lose both eyes to the disease.

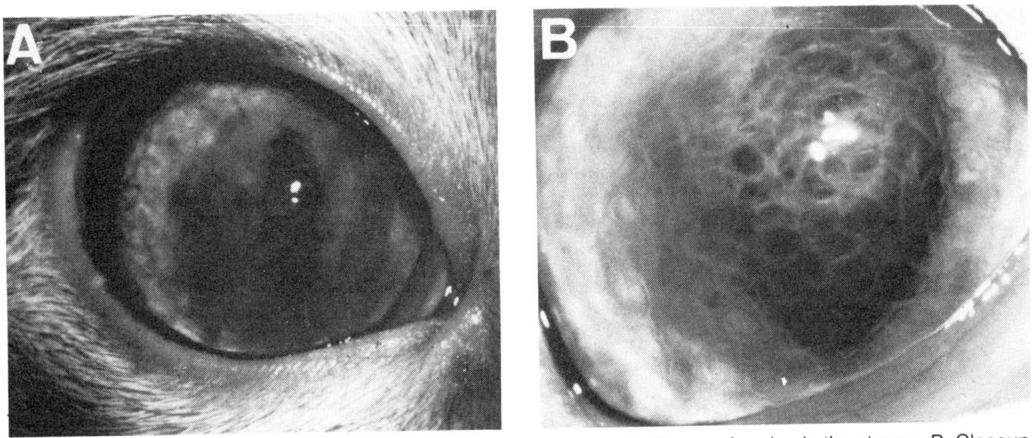

Fig 3. A. Corneal dystrophy in a Manx. The cornea is edematous and bullae are forming in the stroma. B. Closeup of the eye of the cat in Figure A. (Courtesy of Dr S.I. Bistner and Lea & Febiger)

The second type of corneal dystrophy unique to cats is a polysaccharide-glycolipid storage disease known as GM_1-gangliosidosis.[16] The disease seems to exclusively affect newborn kittens. Affected kittens have a mild corneal haze and are ataxic. The corneas are clear enough to visualize the anterior segment, but the haziness often precludes observation of the retina, which may have small foci of degeneration. The ataxia in this disease should be differentiated from that seen with cerebellar hypoplasia caused by panleukopenia virus infection. Kittens with cerebellar hypoplasia usually have no corneal lesions as in GM_1-gangliosidosis. Histologically, the cornea contains vacuolated endothelial cells and the retina contains ganglion cells full of lamellated inclusions typical of glycolipid storage diseases. This disease is rare and no effective treatment is available.

Interstitial Keratitis

Infiltration of the deeper layers of the corneal stroma with vessels is the classic sign of interstitial keratitis. The presence of vessels deeper in the cornea is more often associated with an active inflammatory process of the anterior uveal tract rather than primary corneal disease (Fig C8). Most cats with interstitial keratitis have no corneal ulceration or other corneal disease. Close examination may reveal keratic precipitates on the endothelium, miosis and increased protein in the anterior chamber (flare). Corneal opacification secondary to interstitial edema and endothelial decompensation is also common. Diagnosis and treatment should be directed at establishing the cause of and eliminating the underlying uveitis.

THE UVEAL TRACT

Anatomy

The uvea consists of the iris and ciliary body in the rostral aspect and the choroid in the caudal aspect. These tissues provide the major vascular supply to the interior of the globe.

The iris histologically has, rostral to caudal, a surface epithelium, a stroma containing vessels, sphincter muscles, and 2 layers of pigmented epithelium. The iris is the division between the anterior chamber, which is the space from the corneal endothelium to the face of the iris, and the posterior chamber, which is the space from the caudal aspect of the iris to the face of the vitreous. The iris contains 2 sets of smooth muscle fibers. The constrictor fibers are located parallel to the pupillary slit and are controlled by the parasympathetics of the oculomotor nerve (cranial nerve III). These fibers cause the pupil to constrict or become miotic.

Peripherally in the iris stroma are the radially placed dilator fibers, which are under sympathetic control. Stimulation of these fibers causes mydriasis or dilation of the pupil. In the rostral aspect, the base of the iris joins the cornea and sclera to form the iridocorneal angle, through which aqueous humor drains from the eye.

In the posterior chamber and caudal to the iris is located the ciliary body. The ciliary body contains 3 muscles that play a minor role in ad-

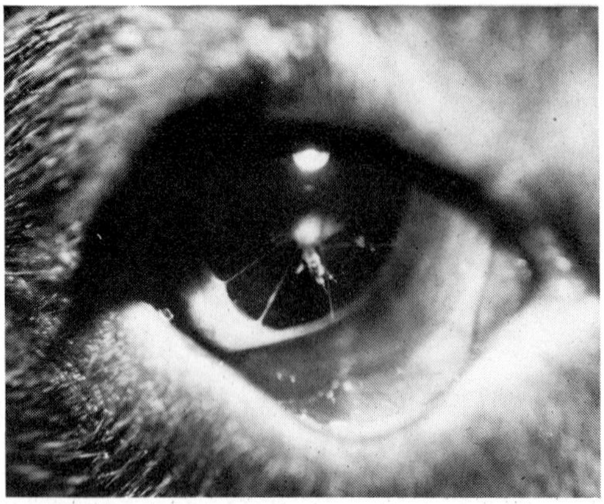

Fig 4. Persistent pupillary membranes. The pupil is mid-sized and bands of membrane emanate from the collarette. The central cornea is opaque where the bands adhere to the endothelium.

justing tension on the lens zonules emanating from the ciliary body, thus assisting in accommodation. Accommodation, the mechanism by which the eye focuses on an object at various distances, is thought to be relatively well developed in cats as compared with other domestic animals.

The choroid is the caudal extension of the uveal tract and lies deep to the retina. Going from the retina toward the sclera, it consists of the choriocapillaris, the tapetum (dorsad only) and the major vascular layer.

The choroid's main function is to provide a vascular supply to the outer layers of the retina. The tapetum is a cellular layer 60-80 μ thick and is the highly reflective tissue observed in the dorsal half of the retina of most cats. Its function is not clearly understood but one common hypothesis is that it aids nocturnal animals by additionally stimulating the retina with the light reflected from its surface.

Diseases of the Uveal Tract

The uveal tract can be affected by congenital or acquired diseases. Congenital defects in formation of the uveal tract, such as aniridia and colobomas of the iris, are rare.

Persistent Pupillary Membrane

This disease represents a developmental anomaly involving the iris. During embryologic development, the face of the iris is a solid structure. Shortly before birth, and continuing for about the first 10 days of life, the center of the iris atrophies, creating the pupil. Small strands of this mesodermal remnant may remain. These strands of pupillary membrane always emanate from the junction of the constrictor and dilator fibers, the collarette. Generally the persistent strands of membrane are few in number and simply cross the pupil or traverse the face of the iris without impairing visual function. Occasionally a strand of this persistent membrane adheres to either the anterior lens capsule or the endothelium of the cornea (Fig 4).

The diagnosis of persistent pupillary membrane is based on locating the emanating point of the strand on the collarette. This allows the clinician to differentiate this condition from iris prolapse and anterior or posterior synechiation, which involve only the pupillary border. There is no medical therapy and surgery is rarely attempted to resolve any problems associated with persistent pupillary membranes.

Albinism

In mostly white or pure white cats, the albinotic trait may be expressed by the lack of pigment in one or both irides. Heterochromia is the term used to describe irides of different colors without implying any disease state. In cats with multicolored or pink irides, there is also a tendency for deafness.

Hyphema

The presence of frank blood in the anterior chamber is termed hyphema. Blood dyscrasias, warfarin poisoning, retinal detachments and intraocular tumors may cause hyphema. However, trauma to the anterior uveal tract, with resultant bleeding, is the most common cause of hyphema in cats.

The amount of blood present in the anterior chamber may vary from a small spot to total filling of the anterior chamber. Small amounts of blood usually clot and dissipate within a week. Persistent hyphema that remains unclotted indicates a more severe underlying problem and warrants a poor prognosis for recovery of vision.

Treatment for hyphema is a controversial topic. Topical or intraocular use of enzymes does not speed clot resorption. The fact that red cells, once released from the clot matrix, simply flow out of the iridocorneal angle has led some investigators to propose use of 1% pilocarpine to open the angle. However, concern for patient comfort and possible formation of posterior synechiae as a sequela has led to use of atropine for its cycloplegic and mydriatic action.

In my experience, topical use of corticosteroids, in the absence of any corneal lesions, in combination with atropine ointment twice daily has been adequate therapy. All cases of hyphema should be followed until their complete resolution to avoid complications, such as iris bombe and secondary glaucoma.

Uveitis

The result of any traumatic or infectious process that causes inflammation of the iris, ciliary body or choroid is uveitis. Although the inflammatory process may appear to involve only the anterior segment, the entire uveal tract generally is involved.

Signs of anterior uveitis include aqueous flare, miosis and subnormal intraocular pressure. Additionally, the iris may become hyperemic and hypopyon may occur in the ventral anterior chamber (Figs C9, 5). Clumps of inflammatory cells may be attached to the corneal endothelium. The conjunctiva is typically congested, and blepharospasm and photophobia may be present.

Anterior uveitis, also referred to as iridocyclitis, may be classified as endogenous or exogenous. Exogenous anterior uveitis usually is unilateral and almost always the result of blunt or penetrating traumatic injury to the globe. Uveitis as a result of blunt trauma may be treated conservatively with topical corticosteroids and atropine 2-4 times a day. Penetrating wounds can lead to bacterial endophthalmitis and should be treated vigorously with topical antibiotics and atropine 4-8 times a day. Systemic antibiotics, such as chloramphenicol or amoxicillin, should be given if a penetrating wound is diagnosed or suspected.

Endogenous anterior uveitis is almost always a reflection of some systemic disease. Establishing the diagnosis of the underlying cause for bilateral anterior uveitis can be one of the most challenging tasks in feline medicine. The primary differential diagnosis of acute or chronic anterior uveitis should include the feline leukemia complex, feline infectious peritonitis and toxoplasmosis.[17,18] Less common causes of anterior uveitis include cryptococcosis, blastomycosis, histoplasmosis and septicemia. The diagnosis and management of these diseases are covered in the appropriate chapters of this text. Often the prognosis for recovery is poor.

Although an etiologic diagnosis, such as systemic mycosis, may preclude systemic use of corticosteroids, topical use of these drugs would be

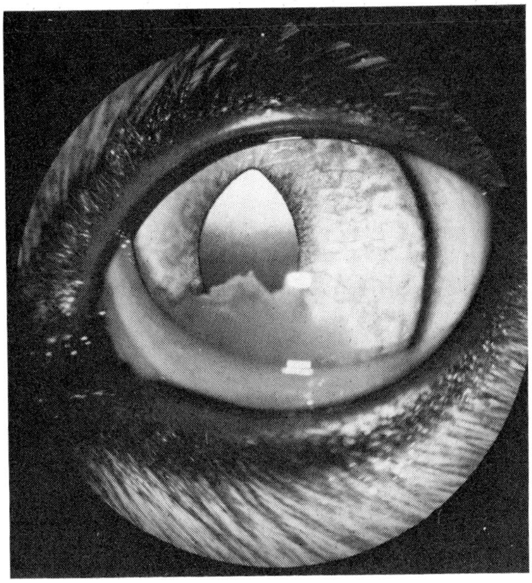

Fig 5. Anterior uveitis in a cat with hypopyon.

the treatment of choice for anterior uveitis. Topical dexamethasone applied hourly or a subconjunctival injection of triamcinolone acetonide can be beneficial in a short period. Posterior synechia and cataract formation are common in eyes that have recovered from anterior uveitis.

Posterior Uveitis and Retinitis

Those diseases associated with anterior uveitis are also most commonly involved in posterior uveitis (choroiditis). The retina, because of its intimate contact with the choroid, is almost always involved in active choroiditis. The result is chorioretinitis, which can be diagnosed with careful ophthalmoscopic examination. The clinical appearance of active chorioretinitis varies with the disease and location in the retina. In early stages, areas of the tapetal retina may appear hazy and do not come into focus on the same plane as the rest of the retina. This is due to edema, either subretinal or within the retina. In major infectious systemic diseases, the hazy areas eventually become white to black granulomatous lesions as the inflammatory cells attempt to wall off the offending organism. In the nontapetal area, the lesions appear as light spots or depigmented areas. It is important to differentiate active from inactive lesions. Inactive chorioretinitis lesions are actually scars on the retina and usually are characterized in the tapetal area by a dark center, representing pigment infiltration, with an area of surrounding

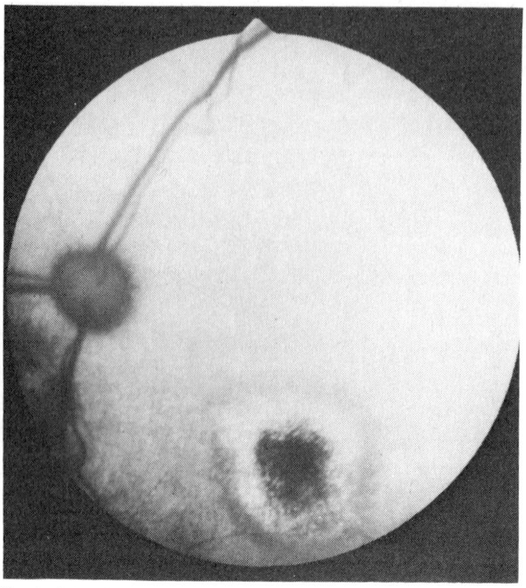

Fig 6. Inactive chorioretinitis lesion dorsomedial to the optic nerve and characterized by a rim of central atrophic retina with central pigment infiltration.

retinal atrophy (Fig 6). These lesions have very distinct borders and are not elevated.

As topical and subconjunctival corticosteroids do not penetrate the caudal portion of the globe at therapeutic levels, treatment of chorioretinitis involves use of high levels of systemic corticosteroids. Systemic use of corticosteroids, however, may be contraindicated in the face of many, if not most, diseases reflected by chorioretinitis. Therefore, as definitive a diagnosis as possible should be made before their use.

Glaucoma

The elevation of intraocular pressure above 15-25 mm Hg is defined as glaucoma. The disease is associated with obstruction of the iridocorneal angle rather than overproduction of aqueous humor. Peripheral anterior synechiation secondary to uveitis, intraocular tumors, anterior lens luxation or posterior synechia leading to iris bombe all can result in glaucoma. Clinical signs of glaucoma include a fixed, dilated pupil, subluxated or luxated lens, retinal atrophy and cupping of the optic nerve head. Buphthalmos generally is seen in chronically affected eyes (Fig 7), which are usually blind.

Glaucoma often reflects systemic disease. Cryptococcosis and ocular lymphoma associated with the feline leukemia complex may cause glaucoma without showing any other clinical signs. The glaucoma may persist for several months to a year before the cat shows signs of the primary disease. Therefore, as with anterior uveitis and chorioretinitis, a complete diagnostic work-up is warranted in most cases of glaucoma.

Topical use of 4% pilocarpine 4 times daily and oral administration of dichlorphenamide (Daranide:Merck), a carbonic anhydrase inhibitor, at 0.5 mg/kg (1 mg/lb), satisfactorily reduce intraocular pressure in most cases. However, medical therapy cannot benefit a buphthalmic, blind eye; cyclocryosurgery, an intraocular prosthesis, or enucleation may be indicated.[19]

THE LENS

Anatomy

The crystalline lens is surrounded by a capsule and suspended in the posterior chamber by the lens zonules attached to its equator. The lens capsule completely surrounds the lens and is considered to be a basement membrane. The epithelium of the lens lines the inside of only the anterior lens capsule. These epithelial cells migrate toward the equator throughout life and become lens fibers. The lens can be divided into the nucleus or central portion and the cortical regions. The lens grows throughout life and is nourished by aerobic metabolism.

Diseases of the Lens

Congenital disease of the lens is rare in cats and such conditions as congenital aphakia and

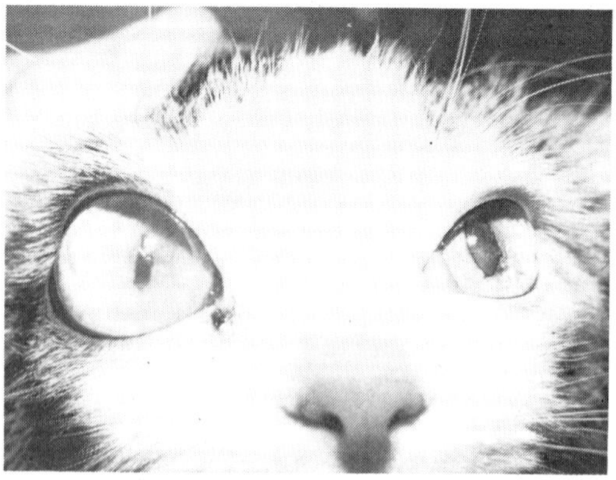

Fig 7. Buphthalmos secondary to chronic glaucoma of unknown etiology. The pupil has been constricted by instillation of a miotic.

lenticonus have not been reported. Likewise, no hereditary trait for cataracts has been reported.

Cataract

An opacity on the lens capsule or within the lens itself is a cataract (Fig 8). The causes of cataracts can include trauma, diabetes mellitus and senile degeneration. Cataract formation also is a common sequela to anterior uveitis. Clinical evaluation of a cataract should include a complete history, careful examination of pupillary responses to light, determination of intraocular pressure, examination of the lens after mydriasis, and funduscopic examination if the retina can be visualized.

Classification of cataracts is based on their location in the lens, age or underlying cause. Bilateral cataracts are associated with congenital and diabetic causes and are uncommon in cats. Unilateral cataracts, as a result of trauma, are the most common type in this species.

Trauma to the lens, by a penetrating wound or by blunt force, can cause degeneration of the lens capsule. Once the capsule is compromised, the highly antigenic, soluble lens proteins can leak from the capsule and incite a "foreign-body" uveitis. This phakoanaphylactic uveitis is easily treated with topical corticosteroids. Monitoring intraocular pressure, which is subnormal in uveitis and returns to normal as the uveitis subsides, is the best method of determining when to discontinue treatment.

Surgical removal of monocular cataracts is usually contraindicated since the purpose of cataract surgery is to restore functional vision. Surgical removal of one or both lenses in the case of bilateral cataracts re-establishes vision if the underyling retina is in good health.[20] This can be determined by the history, the presence of good pupillary responses to light, and electroretinography. If the cataract has affected only the central portion of the lens, as with some congenital cataracts, the use of atropine as a mydriatic may re-establish vision and eliminate the need for surgery.

Nuclear Sclerosis

As the lens grows throughout life, the lens fibers in the nucleus become compacted. This change may impart a hazy appearance to the lens on gross examination; however, no opacities are evident in the lens after dilation of the pupil. The nucleus may appear as a clear sphere within the lens. Nuclear sclerosis is easily differentiated from cataracts in that the retina is clearly visible and there are no visual deficits in cats with nuclear sclerosis.

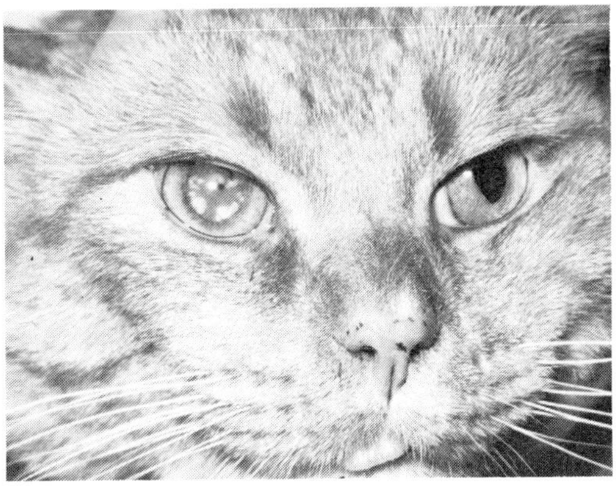

Fig 8. Unilateral cataract secondary to trauma in a 5-year-old male.

Lens Luxation

Displacement of the lens from its normal position is a relatively common sequela to trauma or glaucoma. A lens that has lost a portion of its zonular connections yet remains in a relatively normal position can be considered subluxated. Confirmation of the diagnosis of subluxation can be based on 2 findings. First, as the gaze or position of the head changes rapidly, the iris appears to tremble over the area from which the lens is displaced. This is termed iridodenesis. Second, on dilation of the pupil, a clear crescent, the aphakic crescent, appears peripheral to the equator of the lens. This is absolute evidence of a subluxated lens. A subluxated lens warrants no treatment and only periodic evaluation. In cases of glaucoma or trauma, the underlying cause should be treated.

Completely luxated lenses generally occur in association with chronic glaucoma after a globe has become buphthalmic. If the lens has become displaced caudad into the vitreous, there is no indication for surgical removal. However, if the lens has luxated into the anterior chamber, it may cause glaucoma from pupillary block or physical damage to the endothelium of the cornea. Surgical removal of the lens is the treatment of choice for anterior lens luxation. This procedure is far more difficult than it would appear and should be performed only by an accomplished ophthalmic surgeon. As is the case with subluxated lenses, any underlying disease should be treated. Generally, a lens that has lost all zonular attachment becomes cataractous in time.

This may be of little consequence if the luxated lens is no longer in the visual axis.

THE RETINA

Anatomy

The feline retina is anatomically similar to that of most other carnivores. The dorsal portion has a brightly colored tapetal area that usually surrounds the optic nerve. The retinal vessels emanate from the periphery of the optic nerve. The retina has a clearly visible, avascular area, the area centralis, located lateral to and slightly dorsal to the optic nerve. This area is composed mainly of cone photoreceptors.

Diseases of the Retina

Congenital and Hereditary Diseases

Cats are relatively free of hereditary and congenital retinal defects. Progressive retinal atrophy, with its decreased retinal vascularity, atrophic neurosensory retina and eventual blindness, has been documented in only 2 litters of related Persian cats.[5] The mode of inheritance appears to be autosomal recessive.

Prenatal panleukopenia virus infection produces areas of focal retinal dysplasia and atrophy in kittens.[21] Congenital retinal atrophy often occurs in kittens with cerebellar hypoplasia.

Retinal Hemorrhage

Retinal hemorrhages are a common ophthalmoscopic finding in hemobartonellosis, thrombocytopenia, hypertension, uremia and the feline leukemia complex. The hemorrhagic areas generally are intraretinal and recognized as small focal spots of hemorrhage. The small areas of hemorrhage resolve as the underlying problem is corrected.

Central retinal degeneration, progressive retinal atrophy and diffuse retinal atrophy were all terms previously used to describe various stages of what is now known to be a single disease.[22-24]

Taurine, an amino acid nonessential in other species and endogenously produced from cysteine, is required for normal retinal health in cats. Cats apparently cannot produce enough taurine and require dietary supplementation of this amino acid. In experimental studies, cats fed a taurine-free diet developed retinal deficiencies, photoreceptor cell malfunctions and subsequent photoreceptor cell death after about 23 weeks.[25] Clinical reports of numerous cats fed dog food diets and subsequently developing classic lesions of feline central retinal degeneration have also appeared in the literature. Investigations of both dog and cat foods showed variable and sometimes inadequate taurine levels.[22] It is now recognized that a dietary deficiency of taurine is responsible for central retinal degeneration in cats.

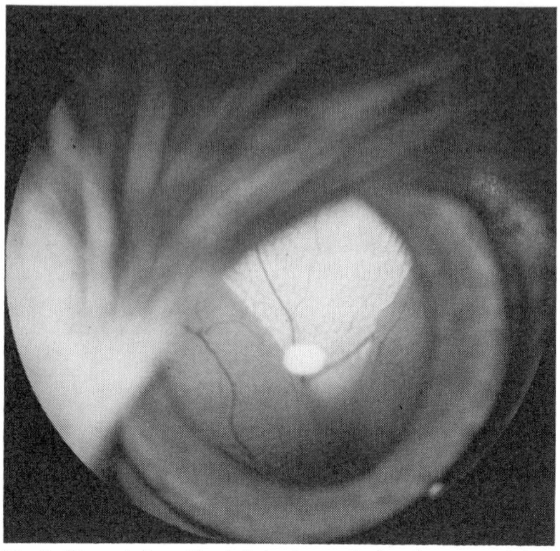

Fig 9. Complete retinal detachment of unknown origin. The retina is floating in the vitreous cavity.

The retinal changes observable ophthalmoscopically begin with a subtle granularity in the center of the area centralis (Fig C10). The lesion progresses to an elliptical area of focal hyperreflectivity representing photoreceptor cell loss. As the process continues, the area of hyper-reflectivity increases in size and encompasses the retina from the area centralis to the nasal side of the optic disc (Fig C11). The end stage of the disease is complete retinal atrophy, with loss of retinal vessels and generalized hyper-reflectivity (Fig C12). During the course of degeneration, the pupillary reflex to light changes from normal in the early stages to a fixed mydriatic state with complete degeneration. Vision degenerates to blindness as the entire retina is affected.

If the disease is recognized in its early stages, it can usually be arrested by dietary supplementation of 100 mg taurine daily or by increasing the intake of seafood, which is rich in taurine.

Retinal Detachment

Detachment of the neurosensory retina from the retinal pigment epithelium is common in cats. As with chorioretinitis, retinal detachment is often associated with generalized systemic disease, and a complete medical work-up should follow diagnosis of this condition. Such diseases as lymphosarcoma, FIP, cryptococcosis, histoplasmosis, glomerulonephritis and hypertension can all cause retinal detachment.

Retinal detachment, in its early stages, may appear ophthalmoscopically as small bullae on the retinal surface. In complete retinal detachment, a white veil of retinal tissue floats in the vitreous cavity. The retina may become totally detached from the ora serrata and can be found lying in the ventral vitreous (Fig 9). Complete detachment often obscures the optic nerve.

The condition may resolve spontaneously or may require medical treatment. Treatment consisting of oral prednisolone at 0.25 mg/kg and oral furosemide at 1 mg/kg given BID for a week results in reattachment in most cases. Treatment instituted early in the disease warrants a much more favorable prognosis. Surgical treatment of detachments is not recommended. Reattachment of a retina, either spontaneously or with treatment, may result in retinal folds or atrophic areas.

NEUROPHTHALMOLOGIC DISEASES

Anisocoria

Unequal pupil size is termed anisocoria. This condition is associated with diseases affecting both the parasympathetic and sympathetic innervation to the pupil. The first problem in assessing anisocoria is to determine which pupil is affected.

Causes of a single dilated pupil include exposure to a mydriatic, glaucoma, interruption in the parasympathetic innervation (Addi's tonic pupil) or rupture of the optic nerve. The iris is innervated with parasympathetics that travel through the ciliary ganglion and short ciliary nerves. The lateral and medial halves of the iris have separate or branching innervation by the parasympathetics and a lesion in these fibers can cause a unique D-shaped pupil on the affected side.

Causes of a constricted pupil include exposure to a miotic, uveitis, synechia or interruption in sympathetic innervation (Horner's syndrome).

Loss of sympathetic tone to the pupil and ocular structures results in miosis, slight ptosis and enophthalmos, with elevation of the nictitating membrane (Fig 10). This triad of signs is classic for Horner's syndrome. A diagnosis of Horner's syndrome can be confirmed by pharmacologic testing. Placing a drop of 10% cocaine in each eye and measuring the pupil diameter at 5-minute intervals for 30 minutes reveals moderate dilation in the normal eye and no dilation in the affected eye. As most feline cases of Horner's syndrome involve interruption of the sympathetic pathway in the cervical area from some form of trauma, further testing to localize the lesion may be unnecessary. Treatment of Horner's syndrome is not indicated since vision is unimpaired.

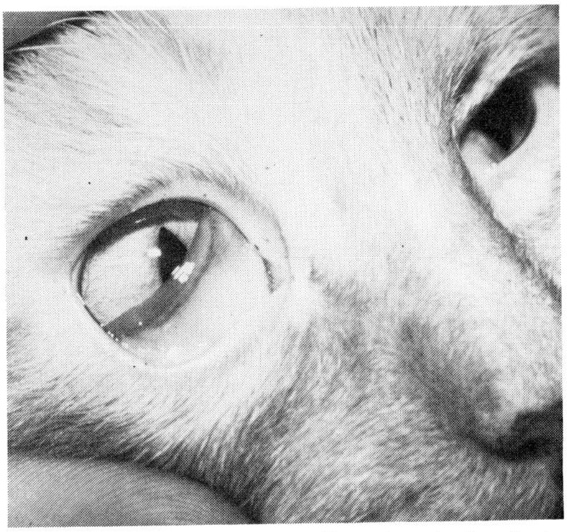

Fig 10. Horner's syndrome manifested as ptosis, miosis and elevation of the third eyelid. A cervical tumor had been removed on the affected side.

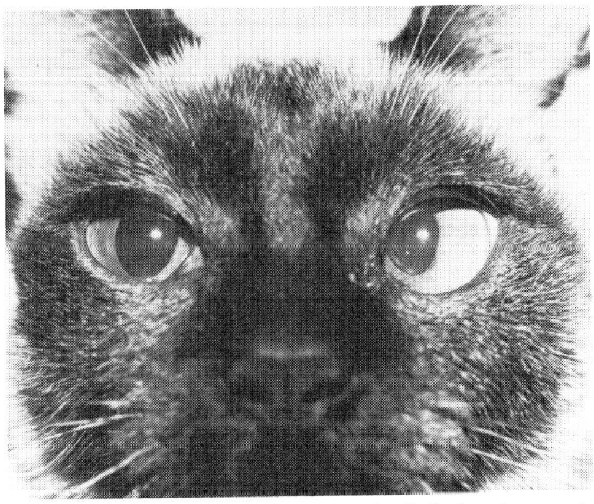

Fig 11. Anisocoria secondary to metastatic involvement of the parasympathetics of cranial nerve III in an adult Siamese with thymic lymphosarcoma.

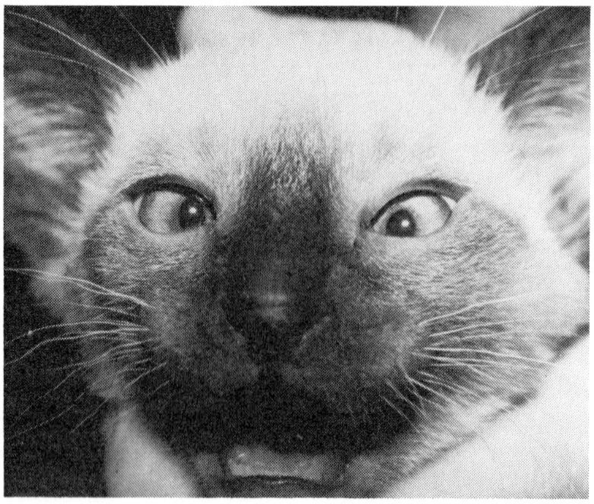

Fig 12. Esotropia in a Siamese kitten with no detectable visual problems.

Anisocoria that seems intermittent and affects a different eye on each episode has been observed in cases of thymic lymphosarcoma associated with the feline leukemia complex (Fig 11).

Strabismus

Esotropia is a type of strabismus in which the visual axis of one eye is deviated toward that of the other eye. It is common in Siamese cats (Fig 12).[26] The underlying cause seems to be associated with abnormal development of the optic pathways. The genotypic trait is present in all Siamese cats and apparently is related to the tendency toward albinism. The expression of this trait seems to be inherited as an autosomal recessive. In normal retinal pathways, 60% of the fibers decussate at the optic chiasm and go to distinct layers in the lateral geniculate bodies.[9] Affected cats may have minor visual disturbances from this condition but are able to function normally. Because of the congenital abnormality in the optic tracts, corrections of the defect by surgery on the extraocular muscles does not improve vision and is not recommended.

Protrusion of the Nictitating Membrane

Cats occasionally are affected by protrusion of one or both nictitating membranes. After close examination and elimination of such diagnoses as Horner's syndrome, loss of orbital fat due to trauma, or infection, a diagnosis of protrusion of the nictitating membrane can be made.

Extensive medical and neurologic work-ups have failed to define a cause. Application of a single drop of 2% epinephrine causes the nictitating membrane to recede to a normal position. This is only a temporary cure, but generally the condition resolves itself in several weeks to a month. Based on these facts, it is hypothesized that the lesion is either a temporary interruption of sympathetic innervation or an irritation of parasympathetic innervation supplying the musculature of the nictitating membrane.

References

1. Prince, J *et al:* Anatomy and Histology of the Eye and Orbit in Domestic Animals. Charles C Thomas, Springfield, IL, 1960.
2. Roberts and Lipton, in Catcott: Feline Medicine and Surgery. 2nd ed , American Veterinary Publications, Santa Barbara, 1975.
3. Severin, G: Veterinary Ophthalmology Notes. 2nd ed. Colorado State Univ Press, Fort Collins, 1976.
4. Slatter, D: Fundamentals of Veterinary Ophthalmology. WB Saunders, Philadelphia, 1981.
5. Peiffer, in Gelatt: Veterinary Ophthalmology. Lea & Febiger, Philadelphia, 1981.
6. Soulsby, E: Helminths, Arthropods and Protozoa of Domesticated Animals. 6th ed. Williams & Wilkins, Baltimore, 1968.
7. Martin, C. Proc 48th Ann Mtg AAHA, 1981.
8. Bistner, S *et al:* Atlas of Veterinary Ophthalmology. WB Saunders, Philadelphia, 1977.
9. Guillery, R. Sci Am **230(5)1** (1974) 44.
10. Cello, RM. Am J Ophth **63** (1967) 244.
11. Bistner, S *et al.* JAVMA **159** (1971) 1223.
12. Campbell, L *et al.* JAVMA **163** (1973) 991.
13. Knecht, C *et al.* JAVMA **149** (1966) 1192.
14. Brightman, A *et al.* Feline Pract **9(3)** (1979) 21.
15. Bistner, S *et al.* Invest Ophth **15** (1976) 15.
16. Murray, J *et al.* J Sm Anim Pract **18** (1977) 1.
17. Doherty, M. JAVMA **159** (1971) 417.
18. Vasinisi, S and Campbell, L. JAVMA **154** (1969) 141.
19. Vestre, W *et al.* Feline Pract **8(4)** (1978) 23.
20. Peiffer, R and Gelatt, K. Feline Pract **4(1)** (1974) 34.
21. Percy, D. JAVMA **167** (1975) 935.
22. Aguirre, G and Schmidt, S. Proc 7th Ann Mtg Am Coll Vet Ophth, 1976.
23. Morris, M. Cornell Vet **55** (1965) 295.
24. Rubin, L and Lipton, D. JAVMA **162** (1973) 467.
25. Schmidt, S *et al.* Invest Ophth **15** (1976) 47.
26. Blake, R and Crawford, M. Brain Res **77** (1974) 492.

18

the ear

W.R. ROSE

Feline ear diseases are a major problem in veterinary practice.[1] Due to the subtle nature of the symptomatology and incomplete evaluation procedures, the early stages of ear diseases can go undetected. Veterinary otology, the study of animal ear diseases, encompasses many diverse disciplines in an effort to meet the practitioner's needs. The otologist must draw on the disciplines of pharmacology, parasitology, embryology, oncology, pathology, bacteriology, neurology, mycology, dermatology, audiology, radiology, cytology and surgery, and must have a thorough understanding of the anatomy and physiology of the feline ear. The specialized information taken from these diverse fields must be organized in a logical and rational manner to be applied in clinical practice.[2]

A complete examination of the patient is essential and should include behavior and function tests, as well as physical examination and laboratory tests (Table 1). Ears are highly specialized, delicate sense organs that require specialized diagnostic procedures.

Another area of concern in feline otology is communication with and education of the client. The client's assistance is needed in formulation of an accurate medical history, administering medication, and keeping the practitioner informed as to the progress of disease resolution. The client must be aware of the complexities of feline ear diseases and the value of diagnostic tests, and that treatment may be protracted.

Anatomy and Physiology

Pinna

The pinna is a rather large structure in cats, with its base often hidden by the haircoat. It is well endowed with muscles (preauricular, postauricular, ventroauricular) that allow for very fine movement of the external ear to facilitate location of sound.[3]

The auricular cartilage contains numerous foramina through which vessels abundantly supply blood to all parts of the pinna (Fig 1). The perichondrium covers both surfaces of the pinna. In cases of severe inflammation, with shaking of the head, rubbing the ears on the ground or scratching, this cartilage may be injured, resulting in hemorrhage. Blood from such trauma accumulates in the space between the perichondrium and skin. Lacerations or bite wounds of the pinna usually result in copious bleeding.

External Ear Canal

The external ear canal consists of a vertical portion that terminates externally at the base of the pinna, and a horizontal portion that extends mediad to the tympanic membrane. On cross section it is oval or round and is lined with skin containing ceruminous and sebaceous glands, the secretions of which constitute cerumen.

Table 1. Complete Otologic Examination

History and Clinical Signs
↓
Otoscopic Examination and Ear Cleaning
↓
Laboratory Evaluation
↓
Radiographic Examination
↓
Neurologic Examination
↓
Audiologic Examination
↓
Diagnosis and Treatment
↓
Client Instructions

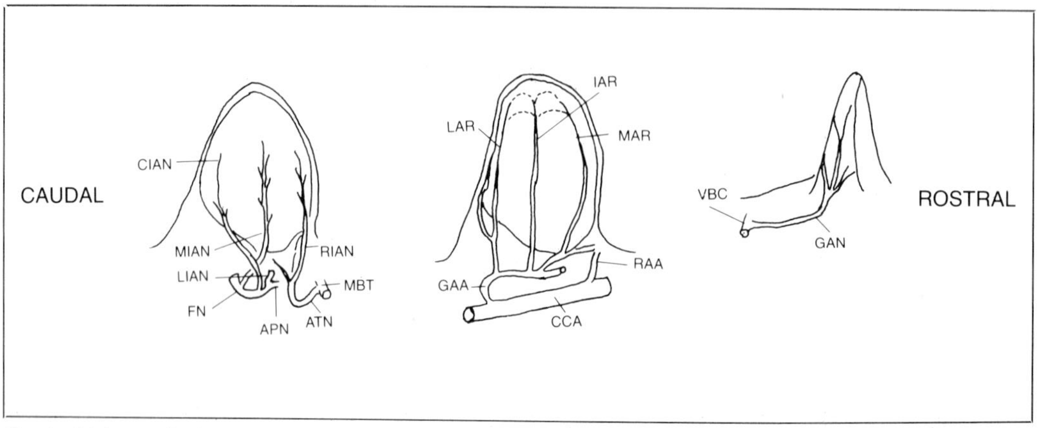

Fig 1. Major auricular arteries and nerves. CCA = common carotid artery, GAA = great auricular artery, LAR = lateral auricular ramus, IAR = intermediate auricular ramus, MAR = medial auricular ramus, RAA = rostral auricular artery, FN = facial nerve (VII), MIAN = middle internal auricular nerve, CIAN = caudal internal auricular nerve, APN = auriculopalpebral nerve, LIAN = lateral internal auricular nerve, MBT = mandibular branch of trigeminal nerve (V), ATN = auriculotemporal nerve, RIAN = rostral internal auricular nerve, VBC_2 = ventral branch of the 2nd cervical nerve, GAN = great auricular nerve.

Tympanic Membrane

The tympanic membrane separates the external ear canal from the middle ear and is composed of 3 layers: the dermal layer, which faces the external acoustic meatus, the fibrous layer, and the mucous layer, which is continuous with the middle ear (tympanic cavity). The margin of the greater part of the tympanic membrane attaches to a narrow groove (sulcus tympanicus ossis temporalis) in the medial part of the external acoustic meatus of the temporal bone. The groove is part of the tympanic ring (annulus tympanicus).[4]

The membrane is pearl grey, oval and drawn mediad toward the tympanic cavity at its ventral aspect (Fig 2). The point of greatest concavity is at the umbo, the end of the handle (manubrium) of the hammer (malleus). The rostrodorsal extent is marked by the pars flaccida (Shrapnell's membrane), radiating out as the anterior mallear plica fold and the posterior mallear plica fold. The radiating tension lines from the manubrium at the point of greatest concavity is called the pars tensa.[5,6]

For purposes of recording findings of otoscopic examinations, the tympanic membrane can be divided into quadrants. When lines are drawn at right angles to each other, one bisects the long axis of the malleus and the other transects the first at a point one-third the distance up the manubrium. The quadrants thus formed are the rostrodorsal, caudodorsal, rostroventral and caudoventral quadrants (Fig 3). These landmarks are useful in describing the location of perforations, scars and hemorrhages, and serve as landmarks for surgical procedures.

Middle Ear

The middle ear (cavum tympani) is a bony cavity lined with a mucous membrane partially covered by a double-layered, ciliated columnar epithelium and partially by a single layer of squamous epithelium. The cavity is divided into the recessus tympanicus, a small dorsal cavity containing the head of the malleus and most of the incus, the mesotympanum, the middle section including the ossicula auditus (ossicles) and the opening to the Eustachian tube (tuba auditiva), and the hypotympanum (tympanic bulla), the large ventral cavity communicating with the mesotympanum via a dorsal opening.

The muscles of the middle ear include the tensor tympani, which originates in the cartilaginous portion of the Eustachian tube and inserts on the manubrium of the malleus. Its function is to tense the tympanic membrane. The stapedius muscle, the smallest muscle in the body, originates from inside the pyramid of the middle ear and inserts on the neck of the stapes, the smallest bone in the body. Its function is to control stapedial activity. The center ossicle, the incus, articulates with the malleus and the head of the stapes, and is attached to the walls of the tympanic cavity by means of 2 crura (Fig 4).

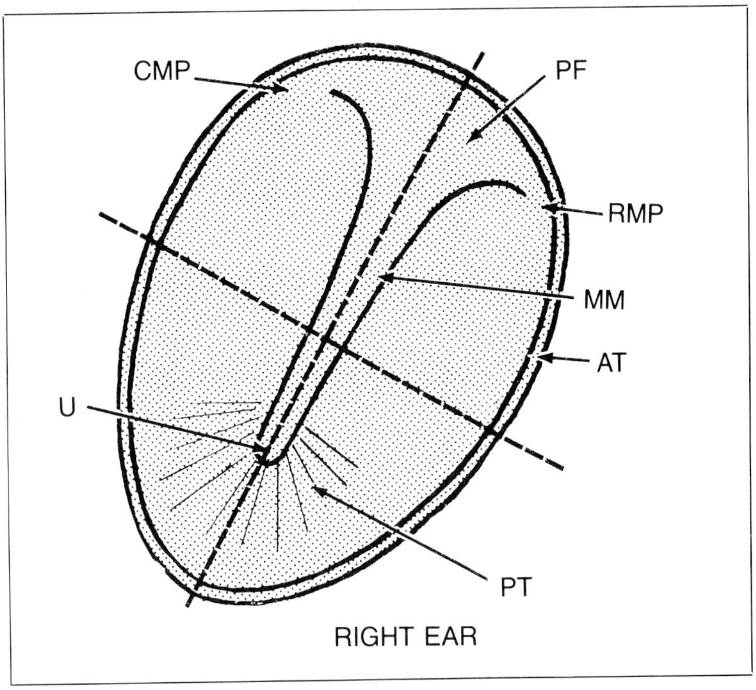

Fig 2. Division of the tympanic membrane as an aid in describing the location of lesions during otologic examination. CMP = caudal mallear plica (fold), PF = pars flaccida (Shrapnell's membrane), RMP = rostral mallear plica (fold), MM = manubrium of the malleus, AT = annulus tympanicus, PT = pars tensa (membrane ventral to umbo), U = umbo. (Courtesy of VM/SAC)

The oval footplate of the stapes, the innermost auditory ossicle, covers the oval window (fenestra vestibule) and its cartilaginous margin. Its action against the oval window stimulates motion of the perilymph of the cochlea.

The nerves serving the middle ear include a branch of the mandibular division of the trigeminal (fifth cranial) nerve to the tensor tympani muscle, the stapedial branch of the facial (seventh cranial) nerve to the stapedius muscle, and the chorda tympani nerve.

Inner Ear

The inner ear consists of an auditory unit, responsible for hearing, and a vestibular unit, responsible for balance and orientation. The auditory unit functions by movement of the stapes against the oval window, which activates the fluid wave in the vestibular canal. This wave causes movement of Reissner's membrane and the tectorium (membrana tectoria ductus cochlearis), activating the hair cells and the auditory nerve. The fluid wave passes back to the round window for equalization of pressure and the cycle is repeated. The initiated impulse then travels along the acoustic fibers of the eighth cranial nerve to the medulla, midbrain and cerebral cortex. At each stage of the auditory system, ascending toward the brain, the number of nerve fibers increases. For each fiber leaving the cochlea, there are about 40 in the auditory cortex. The pathways are ipsilateral and contralateral.

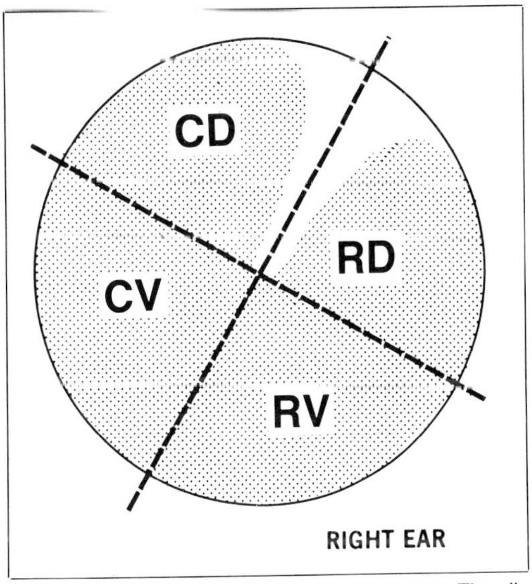

Fig 3. Quadrants of the tympanic membrane. The dividing lines intersect at the umbo. CD = caudodorsal, RD = rostrodorsal, CV = caudoventral, RV = rostroventral. (Courtesy of VM/SAC)

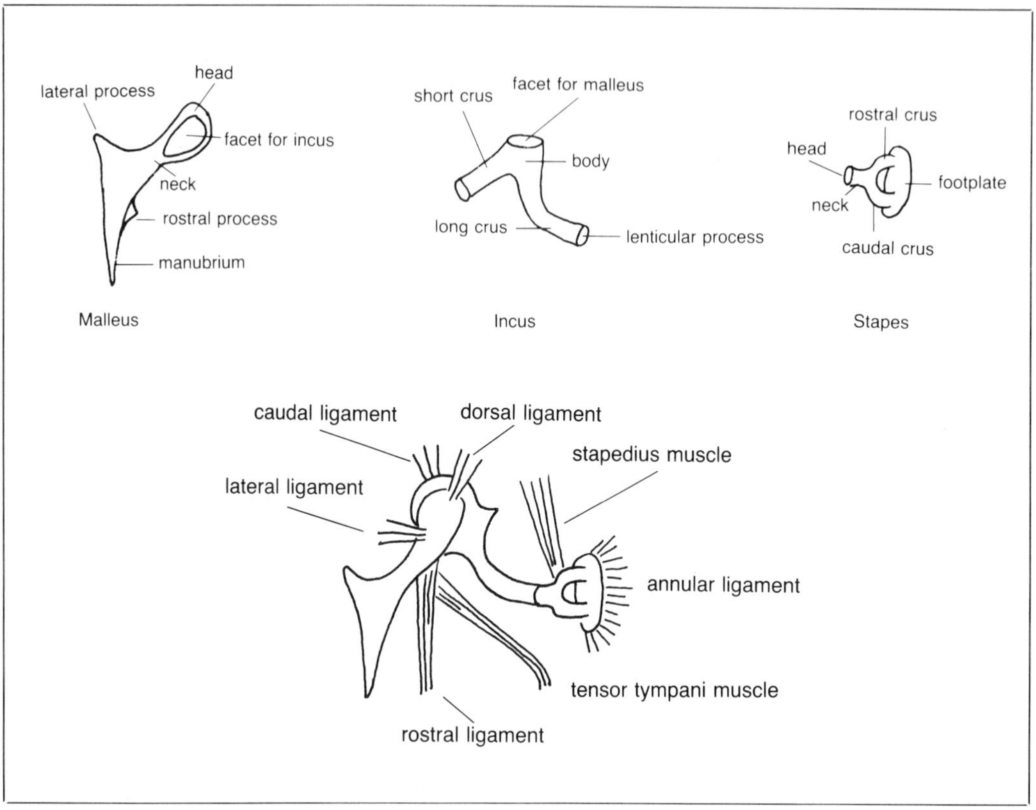

Fig 4. Ossicles, muscles and ligaments of the middle ear.

Inside the osseous labyrinth is a series of thin-walled tubes and sacs comprising the membranous labyrinth that contains endolymph. Between the osseous labyrinth and the membranous labyrinth is the perilymph, which acts as a shock absorber for the delicate structures of the membranous labyrinth. Perilymph, similar to extracellular fluid, contains high levels of Na and low levels of K. Endolymph, similar to intracellular fluid, contains high levels of K and low levels of Na. The differences in concentrations of these Na and K ions is related to drug toxicity, which tends to alter their relative concentrations.[7]

The vestibular component contains the saccule, utricle and semicircular canals, which are all part of the same fluid-filled labyrinth. The sensory endings of the maculae acusticae, in the utricle and saccule, and the crista acustica, in the semicircular canal, are concerned with balance and body position. The action of endolymph on these structures sends impulses along the vestibular pathways to the brain and extrinsic eye muscles. There are also connections with the autonomic nervous system, as indicated by nausea, vomiting and vertigo associated with ear disease. The vestibular nuclei and the nuclei of the third, fourth and sixth cranial nerves are also involved in the production of nystagmus in the caloric test (see Audiologic Examination).[8]

Eustachian Tube

The Eustachian tube, which connects the middle ear to the caudal nasopharynx, branches from the mesotympanicum. In the cat, the Eustachian tube is oval and short, with a maximum length of about 10 mm and diameter of 1-3 mm. It is composed of 2 portions. A long cartilaginous portion is collapsed and slit-like in the resting state. It is opened by the action of the levator and tensor veli palatini muscles, and is closed by the elasticity of the cartilage. The second is a short bony portion, without cartilage or muscle, that is a continuation of the cartilaginous portion. The tympanic end remains open and is composed of bone of the mesotympanicum, covered with respiratory epithelium (Fig 5).[9,10]

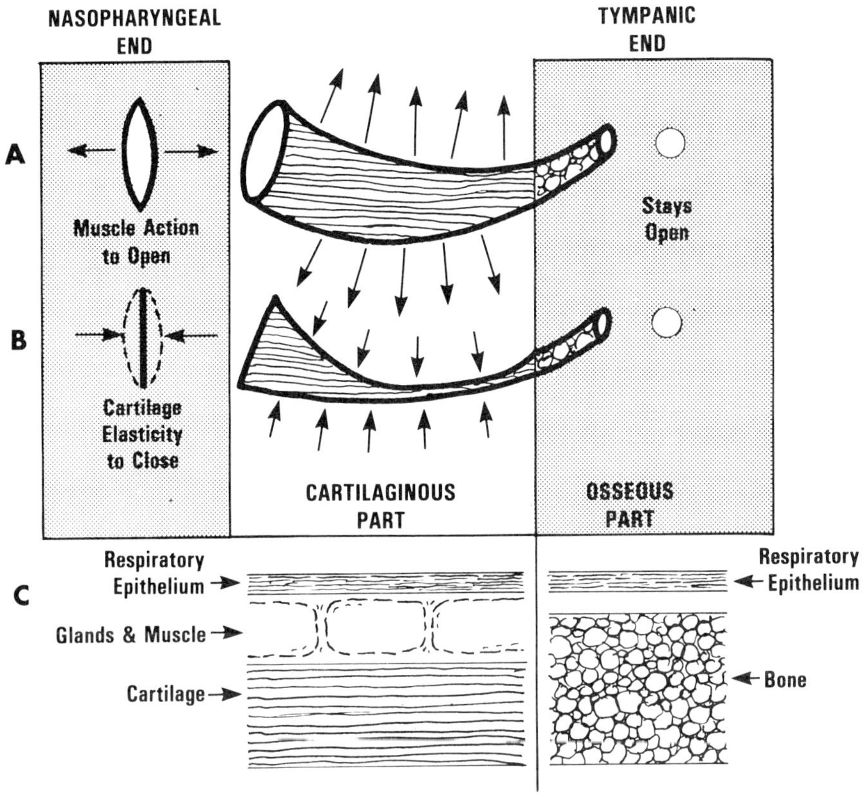

Fig 5. Function of the Eustachian tube. A. The tympanic ostium remains open and the nasopharyngeal ostium is opened by contraction of the pharyngeal muscles. B. While the tympanic ostium remains open, the nasopharyngeal ostium closes through recoil of the cartilage during relaxation of the pharyngeal muscles. C. Structure of the cartilaginous and osseous portions of the Eustachian tube. (Courtesy of VM/SAC)

The Eustachian ostia are situated in the middle of the soft palate, midway between the caudal nares and the caudal border of the soft palate. These openings face rostroventrad on the lateral walls of the nasopharynx. Between the openings is a strip of lymphoid tissue similar to the pharyngeal tonsil in people.

The functions of the Eustachian tube are to equalize air pressure in and eliminate fluids from the middle ear.

Diagnosis of Ear Diseases

Clinical Signs

It must be ascertained if ear disease actually exists, what regions of the ear are involved, and whether the disease is acute or chronic. The routes by which infections can spread from one part of the ear to another can aid in determining the etiology. One of the most common routes of spread is from the pinna, to the external auditory canal, to the middle ear, and then to the inner ear and brain. A second route is via the Eustachian tube, to the middle ear, and then to the auditory canal or inner ear. Finally, infections can be spread hematogenously.

The clinical signs of feline ear disease can be divided into those of otitis externa, which affects the pinna and external auditory canal, otitis media, which affects the middle ear, tympanum and Eustachian tube, and otitis interna, which affects the inner ear and eighth cranial nerve.

Table 2. Questions Asked in Obtaining a History of Ear Disease*

1. When was the problem first noticed?	10. Has the cat's behavior changed? (otalgia, headache)
2. What brought the problem to your attention?	11. Does noise irritate the cat? What type of noise? (pain, distorted perception of sound)
3. How has the condition changed since it was first noticed?	12. Does the cat appear to listen with one ear more than the other? (autophony, hearing loss)
4. Has there been a change in the cat's eating habits or interest in food? (nausea, pain)	13. Does the cat stand or wander as though lost? (disorientation)
5. Has the cat vomited or tried to vomit? (nausea)	14. Does the cat fail to respond when called? (loss or impairment of hearing)
6. Is the cat reluctant to move its head? (otalgia)	15. Does the cat avoid being touched on one ear or scratch or rub one ear? (pain, difference in severity of bilateral infection, unilateral infection)
7. Does the cat periodically lose its balance, stumble or fall? (vertigo)	16. Does the cat sleep more than usual? (fatigue)
8. Does the cat have running fits or cry out? (pain)	17. Does the cat sleep less than usual? (otalgia)
9. Does the cat behave differently in a quiet environment, or appear to be listening to nonexistent sounds? (tinnitus, increased perception of body sounds)	

* (Courtesy of VM/SAC)

Some of the major clinical signs encountered in each category are as follows:[11]

Otitis Externa: Signs of otitis externa include mild to intense scratching, head shaking, aural discharge and/or odor, increased temperature of the pinna, and periodic personality changes, including running fits and irritability. Pain can be mild to very severe, especially on movement of the pinna.[12-14] Vomiting and/or anorexia can be present in severe cases.

Otitis Media: Clinical signs of otitis media include personality changes, hanging of the head, nausea and vomiting, pain on manipulation of the head or jaw, increased or distorted perception of sound, restlessness, insomnia, vertigo and fever. Many of these signs are eliminated by release of pressure in the ear.

Otitis Interna: Otitis interna is characterized by many signs similar to those of otitis media, with the addition of ataxia, nystagmus, circling, lateropulsion, disorientation, and loss or impairment of hearing.

In addition to the overt clinical signs listed above, a range of signs, present in human otologic disease, may also be present in feline ear disease. Some examples of implied signs usually associated with otitis media and otitis interna are headache, tinnitus and increased perception of normal sounds.

History

When more than one region of the ear is diseased, accurate assessment of clinical signs becomes even more critical to determine if the disease has spread. Careful questioning of the client can aid in determining the rate of spread by providing information on behavioral changes, when such changes were first noticed, increasing severity, and whether the signs are continuous or intermittent in nature. Has the animal's behavior pattern changed, as indicated by play, sleeping, withdrawal, irritability, restlessness or insomnia? Does the animal fail to respond when called or does it stand or wander as though lost? Through carefully structured questions, an accurate assessment of the type, duration and severity of the otitis can be obtained (Table 2).[15-17]

Physical Examination

An accurate record of case histories and examination results is essential in otologic cases. A special otologic examination form can be used to ensure that all pertinent information is recorded (Fig 6).

Physical examination should begin by visual inspection and palpation of the pinna and surrounding tissue. The pinna should be examined for cartilage irregularities, scars, trauma, fluid, nodules, cysts, polyps, ulcers, excoriation, hyperkeratosis, fistulas, neoplasms, granulation, loss of hair, insect bites and parasites.

Next, the vertical and the horizontal portions of the external auditory canal should be examined. A 3.5-volt quartz halogen otoscope (Welch Allyn), with veterinary specula, provides an excellent source of illumination. Human endaural specula can be used on kittens and human nasal specula can be used on the vertical canal of adult cats (Fig 7). The pinna should be lifted dorsad and the cone inserted to the angle of the canal. The pinna is then pulled laterad and the cone is passed until the tympanic membrane can be seen clearly. The examiner should observe through the otoscope during its insertion. Care should be taken not to traumatize the wall of the auditory canal or the tympanic membrane during examination.[18]

Otoscopic specula should be disinfected after each use to prevent transmission of contaminants from one ear or animal to another. Specula can be cold-sterilized in a disinfectant solution. Disinfected specula should then be rinsed in sterile water and allowed to dry. It is convenient to have several sets of specula that can be rotated as used. Stainless-steel specula are available and can be autoclaved for use in surgery and other ear procedures.

Before the ear is cleaned, the ear canal should be given a preliminary otoscopic examination to detect any pathologic processes. This procedure is useful for the vertical portion of the external auditory canal but is of little benefit in the horizontal part of the canal if much debris is present. It is nearly impossible to examine a debris-filled ear canal, much less venture a diagnosis based on that examination. Cat ears are notorious for the amount of debris they can contain.

Before the ears are cleaned, swabs of any debris or exudate should be obtained for laboratory analysis. This procedure provides better and more reliable results on microbiologic evaluation than if samples are obtained after cleaning.

The preliminary examination is also used to determine the ear-cleaning procedure to be used. The method used to clean the canal varies, depending on the sensitivity of the ear, the degree of any erosion or inflammation, the nature of any exudate, the degree of any impaction, and the presence of trauma.

Sensitive tissues should be cleaned carefully to minimize trauma and pain. Excessive stimulation of the middle and inner ear can be avoided by using cleaning solutions at room or body temperature (25-37 C). The external ear canal can be cleaned in 3 ways.[19-22]

Manual Massage: A ceruminolytic agent is introduced into the ear canal in accordance with the manufacturer's directions and the base of the ear is gently massaged for 3-5 minutes (Table 3). If possible, the agent is allowed to remain in the ear for 5-10 minutes. This gives the agent time to penetrate and dissolve cerumen, oil, fats, crusted debris and pus. The cat is allowed to shake its head to remove as much medication and debris as possible after the massage. Gauze sponges and cotton-tipped swabs are then used to complete the process of cleaning. This process may have to be repeated several times to thoroughly clean the ear.

Syringe Method: A hexachlorophene solution (pHisoHex:Winthrop) of 15 parts water to 1 part pHisoHex, at body temperature, is drawn into a 20- to 50-ml syringe to which is attached sterile flexible tubing. The tubing is passed into the external auditory canal to the entrance of the

Table 3. Commercial Ceruminolytic Agents*

Cerusol (Burns-Biotec): Contains dioctyl sodium sulfosuccinate, a surfactant for reducing surface tensions and dissolving debris, wax and pus in the ear canal. Do not use if ear drum is damaged.

Oticol (Hart-Delta): A urea-peroxide solution that dissolves pus, wax and scales, and debrides dead tissue in the ear canal.

Sebumsol (Parlam): Contains hexamethyltetracosane, a saturated hydrocarbon that is miscible with cerumen, as well as with other oils, fats and waxes of the skin.

Surfak (National Labs): Contains dioctyl calcium sulfosuccinate, a surfactant for lowering surface tension and dissolving debris, wax and pus in the ear canal. Do not use if ear drum is damaged.

pHisoHex (Winthrop): Contains hexachlorophene. Used in solution (1 part pHisoHex: 15 parts water) for flushing and disinfecting the ear canal.

* (Courtesy of VM/SAC)

STANDARD OTOLOGIC EVALUATION FORM

Case Number ____________

Date ____________

Name (Owner) ____________

Address ____________ Telephone ____________

Animal's Name ____________ Species ______ Breed ____________ Age ____ Sex ____

HISTORY AND CLINICAL SIGNS (head tilt, pruritus, pain, etc.): ____________

EXAMINATION

External Ear (Pinna)	Right Ear	Left Ear
Margin		
Lacerations		
Swelling (hematoma)		
Hyperemia		
Desquamation		
Tumor		
Parasites		
Other		

External Auditory Canal	Right Ear	Left Ear
Debris		
Cerumen (yellow, crusty, etc.)		
Parasites		
Hyperemia		
Ulceration		
Hyperplasia		
Exudate (pus, blood, etc.)		
Other		

Fig 6. Standard otologic evaluation form. (Courtesy of VM/SAC)

Tympanic Membrane

(color, transparency, edema, bulging, retraction, perforations, scars, deposits)

Description: ____________________

____

____

____

____

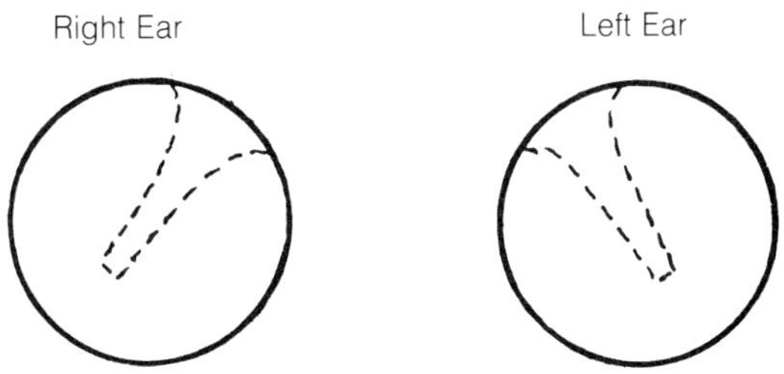

Middle and Inner Ear

Test	Results
___ Vestibular and Neurology	____________________
___ Microscopy	____________________
___ Culture	____________________
___ Cytology	____________________
___ Radiology	____________________
___ Audiology	____________________
___ Other	____________________

DIAGNOSIS AND TREATMENT: ____________________

____

____

____

PROCEDURES:

____________ Cleaning ____________________

____________ Surgery ____________________

____________ Other ____________________

RESULTS (follow-up): ____________________

____

____

____

Fig 6, continued.

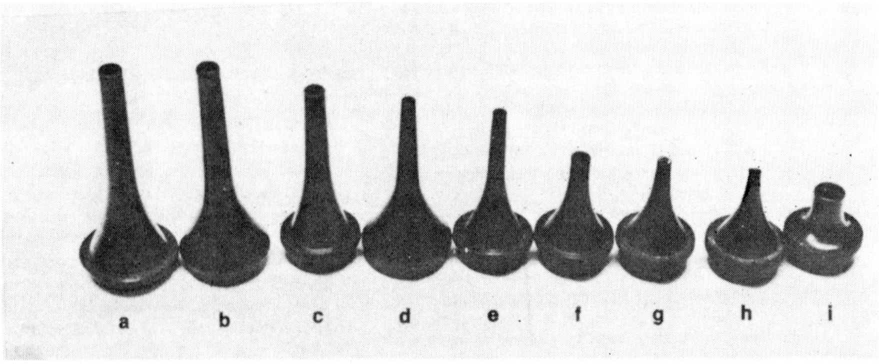

Fig 7. Otoscopic specula. A, B, C. Adult size for veterinary use. D, E. Juvenile sizes for veterinary use. F. Adult size for human use. G. Juvenile size for human use. H. Pediatric cone for human use. I. Nasal cone for human use. (Courtesy of VM/SAC)

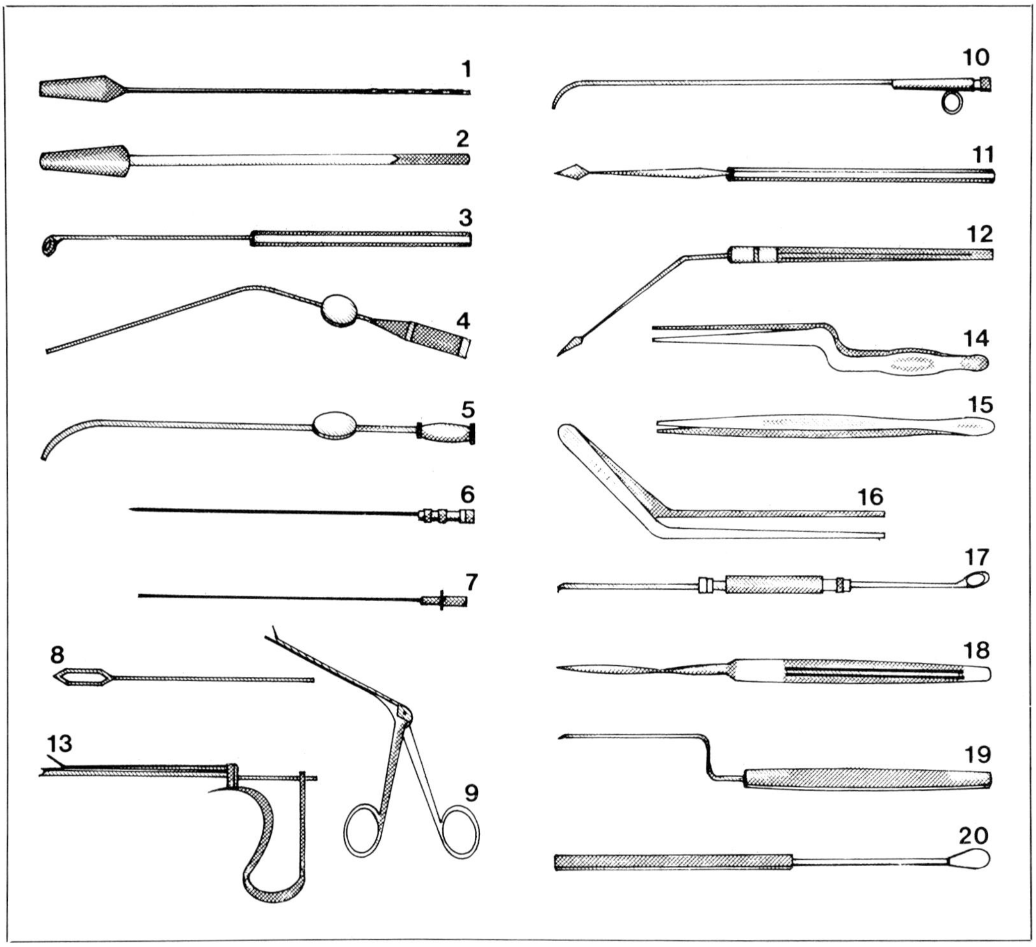

Fig 8. Instruments used to remove pus, blood, serum and cleaning agents from the external auditory canal and middle ear. The tip of these instruments must be small enough to pass through the end of the speculum and still allow adequate visualization. 1. Allen ear applicator with knurled tip. 2. Brown ear applicator with triangular tip. 3. Buck ear curette. 4. Frazier curved suction tip. 5. Frazier straight suction tip. 6. Special-purpose needle with sharp tip. 7. Aspirating needle with blunt tip. 8. Probe. 9. Delicate alligator forceps. 10. Hartman Eustachian catheter. 11. Lempert spear perforator. 12. Politzer perforator. 13. Quire foreign body remover. 14. Lucae bayonet forceps. 15. Dressing forceps. 16. Wilde ear forceps. 17. Yankauer ear probe with hook and blunt tip. 18. Gerzog and Sexton ear knife. 19. Buck ear knife. 20. Billeau ear loop. (Courtesy of VM/SAC)

vertical canal. The tubing should never be forced against the tympanic membrane and the space around the tube should be sufficient to permit the solution to flow back through the vertical canal and out of the ear. Excess solution is aspirated by a syringe or suction apparatus or is removed with cotton-tipped swabs.

Pulsating Fluid Current: A dilute hexachlorophene (pHisoHex) or povidone iodine (Betadine:Purdue Frederick) solution is put in the reservoir of a dental Water Pik. The control is set at low water pressure and the nozzle is passed part way down the vertical canal. Care must be taken against directing a strong stream of water against the tympanic membrane since this can cause temporary or permanent deafness. After flushing for 3-5 minutes, the excess solution is aspirated or swabbed from the ear canal. The procedure is repeated if needed.

Deposits not flushed out by the above technics can be removed with Buck curettes or Billeau ear loops (Fig 8). Foreign bodies can be removed with Wilde or fine alligator forceps. These procedures should be done through an otoscope.

Laboratory Evaluation

Several types of laboratory tests can be performed in an otologic examination. Sterile cotton-tipped swabs (Culturette:Marion Scientific) are used to obtain samples for bacterial and mycotic isolation and drug sensitivity testing. Pathogens are usually identified by their culture characteristics and by staining and microscopic examination.[23]

Exudates or ear washings can be examined microscopically for parasites and their eggs. Microscopic examination of skin scrapings or biopsies from the ear canal may reveal indications of neoplasia, hyperplasia, parasitism or fungal infection.[24-26]

Gross or histopathologic examination of necropsy specimens can confirm a diagnosis.

Radiographic Examination

Radiographic examination is very useful in the diagnosis of otitis media or otitis interna. Radiographs can reveal fistulas, senile calcification, congenital anomalies, radiopaque foreign bodies, fractures and chronic infections. The key to successful radiographic diagnosis is proper positioning, for which tranquilization or sedation of the patient is usually necessary. The standard radiographic views are ventrodorsal, dorsoventral, lateral, oblique and anteroposterior (open mouth). Several views should be obtained for an accurate assessment.

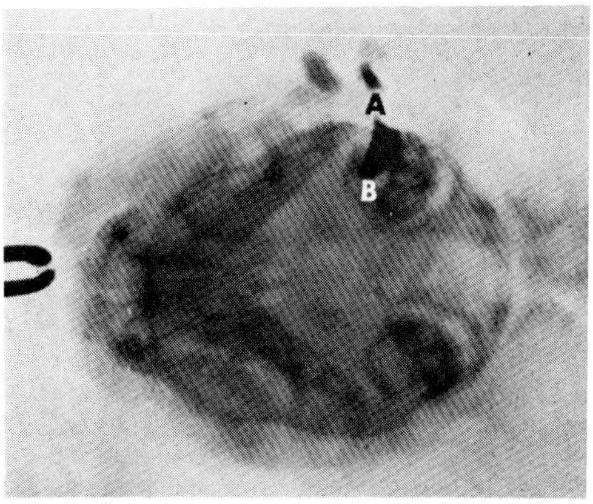

Fig 9. Dorsoventral radiograph of the skull obtained 5 minutes after instillation of Hypaque in the external auditory canal. The presence of the medium in the middle ear indicates an incomplete tympanic membrane. A = external auditory canal. B = middle ear. (Courtesy of VM/SAC)

The external auditory canal can be examined and patency of the tympanic membrane determined with the use of radiopaque media, such as barium solution or sodium diatrizoate (Hypaque:Winthrop). The instruments required include a long, blunt-tipped needle, disposable 3-ml syringe, mosquito forceps, sterile cotton sponges and nonabsorbent swabs. The long needle is used to instill the medium deep into the external auditory canal to reduce the chance of spillage, which could obscure the area on radiographs. Although the procedure is not painful, the patient may require sedation to avoid spillage of the medium and movement while obtaining the radiographs.

With the cat in lateral recumbency and the affected ear up, 1-3 ml medium are instilled in the external auditory canal. Excess medium is sponged from the outer ear and the ear canal is occluded with nonabsorbent swabs. Radiographs subsequently obtained reveal fistulas, constrictions and ulcers of the canal, and can locate perforations of the tympanic membrane that were unobserved on otoscopic examination. The presence of radiopaque medium in the middle ear indicates a patent tympanum (Fig 9).

Radiographs of the ear can be enhanced by making contact or enlarged prints on photographic paper, using the radiograph as a negative (Fig 10). This converts a white-on-black image to a black-on-white image. Such black-on-white prints make structures of the ear easier to identify, and eliminate glare and magnifier distortion. An additional benefit is that the small print can be attached to the patient's record for quick reference and referral.

Neurologic Examination

Evaluation of the auditory and vestibular pathways is indicated when otitis media or otitis interna is suspected. The causes of pathologic changes in the inner ear are many and diverse: spread of otitis media to the inner ear, fractures of the skull with intracranial hemorrhage, meningitis, toxic reactions to heavy metals or drugs, and tumors. Of the many neurologic tests used to evaluate various nerve pathways, several are of particular value in otologic examination. Figure 11 illustrates a worksheet to record the findings of neurologic examination.

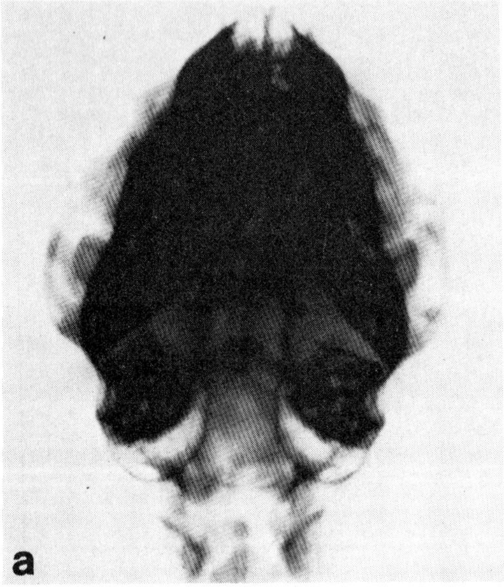

a

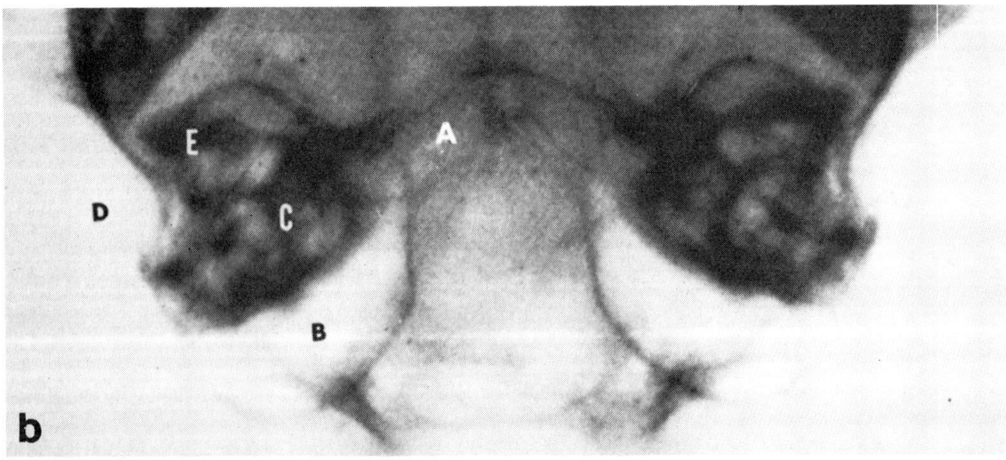

b

Fig 10. a. Ventrodorsal radiograph of a normal young cat. b. In this enlargement of the same radiograph, the Eustachian tube (A), evident radiographically only in young animals, tympanic bulla (B), cochlea (C), opening into the external auditory canal (D), and epitympanicum (E) are evident. (Courtesy of VM/SAC)

Righting Reflex (Without Vision): The blindfolded cat is turned upside down and dropped from a distance of twice its standing height. A normal cat lands on its feet. If the animal lands on its side or back, a lesion may exist in the eighth cranial nerve, vestibular apparatus or cerebellum.

Righting Reflex (With Vision): The cat is held upside down and released from a distance twice its standing height. It should land on its feet. If the animal lands on its back or side, lesions may exist on the eighth cranial nerve, vestibular apparatus, cerebellum, eye or spinal cord.

Walking Test: The cat is blindfolded and called by its owner. If hearing is present, abnormal body positions and movements, such as lateropulsion, circling and rolling, are magnified without the aid of vision. If the cat cannot hear, there is no response to sound at any level. Lesions may exist in the eighth cranial nerve, semicircular canal or cerebellum.

Hearing Test: This evaluation is considered separately later in this chapter (see Audiologic Examination).

Caloric Test: The caloric test is a simple test of vestibular apparatus function using irrigation of the external auditory canal with cold and warm water. The resultant nystagmus indicates the degree of dysfunction, if any.

Nystagmus consists of 2 components: slow movement of the eyes in one direction, followed by rapid movement (beat) in the opposite direction. Since the rapid beat is easier to detect, traditionally it is considered to indicate the direction of nystagmus. Most nystagmus is hori-

Owner ______________________ Case Number ______________

Address ______________________ Telephone ______________

Animal's Name ____________ Species ______ Breed ________ Age ____ Sex ____

1. Righting Reflex (with vision): Back ________ Side ________ Feet ________ Chest ________

2. Righting Reflex (without vision): Back ________ Side ________ Feet ________ Chest ________

3. Blindfold Walking Test: Body Position ________ Circling ________ Incoordination ________ Rolling ________

4. Centrifugal Test (same as number 3), including duration of signs: ________

5. Caloric Test: O = Opposite S = Same

TEST	EAR IRRIGATED	WATER TEMP.		DIRECTION OF NYSTAGMUS	DURATION OF NYSTAGMUS	TYPE OF NYSTAGMUS
A	LEFT	COLD	(30 C)			
B	RIGHT	COLD	(30 C)			
C	LEFT	WARM	(44 C)			
D	RIGHT	WARM	(44 C)			

Directional Preponderance Calculations:

6. Audiologic Examination:
Normal ________ Abnormal ________

7. Notes:

Fig 11. Neurologic examination worksheet.

zontal; however, in rare instances vertical nystagmus occurs and usually indicates a lesion central to the vestibular nuclei.

The vestibular apparatus consists of the saccule, utricle and semicircular canals, all of which are part of the same fluid-filled labyrinth (Fig 12). These structures are all concerned with balance and body position through sensory endings: the maculae (in the utricle and saccule) and the crista (in the semicircular canals). The action of endolymph movement on these sensory structures sends impulses through the vestibular pathways to the brain and extrinsic eye muscles.

Connections with the autonomic nervous system are indicated by the nausea and vomiting associated with vertigo. The vestibular nuclei and nuclei of cranial nerves III, IV and VI are all involved in production of nystagmus upon stimulation (Fig 12).

During caloric stimulation, the endolymph nearest the external auditory canal is cooled or heated more than the rest of the fluid. This lo-

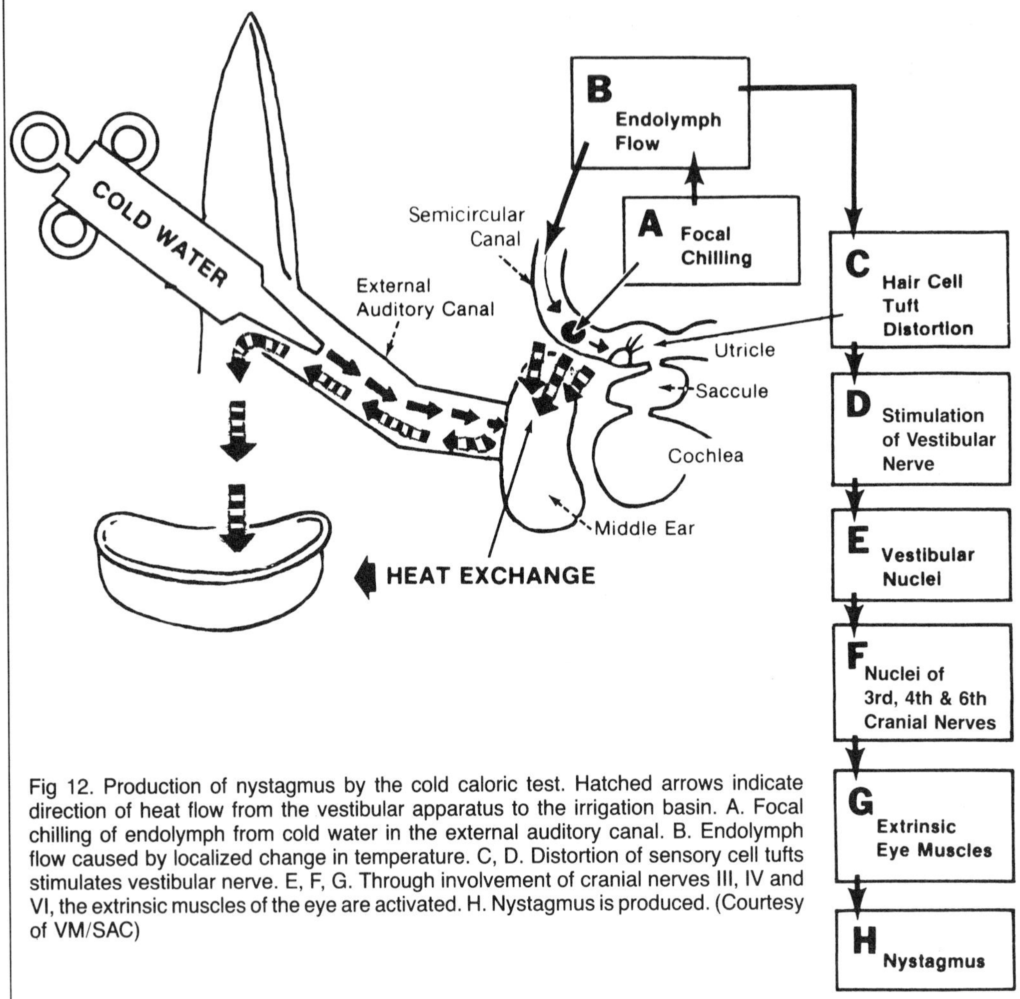

Fig 12. Production of nystagmus by the cold caloric test. Hatched arrows indicate direction of heat flow from the vestibular apparatus to the irrigation basin. A. Focal chilling of endolymph from cold water in the external auditory canal. B. Endolymph flow caused by localized change in temperature. C, D. Distortion of sensory cell tufts stimulates vestibular nerve. E, F, G. Through involvement of cranial nerves III, IV and VI, the extrinsic muscles of the eye are activated. H. Nystagmus is produced. (Courtesy of VM/SAC)

calized change in temperature causes flow of the endolymph (convection current) and stimulation of the sensory endings, resulting in nystagmus. Cold-water stimulation of the endolymph normally results in nystagmus to the contralateral side, *ie,* cold-water irrigation of the right ear results in the fast component of the nystagmus (beat) to the left, and vice versa. Warm-water stimulation of the endolymph causes nystagmus to the ipsilateral side, *ie,* warm-water irrigation of the right ear results in nystagmus to the right. The direction of nystagmus should be recorded during caloric stimulation.

Because sensitivity of patients to caloric stimulation varies, it is best to start with a mild stimulus on a patient with an empty stomach. This reduces the chances of autonomic stimulation and nausea. An ear syringe or a 20-ml syringe with a 15-ga needle with a rubber tip is filled with cold water (30 C). The animal is allowed to stand or is restrained in lateral recumbency. The ear is irrigated at a rate of 1 ml/sec. The cold water should contact the tympanic membrane for 20 seconds (accurately timed). The direction of the beat (normally contralateral), frequency of the beat (3-5 beats/sec normal), duration of the nystagmus (in seconds), and severity of the nystagmus should be recorded. The other ear is checked after the patient is rested for 5 minutes. If mild stimulation fails to cause nystagmus, the procedure should be repeated, with the cold water left in contact with the tympanum for 30 seconds.

The results obtained from this simple test can help determine if the labyrinths are normal, hypofunctional or nonfunctional. In normal animals, nystagmus is horizontal, with the duration about the same for both ears. In animals with hypofunction of the labyrinth, the nystagmus is of shorter duration on the affected side. Absence of nystagmus upon cold-water irrigation of the ear indicates a nonfunctioning labyrinth. When accurately timed, a difference of 40-60 seconds' duration of nystagmus upon stimulation of each ear indicates labyrinth disease. If one eye moves while the other remains still, only moves slightly, or moves in the opposite direction, a central lesion should be suspected.

A more accurate determination of labyrinth function can be obtained by determination of directional preponderance. This procedure helps distinguish central lesion from a hypofunctioning labyrinth. If each ear is tested with warm and cold water, one can determine the side on which these stimuli cause the greater duration of nystagmus (directional preponderance). The directional preponderance usually is toward the side of a central lesion and away from the side of a labyrinth lesion.

In the test for directional preponderance, 250 ml cold water (30 C) are placed in an irrigation can. The left ear is irrigated with the cold water for 40 seconds and the duration of nystagmus is recorded (Table 4). The right ear is similarly tested and the duration of nystagmus recorded. Each ear is rested for 5 minutes after each test. Then, 250 ml warm water (44 C) are placed in the prewarmed irrigation can. The left ear is irrigated with the warm water for 40 seconds and, after a 5-minute rest, the right ear is similarly irrigated. The time is recorded in seconds from the beginning of irrigation until the nystagmus stops.

Calculations for interpretation of the caloric test are listed in the example below. The first set of calculations is for interpretation of the cold-water test only. The second set is for interpretation of both warm- and cold-water tests. The third set illustrates calculations of directional preponderance.

1. Cold-water irrigation only:

$$\begin{array}{r} 200 \text{ sec (left)} \\ -\,100 \text{ sec (right)} \\ \hline 100 \text{ sec} \end{array} = \text{difference in duration of nystagmus}$$

A difference of 40 seconds or greater indicates hypofunction of the right labyrinth.

2. Cold- and warm-water irrigation:

$$\begin{array}{l} 200 \text{ sec} + 180 \text{ sec} = 380 \text{ sec (both left ear times)} \\ 100 \text{ sec} + 110 \text{ sec} = 210 \text{ sec (both right ear times)} \\ \hline 170 \text{ sec} = \text{difference in duration of nystagmus between ears} \end{array}$$

Combining the cold- and warm-water test times provides a more accurate indication of labyrinth function. Note the greater difference as compared with the calculations in number 1.

3. Directional preponderance:

$$\begin{array}{l} 200 \text{ sec} + 110 \text{ sec} = 310 \text{ sec (both right nystagmus times)} \\ 100 \text{ sec} + 180 \text{ sec} = 280 \text{ sec (both left nystagmus times)} \\ \hline 30 \text{ sec} = \text{difference in duration of nystagmus} \end{array}$$

A difference of 40 sec or greater indicates directional preponderance to one side or the other. In this example, there is no directional preponderance; therefore, the lesion is more likely peripheral than central.

Table 4. Caloric Test to Determine Directional Preponderance[51]

Ear Irrigated	Water Temperature	Direction of Nystagmus	Duration of Nystagmus (seconds)
left	cold (30 C)	right or left (normally opposite)*	
right	cold (30 C)	right or left (normally opposite)	
left	warm (44 C)	right or left (normally same)**	
right	warm (44 C)	right or left (normally same)	

(Courtesy of VM/SAC)
* Cold-water stimulation usually produces nystagmus toward contralateral ear.
** Warm-water stimulation usually produces nystagmus toward ipsilateral ear.

Audiologic Examination

Audiologic testing is a practical way to detect hearing loss and determine the type of hearing loss, the progress of middle or inner ear disease and the efficacy of treatment. The causes of hearing loss in cats include the following: impacted external auditory canal or perforated or thickened tympanum; damage to the cochlea by trauma, drug toxicity or infection; brain and nerve damage from drug toxicity, trauma or infection; hereditary and developmental causes; neoplasms of the middle and inner ear; and miscellaneous or unknown causes.[27-30]

There are 5 types of hearing loss:[31]

Conductive: Conductive hearing loss is caused by interruption of the transmission of sound from the external auditory canal to the oval window. These conditions may involve the tympanic membrane and/or the ossicular chain.

Nerve Deafness: Nerve deafness (sensorineural hearing loss) is caused by factors that interrupt transmission in the inner ear and auditory nerve. Damage to hair cells and the cochlea are common causes.

Central Deafness: Causes of central deafness are those that interfere with conduction of impulses to the cerebral cortex, such as brainstem lesions.

Congenital Deafness: Deafness from birth usually is caused by malformations of the external, middle or inner ear and neural pathway.

Mixed Hearing Loss: Mixed hearing loss includes both conductive and neural components. This type is frequently seen in older animals.

The hearing range of the cat is estimated to be from 60 hertz (Hz) to over 50,000 Hz. This range is far broader than that for people.

Several hearing tests can be used to quantitate hearing capacity.

Pure-Tone Audiometer and Sound Box: Pure sound of different frequencies is introduced, by earphones, into a soundproofed box containing the animal (Fig 13). The cat's response to each frequency at varying decibel levels is noted (Fig 14). Overt physical responses include head, eye, ear and body movement. Each positive response is recorded on an audiogram for each ear.

This type of testing is called air-conduction testing, which tests the external, middle and inner ear. A second test, using the audiometer, is called the bone-conduction test, which tests the inner ear and neural pathways.[32-36]

Startle Test: A brief, loud sound, with a narrow frequency range, such as a hand clap, should elicit a response in the animal. This is not a quantitative test.

Tuning Fork Test: Using a standard set of tuning forks, sound can be produced at predetermined frequencies of 128, 256, 512, 1024, 2048 and 4096 Hz.[37]

Ultrasonic Testing: A silent dog whistle or Galton whistle can be used to determine if the cat can hear in the ultrasonic range.

Natural Sound Test: Tapes of natural sounds that have meaning to a cat, such as threatening sounds or prey sounds, are played into a sound box and the animal's reaction to each sound is observed.[38]

The major drawback of audiologic testing of animals is the interpretation of the responses of an animal when exposed to a given sound frequency. Many single and combination reactions can be used; however, from the author's experience, the movement of the ears, eyes and head

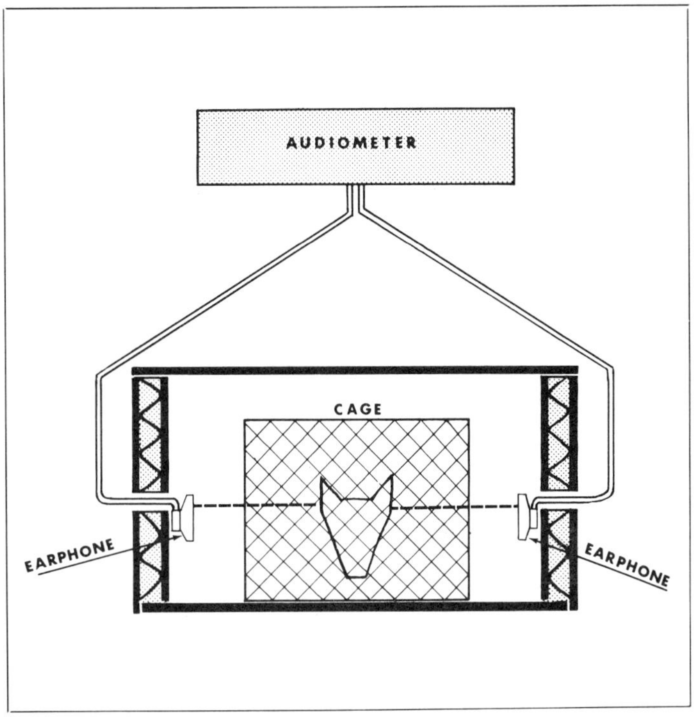

Fig 13. Diagram of the soundbox test chamber and placement of the earphones. A wire cage may be placed within the chamber to restrict the cat's movement. (Courtesy of VM/SAC)

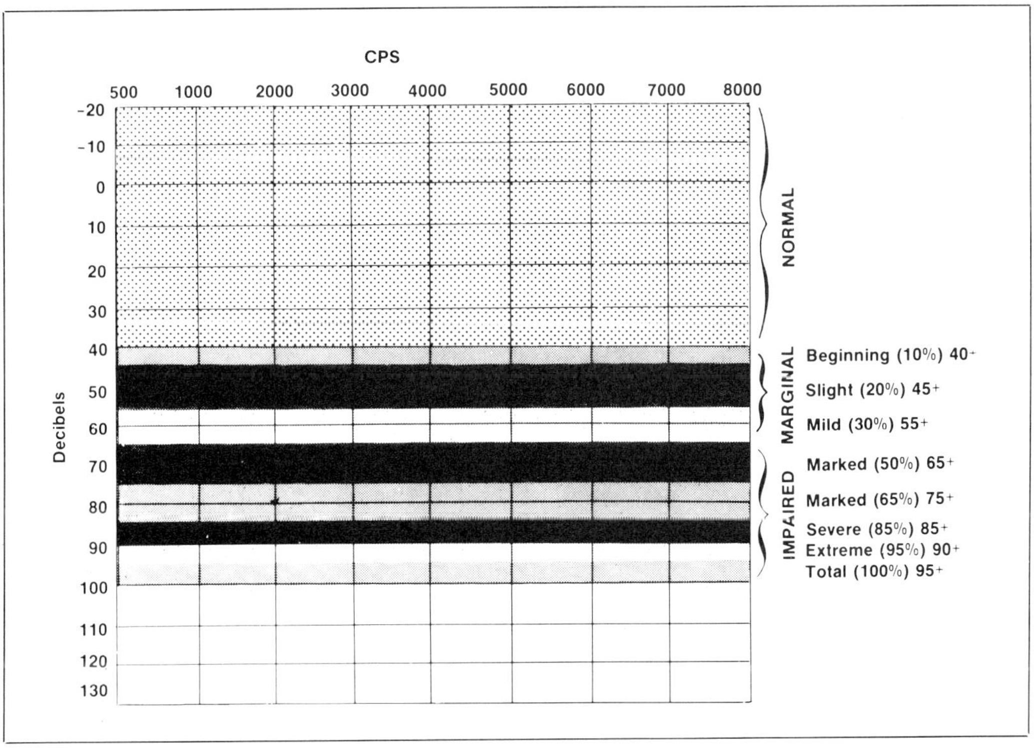

Fig 14. Hearing threshold scale. The degree of any hearing impairment can be determined by relating response points on the audiogram to the scale. (Courtesy of VM/SAC)

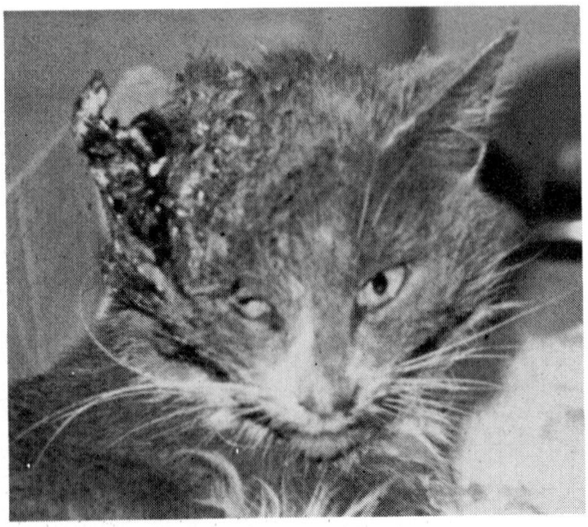

Fig 15. Untreated lacerations of the pinna of a 4-year-old domestic shorthaired cat resulted in degeneration of the auricular cartilage. *Pseudomonas* and *Clostridium* were isolated from the wound.

seem to be the most reliable reactions. The simplest method of checking the validity of observations is repeated testing. The observer simply records the reactions and reports them to the audiometrist. The observer does not know the decibel levels until the test is over.

Diseases of the Pinna

Severe pain and an extreme reluctance to be touched is one of the first signs of disease of the pinna, the abundant nerve supply to the ear, of course, being the reason for this phenomenon (Fig 1). Use of ultrashort-acting barbiturates may be required to prevent self-mutilation and allow complete examination, including the manipulation of the structure.

The concave and convex aspects of the pinna should be examined for size, shape, evidence of previous trauma, temperature, color, odor, swelling, desquamation, hematomas, parasitic infestations, cysts, nodules, polyps, alopecia and congenital defects. Microabscesses or other small lesions can be easily overlooked unless magnification is used in conjunction with good lighting.

Lacerations

Lacerations and perforations from fighting usually involve the tip of the pinna and are usually heavily contaminated (Fig 15). Immediate treatment with systemic and topical antibiotics is always indicated. General anesthesia may be required for treatment of severe wounds. The affected area should be cleaned with an antiseptic solution, such as povidone iodine, and a topical antibiotic ointment applied. Partial amputation may be required when gangrene or ischemia complicates the case. Amputation may be required in severe cases of photodermatitis (see Chapter 16).

Injury of the base of the ear may result in abscess formation. Injuries to the apical portion of the pinna may result in ulcer formation. In some cases, fistulous tracts lead from the base of the ear to the maxilla, forming large pus pockets that must be drained and flushed. Small puncture wounds often initiate this process, which continues long after the initial wound has healed. For this reason, the pinna and especially the base of the pinna always should be carefully examined.

Lacerations of the pinna should be treated with systemic antibiotics for 5-10 days and topical antibiotic ointment when appropriate.

Hematomas

Hematomas are the second most common pathologic change of the pinna. These usually result from injury inflicted by the ipsilateral rear claws in scratching initiated by acute otitis externa, especially otoacariasis. The hematoma is the result of the tearing of small blood vessels between the skin and cartilage, usually on the concave surface of the pinna. Aspiration may be required to differentiate an abscess from a hematoma. Hematomas can be lanced or aspirated and injected with antibiotics and corticosteroids. However, the most important consideration is elimination of the underlying cause. Without resolution of the causative irritation, the hematoma can become chronic, leading to abscessation, ulceration or disfiguration of the pinna. Chronic ulceration may require curettage, excision or cautery for resolution.

Diseases of the External Ear Canal

Otitis Externa

The most common type of ear disease in cats is otitis externa or inflammation of the external ear canal. Otitis externa seems to occur most frequently in the American domestic breeds, followed by the Siamese and Persian breeds. This observation, however, may only reflect the greater population of domestic breeds. The prevalence of otitis externa is significantly higher among cats under a year of age; cats over 7 years old seem relatively refractory, with the prevalence dropping markedly as animals age.

Table 5. Bacteria Isolated in Otitis Externa*

Pathogen	Morphology	Colony	Exudate	Other Tests
Pseudomonas (Gram-negative)	Slender rod; very motile	Gray, shiny, moist spreading colony	Green pus from pyocyanin	Lactose-positive; VP (Voges-Proskauer)-negative
Escherichia (Gram-negative)	Small rod; varies with conditions; slow motility	Smooth, glistening, unpigmented-to-white	Creamy pus	Lactose-positive; VP-negative (related *Klebsiella* differentiation by VP test)
Klebsiella (Gram-negative)	Encapsulated rod	Moist, white-to-yellow	May or may not produce pus	Lactose-positive; VP-positive
Proteus Gram-negative)	Motile rod	Thin, confluent growth	May or may not produce pus	Lactose-negative; VP-negative; Urease test broth
Streptococcus (Gram-positive)	Chains of cocci	White pigment on blood; beta hemolytic = clear zone; alpha hemolytic = green zone	May or may not produce pus	Lactose-negative
Staphylococcus (Gram-positive) (Gram-negative)	Grape-like clusters	White-to-yellow orange *S. aureus* = deep golden yellow *S. albus* = white	A pus-former	Lactose-negative

* (Courtesy of VM/SAC)

Cause: Approximately 30% of cases of otitis externa are associated with ear mite infestation (see Otoacariasis). Mixed bacterial infections are as common as those from one bacterial species. *Staphylococcus* spp, *Streptococcus* spp, *E coli*, *Proteus* spp and *Pseudomonas* spp are common bacterial isolates in acute cases of otitis externa (Table 5).

Clinical Signs: The condition is more often bilateral than unilateral. The most common clinical signs are pruritus, erythema, edema, pain, ulceration and discharge.

Treatment: Many cases of otitis externa are of mixed etiology. Because about 50% of external ear infections are caused by mixtures of bacterial types, mixtures of bacteria and fungi, mixtures of bacteria and mites, or any combination, treatment strategy is heavily dependent on laboratory results.

When possible, treatment is more effective when debris and cerumen have been removed. Systemic therapy should be coupled with topical therapy, especially in chronic cases. During extended periods of treatment, topical treatment should be discontinued intermittently to allow the external ear canal to dry. For example, if a topical ointment or liquid is used for 5-7 days, at the end of that period a 3- to 5-day drying period should be allowed. This cycle can be repeated if necessary. However, systemic therapy is maintained for the entire period. Excess glandular secretions that accumulate during the

Table 6. Characteristics of Pathogenic Fungi*

Trichophyton mentagrophytes
1. Does not fluoresce.
2. Colony: white, cotton-like or powdery; bright red pigment (some yellow or brown) on underside.
3. Morphology: grape-like clusters of spherical microconidia (microaleuriospores) on coiled hyphae. Macroconidia are rare. When present, they are cigar-shaped, septate, and thin-walled.
4. Hair: ectothrix—chains of spores on outside of hairshaft.

Trichophyton rubrum
1. Does not fluoresce.
2. Colony: white, velvety to fluffy; dark red pigment (some purple) on underside.
3. Morphology: small tear-shaped microconidia (microaleuriospores) alternating along sides of the hyphae. Macroconidia are narrow, septate, long and terminal.
4. Hair: ectothrix—chains of spores on outside of hairshaft.

Microsporum canis
1. Yellow-green fluorescence.
2. Colony: white, coarsely fluffy; yellow pigment (some orange) on underside.
3. Morphology: numerous macroconidia; spindle-shaped with knob at the tip, multiseptate (with seven or more cells), and thick-walled.
4. Hair: ectothrix—masses of spores on outside of hairshaft.

Microsporum gypseum
1. Dull fluorescence, if any.
2. Colony: cinnamon, powdery.
3. Morphology: numerous macroconidia; spindle-shaped, rough surface, 6 or less cells, thin-walled. Microconidia, if present, are not diagnostic.
4. Hair: ectothrix—sparse chains of spores may or may not be present.

Candida albicans
1. Does not fluoresce.
2. Colony: cream-colored, yeast-like, mucoid.
3. Morphology: yeast-like fungus with budding forms, chlamydospores on tip of pseudomycelium, spherical.
4. Gram-positive.

* (Courtesy of VM/SAC)

drying period can be controlled with powders (*eg*, sulfur, neomycin, nitrofurazone, zinc oxide or talc preparations) used sparingly in single applications every other day during the drying period. Drying agents should not be used if the tympanic membrane is perforated.

There is no single universal treatment for otitis externa in the cat. Rather, the selection of topical preparation must be based on otoscopic examination, laboratory results and clinical signs. The categories of drugs used include antibacterials, antifungals, anthelmintics, analgesics, anti-inflammatories and ceruminolytics (Table 7). Some otic preparations contain drugs in all of these categories! In certain cases, unneeded compounds, such as ceruminolytics, can irritate the ear canal and prolong recovery time. Anti-inflammatory and analgesic compounds may mask clinical signs. To be effective, each type of drug must be used only when indicated.[39]

If thorough cleaning of the ear canal is not possible, ceruminolytics may be used to allow penetration of the drug to the site of action. Anti-inflammatories and analgesics should be used if intense pain or self-mutilation due to pruritus is a problem.

Pyrethrum and rotenone compounds should be used only after thorough cleaning of the ear canal. The base of the ear should be massaged with each application to ensure penetration of the horizontal portion of the auditory canal. Treatment BID for 4 days is usually sufficient. Because insecticide compounds are usually irritating, short treatment periods are advisable. Only compounds specified for cats should be used. Such compounds as benzene hexachloride (hexachlorocyclohexane) are very toxic to cats, as is methoxychlor to very young animals. These compounds should not be used if the tympanic membrane is perforated.

Use of topical antifungal agents should be reinforced by systemic antifungals when possible because of the refractory nature of fungal infections. Griseofulvin, nystatin, thiabendazole and cuprimyxin, in preparations recommended for cats, should be used beyond the point at which clinical signs disappear. Systemic therapy for 3-6 weeks is not uncommon. If signs of toxicity appear during systemic therapy, a 4- to 7-day break in treatment is indicated. Periodic cultures should be taken as a routine follow-up.[40]

Client education should be thorough in all cases of otitis externa. Routine ear hygiene, signs of reinfection or toxicity, the importance

Table 7. Topical Otic Preparations and Their Properties*

Product	AP	AB	AM	AI	AN	CE
Aurimite (Burns-Biotec)	+	+		+	+	
Cankerine (Norden)		+				
Canolene (Norden)	+	+	+			
Cerumite (EVSCO)	+					+
Cerusol (Burns-Biotec)						+
Demolene (Hart-Delta)	+					
Forte-Topical Upjohn)		+		+		
Fulvidex (Schering)		+	+	+		
Furacin-Micofur (Eaton)		+				
Furacin (Eaton)		+			+	
Furacort (Eaton)		+		+		
Gentocin Otic (Schering)		+		+		
Liquichlor (EVSCO)		+		+	+	+
Mitecide (Lilly)	+	+				
Mitox (Norden)	+	+				
Mycodex (Beecham)		+	+	+		
Neo-Cortef (Upjohn)		+		+	+	
Neo-Delta-Cortef (Upjohn)		+		+	+	
Neo-Predef (Upjohn)		+		+		
Oticol (Hart-Delta)						+
Otomite (Carson)	+					
Otosol (Trico)						+
Panolog (Squibb)		+	+	+		
Ridamite (Parlam)	+					
Sebumsol (Parlam)						+
Sulfacaine (Norden)		+			+	
Stereocaine (Jen-Sal)		+	+		+	
Synotic (Diamond)				+	+	
Toptic (Lilly)		+	+	+		
Tresaderm (Merck)		+	+	+		
Trikicide (Haver-Lockhart)		+	+			
Tympacaine (Affiliated)		+			+	
Unitop (Hoffmann-La Roche)		+	+			
Virmyxin (Norden)		|				

AP = antiparasitic AB = antibacterial AM = antimycotic
AI = anti-inflammatory AN = analgesic CE = ceruminolytic
* (Courtesy of VM/SAC)

of environmental hygiene, and the need for examination of other animals on the premises to prevent cross-infection or reinfection should be discussed with the client.

Meticulous records should be kept of drug resistance by certain strains of bacteria to facilitate the use of effective drugs. *Pseudomonas* and *Staphylococcus* are noted for their resistance to certain antibiotics. Fungal infections may also present a problem of resistance.

Otomycosis

Otomycosis, fungal infection of the ear, is most prevalent in young animals. Fungal infections of the external ear canal are often complicated by secondary bacterial infection. The most common fungal pathogens in otitis externa are *Trichophyton mentagrophytes*, *Microsporum gypseum*, *Trichophyton rubrum*, *Microsporum canis* and *Candida albicans* (Fig 16, Table 6). Other species of questionable pathogenic status or secondary contaminants include *Alternaria* spp, *Aspergillus* spp, *Penicillium* spp, *Rhizopus* spp and several species of yeast.[41]

Seasonal variants and climatic factors, such as rainfall, high temperature and high humidity, often contribute to the incidence.

Clinical Signs: Clinical signs of otomycosis may vary in degree from none to severe. Lesions may be dry and crusty or moist and painful. A definitive diagnosis is usually made by isolation

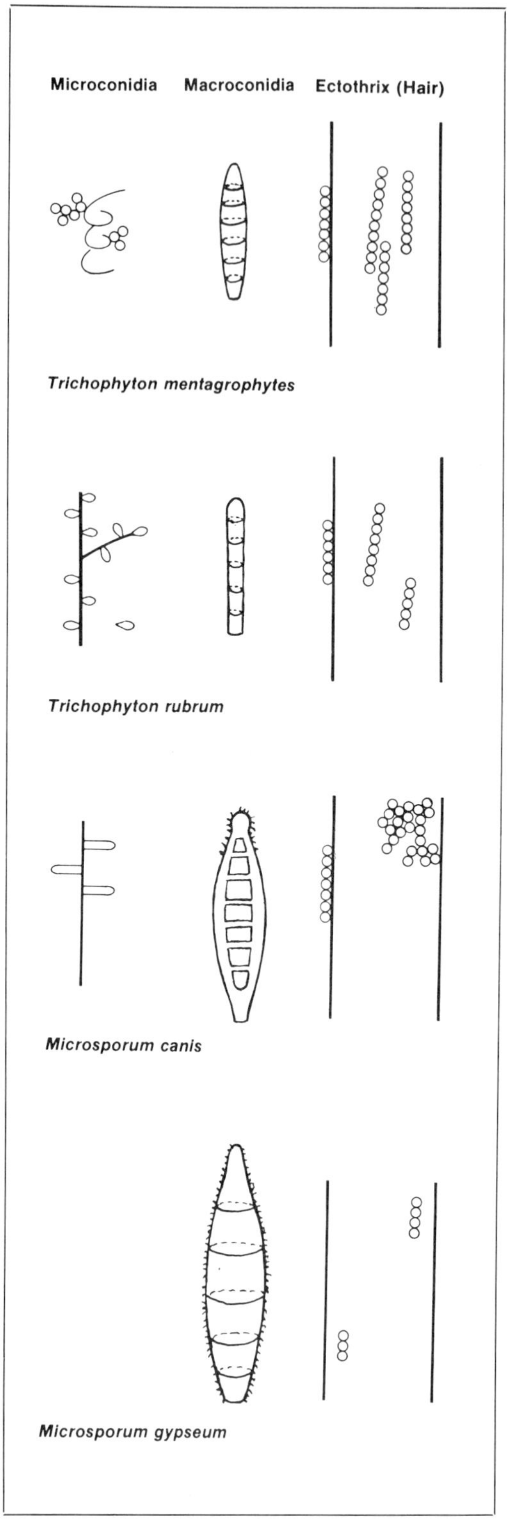

Fig 16. Common pathogenic fungi in otitis externa. (Courtesy of VM/SAC)

of the organism in dermatophyte culture medium. Chapter 16 contains a discussion of culture of dermatophytes.

Parasitic Otitis

Cause: The most common cause of parasitic otitis is the ear mite, *Otodectes cynotis* (Fig 17). Other mites that may infest the feline ear include *Sarcoptes scabiei, Notoedres cati, Demodex felis* and *Trombicula alfreddugesi.* The external ear canal may also offer temporary shelter to ticks, including *Dermacentor variabilis, Rhipicephalus sanguineus, Amblyoma* spp, *Ixodes* spp and *Otobius megnini.*[42-44]

Transmission of mites is usually direct or by environmental contamination. Otoacariasis, infestation with *Otodectes cynotis,* in one member of a litter soon spreads to the littermates. People, especially children, can become temporarily infested with *Sarcoptes scabiei* and *Notoedres cati.* Clients should also be warned of the possibility of zoonoses transmitted by the American brown dog tick, *Dermacentor variabilis.*

Clinical Signs: Otoacariasis affects cats of all ages but young animals seem to be especially susceptible. The decreased incidence in older cats is apparently due to acquired immunity.

The life cycle of *Otodectes cynotis* requires 3-4 weeks. The eggs are laid on the epithelium of the ear canal and, after a 4-day incubation period, the eggs hatch into 6-legged larvae. The larvae feed for 5 days and rest for 24 hours before undergoing progressive changes to protonymph and deutonymph. A deutonymph attaches to an adult male and matures into an 8-legged adult within 5-6 days. Adult females live about 2 months, during which an egg is laid to renew the cycle.[45]

Clinical signs of parasitic otitis vary from twitching of the ears and shaking of the head to epileptiform seizures. Severely infested cats may run wildly about or display other escape behavior. Uncomplicated acute infestations can progress to uncomplicated chronic infestations or may be complicated by secondary bacterial infection.

Treatment: As previously outlined in the section on treatment of otitis externa, parasitic otitis is treated by instillation of oily insecticide otic preparations into the external ear canal. Excess waxy deposits should first be removed with ceruminolytics. Preparations containing anti-inflammatory agents should be used if the ear canal is very inflamed. Bland oils, such as mineral oil, may be used on cats that have a severe inflammatory reaction to instillation of insecticide preparations. Treatment should be repeated after 14 days to remove immature forms unaffected by the initial treatment.

Ticks should be carefully removed with forceps and an antibiotic otic preparation instilled.

Disease of the Middle Ear

Otitis Media

Cause: Inflammation of the middle ear can be initiated by extension of otitis externa across a perforated tympanic membrane, ascent of a pharyngeal infection up the Eustachian tube, and hematogenous spread of infectious organisms.

Because of the delicate tissues comprising the middle ear, otitis media typically causes severe pathologic changes, including swelling and occlusion of the Eustachian tube, erosion of the mucosa of the tympanic cavity, degeneration or proliferative changes of such bony structures as the tympanic bulla, auditory ossicles or oval or round window, accumulation of inspissated pus in the tympanic bulla, inflammation and rupture of the tympanic membrane, and hearing loss from ossicular change.

Clinical Signs: Signs of otitis media vary in severity and usually develop progressively. One of the most common signs is a head tilt toward the affected side, which affects locomotion. Severely affected cats may have convulsions or crouch down and remain immobile. Others exhibit signs of pain when handled about the head.

Diagnosis: Cats with otitis externa should always be examined for concurrent otitis media. Careful examination of the tympanic membrane is required to help establish a diagnosis.

The tympanic membrane should be examined for the following characteristics.

Transparency: The normal tympanic membrane is translucent. Cloudiness or opacity indicates pathologic change.

Luster and Color: Normally the membrane is pearl-grey and glistening. The luster is lost and the color changes in most diseases of the middle ear. A bluish translucence indicates intratympanic hemorrhage. The short process and handle of the malleus may be injected, with isolated hemorrhages in the tympanic membrane. A red color indicates acute otitis media. Retraction of the membrane may be apparent. A diffuse, opaque white area, surrounded by a red area, suggests accumulation of pus within the tym-

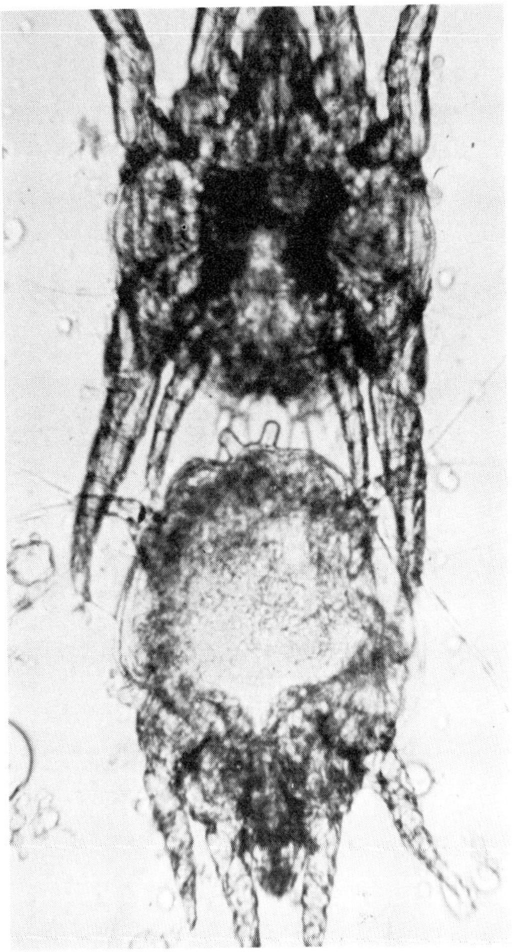

Fig 17. Male and female *Otodectes cynotis*.

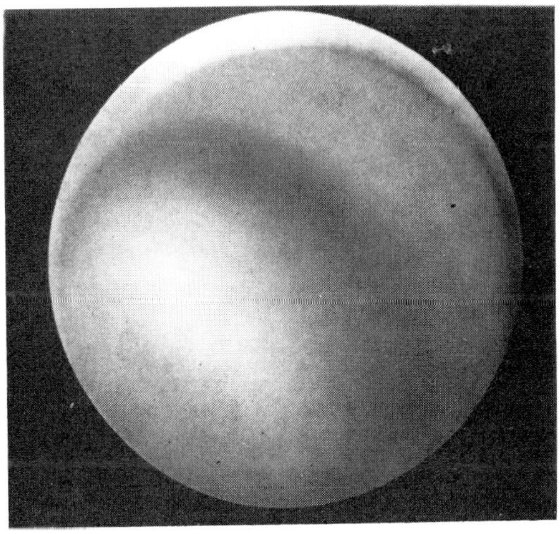

Fig 18. Bulging and loss of detail of the tympanic membrane caused by suppurative otitis media. Myringotomy is indicated to relieve pressure.

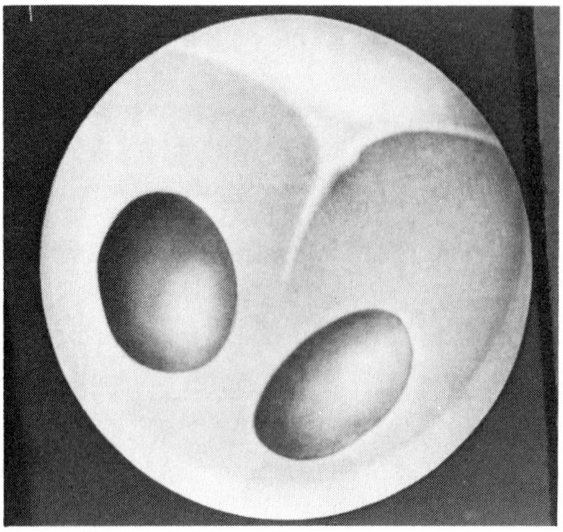

Fig 19. Two large perforations of the tympanic membrane expose the middle ear to infection or indicate middle ear infection.

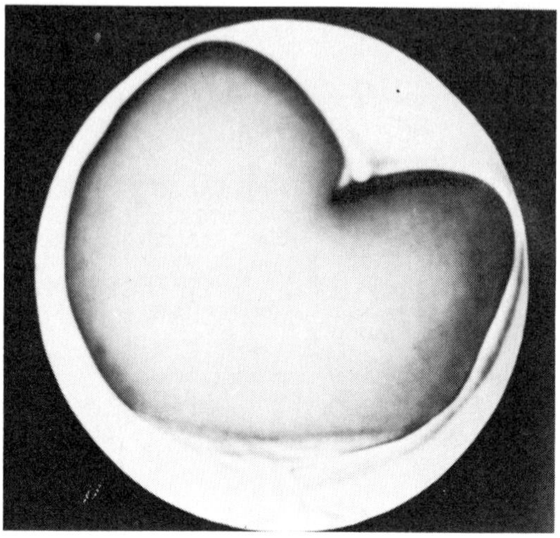

Fig 20. Tympanic membrane completely eroded from otitis media.

panic cavity (acute purulent otitis media). There may be marked bulging of the membrane (Fig 18). A translucent amber color characterizes the presence of serous transudate. Air bubbles sometimes can be seen in the serum.

Tension: The normal tympanic membrane is slightly concave. Bulging occurs when blood, pus or serum accumulates behind the membrane (Fig 18). Retraction of the membrane suggests a partially filled tympanic cavity and an obstructed Eustachian tube.

Perforation: Seen otoscopically, disruptions of the tympanic membrane appear as dark spots (Figs 19, 20).

Thickenings, Scars and Deposits: Those indicate previous inflammatory processes.

Radiographic examination is indicated if otitis media is suspected (Figs 9, 10).

Treatment: Relief of pressure and pain are the prime considerations in treating otitis media. Sedatives and analgesics are given to reduce pain. Antibiotics and corticosteroids, systemic and topical, are given to reduce inflammation and swelling. A myringotomy should be performed if pressure in the middle ear is excessive, as indicated by a bulging tympanic membrane and manifestation of severe pain.[46]

Tympanic

A bulla osteotomy may be warranted in chronic cases or when radiographs indicate filling of that structure with purulent material. The reader is referred to surgery texts for details on myringotomy and bulla osteotomy.

Surgery, in conjunction with systemic and topical medication, is the best course of action in most cases. Drainage of the middle ear, removal of inspissated or organized material, and topical antibiotics instilled into the middle ear cavity are essential for resolution (Fig 21).

Disease of the Inner Ear

Otitis Interna

Cause: Otitis interna is the term used to indicate any pathologic process of the inner ear. Some causes of these pathologic changes include spread of otitis media to the inner ear, fractures and hemorrhage, meningitis, drug toxicity, congenital defects, systemic infection, neoplasia, degenerative disease in older animals, allergic reactions resulting in edema, and acoustic trauma.

The labyrinths of the vestibular and cochlear systems are all connected by ducts, forming a continuous, closed fluid environment. Consequently, when one part of the system is damaged or changed, the whole system may be affected. Congestion and defects in fluid circulation can complicate an inner ear problem. The small size and delicate components of the inner ear, with their rich nerve supply and close proximity to the brain, explain the rapid spread of infection from the inner ear to the brain. If the infection follows the internal acoustic meatus and the eighth cranial nerve to the brain, a fatal brain abscess can result.

Clinical Signs: The clinical signs of otitis interna range from pain that rapidly increases in

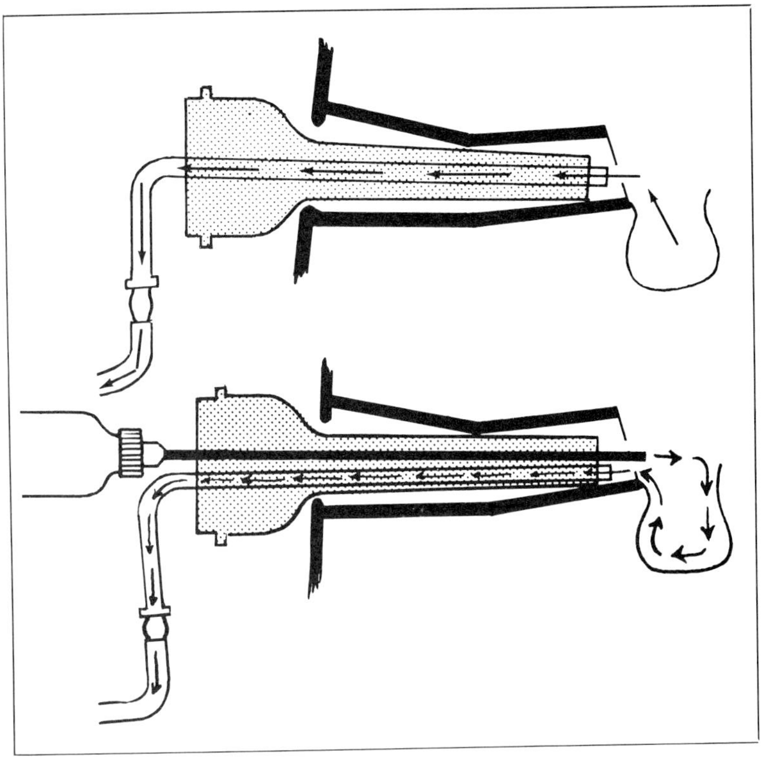

Fig 21. Top. The suction apparatus is in position after myringotomy. Bottom. The middle ear is flushed with antibiotic solution with a special-purpose, blunt-tipped needle attached to a 20-ml syringe.

severity, to vertigo and disturbances of equilibrium (nystagmus, nausea, and vomiting), hearing loss, ataxia, convulsions and death. Nystagmus, with the slow movement toward the affected side, may be present. Clinical signs vary, depending on the type of lesion, its location, and the amount and extent of inflammation and swelling.

Diagnosis: Diagnosis of otitis interna is based on consideration of the history, observation of clinical signs, and findings of otoscopic, neurologic, radiographic and audiologic examinations.

Ototoxicity should be a factor considered in the medical history and selection of a treatment regimen. Cats are very susceptible to drug ototoxicity. Some drugs implicated in causing ototoxicity in cats are streptomycin, dihydrostreptomycin, kanamycin, neomycin, salicylates, mercurials, arsenic and lead.

Neurologic examination should include evaluation of the cochlea, semicircular canals, utricle, eighth cranial nerve, and flocculonodular lobe of the cerebellum (see Chapter 14).

Treatment: Due to the close relationship of the components of the inner ear, therapeutic measures must begin immediately. These include use of antibiotics to combat infection, corticosteroids to reduce swelling, diuretics to remove excess fluid, and sedatives and analgesics to reduce neurologic complications and pain. Topical treatment is indicated after a myringotomy is performed to relieve pressure and treat concurrent otitis media. As in otitis media, tympanic bulla osteotomy may be required.

Systemic

Antihistamines may be of value in otitis interna of allergic origin. Vitamin A, with B-complex and citrus bioflavonoid, is commonly used to treat people for nerve deafness.

Disease of the Eustachian Tube

Conditions that usually necessitate Eustachian tube therapeutics include otitis media, pharyngitis and nasal congestion. The tympanic end of the tube can become occluded with exudates from the middle ear, the midsection can collapse or can be restricted by inflammation or trauma, and the pharyngeal end can be constricted by inflammation.

Diagnosis: The Eustachian pharyngeal orifice can be examined by direct observation with min-

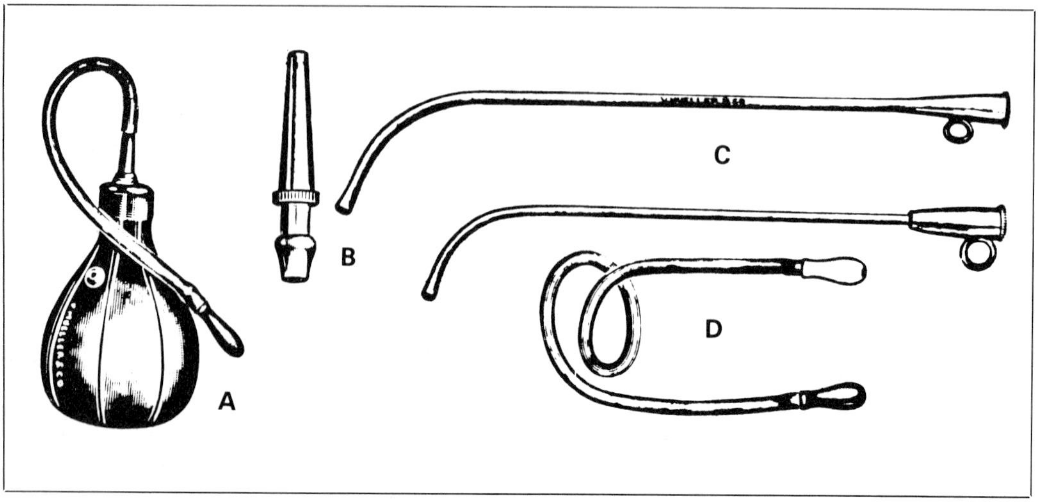

Fig 22. Instruments used to test for Eustachian tube patency (available from V. Mueller, Garland, TX). A. The 8-oz Politzer air bag, with valve, tubing and nasal tip. This device allows inflation of the Eustachian tube without catheterization. B. Metal connector to connect Eustachian catheter to air bag. C. Eustachian catheters for use with Politzer air bag. D. Diagnostic tube (auscultation tube), with ear tips. (Courtesy of VM/SAC)

imum manipulation of the soft palate, direct observation with retraction of the soft palate, and direct observation employing nasal intubation. Sedation is required and a good light source is mandatory.

Because of the lack of a reliable test for patency of the Eustachian tube, in cases of otitis media the practitioner is unable to determine if patency exists, the degree of any occlusion, and the portion of the tube occluded. The following methods help assess Eustachian tube patency:

Indirect Function Test: Water is injected into the oral cavity, causing the animal to swallow while the tympanum is observed otoscopically. If the membrane bulges slightly into the oral cavity at the moment of swallowing, the Eustachian tube can be considered patent.

Politzer Test: With one nostril occluded, the nasal tip of a Politzer bag is inserted in the antrum of the other nostril while an auscultation tube is passed into the external auditory canal (Fig 22). A popping sound is created by air rushing into the Eustachian tube, indicating patency.

Catheter Inflation Test via the Nasal Cavity: The nasal passage is sprayed with a vasoconstrictor and topical anesthetic (*eg*, Afrin Nose Drops 0.05%:Schering). A urethral catheter is passed along the floor of the nasal cavity to the nasopharynx. When the catheter has been positioned, a bulb syringe is attached to the catheter and an auscultation tube is attached to the ear canal. Air is introduced into the opening of the Eustachian tube by gentle pressure on the bulb. If the tube is open, the sound of air rushing against the membrane can be heard. Fluid in the middle ear causes a crackling sound.

Catheter Inflation Test via the Oral Cavity: This is a variation of the preceding test, with the catheter and viewing instruments introduced through the oral cavity.

External Ear Canal Inflation Test: A tube that snugly fits the external ear canal is attached to a bulb or syringe, air is gently forced into the external ear canal by pressure on the bulb or syringe, and the Eustachian tube orifice is observed by a laryngeal mirror or endoscope in the pharynx. This test is not very reliable because of the difficulty of opening the Eustachian orifice by this method.

Fluorescein Clearance Test: This is the most valuable test of Eustachian tube patency. It is used when the tympanic membrane has been perforated and occlusion of the Eustachian tube is suspected. A 17- or 18-ga, 7-inch blunt-tipped needle is used to inject 1-2 ml sterile fluorescein dye through the tympanic membrane into the middle ear. The pharynx is then periodically examined with a Wood's light for the presence of the fluorescent dye over the next several hours. Dye in the pharynx indictes patency of the Eustachian tube. Corticosteroids, antihistamines and antibiotics should be given systemically to decrease inflammation and reduce the chance of infection.

Fluorescein-Radiopaque Medium Clearance Test: The only difference between this test and the preceding one is that a mixture of fluorescein and contrast medium (Hypaque:Winthrop) is injected through the tympanic membrane. The presence of the fluorescein dye and radiopaque medium makes possible Wood's light examination and contrast radiography with only one injection. As with the preceding test, corticosteroids, antihistamines and antibiotics should be given to decrease inflammation and reduce the chance of infection.

Treatment: Topical medications are effective in treating the pharyngeal end of the Eustachian tube. Most occlusions of the pharyngeal end of the Eustachian tube result from isolated otologic problems, allergy, nasal congestion, pharyngitis or a systemic infection. Symptomatic treatment is directed toward alleviation of congestion. Most medications used for this purpose are sympathomimetic, constricting the surface vasculature of the mucosa and thus reducing edema. These drugs interfere with or shield the cells from the action of histamine, which reduces blood pressure by dilating capillaries and constricting small arteries. Side effects are drowsiness and frequent urination.

When a nasal (or pharyngeal) spray is used, pH must be considered. Mucus from the nasal mucosa is usually acidic (pH 5.5-6.5) and bacteriostatic. In cases of allergy, infection or trauma, the secretions become alkaline, which slows ciliary action. Therefore, nasopharyngeal sprays should be slightly acidic, have high buffering capacity, and not impair ciliary activity. Because nose drops do not spread easily, dangerous doses can be ingested. This is why most nasal medications are in the form of a liquid spray.

Sprays that reduce edema of the nasopharynx and Eustachian orifice are phenylephrine HCl (Neo-Synephrine:Winthrop, Isophrin:Riker), oxymetazoline HCl (Afrin:Schering), and tetrahydrozoline HCl (Tyzine:Pfizer). Most medications used to treat the pharyngeal area are atomized. They are unstable suspensions that cannot be taken into the lungs. Special applicator nozzles may be used with atomized sprays to ensure saturation of the caudal nasopharynx. Many sprays can be administered directly into the external nares of cats.

Neoplasms of the Ear

Neoplasms of the ear can be classified as those involving the skin, subcutaneous tissues and cartilage of the pinna, those involving the secretory glands and wall of the external auditory canal, and those involving the inner ear and nerves.

Types: The pinna is subject to the same types of tumors that affect other areas of the skin. Skin tumors are most prevalent in cats over 4 years of age. Squamous-cell carcinomas are malignant tumors that form spreading nodules covered with a loose crust. The margin of the pinna is usually inflamed and alopecic. This condition is aggravated by solar radiation and is most common in white-haired, blue-eyed cats.[47]

The basal-cell carcinoma originates in the basal-cell layer of the skin. The mass is circular, usually firm and ulcerates in the late stages. This type of tumor is usually found at the base of the pinna.

Tumors of the external auditory canal are usually associated with the ceruminous glands lining the ear canal. The most common type is the adenoma, which may become a carcinoma. Squamous papillomas and adnexal tumors are also found in the ear canal. The ceruminous-gland adenoma or adenosarcoma is usually obscured as a single mass in the external ear canal. It occurs most frequently in old animals with chronic ear disease.

The third group of tumors are those involving the middle and inner ear. Neurofibromas and cholesteatomas are rare in cats. The neurofibroma is a tumor of the nerve sheath and may be benign or malignant, solitary or multilobulated. It is associated with the neural structures of the inner ear and eighth cranial nerve. Cholesteatomas are rare and appear as a cystic mass lined with stratified squamous epithelium. These benign tumors are usually associated with chronic ear disease.

Diagnosis: On clinical examination, tumors must be differentiated from inflammatory lesions, granulomas, abscesses, encysted parasites and foreign bodies. The size, location and appearance of the growth, coupled with the age and breed of animal, are important indicators. Characteristically, skin tumors are chronic, proliferative growths that may form nonhealing ulcers or become secondarily infected. They often are inflamed and have a rich blood supply. An accurate diagnosis of the type of neoplasm depends largely on histopathologic examination.

Treatment: Methods of treating neoplasms include surgery, chemotherapy and radiotherapy. The method used is dictated by the site and type of the tumor. Surgical options include conventional excision of localized tumors, electrosurgery for small benign tumors, such as papillomas and adenomas, cryosurgery for multicentric or generalized tumors restricted to the pinna, because of the large area of tissue which is destroyed, and chemosurgery with chloroacetic acid or silver nitrate, restricted to the pinna.[48,49]

Chemotherapy is used for multicentric or generalized tumors. It may be used as an adjunct to surgery or as the sole treatment in the case of inoperable or highly malignant tumors. Anticancer drugs, such as vinblastine and cyclophosphamide, are used in conjunction with hormones, such as diethylstilbestrol, and corticosteroids.

Radiotherapy is used for multicentric or generalized tumors. Its use is restricted to medical centers because of the expensive equipment required, but it is warranted when life-threatening metastasis is suspected.[50]

References

1. Rose, WR. VM/SAC **71** (1976) 638.
2. Rose, WR. VM/SAC **71** (1976) 308.
3. Stevens, SS and Newman, EB. Am J Psychol **48** (1963) 297.
4. Rose, WR. VM/SAC **71** (1976) 1611.
5. Rose, WR. VM/SAC **71** (1976) 1443.
6. Moltzen, H. Adv Sm Anim Pract **3** (1972) 56.
7. Rose, WR. VM/SAC **71** (1976) 1673.
8. Rose, WR. VM/SAC **72** (1977) 63.
9. Susheston, ME and Cannon, MS. Arch Otolaryng **93** (1971) 58.
10. Miller, GF. Arch Otolaryng **81** (1965) 41.
11. Rose, WR. VM/SAC **71** (1976) 506.
12. Fernando, SDA. Am J Vet Res **28** (1967) 278.
13. Cross, JF. Victoria Vet Pract 1968-1969 (1969) 47.
14. Fernando, SDA. Am J Vet Res **26** (1965) 1157.
15. Erlewein, DL *et al:* Instructions for Veterinary Clients. WB Saunders, Philadelphia, 1975.
16. Ear Diseases in Cats. Client Information Series, Veterinary Practice Publishing, Santa Barbara, 1978.
17. Rose, WR: Hearing and Ear Problems of Dogs and Cats. Southern Calif VMA, Pico Rivera, 1976.
18. Rose, WR. VM/SAC **71** (1976) 31.
19. Baker, E. Sm Anim Clin **1** (1961) 387.
20. Rose, WR. VM/SAC **71** (1976) 151.
21. Ryan, RE *et al:* Synopsis of Ear, Nose and Throat Diseases. 2nd ed. CV Mosby, St. Louis, 1963.
22. Strickland, JH. Am J Vet Res **21** (1960) 845.
23. De Weese, DD and Saunders, WH: Textbook of Otolaryngology. 4th ed. CV Mosby, St. Louis, 1973.
24. Rose, WR. VM/SAC **71** (1976) 695.
25. Rose, WR. VM/SAC **71** (1976) 1025.
26. Rose, WR. VM/SAC **71** (1976) 1280.
27. Wolfsen, RD *et al:* Clinical Symposia Anthology. Ciba Pharmaceutical, 1966.
28. Brodey, RS. Adv Vet Sci Comp Med **14** (1970) 309.
29. Miller, JC *et al.* Acta Otolaryng **Suppl 176** (1963) 1.
30. Watson, CS. J Acoust Soc Am **35** (1963) 167.
31. Rose, WR. VM/SAC **72** (1977) 281.
32. Rose, WR. VM/SAC **72** (1977) 422.
33. Rose, WR. VM/SAC **72** (1977) 624.
34. Rose, WR. VM/SAC **72** (1977) 863.
35. Rose, WR. VM/SAC **72** (1977) 1090.
36. Allen, GW and Fernandez, C. Ann Otol **69** (1960) 5.
37. Rose, WR. VM/SAC **72** (1977) 1295.
38. Rose, WR. VM/SAC **72** (1977) 1165.
39. Rose, WR. VM/SAC **71** (1976) 755.
40. Blakemore, JC. VM/SAC **66** (1971) 357.
41. Toplin, D: Dermatophytes: Their Recognition and Identification. Univ Miami Press, Coral Gables, 1970.
42. Gilbride, AP. Norden News **44(2)** (1969) 24.
43. Sweatman, GK. Can J Zool **36** (1958) 363.
44. Weisbroth, SH *et al.* JAVMA **165** (1974) 1088.
45. Senturia, B: Diseases of the External Ear. Charles C Thomas, Springfield, IL, 1957.
46. Rose, WR. VM/SAC **72** (1977) 1646.
47. Cotchin, E. Vet Rec **69** (1957) 425.
48. Kirchner, FR. Otolaryng Clin No Am **10** (1977) 59.
49. Bostock, DE and Owen, LN. J Sm Anim Pract **13** (1972) 359.
50. Banks, WC *et al.* JAVMA **160** (1972) 446.

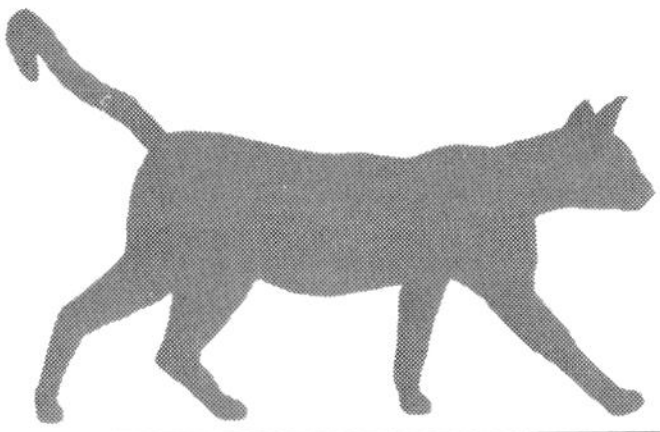

19 behavior

V.L. VOITH AND P.L. BORCHELT

Behavior is what an animal does. It is the outcome of the relationship between the animal and its environment, and is influenced by an infinitude of variables from the time of conception to death. This chapter focuses on behaviors of cats that pose problems for people, other cats or themselves. To understand a problem behavior and effectively treat it, one must understand behavior in general. Most behavior problems of cats consist of essentially normal behaviors that are undesirable from the owner's viewpoint.

FACTORS INFLUENCING BEHAVIOR

Development

The gene-environment interaction is ubiquitous among all of the systems of an organism. Morphology, physiology and behavior are genetically based but continuously shaped and influenced by environmental factors. Morphology is most susceptible to environmental factors early in development. The environment continues to have profound effects on physiology and particularly behavior throughout life.

Some gene-environment interactions cause effects that cannot be modified. These interactions usually are associated with critical periods in the development of an animal. Early experiences tend to set a physiologic and behavioral baseline for an animal throughout life.

An example of the impact of experience on morphology during a critical period is the presence or absence of the stimulus of light on the retina of a cat.[1-3] This experience, within a restricted period after birth, influences the neurologic organization and function of the visual system. Cats raised in the dark or in diffuse light from birth to 3 months of age have thinner lateral geniculate laminae, reduced thickness of the inner plexiform layer of the retinal ganglion, less higher-order dendritic branching in stellate cells of layer IV in the visual cortex and alterations in recordings from single cells in the lateral geniculate and visual cortex. Unilateral light deprivation results in more marked alterations than bilateral deprivation.

When the kittens are allowed to "see" with the eye(s) that has(have) experienced light deprivation, they cannot visually follow objects, frequently collide with objects, cannot jump from one location to another, have no menace (eye blink) response, and have difficulty with visual placing tests and avoidance of "visual cliffs." With time the behavior impairments diminish but the morphologic changes appear to remain. Current research is investigating if visual and behavioral systems temporarily deprived of light can develop after re-exposure to light on a delayed, slowed or different time course.

Rats reared in barren, isolated environments have lower cortical weights and different neurologic configurations than do animals raised in a more normal environment.[4]

The perinatal exposure to certain hormones influences the morphology, physiology and behavior of the individual postnatally. For example, female mammals exposed perinatally to androgens display more masculine behavior traits and morphologic characteristics (somatically and neurologically) than do females unexposed to androgens during this sensitive period.[5,6]

Rats handled (stroked) or exposed to short periods of cold early in life show different adrenal-pituitary and behavioral responses to stress in adulthood than do rats not so manipulated. In adulthood the handled rats appear less frightened in novel situations and are more resistant to many diseases and other environmental stress.[7,8]

There have been few experiments involving the effects of handling or early experience on the behavior of cats. Siamese kittens stroked daily in the first 10 days of life open their eyes sooner, weigh more at weaning, develop adult haircoat coloring earlier and behave differently during learning tasks than kittens not handled.[9] Kittens weaned at 4, 6 and 12 weeks and subsequently raised in isolation differ in their response to novel environments, fearful stimuli and behavior on learning tasks.[10] The earlier the cat was isolated, the more extreme and frightened its behavior in adulthood. Cat owners report that kittens rarely handled before weaning at 8-12 weeks generally are more "skittish," difficult to handle and less friendly to people as adult cats than are cats handled frequently during early kittenhood.

Internal States and External Stimuli

Environmental factors influence an organism's behavior throughout life. For example, spraying urine is a genetically based behavior, the expression of which is influenced by a number of internal and external variables (Fig 1). Androgens facilitate spraying behavior. Castration, treatment with antiandrogens or cessation of treatment with androgen anabolic agents results in reduction or cessation of spraying behavior. Estrous females spray more often than do anestrous females. The percentage of households in which spraying occurs is directly proportional to the number of cats in the household.[11] Owners report a correlation between spraying in the house by resident cats and the number of visiting cats in the neighborhood. Some resident cats only begin spraying after they have fought with an outside cat.

Ethologists have traditionally focused on the study of instinctive, species-typical behaviors that are reactions to stimuli or signals in the environment. These behaviors, through the process of evolution, have helped the animal adapt to its environment. Behaviors generally have evolved under specific conditions and are elicited by certain stimuli in the environment.

In cats, stimuli that elicit species-typical behavior can be complex. To understand complex stimulus-response relationships, it is beneficial to look at some examples in other species that involve simpler stimuli and responses. A classic example is the male robin's aggressive response to the intrusion of another male robin entering its territory during the breeding season.[12] It is not the entire visual configuration of a male robin that elicits the aggressive response to the resident robin. The resident male robin also attacks a small tuft of red cotton. A male robin with its red feathers dyed another color does not elicit an attack. Since no other birds with red body coloration inhabit the areas where robins evolved, an item with red coloration entering the robin's territory has a high likelihood of being another male robin. Therefore, the resident male robin only needs the color red to effectively trigger an attack that leads to chasing the competitor out of its territory. Territorial aggression by male robins in the breeding season is elicited by only one of the characteristics of a male robin, *ie,* the red color.

There are numerous examples in the ethology literature of behavior elicited by only a small part of the stimulus complex. Male stickleback fish in reproductive condition approach a variety of red objects.[13] The males' behavior is more threatening if the color red is restricted to the lower half of an oblong object. In this example, the color red, the position of the color and shape of the object act in an additive fashion to elicit aggressive behavior of the male stickleback, but only when the males are in a reproductive state. This experiment demonstrated the additive effects of components of a stimulus or subsets of a stimulus and the influence of the physiologic state of the individual.

An example of the influence of physiologic states on a cat's response to environmental stimuli is the response of a female cat to being grasped by the nape of the neck or stroked in the anogenital region by a person. When in estrus, female cats are highly likely to respond by lowering the front portion of the body and treading with the back feet. When in anestrus, the same cat usually does not exhibit such behavior. This interaction between hormones and the external environment may be additionally influenced by the cat's experience, such as familiarity with the person stroking it.

Cats approach and investigate cardboard silhouettes in the shape of a cat.[14] Usually the investigating cat sniffs the nose and anogenital areas of the cardboard silhouette. The cat is responding to the configuration of the silhouette and, in a more refined way, to specific areas of the silhouette. These are examples of configurational visual releasers or eliciting stimuli.

Sometimes more than one type of behavior is elicited simultaneously. In these situations, the animal's responses may be ambiguous. The animal either rapidly alternates its responses to the different stimuli or responds with a behavioral composite, incorporating components of several different types of behavior. For example, in preliminary courtship behavior there is an inherent conflict between approach for sexual purposes and withdrawal because of fear of attack by the other animal. The approaching animal may, therefore, demonstrate a composite expression by combining features of both behaviors simultaneously or may rapidly alternate between expressions of intention to approach and flee. Ambivalent behavior frequently occurs when an animal meets an unfamiliar animal of the same species near the boundaries of its territory. If far from home, the animal may readily flee and/or assume a submissive expression. However, on its own territory it is likely to immediately engage in an offensive sequence of behavior and confront the approaching animal. If the animal is at the boundary of its territory, it is likely to exhibit ambivalent behavior.

The threatening, offensive stance of cats consists of the head held forward, ears erect and turned sideways, pupils constricted and mouth closed. A cat's defensive position is head drawn back, ears flattened tightly against the head, pupils dilated and mouth held wide open. A cat in an ambivalent state may rapidly switch back and forth between the extremes of these expressions or assume an intermediate or composite expression. The ears may be held horizontally, with the pupils moderately dilated and mouth partially open.[14]

Sometimes when an animal is motivated to engage in a behavior but is prevented from directing that behavior toward the appropriate target, the animal redirects the behavior to another target. Aggression often is redirected. An indoor cat may see, through a window, a cat approaching its territory. The indoor cat may then turn and attack another indoor cat sitting nearby. Sometimes this is how fighting between cats in a household is initiated. An owner intervening in a fight between cats may be bitten and scratched. This is another example of redirected aggression.

A cat in a conflict may engage in a displacement activity, which is seemingly irrelevant behavior. Displacement activities can occur when 2 behavioral systems are stimulated simultaneously or when the expression of a behavior system is prevented. For example, a cat motivated to approach an owner but inhibited because of the presence of a stranger instead may sit and groom itself. Grooming is a common displacement activity. A bird on the edge of its territory may preen when confronted with an intruder. When nervous, people engage in grooming behavior, such as running fingers through their hair, rubbing their arms or hands, and scratching or picking at scabs or scars.

Prolonged conflict situations in cats may result in excessive grooming, hair loss and self-inflicted injuries. Birds may progress to feather picking. People may excessively scratch their head or bite their fingernails.

Experience

Species-typical behavior generally is an immediate response to specific stimuli and evolved for specific functions of an animal in its environment. Rapidly changing environments limit the usefulness of rigidly programmed behavior. Many species live in changing environments that dictate flexibility in stimulus-response conditions to ensure survival. In other words, they must incorporate experiences to shape their behavior; they must learn.

One of the simplest forms of learning is habituation, the loss or reduction of the performance of a response as a result of exposure to a stimulus without any consequences to the animal. For example, a cat initially may be frightened when it enters a familiar room with rearranged furniture. Continued or repeated exposure to the room leads to a decrease in the fearful behavior. Another common example of habituation is a loss of the fearful and defensive/aggressive behavior of kittens when they first encounter a passive dog. The kittens gradually habituate to the presence of the dog even if there are no positive consequences.

Habituation is influenced by a number of variables, such as the interval between exposures to stimuli or the intensity of the response elicited by the stimulus. For example, the more intense the stimulus, the more intense the response and consequently the more exposure is necessary for habituation.

When a behavior is followed by a positive or negative consequence, subsequent performance of that behavior may change. For example, if a cat is consistently and immediately scolded for jumping onto a table, the frequency of jumping onto the table is reduced. This is an example of punishment. If a cat is frequently fed at a certain time of day after the sound of a refrigerator door opening or the sound of a can opener operating, it will probably run into the kitchen when it hears these sounds at that time of day. This is an example of positive reinforcement or reward.

If the cat is consistently no longer fed after it hears the sound of the refrigerator door or can opener, the cat ceases to respond to the sounds. This is an example of extinction. If the cat had been fed periodically after it heard the sounds of the refrigerator and can opener, the response would take longer to extinguish. Periodic rewards (intermittent schedules of reinforcement) result in very persistent behavior. Some undesirable behaviors of cats are unwittingly reinforced by the owners on an intermittent schedule. For example, an owner awakened early in the morning by cats may feed them so he can resume sleeping. This intermittently rewards the cats for awakening the owner. When the owner ceases the feeding behavior, the cats persist in the early morning activities for a long time.

Definitions

Through the rest of the chapter, a number of terms from the animal behavior and learning literature will be used. The following is a list of abbreviated definitions of these terms.

Experience: Exposure to an environment or stimulus that can have a general effect, either immediately or later, on behavior. Experience is not necessarily identical to learning.

Learning: A more or less permanent change in an animal's response to an environmental stimulus as a result of experience with that stimulus. Learning involves the pairing of specific stimuli with specific responses.

Habituation: Loss or reduction in the frequency, magnitude or duration of a response as a result of repeated exposure to a stimulus that leads to no positive or negative consequences.

Reinforcement: A stimulus or event that increases the future probability of performance of a behavior.

Positive Reinforcement or Reward: A stimulus or event that, after a response, leads to an increase in frequency of that response.

Extinction: Reduction of a response initially acquired by positive reinforcement, following withdrawal of that positive reinforcement.

Negative Reinforcement: An aversive event or stimulus that increases the frequency of performance of a behavior. The animal performs the behavior to escape or avoid the negative reinforcement.

Punishment: A stimulus or event that, after a response, leads to a decrease in the frequency of that response. Punishment usually consists of aversive stimuli.

Generalization: The process by which a response to a specific stimulus is elicited by similar stimuli. The more similar the other stimuli are to the original stimulus, the more similar the responses are to the original response.

Schedules of Reinforcement: The time or frequency relationships between responses and reinforcement. An animal rewarded every time it performs a behavior is on a continuous reinforcement schedule. An animal rewarded periodically is on an intermittent schedule of reinforcement. Behaviors reinforced on intermittent (especially random) schedules are harder to extinguish than behaviors continuously reinforced.

Eliciting Stimulus: A stimulus that elicits a behavior.

Sign Stimulus: Usually a small portion of a stimulus complex that elicits species-typical behavior (instinctive behavior patterns).

Species-Typical Behavior: Behavior that is not learned and that occurs in all members of the species in similar environmental conditions. Species-typical behaviors can be influenced by the physiologic status of the animal and to some degree by experience.

Unconditioned Stimulus: A stimulus that elicits reflexes or species-typical behavior.

Unconditioned Response: A reflex or a component of species-typical behavior evoked by unconditioned stimuli.

Conditioned Stimulus: A stimulus that previously did not elicit reflexes or species-typical behavior, but which does so after being repeatedly paired or associated with an unconditioned stimulus.

Conditioned Response: A response evoked by a conditioned stimulus. The conditioned response is similar to and sometimes nearly identical to the unconditioned response.

Behavior Modification: The application of learning principles to the treatment of problem behavior. Behavior modification generally uses positive reinforcement, desensitization and counterconditioning rather than punishment.

Desensitization: A method of treating anxiety, fears and phobias that involves a gradual exposure to the eliciting stimuli without evoking anxiety or fear responses.

Counterconditioning: A method of ameliorating undesirable behavior by conditioning the animal to engage in a response incompatible with the undesirable response in the same circumstance(s) as that which elicits the undesirable response. Counterconditioning is frequently used in conjunction with desensitization.

BEHAVIOR SYSTEMS

Behavior systems are composed of sequences of species-typical behaviors coordinated to serve a specific function that has adaptive value. The concept of behavior systems is useful in differential diagnosis and treatment of behavior problems. Some behavior problems involve more than one behavior system.

The following list of behavior systems of cats is derived from traditional ethologic classifications. Incorporated in the descriptions of these behavior systems are important general principles of animal behavior and behavior therapy. These principles are introduced in behavior systems that provide good teaching examples. However, it is important that these principles are potentially useful in a multitude of situations and are critical for understanding the next section on treating behavior problems of cats.

Feeding

The feeding behavior system of a predator, such as the cat, can encompass a range of behavior, including searching, chasing, catching, killing and then consuming the prey. In such long sequences of behavior there is considerable flexibility regarding learning in the early stages of the sequence and less at the later stages. The early part of the predatory sequence, such as searching for prey, involves learning where and when prey is likely to be available, learning to stalk accurately, etc. As the cat nears the end of the feeding sequence, its behavior becomes more stereotyped and less amenable to modification by experience or learning. Cats typically catch a small mammal at the nape of the neck, sliding their teeth between the vertebrae to pierce the spinal cord. Whereas the beginning of the sequence requires flexibility and learning, the end of the sequence does not. The end of the sequence requires behavior that leaves little room for error and usually is programmed genetically. The behavior must be performed correctly to ensure survival of the animal.

Elimination

By 4 weeks of age kittens scratch and then eliminate in a suitable substrate, such as "kitty litter" or sand. They do this without having ever seen their dam or other cats use such material and they use a suitable substrate even if it has never been used by another cat.

Urination and defecation involve finding a suitable place and surface on which to eliminate. The typical pattern involves scratching, making a depression in the material, eliminating and scratching the material over the feces or urine. Sometimes the cat simply scratches nearby without covering the feces or urine.

Urine Marking

Urine marking apparently has a communicative function and usually occurs in the context of territorial, agonistic and sexual behavior. Agonistic behavior refers to all aspects of competitive encounters between animals, usually of the same species. Cats most often urine mark in a spraying position. Spraying usually involves expulsion of small amounts of urine on easily noticed objects. A spraying cat stands with a quivering erect tail, alternately steps with the back feet, and expels urine backward onto a vertical surface (Fig 1). Scratching behavior usually does not precede or follow spraying. Occasionally cats squat and expel small amounts of urine in locations and situations similar to those in which spraying occurs; this might be considered marking behavior. To categorize voiding urine in a squatting posture as urine marking requires that it be manifested in the same circumstances as spraying behavior. If a cat frequently performs urine marking, it may never squat and urinate in the litterbox.

Spraying behavior classically demonstrates the dynamic relationship between internal and external stimuli that can facilitate the behavior. Spraying is undoubtedly a genetically based behavior, but whether the animal expresses this behavior depends on a variety of factors. Androgens, endogenous or exogenous, facilitate spraying behavior. Removal of these substances, by castration or cessation of medication, usually results in cessation or reduction of spraying behavior. Treatment with antiandrogens and pro-

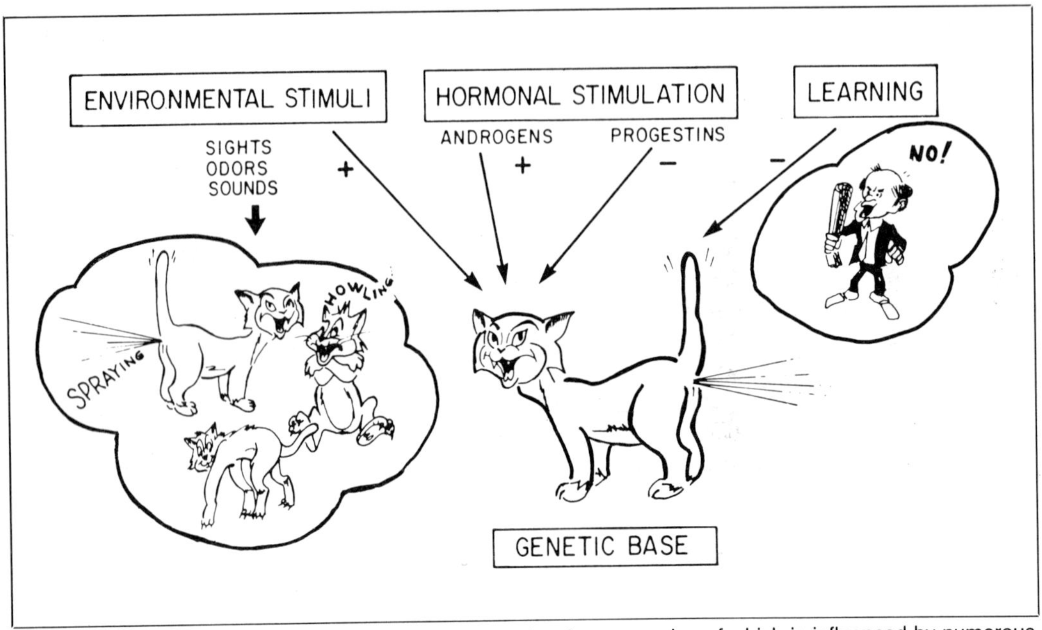

Fig 1. Spraying by male cats is genetically based behavior, the expression of which is influenced by numerous stimuli. (Courtesy of the California Veterinarian)

gestins also tends to suppress spraying behavior. Male cats are more likely to spray than female cats; females in estrus are more likely to spray than anestrous females. Intact males are more likely to spray than castrated males.

A number of environmental variables affect spraying behavior. The probability of spraying by at least one cat increases linearly from 25% in a single-cat household to 100% in households of more than 10 cats (Fig 2).[11] The presence or increase in number of cats invading the yard or perimeter of the area where a housecat lives may precipitate spraying behavior. When the number of cats in a household is reduced or outside cats are prevented from approaching the home of the resident cat, spraying behavior in the home often subsides.

Grooming

Grooming behavior helps maintain the condition of the integument. It involves licking, washing, nibbling or removing hairs or objects from the coat and from between the toes. Cats also remove sloughing sheaths from their nails by scratching. Interestingly, even after a cat is declawed it continues "claw-sharpening" behavior. Cats do not appear to suffer "psychological damage" as a result of proper declawing. They continue to behave as if they still had claws and do not appear "distressed" or "frustrated."

Cats frequently engage in mutual grooming and often groom parts of the body on other cats that are hard for individuals to reach themselves. Grooming also may serve a communicative function in social behavior, such as attachment and subordinance/dominance relationships. Grooming behavior often serves as displacement activities in cats; when carried to an extreme, self-injury can result.

Sleep

Most mammals require sleep or rest periods. Cats often engage in considerable amounts of sleep. Sleep may be a restorative process or an alternative behavior when there is nothing else to do. Cats often seek out warm places to sleep and often sleep with people or other cats. In fact, when they are preparing to sleep, many pet cats seek out their owners.

Play

One of the characteristics of mammals, particularly the young, is play behavior. Play is difficult to define but easy to recognize. Play apparently has no immediate goal other than play itself; although it may ultimately result in benefits, such as sharpening skills of hunting, fighting, social signaling and establishment of social hierarchies. Play is composed of sequences of other behavior systems, particularly aggressive and predatory systems. Owners sometimes misinterpret the playful behavior of cats as abnormal aggressive behavior.

Exploration

Cats often investigate novel or unfamiliar situations, ranging from paper bags to new individuals. Exploration can lead to learning more about the environment. This information can be used for hunting and finding prey, establishing escape routes or discovering new feeding or drinking resources. Relatively solitary animals, such as cats, may engage in more exploratory behavior than do social animals living in groups that benefit from the experience of others.

Sexual Behavior

Sexual behavior involves finding a potential mate, courtship, copulation and postcopulatory behavior. Feline sexual behavior has been more extensively researched than other behavior systems and more is known about its physiologic components.

The cat is a polyseasonal, induced ovulator (see Chapter 15). In the northern hemisphere, queens usually come into estrus in early spring and late summer.[15] Queens remain in heat 4-8 days and, if conception does not occur, cycle at 2-week intervals during that breeding season. Domestic cats can produce 2-3 litters a year. Feral queens usually have only one litter a year unless the first litter is lost.[16]

Feral cats tend to live by themselves, although they may congregate at specific locations, such as a barn, and frequently communicate via auditory, olfactory and visual signals. Estrous queens usually increase their vocalization and may spray urine.

Queens may not always breed with any available male.[14] Female cats, like dogs, may have preferences and reject normal, fertile males.

A female cat may mate with more than one male. Consequently, a litter may be sired by more than one tom (see Chapter 15).

A female cat might solicit a male by approaching, touching noses, crouching on her elbows, elevating her pelvis and treading with the back feet before the male mounts her. More frequently, a male cat initiates most of this behavior by grasping the female by the back of the neck with his teeth.

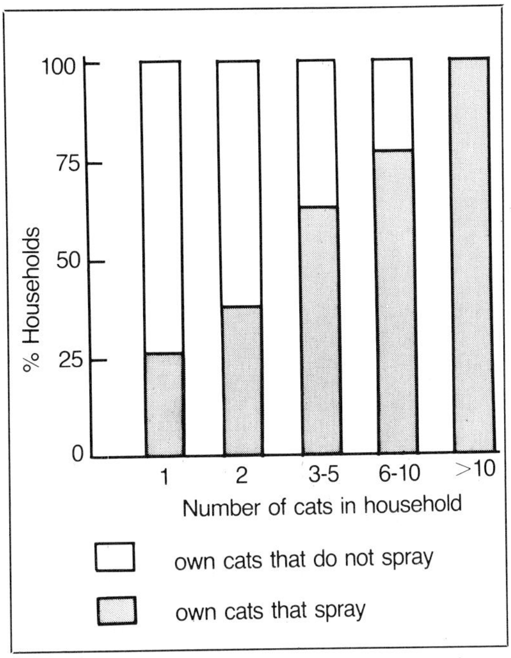

Fig 2. Relationship of spraying and the number of cats in the household. (Courtesy of Drs J.E. Jemmett and G. Skerritt)

Courtship behavior in feral cats has not been described. In laboratory situations, the male and female, upon introduction, usually approach each other and sniff noses. The male, depending upon his experience, then grasps the female by the back of the neck and mounts her. The neck bite often elicits the elevated pelvis and deviated tail. The female's treading motions may not be elicited until the male cat starts strumming her thorax with his front feet. Upon intromission, the female cries and begins to pull away. Unless he holds on with his teeth, the male is actively displaced. Shortly after the female cries, the male voluntarily releases or is forced to release the neck bite by the female's twisting motions.

Upon release, the female usually turns and swats at the male, often forcing him to retreat. She then usually engages in rolling and rubbing behavior. During this postcopulatory display, the female lies on the ground and rubs her sides or rolls over repeatedly. Owners sometimes misinterpret this as abnormal behavior. The female may direct aggression (biting and scratching) toward the male cat or a person who tries to interrupt this behavior. When the rubbing and rolling subside, the female then usually licks her vulva. The male, in a laboratory situation, watches from a distance, usually licks his genitalia and waits for an opportunity to again breed the female. If the male does not take the initiative after some time, the female may then again solicit the male for breeding.

Housecats in estrus might become more aggressive or more friendly toward people. A person familiar with a specific cat might be able to elicit signs of estrus with tactile stimulation approximating that of a male cat. By grasping the cat by the nape of the neck and stroking the back and pelvic area, a person can cause her to elevate her pelvis, deviate her tail and tread with her back legs. This behavior can be facilitated by stroking the cat in the perineal area.

Female cats that are very attached to their owners may delay parturition unless the owner remains with them. Some cats cease attending to the birth process and follow when the owner leaves the room. However, after several kittens are born, the cat becomes engrossed in her maternal activities and stays with the kittens (see Chapter 15).

Parental Behavior

Parental behavior can encompass nesting, parturition, raising the young and training the young to hunt. Raising the young includes nursing, grooming, retrieval of wandering kittens, moving the kittens, defending the kittens, etc. Male cats usually do not participate in raising the young.

Queen-kitten nursing interactions occur in 3 phases.[17] In the first phase, which lasts about 3 weeks, the queen initiates all contact with the offspring. During the first several days after parturition, the queen may stay with the kittens constantly. Thereafter, her departures become more frequent and longer. In the second phase, from 3 to 6 weeks, both queen and kittens initiate contact equally often. In the third phase, only the kittens initiate nursing contact and the queen begins to wean them. Females reared together or that live together under friendly circumstances may share nursing responsibilities of litters. Some queens deposit their kittens with another litter, abandoning them to the care of another queen.[16]

Killing of kittens by tom cats is a commonly held belief but has rarely been observed by researchers in the field. Nomadic male lions have been observed killing infant cubs in prides they have not sired.[18,19] In domestic cats, nursing queens are more nervous than other females when a new male enters their territory.[16]

Queens bring prey back to their offspring when the kittens reach about 16 weeks; thereafter, they may take one or all of the kittens on foraging expeditions away from the home area.[16] Kittens undisturbed by people may continue to periodically nurse until 6 months of age or older. The abnormal sucking and chewing behavior seen in some domestic cats may be a result of genetic/early weaning experience interactions.[20]

Attachment

Mammals engage in varying degrees of interaction with animals of the same species. Some remain in highly coordinated social groups throughout their entire lives; others openly associate with those of the same species only during the reproductive season, and some are in social groups only from birth to weaning. Cats belong to a variable system. Many housecats live amicably together throughout their entire lives. If outdoor cats are well provisioned by people, large matriarchal social groups may form. These units are comprised of adult females, usually related, and their female offspring. At about a year of age, males become targets of attacks by older males patrolling that territory. Shortly thereafter, the young males emigrate. At 2-3 years of age, they may begin to challenge older males.[30] In other, probably less well-provisioned rural areas, the kittens may disperse or the queen may leave her grown kittens and seek a new territory for herself. The kittens then divide up her former territory.[16] In the feral state, adult cats are relatively solitary. However, even these cats may congregate periodically at certain places, such as feeding stations (*eg*, a barn) or rendezvous points (*eg*, alley or backyard), where singing or vocalization takes place.[14] Despite the fact that cats do not live continuously in groups, they probably are in frequent communication by vocalization and olfactory signals.

The wide range of facial and body expressions implies that cats engage in social visual signals, which in turn implies a degree of sociality. Pet cats often live compatibly in groups within a house and display attachment behaviors to each other and to people. Cats may follow each other or the owner from room to room and constantly seek contact, to the point of pestering the owner. Cats may insist on the owner being with them during parturition. Some vocalize when the own-

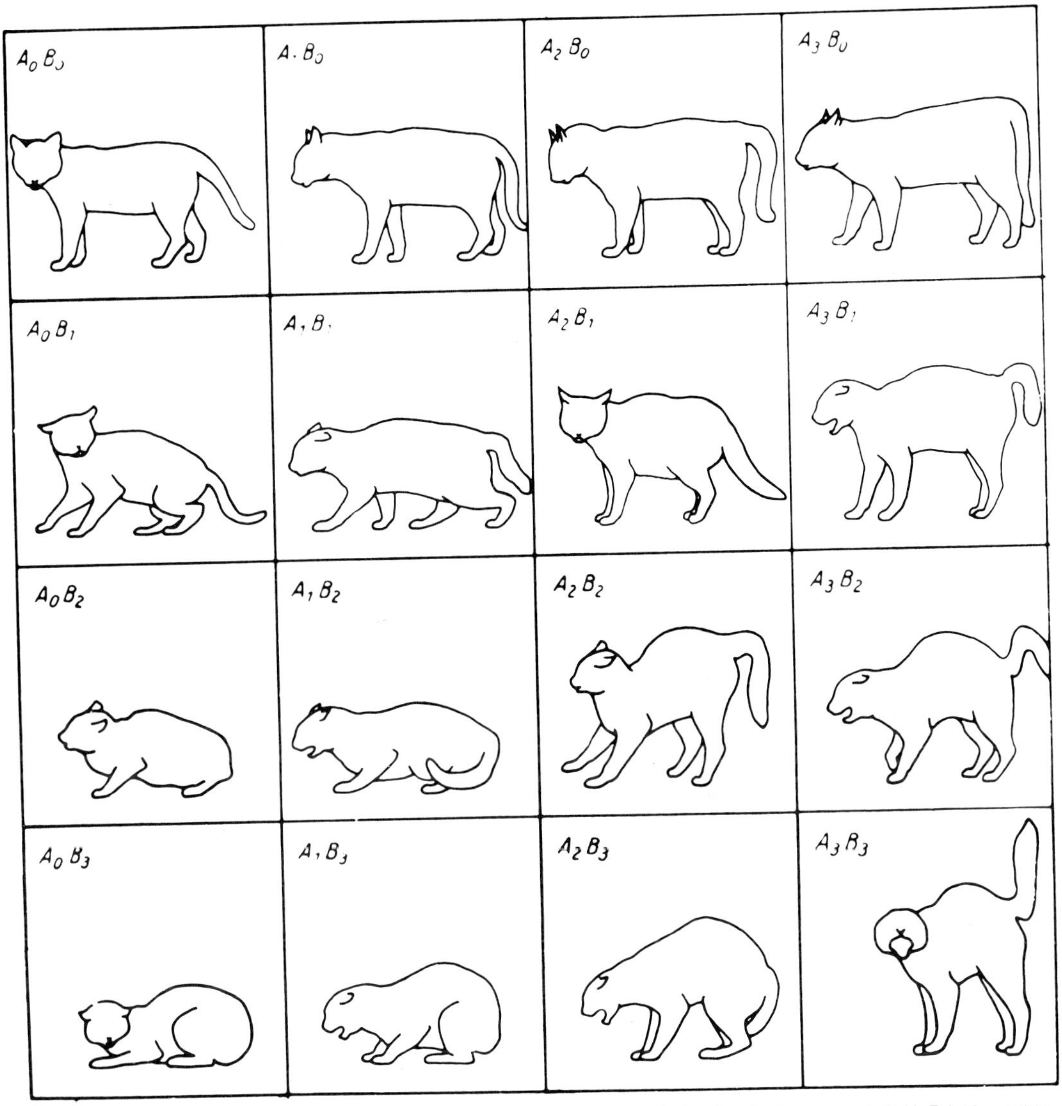

Fig 3. Body posture in varying degrees of aggressive and defensive behavior. In the upper left (A_0B_0), the cat is in a "neutral" state, neither aggressive or defensive. Moving along the top row to the right, the posture reflects an increasing degree of aggression. Moving from the neutral state down the left column, the posture becomes increasingly defensive. Moving from the neutral posture down and to the right, the postures become increasingly a combination of aggression and defense. A_3B_3 illustrates an equally high intensity of aggressive and defensive posturing. (Courtesy of Dr P. Leyhausen and Garland STPM Press)

ers depart or show other apparent separation-anxiety behaviors.

Agonistic Behavior

Agonistic behavior is on a continuum, from highly offensive behavior (attacks, threats, signals of attack) to purely defensive behavior (defensive aggression, submissive behavior, fleeing). The range of facial expressions and body postures of cats have been correlated with the various motivational states.[14] Observations or detailed descriptions of the expressions of a cat when engaging in an aggressive situation should help the clinician determine why the cat is acting as it is and, therefore, facilitate treatment. Cats often rapidly move from one set of expressions to another in conflict situations.

Aggression in domestic cats involves biting, scratching and threats, such as hissing, spitting and growling, directed to a person or another animal. To understand the kinds of aggressive behavior problems owners typically encounter with pet cats, one must understand the elements of offensive or attack behavior, the elements of defensive or "fear behavior," and how these elements are combined during aggression (Fig 3). Most of the information about social and aggressive signals and postures of free-ranging cats is based on observations and experiments.[14]

Intermale Aggression

Aggression between 2 tom cats may include "pure attack," *ie,* without any signs of defensive or fear behavior. These postures have been described as "rival fighting" (Fig 3 A_3B_0). The attacking male draws itself up on its legs, with the back straight. The back is held higher than the front; the forward-facing slope of the back is accentuated by piloerection along the dorsum. The tail continues these lines for an inch or so, then bends down sharply. The tail is stiff and the end may twitch back and forth.

The pupils are not dilated and may even be somewhat constricted. The head is stretched forward and the cat stares at the opponent. The ears are not flattened back but are raised and turned outward so the back of the ear is visible to the opponent. The cat moves forward very slowly and deliberately, alternately meowing, howling or growling.

When close, the attacker raises and tilts the head at an angle of about 45° while continuing to stare at the opponent. The attacker slowly turns its tilted head from side to side. As the cats get closer, the steps taken become shorter and slower. The cats might remain facing each other for many minutes before suddenly one bites toward the nape of the other's neck, whereupon they usually roll around on the ground biting at each other, scratching and clawing with the rear legs. Such wrestling may be interrupted several times by a resumption of threat behavior.

The victorious cat usually walks away or sniffs the ground. Immediate fatalities are not usual, although many wounds may be inflicted. Victorious cats do not always move in and take over another cat's territory.

Territorial Aggression

A cat's territory consists of a home area and a home range. In free-ranging cats, the home area may be a house, barn or garage, and the home range an area of 0.5 to several square kilometers.[14] Territories of females usually are smaller than the territories of males. Free-ranging cats seem to regulate their comings and goings by visual and olfactory contact. Cats that see another cat on a path usually avoid a confrontation. If they have fought in the past, the previous loser is chased away by the victor. Spraying behavior, by either males or females, apparently is another source of information related to territory and social structure. The odor does not seem to intimidate the approaching cat, but seems to serve as a signal indicating who is where in the territory and how long ago they passed the sprayed location. The home range of housecats usually is the entire house.

The relationship between territory and social rank in domestic cats is very complex. Cats do not form a rigid social hierarchy or linear "pecking order," in which the "top cat" dominates all others, a second cat dominates all but the first, and so on down the line. Instead, they form a "relative social hierarchy," in which social superiority is relative to place and time.[14] For example, the cat that arrives first at a location may have priority over a cat arriving later. If 2 cats have had a confrontation, the winner may assume priority over the loser when they subsequently meet at the same time of day in that location.

Cats, usually thought of as being asocial, often gather together at night, when they engage in such group activities as mutual grooming, sitting in contact, or perhaps just sitting and watching other cats. These gatherings are friendly and sociable even though at other times and places the cats may be very territorial.

As a young intact male matures, he is challenged by other adult tom cats in the population. This social "testing" may lead to intense fighting, followed by the youngster fitting into the social hierarchy or leaving. Territorial aggression frequently occurs between adult tom cats meeting for the first time. In a typical household, male cats routinely are castrated, which significantly reduces intermale aggression.

Female cats, even when spayed, frequently engage in territorial aggression. Females with young also are very territorial.

Territorial aggression seems to occur after cats have fully matured at about 2-3 years of age. Siblings may be compatible for several years before territorial disputes occur. Aggression also can occur when a new cat is introduced into the house. Occasionally, a new cat elicits from the resident cat fear or defensive aggression, which usually disappears within a few days or weeks. However, if the resident cat is territorial, the aggression continues and involves more attack than defensive components. In territorial disputes, the resident charges the intruder and chases it away. The intruder usually runs away; if not, the 2 cats may rear up and box at each other with their paws.

When many unrelated adult cats are kept together, particularly in relatively confined areas (homes or apartments), typically 1-2 cats take over the most desirable resting places, go first to the food bowl and in general "rule the roost." Sometimes a cat is tolerated only as long as it stays away from the others and does not interact with them.

There appears to be a direct relationship between the degree of crowding and the rigidity of social hierarchies. The greater the density of cats, the more the hierarchy becomes absolute rather than relative. However, cats in extremely crowded situations paradoxically do not fight as intensely. Rather, cats in crowded situations continuously display low-intensity aggression, such as hissing, swatting with paws and piloerection, which appears to prevent frequent, intensive fighting. A cat's social position does not always appear to be determined by size, strength or sex.[14] However, in rural areas, the older and largest feral tom cats maintain territories and engage in most of the breeding.[30]

Defensive/Fear-Induced Aggression

In contrast to attack behavior, of which biting and clawing with the rear feet are the principal characteristics, the major feature of defensive aggression is blows with the front paws. The head is drawn back, the cat crouches, the pupils are dilated and the hair is erect. These defensive postures are not so much behavior of submission but rather a means by which the cat defends itself, particularly the nape of its neck, from its opponent. They are meant as serious threats to intimidate the attacker. It is typical for a cat to alternate between attack and defense, depending on the circumstances and the behavior of the other cat.

A common aggressive behavior problem in cats in the home involves defensive aggression in the context of fear. For instance, a cat confronted with a new dog, cat or person in the home may hiss, spit, erect the hair on its dorsum and arch its back (Fig 3 A_3B_3). As the fear subsides, the level of aggression usually wanes.

Redirected Aggression

A cat in an aggressive "mood," due to defensive, intermale or territorial aggression, readily redirects its aggression to other stimuli. For instance, a cat may be sitting at the window, looking and hissing at another cat outside. If the owner then picks up the pet cat to take it away, the cat may attack the owner. The cat redirects its aggression from the stimulus outside the window to another object nearby.

BEHAVIOR PROBLEMS

Differential Diagnostic Categories

There are several classification schemes involved in the diagnosis of behavior problems. These divisions are not mutually exclusive.

Etiologic Classification

A behavior problem might stem from normal or abnormal behavior. Normal behavior is species-typical and learned behavior that is advantageous to the animal in its present circumstance. Most behavior problems in animals involve normal behavior that poses problems to the owner.

Abnormal behavior may result from disease, aberrant environments or experiences. For example, restricted environments early in life can lead to pervasive fears and unusual reactions to novel situations throughout adult life. Phobias, intense fears out of proportion to the real threat of the stimulus, and psychosomatic disorders are acquired as a result of experience.

Descriptive Classification

Behavior also can be descriptively classified. For example, hissing, scratching, biting, urination and defecation are all specific responses. The description of the actual behavior problem contains elements or entire sequences of species-typical behavior.

Functional Classification

Once a description of the behavior and the context in which the behavior occurs are obtained, the behavior can be categorized according to a function, motivational set or behavioral system of the animal. For example, a cat is described as attacking the owner. The description of the behavior reveals that the cat swats at, lightly scratches and lightly bites the ankles of the person as he or she goes up and down the steps. Sometimes the cat approaches the owner, hopping sideways with an arched back. Although several people live in the household, the cat only directs this behavior to the person to whom the cat is most attached. The description of this behavior is compatible with a cat engaging in play behavior. Play, particularly in cats, involves many components of aggression. This case would be diagnosed as play-motivated aggressive behavior and is treated differently than territorial or fear-related aggressive problems.

Diagnosis and Treatment of Specific Behavior Problems

Ingestive Behavior Problems

Ingestion of normally inedible objects is not an uncommon complaint by owners of purebred and mixed-breed Siamese cats. The etiology of this behavior is not known. These cats often consume woolen objects and sometimes other cloth items. Punishment, using aversive tastes and alterations in diet, have been tried with only occasional success. It has been hypothesized that wool-chewing results from an interaction of genetic predisposition and weaning before 6-8 weeks, the age at which cats are weaned by the undisturbed dam.[20] Wool-chewing is a trait that is potentially detrimental to both the cat and the owner's property.

Ingestion of grass, plants and growing vegetables is normal in cats of all breeds, sexes and ages. The cat may vomit after ingesting plant material. The plants may afford some nutritional ingredients or serve as emetics that facilitate expulsion of hair balls.

Anorexia is the reduction or cessation of normal eating. Disease usually is the cause of anorexia. However, cats may stop eating in anxious or psychologically depressing situations, such as when separated from an owner or another animal.[20] If specific stimuli can be identified as eliciting the anxiety behavior, the cat can be desensitized and counterconditioned.[21]

Elimination Behavior Problems

The most common behavioral problem is urination, defecation or spraying outside the litterbox. When a cat is presented for "wetting" in the house, the clinician's first task is to determine if the cat is squatting or spraying. The clinician should not assume the owner knows what the term "spraying" means, even if the client uses the term. If the client cannot describe the posture of the cat, the clinician should obtain a precise description of where the urine is found. Cats that spray deposit urine on vertical surfaces, several inches to a foot off the floor. Squatting cats deposit urine on horizontal surfaces. If the cat is squatting, voiding large amounts, does not have a urogenital disease and is not voiding urine in contexts similar to those in which spraying occurs, it can be assumed that the cat is simply urinating.

Inappropriate Urination and Defecation: Urination and defecation outside the litterbox are treated similarly and are discussed together below. Some cats only defecate or only urinate outside the box; some eliminate on specific surfaces, such as carpet or linoleum. Some cats have never consistently used litterbox material; from the time they were kittens, they periodically eliminated outside the box. For whatever reason, some cats develop a preference for eliminating in locations and on materials other than those provided for them by the owners.

Treatment consists of making the litterbox area more attractive and decreasing the attractiveness of eliminating elsewhere. Implementation of these objectives encourages the cat to resume using the litterbox and re-establishes the habit of consistently eliminating there. Treatment of the problem first necessitates an evaluation of all characteristics of the litterbox, *eg,* where it is, how it is maintained and how it is constructed. Detailed descriptions must also be obtained of the inappropriate areas the cat uses, the amount of urine expelled and, if possible, the time of day the behavior occurs.

One of the first approaches in treating an elimination problem is to determine the relative attractiveness of the litterbox or litter material. Some cats do not care to eliminate in boxes that are too small, covered with a lid that traps odors within the box, frequently used by other cats, not cleaned frequently, kept in a noisy or heavily trafficked area, or that contain specific types of litter material, such as chlorophyll tablets or pellets. A cat may avoid the litterbox area if it is frequently disturbed there by people.

Sometimes inappropriate punishment employed in attempts to treat elimination problems make the litterbox area more aversive. If an owner punishes a cat some time after it has eliminated in an inappropriate area and then immediately takes the cat to the litterbox, there is actually a closer temporal pairing of punishment with the litterbox than with the other area!

If a cat is eliminating in only a few places outside the litterbox, changing the significance of these locations from elimination to another behavior system may stop the cat from eliminating there and consequently force it back to the litterbox. Sometimes placing food or playthings in such locations or making the area aversive with mothballs or a repellent stops the cat from eliminating there. Covering the area with something a cat does not like to walk or scratch

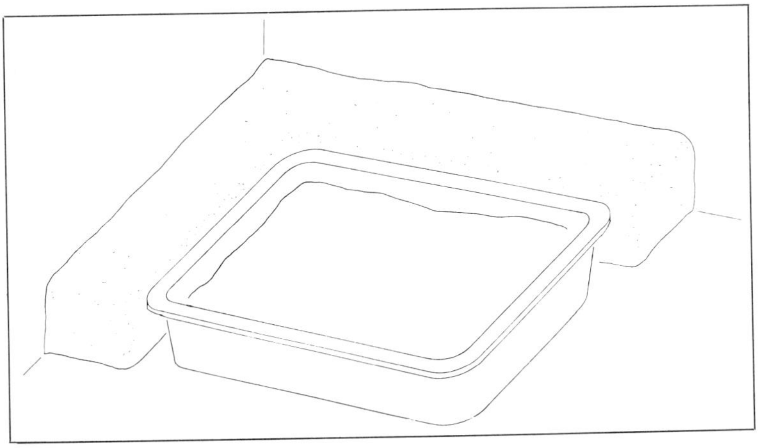

Fig 4. Carpeted shelf around the litterbox encourages the cat to eliminate in the box.

on also often discourages a cat from eliminating in that location.

One should, of course, clean the inappropriate area where the cat eliminates with a substance that masks or deactivates the odoriferous properties of urine or feces. The odor of previous elimination may attract the cat back to the area. Since one of the degradation products of urine is ammonia, use of cleaning products containing ammonia should be avoided because they might attract the cat. It should be noted that cats may continue to eliminate in an area even though the urine odor has been completely removed.

The species-typical sequence of elimination behavior of cats involves scratching before and after elimination. Pre-elimination scratching usually includes digging behavior; postelimination scratching usually includes covering behavior. Scratching behavior and scratching preferences provide clues as to the type of material upon which a cat prefers to eliminate. For example, many cats consistently eliminate outside of the litterbox upon specific types of carpet, often the plushest carpeting in the house. Other cats prefer throw rugs, clothing or mattresses. Cats that eliminate outside the litterbox often have histories of frequently scratching on other substances shortly before or after eliminating in the litterbox. Many of these cats rarely scratched in the litter to cover their feces.

One step in treating these problems is to place materials associated with elimination around the litterbox, such as on a platform surrounding the box, tacked over the sides or in the bottom of the litterpan (Fig 4). This increases the probabilty that the cat will scratch on the material attached to the litterbox and also eliminate in the litterbox. However, this technic must be coupled with keeping the cat from eliminating in the inappropriate area. Repeated elimination in the litterbox re-establishes the habit of eliminating there.

A cat usually can be prevented from eliminating on carpeted areas by picking up the carpet, covering the carpeted area with aluminum foil or plastic, or prohibiting access to that particular room. Regardless of the preventive technic, the cat must eventually be allowed access to these areas without eliminating on them. After the cat has resumed using the litterbox for several weeks, the room should be gradually changed back to its original appearance. If the cat has been eliminating at the perimeter of the room, the first portion of the floor to be uncovered should be the center. Once the cat has demonstrated that it can spend time in the room without eliminating, the central exposed area can be gradually expanded several inches a day until the entire room is again uncovered.

If the cat has demonstrated a preference for eliminating on smooth surfaces, such as bathtubs, tile or linoleum, a smooth substrate for elimination can be provided by using a large, empty litterbox. Again, care must be taken to prevent the cat from eliminating on the inappropriate smooth surfaces. The floor might be covered with paper or throw rugs, and tubs and sinks filled with water. Slightly tilting the litterbox allows the urine to run to one end and facilitates cleaning. The cat should be allowed to use the smooth-surfaced empty litterbox for several weeks before the owner begins adding litter. Litter should gradually be added (no more than a few tablespoons a day). Cats that eliminate on smooth surfaces in the house often have histories of having scratched smooth surfaces, such as floor, walls or the toilet bowl, before or after using the litterbox.

When the above tactics do not discourage the cat from eliminating in inappropriate places, this indicates the cat may have a strong location preference for elimination. This is graphically demonstrated when owners rotate a rug 180° and the cat continues to eliminate in the same location even though the area on the rug where it had been eliminating is now at the opposite end of the room. When a cat has a strong location preference, it will eliminate on top of plastic, aluminum foil, near food, etc. In such cases, the most effective treatment is to put the litterbox where the cat is eliminating. Usually the cat uses the box. Then the box can be slowly and gradually moved from that area to a location that the owner wishes. As the box is moved away, one might implement other technics to keep the cat from eliminating in the old location. If the box is moved gradually and steps have been taken to make the litterbox more attractive, the cat usually follows the box back to where the owner wishes it to be kept.

Occasionally a cat may begin eliminating outside the litterbox because of a change in environmental situations. A cat apprehensive of a new person or animal in the house may be afraid to traverse open areas and travel to the litterbox. This problem could be corrected with desensitization and counterconditioning or by moving the litterbox to where the cat can easily reach it. Some cats appear to eliminate outside the litterbox when the owner is away for a prolonged time. In some cases this is because the litterbox becomes dirtier than usual, but other times this factor is not a consideration. Interestingly, under such circumstances, the cat may eliminate upon a very personal item of the owner, such as the bed, pillows or clothing. It is unclear whether to label this type of elimination pattern as marking behavior.

If the cat is upset due to the presence of other persons or animals, desensitization and counterconditioning may be effective ways of treating the problem. If the cat is reacting to prolonged absences of the owner, a more effective treatment may be temporary use of drugs that reduce anxiety, such as amitriptyline, benzodiazepines and progestins. It should be remembered, and owners advised, that these drugs are not approved for use in cats. Clinicians should be familiar with possible side effects and consequences of such drug therapy. The rationale in using antianxiety drugs is to allow the animal experience in the situation without anxiety or fear. The goal is to gradually withdraw the drug and maintain the animal in a drug-free state. The drug should be withdrawn gradually so the animal gradually perceives the environment in an unemotional state. We have not treated a sufficient number of cats, according to a specific regimen, to confidently recommend specific drug dosages and therapeutic schedules of treatment. We have been treating animals with an initial dosage for 2 weeks, reducing the dosage by half over the next 2 weeks, and then stopping administration or continuing to reduce the dosage over the following several weeks. The duration of administration depends on the severity of the problem, environmental factors and how rapidly the problem is responding to treatment.

Marking: Cats may mark in a spraying or squatting posture. If it uses a squatting posture, the amount of urine expelled usually is small and in the same circumstances or location that an animal would spray. For example, marking behavior is suggested if a cat eliminates inside the box and also voids urine in small amounts near the door or windows.

There are several therapeutic approaches for spraying or marking. Some clinicians believe there is a correlation between cystitis and spraying, but this has not been documented. Spraying is performed most frequently by intact male cats. Of cats castrated for this problem, 90% stop or greatly reduce spraying.[22]

Some cats cease marking behavior if the environment is manipulated. For example, spraying is correlated with the number of cats in a household. If the spraying cat becomes a solitary housecat, the problem may stop. The presence of transient outdoor cats might elicit spraying in a resident cat. Preventing cats from visiting may reduce spraying. This can sometimes be accomplished by redirecting the visitor's route around the owner's yard with fencing or barriers. If a cat is spraying or urine marking in only a few locations, changing the significance of the location may stop the problem. Converting these areas to feeding stations, by placing small amounts of food in the area, or play stations, by placing toys or strips of aluminum foil in the vicinity, may prevent the cat from spraying there. Sometimes the same effect can be accomplished by making these areas aversive, by placing mothballs in the area. These technics are not likely to work if the cat sprays in a number of places in the home.

If the cat is spraying or urine marking in several locations, the alternatives available are neutering, reducing the number of cats in the household, reducing contact with outside cats and removing constant sources of stress that may be precipitating the behavior. If these alternatives are not feasible or do not work, progestin therapy and olfactory tractotomy are 2 remaining alternatives. Megestrol acetate (Ovaban:Schering) and medroxyprogesterone acetate (Depo-Provera:Upjohn) are the most commonly used drugs to suppress spraying.

Megestrol acetate generally is used initially at 5 mg/day given PO for 1-2 weeks. If the spraying does not stop, use of the medication should be stopped. If the spraying ceases, the dose should be gradually reduced to a minimum effective level. Maintenance doses vary considerably. Use of the medication should be periodically stopped to determine if the cat is still motivated to spray. Repository injections of 100 mg medroxyprogesterone acetate can be repeated a few times a year. Frequent administration is likely to result in adverse side effects. The progestins should not be used in intact females for treatment of spraying behavior. The progestins are not approved for use in cats and their use in cats must be considered experimental.

Owners also should be made aware of the possible side effects from use of progestins. The synthetic progestogens can cause increases in appetite, mammary gland hyperplasia and hyperglycemia. Research in dogs also indicates elevated plasma insulin levels, elevated plasma growth hormone levels, acromegaly, glucose intolerance/diabetes mellitus, polyuria, suppression of adrenal cortex activity, decreased PCV, reduced exercise tolerance, thickening of the gall bladder epithelium and possible jaundice, and, in intact females, chronic endometrial hyperplasia or pyometra.[23-25] Prolonged treatment with medroxyprogesterone caused adenocarcinomas in female cats.[26] The use of synthetic progestins should not be taken lightly.

In dogs, the probability of developing most of these side effects increases with age. Therefore, older animals should be considered at more risk than younger animals. The possibility of side effects should be weighed by the practitioner and owner against the probability of the drug working, the side effects that may occur relative to the cat's age and the possibility of euthanasia if the cat continues to engage in the behavior problem.

Oral progestins have the advantage of immediate cessation of administration if side effects result. Repository injections cannot be easily retrieved.

There are advantages to periodically stopping progestin administration. The factors that influence spraying may no longer be present or may have waned in importance and the drug may no longer be necessary. Intermittent use of the medication also may reduce the probability of side effects. In younger animals, if side effects are detected early, withdrawal of the drug should result in reversal of the side effects.

Olfactory tractotomy has reduced or stopped marking or spraying in male and female cats.[27] No objectionable side effects from the surgery have been reported. The advantages and disadvantages of the neurosurgery should be weighed against the probability of euthanasia or side effects from prolonged use of progestins.

Medial preoptic lesions resulted in suppression or cessation of spraying in most male cats but did not affect spraying in female cats.[28] The side effects of this lesion were hyperphagia and a "startle reaction" during sleep. Because of these side effects, this procedure is not recommended for clinical treatment of spraying.

The efficacy of such drugs as diazepam and phenobarbital has not been evaluated in treatment of spraying. In the authors' experience, such drugs usually are not effective.

Reward and Punishment: Elimination problems do not lend themselves readily to treatment with positive reinforcement and punishment. For punishment to be effective, it must be administered immediately upon the onset of the behavior and every time the behavior occurs. For reward to be effective, it should be administered within a few seconds of performance of a behavior. Both of these constraints are hard for the average cat owner to meet. Punishing the cat, even a few seconds after it has eliminated in an area, by bringing it back, rubbing its nose in the spot, hitting it or severely scolding it, does not meet the requirements of effective punishment. Many cat owners have tried punishment and found it has not corrected the problem. If a cat stops eliminating in an area after the application of such a procedure, it usually is a cat with a very location-specific elimination pattern. The punishment may have made the entire area aversive and the cat, therefore, avoids it and does not eliminate there. The cat has not stopped eliminating in this area because it has associated elimination in that location with punishment.

Punishment often makes the problem worse. Most owners, after punishing the cat, take it back and place it in the litterbox. In actuality, there is a closer time contingency between the punishment and the litterbox than between punishment and the act of eliminating in the inappropriate area. Cats frequently punished also begin avoiding the owner and engaging in fearful behavior.

It may be true that a cat "looks guilty" or hides when the owner returns home only if it has eliminated outside of the litterbox. However, it is not necessarily true that the cat knows it has done something wrong. A simpler, more logical explanation is that the cat has learned to associate the presence of 2 stimuli (return of owner and elimination products outside of the litterbox) with punishment. Whenever these 2 stimuli appear together, the cat has learned that it is going to be disciplined and, therefore, acts in a fearful way.

Grooming Behavior Problems

Grooming behavior is a frequent displacement activity in animals. The authors have observed several cases in which cats have groomed excessively to the point of pulling out hair and causing skin lesions. In some of these situations, stress has been correlated with the onset of excessive grooming. Examples of such stress are the addition of new people in the household (who sometimes actually like, but inadvertently frighten the cat) and the presence of another animal that harasses the cat. Desensitizing or counterconditioning the cat to these situations might be appropriate. Sometimes, however, it is difficult or impossible to eliminate the sources of stress. These cats often respond to drugs that tend to alleviate anxiety, such as amitriptyline, benzodiazepines or progestins. These drugs are not marketed for cats; they must be considered experimental and the owner should be warned of this and of potential side effects.

Chapter 16 contains a discussion of self-induced skin lesions.

Reproductive Behavior Problems

Behavioral idiosyncrasies may prevent mating. Inexperienced males may grab the head or neck area inappropriately, release the neck grip too soon, mount in the wrong position or engage in pelvic thrusting without intromission. If a male's initial experience with a female is traumatic, he may be inhibited about breeding for a long time thereafter.

As a male gains experience, he orients and mounts correctly, and shortens the time engaged in pelvic thrusting. If a reliable stud begins to engage in excessive pelvic thrusting but does not achieve intromission, his penis should be inspected for a hair ring (see Chapter 15).[29] Sometimes the hairs of the cat accumulate around the penis during breeding and may eventually prohibit breeding. Another reason for prolonged pelvic thrusting without intromission is anatomic incompatibility, such as a shorter male attempting to breed a long-bodied female.

As with other species, it is more important for the male than the female to be habituated and comfortable in his surroundings in order to breed. Therefore, the female should be taken to a location with which the male is familiar. Routinely taking a male to a specific location for breeding eventually conditions him to anticipate this event and breed a receptive female within a few minutes.

Females may not breed with specific males. Mate selection is a phenomenon recognized in many species, and probably in cats. If a female pulls away too rapidly from a male, thereby preventing intromission, a person familiar with the cat can easily hold her head and immobilize her. If both cats are familiar with the handler, they proceed with breeding. Sometimes male cats do not hold on with a neck grip because of malocclusion or other dental problems.

Some queens are so attached to their owners that they delay parturition or cease tending the kittens if they are separated from the owners. The easiest solution to this problem is for the owner to remain with the cat until she becomes fully occupied with caring for the kittens (see Chapter 15).

Aggressive Behavior

There are several common types of aggressive behavior in cats, including intermale aggression, aggression related to territorial behavior, defensive aggression, play aggression and redirected aggression. An accurate description of the postures the cat assumes before or during the aggression is important for diagnosis. These postures and the context in which each problem occurs have been described above. The general treatments are discussed below.

Intermale Aggression: Intermale aggression is more likely to occur in intact males than in castrated males. Thus, castration is often an effective step in prevention and treatment.[22] Synthetic progestin therapy, at the same dosage regimen used to treat spraying, may suppress intermale aggression even when castration is not effective. Sometimes counterconditioning is an appropriate treatment (see below).

Territorial Aggression: Territorial aggression is extremely difficult to treat. This type of aggression often does not respond to synthetic progestin therapy or counterconditioning. Often the best solution is to place one of the cats in another home.

Defensive/Fear-Induced Aggression: Another common problem involves defensive or fear-induced aggression. A frightening event can elicit a full complement of defensive aggression postures, which in turn elicits an aggressive reaction from another cat. For instance, in one case, a cat was sitting at the window when a rock thrown by a neighbor child crashed through the glass. The cat jumped up, hissed and ran out off the room with the hair raised on its tail and back. The second cat happened to enter the room at the same time. It was frightened by the behavior of the first cat and, in response, hissed, spat and swatted at the first cat. In return, the first cat became aggressive to the second cat. The consequence of this brief, but intense, interaction was that each cat learned, in one trial, to anticipate aggression from the other, and would hiss, spit and growl when it saw the other. If they got too close, they would fight. The owner managed the problem by keeping them in different rooms.

This type of problem is common and involves "misperception" by one cat of the signals of another cat. The problem often occurs among cats that have been "best friends" for years, with much social grooming, play and eating behavior between them. This paradox may be explained by the fact that the cat's history involves little or no experience with aggressive or defensive aggression signals. Thus, when confronted, perhaps for the first time, with a cat in a full-blown defensive-aggressive posture, the cat misinterprets it as an attack. Of course, as in the case described above, this misperception usually is by both cats (or more) and, thus, the entire problem is a self-perpetuating mistake.

Although this problem may develop in only a few seconds, it often takes weeks or months to resolve. Sometimes the aggression wanes by itself as the cats gradually are exposed to each other during periods of little or no aggression. However, in other cases the problem may escalate. The problem may generalize from the place or time when and where it first occurred to other locations and times.

If the problem does not gradually resolve itself within a few weeks, desensitization or counterconditioning can be employed. The idea is to gradually expose one cat to the other in such a manner that no fear or aggression is elicited. In simple cases, this may be accomplished by the owner picking up one cat and holding it, stroking it, and keeping it calm as the 2 cats gradually see each other. This can be done by presenting one cat to the other at a distance and then gradually, over many trials, reducing the distance between them or by using a time gradient whereby very short exposures are gradually lengthened. It is critical that the process be conducted slowly and carefully so that no fear or aggression occurs. Any fear or aggression allows the cats to quickly associate the possibility of further aggression with the place or circumstances in which the treatment occurs. The cats should also be completely isolated from each other except during actual time of treatment, to prevent self-perpetuation of the aggression.

Counterconditioning requires associating the sight, movement or proximity of the other cat(s) with a behavioral system that tends to inhibit fear or aggression. Examples of competitive behavioral systems are eating, grooming, play and affection. These systems can be elicited with a high enough intensity to overcome a very weak fear or aggression tendency. To keep the tendency toward fear or aggression low, the cats either must be far apart or somehow partially blocked from each other's view. For instance, the cats may be fed very small meals on each side of a door. In other cases, it may be possible to get one or both cats playing with a string or moving toys on each side of the partially opened door. Sometimes it is possible to facilitate mutual grooming. This can be done by getting one or more of the cats wet or by applying a substance, such as vegetable or mineral oil, to the fur.

Play Aggression: Another common aggressive behavior problem of cats involves play behavior, which has such predatory and aggressive components as stalking attack, clawing or biting.

Play and predatory behavior in cats share many common features, such as stalking, pouncing on and biting at moving objects. The most important stimulus that elicits play or predatory behavior appears to be movement. A play-aggression behavior problem often may occur when the cat is left alone for a long time during the day or is not played with very much by the owner. When the owner comes home or begins to play with the cat, it stalks the owner in a predatory manner. Thus, a cat that is somewhat deprived of play may attend very closely to the movement of the owner or other people walking around the apartment. A cat may stalk, chase and bite at moving feet or legs. Owners are confronted with a time-consuming or even frightening situation of having to watch for the cat so it does not attack them. Cats readily associate their behavior with the time and place at which various eliciting stimuli occur. Thus, many owners report that the cat only bites their feet at certain times and locations, for example, when they are stepping out of the shower or going up and down the stairs.

Play aggression problems usually are treated successfully by redirecting the cat's play and predatory behavior to other moving objects. It is not sufficient to buy the cat toys that lie around the house immobile. Usually toys have been available but the owner fails to realize that moving toys are required. In some cases, it is helpful for the owner to temporarily carry a toy to which the cat can redirect its play/predatory behavior. A simple toy that effectively redirects aggressive play is a long piece of string with a small object tied to one end.

After many trials, the cat learns to associate aggressive play behavior with the moving toy, rather than with the owner's legs, feet or arms. Some cats have a very high level of play behavior and the owner may be obliged, at least at the beginning of treatment, to spend considerable time playing with the cat. If the owners initiate appropriate play first, they may reduce the frequency of the cat aggressively initiating inappropriate play. Providing a playful companion cat or toys that a cat can easily chase by itself, such as ping-pong balls, may lower the cat's motivation to play aggressively with the owner.

Redirected Aggression: When a cat is aggressive, it is potentially dangerous to pick it up or interact with it in any significant way because the cat may redirect its aggressive behavior to the person. Some cats maintain a certain level of arousal or aggression for many hours after an aggressive display. To reduce the likelihood of redirected aggression, it is best not to approach such a cat until it first engages in a non-aggressive behavior.

References

1. Wiesel, TN and Hubel, DH. J Neurophysiol **28** (1965) 1060.
2. Riesen, AH. Prog Physiol Psychol **1** (1966) 117.
3. Grobstein, P and Chow, KL: Neural and Behavioral Specificity: Studies on the Development of Behavior and the Nervous System. Vol 3. Academic Press, New York, 1976.
4. Rosenzweig, in Tobach *et al:* The Biopsychology of Development. Academic Press, New York, 1971.
5. MacLusky, NJ and Naftolin, F. Science **211** (1981) 1294.
6. McEwen, BS. Science **211** (1981) 1303.
7. Ader, R: Hormonal Correlates of Behavior. Plenum Press, New York, 1975.
8. Levine, S *et al.* Physiol Behav **2** (1967) 55.
9. Meier, GW. J Comp Physiol Psychol **54** (1961) 284.
10. Seitz, PFD. Psychosom Med **21** (1959) 353.
11. Jemmett, JE and Skerritt, G. Display at 116th AVMA Mtg, 1979.
12. Lack, D: The Life of the Robin. Cambridge Univ Press, London, 1943.
13. Tinbergen, N: The Study of Instinct. Oxford Univ Press, London, 1951.
14. Leyhausen, P: Cat Behavior. STPM Press, New York, 1979.
15. Scott, in Hafez: Cats. Lea & Febiger, Philadelphia, 1970.
16. Wolski, T. Vet Clin No Am **12** (1982) 563.
17. Schneirla *et al,* in Rheingold: Maternal Behavior in Mammals. J. Wiley and Sons, New York, 1963.
18. Schaller, GB: The Serengeti Lions: A Study of Predatory-Prey Relations. Univ Chicago Press, Chicago, 1972.
19. Bertram, BCR. E Afr Wildlife J **11** (1973) 215.
20. Houpt, K. Vet Clin No Am **12** (1982) 563.
21. Wolpe, J: Psychotherapy by Reciprocal Inhibition. Stanford Univ Press, Stanford, CA, 1958.
22. Hart, BL and Barrett, RE. JAVMA **163** (1973) 290.
23. Eigenmann, JE. JAAHA **17** (1981) 805.
24. Eigenmann, JE and Venker-van Haagen, AJ. JAAHA **17** (1981) 813.
25. Eigenmann, JE and Eigenmann, RY. Acta Endocrin **98** (1981) 599.
26. Hernandez, FJ *et al.* Feline Pract **5(5)** (1975) 45.
27. Hart, BL. JAVMA **179** (1981) 231.
28. Hart, BL and Voith, VL. Brain Res **145** (1978) 405.
29. Hart, BL and Peterson, DM. Lab Anim Sci **21** (1971) 422.
30. Liberg, O. Doctoral dissertation, Univ Lund, Sweden, 1981.

index

A

B

C

D

E

F

G

H

I

J

K

L

M

N

O

P

R

S

T

U

V

W

Y

Z